CURRENT THERAPY OF

TRAUMA AND SURGICAL

CRITICAL CARE

CURRENT THERAPY OF TRAUMA AND SURGICAL CRITICAL CARE

2nd EDITION

JUAN A. ASENSIO
MD, FACS, FCCM, FRCS, KM

Professor of Surgery
Chief, Division of Trauma Surgery and Surgical Critical Care
Director, Trauma Center and Trauma Program
Department of Surgery, Creighton University School of Medicine
Creighton University Medical Center
Omaha, Nebraska

DONALD D. TRUNKEY
MD, FACS

Professor Emeritus
Department of Surgery
Division of Trauma
Oregon Health and Science University
Portland, Oregon

ELSEVIER

ELSEVIER

1600 John F. Kennedy Blvd.
Ste 1800
Philadelphia, PA 19103–2899

CURRENT THERAPY OF TRAUMA AND SURGICAL
CRITICAL CARE, SECOND EDITION

ISBN: 978-0-323-07980-8

Library of Congress Cataloging-in-Publication Data

Current therapy of trauma and surgical critical care / [edited by] Juan A. Asensio, Donald D. Trunkey.
– 2nd edition.
    p. ; cm. – (Current therapy)
  Includes bibliographical references and index.
  ISBN 978-0-323-07980-8 (hardcover : alk. paper)
  I. Asensio, Juan A., editor.   II. Trunkey, Donald D., editor.   III. Series: Current therapy series.
0831-8689
[DNLM: 1. Wounds and Injuries–therapy. 2. Critical Care–methods. 3. Emergency Medical
Services–organization & administration. 4. Emergency Treatment–methods. 5. Surgical Procedures,
Operative–methods. 6. Trauma Centers–organization & administration. WO 700]
  RD93.95
  617.1–dc23
                                                                                            2015008890

Publishing Manager: Michael Houston
Content Development Specialist: Lauren Boyle
Publishing Services Manager: Patricia Tannian
Project Manager: Amanda Mincher
Designer: Ryan Cook

Printed in China
Last digit is the print number: 9 8 7 6 5 4 3 2 1

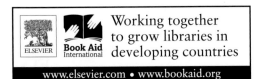

Working together
to grow libraries in
developing countries

www.elsevier.com • www.bookaid.org

CONTRIBUTORS

Kareem R. AbdelFattah, MD
Fellow in Burns, Trauma, and Critical Care, University of Texas Southwestern Medical Center, Dallas, Texas

Michel B. Aboutanos, MD, MPH, FACS
Associate Professor of Surgery, Director, Injury Prevention Program, Director, International Trauma System Development Program, Division of Trauma Critical Care and Emergency General Surgery, Department of Surgery, Virginia Commonwealth University, Richmond, Virginia

Louis A. Aliperti, MD
Department of Surgery, Division of Trauma and Critical Care, Tulane University School of Medicine, New Orleans, Louisiana

John T. Anderson, MD, FACS
Associate Professor, Department of Surgery, Division of Trauma and Emergency Surgery, University of California Davis, Sacramento, California

Devashish J. Anjaria, MD, FACS
Assistant Professor of Surgery, Trauma, Surgical Critical Care and General Surgery, Rutgers New Jersey Medical School, Newark, New Jersey

Juan A. Asensio, MD, FACS, FCCM, FRCS
Professor of Surgery, Chief, Division of Trauma Surgery and Surgical Critical Care, Director, Trauma Center and Trauma Program, Department of Surgery, Creighton University School of Medicine, Creighton University Medical Center, Omaha, Nebraska

Morad Askari, MD
Assistant Professor of Plastic and Reconstructive Surgery, Assistant Professor of Orthopedic Surgery, Division of Hand Surgery, Department of Surgery, Department of Orthopedic Surgery, University of Miami, Miami, Florida

Jeffrey A. Bailey, MD, MPA, FACS
Emeritus Director, Joint Trauma System, Associate Professor of Surgery, Uniformed Services University of the Health Sciences, Bethesda, Maryland

Marcus Balters, MD
Assistant Professor of Surgery, Division of Cardiovascular Surgery, Creighton University School of Medicine, CHI-Health Alegent Creighton Clinic, Omaha, Nebraska

Ron Barbosa, MD
Medical Director, Trauma Intensive Care Unit, Legacy Emanuel Hospital, Portland, Oregon

Philip S. Barie, MD, MBA, MCCM, FIDSA, FACS
Professor of Surgery, Division of Burns, Critical Care and Trauma, Professor of Public Health in Medicine, Division of Medical Ethics, Weill Medical College of Cornell University, New York, New York

Edward J. Bedrick, PhD
Professor of Biostatistics, Department of Mathematics and Statistics, Department of Internal Medicine, University of New Mexico, Albuquerque, New Mexico

John D. Berne, MD, FACS
Clinical Assistant Professor of Surgery, University of Texas at Houston, Houston, Texas

Stepheny D. Berry, MD
Co-Medical Director for Trauma, Assistant Professor of Surgery, The University of Kansas Medical Center, Kansas City, Kansas

Robert Bertelotti, MD
Resident, General Surgery, Creighton University, Omaha, Nebraska

Pulkesh Bhatia, MBBS
Surgical Resident, Creighton University Medical Center, Omaha, Nebraska

Walter L. Biffl, MD, FACS
Associate Director of Surgery, Denver Health Medical Center, Professor of Surgery, University of Colorado, Denver, Colorado

Brian Biggerstaff, MD
Surgical Resident, Creighton University Medical Center, Omaha, Nebraska

John K. Bini, MD, FACS, LtCol, USAF MC
Assistant Professor of Surgery, Boonshoft School of Medicine, Wright State University; Assistant Professor of Surgery, Uniformed Services University of Health Sciences; Trauma Surgeon, Wright Patterson Medical Center, Dayton, Ohio

F. William Blaisdell, MD, FACS
Professor, Department of Surgery, University of California Davis, Sacramento, California

Matthew C. Bozeman, MD
Assistant Professor, Hiram C. Polk, Jr. Department of Surgery, University of Louisville, Louisville, Kentucky

Steven B. Brandes, MD
Professor of Urologic Surgery, Director of Reconstructive Urology, Division of Urologic Surgery, Washington University School of Medicine, St. Louis, Missouri

Karen J. Brasel, MD, MPH
Oregon Health and Science University, Portland, Oregon

Benjamin M. Braslow, MD
Associate Professor of Clinical Surgery, Division of Traumatology, Surgical Critical Care and Emergency Surgery; Section Chief, Emergency Surgery Service, Department of Surgery, Perelman School of Medicine, University of Pennsylvania, Philadelphia, Pennsylvania

L.D. Britt, MD, MPH, FACS
Henry Ford Professor and Edward J. Brickhouse Chairman, Department of Surgery, Eastern Virginia Medical School, Norfolk, Virginia

Susan I. Brundage, MD, MPH
Section Chief, Acute Care Surgery, Director, Surgical Critical Care, Department of Surgery, New York University School of Medicine; NYU Langone Medical Center, Tisch Hospital; Department of Surgery, Bellevue Hospital, New York, New York

Thomas P. Brush, MD
Resident, Department of Surgery, Creighton University, Omaha, Nebraska

Clay Cothren Burlew, MD, FACS
Director, Surgical Intensive Care Unit, Program Director, SCC and TACS Fellowships, Department of Surgery, Denver Health Medical Center; Professor of Surgery, University of Colorado School of Medicine, Denver, Colorado

Patricia Marie Byers, MD, FACS
Chief, Surgical Nutrition, Division of Trauma and Surgical Critical Care, The DeWitt Daughtry Family Department of Surgery, University of Miami Miller School of Medicine, Miami, Florida

Kim M. Caban, MD
Assistant Professor of Radiology, University of Miami Miller School of Medicine, Jackson Memorial Hospital–Ryder Trauma Center, ER-Trauma Radiology Division, Miami, Florida

Jeremy Cannon, MD, SM, FACS, LtCol, USAF MC
Chief, Trauma and Critical Care, San Antonio Military Medical Center, San Antonio, Texas; Associate Professor of Surgery, Uniformed Services University of the Health Sciences, Bethesda, Maryland

Shawn M. Cantie, MD
Clinical Instructor of Anesthesiology, The University at Buffalo, State University of New York, Erie County Medical Center, Buffalo, New York

José Ceballos Esparragon, MD
Surgical Resident, Creighton University Medical Center, Omaha, Nebraska

Howard R. Champion, FRCS, FACS
Professor of Surgery, Uniformed Services University of the Health Sciences, Bethesda, Maryland

Benjamin Chandler, MD
PGY-4 Resident, Department of Surgery, Rutgers New Jersey Medical School, University of Medicine and Dentistry of New Jersey; Resident, Department of Surgery, University Hospital, Newark, New Jersey

David C. Chang, PhD, MPH, MBA
Associate Professor of Surgery, Massachusetts General Hospital, Harvard Medical School, Boston, Massachusetts

Steven Cheung, MD
Resident, General Surgery, Creighton University Medical Center, Omaha, Nebraska

William C. Chiu, MD, FACS, FCCM
Associate Professor of Surgery, Director, Surgical Critical Care Fellowship Program, R Adams Cowley Shock Trauma Center, University of Maryland School of Medicine, Baltimore, Maryland

A. Britton Christmas, MD, FACS
Associate Professor of Surgery, Trauma, Surgical Critical Care, and Emergency General Surgery, Carolinas Medical Center, Charlotte, North Carolina

David J. Ciesla, MD
Professor of Surgery, Director of Acute Care Surgery Division, University of South Florida Morsani College of Medicine; Medical Director, Regional Trauma Program, Tampa General Hospital, Tampa, Florida

William G. Cioffi, MD, FACS
J. Murray Beardsley Professor and Chairman, Alpert Medical School of Brown University

Department of Surgery; Surgeon-in-Chief, Rhode Island Hospital and The Miriam Hospital, Providence, Rhode Island

Christine S. Cocanour, MD, FACS, FCCM
Professor of Surgery, UC Davis Medical Center, Sacramento, California

Mitchell J. Cohen, MD
Assistant Professor in Residence, Department of Surgery, University of California San Francisco, San Francisco, California

Raul Coimbra, MD, PhD, FACS
The Monroe E. Trout Professor of Surgery, Surgeon-in-Chief, Executive Vice-Chairman, Department of Surgery, Chief Division of Trauma, Surgical Critical Care, Burns, and Acute Care Surgery, University of California San Diego Health System, San Diego, California

Peter Collister, MD
Resident, General Surgery, Creighton University, Omaha, Nebraska

Edward E. Cornwell, III, MD, PhD, FACS
Chairman and Professor of Surgery, Howard University, Washington, D.C.

Thomas B. Cox, BS
President, Cox Business Consulting, Inc., Beaverton, Oregon

Martin A. Croce, MD
Professor, Department of Surgery, University of Tennessee Health Science Center; Chief of Trauma and Critical Care, Trauma Division Regional One Health, Memphis, Tennessee

Gary H. Danton, MD, PhD
Medical Director of Radiology, Trauma/ER Radiology, Jackson Memorial Hospital; Director, Radiology Residency Training Program, Assistant Professor of Clinical Radiology, Jackson Health System, Jackson, Florida; Chief, Section of Imaging Informatics, Trauma/ER Radiology, University of Miami, Miami, Florida

Kimberly A. Davis, MD, MBA
Professor of Surgery, Vice Chairman of Clinical Affairs, Chief of the Section of Trauma, Surgical Critical Care, and

Surgical Emergencies, Yale University School of Medicine; Trauma Medical Director, Surgical Director, Quality and Performance Improvement, Yale-New Haven Hospital, New Haven, Connecticut

Elias Degiannis, MD, PhD, FRCS (Glasg), FCS (SA), FACS
Professor of Surgery, University of the Witwatersrand; Head, Trauma Directorate, Chris Hani Baragwanath Academic Hospital, Johannesburg, South Africa

Edwin A. Deitch, MD
Professor and Chairman, Rutgers New Jersey Medical School, University of Medicine and Dentistry of New Jersey; Chief of Surgery, University Hospital, Newark, New Jersey

Richard Denney, MD
Chief Resident, General Surgery, Creighton University, Omaha, Nebraska

Christopher J. Dente, MD, FACS
Associate Professor of Surgery, Emory University; Associate Director of Trauma, Grady Memorial Hospital, Atlanta, Georgia

Urmen Desai, MD, MPH
Plastic, Aesthetic, and Cosmetic Surgeon, Desai Plastic Surgery of Beverly Hills, Beverly Hills, California

Rochelle A. Dicker, MD
Associate Professor of Surgery and Anesthesia, University of California San Francisco, San Francisco General Hospital, San Francisco, California

Lawrence N. Diebel, MD, FACS
Professor, Department of Surgery, Wayne State University, Detroit, Michigan

Karev Dimitryi, MD, FACS
Professor, Department of Surgery, Wayne State University, Detroit, Michigan

Andrew R. Doben, MD
Associate Professor of Surgery, Department of Surgery, Tufts University School of Medicine, Boston, Massachusetts; Director, Surgical Intensive Care Unit, Division of Trauma and Acute Care Surgery, Department of Surgery, Baystate Medical Center, Springfield, Massachusetts

Jay Doucet, MD, MSc, FRCSC, FACS, RDMS
Professor of Clinical Surgery, Director, Surgical Intensive Care Unit, Director, Emergency Preparedness and Response, Division of Trauma, Surgical Critical Care, and Burns, Department of Surgery, University of California San Diego Health System, San Diego, California

Therese M. Duane, MD, FACS, FCCM
Vice-Chair, Department of Surgery for Quality and Safety, Medical Director for Acute Care Surgery Research, John Peter Smith Health System, Fort Worth, Texas

Joe DuBose, MD, FACS
Associate Professor of Surgery, Uniformed Services University of the Health Sciences, Baltimore, Maryland; Vascular Fellow, University of Texas Health Sciences Center–Houston, Houston, Texas

Wayne Dubov, MD
Board Certified by the American Board of Physical Medicine and Rehabilitation (ABPMR), Subspecialty–Spinal Cord Injury Medicine, Diplomate of the American Board of Electrodiagnostic Medicine, Lehigh Valley Health Network, Allentown, Pennsylvania; Clinical Assistant Professor, University of South Florida, Morsani College of Medicine, Tampa, Florida

Juan C. Duchesne, MD, FACS, FCCP, FCCM
Trauma Medical Director, GME Medical Director, North Oaks Health System, Hammond, Louisiana; Associate Professor of Surgery, Tulane University, Louisiana State University Health Sciences Center; Chairman, Louisiana Committee of Trauma, New Orleans, Louisiana

Stanley J. Dudrick, MD, FACS, FACN, CNS
Professor of Surgery, The Commonwealth Medical College, Scranton, Pennsylvania; Edward S. Anderson Endowed Chair, Professor and Medical Director of Physician Assistant Studies, School of Arts and Sciences, Misericordia University, Dallas, Pennsylvania; Professor of Surgery, Emeritus, Yale University Medical School, New Haven, Connecticut

Rodney Durham, MD, FACS
Professor of Surgery, University of South Florida, Tampa, Florida

Anthony M. Durso, MD
Assistant Professor of Radiology, University of Miami Miller School of Medicine, Jackson Memorial Hospital, Miami, Florida

Soumitra R. Eachempati, MD, FACS, FCCM
Professor of Surgery, Professor of Medicine, Division of Medical Ethics, Weill Cornell Medical College, New York, New York

Colonel (Ret.) Brian Eastridge, MD
Trauma and Surgical Critical Care, Director Emeritus, Joint Trauma System Program; Trauma Consultant, U.S. Army Surgeon General, Institute of Surgical Research, Houston, Texas

Aileen Ebadat, MD
Resident, Department of Surgery, University of Texas Southwestern, Austin, University Medical Center Brackenridge, Austin, Texas

David T. Efron, MD, FACS
Associate Professor of Surgery, Anesthesiology and Critical Care Medicine, Emergency Medicine, Chief, Division of Acute Care Surgery: Trauma, Critical Care, Emergency, and General Surgery, Director of Adult Trauma, Department of Surgery, The Johns Hopkins Hospital, Baltimore, Maryland

Eric Elster, MD, FACS, CAPT MC USN
Professor and Chairman, Norman M. Rich Department of Surgery, Uniformed Services University of the Health Sciences, Bethesda, Maryland

Michael Englehart, MD
Billings Clinic, Billings, Montana

Thomas J. Esposito, MD, MPH
Professor, Department of Surgery, Loyola University Chicago, Stritch School of Medicine, Chicago, Illinois; Chief, Division of Trauma, Surgical Critical Care and Burns, Department of Surgery, Loyola University Medical Center, Maywood, Illinois

Glyn Estebanez, MD, MRCS
Surgical Registrar, Wessex School of Surgery,
United Kingdom; Trauma Research Fellow,
MEDITECH, Neiva, Colombia

Susan Evans, MD, FACS, FCCM
Associate Professor of Surgery, Division of
Acute Care Surgery, Carolinas Medical
Center, Charlotte, North Carolina

Samir M. Fakhry, MD, FACS
Charles F. Crews Professor and Chief,
General Surgery, Medical University of South
Carolina, Charleston, South Carolina

Anthony Falvo, DO, FACOS, FACS
Clinical Educator, Wayne State University
School of Medicine, Detroit, Michigan

David V. Feliciano, MD
Battersby Professor and Chief, IU Division
of General Surgery, Chief of Surgery,
Indiana University Hospital, Indianapolis,
Indiana

**Luis G. Fernández, MD, KHS, FACS,
FASAS, FCCP, FCCM, FICS**
Assistant Clinical Professor of Surgery/Family
Practice, University of Texas Health Science
Center, Tyler, Texas; Adjunct Clinical
Professor of Medicine and Nursing,
University of Texas, Arlington, Texas;
Chairman, Division of Trauma Surgery/
Surgical Critical Care, Chief of Trauma
Surgical Critical Care Unit, Trinity Mother
Frances Health System, Tyler, Texas; Brigadier
General, Past Commanding General, TXSG
Medical Brigade, (Ret/HR), Austin, Texas

Mitchell Fink, MD
University of Pittsburgh, Pittsburgh,
Pennsylvania

Lewis M. Flint, MD, FACS
Editor-in-Chief, Selected Readings in General
Surgery, Division of Education, American
College of Surgeons, Chicago, Illinois

Donald E. Fry, MD, FACS
Adjunct Professor of Surgery, Northwestern
University Feinberg School of Medicine,
Chicago, Illinois; Emeritus Professor of
Surgery, University of New Mexico School
of Medicine, Albuquerque, New Mexico

Takashi Fujita, MD, PhD, FACS
Associate Professor, Trauma and
Resuscitation Center, Teikyo University
Hospital, Tokyo, Japan

Joseph M. Galante, MD
Associate Professor and Vice Chair,
Education, Department of Surgery,
University of California, Davis; Division of
Trauma, Acute Care Surgery, and
Surgical Critical Care, UC Davis,
Medical Center, Sacramento, California

**Richard L. Gamelli, MD, FACS,
FRCSEd (Hon)**
Editor-in-Chief, Journal of Burn Care and
Research; Professor Emeritus, Stritch School
of Medicine, Loyola University Chicago,
Chicago, Illinois

**Luis Manuel García-Núñez, MD,
FACS, FAMSUS**
General and Trauma Surgeon, Chief,
Emergency Department, Military Central
Hospital, National Defense Department,
Mexico City, Mexico

Larry M. Gentilello, MD
Professor of Surgery, Adjunct Professor of
Management, Policy, and Community
Health, Department of Surgery, University of
Texas, Austin, Texas

Ramyar Gilani, MD
Assistant Professor, Michael E. DeBakey
Department of Surgery, Division of Vascular
Surgery, Baylor College of Medicine; Chief of
Vascular Surgery, Ben Taub General
Hospital, Houston, Texas

Laurent G. Glance, MD
Vice-Chair for Research, Department of
Anesthesiology, Professor of Anesthesiology,
Professor of Public Health Sciences, Senior
Scientist, RAND (adjunct), University of
Rochester School of Medicine, Rochester,
New York

Nestor R. Gonzalez, MD
Assistant Professor, Neurological Surgery
and Radiological Sciences, UCLA Medical
Center, Los Angeles, California

Daniel J. Grabo, MD
Fellow, Division of Traumatology, Surgical
Critical Care and Emergency Surgery,
Hospital of the University of Pennsylvania,
Philadelphia, Pennsylvania

Gerald Gracia, MD

Vincente H. Gracias, MD
Interim Dean, CEO, Robert Wood Johnson
Medical Group; Professor and Chief,
Department of Surgery, Rutgers Robert
Wood Johnson Medical School, Robert
Wood Johnson University Hospital,
New Brunswick, New Jersey

Kirby R. Gross, MD
Colonel, Medical Corps, United States Army;
Director, Joint Trauma System, San Antonio
Military Medical Center, San Antonio, Texas;
Associate Professor, Uniformed Services
University of the Health Sciences, Bethesda,
Maryland

Ronald I. Gross, MD
Associate Professor of Surgery, Tufts
University School of Medicine, Boston,
Massachusetts; Chief, Division of
Trauma, Acute Care Surgery, and
Surgical Critical Care, Baystate Medical
Center, Springfield, Massachusetts

Chrissy Guidry, DO
Trauma and Critical Care, Tulane
University School of Medicine, New
Orleans, Louisiana

Oliver L. Gunter, Jr., MD, MPH, FACS
Vanderbilt University School of Medicine,
Section of Surgical Sciences, Department
of General Surgery, Division of Trauma
and Surgical Critical Care, Nashville,
Tennessee

Joseph M. Gutmann, MD
University of South Florida, Tampa, Florida

Erin Hale, MD
Resident, General Surgery, Creighton
University, Omaha, Nebraska

S. Morad Hameed, MD, MPH
Associate Professor and Chief, Section of
Trauma, Acute Care Surgery, and Surgical
Critical Care, Department of Surgery,
University of British Columbia Trauma
Services VGT, Vancouver, British Columbia

Molly Hartmann, MD
Resident, General Surgery, Creighton
University, Omaha, Nebraska

Carl Hauser, MD, FACS, FCCM
Professor of Surgery, Harvard University;
Attending Surgeon, New England Deaconess
Medical Center, Boston, Massachusetts

Sharon Henry, MD, FACS
Anne Scalea Professor of Trauma Surgery, University of Maryland School of Medicine, University of Maryland Medical Center, R Adams Cowley Shock Trauma Center, Baltimore, Maryland

Mathilda Horst, MD, FACS, FCCM
Medical Director, Surgical Critical Care; Henry Ford Hospital; Professor of Surgery, Wayne State School of Medicine, Detroit, Michigan

Ari Hoschander, MD
Department of Surgery, Division of Plastic Surgery, University of Miami Hospital, Jackson Memorial Hospital, Miami, Florida

Herman P. Houin, MD
Senior Staff Surgeon, Department of Plastic Surgery, Henry Ford Health System, Detroit, Michigan

David Hoyt, MD, FACS
Executive Director, American College of Surgeons, Chicago, Illinois

Jared M. Huston, MD
Department of Surgery, Division of Trauma and Acute Care Surgery, North Shore University Hospital, North Shore-LIJ Health System, Manhasset, New York

Kyros Ipaktchi, MD
Associate Professor of Orthopedic Surgery, Chief of Hand-Microvascular Surgery, Department of Orthopedic Surgery, Denver Health Medical Center, University of Colorado, Denver, Colorado

D'Andrea Joseph, MD, FACS
Assistant Professor of Surgery, Associate Director of Trauma, Program Director of Acute Care Fellowship, Department of Surgery, Hartford Hospital/University of Connecticut, Hartford, Connecticut

Gregory J. Jurkovich, MD, FACS
Chief of Surgery, Denver Health and Hospitals; Rockwell Distinguished Professor of Trauma Surgery, University of Colorado, Denver, Colorado

Steven Kalandiak, MD
Assistant Professor of Clinical Orthopedics, University of Miami Miller School of Medicine, Miami, Florida

Riyad Karmy-Jones, MD
Chief of Trauma, Thoracic and Trauma Surgery, Legacy Emanuel Medical Center, Portland, Oregon

Larry T. Khoo, MD
Director of Minimally Invasive Neurological Spinal Surgery, Los Angeles Spine Clinic at Good Samaritan Hospital, The Los Angeles Spine Clinic, Los Angeles, California

Laszlo Kiraly, MD, FACS
Associate Professor, Department of Surgery, Oregon Health and Science University, Portland, Oregon

Orlando C. Kirton, MD, FACS, MCCM, FCCP
Professor of Surgery, Vice Chair, Department of Surgery, University of Connecticut School of Medicine, Farmington; Ludwig J. Pyrtek, MD Chair in Surgery, Chief, Department of Surgery, Chief, Division of General Surgery, Interim Director, Trauma Service, Hartford Hospital, Hartford, Connecticut

Michael Ksycki, DO
Chief of Surgery, Browning Community Hospital, HIS, Billings, Montana

Anastasia Kunac, MD, FACS
Assistant Professor of Surgery, Division of Trauma Surgery and Surgical Critical Care, Rutgers New Jersey Medical School, Newark, New Jersey

Kulsoom Laeeq, MD
Resident, General Surgery, Creighton University, Omaha, Nebraska

Anna M. Ledgerwood, MD, FACS
Professor, Michael and Marian Ilitch Department of Surgery, Wayne State University, Detroit, Michigan

Benjamin T. Lemelman, MD
University of Chicago Medical Center, Section of Plastic and Reconstructive Surgery, Chicago, Illinois

Ari Leppäniemi, MD, PhD, MDCC
Professor of Surgery, Chief of Emergency Surgery, Meilahti Hospital, University of Helsinki, Finland

David H. Livingston, MD, FACS
Wesley J. Howe Professor and Chief of Trauma and Surgical Critical Care, Rutgers New Jersey Medical School, Newark, New Jersey

Jason Loden, DO
Department of Surgery, Creighton University, Omaha, Nebraska

Gary Lombardo, MD, FACS
Assistant Professor of Surgery, New York Medical College, Westchester Medical Center, New York, New York

Andrew Loukas, MD
Clinical Anesthesiologist, South Miami Hospital/Baptist Health, Miami, Florida

Charles E. Lucas, MD
Professor Michael and Marian Ilitch Department of Surgery, Wayne State University, Detroit, Michigan

Fred A. Luchette, MD, MSc
Chief of Surgical Services, Edward Hines, Jr. VA Medical Center; Vice-Chair, VA Affairs; Professor of Surgery, Stritch School of Medicine, Loyola University of Chicago, Hines, Illinois

Charles D. Mabry, MD, FACS
Associate Professor, Department of Surgery, College of Medicine, University of Arkansas for Medical Sciences, Little Rock, Arkansas

Robert C. Mackersie, MD, FACS
Professor of Surgery, University of California San Francisco; Director of Trauma Services, San Francisco General Hospital and Trauma Center, San Francisco, California

Paul M. Maggio, MD, MBA, FACS
Assistant Professor of Surgery, Co-Director, Critical Care Medicine, Stanford University Medical Center, Stanford, California

Louis J. Magnotti, MD, FACS
Associate Professor, Department of Surgery, University of Tennessee Health Science Center, Memphis, Tennessee

John W. Mah, MD, FACS
Associate Professor, Department of Surgery, University of Connecticut School of Medicine, Farmington, Connecticut; Associate Director, Surgery Critical Care, Hartford Hospital, Hartford, Connecticut

Ajai K. Malhotra, MBBS (MD), MS, DNB, FRCSEd, FACS
Professor of Surgery, Virginia Commonwealth University, Richmond, Virginia

Darren Malinoski, MD, FACS
Assistant Chief of Surgery–Research and Education, Chief, Section of Surgical Critical Care, VA Portland Health Care System; Associate Professor of Surgery, Oregon Health and Science University, Portland, Oregon

Brittney J. Maloley-Lewis, DO, MBA
Surgical Resident, Creighton University Medical Center, Omaha, Nebraska

Corrado Paolo Marini, MD, FACS
Chief of Trauma, Surgical Critical Care and Emergency Surgery; Director of Surgical Critical Care Fellowship, Department of Surgery, Westchester Medical Center, Valhalla, New York

Colonel Matthew J. Martin, MD, FACS
Trauma Medical Director, Madigan Army Medical Center, Tacoma, Washington; Director of Trauma Informatics, Legacy Emanuel Medical Center, Portland, Oregon; Associate Professor of Surgery, Uniformed Services University of the Health Sciences, Bethesda, Maryland

Leonard Mason, MD
PGY-3 General Surgery Resident, Department of Surgery, Rutgers New Jersey Medical School, Newark, New Jersey

Kenneth L. Mattox, MD
Distinguished Service Professor, Michael E. DeBakey Department of Surgery, Baylor College of Medicine; Chief of Staff and Chief of Surgery, Ben Taub General Hospital, Houston, Texas

Kimball Maull, MD, FACS
Adjunct Professor of Surgery, University of Pittsburgh Medical Center, Pittsburgh, Pennsylvania

John C. Mayberry, MD
Professor of Surgery, Division of Acute Care Surgery, Oregon Health and Science University, Portland, Oregon

Federico N. Mazzini, MD
Surgical Resident, Creighton University Medical Center, Omaha, Nebraska

Christopher McFarren, MD
Assistant Professor of Medicine, Division of Nephrology and Hypertension, Department of Internal Medicine, University of South Florida College of Medicine, Tampa, Florida

Norman E. McSwain, Jr., MD
Trauma and Critical Care, Tulane University School of Medicine, New Orleans, Louisiana

Mario A. Meallet, MD
A Center for Vison Care, LAC and USC Medical Center, Los Angeles, California

J. Wayne Meredith, MD, FACS
Richard T. Myers Professor and Chair, Department of Surgery, Wake Forest University School of Medicine; Chief of Surgery, Wake Forest University Baptist Medical Center, Winston Salem, North Carolina

Christopher P. Michetti, MD, FACS, FCCM
Medical Director, Trauma ICU, Inova Fairfax Hospital; Associate Professor of Surgery, VCU School of Medicine, Inova Campus, Falls Church, Virginia

Keith R. Miller, MD
Assistant Professor of Surgery, University of Louisville, Louisville, Kentucky

Preston R. Miller, MD
Associate Professor, Department of Surgery, Wake Forest University, Winston-Salem, North Carolina

Richard S. Miller, MD, FACS
Vanderbilt University School of Medicine, Section of Surgical Sciences, Department of General Surgery, Division of Trauma and Surgical Critical Care, Nashville, Tennessee

Joseph P. Minei, MD, MBA
Professor and Chair, Division of Burn, Trauma, and Critical Care, C. James Carrico, MD, Distinguished Chair in Surgery for Trauma and Critical Care, University of Texas Southwestern Medical Center; Surgeon-in-Chief, Parkland Health and Hospital System, Dallas, Texas

Haaris Mir, MD
Plastic and Reconstructive Hand Surgery, Joseph M. Still Burn Center and Burn Centers of Florida, Miami, Florida

Frank L. Mitchell, MD
Medical Director, Trauma and Surgical Critical Care, St. John Medical Center, Tulsa, Oklahoma

Alicia M. Mohr, MD, FACS
Associate Professor of Surgery, Division of Acute Care Surgery, University of Florida, Gainesville, Florida

Ernest E. Moore, MD
Professor and Vice Chairman for Research, Department of Surgery, University of Colorado Denver; Editor, Journal of Trauma and Acute Care Surgery, Denver, Colorado

Anne C. Mosenthal, MD, FACS
Professor and Chair, Department of Surgery, Rutgers New Jersey Medical School, Newark, New Jersey

Felipa Munera, MD
Associate Professor of Radiology, Chief, Department of Radiology, University of Miami Hospital, University of Miami Hospital and Clinics, and Sylvester Comprehensive Cancer Center; ER-Trauma Radiology Division, University of Miami–Miller School of Medicine, Jackson Memorial Hospital–Ryder Trauma Center, Miami, Florida

Alan D. Murdock, MD
Consultant to the Surgeon General for Trauma and Surgical Critical Care, Department of Trauma and General Surgery, University of Pittsburgh Medical Center, Pittsburgh, Pennsylvania; Consultant to the Surgeon General for Surgical Services, Air Force Medical Operations Agency, Lackland-Kelly Air Force Base, Texas

Mamoun Nabri, MD, FRCSI, FACS
Trauma Surgery/Surgical Critical Care Surgeon, Assistant Professor, Department of Surgery, Faculty of Medicine, University of Dammam, Dammam, Saudi Arabia

Lena M. Napolitano, MD, FACS, FCCP, FCCM
Professor of Surgery, Division Chief, Acute Care Surgery (Trauma, Burn, Critical Care, Emergency Surgery), Associate Chair of Surgery, Director, Trauma and Surgical Critical Care, University of Michigan Health System, Ann Arbor, Michigan

Nicholas A. Nash

Scott H. Norwood, MD, FACS
Clinical Professor of Surgery, Morsani College of Medicine, University of South Florida, Tampa, Florida; Trauma Service, Regional Medical Center, Bayonet Point, Hudson, Florida

John Oeltjen, MD, PhD
Associate Professor of Surgery, University of Miami, Miami, Florida

Chris Okwuosa, MD
Surgical Resident, Creighton University Medical Center, Omaha, Nebraska

Turner M. Osler, MD, MSc, FACS
Research Professor, Department of Surgery, University of Vermont, Burlington, Vermont

Angela Osmolak, MD
Surgical Resident, Creighton University Medical Center, Omaha, Nebraska

Yasuhiro Otomo, MD, PhD
Director, Trauma and Acute Critical Care Center, Tokyo Medical and Dental University Hospital of Medicine, Tokyo, Japan

Patrick Owens, MD
Associate Professor of Clinical Orthopedics, Associate Professor of Surgery, University of Miami, Miami, Florida

John T. Owings, MD, FACS
Director of Trauma Services, University Health, Professor of Surgery, Chief of Trauma and Critical Care, Louisiana State University School of Medicine, Shreveport, Louisiana; Professor Emeritus, University of California Davis, School of Medicine, Sacramento, California

H. Leon Pachter, MD, FACS
The George David Stewart Professor and Chair, Department of Surgery, New York University School of Medicine, New York, New York

David Palange, DS
Doctor of Osteopathic Medicine, University Hospital–UMDNJ, Newark, New Jersey

Zubin Jal Panthaki, BEng, MD, CM, FACS
Professor of Clinical Surgery, Division of Plastic Surgery, Professor of Clinical Orthopedics, Director, Hand Surgery Fellowship Program, Associate Director, Plastic Surgery Residency Program, The University of Miami, Leonard M. Miller School of Medicine; Chief of Plastic Surgery, Chief of Hand Surgery, Miami Veterans Administration Hospital; Chief of Plastic Surgery, Sylvester Comprehensive Cancer Center; Chief of Hand Surgery, University of Miami Hospital, Miami, Florida

Manish S. Parikh, MD
Associate Professor of Surgery, New York University School of Medicine, New York, New York

Michael D. Pasquale, MD, FACS, FCCM
Chair, Department of Surgery, Lehigh Valley Health Network, Allentown, Pennsylvania; Professor of Surgery, University of South Florida, Morsani College of Medicine, Tampa, Florida

Andrew B. Peitzman, MD
Distinguished Professor of Surgery, Mark M. Ravitch Professor and Vice-Chair, Vice-President for Trauma and Surgical Services, University of Pittsburgh School of Medicine, Pittsburgh, Pennsylvania

Alejandro Perez-Alonso, MD, PhD
International Doctor in Medicine and Surgery, General and Digestive Surgeon, Master in Tissue Engineering, Master in Trauma Surgery, Assistant Professor of Surgery, Senior Researcher, Department of Experimental Surgery, University of Granada; Attending Physician, Trauma and General Surgery, Hospital Universitario San Cecilio, Granada, Spain

Christopher H. Perkins, MD
Assistant Professor, Orthopedic Trauma, Baylor College of Medicine, Houston, Texas

Austin Person, MD
Resident, General Surgery, Creighton University, Omaha, Nebraska

Patrizio Petrone, MD, MPH, MHA, FACS
Director of Research, Program Director, International Visiting Scholars/Research

Fellowship; Division of Trauma Surgery, Surgical Critical Care, and Acute Care Surgery, Department of Surgery, New York Medical College; Westchester Medical Center University Hospital, Valhalla, New York

K. Shad Pharaon, MD
Division of Trauma, Critical Care, and Acute Care Surgery, Department of Surgery, Oregon Health and Science University, Portland, Oregon; Division of Trauma and Acute Care Surgery, Surgical Critical Care, PeaceHealth Southwest Medical Center, Vancouver, Washington

Allan S. Philp, MD, FACS, FCCM
Trauma Medical Director, Allegheny General Hospital; Associate Professor of Surgery, Temple University, Pittsburgh, Pennsylvania

Edgar J. Pierre, MD
Volunteer Associate Professor, Department of Anesthesia and Surgery, University of Miami Miller School of Medicine, Miami, Florida

Greta L. Piper, MD
Assistant Professor of Surgery, NYU Langone Medical Center, New York, New York

Frank Plani, MD, FCS(SA), FRACS, Trauma Surgery (SA)
Principal Specialist and Deputy Head, Chris Hani Baragwanath Academic Hospital Trauma Directorate, Division of Surgery, Soweto; Adjunct Professor, Department of Surgery, Clinical School of Medicine, University of the Witwatersrand, Johannesburg, South Africa

Patricio Polanco, MD
Department of Surgery, University of Pittsburgh Medical Center, Pittsburgh, Pennsylvania

Anthony Policastro, MD, FACS
Department of Surgery, New York Medical College; Associate Professor of Surgery, Westchester Medical Center University Hospital; Division of Trauma and Surgical Critical Care, Associate Director of Surgical Critical Care, Director of Surgical and Trauma Intensive Care Units, Valhalla, New York

Nathan J. Powell, DO, FACOS
Attending Surgeon, Trauma/Acute Care Surgery, St. Francis Trauma Institute, Tulsa, Oklahoma

Riaan Pretorius, MBChB(Pta), FCS (SA), Certificate in trauma surgery (SA)
Trauma Consultant, Chris Hani Baragwanath Academic Hospital; Junior Lecturer, University of Witwatersrand, Johannesburg, South Africa

Brandon Propper, MD

G. Daniel Pust, MD
Assistant Professor of Surgery, Division of Trauma and Surgical Critical Care, The DeWitt Daughtry Family Department of Surgery, Ryder Trauma Center/Jackson Memorial Hospital, University of Miami Miller School of Medicine, Miami, Florida Miami, Florida

Bradley S. Putty, Lt Col, USAF, MC
Assistant Professor, Department of Surgery, Division of Trauma and Critical Care, St. Louis University Hospital, St. Louis, Missouri

Juan Carlos Puyana, MD, FACS
Associate Professor of Surgery and Critical Care Medicine, University of Pittsburgh; Chief Medical Officer, Innovative Medical Information Technologies Center, University of Pittsburgh Medical Center, Pittsburgh, Pennsylvania

Stephen M. Quinnan
University of Miami Miller School of Medicine, Jackson Memorial Hospital, Miami, Florida

David J. Quintana, MD
Emory University School of Medicine, Department of Radiology, Division of Interventional Radiology and Image-Guided Medicine, Atlanta, Georgia

R. Lawrence Reed II, MD, FACS, FCCM
Professor of Surgery, Indiana University; Director of Trauma Services, Indiana University Health Methodist Hospital, Indianapolis, Indiana

Bibiana J. Reiser, MD, MS
Children's Hospital of Los Angeles, University of Southern California, Los Angeles, California

Peter Rhee, MD, MPH, FACS, FCCM, DMCC
Martin Gluck Professor of Surgery, University of Arizona; Director of Trauma, Critical Care, Burns, and Emergency Surgery, University of Arizona Medical Center, Tucson, Arizona

Michael Rhodes, MD, FACS, FCCM
Professor of Surgery, Thomas Jefferson University; Value Institute Senior Consultant for Advances in Medicine; Chair Emeritus, Department of Surgery, Christiana Care Health Systems, Wilmington, Delaware

Norman M. Rich, MD, FACS, DMCC, COL, MC
Leonard Heaton & David Packard Professor, Senior Advisor to the Chairman, Norman M. Rich Department of Surgery, F. Edward Hebert School of Medicine, Uniformed Services University of the Health Sciences, Bethesda, Maryland

J. David Richardson, MD
Professor of Surgery, University of Louisville, Louisville, Kentucky

Charles M. Richart, MD, FACS
Associate Professor, Department of Surgery, University of Missouri—Kansas City; Associate Director, Trauma Surgical Critical Care, Director, Surgical Critical Care Research and Surgical ANH Program, Saint Luke's Hospital of Kansas City, Kansas City, MO

Luis A. Rivas, MD
Associate Professor of Radiology, Chief, Trauma and Emergency Radiology, University of Miami, Jackson Memorial Medical, Miami, Florida

Jennifer C. Roberts, MD
Marshfield Clinic, Marshfield, Wisconsin

Aurelio Rodríguez, MD, FACS
Trauma and General Surgeon, Associate Director, Division of Trauma, Sinai Hospital, Baltimore, Maryland; Director Emeritus, Allegheny General Hospital, Shock Trauma Center, Pittsburgh, Pennsylvania

Jorge L. Rodríguez, MD
University of Louisville, Louisville, Kentucky

Erwin Rodriguez-García, MD
Department of Surgery, Hospital Militar Central–Universidad Militar Nueva Granada, Bogota, Colombia

Rosaine Roeder, MD, MPH
Lahey Hospital and Medical Center, Burlington, Massachusetts

David Rojas-Tirado, MD
Department of Surgery, Hospital Militar Central–Universidad Militar Nueva Granada, Bogota, Colombia

Michael F. Rotondo, MD, FACS
Chief Executive Officer, University of Rochester Medical Faculty Group; Vice Dean for Clinical Affairs, School of Medicine, Professor of Surgery, Division of Acute Care Surgery, Vice President of Administration, Strong Memorial Hospital, University of Rochester Medical Center, Rochester, New York

Susan Rowell, MD, MCR
Associate Professor of Surgery, Program Director, Surgical Critical Care Fellowship, Department of Surgery, Division of Trauma, Critical Care, and Acute Care Surgery, Oregon Health and Science University, Portland, Oregon

Jerry A. Rubano, MD
Department of Surgery, Division of Trauma, Critical Care, and Burns, State University of New York, Stony Brook University Health Sciences Center, Stony Brook, New York

Andrés M. Rubiano, MD, PhD, FACS
Medical and Research Director, MEDITECH Foundation; Professor of Neurosciences, South Colombian University; Neurosurgeon, Trauma and Emergency Service, Neiva University Hospital, Neiva (Huila), Colombia

Amy Rushing, MD
Assistant Professor of Surgery, Division of Trauma, Critical Care, and Burn, Wexner Medical Center, The Ohio State University, Columbus, Ohio

Irony C. Sade, MD
Resident, 3rd Year, General Surgery, Westchester Medical Center, Valhalla, New York

Christopher Salgado, MD
Professor of Surgery, Division of Plastic Surgery, Section Chief, University of Miami Hospital; Editor in Chief, Journal of Anaplastology, Miami, Florida

Ali Salim, MD, FACS
Professor of Surgery, Harvard Medical School; Chief, Division of Trauma, Burns, and Surgical Critical Care, Boston, Massachusetts

Noelle Salliant, MD
Division of Traumatology, Department of Surgery, Critical Care and Acute Care Surgery, The Trauma Center at Penn, University of Pennsylvania, Philadelphia, Pennsylvania

Jason Salsamendi, MD
Assistant Professor of Clinical Radiology, Department of Radiology, Assistant Professor of Clinical Surgery, Department of Surgery, University of Miami Miller School of Medicine, Miami, Florida

James B. Sampson, MD, FACS
David Grant Medical Center, Travis Air Force Base, Fairfield, California; University of California Davis, Sacramento, California

Juan A. Sanchez, MD, MPA, FACS, FACC
Associate Professor of Surgery, Johns Hopkins University School of Medicine; Chairman, Department of Surgery, Baltimore, Maryland

William Sánchez Maldonado, MD, FACS
Department of Surgery, Hospital Militar Central–Universidad Militar Nueva Granada, Bogota, Colombia

Thomas M. Scalea, MD
Physician in Chief, R Adams Cowley Shock Trauma Center, Francis X. Kelly Distinguished Professor of Trauma, University of Maryland School of Medicine, Baltimore, Maryland

William P. Schecter, MD
Professor of Clinical Surgery, University of California San Francisco, San Francisco General Hospital, San Francisco, California

Paul Schipper, MD, FACS, FACCP
Professor of Surgery and Program Director, Cardiothoracic Surgery Residency, Oregon Health and Science University and Portland Veterans Administration Medical Center, Portland, Oregon

Martin Schreiber, MD, FACS
Professor of Surgery, Chief, Division of Trauma Critical Care, and Acute Care Surgery, Department of Surgery, Oregon Health and Science University, Portland, Oregon

John T. Schulz III, MD, PhD
Medical Director, Sumner Redstone Burn Center, Massachusetts General Hospital, Boston, Massachusetts

C. William Schwab, MD, FACS
Professor of Surgery, Perelman School of Medicine, University of Pennsylvania; Division of Traumatology, Surgical Critical Care and Emergency Surgery, Hospital of the University of Pennsylvania, Philadelphia, Pennsylvania

Stephen Serio, MD
Surgical Resident, Creighton University Medical Center, Omaha, Nebraska

Parth Shah, MD
General Surgery Resident, Department of Surgery, CHI Health Alegent Creighton Clinic, Omaha, Nebraska

Marc J. Shapiro, MD
Professor of Surgery and Anesthesiology, Chief of General Surgery, Trauma, Critical Care, and Burns, Department of Surgery, SUNY-Stony Brook, Stony Brook, New York

David Shatz, MD
Professor, Department of Surgery, Division of Trauma and Emergency Surgery, University of California Davis, Sacramento, California

Shreya Shetty, MD
Resident, General Surgery, Creighton University, Omaha, Nebraska

Adam M. Shiroff, MD, FACS
Chief of Trauma, Jersey Shore University Medical Center, Assistant Professor of Surgery, Rutgers Robert Wood Johnson Medical School, New Brunswick, New Jersey

Ziad C. Sifri, MD
Associate Professor of Surgery, Division of Trauma, Rutgers New Jersey Medical School, Newark, New Jersey

Ronald Sing, DO, FACS, FCCM
Professor of Surgery, Division of Acute Care Surgery, Carolinas Medical Center, Charlotte, North Carolina; Adjunct Professor of Surgery, University of North Carolina School of Medicine at Chapel Hill, Chapel Hill, North Carolina

Amy C. Sisley, MD, MPH
Division Chief, Acute Care Surgery, Department of Surgery, Henry Ford Hospital, Detroit, Michigan

R. Stephen Smith, MD
System Chief, Division of Trauma, Burn, and Acute Care Surgery, West Penn Allegheny Health System; Professor of Surgery, Temple University School of Medicine, Pittsburgh, Pennsylvania

Eduardo Smith-Singares, MD, FACS
Chief, Division of Surgical Critical Care, Department of Surgery, University of Illinois at Chicago College of Medicine; Co-Director SICU, University of Illinois Hospital and Health Sciences System, Chicago, Illinois

David A. Spain, MD, FACS
Carol and Ned Spieker Professor and Chief of Acute Care Surgery, Department of Surgery, Stanford University, Stanford, California

Nicholas Spoerke, MD
Surgical Critical Care Fellow, Oregon Health and Science University, Portland, Oregon

Ananth Srinivasan, MBBS
Creighton University School of Medicine, Omaha, Nebraska

Deborah M. Stein, MD, MPH
Associate Professor of Surgery, University of Maryland School of Medicine; Chief of Trauma, R Adams Cowley Shock Trauma Center, Baltimore, Maryland

Joseph J. Stirparo, MD
Trauma, Surgical Critical Care, Lehigh Valley Health Network, Allentown, Pennsylvania; Assistant Professor of Surgery, University of South Florida, Morsani College of Medicine, Tampa, Florida

Lance E. Stuke, MD, MPH, FACS
Associate Professor of Surgery, Louisiana State University, Spirit of Charity Trauma Center, New Orleans, Lousiana

Mithran Sukumar, MD
Assistant Professor of Surgery, Oregon Health and Science University; Section Head, General Thoracic Surgery, Division of Cardiothoracic Surgery, Portland Veterans Administration Medical Center, Portland, Oregon

Abhishek Sundaram, MD
General Surgery Resident, Department of Surgery, Creighton University, Omaha, Nebraska

Wendy Jo Svetanoff, MD
HO4, Department of Surgery, Creighton University Medical Center, Omaha, Nebraska

⚜Kenneth G. Swan, MD
Professor of Surgery, Director, Third Year Surgical Clerkship, Department of Surgery, New Jersey Medical School, University of Medicine and Dentistry of New Jersey, Newark, New Jersey

Vartan S. Tashjian, MD, MS
Resident Surgeon, Division of Neurological Surgery, University of California, Los Angeles, Los Angeles, California

Thomas Templin, MD
Resident Physician, Creighton University School of Medicine, Creighton University Medical Center, Omaha, Nebraska

Erwin Thal, MD, FACS, FRACS (Hon.)
Professor of Surgery, Department of Surgery, University of Texas Southwestern Medical Hospital; Attending Surgeon, Department of Surgery, Parkland Hospital; Attending Surgeon, Department of Surgery, University of Texas Southwestern University Hospital–St. Paul; Attending Surgeon, Department of Surgery, University of Texas Southwestern University Hospital–Zale Lisphy, Dallas, Texas

Seth R. Thaller, MD, DMD, FACS
Chief and Professor, Division of Plastic Surgery, The DeWitt Daughtry Family Department of Surgery, University Of Miami Health System, Miami, Florida

Gregory Tiesi, MD
Department of General Surgery, Rutgers New Jersey Medical School, Newark, New Jersey

Brandon Tieu, MD, FACS
Assistant Professor of Surgery, Division of Cardiothoracic Surgery, Department of Surgery, Oregon Health and Science University and Portland Veterans Administration Medical Center, Portland, Oregon

Areti Tillou, MD, FACS, MsEd
Associate Professor, Vice Chair for Education, UCLA David Geffen School of Medicine, Los Angeles, California

Glen Tinkoff, MD, FACS, FCCM
Associate Vice Chair, Department of Surgery, Christiana Care Health System, Newark, Delaware; Clinical Professor of Surgery, Jefferson Medical College, Philadelphia, Pennsylvania

Samuel Tisherman, MD, FACS, FCCM
R Adams Cowley Shock Trauma Center, University of Maryland, Director, Surgical Intensive Care Unit, Baltimore, Maryland

S. Rob Todd, MD
Associate Professor of Surgery, New York University Langone Medical Center; Director, Bellevue Emergency Surgery Service, Department of Surgery, Bellevue Hospital Center; Faculty, Department of Surgery, Tisch Hospital, New York, New York

Zachary Torgersen, MD
Surgical Resident, Creighton University Medical Center, Omaha, Nebraska

Peter G. Trafton, MD, FACS
Professor and Vice Chair, Department of Orthopedic Surgery, Brown University School of Medicine, Providence, Rhode Island

Mark Traynham, MD
Creighton University Medical Center, Omaha, Nebraska

L.R. Tres Scherer, MD, FACS
Volunteer Clinical Professor of Surgery, Indiana University School of Medicine, Carmel, Indiana

Donald D. Trunkey, MD, FACS
Professor Emeritus, Department of Surgery, Division of Trauma, Oregon Health and Science University, Portland, Oregon

Peter I. Tsai, MD, MA
Assistant Professor of Surgery, Division of Cardiothoracic Surgery, Michael E. DeBakey Department of Surgery, Baylor College of Medicine/Texas Heart Institute; Medical Director, Department of Cardiothoracic Surgery, Ben Taub General Hospital, Houston, Texas

David W. Tuggle, MD
Associate Trauma Medical Director, Dell Children's Medical Center of Central Texas, Austin, Texas

Anthony M. Udekwu, MD, FRCS(C), FACS

Alex B. Valadka, MD, FAANS, FACS
Chairman and Chief Executive Officer, Seton Brain and Spine Institute, Austin, Texas

Nicole VanDerHeyden, MD, PhD
Trauma Medical Director, Trauma Services, Salem Hospital, Salem, Oregon

Thomas K. Varghese, Jr., MD
Assistant Professor, Associate Program Director–Cardiothoracic Surgery Residency, University of Washington; Director of Thoracic Surgery, Department of Surgery, Harborview Medical Center, Seattle, Washington

Michel Wagner, MD, FACS
Assistant Professor, Division of Trauma, Creighton University School of Medicine, CHI–Creighton University Medical Center, Omaha, Nebraska

Matthew J. Wall, Jr., MD
Professor, Michael E. DeBakey Department of Surgery, Baylor College of Medicine; Deputy Chief of Surgery, Chief of Cardiothoracic Surgery, Department of Surgery, Ben Taub General Hospital, Houston, Texas

Anthony Watkins, MD
Clinical Instructor in Surgery, Department of Transplantation, Columbia University/New York Presbyterian Hospital, New York, New York

John Weigelt, MD
Medical College of Wisconsin, Milwaukee, Wisconsin

⚜Deceased.

Leonard J. Weireter, Jr., MD, FACS
Arthur and Marie Kirk Family Professor of Surgery, Department of Surgery, Eastern Virginia Medical School, Norfolk, Virginia

David R. Welling, MD, FACS, FASCRS, DMCC
Professor of Surgery, Uniformed Services University of the Health Sciences, Walter Reed National Military Medical Center, Bethesda, Maryland

Paul W. White, MD, FACS
LTC, Medical Corps, United States Army; Program Director, Vascular Surgery Fellowship, Walter Reed National Military Medical Center; Associate Professor of Surgery, Uniformed Services University of the Health Sciences, Bethesda, Maryland

Lucas R. Wiegand, MD
Assistant Professor of Urology, University of South Florida, Tampa, Florida

Harry E. Wilkins, MD
Associate Professor, Department of Surgery, University of Missouri–Kansas City; Medical Director, Trauma and Surgical Critical Care, Saint Luke's Hospital of Kansas City, Kansas City, Missouri

Robert F. Wilson, MD, FACS, MCCM
Professor of Surgery, Wayne State University School of Medicine; Director, Surgical Intensive Care Unit, Detroit Receiving Hospital, Detroit, Michigan

David H. Wisner, MD
Professor and Vice Chair, Department of Surgery, University of California Davis; Chief of Surgery, UC Davis Medical Center Sacramento, California

D. Dante Yeh, MD, FACS
Massachusetts General Hospital, Harvard Medical School, Boston, Massachusetts

FOREWORD

Traumatic injury is the leading cause of death and disability for young adults and affects the lives of people all over the world. Comprehensive trauma surgical management must address prevention, the immediate needs of one victim or the sudden arrival of mass casualties, as well as rehabilitation and end-of-life care. The second edition of Current Therapy of Trauma and Surgical Critical Care is an invaluable resource for all who participate in the care of trauma patients, including military personnel and medical consultants.

Noted experts who are practicing academic trauma surgeons author the chapters and address controversies in an objective manner. Evidence-based guidelines are presented and discussed as are best practice recommendations based on years of busy clinical and operative experience. The critical care section of the book is well written and masterfully bridges basic physiology to the bedside evaluation of the patient.

New chapters in this edition address areas of growing importance including triage in civilian as well as military facilities, vascular injuries, difficult and complex injuries, recent lessons learned from the care of combat casualties, brain death, and organ donation.

The editors, Drs. Juan A. Asensio and Donald D. Trunkey, are visionary leaders who have spent their careers changing the way we view trauma care. They have revised and expanded this edition of Current Therapy of Trauma and Surgical Critical Care to help trauma systems meet new challenges in an increasingly global society.

ROBERT DUNLAY, MD
Dean
Creighton University School of Medicine

"If you get him to the operating room with a blood pressure, I will come in"

Growing up and training on the South Side of Chicago, I distinctly remember these words being spoken to me by my mentor during my cardiothoracic surgery residency.... I called him twice in 2 years. Trauma care has come a long way since that time and though many of the principles of management are the same and our focus always remains on the injury at hand, I now know that there is an ever evolving, complex, and sophisticated "trauma system" in place coordinating the efforts of many professionals and necessary to have that patient arrive on my operating table with a "blood pressure."

As *Current Therapy of Trauma and Surgical Critical Care* now enters its second edition, it is already one of the leading references for anyone involved in trauma. This current edition continues in the tradition of the *Current Therapy* series by updating, revising and expanding sections. There are new and updated sections on vascular injuries, developments in imaging technology, and up-to-date information on the newer ventilatory techniques. Edited by Dr. Juan Asensio and Dr. Donald Trunkey, two of the most well recognized names in trauma, it represents a comprehensive and authoritative text that covers the complete continuum of care with an emphasis on operative techniques for even the most complex of injuries.

The list of contributors represents a virtual "who's who" in trauma and critical care and is formatted to give the practicing professional practical, concise, and updated information focusing on organ systems and operative techniques. It is a compendium of what is considered common and accepted practice that is evidence based and clinically relevant, expert opinion, and discussion of controversial areas and challenges. There is something for everyone involved in trauma care, beginning with the history of trauma, the development of trauma systems, and the latest information regarding specific organ injury management, prevention, ICU care, mass casualty events, palliative care, rehabilitation, and outcomes.

Current Therapy of Trauma and Surgical Critical Care clearly represents a labor of love for Dr. Trunkey and now Dr. Asensio with a vision to create a comprehensive yet practical and concise reference for the trauma community. I would recommend it as worthwhile reading and a valuable reference for anyone involved in the care of the trauma patient

JEFFREY T. SUGIMOTO, MD
Dr. and Mrs. Arnold Lempka Chair in Surgery
Professor and Chairman
Chief, Cardiothoracic Surgery
Department of Surgery
Creighton University School of Medicine
Creighton University

It is now the dawn of the twenty-first century, and what a turbulent century it threatens to be. Once again it is a privilege and an honor to serve as the editor of *Current Therapy of Trauma and Surgical Critical Care*. This is actually the sixth edition; however, the editors have renumbered it as the second edition because we have added surgical critical care to this noble textbook.

One thing is constant: our world is turbulent and dangerous and will continue to be so for many future generations. A quick scan of the media, whether it is television, digital news, or the printed word, reveals that our world is currently experiencing multiple armed conflicts, with a large number of casualties from these conflicts. Our profession, perhaps the most godly of all professions, continues to be under siege; economic and market forces continue to encroach on the ability of doctors, and of course surgeons, to deliver the most optimum of care, especially, as it is often said, "To the least of these. . .," which means to the poorest of our brethren.

Amidst all of this turmoil, trauma surgeons and surgical critical care specialists have risen to the occasion by also taking on the burden of the management of acute care surgery. Once again trauma surgeons stand as pillars of strength, the quintessential "band of brothers." I rise to quote Shakespeare in describing trauma surgeons:

"That he which hath no stomach to this fight,
Let him depart. His passport shall be made,
And crowns for convoy put into his purse.
We would not die in that man's company
That fears his fellowship to die with us.
From this day to the ending of the world,
But we in it shall be remembered—
We few, we happy few, we band of brothers;
For he today that sheds his blood with me
Shall be my brother." (Henry V, Act IV, Scene 3)

It is my strong belief that the honor and the privilege of attempting to save a life not only in an operating room but also by counseling patients is indeed a noble task in the effort to eliminate trauma as a disease. We continue to hold on to the dream that we as leaders will eventually see a world in which there will be no wars and there will be greater understanding and more time and effort dedicated to the improvement of the human condition. We continue to believe that with our dedication we will make a difference, hoping to create bridges between people, leading to greater understanding and cooperation in human relations and in the field of scientific research. These ideals and goals remain lofty, but in speaking to my colleagues, this belief is strong and continues to motivate us all. I strongly believe that the alleviation of pain and suffering and the saving of lives remains a most important commitment for those who belong to this elite fraternity, the "band of brothers."

Once again I challenge, I urge, I beseech all of my colleagues in trauma surgery to go beyond the walls of academia to serve those who must be served, to use the power of our professions to exercise our consciences, to serve as leaders and advocates for human rights, to heal the wounded, and to teach the future generations of those who will be given the great gift to perform trauma surgery. We must be prepared to take the challenge to create peace and to heal wounds because it is we and those who have come before us who have been there, holding the hands of the wounded and injured, filled with pain and crying, often inwardly, when a life is lost, and continuing to struggle to save other lives.

IF—

By Rudyard Kipling

If you can keep your head when all about you
    Are losing theirs and blaming it on you,
If you can trust yourself when all men doubt you,
    But make allowance for their doubting too;
If you can wait and not be tired by waiting,
    Or being lied about, don't deal in lies,
Or being hated, don't give way to hating,
    And yet don't look too good, nor talk too wise:

If you can dream—and not make dreams your master;
    If you can think—and not make thoughts your aim;
If you can meet with Triumph and Disaster
    And treat those two impostors just the same;
If you can bear to hear the truth you've spoken
    Twisted by knaves to make a trap for fools,
Or watch the things you gave your life to, broken,
    And stoop and build 'em up with worn-out tools:

If you can make one heap of all your winnings
    And risk it on one turn of pitch-and-toss,
And lose, and start again at your beginnings
    And never breathe a word about your loss;
If you can force your heart and nerve and sinew
    To serve your turn long after they are gone,
And so hold on when there is nothing in you
    Except the Will which says to them: 'Hold on!'

If you can talk with crowds and keep your virtue,
    Or walk with Kings—nor lose the common touch,
If neither foes nor loving friends can hurt you,
    If all men count with you, but none too much;
If you can fill the unforgiving minute
    With sixty seconds' worth of distance run,
Yours is the Earth and everything that's in it,
    And—which is more—you'll be a Man, my son!

From *A Choice of Kipling's Verse* (1943)

JUAN A. ASENSIO, MD, FACS, FCCM, FRCS, KM

CONTENTS

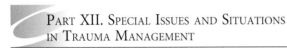

PART XII. SPECIAL ISSUES AND SITUATIONS IN TRAUMA MANAGEMENT

PART XIII. CRITICAL CARE I: MANAGEMENT OF ORGAN FAILURES AND TECHNIQUES FOR SUPPORT

PART XIV: CRITICAL CARE II: SPECIAL ISSUES AND TREATMENTS

PART XV: REHABILITATION AND QUALITY OF LIFE AFTER TRAUMA AND OTHER ISSUES

TRAUMA SYSTEMS

DEVELOPMENT OF TRAUMA SYSTEMS

Donald D. Trunkey

Modern trauma care consists of three primary components: prehospital care, acute surgical care or hospital care, and rehabilitation. Ideally, a society, through state (department, province, regional, etc.) government, should provide a trauma system that ensures all three components. The purpose of this chapter is to show how trauma systems have evolved, to discuss whether or not they work, and to define current problems.

From an historical viewpoint, it is an accepted concept that trauma care and trauma systems are inextricably linked to war. What is not appreciated is that trauma systems are not recent concepts. They date back to centuries before the Common Era. It is not known for certain whether the wounds of prehistoric humans were due primarily to violence or to accident. The first solid evidence of war wounds came from a mass grave found in Egypt and date to approximately 2000 BC. The bodies of 60 soldiers were found in a sufficiently well-preserved state to show mace injuries, gaping wounds, and arrows still in the body. The Smith Papyrus records the clinical treatment of 48 cases of war wounds, and is primarily a textbook on how to treat wounds, most of which were penetrating. According to Majno, there were 147 recorded wounds in Homer's *Iliad*, with an overall mortality rate of 77.6%. Thirty-one soldiers sustained wounds to the head, all of which were fatal. The surgical care for a wounded Greek soldier was crude at best. However, the Greeks did recognize the need for a system of combat care. The wounded were given care in special barracks (*klisiai*) or in nearby ships. Wound care was primitive. Barbed arrowheads were removed by enlarging the wound with a knife or pushing the arrowhead through the wound. Drugs, usually derived from plants, were applied to wounds. Wounds were bound, but according to Homer, hemostasis was treated by an *"epaoide,"* that is, someone sang a song or recited a charm over the wound.

The Romans perfected the delivery of combat care and set up a system of trauma centers throughout the Empire. These trauma centers were called *valetudinaria* and were built during the first and second centuries AD. The remains of 25 such centers have been found, but significantly, none were found in Rome or other large cities. Of some interest, there were 11 trauma centers in Roman Britannia, more than currently exist in this area. Some of the *valetudinaria* were designed to handle a combat casualty rate of up to 10%. There was a regular medical corps within the Roman legions, and at least 85 army physicians are recorded, mainly because they died and earned an epitaph.

From elsewhere in the world came other evidence that trauma systems were provided for the military. India may well have had a system of trauma care that rivaled that of the Romans. The *Artasastra*, a book written during the reign of Ashoka (269–232 BC) documented that the Indian army had an ambulance service, with well-equipped surgeons and women to prepare food and beverages. Indian medicine was specialized, and it was the *shalyarara* (surgeon) who would be called upon to treat wounds. *Shalyarara* literally means "arrow remover," as the bow and arrow was the traditional weapon for Indians.

Over the next millennium, military trauma care did not make any major advances until just before the Renaissance. Two French military surgeons, who lived 250 miles apart, brought trauma care into the Age of Enlightenment.

Ambrose Paré (1510–1590) served four French kings during the time of the French-Spanish civil and religious wars. His major contributions to treating penetrating trauma included his treatment of gunshot wounds, his use of ligature instead of cautery, and the use of nutrition during the postinjury period. Paré was also much interested in prosthetic devices, and designed a number of them for amputees.

It was Dominique Larrey, Napoleon's surgeon, who addressed trauma from a systematic and organizational standpoint. Larrey introduced the concept of the "flying ambulance," the sole purpose of which was to provide rapid removal of the wounded from the battlefield. Larrey also introduced the concept of putting the hospital as close to the front lines as feasible in order to permit wound surgery as soon as possible. His primary intent was to operate during the period of "wound shock," when there was an element of analgesia, but also to reduce infection in the postamputation period.

Larrey had an understanding of problems that were unique to military surgery. Some of his contributions can best be appreciated by his efforts before Napoleon's Russian campaign. Larrey did not know which country Napoleon was planning to attack, and there was even conjecture about an invasion of England. He left Paris on February 24, 1812, and was ordered to Mentz, Germany. Shortly thereafter, he went to Magdeburg and then on to Berlin, where he began preparations for the campaign, still not knowing precisely where the French army was headed. In his own words, "Previous to my departure from the capital, I organized six divisions of flying ambulances, each one consisting of eight surgeons. The surgeons-major exercised their divisions daily, according to my instructions, in the performance of operations, and the application of bandages. The greatest degree of emulation, and the strictest discipline, were prevalent among all the surgeons."

The 19th century may well be described as the century of enlightenment for surgical care in combat. This was partly because of better statistical reporting, but also because of major contributions to patient care, including the introduction of anesthesia. During the Crimean War (1853–1856), the English reported a mortality rate of 92.7% in cases of penetrating wounds of the abdomen, and the French had a rate of 91.7%. During the American War Between the States, there were 3031 deaths among the 3717 cases of abdominal penetrating wounds, a mortality rate of 81.5%.

The Crimean War was noteworthy in having been the conflict in which the French tested a number of local antiseptic agents. Ferrous chloride was found to be very effective against hospital-related gangrene, but the English avoided the use of antiseptics in wounds. It was also during the Crimean War that two further major contributions to combat medicine were introduced when Florence Nightingale emphasized sanitation and humane nursing care for combat casualties.

The use of antiseptics was continued into the American War Between the States. Bromine reduced the mortality rate from hospital gangrene to 2.6% in a reported series of 308 patients. This contrasted with a mortality rate of 43.3% among patients for whom bromine was not used. Strong nitric acid was also used as an antiseptic in hospital gangrene, with a mortality rate of 6.6%. Anesthetics were used by federal military surgeons in 80,000 patients. Tragically, mortality rate from gunshot wounds to the extremities remained high, paralleling that reported by Paré in the 16th century. The mortality rate from gunshot fractures of the humerus and upper arm was 30.7%; those of the forearm, 21.9%; of the femur, 31.7%; and of the leg, 14.4%. The overall mortality rate from amputation in 29,980 patients was 26.3%.

The Franco-Prussian War (1870–1874) was marked by terrible deaths and the reluctance of some surgeons to use the wound antiseptics advocated by Lister. The mortality rate for femur fractures was 65.8% in one series, and ranged from 54.2% to 91.7% in other series. Late in the conflict, surgeons finally accepted Lister's recommendations, and the mortality rate fell dramatically.

During the Boer War (1899–1902), the British advised celiotomy in all cases of penetrating abdominal wounds. However, early results were abysmal, and a subsequent British military order called for conservative or expectant treatment.

During the early months of World War I, abdominal injuries had an unacceptable 85% mortality rate. As the war progressed, patients were brought to clearing stations and underwent surgery near the front, with a subsequent decrease in mortality rate to 56%. When the Americans entered the conflict, their overall mortality rate from penetrating abdominal wounds was 45%. One of the major contributions to trauma care during World War I was blood transfusion.

Since World War II, many contributions to combat surgical care have led to reductions in mortality and morbidity. Comparative mortality rates for various conflicts are listed in Table 1. Surgical mortality rates are shown in Table 2. The introduction of antibiotics and improvements in anesthesia, surgical techniques, and rapid prehospital transport are just a few of the innovations that have led to better outcomes.

MODERN TRAUMA SYSTEM DEVELOPMENT

Between the two world wars, some significant advances were made in civilian trauma care. Lorenz Böhler formed the first civilian trauma system in Austria in 1925. Although initially directed at work-related injuries, it eventually expanded to include all accidents. At the onset of World War II, the Birmingham Accident Hospital was founded. It continued to provide regional trauma care until recently. By 1975, Germany had established a nationwide trauma system, designed so that no patient was more than 15 to 20 minutes from one of these regional centers. Due to the work of Harald Tscherne and colleagues, this system has continued into the present, and mortality rate has decreased by over 50% (Fig. 1).

In North America, foundations for modern trauma systems were being undertaken. In 1912, at a meeting of the American Surgical Association in Montreal, a committee of five was appointed to prepare a statement on the management of fractures. This led to

TABLE 1: Percentage of Wounded American Soldiers Who Died from Their Wounds

War	Years	Number of Wounded Soldiers	Percentage of Wounded Soldiers Who Died of Wounds
Mexican War	1846–1848	3,400	15
American War Between the States	1861–1865	318,200	14
Spanish-American War	1898	1,600	7
World War I (excluding gas casualties)	1918	153,000	8
World War II	1942–1945	599,724	4.5
Korean Conflict	1950–1953	77,788	2.5
Vietnam Conflict	1865–1972	96,811	3.6

TABLE 2: Surgical Mortality Rates for Head, Chest, and Abdominal Wounds in Soldiers from U.S. Army

	Head	Thorax	Abdomen
World War I			
Number of soldiers	189	104	1816
Mortality rate (%)	40	37	67
World War II			
Number of soldiers	2051	1364	2315
Mortality rate (%)	14	10	23
Korean Conflict			
Number of soldiers	673	158	384
Mortality rate (%)	10	8	9
Vietnam Conflict			
Number of soldiers	1171	1176	1209
Mortality rate (%)	10	7	9

a standing committee. One year later, the American College of Surgeons was founded, and in May 1922, the Board of Regents of the American College of Surgeons started the first Committee on Fractures with Charles Scudder, MD, as chair. This eventually became the Committee on Trauma. Another function begun by the college in 1918 was the Hospital Standardization Program, which evolved into the Joint Commission on Accreditation of Hospitals. One function of this standardization program was an embryonic start of a trauma registry with acquisition of records of patients who were treated for fractures. In 1926, the Board of Industrial Medicine and Traumatic Surgery was formed. Thus, it was the standardization program by the American College of Surgeons, the Fracture Committee

TRAUMA DEATHS

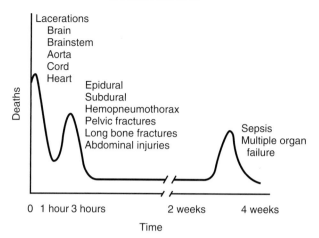

FIGURE 1 Trauma deaths have a trimodal distribution. The first death peak (approximately 50%) is within minutes of the injury. The second death peak (approximately 30%) occurs within a few hours to 48 hours. The third death peak (approximately 15%) occurs within 1 to 4 weeks and represents those patients who die from the complications of their injury or treatment. From a public health perspective, the first death peak can be addressed only by prevention, which is difficult, because part of this strategy means dealing with human behavior. The second death peak is best addressed by having a trauma system, and the third death peak requires critical care and research.

appointed by the American College of Surgeons, the availability of patient records from the Hospital Standardization Program, and the new Board of Industrial Medicine and Traumatic Surgery that provided the seeds of the trauma system.

In 1966, the first two trauma centers were established in the United States: William F. Blaisdell at San Francisco General Hospital and Robert Freeark at Cook County Hospital in Chicago. Three years later, a statewide trauma system was established in Maryland by R. A. Cowley. In 1976, the American College of Surgeons Committee on Trauma developed a formal outline of injury care called Optimal Criteria for Care of the Injured Patient. Subsequently, the task force of the American College of Surgeons Committee on Trauma met approximately every 4 years and updated their optimal criteria, which are now used extensively in establishing regional and state trauma systems and have recently been exported to Australia. Other contributions by the American College of Surgeons Committee on Trauma include introduction of the Advanced Trauma Life Support courses, establishment of a national trauma registry (National Trauma Data Bank), and a national verification program. The latter is analogous to the old hospital standardization program, and "verifies" by a peer review process whether a hospital's trauma center meets American College of Surgeons guidelines.

ARE TRAUMA SYSTEMS EFFECTIVE?

Since 1984, more than 15 articles have been published showing that trauma systems benefit society by increasing the chances of survival when patients are treated in specialized centers. In addition, two studies have shown that trauma systems also reduce trauma morbidity. In 1988, a report card was issued on the current status and future challenges of trauma systems. At that time, an inventory was taken of all state emergency medical service directors or health departments having responsibility over emergency and trauma planning. They were contacted via telephone survey in February 1987, and then were asked eight specific questions on their state trauma systems. Of the eight

criteria, only two states, Maryland and Virginia, were identified as having all eight essential components of a regional trauma system. Nineteen states and Washington, D.C. either had incomplete statewide coverage or lacked essential components. Not limiting the number of trauma centers in the region was the most common deficient criterion.

In 1995, another report card was issued in the *Journal of the American Medical Association*. This report card was an update on the progress and development of trauma systems since the 1988 report. It was a more sophisticated approach, as it expanded the original eight criteria and was more comprehensive. According to the 1995 report, five states (Florida, Maryland, Nevada, New York, and Oregon) had all the components necessary for a statewide system. Virginia no longer limited the number of designated trauma centers. An additional 15 states and Washington, D.C. had most of the components of a trauma system.

The 1995 report card was upgraded at the Skamania Conference in 1998. There are now 35 states across the United States actively engaged in meeting trauma system criteria. In addition to the report card, the Skamania Conference evaluated the effectiveness of trauma systems. The medical literature was searched and all available evidence was divided into three categories: reports resulting from panel studies (autopsy studies), registry comparisons, and population-based research. Panel studies suffered from wide variation and poor inter-rater reliability, and the autopsies alone were deemed inadequate. This finding led to the general consensus that panel studies were only weak class III evidence. Despite these limitations, however, MacKenzie et al. concluded that when all panel studies are considered collectively, they do provide some face validity and support the hypothesis that treatment in a trauma center versus a nontrauma center is associated with fewer inappropriate deaths and possibly even disability. Registry evaluation was found to be useful for assessing overall effectiveness of trauma systems. Jurkovich and Mock concluded the data clearly did not meet class I evidence. Their critique of trauma registries included the following: there are often missing data, miscodings occur, there may be inter-rater reliability factors, the national norms are not population-based, there is little detail about the cause of death, and they do not take into account prehospital deaths. Despite these deficits, conference participants reached consensus, concluding that registry studies were better than panel studies but not as good as population studies. Finally, population-based studies were evaluated and found to comprise class II evidence. An advantage over registry studies is attributed to studying and evaluating a large population in all aspects of trauma care, including prehospital, hospital, and rehabilitation. Unfortunately, only a limited number of clinical variables can be evaluated, and it is difficult to adjust for severity of injury and physiologic dysfunction. Despite disadvantages with all three studies, the advantages may be applied to various individual communities to help influence public health policy with regard to trauma system initiation and evaluation.

Two recent studies document the effectiveness of trauma systems. The first is a comparison of mortality rates between Level I trauma centers and hospitals without a trauma center. The in-hospital mortality rate was significantly lower in trauma centers than in nontrauma centers (7.6% vs. 9.5%). This 25% difference in mortality rate was present 1 year after injury with a 10.4% mortality rate connected to trauma centers and 13.8% to nontrauma centers. The second study was an assessment of the State of Florida's trauma system, and this study confirmed a 25% lower mortality rate in designated trauma centers.

WHAT ARE THE CURRENT PROBLEMS?

In the global burden of disease study by Murray and Lopez, the world is divided into developed regions and developing regions. They also examine various statistics on a global level. The most useful statistic or means of measuring disability is the disability-adjusted life year

(DALY). This is the sum of life years lost due to premature death and years lived with disability adjusted for severity. By 2020, road traffic accidents will be the number 3 overall cause worldwide of DALYs. This does not include DALYs from war, which is number 8. In developed countries, road traffic accidents are the fifth highest cause of DALYs, and in developing regions, the second highest cause. One of the most difficult problems that we face in the coming years is how to provide reasonable trauma care and trauma system development in the developing regions of the world. Prehospital care is currently nonexistent in most of these developing countries. There are few, if any, trauma centers in the urban areas, and certainly none in the rural areas of the same countries. Even if there were such centers or a trauma system, rehabilitation is almost totally lacking, and therefore, the injured person would rarely be able to return to work or productivity after a severe injury.

As noted earlier, Europe has in the last century developed some statewide trauma systems. However, there is no concerted effort by the European Union (EU) to establish criteria for trauma systems or to coordinate trauma care among countries within the EU. Similarly, the EU does not have standards for prehospital care, nor is there a network of rehabilitation facilities that have standards and are peer reviewed. In theory, surgeons trained in one EU country should be able to cross the various national borders and to practice surgery, including trauma care, within these different EU countries. Again, there are no standards for what constitutes a trauma surgeon, and in fact, trauma surgery is a potpourri of different models. One model is exemplified by Austria, where trauma surgery is an independent specialty. Another model incorporates trauma surgical training into general surgery, and this includes France, Italy, The Netherlands, and Turkey. In a third model, the majority of trauma training is given with orthopedic surgery residency training. Belgium and Switzerland follow this model. The largest model provides trauma surgery training within specific specialties without any single specialty having any major responsibility for trauma training, and this model prevails in Denmark, Germany, Portugal, Estonia, Iceland, England, Norway, Finland, and Sweden.

Some of the most vexing problems in trauma surgery occur now in North America, particularly in the United States. This is in part due to changes in general surgery. It is predicted that there will be a *major* shortage of general surgeons in the United States within the next few years. General surgeons are now older, and more importantly, general surgeons are now subspecializing. We now have foregut, hepatobiliary, vascular, breast, and colorectal surgeons. The one thing they all have in common is they do not want to take trauma calls. Our medical specialty colleagues' night call is now in transition and hospitals are hiring so-called "hospitalists," who are trained in family medicine or internal medicine. In many instances, the hospital will pay their salaries to provide 24/7 calls, usually on a 12-hour shift basis. In some instances, possibly up to one third, various practice groups will pay these hospitalists to take their calls in hospital. Another trend affecting general surgery is the rapid transition to nondiscrimination regarding gender. At least 50% of entering medical students are now female, but only 7% (approximately 500 individuals) apply to surgery. The reasons given are long hours and poor lifestyle, as these women wish to combine professional careers with parenting responsibilities. There is an overall decrease in applications to general surgery, and the reasons for this are complex and multifaceted. One important reason is that general surgeons' incomes are approximately 50% less than those of some specialty surgeons. A more concerning reason, however, is lifestyle perceptions. Younger medical students and physicians tend to opt out of surgery, and they particularly abhor trauma surgery, because of the time commitment and related lifestyle issues. Another problem, which may be unique to the United States, is the decrease in operative cases in trauma. There has been a shift from penetrating trauma to blunt trauma and another shift to nonoperative management, particularly of liver and spleen injuries. General surgeons have compounded the problem by referring cases to surgeons who specialize in vascular surgery or chest surgery. Interventional radiologists also participate in management of certain traumatic injuries.

Another vexing problem in trauma care in the United States is the current demand for on-call pay by specialty surgeons. This is particularly true in orthopedics and neurosurgery. This on-call pay ranges from $1000 to $7000 a night. On average, a neurosurgeon in a Level I hospital would only be called in 33 times in the course of a year. In contrast, orthopedic surgeons average approximately 275 emergency cases during the year. Obviously, this responsibility could be shared between groups. Nevertheless, hospitals are being asked to pay on-call stipends to neurosurgeons that are quite large, considering the relatively low probability of being called in.

Other factors affecting trauma availability by specialty surgeons are freestanding ambulatory surgery centers where the surgeons can often avoid government regulations, do not have to take calls, and have hospitalists care for their patients at night.

These problems will be accentuated in the next few years as the elderly population (aged 65 and older) reaches 30% of the total population. Studies in the United States show that the mortality rate for people aged 65 and older in the intensive care unit is 3.5 times greater than that of younger people, and length of stay is longer. Unfortunately, the majority of these elderly patients who are seriously injured do not return to independent lifestyles following acute care.

SOLUTIONS

Correcting the problems in developing countries may be the most difficult. Most of these countries are totally lacking in the infrastructure for provision of a trauma system, including prehospital care, sufficient adequately trained surgeons, and rehabilitation services. International institutions such as the World Bank and World Health Organization would have to take a leading role in providing financial resources and training for prehospital care. This would be a potentially huge sum, because it would require creating and developing adequate communications, ambulances, and properly trained prehospital personnel. Similarly, provision of appropriately trained surgeons is equally problematic. Bringing surgeons to Western countries for training has been a problem because many of them do not return to their countries of origin. In my opinion, the optimal way to train these individuals would be for surgical educators from countries with mature trauma systems to spend time educating surgeons in the appropriate medical schools in their home countries. This is also problematic, because the quality of medical schools varies tremendously in developing nations. Furthermore, in addition to surgeons, anesthesiologists, critical care physicians, and nurses would have to be educated as well. The third component of a trauma system, rehabilitation, is almost totally lacking in developing countries. This element may not be as resource-dependent or costly as other components, but it would have to be developed concomitantly with prehospital and acute care.

The fundamental problem in developing regions is setting priorities. If we accept that DALYs are a reasonable approach to developing sound health care policy, then we can examine the 10 most common causes of DALYs. A rank order of the 10 most frequent DALYs in developing countries are: (1) unipolar major depression, (2) road traffic accidents, (3) ischemic heart disease, (4) chronic obstructive pulmonary disease, (5) cerebrovascular disease, (6) tuberculosis, (7) lower respiratory infections, (8) war, (9) diarrheal diseases, and (10) HIV (human immunodeficiency virus) infection. I am biased, but I believe that road traffic accidents may be the most cost-effective DALY to try to address. Prevention would clearly play a major role in chronic obstructive pulmonary disease, ischemic heart disease, and cerebrovascular disease, if the United States (among others) simply quit making and exporting cigarettes. I would also argue that as the world economy becomes more globalized and developing countries become economic powers in their own right, it is important for us to be involved early on in providing the infrastructure for managing health care in general and trauma care in particular.

The solutions in Europe are also somewhat problematic. I believe it is safe to say there are no standards being developed by the EU to address what constitutes optimal prehospital care. I think it is also safe to say that medical education, and specifically surgical training, varies markedly from country to country. The same could be said regarding critical care standards. The current approach to training a trauma surgeon in the EU is variable, and various specialists tend to provide this training. This approach is not necessarily negative, but there should be some standards that constitute the bare minimum in order for surgeons to come and go across borders and meet this standard of care. Within the EU, rehabilitation is also variable. One of the best examples of an excellent trauma rehabilitation program exists in Israel, which might represent a model for the EU. The best place to start would be for the EU to develop a document similar to the American College of Surgeons Optimal Criteria that would apply to all countries. It cannot be overemphasized that some type of review and verification must be applied to all three components of a trauma system—prehospital, acute care, and rehabilitation.

The solutions for the United States may be even more problematic than for developing countries. The reason is quite simple: the U.S. health care system is broken. A system that was historically "not for profit" has become "for profit." Forty-four million individuals have no insurance, tens of millions are underinsured, and health care cost inflation is such that health care in the United States now accounts for a larger proportion of gross domestic product than in any other developed nation. Solving these issues obviously takes priority over solving the problems within trauma care, and yet they may be related.

There are many possible solutions to the health care problems in the United States from a global standpoint. Most economists argue that health care is a public good, similar to military, fire fighting, and police services. Through a public good model, there could be direct provision of care by government, or it could be contracted to insurance companies. Some have argued that this arrangement would cost more, that there would be loss of incentives, and that the system would continue to be double-tiered, because people could still buy additional insurance or pay extra for their health care. Another solution would be a public utility model, in which health care services would be regulated by local, state, or federal officials. The most positive aspect of this model is that there is public input. The disadvantage, particularly in the United States, is that given recent scandals associated with public utilities (e.g., Enron), there has been gaming of the system.

In anticipation of growth in the global economy, it would be possible to reduce pharmaceutical costs by outsourcing to developing countries. For years, the United States has imported nurses to make up for deficiencies in the training of nurses in the United States. A similar effort could be made by importing health care professionals, such as surgeons. In many ways, this model is completely unrealistic, because it removes professionals from countries, especially resource-poor countries, that need them the most.

The most reasonable model for the public would be to have universal health care with either a single payer or a multiple payer system. There would be a defined level of basic care, flexible co-payments, and catastrophic care, and freedom of choice to select professionals and hospitals would be maintained. Such a system would also emphasize disease prevention, patient education, and oversight of insurers. Malpractice would be arbitrated, and overdiagnosis and overtreatment would be curtailed. Although this last solution has merit, it is going to take time to bring about such changes.

The problems in trauma care in the United States are such that it is not possible to wait for a change in the overall health care system. Recently, a combined committee of the American College of Surgeons Committee on Trauma (ACS-COT) and the American Association for the Surgery of Trauma (AAST) has recommended a set of solutions for trauma systems. They have proposed that the American Board of Surgery (ABS) establish a primary board titled "The American Board of Emergency and Acute Care Surgery." The curriculum would comprise 4 years of general surgery, followed by 2 years of trauma surgery, including some of the specialties within trauma. It would include critical care and vascular and noncardiac thoracic surgery. An opportunity would also include additional training in emergency orthopedics, neurosurgery, minor plastic surgery, and some interventional radiology as well. Essentially, the proposed curriculum would create a surgical hospitalist who would perform shift work and provide 24/7 coverage of nearly all surgical emergencies. One of the problems yet to be solved is how to provide continuity of care, particularly at shift change.

Prehospital care and rehabilitation are also problems that need to be solved. The committee has recommended that we develop optimal criteria standards for prehospital care that would include peer review and verification. Similarly, rehabilitation care needs development of optimal criteria standards with peer review and verification.

Trauma care and trauma systems in the Western Hemisphere are a microcosm of the rest of the world. Canada has provincial trauma systems and centers, but lacks a nationwide trauma system. Mexico, Central America, and South America have embryonic components of the trauma system, including trauma centers in many academic hospitals, but lack prehospital care, rehabilitation, and statewide trauma systems. This arrangement is particularly problematic for countries such as Colombia, where violence is a major contributor to trauma injuries. One could argue that as the economy becomes globalized, it will be important to have worldwide standards for trauma management and peer review. I consider this a challenge and an opportunity.

For the chapter's Suggested Readings list, please visit the book at www.ExpertConsult.inkling.com.

TRAUMA CENTER ORGANIZATION AND VERIFICATION

Colonel (retired) Brian Eastridge and Erwin Thal

Please visit the book at www.ExpertConsult.inkling.com to read this chapter in full.

Injury Severity Scoring: Its Definition and Practical Application

Turner M. Osler, Laurent G. Glance, and Edward J. Bedrick

Please visit the book at www.ExpertConsult.inkling.com to read this chapter in full.

Role of Alcohol and Other Drugs in Trauma

Larry M. Gentilello and Thomas J. Esposito

Please visit the book at www.ExpertConsult.inkling.com to read this chapter in full.

Role of Trauma Prevention in Reducing Interpersonal Violence

Edward E. Cornwell and David C. Chang

Please visit the book at www.ExpertConsult.inkling.com to read this chapter in full.

Trauma Scoring

Nicole VanDerHeyden and Thomas B. Cox

Please visit the book at www.ExpertConsult.inkling.com to read this chapter in full.

RESULTS OF THE MEDICAL STRATEGY FOR MILITARY TRAUMA IN COLOMBIA

William Sánchez Maldonado, Erwin Rodriguez-García, David Rojas Tirado, and Juan A. Asensio

Throughout history, wars have resulted in the development of medical and surgical techniques for the care of the wounded that have been later adopted successfully in civilian trauma. Colombia has faced more than 50 years of irregular armed conflict with the result of multiple experiences gained, particularly regarding the management of complex trauma. We present our care plan in military trauma and our results of the project.

The impact on medical care of the many wounded from a long-standing irregular war with guerrillas, and more recently with drug dealers and criminal gangs, prompted the development of a medical care strategy designed to ensure fast, effective, and optimal treatment with the highest probability of survival of the wounded and a satisfactory rehabilitation.

The finding that fueled the strategic plan was an analysis conducted in early 2000 that revealed a worrying figure of 32% average immediate mortality rate in the battlefield, the absence of specialized medical care after the traumatic event, and deficient medical transportation logistics with long evacuation delays, but at the same time there was a higher probability of survival (6% mortality rate) at the Hospital Militar Central, as a result of high-level specialized medical care.

The initial design of the strategy was developed by Lieutenant Colonel Erwin Rodríguez García, MD, and Major David Rojas Tirado, MD, with the support of the U.S. Army Southern Command. The plan received the name of PANTERA and was based on the model by William Haddon, who described in New York in 1970 a matrix for analyzing trauma care in which the injury-promoting factors were interrelated—human, environmental, and technical—in each of the three possible phases of the event—before, during, and after trauma. After 1 year of strategic planning, the PANTERA project was implemented in February 2004 with the participation of multiple players from the administrative, military, training, and medical areas. Eight years later, it is still active.

Seven consecutive steps are described in the planning and action flowchart (Fig. 1).

KNOWING THE PRIMARY ENEMY

The main characteristic of the primary enemy (guerrillas, drug traffickers, and criminal gangs) is lack of respect for the principles of international humanitarian law in their criminal warfare:

1. Many of their combatants are children who are drafted by force and who suffer from profound psychological disorders as a result of their abnormal development amidst violence during their childhood and adolescence, further aggravated by social rejection.
2. The use of nonconventional elements of war is also characteristic, including land mines, biologic contamination of weapons, and nontraditional explosives.
3. The use of extortion, kidnapping, and torture as social intimidation maneuvers is also characteristic.

Consequently, the military actions of the primary enemy are insane by nature and the secondary wounds resulting from this irregular warfare are usually high-energy injuries with great tissue destruction, a high proportion of limb amputation and dismemberment, and high levels of contamination (Fig. 2). Therefore, medical care must be planned around critically injured patients with considerable trauma and a high probability of morbidity and mortality.

FIGURE I Military medical care plan.

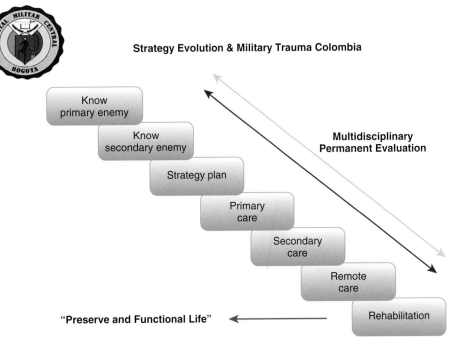

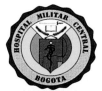

Wounded Soldiers

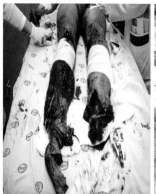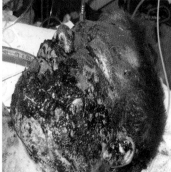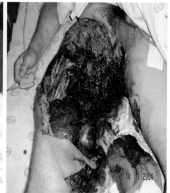

FIGURE 2   Soldiers wounded in combat with amputations, burns, and severe soft tissue injury.

KNOWING THE SECONDARY ENEMY

Immediately after the attack, the enemy for the victims and the medical team changes, and bleeding and infection become the new foes.

After trauma in the battlefield or after military action, control of acute bleeding becomes a priority in primary care. All measures of medical care must focus on controlling continuous persistent bleeding that may lead to shock and exsanguination. Our management guidelines are based on five sequential components:

1. The first immediate step is an attempt at controlling local acute bleeding with external compression or a tourniquet in the case of injured limbs. All military personnel are trained in first aid, and a team of medics is always present to provide support in every military operation. In some critical situations, good medical judgment may lead to considering risking the viability of an extremity rather than risking the patient's life.
2. The second step is the use of local hemostatic agents such as matrices or thermal coagulants by the primary care team. These elements are always part of the first aid kit.
3. The third step is to secure venous access and initiate fluid resuscitation under a hypotensive technique, preferably with hypertonic solutions.
4. After evacuation, the patient is received at the combat hospital (GATRA), where whole blood transfusion is initiated, if necessary, always considering the possibility of autotransfusion, if indicated.
5. Finally, we have developed for each military unit a database of potential, immediately available blood bank donors, and each medical support team must check the availability of blood or donors for all soldiers going into action.

The second new enemy is infection. Our guidelines for the management of war injury infections include the following:

1. Immediate irrigation and cleaning of the wound with saline solution in the battlefield. This is done simultaneously with the control of bleeding.
2. Coverage and isolation of the wound with aseptic dressings. Some rescue teams and all combat hospitals (GATRA) have negative pressure VAC (vacuum-assisted closure) systems that are very useful for the management of wounds with significant tissue losses, bearing in mind that the selection of foams and

pressure variables must be tailored to the needs of the individual patient.
3. A golden rule for us is to consider that all war injuries are contaminated or potentially infected. This consideration is based on the observation of guerilla tactical operations (biologic contamination of weapons) and a prospective study that we conducted, which included 18,627 cultures in order to determine the most frequent bacteria responsible for infections in our patients; The first was *Escherichia coli* (30%) followed by *Staphylococcus aureus* and *Klebsiella pneumoniae*. *E. coli* infection accounted for 50% of all gram-negative infections (Table 1). Consequently, antibiotic therapy is therapeutic and focuses mainly on the treatment of gram-negative infections.

TABLE 1: Top Ten Microorganisms That Cause Infection in Hospital Militar Central, 2010–2012

Microorganism	NO. OF ISOLATES/YEAR		
	2012	2011	2010
Escherichia coli	1869	1769	1868
Staphylococcus aureus	352	340	434
Klebsiella pneumoniae	428	413	412
Staphylococcus epidermidis	274	271	378
Pseudomonas aeruginosa	212	262	319
Proteus mirabilis	253	296	303
Enterococcus faecalis	300	336	277
Candida albicans	142	165	171
Enterobacter cloacae	142	165	151
Serratia marcesens	84	108	116

From Hospital Militar Central, Bogota.

STRATEGIC PLAN FOR MEDICAL CARE

Our medical care plan was named PANTERA and it was built around levels and types of care teams (Fig. 3):

Level I: This team is called **EMEREVAC** in Spanish (Combat Rescue and Evacuation Medical Team) and consists of one physician, one licensed practical nurse, and two soldiers who are experts in rescue. The main goals of this team are to ensure survival of the wounded in the battlefield by providing first aid support in the form of control of acute bleeding, infection prophylaxis, and immediate evacuation (Fig. 4).

Level II: This level comprises combat hospitals. It is called **GATRA** in Spanish (Air-Transport Trauma Life Support Team) and consists of one general surgeon, one orthopedic surgeon, one anesthetist, one medical assistant, one head nurse, one laboratory technician, and four licensed practical nurses. This team receives the wounded from the EMEREVAC within less than 1 hour and performs all the procedures necessary to resuscitate and stabilize them, including resuscitation and damage control surgery. If necessary, this team also initiates basic intensive care and prepares the patients for evacuation to a higher-complexity center in a condition that enables them to survive long distances and undergo major reconstructive surgery. Patients must not remain in a GATRA unit for more than 6 hours (Fig. 5). Every combat hospital has the number of GATRA units that are required depending on the needs of the military operation.

Level III: After receiving treatment in the combat hospital for damage control, the wounded patient is transferred to the next level, namely, the distant evacuation team behind the lines, in Spanish **ECCAT** (Air-Transport Critical Care Team). This team's mission is to transport the wounded in optimal conditions, maintaining hemodynamic stability. The basic team consists of a physician with training in critical care, a head nurse, and two licensed practical nurses. The number of team members grows depending on the number of victims that require transportation, as is also the case with the type and number of aircraft (Fig. 6).

Level IV: The highest level of care is provided at the Hospital Militar Central, a university institution equipped with high-technology infrastructure and wards dedicated only to the wounded in combat. All the hospital staff members, regardless of their specialty, are trained in trauma and this multidisciplinary approach to care allows for comprehensive treatment, ranging from repair surgery to complete rehabilitation, including psychological rehabilitation. The university hospital provides care to the wounded in a setting of continuing medical education and research projects centered on the issue of war trauma, using all the current teaching aids (basic and clinical research, simulation, telemedicine, etc.). This ensures high-level training in trauma for the benefit of the patients.

Results of the Strategy

The PANTERA plan has made it possible to provide highly specialized medical care from the very moment an event occurs and a soldier is wounded in action. An analysis of the warfare techniques used by the irregular combatants between 2000 and 2005 revealed that 80% of the military casualties were wounded by large-caliber high-speed firearms, at a time when the war was fought with conventional weapons and in direct confrontation. The warfare technique evolved to avoid direct engagement, and by 2009–2010, 75% of the casualties were the

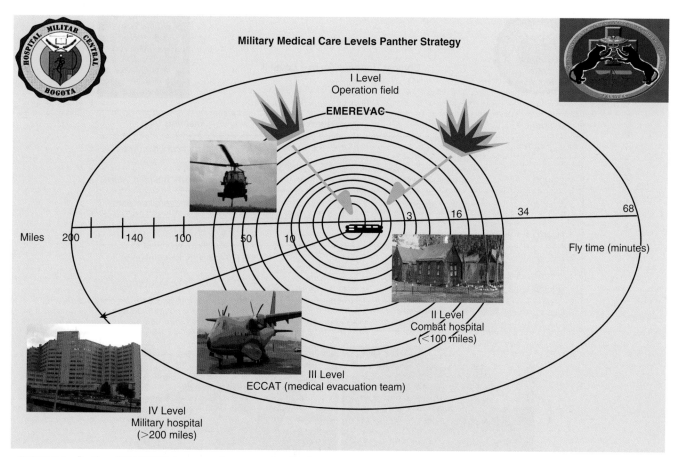

FIGURE 3 Panther (PANTERA) strategy—three operation levels.

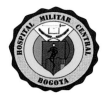
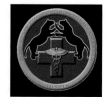

EMEREVAC TEAM

Evacuation – Battlefield Team Level I

Grade	Profile	Number	Training
TE–CT	MD	1	ATL, Military hospital course
C3–SV	Nurse	1	PHTLS, Military hospital course
SLP	Paramedic	2	CSAR Rescue techniques Military hospital course

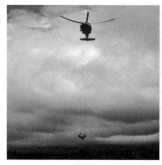
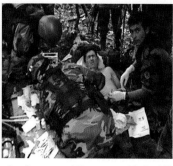
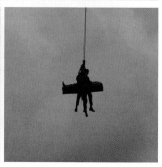

FIGURE 4   EMEREVAC team (Combat Rescue and Evacuation Medical Team)—Level I.

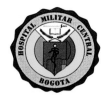
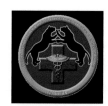

GATRA TEAM

Combat Hospital Team – Level II

Grade	Profile	Number	Training
CT–CR	General surgeon	1	ATLS, Military hospital course
CT–CR	Anestesiologic	1	ATLS, ACLS, Military hospital course
CT–CR	Traumatologic	1	ATLS, Military hospital course
TN–CR	MD (assistant)	1	ATLS, Military hospital course
ST–TC	Nurse chief	1	PHTLS, Military hospital course
S3–SP	Nurse crew	2	PHTLS, Military hospital course
C3–SP	Nurse	3	PHTLS, Military hospital course

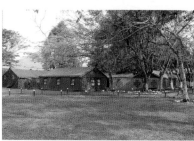
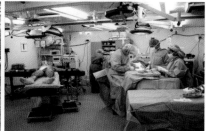

FIGURE 5   GATRA team (Air-Transport Trauma Life Support Team)—Level II.

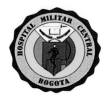

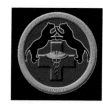

ECCAT TEAM

Medical Evacuation Team – Level III

Grade	Profile	Number	Training
CT–CR	Anestesiologic, critical care	1	ATLS, ACLS, Military hospital course
TN–CR	MD (assistant)	1	ATLS, Military hospital course
C3–SP	Nurse	1	PHTLS, Military hospital course

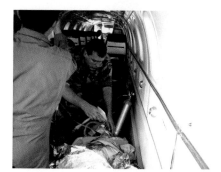
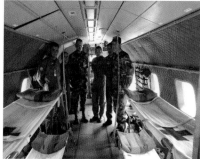

FIGURE 6   ECCAT team (Air-Transport Critical Care Team)—Level III.

result of nonconventional explosives and land mines. This explains the change in the epidemiology of the wounds, with the emergence of injuries with significant tissue loss, a high potential for infection, and a high rate of amputations and dismemberments.

The three primary causes of immediate fatality in the battlefield were chest wounds (34%), dismemberment caused by land mines (31%), and head injuries (17%). In medical prophylactic strategy, emphasis is placed on the use of bulletproof vests, helmets, and means for detecting and dismantling nonconventional explosives during the operations. However, these measures are not easy to implement in the tropical jungle where the armed conflict takes place in Colombia.

The first important favorable result of this medical strategy was reflected in the morale and patriotism of the soldiers who feel backed by a highly qualified medical rescue team that can ensure immediate care and offer the highest probability of survival.

Between January 2005 and December 2010, 8631 Colombian soldiers were wounded in action, and there were 2462 deaths in the field

of military operations (28.5%). Through their action, the EMERE-VAC and GATRA teams contributed to a significant reduction in mortality rate in the battlefield. In 2005, there were 531 deaths (35%) and this figure dropped to 425 (17%) in 2010 (Table 2). Training of the military personnel in first aid and resuscitation, together with the application of management guidelines for controlling acute bleeding and the use of prophylaxis for infection have been critical in improving the probability of survival of wounded soldiers. Another factor that has also contributed to these results is the support from the EMEREVAC team, with professional treatment, resuscitation, and evacuation within a period of time not greater than 1.30 hours, a critical determinant of patient survival.

Between January 1999 and December 2010, the Hospital Militar Central received 4233 critically injured (Injury Severity Score [ISS] > 15) patients of a total of more than 15,000 wounded in action. The analysis of the data for three time periods of this special group of patients revealed that hospital mortality rate decreased progressively

TABLE 2: Wounded in Combat in the Military Forces of Colombia, 2005–2010: Analysis of Mortality

	2005	2006	2007	2008	2009	2010
Total wounded	1543	1538	1419	1248	1355	2500
No. surviving	1002	1080	1042	943	999	2075
No. deaths	541 (35%)	458 (30%)	377 (26%)	305 (24%)	356 (26%)	425 (17%)
Transferred to HMC	433	290	171	227	297	188

Mean age: 24 years
   Total wounded in combat: 8631
   Deaths: 2462 (28.5%)
   Transferred to HMC, ISS > 15: 1606 (26.3%)

From Hospital Militar Central in Bogota.
HMC, Hospital Militar Central; ISS, Injury Severity Score.

TABLE 3: Hospital Militar Central War Trauma—Analysis of In-Hospital Mortality Rate of 4233 Patients Injured in Combat Over Three Periods of Time

Period	No. of Patients	No. of Deaths	Mortality Rate (%)
1999–2003	1572	82	5.2
2004–2008	1531	49	3.4
2009–2010	1130	27	2.3

Global hospital mortality rate: 3.6%
  Total of 4233 patients, Injury Severity Score (ISS) > 15

From Hospital Militar Central, Bogota.

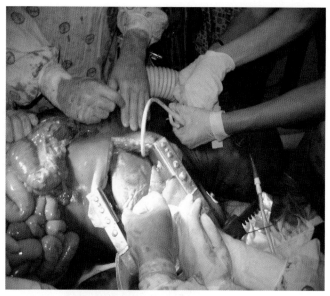

FIGURE 7 Soldier wounded in combat, requiring thoracotomy and laparotomy of damage control and cannulation of right atrium to replace blood volume.

from 5.2% to 2.3%. These results reflect the high degree of expertise in providing care to trauma patients with a multidisciplinary approach, without forgetting the process of physical, psychological, and social rehabilitation as a fundamental pillar of comprehensive patient care (Table 3).

Infection is the main cause of nonacute hospital morbidity and fatality of patients wounded in action, except for the immediate sequelae of exsanguination. At our institution, war injury–associated infections are caused mainly by gram-negative bacteria. E. coli is the primary cause of infection globally (35%), requiring knowledge of the local biologic behavior of the microorganisms, in terms of antibiotic

resistance, in order to determine the best therapeutic selection. In our prospective analysis for 2010–2012, which included 5506 patients with positive cultures for E. coli, the percentage of resistance to ampicillin/sulbactam, trimethoprim-sulfamethoxazole, and ciprofloxacin was 42.9%, 37.1%, 26%, respectively, which means that the selection of antibiotics has to exclude these options and must be based on the result of the sensitivity and bacterial resistance (Table 4).

The following are clinical examples of refined damage control techniques in military trauma care:

1. Patient with penetrating thoracoabdominal gunshot wound that injured the jejunum, colon, spleen, diaphragm, left lung, and the thoracic aorta. The GATRA team performed a resuscitation thoracotomy with cannulation of the right atrium in order to recover intravascular volume and then repair the aorta and the lung injury, combined with laparotomy for damage control of the abdominal injuries (Fig. 7).

TABLE 4: Analysis of Antibiotic Resistance in 5506 Patients with *Escherichia coli* Infections, 2010–2012

Antibiotic Resistance Markers	RESISTANCE (%)					
	2010		2011		2012	
	No. UCI	UCI	No. UCI	UCI	No. UCI	UCI
Amikacin	0.4	1.7	1.6	0.0	0.8	0.0
Ampicillin/sulbactam	31.2	44.8	35.7	41.0	27.6	42.9
Beta-lactamase (BLEE)	11.7	22.4	12.5	15.4	11.6	17.1
Cefoxitin (AmpC marker)	3.2	0.0	4.8	5.1	4.2	8.6
Ciprofloxacin	22.9	29.3	30.6	23.1	27.8	25.7
Gentamicin	13.7	19	16.3	23.1	17.6	15.7
Imipenem	0.4	0.0	0.0	0.0	0.2	0.0
Piperacillin-tazobactam	10.5	24.1	11.3	15.4	6.5	12.9
TMP/SXZ (trimethoprim-sulfamethoxazole)	41.4	42.0	48.0	30.3	39.3	39.2

From Hospital Militar Central in Bogota.
UCI, Urinary catheter infection.

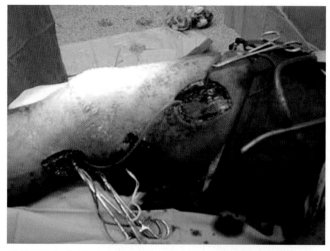

FIGURE 8 Soldier wounded in combat, requiring femoral arterial bypass as a temporary measure to allow the viability of lower limb.

Combat Wounded & VAC®

Liver, Kidney, Ileum, Colon, Stomach, Lung

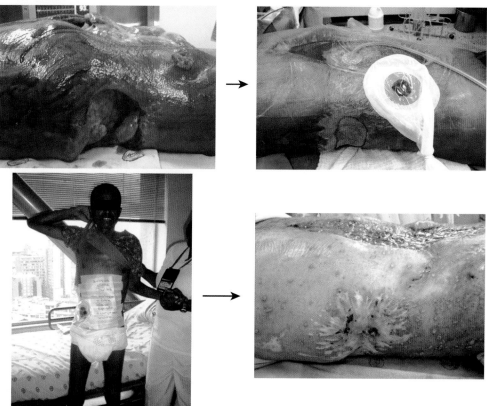

FIGURE 9 Soldier wounded in combat, with injury of multiple intra-abdominal organs and abdominal wall. Sequence of treatment with VAC (vacuum-assisted closure) therapy.

2. Patient injured by a grenade fragment in the right lower limb causing femoral fracture and popliteal-femoral artery lesion. Acute bleeding was controlled by the combat nurse of the EMEREVAC team using local compression and a tourniquet. Later, in the rescue helicopter, the EMEREVAC physician performed an external vascular bypass, securing the viability of the limb before final repair at the Hospital Militar Central (Fig. 8).

3. An additional example of multidisciplinary management using modern technologies is that of a patient wounded in action by an assault rifle grenade causing multiple severe injuries to the liver, right kidney, jejunum, colon, stomach, lung, and abdominal wall. The patient required multiple surgical interventions and treatments by a multidisciplinary team, including VAC therapy, in order to save his life and promote his recovery (Fig. 9).

CONCLUSIONS

1. The strategy for developing the medical care plan for patients wounded in action must consider all possible variables to include in the Haddon matrix analysis.
2. The PANTERA plan, as a pillar of care in the Colombian armed forces, has been shown to be successful in improving the probability of survival of war victims.
3. Every medical care plan for trauma and critically ill patients, and in particular in military medicine, must be based on strong continuing academic training and education of each and every one of the team members.

For the chapter's Suggested Readings list, please visit the book at www.ExpertConsult.inkling.com.

INFLUENCE OF EMERGENCY MEDICAL SERVICES ON OUTCOME AT TRAUMA CENTER

David Shatz

Since the proven effectiveness of trauma systems in the 1970s, the evaluation, treatment, and transport of trauma victims in the prehospital arena have played an important role in the overall management of those victims. Although some aspects of that role have raised controversy, the rapid and effective transport of severely injured patients leaves little room for doubt. Though standardized by the National EMS Scope of Practice Model, actual paramedic and emergency medical technician (EMT) medical care varies across the country and has changed dramatically since codification by the U.S. Department of Transportation in the early 1970s. And although prehospital care has absolutely improved trauma outcomes since the early days of advanced life support in the field, some practices have been less positive than others.

GOLDEN HOUR OR GOLDEN OPPORTUNITY?

"There is a golden hour between life and death. If you are critically injured you have less than 60 minutes to survive." And hence was born the much-quoted dogma of the golden hour of trauma, in a simple interview with Dr. R. Adams Cowley, in 1976. Although there was no scientific evidence to support that statement, it was intuitively obvious to most that the essence of the statement was true. But the blanket acceptance of that concept has not been without cost and risk, and more recent science has brought that concept into question.

Much of our current trauma system structure is based upon the golden hour concept, with patients transported to trauma centers as rapidly as possible, even if that includes helicopter and lights-and-siren ground ambulance transport. Helicopter evacuation of combat casualties became synonymous with the Korean and Vietnam wars with the help of the television, movie, and news industries. Translation to civilian trauma use was easy, with an explosion of helicopter emergency medical services (EMS) providers in recent

decades. In the state of Missouri alone, nine helicopters provided coverage for the state's 5 million citizens in 1989, and 33 helicopters now cover the 6 million people residing in that state. The justification, of course, is the more rapid transport of the trauma victim from the scene to the trauma center. But helicopter transport has been deadly for some. In one 2-year period of the Vietnam War, 39 crew members were killed and 210 were wounded in unarmed medical evacuation missions. Four decades later, civilian EMS helicopters crashed 85 times, killing 77 patients and crew members, between 2003 and 2008.

Transporting patients by ground is also not completely risk free. Several studies have delineated the risks to patients, ambulance crew members, and citizens not directly involved with the ambulance itself. Not surprisingly, the majority of ambulance accidents occurred during emergency calls. And although only 40% of the ambulance occupants of a fatal crash were riding in the rear patient compartment, 72% of the unrestrained occupant fatalities involved those in that compartment. The most common explanation of these fatal injuries is the fact that EMS workers providing active patient care during transport believe they are unable to provide that care effectively while restrained with seatbelts. Extensive work has been done to study this problem, but the solutions are not universal. The highest risk of on-duty fatality for EMS personnel is associated with vehicle crashes. However, not all ambulance crash-related injuries are isolated to EMS providers. In a 10-year study conducted by the National Institute for Occupational Safety and Health (NIOSH), in 300 fatal occupied ambulance crashes, 27 EMS workers perished, as did 55 other ambulance occupants, and 275 occupants of other vehicles and pedestrians. Interestingly, although the Federal Aviation Administration attributes up to 80% of all aircraft accidents to pilot error, 60% of the ambulance crashes seen in the NIOSH study were due to driver error. None of these studies delineated the reason for patient transport, but one can extrapolate these findings to the stress and perceived need for rapid transport of a trauma victim, under the guise of the golden hour.

In a study done by Newgard et al, neither time of transport nor expertise of responding personnel affected the outcome of trauma patients with severe physiologic derangement. One hundred forty-six EMS agencies, including air and ground, transported 3656 trauma patients to 51 U.S. and Canadian Level I and II trauma centers. Study patients were severely injured, as evidenced by inclusion criteria of either a systolic blood pressure less than or equal to 90, Glasgow Coma Scale score less than or equal to 12, respiratory rate less than 10 or greater than 29 breaths per minute, or need for an advanced airway intervention. Median response times (4.28 minutes), on-scene times (19 minutes), and transport times (10 minutes) resulted in total times ranging from 28.4 minutes to 47 minutes, with a median total time of 36.3 minutes. In all variations of time analysis, no mortality difference could be found based on field times. These findings persisted not only with prehospital times, but also for mode of transport, level of first responding EMS provider, patient age, and mechanism of injury.

On the other hand, it would make empiric sense that patients such as those actively bleeding from injuries to the spleen, liver, or pelvis would do better with rapid transport and definitive treatment. Early studies showed an increase in fatality when more than 60 minutes were spent in the prehospital arena. In Trunkey's early description of trauma fatality in 1983, a trimodal distribution of death was identified. More recently, a bimodal distribution has been described, with near elimination of late deaths and a shift in the time of early deaths. Early deaths in Gunst et al's study occurred with a median time of 52 minutes (compared to Trunkey's 120 minutes), and patients arrived to a trauma center at a median time of 42 minutes from the time of injury. With 24% of patients having potentially survivable injuries, yet succumbing in less than an hour after injury, the golden hour may indeed be real.

In the end, there is little disagreement that the likelihood of an improved outcome is probably greater the sooner a severely injured patient can begin definitive care. Dr. Cowley likely was very aware that he was making a scientifically unproven statement, but if his intent was to teach a very important lesson in the early days of civilian trauma care, for that he has been wildly successful. But most importantly, the trauma victim should arrive to that definitive care without incident, and with the safety of the patient, the transporting prehospital crew, and innocent bystanders of foremost concern.

PREHOSPITAL FLUIDS

The debate over whether field paramedics should establish venous access for fluid resuscitation in trauma is not new. For years, Prehospital Trauma Life Support, in cooperation with the American College of Surgeons, has emphasized the importance of field intravenous (IV) access and fluid resuscitation, though that concept is now changing. But what practice is the safest for trauma victims?

Placement of venous lines early in the care of trauma patients has long been considered important, both for fluid and drug administration and while vein diameter still permitted cannulation before hypovolemia was severe enough to collapse peripheral access. However, few if any drugs are indicated in the prehospital environment of the trauma victim, and ready availability of intraosseus access devices now enables venous access in even the most severely volume-depleted patient. Placement of lines should never delay transport to a trauma center. So the question then becomes, does fluid resuscitation during transport affect the outcome in an injured victim?

Animal studies in the early 1990s suggested that though saline resuscitation increased blood loss, mortality rate was not affected. And Advanced Trauma Life Support doctrine has advocated a 2-L bolus of lactated Ringer's solution as needed. This emergency department teaching was subsequently carried into the prehospital environment and became common practice, but with few options for monitoring adequacy of resuscitation. Concerns for underresuscitation included the risks of diffuse organ ischemia, especially in the brain-injured patient. Additionally, at what point would hypovolemia turn from acceptable to lethal?

Despite these concerns, the overwhelming current consensus favors limited to no field resuscitation, even in the emergency department, until control of active, or potentially active, bleeding sites can be obtained. Arguments against normotensive resuscitation include dilution of clotting factors, increase in bleeding and hemoglobin loss, dislodgement of established clot, extravascular fluid overload, and the potential to worsen hypothermia with room temperature fluids. A large 2011 National Trauma Data Bank review showed that patients with a prehospital IV had a significantly higher mortality rate than those who did not. Though one might argue that a selection bias existed, the increase in mortality rate was seen in nearly all subsets of patients. This cohort included both blunt and penetrating injuries, though the mortality rate increase was more pronounced in the latter.

Mortality rate was not affected in normotensive patients, but was significantly increased in the hypotensive ones, and severely brain-injured patients had a 34% increase in risk of death. Low-injury severity patients did not exhibit a difference in mortality rate.

Recent combat experience has further supported the abandonment of normotensive field resuscitation. Though injury patterns are admittedly different in the civilian versus battlefield setting, hemorrhage control is paramount in both. Judicious versus overzealous use of resuscitation fluids is now recommended. The use of crystalloid versus low-volume colloid remains in question.

If the concept of limited fluid resuscitation, or permissive hypotension, is to be embraced by prehospital personnel, what is the limit of permissive? In patients with hemorrhagic shock, in whom bleeding has temporarily ceased, Israeli Defense Force guidelines recommend fluids aimed at restoration of a radial pulse, sensorium, or a systolic blood pressure of 80 mm Hg. Because of the concern for cerebral perfusion in the setting of central nervous system injuries, a systolic blood pressure of 100 mm Hg is recommended. Tactical Combat Casualty Care Fluid Resuscitation Guidelines 2009, now adopted by all services in the U.S. Department of Defense, recommend no IV fluids in patients not in shock, and fluid resuscitation of those in uncontrolled hemorrhagic shock, with shock determined by the absence of a palpable radial pulse.

Despite decades of publications refuting prehospital fluid administration in the prehospital setting, the practice continues. The administration of crystalloid, with "normal" vital signs being the goal, should be abandoned. Although crossing the line of permissive hypotension to death is not a desirable outcome, evidence of adequate, albeit not normal, resuscitation should be the desired end point. At this writing, measures of adequate perfusion include a palpable radial artery pulse and systolic blood pressure of 80 mm Hg (100 mm Hg in suspected traumatic brain injury patients), and should be the preferred end point of field resuscitation. This goal should be accomplished with low-volume (250-mL) boluses, rather than the previous practice of 2-L boluses.

TO BLEED OR NOT TO BLEED—SHOULD TOURNIQUETS BE STANDARD CARE?

Every trauma surgeon has witnessed patients with extremity injuries who arrive in the trauma rooms, with bulky dressings covering the wound, and a trail of blood between the ambulance and the trauma room bed. Paramedic and EMT training dictates that bleeding extremity wounds be covered with bulky dressings and wrapped. If bleeding continues, more bulky dressing and more wrapping is to be applied. But it is obvious that bulky dressings and wrapping cannot reach supra-arterial pressures, and more blood loss is to be expected in those with arterial injuries. In fairness, medics find themselves occupied in transporting and other patient-care duties and often cannot dedicate one person to hold direct pressure over a bleeding wound. A third hand is needed, and that can be provided in the form of tourniquets.

Ambrose Paré has been credited with the first use of the word *tourniquet*, though their use on the battlefield has been dated as early as ancient Rome. With a few modifications since that time, use of pneumatic tourniquets in the operating room has been common practice for decades. The acceptance of the use of tourniquets in combat applications has waxed and waned, but has gained a resurgence in popularity in recent conflicts. With experience gained over the past few years, primarily in combat, use of tourniquets is extending into civilian prehospital trauma care.

Tourniquets fell out of favor largely due to perceived, or observed, tissue ischemia and increased blood loss. But tourniquets of a decade ago were mostly rubber tubing or wide rubber bands, neither one of which was designed to occlude arterial inflow. Instead, these rubber tourniquets, which were designed to assist in IV catheter placement, occluded the venous outflow only. As a result, and not unexpectedly, bleeding did increase, as did interstitial pressure, and tissue ischemia resulted. Additionally, with rubber tubing, the pressure was concentrated over such a small area that nerve compression was more likely, and it was simply very painful for the patient. Tourniquets now commercially available and used extensively by the U.S. military are wider and more evenly distribute the pressure, with the ability to titrate the pressure needed to occlude arterial inflow.

Large-scale military conflicts in recent years have produced renewed experience with exanguinating injuries, including extremity wounds. Although the majority of modern battlefield deaths are nonsurvivable, a review of U.S. military Special Operations Forces deaths revealed that 13% of potentially preventable deaths were due to hemorrhage amenable to tourniquet control. In a subsequent study of Operation Iraqi Freedom casualties, 67 patients had prehospital tourniquets placed for an average duration of 70 minutes, with more than half of the severely injured found to have improved hemorrhage control. Concerns for tourniquet-induced morbidity have fueled the controversy over their use, but Beekley et al and Kragh et al found little to no morbidity with properly placed tourniquets. Tourniquet use of under 2 hours, placed proximal to the wound(s), were important caveats in these studies. Israeli Defense Force experiences have been similar, with over 2 decades of use. Adverse outcomes have been largely limited to nerve injury (5.5% of patients), with the vast majority being in patients with tourniquet ischemia times in excess of 150 minutes. Overall, military experience has shown tourniquet use in severe, bleeding extremity injuries to be lifesaving, and with no limb loss attributable to their use.

Although virtually all U.S. soldiers now carry a tourniquet in their personal first aid kits, the same widespread availability is not present in civilian EMS systems. Because of this, their civilian use is limited, and hence, so is the published data. As opposed to combat injuries, fatal isolated extremity injuries in the civilian setting are rare. However, these are potentially preventable deaths, and should not be ignored. In a study conducted in Houston, Texas, 14 such patients succumbed to their injuries, despite all having signs of life at the scene.

No tourniquets were used. Half of the injuries were due to gunshot wounds, and the other half resulted from knife wounds and lacerations, all of which are presumably amendable to control and repair. Most of the injuries (71%) were to the lower extremity. The Boston EMS system liberalized the use of tourniquets in the 1990s as a result of what was considered potentially preventable extremity injury deaths. With a similar injury pattern, they described 11 patients for whom tourniquets were placed for penetrating extremity wounds. All were found to have major vascular injuries, and all but one survived (the single fatality was pulseless at the scene).

Although most civilian trauma victims lack the protective body armor worn by soldiers, and with the fortunate rarity of explosive devices as a source of civilian injuries, the pattern of those injuries is much different from those experienced during combat. And although it is therefore expected that tourniquet use among EMS providers should be significantly less compared to our military colleagues, their use can be no less lifesaving with proper training and when used in the appropriate setting. From the battlefield to city streets, prehospital tourniquets have without doubt saved lives.

CONCLUSION

The institution of street-level emergency medical care decades ago has saved countless lives. Bringing that care to the field are highly trained, skilled, and motivated professionals who perform those tasks in some of the most difficult settings imaginable. Their skill sets have been modified and expanded over the years, most with good results. However, some of those skills in the treatment of trauma victims have proved harmful, and should be modified, with the absolute goal of expedited delivery of the injured patient to definitive trauma care.

For the chapter's Suggested Readings list, please visit the book at www.ExpertConsult.inkling.com.

FIELD TRIAGE IN THE MILITARY ARENA

Jeffrey A. Bailey and Alan D. Murdock

Please visit the book at www.ExpertConsult.inkling.com to read this chapter in full.

FIELD TRIAGE IN THE CIVILIAN ARENA

Karen J. Brasel, John Weigelt, and Jennifer C. Roberts

Please visit the book at www.ExpertConsult.inkling.com to read this chapter in full.

Prehospital Airway Management: Intubation, Devices, and Controversies

Raul Coimbra, Jay Doucet, and David Hoyt

Prehospital trauma airway management is probably the biggest challenge faced by prehospital providers. These professionals must not only acquire but also maintain essential skills to adequately manage airway problems at the scene and during transport of trauma victims to trauma centers.

Endotracheal intubation is the definitive method of airway management. However, to acquire such skill requires significant training and practice. Although the emergency medical technician (EMT) basic curriculum contains an advanced airway module, the low frequency of these procedures makes it difficult for these professionals to maintain proficiency. In most systems, paramedics and flight nurses are the only professionals allowed to perform rapid sequence intubation (RSI). Therefore, there is a need for simpler ways to maintain a patent airway by EMTs until the patient is delivered to a hospital. Several devices are now available and have been used by prehospital personnel when endotracheal intubation is not practical or possible. These alternate methods include bag-valve-mask with oral or nasopharyngeal airway, or supraglottic airways such as the laryngeal mask, the esophageal-tracheal double lumen tube (Combitube), and the laryngeal-tracheal airway (King) airway. There are also devices that may increase the likelihood of success for EMT-performed RSI, such as the Eschmann tracheal tube introducer (ETTI) and videolaryngoscopes. In some jurisdictions and situations such as tactical combat casualty care, EMTs may be trained in some types of surgical airways such as open or needle cricothyroidotomy.

In this chapter, the indications for airway management in the prehospital arena, the different modalities, devices and techniques, the recognition of a difficult airway, and associated pitfalls will be discussed.

DIAGNOSIS

Who Needs an Airway?

Before we define who needs an airway in the prehospital arena, it is important to clarify that few studies to date have shown efficacy of advanced airway management in trauma prior to arrival at a trauma center.

The goal of airway management is to provide adequate oxygenation and ventilation as part of the overall resuscitation effort. Candidates include those with decreased or absent respiratory movements, signs of airway obstruction, and cardiopulmonary resuscitation in progress. Severe traumatic brain injury (TBI) as an indication for prehospital intubation will be discussed later. In trauma, it has been shown that moribund patients would benefit from an airway, particularly those who are candidates for a resuscitative thoracotomy upon arrival at the hospital (Durham and associates).

Assessing the Airway

Obstruction of the airway in a trauma patient may occur rapidly or insidiously, may be partial or complete, and may be progressive or intermittent. Assessment of the airway is a basic EMT skill. Management of the airway takes precedence over all other civilian prehospital interventions, as loss of the airway will result in an unsalvageable patient. The airway is assessed by looking for signs of direct airway trauma such as maxillofacial, neck, or laryngeal trauma. The mouth is examined for foreign objects such as loose teeth, blood, and vomitus. Soot, singed nasal hairs, and carbonaceous sputum suggest thermal trauma to the airway, which may cause progressive airway obstruction. Listening carefully to the patient who is able to talk yields information about the patency and quality of the airway—the patient who can speak normally provides some reassurance the airway is patent and mentation is normal. Patients who are confused or agitated may have TBI, intoxication, hypoxia, or hypocarbia, and may have or may progress to airway obstruction. Abnormal sounds such as stridor, gurgling, wheezing, or snoring may be associated with partial airway obstruction. Palpation of the neck can reveal crepitus from subcutaneous air due to direct airway trauma, loose cartilage from laryngeal fracture, or hematomas that can compress the airway.

Initial airway maintenance techniques include the chin-lift or jaw thrust maneuvers, done while maintaining cervical spine immobilization in the suspected blunt trauma patient. These maneuvers can both open an airway and reveal whether the airway is being obstructed by the tongue falling back to obstruct the airway in a supine patient. Oropharyngeal airways can be inserted in unconscious patients to ensure a patent upper airway. Tolerance of an oropharyngeal airway usually indicates the patient will require a definitive airway at the trauma center. The majority of unconscious trauma patients are managed with an oropharyngeal airway combined with the bag-valve-mask ventilation. Conscious and some semiconscious patients will not tolerate an oropharyngeal airway but will tolerate a nasopharyngeal airway. Trauma patients need supplemental oxygen, and providing a good seal with the face mask to allow 100% oxygen delivery can be difficult in patients with facial hair, a large face, a small chin, or obesity. It may require the effort of two or three prehospital personnel to maintain a good face mask seal, bag the patient, and maintain in-line cervical spine immobilization. In patients in whom bag-valve-mask and an oral or nasal airway do not provide adequate oxygenation and ventilation, or when transportation precludes optimal use of the bag-valve-mask, a supraglottic or definitive airway may be required.

Assessment of the airway for difficulty of intubation is performed using the LEMON assessment (Table 1). The first step is to *Look* for characteristics that are known to cause difficult intubation or ventilation such as small chin, protruding teeth, or large face. Next the patient is *Evaluated* using the 3-3-2 rule—which indicates that the distance between the patient's incisor teeth should be at least 3 fingerbreadths, that between hyoid bone and the chin should be 3 fingerbreadths, and that between the thyroid notch and the floor of the mouth should be at least 2 fingerbreadths. Third, the *Mallampati* classification is used to assess the oropharynx and hypopharynx in conscious patients (Fig. 1). Fourth, look for evidence of *Obstruction*, including visible and audible signs of conditions that will make laryngoscopy and ventilation difficult, such as direct trauma or burns. Finally, *Neck mobility* is assessed. In the blunt trauma patient wearing a cervical spine collar, it can be anticipated that there will be no neck movement and intubation will be more difficult.

Identifying a difficult airway prevents patient deterioration and possibly death. Alternative devices and strategies should be used when the diagnosis of a difficult airway is made. These include the supraglottic airways such as the laryngeal mask airway (LMA), Combitube, and King airway. RSI using paralytics in a patient with a difficult airway may result in a "can't intubate–can't ventilate" scenario

TABLE 1: LEMON Airway Assessment

L	Look externally	Look at the patient externally for characteristics that are known to cause difficult laryngoscopy, intubation, or ventilation.
E	Evaluate the 3-3-2 rule	In order to allow alignment of the pharyngeal, laryngeal, and oral axes and therefore simple intubation, the following relationships should be observed. The distance between the patient's incisor teeth should be at least 3 fingerbreadths (3), the distance between the hyoid bone and the chin should be at least 3 fingerbreadths (3), and the distance between the thyroid notch and the floor of the mouth should be at least 2 fingerbreadths (2).
M	Mallampati	The hypopharynx should be visualized adequately. This has been done traditionally by assessing the Mallampati classification (see Fig. 1). The patient is sat upright, told to open the mouth fully and protrude the tongue as far as possible. The examiner then looks into the mouth with a light torch to assess the degree of hypopharynx visible. In the case of a supine patient, Mallampati score can be estimated by getting the patient to open the mouth fully and protrude the tongue and a laryngoscopy light can be shone into the hypopharynx from above.
O	Obstruction?	Any condition that can cause obstruction of the airway will make laryngoscopy and ventilation difficult. Such conditions are epiglottis, peritonsillar abscesses, and trauma.
N	Neck mobility	Neck mobility is a vital requirement for successful intubation. It can be assessed easily by getting the patient to place the chin down onto the chest and then to extend the neck, looking toward the ceiling. Patients in hard collar neck immobilization obviously have no neck movement and are therefore harder to intubate.

From Reed MJ, Dunn MJ, McKeown DW: Can an airway assessment score predict difficulty at intubation in the emergency department? *Emerg Med J* 22:99–102, 2005.

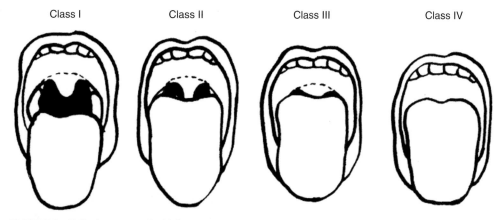

Class I   Class II   Class III   Class IV

FIGURE 1   Difficult airway—the Mallampati score modified by Samsoon and Young. *(From Mallampati SR, Gatt SP, Gugino LD, et al: A clinical sign to predict difficult tracheal intubation: a prospective study. Can Anaesth Soc J 32:429–435, 1985.)*

that may require a surgical airway or may even be impossible to salvage in the prehospital environment.

MANAGEMENT

Which Strategy Should Be Used?

The strategies described here are alternatives to conventional bag-valve-mask ventilation with either a supraglottic or definitive airway.

Laryngeal Mask Airway

The LMA is one alternative to endotracheal intubation (Fig. 2). Its use is particularly important in patients with difficult airways and in patients treated in "unfriendly" environments (rain, dark, prolonged extrication, etc.). It also can be used as a rescue strategy following a

failed RSI. Additionally, it can be used to facilitate intubation, which is obtained by passing the endotracheal tube through the LMA.

The insertion of the LMA is done blindly into the oropharynx, and it is usually tolerated without the need of neuromuscular blockade. The LMA lies in the hypopharynx in the supraglottic position. The successful placement of the LMA is independent of the Mallampati score, presence of a cervical spine collar, or in-line immobilization of the neck. Spontaneous ventilation through the LMA is possible, and manual ventilation through the LMA is superior to bag-valve-mask ventilation, because the latter often requires two hands to maintain a good seal. Studies comparing the success rates have shown that paramedics achieve higher levels of successful placement with the LMA compared to endotracheal intubation. The LMA may be particularly useful in patients with a difficult airway because direct visualization of the cords is not required and neuromuscular blocking agents are not necessary. The advantages of the LMA over the Combitube (described next) include lower risk of malpositioning, no risk of esophageal intubation,

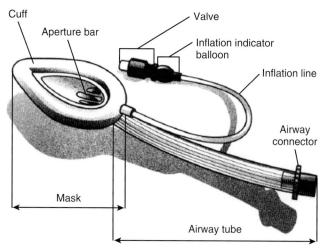

FIGURE 2 Laryngeal mask airway.

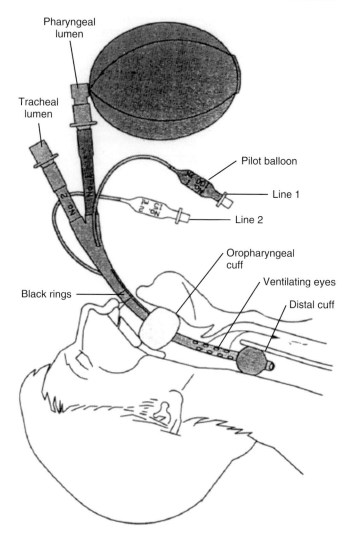

FIGURE 3 Combitube with distal end in the esophagus.

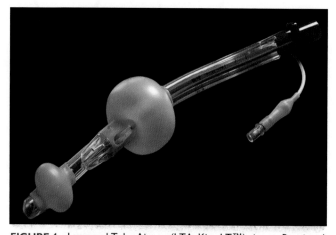

FIGURE 4 Laryngeal Tube Airway (LTA, King LT™) airway. Reprinted with permission from Ambu A/S.

and less trauma to the oropharynx. A major disadvantage of the LMA is that it does not protect against aspiration, which may carry significant risk in patients with intact airway reflexes. Another limitation of LMA is related to the difficulty in generating high airway pressures, which may lead to ineffective ventilation.

Combitube

The Combitube consists of a device with two lumens. One of the lumens has an open distal end similar to an endotracheal tube, whereas the other lumen has a closed distal end, with several holes proximal to its balloon cuff. A second balloon of higher volume is located more proximally to the side holes, and it is used to secure the tube in position. The Combitube is inserted blindly and allows ventilation through either lumen. Following blind insertion, the distal tip is usually located in the esophagus. After inflating the oropharyngeal balloon, the esophageal cuff is inflated. Attempts to ventilate through the pharyngeal lumen will determine whether the distal tip is in the esophagus or trachea. If there is no change in the colorimetric, end-tidal carbon dioxide detector, or if breath sounds are absent, then the distal tip is in the trachea and the patient should be ventilated through the tracheal lumen (Fig. 3).

The Combitube is a useful alternative to endotracheal intubation when an airway is not obtained after multiple attempts, when the airway is considered a difficult one, when direct visualization of the vocal cords by laryngoscopy is not possible at the scene, or when prehospital providers are not trained to perform orotracheal intubation. The great majority of patients brought to trauma centers after insertion of a Combitube will be ventilating and oxygenating well and there is no need for immediate removal of the Combitube and orotracheal intubation. The Combitube is also useful in patients with significant maxillofacial trauma and cervical spine injuries. Because the esophageal cuff is immediately inflated after tube insertion, the Combitube offers protection against aspiration of gastric contents.

The Combitube is contraindicated in patients with intact gag reflex, or when upper airway obstruction is suspected. The Combitube is not available in pediatric sizes. Potential complications include injury to the pharynx and esophagus, and failure to recognize the exact location of the distal end and attempting to oxygenate and ventilate through the wrong lumen.

Laryngeal-Tracheal Airway Device

The laryngeal-tracheal airway, also known as the laryngeal tube airway (LTA) or King airway, is used as an alternative to the Combitube in many jurisdictions (Fig. 4). Like the Combitube or LMA, the LTA is placed without direct visualization of the glottis and does not require significant manipulation of the head or neck for placement. Because it has a single lumen, and is reported to be highly reliable in entering the esophagus with its distal balloon, it offers increased simplicity of use.

It is also available in pediatric sizes, unlike the Combitube. There is also a version that allows passage of a nasogastric tube, which may be used to decompress the stomach and reduce regurgitation. In simulator studies, the success rate in using the LTA is significantly higher than the Combitube or endotracheal intubation. Providers favor the LTA over the Combitube. Like the other supraglottic airways, it is not a definitive airway; it does not provide complete protection from aspiration, it cannot be placed in a conscious patient, and it requires plans for replacement with a definitive airway at the trauma center. Prolonged placement may result in tongue and pharyngeal edema. Vomiting or regurgitation may occur on removal of supraglottic airways. Removal is probably most safely accomplished by exchange of the airway for an endotracheal tube by a skilled airway practitioner in a controlled environment such as in the trauma bay or operating room in the presence of the trauma surgeon and team.

Orotracheal Intubation

Endotracheal intubation (ETI) is the gold standard of airway management. In the prehospital setting, endotracheal intubation without the use of sedatives or neuromuscular blockade is only achievable in deeply comatose patients or patients in cardiac arrest. Because few systems allow paramedics to use RSI, and based on the fact that obtunded patients carry a poor prognosis, endotracheal intubation in those situations may cause more harm than good. Without ideal conditions, endotracheal intubation may be accompanied by an increased number of complications, including hypoxemia, esophageal intubation, and intubation of the mainstem bronchus, with subsequent complete lung collapse, injury to the oropharynx, regurgitation, exacerbation of a potential spinal cord injury, circulatory compromise, increased intracranial pressure, and delay in transport to a trauma center, just to name a few. Inability to recognize a difficult airway may make the intubation impossible and if preceded by RSI may lead to devastating complications and eventually death. Common pitfalls of endotracheal intubation will be discussed.

Adjuncts to Improve Orotracheal Intubation Success

Videolaryngoscopy (VL) devices such as the Glidescope, McGrath, Bullard, Storz CMAC, Kingvision, and others have been modified for use in the prehospital environment. VL can visualize the glottis and vocal cords in cases in which direct laryngoscopy (DL) cannot, such as in difficult airways. VL may require less lifting force than DL, which may reduce cervical spine motion. Failure to intubate and inadvertent injuries are still reported with VL. The relative effectiveness of these devices has yet to be evaluated in clinical trials, and simulator studies have had conflicting results. The relatively high cost and training burden may not yet be justified in many emergency medical services (EMS) systems. Such devices do have the potential to record and transmit video, which may lead to future applications in education and quality control of prehospital airway management.

A low-cost, simple device that can improve first-pass success of endotracheal intubation is the ETTI, sometimes called the gum-elastic bougie, although actual gum-elastic is rarely used now due to the possibility of latex allergies. This device is a 60-cm, 15 F intubating stylet made of a soft synthetic polymer with a coudé tip that is packaged as ready-for-use. It is used when the cords cannot be readily seen on DL. The ETTI is passed under the laryngoscope just behind the epiglottis and its tactile feedback provides information on its location. Tracheal passage is felt as a series of rubs as the coudé tip passes over the tracheal rings, followed by resistance as the tip encounters the carina at about 50 cm. Esophageal passage provides none of these indications. Successful tracheal passage allows passage of an endotracheal tube over the ETTI. There are case reports demonstrating the ETTI allowed intubation of otherwise impossible to intubate prehospital patients.

Confirmation of Orotracheal Tube Placement

Several factors contribute to endotracheal tube malpositioning and include poor lighting, limited access to the patient, insufficient suctioning, difficult airway, intraoral bleeding, vomiting, facial trauma, and airway swelling.

The gold standard for confirmation of adequate placement of an endotracheal tube is the direct visualization of the tube passing through the vocal cords. This is obviously not always possible considering less than ideal conditions at the scene. Auscultation of breath sounds also may be difficult at the scene, particularly in a noisy and chaotic environment.

The colorimetric, end-tidal carbon dioxide detector has been used by prehospital personnel to confirm endotracheal tube placement. In the presence of high levels of carbon dioxide, the device changes color from purple to yellow. The device has been deemed reliable; however, it lacks sensitivity in the setting of cardiopulmonary arrest due to the lack of pulmonary blood flow limiting carbon dioxide delivery. Therefore, approximately 15% of patients properly intubated in that setting would have their endotracheal tubes removed based on the lack of color change in the device. The opposite is also true, and a color change may be observed in patients who have ingested large volumes of carbonated liquids (beer, sodas, etc.), when the tube is in the esophagus or when the stomach has been insufflated with expired gas during bag-valve-mask ventilation.

Another way to determine proper placement of endotracheal tubes is the syringe aspiration technique. If the tube is properly placed in the trachea, the provider should not feel any resistance when attempting to aspirate air from the endotracheal tube (ETT) with airway adaptor fitted to a 60-mL syringe or rubber bulb (Ellick's evacuator). If the tube is in the esophagus, upon negative pressure generated by the syringe, the wall of the esophagus collapses, occluding the openings at the endotracheal tube's tip and resistance to aspiration is felt by the provider.

PREHOSPITAL SURGICAL AIRWAYS

The rate of prehospital surgical airways in U.S. civilian settings is very low, about 4 cricothyroidotomies per 100,000 EMS care events with an 87% success rate. Best practices are difficult to define as there is little published evidence. Lacking a national standard, EMS medical directors and state regulations have considerable variability in practice in allowing EMS personnel to perform such procedures, from jurisdictions with no surgical airways allowed, to some permitting needle cricothyroidotomy only and others also allowing cricothyroidotomy. EMS units may be equipped with open surgical kits or percutaneous Seldinger-type cricothyroidotomy trays. Prehospital cricothyroidotomy is more common in combat casualties; in Operation Iraqi Freedom, the cricothyroidotomy rate was 247 per 100,000 cases with a 77.5% success rate. Given the low experience, critical nature, and "last resort" nature in performing a surgical airway procedure, it represents a considerable training burden for EMS agencies.

CONTROVERSIES IN PREHOSPITAL INTUBATION

Prehospital Intubation in Traumatic Brain Injury

Although an aggressive approach to airway management including endotracheal intubation has been standard of care for patients with severe TBI, it is notable that there is little evidence to support this approach. In fact, several recent studies have demonstrated an increase in mortality rate associated with prehospital intubation. It is not clear whether this represents a selection bias or a true detrimental effect of invasive airway management on outcome. The purported benefits of early intubation include reversal of hypoxia and airway protection from aspiration. However, the morbidity and mortality risks associated with these secondary insults may not be preventable or reversible with invasive airway management 10 to 15 minutes after the initial injury. In addition, there has been a recent increase in awareness of the adverse effects of positive-pressure ventilation on outcome, especially with hyperventilation and hypocapnia.

This makes patient selection for early intubation extremely important so as to maximize the benefit of the procedure. The use of the Glasgow Coma Scale (GCS) score alone to select patients to undergo prehospital intubation has several limitations. An early GCS score appears to have only moderate specificity in identifying severe TBI. In addition, the relationship between GCS score and aspiration is indirect at best. Aspiration events may occur prior to arrival of

EMS personnel or with manipulation of laryngeal structures during intubation. Furthermore, hypoxemia may be reversible with noninvasive airway maneuvers, and oxygen saturation (SpO_2) values with supplemental oxygen may be an important factor in considering prehospital intubation. Although no study has clearly defined a subgroup of head-injured patients who should undergo early intubation, neural network analysis using data from our trauma registry suggests that the most critically injured patients, as defined by GCS score and the presence of hypotension, benefit from the procedure. In addition, intubation does provide additional benefit with regard to the reversal of hypoxemia in some patients.

Who Should Perform Prehospital Rapid Sequence Intubation?

The San Diego Paramedic RSI Trial prospectively enrolled severe TBI patients who could not be intubated without medication. The primary outcome analyses compared trial patients with nonintubated historical control subjects matched for age, gender, mechanism, trauma center, and body region Abbreviated Injury Scale scores. Despite a substantial increase in the percentage of patients arriving with an invasive airway, trial patients had higher mortality rates and a lower incidence of good outcomes. Subsequent analyses suggest that suboptimal performance of the procedure, including hyperventilation and deep desaturations, accounted for at least part of the mortality rate increase. This may reflect the inexperience of paramedics in that system with regard to RSI and the limitations of a single, 8-hour training session.

Other systems providing more intensive training have documented improved success rates, although the link between experience and performance of RSI remains unclear. In the San Diego study, the only subgroup with improved outcomes versus matched historical control subjects was the group undergoing RSI by paramedics and then being transported by air medical crews. The low incidence of hyperventilation in this cohort may explain this somewhat unexpected finding. Subsequent analyses from San Diego and from Pennsylvania document worse outcomes with paramedic intubation but improved outcomes with air medical RSI as compared to emergent intubation in the emergency department. Together, these studies suggest that prehospital RSI may be efficacious when performed by experienced, highly trained individuals. The extent and frequency of initial and ongoing training remain to be defined.

Role of Capnometry in Prehospital Intubation

Quantitative capnometry has several advantages in the management of brain-injured patients. First, capnometry offers accurate confirmation of endotracheal tube placement, both at the time of initial intubation and continuously throughout the prehospital course. Clearly, early recognition of a misplaced endotracheal tube can avoid serious morbidity and even fatality. Systems that have instituted quantitative capnometry as the "gold standard" for endotracheal tube placement have reported unrecognized esophageal intubation rates approaching zero.

Perhaps equally important to the TBI patient is the ability of capnometry to guide ventilation. Data from the San Diego Paramedic RSI Trial established the importance of avoiding hyperventilation and demonstrated the ability of quantitative capnometry to avoid hyperventilation based on arrival P_{CO_2} value. There does appear to be a learning curve, however, as air medical crews who had used

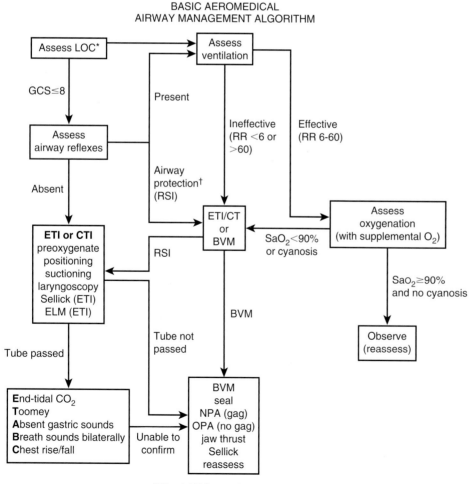

FIGURE 5   Basic aeromedical airway algorithm. BVM, Bag-valve-mask; CTI, Combitube intubation; ELM, external laryngeal manipulation; ETI, endotracheal intubation; FSG, ***; GCS, Glasgow Coma Scale score; LOC, loss of consciousness; NPA, nasopharyngeal airway; OPA, oropharyngeal airway; RR, respiratory rate; RSI, rapid sequence intubation; TBI, traumatic brain injury.

BASIC AEROMEDICAL AIRWAY MANAGEMENT ALGORITHM

*Check FSG, consider Narcan.
†Severe TBI, warning LOC, weak airway reflexes, limited ability to continually reassess.

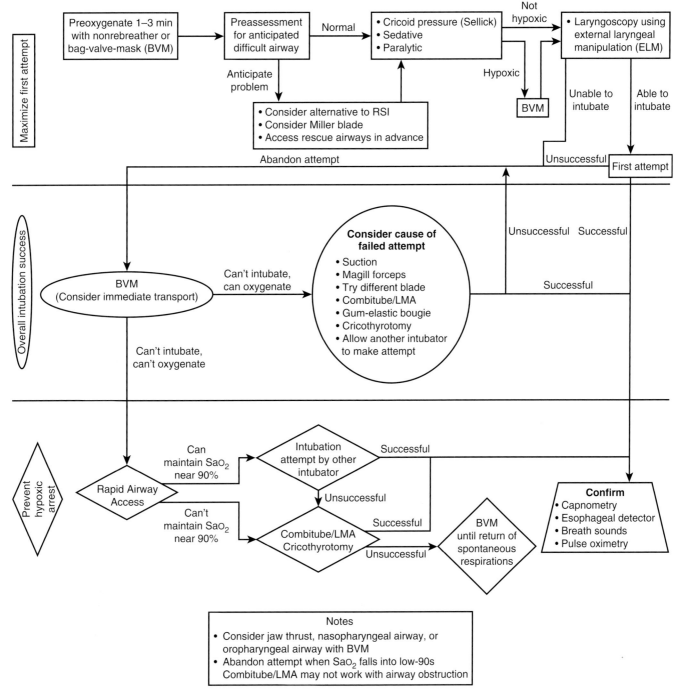

FIGURE 6 Advanced rapid sequence intubation (RSI) algorithm. LMA, Laryngeal mask airway.

capnometry to guide ventilation for many years had better end-tidal carbon dioxide and arrival P_{CO_2} values than paramedics using capnometry. A subsequent registry study from San Diego County demonstrated that patients with moderate to severe TBI do better with intubation, but that prehospital hyperventilations and hypoventilations are associated with worse outcomes. It is our belief that quantitative capnometry should be the standard of care for management of intubated patients in the prehospital environment, especially those with TBI who are especially susceptible to secondary insults.

■ CONCLUSIONS AND ALGORITHMS

Prehospital airway management is a difficult task that requires training and skills. Endotracheal intubation remains the gold standard of

airway management. Specific strategies need to be in place for basic and advanced units (Figs. 5 and 6). Higher success rates will be achieved if endotracheal intubation is attempted after the use of rapid sequence analgesia and paralysis; however, most ground units are not prepared and are not allowed to use such strategy. On the other hand, most aeromedical transport units are facile with RSI and employ this strategy with marked success. A successful RSI program requires medical direction and supervision, training and continuing education, resources for patient monitoring, drug storage and delivery, conformation and monitoring of endotracheal tube placement, standardized protocols, backup airway methods, and continuing quality assurance and performance review.

For the chapter's Suggested Readings list, please visit the book at www.ExpertConsult.inkling.com.

PREHOSPITAL FLUID RESUSCITATION: WHAT TYPE, HOW MUCH, AND CONTROVERSIES

Adam M. Shiroff, Vincente H. Gracias, and Michael F. Rotondo

F luid resuscitation is a vital treatment in the care of hypotensive trauma patients. Restoration of effective circulating blood volume improves oxygen delivery, thereby diminishing the untoward effects of shock at the cellular and organ level. However, fluid resuscitation, in and of itself, is not a panacea. Whereas restoration of effective circulating blood volume is essential, the method of supplying fluid is more controversial and is complicated by several confounding factors. The inability to deliver definitive care in the field, the heterogeneity of patient populations, the variability in mechanism of injury, and the level of in-field hemorrhage control make precise study of the topic challenging. Therefore, the debate persists concerning the type, the amount, and the timing of fluid administration. The purpose of this chapter is to provide insight in the use of fluid resuscitation of trauma patients in the prehospital setting.

EPIDEMIOLOGY

Trauma is the leading cause of civilian death in Americans aged less than 45 years and the fourth leading cause of death in the United States for all ages; hemorrhagic shock is the primary physiologic defect leading to death. Volume deficits develop not only as a result of blood loss, but also due to diffuse capillary-endothelial leak and fluid shifts from the intravascular to the interstitial space. These deficits, and the attendant hypoperfusion, potentially lead to multiple organ dysfunction, failure, and death.

Aggressive fluid administration has been mainstay therapy in trauma patients for over 40 years. Estimates of the numbers of trauma patients in the United Kingdom given prehospital intravenous (IV) fluid range from 8.6 to 65 patients per 100,000 population per year. However, for the last 15 years this practice, especially in the setting of uncontrolled hemorrhage, has been questioned.

CAUSES OF SIGNIFICANT HEMORRHAGE

The causes of hemorrhage vary depending on the mechanism of injury. In blunt trauma, bleeding usually emanates from solid organs such as the spleen and liver, mesenteric blood vessel tears, pelvic and femur fractures, thoracic bleeding from lung lacerations or intercostal vessel bleeding from rib fractures, or external causes such as scalp lacerations. Uncontained bleeding from aortic transection and cardiac rupture usually leads to exsanguination at the scene. When the wounding mechanism is secondary to penetrating trauma, uncontrolled major vascular injury usually is the source of the hemorrhage. External, compressible hemorrhage can be controlled in the prehospital setting with direct compression or tourniquet use; however, cavitary or noncompressbile hemorrhage presents a significant diagnostic and therapeutic problem for the prehospital provider.

DIAGNOSIS AND ASSESSMENT

In the prehospital setting, emergency medical technicians perform an immediate assessment of the trauma victim in the form of a primary and secondary survey. This assessment includes an evaluation of the patient for life-threatening conditions that need to be promptly addressed. The patency of the airway is initially evaluated. This is followed by auscultation of breath sounds assessing for pneumothoraces or hemothoraces. Attention is then turned to the circulation. Central and peripheral pulses are assessed. Obvious sources of external bleeding are controlled. The patient's blood pressure is measured. Because definitive care cannot be rendered at the scene, a "scoop and run" rather than a "stay and stabilize" philosophy should be evoked. Attempts at intravascular cannulation should not delay transfer to the trauma center. Standardized courses such as Prehospital Trauma Life Support are taught throughout the country in an effort to standardize the triage and treatment of life-threatening injuries with the tools available to emergency medical services personnel.

CLASSES OF HEMORRHAGIC SHOCK

Hemorrhage is the most common cause of shock in the injured patient. Shock is defined as the presence of inadequate organ perfusion and tissue oxygenation. In the presence of inadequate oxygen for normal aerobic metabolism, anaerobic metabolism occurs leading to lactic acidosis. If this process continues, cellular membranes lose their integrity leading to cellular swelling, progressive cellular damage, and ultimately, cellular death.

Hemorrhage, an acute loss of circulating blood volume, is classified based on the percentage of blood volume loss. Specific hemodynamic, respiratory, central nervous system, urinary, and integumentary changes occur given the degree of shock (Table 1). Whereas class I hemorrhage is associated with minimal clinical symptoms and requires little, if any, volume replacement, class IV hemorrhage is immediately life-threatening, necessitates blood transfusion, and usually calls for surgical intervention to halt ongoing bleeding.

MANAGEMENT

Access

The basic management principles to follow in hemorrhagic shock are to stop the bleeding and replace the volume loss. Establishing a patent airway with adequate ventilatory exchange and oxygenation is the first priority. Supplemental oxygen is supplied while external bleeding is

TABLE 1: Classification of Hemorrhagic Shock

Parameter	Class 1	Class 2	Class 3	Class 4
Blood loss (%)	<15	15–30	30–40	>40
Blood loss (mL)	<750	750–1500	1500–2000	>2000
Systolic blood pressure	Unchanged	Normal	Reduced	Very low
Diastolic blood pressure	Unchanged	Raised	Reduced	Very low
Pulse	<100	>100	>120	>140

Modified from Advanced Trauma Life Support guidelines.

controlled. Two large-caliber (minimum of 16 G) peripheral IV catheters are inserted, preferably in the antecubital veins. A retrospective study showed that the placement of a second IV line resulted in no clinical improvement, even in hypotensive patients. Another option for access is the intraosseous (IO) catheter, which can be reliably placed in one of three locations: humerus, tibia, and sternum. The IO catheter should be reserved for those situations in which IV access cannot be obtained in the usual fashion. Resuscitative fluids, medications, and even IV contrast material can be administered via the IO catheter. IV access should not delay transport of the patient to the trauma center.

Types of Fluid

Crystalloid

A crystalloid is a solution of small nonionic or ionic particles. They are freely permeable to the vascular membrane and are distributed mainly in the interstitial space. As such, only one third of the volume of crystalloid infused expands the intravascular space. This accounts for the need to provide at least three times more volume of crystalloid than the volume of blood lost. Because of decreased colloid osmotic pressure secondary to decreased serum protein concentration from hemorrhage, capillary leaks, and crystalloid replacement, this ratio of volume of crystalloid infused to blood volume lost may even approach 7:1 to 10:1.

Depletion of both the interstitial fluid volume and the intravascular space following severe injury may be a reason to use crystalloids, which restore volume to both spaces, for fluid resuscitation. Animal and human studies demonstrating improved survival from shock when utilizing isotonic fluid and blood versus blood transfusion alone support this view. Other advantages of crystalloid use in prehospital fluid resuscitation include its negligible cost in comparison to other resuscitative fluids, immediate availability, and long-term storage capacity.

Given the predilection of crystalloid to primarily fill the interstitial space, tissue edema is common and may have deleterious effects. In head-injured patients, increased brain edema may adversely affect outcome. Gas exchange may be impaired secondary to pulmonary edema. Endothelial and red blood cell (RBC) edema impair microcirculation and tissue oxygen exchange, potentially contributing to multiple organ dysfunction.

According to Advanced Trauma Life Support (ATLS) guidelines, fluid resuscitation of the trauma patient begins with a 2-L bolus of crystalloid, usually lactated Ringer's (LR) solution. LR solution is an isotonic fluid that contains L-lactate and D-lactate in a 50:50 mixture. The L-lactate is metabolized in the liver to bicarbonate, thereby providing additional buffer. Although the D-lactate isomer is thought to be a cause of acidosis, studies have shown that resuscitation with LR solution does not lead to increased lactic acid levels. However, normal saline (NS), another isotonic crystalloid, can induce a hyperchloremic acidosis when given in large volumes because of its concentration of chloride ions (154 mEq/L). Healey et al suggest, in their animal model of massive hemorrhage, increased survival rate in animals resuscitated with LR solution and blood relative to those animals that received NS and blood. This difference was thought to be secondary to the profound acidosis occurring in the NS/blood group.

Because LR solution has a lower osmolality than plasma (273 mOsm/L vs. 285–295 mOsm/L), large volumes of it can reduce serum osmolality and contribute to cerebral edema. For this reason, NS may be the preferred resuscitative fluid in head-injured patients.

Hypertonic saline (HS) in concentrations ranging from 3% to 7.5% has been used for the treatment of hypovolemic shock. Because of its elevated osmolality (2400 mOsm/L in 7.5%), HS produces an increase in intravascular volume that far exceeds the infused volume (Table 2). The cardiovascular effects of HS include improved myocardial contractility, decreased systemic and pulmonary vascular resistance, mobilization of tissue edema into the blood compartment,

and reduction in venous capacitance. These effects are transient, however, so HS has been mixed with colloids (dextran or hydroxyethyl starch [HES]) to prolong its efficacy, especially when used for small volume resuscitation.

HS decreases intracranial pressure (ICP), primarily in areas of the brain with an intact blood-brain barrier. Cooper et al, in a double-blind, randomized controlled trial of hypotensive patients with severe traumatic brain injury, studied the effects of prehospital resuscitation with hypertonic saline versus Ringer's lactate on neurologic outcome. These investigators did not find a significant difference in 3- or 6-month extended Glasgow Coma Scale scores between the two groups.

Immunomodulatory effects of HS, either immunostimulatory or immunosuppressive depending on the concentration, have been described. HS affects nuclear activation, protein synthesis and proliferation, polymorphonuclear leukocyte function, and cytoskeleton polymerization. In animal models of hemorrhage, these effects have been associated with reduced organ dysfunction and improved survival.

DuBose et al, described the use of 5% HS on trauma patients within 1 hour of arrival to the trauma center and found a trend toward improved mortality rate with those patients with a Glasgow Coma Scale score less than 8 and a head Abbreviated Injury Scale score of greater than 3.

Despite its benefits, a meta-analysis evaluating the effect of HS compared to isotonic crystalloid on 30-day outcome in trauma patients failed to show a survival advantage. As such, the role of HS in prehospital fluid resuscitation has yet to be defined.

Colloid

Nonbiologically Active

Colloids seemingly have many advantages as resuscitative fluids over crystalloids. Their ability to effectively expand plasma volume exceeds that of crystalloids. End points of resuscitation are met using smaller volumes of colloids, which in turn reduce tissue edema. However, some investigators suggest that colloids potentiate tissue edema. The capillary-endothelial cell leak that develops after severe injury may allow the colloid to pass into the interstitium and exacerbate swelling.

Albumin, a natural colloid, is synthesized in the liver and is responsible for 80% of the oncotic pressure of the plasma. The molecular weight of albumin is approximately 69 kDa. Infusion of the 25% solution expands plasma volume four to five times the volume infused (see Table 2). Derived from pooled human plasma, its risk of transmitting infectious diseases is low because of stringent heating and sterilization. Aside from its volume replacing properties, albumin also possesses a transport function for drugs and endogenous substances

TABLE 2: Effect on Plasma Volume Expansion of Various Solutions

Solution Infused	Volume Infused (mL)	Plasma Volume Expansion (mL)
Dextrose in water (D$_5$W)	1000	100
Lactated Ringer's	1000	250
7.5% hypertonic saline	250	1000
5% albumin	500	375
25% albumin	100	450
6% hetastarch	500	750

Modified from Rizoli SB: Crystalloids and colloids in trauma resuscitation: a brief overview of the current debate. *J Trauma* 54:S82–S88, 2003.

and may have a beneficial effect on membrane permeability secondary to free radical scavenging. These theoretical effects have not been proved clinically.

Disadvantages of albumin include its cost, short supply, and potential disease transmission. Additionally, albumin's use for the resuscitation of critically ill patients has demonstrated either a trend toward or a significant increase in mortality rate. Therefore, the use of albumin cannot be recommended as a resuscitative fluid for hypotensive trauma patients.

Synthetic colloids include dextran, HES, and mixtures of dextran and HES with hypertonic saline solutions. Dextran is a glucose polymer available as 6% dextran 70 (70 kDa) and 10% dextran 40 (40 kDa) solutions. Increase of plasma volume after infusion of 1000 mL of dextran 70 ranges from 600 to 800 mL. Dextran reduces blood viscosity, reduces platelet adhesiveness, and enhances fibrinolysis, resulting in increased bleeding tendency. Severe, life-threatening anaphylactic reactions are also well described. The use of dextran as an exclusive fluid resuscitant is limited by these side effects.

As mentioned previously, dextran has been added to HS to extend its intravascular presence. Its use as a resuscitative fluid was compared with isotonic crystalloid and analyzed via a meta-analysis of several randomized controlled trials of hypotensive trauma patients. Although HS was safe, demonstrated higher increases in blood pressure, and decreased early fluid and blood requirements, no statistically significant survival benefit was attributed to its use. Conversely, in a study by Wade et al, survival to discharge was significantly improved in patients resuscitated with 250 mL of HS who sustained penetrating torso trauma requiring surgical intervention. This suggests a subset of trauma patients may benefit from HS in the prehospital setting.

HES solutions are modified natural polymers of amylopectin. The pharmacokinetic properties of each formulation are determined by its molecular weight, the pattern of hydroxyethylation, and the ratio of C2:C6 hydroxyethylation. These properties influence the plasma expansion, degradation, and side effect profile of HES.

Side effects associated with HES include pruritus and increased bleeding due to reduction of factor VIII and von Willebrand factor. However, most recent studies using modern HES preparations demonstrated no impairment of hemostasis or increased bleeding propensity.

Still, despite the apparent advantages of colloids, meta-analyses suggest a trend toward increased mortality rate when they are used for the resuscitation of trauma patients. Although the methodology of these studies can be questioned, until better designed clinical trials provide irrefutable evidence suggesting improved outcome with the use of colloids for fluid resuscitation, these agents cannot be recommended.

Biologically Active

When considering an ideal resuscitative fluid in hemorrhagic shock, its properties would include volume expansion, oxygen-carrying capacity, universal compatibility, immediate availability, long-term storage capacity, and the absence of vasoactive properties and disease transmission. Although blood transfusion effectively improves volume deficits and provides oxygen delivery, its use in the prehospital setting is limited by expense, short shelf life, short supply, risk of disease transmission, and need for cross-matching. Allogenic RBCs may have adverse immunoinflammatory effects that increase the risk of postinjury multiple organ failure (MOF).

Hemoglobin-based oxygen carriers (HBOCs) are attractive in the prehospital setting, then, for several reasons. Because HBOCs can be heat treated, their risk of disease transmission is low. They have a shelf life of up to 3 years and have oxygen-carrying as well as volume-expansion properties. They are universally compatible, thus eliminating the need for cross-matching. Phase II clinical trials, as well as in vitro and in vivo work, suggest that resuscitation with a HBOC—in lieu of stored RBCs—attenuates the systemic inflammatory response invoked in the pathogenesis of MOF.

Clinical trials with HBOC have shown mixed results. When diaspirin cross-linked hemoglobin (DCLHb) was studied against NS in a U.S. multicenter trial for the treatment of severe traumatic hemorrhagic shock, the 28-day mortality rate was 46% for DCLHb compared to 17% for NS. An increase in systemic and pulmonary vascular resistance leading to decreased cardiac output was felt to be responsible for the higher mortality rate. However, polymerized hemoglobin solutions have shown more promise. In a prospective, randomized trial comparing the therapeutic benefits of Poly-Heme with that of allogenic RBCs in the treatment of acute blood loss, the Poly-Heme group demonstrated similar total hemoglobin concentration after infusion as the RBC group, with less RBC transfusion required through the first day of treatment and without serious or unexpected adverse consequences resulting from Poly-Heme. In a recent subgroup analysis of all deaths in the study, Bernard et al found that the PolyHeme recipients survived longer compared to the control group. This benefit is likely due to the early oxygen-carrying resuscitation of these patients. This oxygenation may allow for the needed time for hemorrhage control in a select group that might otherwise have exsanguinated. In time, it is possible that one or more HBOCs may be used routinely in the resuscitation of hemorrhagic shock.

Resuscitation Targets

Delayed

Studies have begun to scrutinize the potential detrimental effects of raising the blood pressure during uncontrolled hemorrhage. Whereas early work with controlled hemorrhage models was used to support the practice of fluid resuscitation of post-traumatic hemorrhage, these models of resuscitation do not mimic the actual life situation of uncontrolled bleeding and concurrent treatment. In the setting of uncontrolled hemorrhage, fluid administration may disrupt thrombus formation, induce coagulopathy by diluting clotting factors, and lead to increased bleeding. In 1918, Cannon observed increased bleeding induced by rapid fluid infusion prior to hemorrhage control. More recently, in a study of penetrating torso trauma, hypotensive patients were randomized to immediate versus delayed fluid resuscitation with isotonic crystalloid. Prehospital fluid resuscitation was started in the immediate group, but held in the delayed group until control of hemorrhage in the operating room. Compared to patients in the delayed group, patients in the immediate resuscitation group had higher mortality rates and higher rates of postoperative complications. Although the results of this study have been argued, the study rekindled interest and stimulated thought concerning approaches of management for the treatment of uncontrolled hemorrhage.

Hypotensive

This strategy of resuscitation attempts to maintain adequate vital organ perfusion while minimizing further bleeding. A mean arterial pressure (MAP) of 60 mm Hg has been used as a resuscitation target. It is regarded as the lowest safe level because it is the lowest MAP of active autoregulation of cerebral blood flow. No lower limit of hypotensive resuscitation, however, has been firmly established.

Using blood pressure as a guideline simulates prehospital scenarios in which this variable is only one of the hemodynamic parameters available. Dutton et al randomized hypotensive blunt and penetrating trauma patients to a systolic blood pressure (SBP) of 70 mm Hg (hypotensive) or more than 100 mm Hg (normotensive). Crystalloid or blood products were administered to maintain the intended SBP for each group. There was no difference in survival between the two cohorts. This was partly attributed to the difficulty in maintaining the targeted blood pressures. The average SBP for the hypotensive and normotensive groups were 100 mm Hg and 114 mm Hg, respectively. This response suggests spontaneous reduction of bleeding due to inherent hemostatic mechanisms and may validate use of this resuscitation strategy in certain scenarios of uncontrolled hemorrhage.

Normotensive

The traditional approach to the resuscitation of trauma patients in hemorrhagic shock has been to normalize blood pressure by administering large volumes of crystalloid followed by transfusion of blood products. This method of resuscitation developed from animal models of controlled hemorrhage. Restoration of vital organ perfusion improved survival, whereas untreated animals developed organ dysfunction and succumbed. In situations of uncontrolled hemorrhage, animal studies revealed decreased splanchnic perfusion and greater blood loss. In situations in which bleeding has spontaneously resolved, the standard approach to resuscitation is reasonable. It is difficult to predict, however, whether bleeding has spontaneously ceased or may be exacerbated by aggressive resuscitation.

MORBIDITY AND COMPLICATIONS

Prehospital fluid resuscitation is not without its own complications. Exacerbated bleeding, dilution of clotting factors, and dislodgement of thrombi, among other problems, have already been mentioned, and may act to decrease survival of hemorrhagic shock. Additionally, a balance needs to be achieved between underresuscitation and overresuscitation, as both of these concerns contribute to increased morbidity and mortality rates. Whereas the goal of prehospital fluid resuscitation is to preserve blood flow to vital organs (brain, heart) without incurring significant, irreversible damage to other organ systems (renal, splanchnic), excess crystalloid resuscitation may contribute to the development of the abdominal compartment syndrome.

Hypothermia develops commonly after traumatic shock and is exacerbated with the administration of cold fluids. Adverse consequences of hypothermia include impaired coagulation function, reduction of oxygen delivery, and increased rate of infection. The importance of administering warm fluids to avoid the untoward effects of hypothermia cannot be overstated.

SUMMARY

The clinical study of massive hemorrhage and resuscitation is complicated by small numbers, urgency of care, varying goals and end points, and patient heterogeneity with respect to age, comorbid conditions, mechanism of injury, prehospital time and therapy, and complications of resuscitation. Some definite conclusions can be drawn from the vast literature. The rapid transport of the trauma patient to a center where definitive care can be rendered is paramount. Second, the importance of hemorrhage control prior to aggressive fluid resuscitation cannot be overstated. Despite the number of options of resuscitation strategies and fluids, no single choice is perfectly applicable in every trauma scenario. Until human studies can be performed utilizing particular strategies for particular injuries with proven improved outcomes, ATLS guidelines should continue to be practiced.

For the chapter's Suggested Readings list, please visit the book at www.ExpertConsult.inkling.com.

CIVILIAN HOSPITAL RESPONSE TO MASS CASUALTY EVENTS

Rochelle A. Dicker and William P. Schecter

On September 11, 2001, the attack on the Twin Towers stimulated the medical community to better prepare for mass casualty events caused by attacks with both conventional and unconventional weapons. The tsunamis that destroyed coastal areas in Southern Asia in 2004 and Japan in 2011, as well as the flooding of New Orleans after hurricane Katrina in 2005, exposed inadequate responses to loss of infrastructure caused by natural disasters. A thoughtful, coordinated, and well-rehearsed disaster plan is essential. The Tokyo subway sarin gas poisoning is a notable example of problems with early detection of poison gas release and the risk of exposure to the first wave of health care providers.

KEY DEFINITIONS

A *mass casualty event* occurs when the number of patients and the severity of their injuries exceed the capability of the facility to deliver care in a routine fashion. The appropriate initial response is to treat patients sustaining major injuries with the greatest chance of survival first so that valuable resources are not expended on patients with minor injuries or those with little hope of survival.

A *multiple casualty event* occurs when the facility can deliver care in a routine fashion to large numbers of patients by mobilizing additional resources. The goal is to convert a mass casualty event in the field to a multiple casualty event for each receiving hospital by appropriate distribution of victims based on severity to the various receiving facilities.

Triage refers to sorting of patients according to their need for treatment and the available resources. In a mass casualty event, conventional standards of medical care cannot be delivered to all victims. The goal of triage is to optimize care for the maximum number of salvageable patients.

Patients are triaged into four categories at the scene: minor, delayed, immediate, and dead. In military triage systems, a fifth category, expectant care, is used for patients with little chance of survival who would use scarce resources to such an extent as to adversely affect the chance of survival of more salvageable patients. This category is rarely used in civilian situations as mobilization of additional resources is usually possible. Numbers, colors, or symbols may be used to denote the categories (Table 1). *Undertriage* refers to assignment of patients to a level of care inadequate for their level of injury. An undertriage rate greater than 5% is unacceptable as it may lead to unnecessary morbidity and fatality in severely injured patients. *Overtriage* refers to assignment of patients to a level of care greater than required for their level of injury. An overtriage rate of 50% is considered acceptable to minimize undertriage. Excessive overtriage at the

TABLE 1: The Four Colors of Triage

Color	Description
Minor—green	Delayed care/can delay up to 3 hours
Delayed—yellow	Urgent care/can delay up to 1 hour
Immediate—red	Immediate care/life-threatening
Dead—black	Victim is dead/no care required

Modified from Los Angeles Community Emergency Response Team.

scene threatens the response of the entire system due to expenditure of limited resources on patients with relatively minor injuries.

PREHOSPITAL CARE IN A MASS CASUALTY EVENT

The response to a mass casualty event requires the coordinated effort of many agencies with disparate cultures, command structures, and even communications equipment (Fig. 1). Responding agencies should submit to the authority of the incident field commander at the scene. Prior joint training can break down interagency barriers and improve the overall response.

Regardless of the cause, the area of the event must be secured. In the event of a terrorist or military attack with conventional weapons, additional enemy operatives must be identified and neutralized to avoid a "second hit." Second hit also applies to domestic terrorists, as in the Georgia abortion clinic bombings, in which the second bomb was set to involve first responders. Victims must be extracted, concentrated in a safe area, and triaged. Immediate care patients should be transported first after control of external hemorrhage, stabilization of the airway, and decompression of a tension pneumothorax, if present.

Transportation to the hospital may occur by ambulance, bus, or private vehicle. The worried well and patients with minor injuries often self-triage to the hospital, increasing the volume of patients at the receiving hospitals.

Crowd control at the scene is a major problem. Multiple volunteers with various skills arrive to help and hinder. Optimally, the triage area should be secured and individuals inserted to help at the discretion of the incident field commander.

HOSPITAL TRIAGE

All area hospitals must participate in the care of victims of a true mass casualty event to avoid overwhelming one institution. Each hospital should initiate its mass casualty plan upon notification of such an event or the unexpected arrival of a large number of casualties.

All elective surgery must be canceled. Rapid disposition of preexisting patients in the emergency department is required. Depending upon the size of the event, hospitalized patients who are fit may be discharged and patients may be transferred within the hospital to maximize the availability of surgical beds, if required.

The initial hospital triage (Fig. 2) should occur outside the emergency department. Ambulances should pass through a security

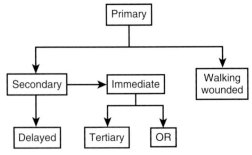

FIGURE 2   Initial triage stations. OR, Operating room.

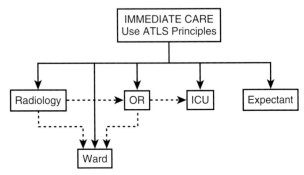

FIGURE 3   Intrahospital traffic flow. ATLS, Advanced Trauma Life Support; ICU, intensive care unit; OR, operating room.

checkpoint prior to entrance to the hospital grounds to identify any terrorists or ordnance that may be on board. Initial triage should be done by a highly experienced clinician. If possible, the walking wounded should be escorted through a separate entrance to avoid overcrowding the resuscitation area.

As soon as stretcher patients enter the emergency department, a senior surgeon should triage each patient to either immediate or delayed care (Fig. 3). The immediate care area should be reserved for salvageable patients with life-threatening problems. The following personnel should be present at each bed in the immediate care area: a senior surgeon for decision making, an anesthesiologist to provide airway control, two emergency department or critical care nurses, and a junior surgeon for vascular access and tube thoracostomy, if necessary.

Treatment in the immediate care area is based upon the principles of Advanced Trauma Life Support. The goals of therapy in the immediate care area are cessation of external hemorrhage, airway control, ventilation, vascular access, and rapid transfer of the patient to the next appropriate treatment station for completion of the secondary survey and additional diagnostic or therapeutic procedures. The next venue of care (the operating room [OR], the intensive care unit [ICU], or the radiology department) is determined by the senior surgeon or incident commander based upon the patient's condition and the number of casualties (Fig. 4).

Prior arrangements should be made to expand the ICU. The postanesthesia care unit is ideal for expansion of ICU services. Because most victims do not require immediate access to the OR (unless they have penetrating trauma due to shrapnel, or traumatic amputations), even empty ORs could be used to temporarily manage critically ill patients in an unusual situation.

Patients with significant but non–life-threatening injuries are triaged to delayed care. A junior surgeon and nurse should be assigned to each of these patients. A senior surgeon, however, should command the delayed care area to provide advice and correct any errors in triage.

Walking wounded patients should be managed in a separate area of the hospital by nurses and physicians. If possible, a surgeon or

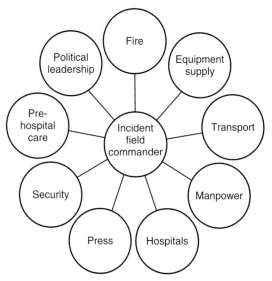

FIGURE 1   Components of disaster response.

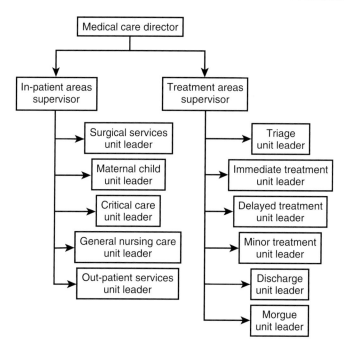

FIGURE 4 Simplified model of Hospital Emergency Incident Command System.

emergency physician should command this area. Most of the walking wounded patients can be discharged from the emergency department after receiving screening for psychological trauma.

HOSPITAL EMERGENCY INCIDENT COMMAND SYSTEM

The basic principle of Hospital Emergency Incident Command System is that one individual supervises no more than five people and reports to only one person. A senior surgeon is the ideal incident commander. This system allows for efficient lines of communication and direct accountability. There are four main section chiefs: planning, logistics, finance, and operations. The operations chief has overall responsibility for the triage of victims, their clinical care, and coordination with other area hospitals (Fig. 5).

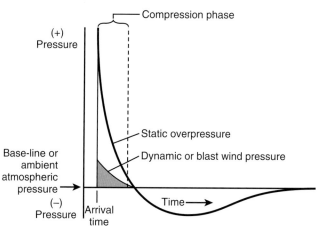

FIGURE 5 Physics of a blast wave.

Each hospital must play its role within a coordinated regional disaster response.

For example, Los Angeles County has 13 Level I and II trauma centers that have a defined catchment area. However, when a mass casualty or multiple casualty event occurs, a Medical Alert Center coordinates distribution of casualties between the trauma centers and community hospitals to provide Level I trauma care to the most severely injured without overburdening any one center.

CAUSES OF MASS CASUALTY EVENTS

Conventional Weapons/Blast Injury

Bombings were responsible for almost 70% of terrorist attacks in the United States and its territories between 1980 and 2001. Many terrorist bombs contain shrapnel, such as nails and bolts, designed to maximize casualties.

Injury patterns from explosions are dependent upon several factors: the materials involved, the surrounding environment (open versus closed space), the distance of the victim from the explosion, and the presence of protective barriers.

A primary blast injury occurs when the pressure wave directly hits the body surface. Organs with air-fluid interfaces are particularly susceptible to injury (lungs, intestines, and ears). Damage to the eye and brain may also occur. Specific injuries are summarized in Table 2. A secondary blast injury occurs as a result of flying debris. It can cause both blunt and penetrating injury. Tertiary blast injury occurs when victims are thrown against solid objects by the blast wave. The term quaternary blast injury encompasses miscellaneous injuries such as burns and crush injuries. Illnesses directly related to the blast such as post-traumatic stress disorder, bronchospasm, angina, or inhalation of toxic fumes are also classified as quaternary blast injuries.

TABLE 2: Spectrum of Explosive-Related Injuries

Organ System	Effect
Auditory	Ruptured tympanic membrane (almost always seen with blast lung), ossicular disruption, foreign body
Eye, orbit, face	Ruptured globe, foreign body, fracture, air embolus
Respiratory	Blast lung, pulmonary contusion, pneumothorax, left-sided air embolism, aspiration
Circulatory	Myocardial contusion, myocardial infarction (air embolism), hemorrhagic shock
Central nervous	Closed or open head injury, stroke or spinal cord injury from air embolism, spinal cord injury from blunt trauma
Renal	Contusion, laceration, acute renal failure from hypotension or rhabdomyolysis
Gastrointestinal	Bowel perforation, hemorrhage, solid organ injury, mesenteric ischemia (air embolus)
Extremity*	Amputation, crush, fracture, compartment syndrome, burns, vascular injury

*Most common system needing operative intervention.

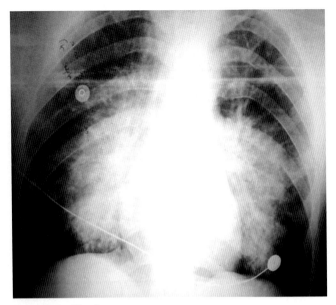

FIGURE 6 Blast lung.

Blast lung injury is a direct injury to the pulmonary parenchyma due to barotrauma. The clinical presentation is similar to that for pulmonary contusion. The most common symptoms and signs are hemoptysis and hypoxia leading to dyspnea, tachypnea, and poor compliance. Unlike pulmonary contusion, blast lung injury does not usually have associated rib fractures. Typical chest radiographic findings (Fig. 6) include a "butterfly" pattern of infiltrates, pneumomediastinum, hemothorax, and pneumothorax.

If mechanical ventilation is required, tidal volumes, peak inspiratory pressures, and positive end-expiratory pressure levels should be kept as low as possible to decrease the risk of ventilator-associated barotrauma. On occasion, a patient with blast lung injury can develop left-sided air embolism due to rupture of the alveolar capillary membrane resulting in neurologic symptoms or coronary artery occlusion.

Biologic Agents

Unlike a conventional mass casualty event, the extent of a biologic attack may not be known for some time. Many victims may initially be unaware that they are infected and contagious. Health care facilities may become contaminated prior to recognition of the attack.

The United States categorizes biologic agents based on their risk to the population. Category A agents can be easily disseminated, have a high mortality rate, cause panic, and require a major public health effort to contain the spread of disease. The four major agents in Category A, their characteristics, and management strategies are listed in Table 3.

Category B agents are moderately easy to disseminate and are associated with a moderate risk of morbidity and mortality. Category B diseases/agents include brucellosis, *Clostridium perfringens*, *Salmonella*, *Escherichia coli*, *Shigella*, glanders, ricin, typhus, streptococcus enterotoxin B, Q fever, psittacosis, water safety threats, and viral encephalitis.

Category C diseases are emerging pathogens that could be engineered as biologic weapons in the future. They have a high potential for morbidity and mortality.

Health Care and Hospital Response to Bioterrorism

In an attack with a Category A biologic weapon, there may be no obvious initial scene. The patient's first contact with the health care system

TABLE 3: Category A Diseases/Agents*

Disease	Agent	Incubation Period	Transmission	Presentation	Treatment	Prevention
Anthrax†	*Bacillus anthracis*	1 day to 8 weeks	Inhalation, skin contact, ingestion	Flulike symptoms then respiratory failure, wide mediastinum on chest radiograph	Fluoroquinolones or doxycycline	Inactivated vaccine, limited availability
Botulism	7 toxins produced by *Clostridium botulinum*	12–72 hours	Ingestion, inhalation of spores (no person-to-person transmission)	Symmetrical cranial neuropathies, descending weakness proximal to distal, respiratory dysfunction	Mechanical ventilation can be for 2–3 months while neurologic function recovers	Investigational pentavalent vaccine
Plague	*Yersinia pestis*	2–8 days (may be shorter if inhaled)	Infected fleas, with bioterror, likely aerosolized	Fever, cough, hemoptysis, chest pain	Doxycycline, second choice is ciprofloxacin	Not available in United States
Small pox	Variola virus	7–17 days	Inhalation, can be person to person, or contact with skin lesion	Fever, myalgias, then rash mostly to face and extremities	Vaccination except if pregnant or immunocompromised	Live virus vaccine, may *not* confer lifetime immunity

*Viral hemorrhagic fevers such as filovirus and arenavirus are also now being considered a potential Category A threat.

may be a doctor's office, a free-standing clinic, or an emergency room. Multiple health care facilities, including hospitals and their staff, will be exposed to the pathogen.

The principles of management of a biologic attack are similar to those of an epidemic: (1) rapid detection and strict isolation of patients, (2) identification and treatment of contacts, (3) strict hospital infection control possibly including hospital lockdown, and (4) avoidance of funeral practices allowing close contact with the bodies. These public health measures are essential but difficult to achieve.

Patients injured in a biologic attack will most likely acquire their infection via the inhalation route. Routine reverse isolation suffices for all of these patients except those with highly contagious, viral hemorrhagic fevers who require strict isolation and care by individuals wearing Level A protective clothing.

Chemical Agents

Four types of chemical weapons can potentially be used in a terrorist attack: nerve agents, cyanide, vesicants, and pulmonary agents. The most likely weapons are nerve agents and cyanide.

Nerve Agents

Nerve agents are organophosphate compounds that inhibit cholinesterase at the synaptic and neuromuscular junctions causing an excess of acetylcholine leading to a cholinergic crisis. Five nerve agents have been produced as weapons: tabun, sarin, soman, GF, and Vx.

Symptoms and Signs of Cholinergic Crisis

Acetylcholine binds to receptors on the postsynaptic cell membrane, the smooth muscle end plates, and secretory glands, causing the muscarinic effects of acetylcholine. These effects include bronchospasm, low pulmonary compliance, nausea, vomiting, diarrhea, miosis, blurred vision, bradycardia, and hypersecretions of the oropharynx, conjunctivae, tracheobronchial tree, and gastrointestinal tract.

Acetylcholine also binds to skeletal muscle end plates and synaptic ganglia, causing the nicotinic effects. The nicotinic effects of acetylcholine include fasciculations, flaccid paralysis, tachycardia, and hypertension. Heart rate during a cholinergic crisis is variable due to the opposing actions of the nicotinic and muscarinic effects. Patients may experience initial tachycardia progressing to bradycardia as the severity of the cholinergic crisis increases.

Treatment of Nerve Agent Injury

There are two separate antidotes for a cholinergic crisis. Atropine is a very effective antidote for the muscarinic effects but has no influence on the nicotinic effects. Atropine competitively binds at the postsynaptic muscarinic receptor thereby displacing acetylcholine. Atropine should be given until secretions abate and pulmonary compliance improves.

The antidote for the nicotinic effects of acetylcholine is a class of drugs called oximes. In the United States, pradiloxime chloride is the oxime of choice. Oximes act as a "molecular crowbar" separating the nerve agent from the cholinesterase thereby allowing acetylcholine breakdown at the nicotinic receptors. Unfortunately, the oximes must be given before irreversible binding of the nerve agent and the cholinesterase occurs, a phenomenon known as aging. The aging half-life varies from 2 minutes for soman to several hours for sarin.

The recommended initial treatment for mild to moderate nerve agent injury is atropine, 2 mg intramuscular (IM) and pradiloxime chloride 600 mg IM. For severe injury, atropine 6 mg IM and pradiloxime chloride 1200 mg IM are recommended.

Cyanide

Cyanide is a highly effective chemical weapon when employed in closed spaces as demonstrated by the criminal efficiency of the gas chambers in Nazi concentration camps during World War II. The high volatility of cyanide makes it an ineffective weapon when employed in open spaces because of rapid dissemination.

Moderate exposure causes a bright red appearance to the skin and venous blood, metabolic acidosis, and the odor of bitter almonds. Severe exposure causes coma, apnea, and cardiac arrest.

The most recent recommended antidotes to cyanide poisoning include "solutions A and B," which are ferrous sulfate dissolved in citric acid and sodium carbonate, both given orally. They are only effective in reducing the absorption of swallowed cyanide. Amyl nitrate can be given by inhalation, but its safety and efficacy record is in question. Dicobalt can be administered intravenously to people with severe toxicity, but it is also quite toxic.

Vesicants

The mustards are liquid chemical weapons that cause burns to the skin and mucous membranes and induce bone marrow suppression. Treatment involves decontamination, management of the burn wounds, and treatment of hematologic abnormalities. At least 40,000 Iranian casualties sustained vesicant injuries when Iraq employed mustard agents during the Iran-Iraq War in the 1980s.

Pulmonary Agents

Chlorine, and later phosgene, were employed as chemical weapons causing pulmonary edema and respiratory insufficiency during World War I. Patients exposed to these agents developed chest tightness progressing to cough, hoarseness, stridor, and hypoxia over a period of 2 to 4 hours depending upon the degree of exposure. The pulmonary parenchymal injury resembles an inhalation injury resulting from exposure to smoke and burning plastic.

Implications of a Chemical Weapon Attack for Scene Management and the Hospital Disaster Plan

If a chemical agent is suspected, individuals providing care at the scene should don protective clothing. Ideally, victims should be decontaminated at the scene before transport to the hospital (Fig. 7).

Experience from the Aum Shinrikyo Japanese sarin attacks demonstrates that nerve agents are more of a "mass hysteria" weapon than a "mass destruction" weapon. Most of the severe cases will be dead in the field. A large number of worried well or mildly exposed patients will flood the hospital. Hospital security and early lockdown are essential to prevent contamination of the facilities and staff, as happened in the Tokyo sarin attack. There probably will not be time to deploy a decontamination facility prior to the arrival of the first patient. At San Francisco General Hospital, it takes a minimum of 1 hour to erect the decontamination tent during prearranged drills occurring in daylight with all key personnel assembled in advance.

Decontamination is a critical part of the treatment. Early decontamination protects the patient from further exposure. Late decontamination protects the medical team. Simple removal of clothing results in decontamination of approximately 80% of a liquid nerve agent. Decontamination showers should be part of a hospital mass casualty event plan in case of a terrorist nerve agent attack. The problem of hypothermia during decontamination in cold climates has yet to be solved.

Patients in severe cholinergic crisis will require resuscitation by health care personnel in the decontamination zone wearing personal

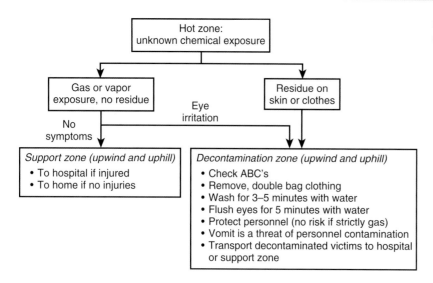

FIGURE 7 Algorithm for chemical decontamination at the scene. ABCs, Airway, breathing, and circulation.

protective equipment. The idea that efficient resuscitation of large numbers of patients with cholinergic crisis due to nerve agent poisoning by staff unpracticed in this procedure wearing bulky unwieldy protective clothing is naïve. Surgeons and anesthesiologists should be aware of the potentiating effect of nerve agents on neuromuscular blockade as well as the effect of hypersecretions and bronchospasm on general anesthesia in the event that surgery is required to treat a trauma patient exposed to nerve agents.

Radiation Injuries

There are three different types of possible exposure to radiation. The first is exposure due to radiation dispersal devices (dirty bombs) that cause conventional blast injury. Radiation levels are not typically high enough to cause acute radiation syndrome (see later). Because 85% of decontamination occurs when clothing is removed, radiation exposure to health care personnel is minimal. The second type of exposure occurs after either unintentional or intentional damage to nuclear power plant reactors. Victims suffer both blast and radiation injury. First responders would be at risk for severe radiation exposure and contamination of the surrounding region is likely. The third scenario, a nuclear detonation, would cause massive destruction and large numbers dead and injured at the scene.

Severe radiation exposure results in hair loss, burns, acute radiation sickness (ARS), and death. Three syndromes are associated with major exposure: the hematopoietic, gastrointestinal, and neurologic/cardiovascular. The initial symptoms of the hematopoietic syndrome are nausea, vomiting, and anorexia. In the latent phase, stem cells in the bone marrow die. Patients with significant exposure (over 120 rads) may die within a few months. Less severely affected patients can make a full recovery.

The initial symptoms of the gastrointestinal syndrome are similar to those for the hematopoietic syndrome with the addition of diarrhea. The LD_{100} (full lethal dose) for this syndrome is about 1000 rads, from which victims die of infection and dehydration. The cardiovascular/central nervous system syndrome is seen at exposures greater than 2000 rads. Initial symptoms are similar to those for the gastrointestinal syndrome with the addition of mental status changes. Convulsions and coma may occur within hours.

First responders should don personal protective equipment. Emergency equipment and decontamination zones should be placed upwind from the contaminated area. Victims without life-threatening blast injuries should be decontaminated at the scene prior to being transported to hospital.

Hospitals should be equipped with a radiation survey device and a separate decontamination area outside the emergency department should be established. As with chemical exposure, decontamination consists of removal of all clothing and thorough washing with water. Open wounds should be washed first. Symptoms consistent with ARS should be treated. After patient decontamination, health care workers are not at risk for radiation injury. The patient is suffering the effects of radiation exposure but is not radioactive. Additional help can be obtained from the Radiation Emergency Assistance Center and Training Site and the Medical Radiobiology Advisory Team.

COMMUNICATION DURING MASS CASUALTY

Cellular phone systems may be shut down by the authorities to prevent a second hit after an explosion causing a mass casualty event or the communication systems may be overwhelmed by the large volume of calls generated by worried family members. Reliance on standard communication equipment immediately following a mass casualty event is unwise. The ADAM (Area Defense Anti-Munitions) System in Israel requires Israeli hospitals to open communication centers when a mass casualty event occurs. Municipal officials, the Ministry of Health, the Forensic Institute, and the police can all easily access information via ADAM.

CONCLUSION

Surgeons should take an active role in preparation for disasters and mass casualty events. A careful plan with efficient triage and resource allocation is critical in order to maximize the number of lives saved. Mass casualty events secondary to terrorist attacks will most likely involve conventional explosive devices. However, hospital disaster plans should be prepared in the event of a chemical, biologic, or radioactive weapon attack.

For the chapter's Suggested Readings list, please visit the book at www.ExpertConsult.inkling.com.

INJURIES FROM EXPLOSIVES

Howard R. Champion

Explosives have been used in every major conflict in which the United States has been involved and today are the primary mechanism of injury among U.S. combatants (Fig. 1). Explosives, most notably improvised explosive devices (IEDs), are also commonly used against civilian targets. After a bomb attack on civilian populations, scene responders are responsible for triage and transport decisions, and then hospital personnel must retriage and reassess all patients who arrive at their facility. Most blast events are mass casualty incidents, and early recognition of symptoms that can point to more significant injury, within the chaos of the patient surge, is key to optimizing patient outcomes.

INCIDENCE

Explosive devices are the most frequently used weapons in combat and by terrorists. In Afghanistan and Iraq, three fourths of the almost 50,000 injuries and deaths among U.S. troops were caused by explo-sive devices, often IEDs.* Among civilians throughout the world, 62% of the close to half million injuries and deaths (317,029 and 157,023, respectively) that occurred in the 77,134 terrorist attacks between January 1990 and April 2011 were caused by explosives.[†]

MECHANISMS OF INJURY AND DIAGNOSIS

A bomb is any container filled with explosive material whose explosion is triggered by a clock or other device. Bombs used by terrorists are primarily IEDs, may use a number of designs or explosives, and are of two types: (1) conventional (filled with chemical explosives containing hydrogen, oxygen, nitrogen, and carbon) or (2) dispersive (filled with chemicals or projectiles such as nails, steel pellets, screws, and nuts). Nuclear devices (outside the scope of this chapter) rely on nuclear fission or fusion. The term "blast injury" refers to the biophysical and pathophysiologic events and the clinical syndromes that occur when a living body is exposed to blast of any origin.

Blast injuries are unique in that they combine several mechanisms of injury including blunt, penetrating, and thermal. Therefore, knowledge of the mechanisms of blast effect and early recognition of the potential injuries are of paramount importance in the management of blast-injured patients. Blast injuries are classified according to their underlying mechanisms into five categories (Table 1).

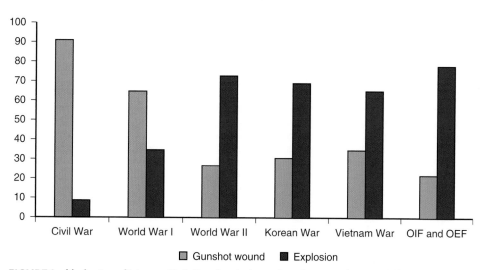

FIGURE I   Mechanism of injury and lethality of explosion and gunshot wounds among U.S. forces from the Civil War to current conflicts. OEF, Operation Enduring Freedom (Afghanistan); OIF, Operation Iraqi Freedom (Iraq). *(Data from Bellamy RF, Zajtchuk R: Assessing the effectiveness of conventional weapons. In Conventional warfare: ballistic, blast, and burn injuries. Washington, D.C., Office of the Surgeon General, 1991, pp 53–82; Beebe GW, DeBakey ME: Death from wounding. In Battle casualties, Springfield, Ill., Charles C Thomas, 1952, pp 74–147; Reister FA: Battle casualties and medical statistics: U.S. Army experience in the Korean war. Washington, D.C., The Surgeon General, Department of the Army, 1973; Hardaway RM: Viet Nam wound analysis. J Trauma 18:635–643, 1978; Global War on Terrorism by Reason, October 7, 2001 through April 4, 2011. Available at http://siadapp.dmdc.osd.mil/personnel/CASUALTY/gwot_reason.pdf. ; Gawande A: Casualties of war—Military care for the wounded from Iraq and Afghanistan. N Engl J Med 351:2471–2475, 2004.)*

---

*Data from October 7, 2001 through April 4, 2011. The category of explosion in this military dataset encompasses the following: weaponry, artillery/mortar/rocket; weaponry, explosive device; weaponry, grenade; and weaponry, rocket propelled grenade. "Weaponry, explosive device" is by far the largest category, encompassing 86% of the explosion-related injuries and deaths.

[†]The category of explosion in this civilian dataset encompasses the following: arson/firebombing, bombing, and suicide. The category of "bombing" encompasses almost 70% of the explosion-related injuries and deaths.

TABLE 1: Explosive Blast: Chain of Interactions and Injuries, Taxonomy, Typical Injuries, and Affected Body Regions

Blast Interactions	Taxonomy of Injury	Typical Injuries
Detonation ↓ Shock front of blast wave created ↓ Shock front dissipates ↓ Blast wind ↓ Blast wind propels fragments, objects, people ↓ Heat, flames, gas, smoke generated; release of bacteria or radiation also possible	**Primary** Injury produced by pressure differential causing direct tissue damage	*Primarily organs with density interfaces, e.g.,* tympanic membrane rupture, blast lung, eye injuries, abdominal hemorrhage, concussion, can also rip through tissue and limbs
	Secondary Injury produced by primary fragments from the exploding device (casing, items packed into the device) and secondary fragments (projectiles from the environment such as debris, glass, vehicular metal, etc.)	*Any/all body regions* Penetrating injuries, traumatic amputations, ocular injuries, lacerations, concussion Multiple injuries, most frequent type of injury
	Tertiary Injury produced by the blast wave propelling individuals into hard objects or hard objects onto individuals; includes injuries caused by structural damage to and collapse of buildings	*Any/all body regions* Blunt injuries, crush and compartment syndrome, fractures, traumatic avulsions and amputations, brain injuries, concussion
	Quaternary Injuries produced by other effects of explosions including heat, toxic gases, and environmental contamination	*Any/all body regions* Burns, inhalation injury, injury from environmental contamination, asphyxiation
	Quinary Injuries produced by elements added to explosive devices such as radiation or bacteria; includes disease transmission from propelled biologic material such as bone fragments	*Any/all body regions* Radiation sickness, increased risk of disease

Data from Federal Emergency Management Agency: Explosive blast. In *Primer to design safe schools projects in case of terrorist attacks*, Washington, D.C., Federal Emergency Management Agency, 2003, 4-1–4-13; Department of Defense Directive. Medical Research for Prevention, Mitigation, and Treatment of Blast Injuries. Number 6025.21E. July 5, 2006 (Defense Technical Information Center website). Available at http://www.dtic.mil/whs/directives/corres/pdf/602521p.pdf. Accessed May 25, 2011; DePalma RG, Burris DG, Champion HR, et al: Blast injuries. *N Engl J Med* 352:1335–1342, 2005; Explosions and blast injuries: A primer for clinicians. CDC Mass Casualties. Reviewed June 14, 2006. Available at http://www.bt.cdc.gov/masscasualties/explosions.asp.

Primary Blast Injury

Primary blast injury results from the effects of pressure differentials (alternating over- and underpressure). Most vulnerable to primary blast injury are organs with density interfaces, namely the ear, lung, and gastrointestinal (GI) tract; effects of a range of pressures are shown in Table 2.

Diagnosis and Management

Patients are at greater risk for primary blast injury when they are close to the point of detonation, are in an enclosed space (regardless of whether the explosion occurred inside or outside the enclosure), or are near a solid surface such as a wall that reflects and amplifies the blast wave. The diagnosis of primary blast injury is complicated by the fact that it can occur with little or no outward signs of injury and that symptoms may not be immediately apparent.

Ears

Ear injury may be suspected when there is bleeding or discharge from the ear; earache; tinnitus; vertigo; or immediate, sometimes transient, loss of hearing. Tympanic membrane rupture is the most common injury to the ear, but high overpressure may cause more significant injury such as dislocation and fracture of the ossicles, cochlear

TABLE 2: Short-Duration Pressure Effects Upon Unprotected Persons

Pressure (psi)	Effect
5	Possible eardrum rupture
15	50% chance of eardrum rupture
30 – 40	Slight chance of lung injury
80	50% chance of lung injury
100 – 200	Slight chance of death
130 – 180	50% chance of death
200 – 250	Almost certain death

Table reproduced from Nursing Mirror with kind permission of EMAP. psi, Pounds per square inch.

damage, and traumatic disruption of the oval or round window and subsequent permanent hearing loss. The Centers for Disease Control and Prevention (CDC) recommends that patients who have been exposed to an explosive blast receive an otologic assessment and audiometry.

The facts that tympanic membrane injury occurs at low pressure and that much more pressure is needed to damage other structures has suggested that tympanic membrane perforation is an indicator of primary blast injury. Recent research, however, has shown tympanic membrane perforation to be an unreliable indicator; thus, all victims of explosions should be assessed for primary blast injury regardless of whether their tympanic membranes are perforated.

In treating tympanic membrane rupture, foreign bodies should not be removed from the ear, nor should water or other nonsterile substances be introduced. Neither prophylactic antibiotics nor otologic suspensions should be introduced, but ophthalmologic gentamicin may be used. Treatment primarily consists of pain management and subsequent referral to an ear, nose, and throat specialist if significant debris is present or if symptoms persist.

Lungs

Primary blast injury to the lung (commonly known as "blast lung") occurs at air pressures of approximately 56 to 76 pounds per square inch (psi). It is sometimes accompanied by a clinical triad of apnea, bradycardia, and hypotension. Signs and symptoms may be evident upon presentation or may manifest as late as 48 hours from the time of the initial incident. Insidious characteristics of blast lung injury include the fact that initial signs and symptoms are easily underestimated or missed and that the patient's condition may deteriorate rapidly to the point of needing mechanical ventilation. Warning signs for clinicians may be grouped into the categories of hemorrhage or escape of air. Nonspecific symptoms common to primary blast injury include chest pain and dyspnea, confirmed on examination by the presence of cyanosis and tachypnea.

The CDC recommends that anyone exposed to explosive blast be given a chest radiograph to rule out blast lung, which may be identified by a characteristic "butterfly" pattern. Computed tomography (CT) and Doppler scanning, and arterial blood gas analysis may also be used to help make the diagnosis if they do not delay treatment. When blast lung is suspected, the CDC also recommends tube thoracostomy prior to air evacuation or administration of general anesthesia.

Management of blast lung injury is similar to that for pulmonary contusion. Treatment options include administration of fluid (without volume overload) and high-flow oxygen, treatment for airway compromise if needed, prompt decompression when evidence indicates hemothorax or pneumothorax, and intubation (being careful to avoid alveolar rupture and air embolism).

Abdomen

Primary blast injury to the abdomen is highly lethal and may have few initial signs. Clinical examination may reveal peritonitis, absent bowel sounds, shock, abdominal tenderness, and ensuing sepsis. Immediate injuries may include mesenteric shear injuries, solid organ lacerations, testicular rupture, hemorrhage (hematoma and subsequent obstruction, GI bleeding, hemoperitoneum), or escape of contents (mediastinitis, peritonitis). Symptoms may include abdominal, rectal, or testicular pain; nausea; vomiting; hematemesis; tenesmus; unexplained hypovolemia; or any indications of acute abdomen. Perforation of the bowel may be immediately apparent or may not be evident for hours. Insidious manifestations of symptoms and the presence of additional life-threatening injuries often make abdominal injury difficult to recognize; thus, repeated clinical examination is warranted.

Head

Other injuries caused by primary blast effects include facial fractures, brain concussion, cerebral air embolism, and eye trauma. Mild

traumatic brain injury (TBI) has become a major issue in the past decade, resulting in massive research efforts to elucidate the mechanisms by which it occurs, the symptoms and cognitive decrement that may affect performance, methods of diagnosis including biometrics, treatment, and long-term consequences. TBI including concussion may be caused by primary blast (e.g., in Iraq and Afghanistan), especially when patients are close to the point of detonation and when they present with constitutional symptoms such as headache, fatigue, problems concentrating, depression, anxiety, or lethargy. Researchers are currently exploring whether the primary blast wave causes brain damage through mechanisms that differ in combat and civilian TBI and whether multiple exposures to low-level blast can lead to long-term sequelae.

Limbs

When primary blast waves run along the long bones, they create a powerful shearing force that can avulse soft tissue and causes comminuted fractures or traumatic amputation of the extremity (although there is some uncertainty about whether the blast wave is solely responsible for this). The latter occurs at counterintuitive locations, that is, one third of the way along the shaft versus through joints. Traumatic amputation may also occur as a result of tertiary blast effects. It carries a high mortality rate (in 50% to 99% of cases). Four-compartment fasciotomy should always be considered in all patients with explosion-related injuries.

Secondary Blast Injury

The most common effect of explosives is caused by the high-velocity dispersal of primary and secondary fragments. Fragment projectiles can travel as fast as 2700 feet per second; which is more than 50 times the speed necessary to penetrate the skin and almost 7 times the speed necessary to enter and damage any major body cavity. They travel much further than the typical IED overpressure blast effect thus causing more injury. Primary fragments include projectiles produced from the destruction of the bomb casing and sharp objects within the bomb casing (added to increase wounding potential). Secondary fragments typically include objects-turned-projectiles and broken pieces of environmental debris including glass.

Secondary blast injury is the most common type of injury associated with explosive blast incidents, regardless of whether they occur among civilian or military populations. A majority of combat casualties in the current conflicts have secondary/fragment injuries (some accompanied by primary blast injuries). Because of combatant body armor, extremity injuries are the most commonly treated explosion-related combat injuries. These typically include large lacerations, multiple small wounds ("peppering"), and mangled extremities. Peppering is caused by high velocity blast missiles, which form projectile pathways that force foreign bodies and contaminants deep within the tissues.

Diagnosis and Management

Unlike primary blast injuries, secondary injuries caused by fragments are diagnosed and treated in the same manner as other penetrating injuries. Although many of these are noncritical soft tissue and skeletal injuries, they may be numerous, extensive, and time-consuming to manage. Important things to keep in mind include the following:

- Wounds that appear innocuous may signal underlying thoracic, abdominal, or vascular injury; small wounds may mask entrance wounds for large fragments.
- In patients with penetrating limb injuries, vascular integrity should be evaluated to rule out delayed vascular occlusion.
- As soon as possible, penetrating wounds should be irrigated and minimally débrided, with dead tissue and easily accessible fragments removed.

■ Delayed primary closure is generally called for, especially in wounds involving muscle or in the buttock or thigh areas; fragments not immediately or easily found may be removed later.

■ Because penetrating ocular trauma from fragments is common among survivors of explosive blasts, eye examinations should be performed; the eye should be covered if any injury is suspected.

■ When multiple penetrating wounds are present, cardiac or vascular injury should be ruled out as a priority.

Tertiary Blast Injury

Tertiary blast injuries are caused by collapse and fragmentation of buildings, vehicles, and other objects, and include crush, amputation caused by blunt-force collision with large projectiles such as chunks of concrete, and whole-body translocation. Building collapse is a frequent cause of death of large numbers of people at the scene of bomb explosions and is a primary predictor of patient outcome. In a comparison of outcomes by bombing types, structural collapse was associated with a 25% immediate mortality rate, compared to 4% in which no structural collapse occurred.

Tertiary blast injuries can also occur when the victims themselves become airborne by the blast wave and collide with nearby objects. These blast victims usually are very close to the point of detonation and therefore frequently sustain multiple injuries such as spinal, orthopedic, head, and solid- and hollow-organ injuries. Any body part may be affected and open fractures, traumatic limb amputations, and brain injuries are not uncommon.

Diagnosis and Management

Tertiary blast injuries follow patterns typical of any blunt trauma, and thus have no special treatment considerations per se. Complicating factors are tertiary injuries presenting in conjunction with other injuries or in the context of a mass casualty incident.

Entrapment under the rubble of collapsed buildings can lead to crush syndrome, which may lead to renal failure and death from acidosis and metabolic derangement. The risk of rhabdomyolysis is higher in patients who have been entrapped for prolonged periods, have an injury or injuries consistent with reperfusion, and dark urine (if any); the diagnosis may be confirmed with elevated serum creatinine kinase or urinary myoglobin, and treatment consists of aggressive hydration, urinary alkalinization, forced mannitol diuresis, renal replacement therapy, and electrolyte adjustment as needed.

The risk of compartment syndrome in injured extremities is elevated in entrapment scenarios as well. Thus, clinicians should be on the lookout for early indications, which include pain out of proportion to injury, pain with passive stretch, and compartmental tension and swelling. Late indications include paresthesia, pulselessness, pallor, and paralysis. Pressure monitoring can be used to confirm the clinical diagnosis, but only if it does not delay treatment if the index of suspicion is high. Compartment syndrome may lead to loss of limb or life if a fasciotomy is not performed to relieve the compartment pressure.

Quaternary Blast Injury

Quaternary blast injuries include burns, inhalation injury, and asphyxia caused by radiation exposure or inhalation of materials such as carbon monoxide, cyanide, toxic dust, or gas. Quaternary blast injury may exacerbate chronic diseases such as asthma, diabetes, hypertension, coronary artery disease, mental health issues, and substance abuse, and trigger behavioral problems.

Burns may be flash/cutaneous burns from the primary blast or full- or partial-thickness burns from the fireball or fires that result from the explosion. Materials used in incendiary bombs can cause severe burns that may affect larger body surface areas in enclosed-space more than in open-space explosions. Burns are more common in explosion-related incidents than in other types of trauma. Burn patients often have other blunt or penetrating injuries, which can present a clinical dilemma. For example, in patients with burns, which call for liberal fluid administration, and blast lung, which calls for fluid restriction, sophisticated invasive monitoring for fluid management is called for.

Aboard ships, inhalation injury may be caused by gas or particle components, and additional insults may result from retardants such as Halon, which can cause hypoxia. Halon is heavier than air, so its carbonic release raises the risk factor for inhalation injury at lower points. In a recent example, a casualty placed on the floor of an evacuation helicopter that had been on fire went into respiratory distress from Halon inhalation.

Diagnosis and Management

Inhalation injury may result from inhalation of chemicals or toxins either from the explosive device itself or from fumes of materials ignited by the explosion. Many variables influence diagnosis and treatment, such as the type and amount of substance inhaled, duration of exposure, and comorbid conditions of the patient (e.g., advanced age, cardiopulmonary conditions).

Quinary Blast Injury

Quinary blast injuries are caused by inhalation or absorption by skin and mucous membranes of toxic substances that are liberated by explosives. These injuries commonly occur after bomb attacks with incendiary devices. They differ from quaternary inhalation injuries in that they are caused by absorption of explosives that have vasodilatory properties (e.g., Detasheet or pentaerythritol tetranitrate) and are characterized by a "hyperinflammatory state," similar to systemic inflammatory response syndrome. This manifests as tachycardia, fever, low central venous pressure, and excessive fluid requirement to maintain adequate tissue perfusion. Another type of quinary blast injury is biologic foreign body injury, largely caused by embedded bone fragments from suicide bombers, which puts victims at risk for bloodborne diseases such as HIV (human immunodeficiency virus) infection and hepatitis B.

ANATOMIC LOCATION OF INJURY

The anatomic pattern of wounding among 100 casualties of roadside IEDs in Iraq is shown in Figure 2. All survivors and nonsurvivors had open wounds; the breakdown of other injuries was as follows (survivors and nonsurvivors, respectively): fractures (39% and 100%), burns (15% and 16%), amputations (7% and 50%), intracranial injuries (2% and 75%), and internal thoracic, abdominal, or pelvic injury (0 and 67%). The high percentage of extremity and head/face/neck wounds may be explained by the fact that soldiers typically wear personal protective equipment (PPE) that provides some thoracic protection.

MORBIDITY AND MORTALITY

In a retrospective review of morbidity and mortality rates in 4765 U.S. military personnel in Iraq and Afghanistan, explosions accounted for 78% of injuries and 77% of deaths. When data from 2003–2004 and 2005–2006 were compared, IEDs were implicated in a higher proportion of explosion-related injuries, and injury severity and the incidence of primary blast injury increased significantly. Increased

FIGURE 2 Anatomic pattern of wounding among survivors and nonsurvivors of roadside improvised explosive devices (IEDs) in Iraq, 2006. Figures are percentages of total, and overlap occurs because most casualties had multiple injuries (an average of 2.6 anatomic locations were affected in survivors and 4.7 in nonsurvivors). *(Modified from Ramasamy A, Harrisson SE, Clasper JC, et al: Injuries from roadside improvised explosive devices. J Trauma 65:910–914, 2008.)*

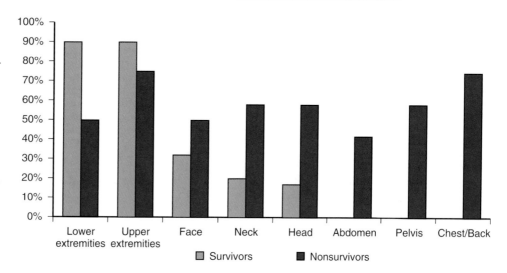

injury severity manifested in a decreased rate of return to duty after treatment (18%), that was less than half of what it had been earlier (40%), although explosion-related mortality rate remained low (1.4% and 1.5%, respectively).

The wounding effects of terrorist bomb attacks is maximized by various strategies such as creating secondary explosions (e.g., cluster bombs), deploying subsequent bombs; deploying the explosive in enclosed spaces to maximize both the wounding potential of the blast wave and the generation and propelling of fragments at close range; inducing structural collapse; and adding chemical, biologic, or radioactive materials to induce quinary effects.

Enclosed-space explosions (e.g., in buildings or vehicles) merit special note here because they are associated with a higher incidence of primary blast injuries and are significantly more deadly than those in open air. Although open-space explosions predominate in the military context, enclosed-space explosions and building collapse predominate in terrorist bomb attacks on civilian populations because terrorists generally target densely populated areas for maximum effect. When compared with open-air bombings, bombings in ultra-confined spaces such as buses are associated with significantly higher injury severity (median Injury Severity Score [ISS] 18 vs. 4) and mortality rate (49% vs. 8%).

SURGICAL MANAGEMENT

Surgical management of patients exposed to injury from explosions is no more technically difficult than trauma surgery in general. The differences lie in the multimechanistic, multisystem nature of injuries from explosions. A full understanding of the mechanisms and kinetics of each patient's injuries, ideally supported by information such as the standoff distance and scenario of injury, greatly aids in treatment prioritization and competent management of these complex injuries. Particular issues include the following:

■ Early recognition and aggressive management of overpressure injury to the lungs and brain
■ Diagnosis of significant occult torsal injury, particularly involving hemorrhage or vascular compromise
■ Adequate débridement of the extensive soft tissue injury that can occur, particularly in casualties wearing PPE, whose exposed limbs were injured by IEDs
■ Early use of fasciotomy in any limb compartment damaged from exposure to overpressure, multiple fragments, or crush

When acquiring history from the patient or prehospital care personnel, it is important to get answers to as many of the following questions as possible:

■ Did the explosion occur in a free field or in an enclosed space? (More risk in the latter.)
■ Was the casualty the occupant of a vehicle? (If yes, less risk but chance of secondary blunt injury from vehicle translocation.)
■ What was the casualty's standoff distance from the source of the explosion (how far was he or she from the point of detonation)? (The greater the distance, the less exposure to blast overpressure.)
■ What was the overall severity of the incident (i.e., what was the location of fatalities relative to the casualty)?
■ Was the casualty at risk of sustaining a crush injury?

These data are essential to understanding the likely pathophysiology and prioritizing the diagnostics and surgical approaches, put forward by Committee on Tactical Combat Casualty Care and Advanced Trauma Life Support principles of the American College of Surgeons Committee on Trauma.

INJURY SEVERITY SCORING

Injury severity scoring is necessary for describing and classifying injuries. Accurate coding of injuries is the cornerstone of injury databases: the repositories upon which enhancements in patient care and protective equipment design, evaluation of care, clinical research, quality assurance, and resource allocation, are often based.

The International Classification of Diseases is one taxonomy that is widely used to describe injury. However, it was not intended to be used as an anatomic injury scoring system, was not developed specifically for trauma, does not characterize injury severity, and is not predictive of outcome. Another scoring system is the Organ Injury Scale, which was developed to classify injuries to single organs by their severity. The Abbreviated Injury Scale (AIS), however, is the most commonly used anatomic scoring system. Developed in the early 1970s as a scoring system for civilian blunt trauma (primarily automobile crashes), the AIS has become an international standard for characterizing anatomic injury. It has not, however, been shown to be up to the task of accurately describing civilian penetrating trauma and combat injuries, which in current conflicts primarily consist of blast-related injuries.

Despite several efforts to modify the AIS to make it more descriptive of combat/explosion-related injuries, AIS-based codes (including the ISS) remain inadequate descriptors of these types of injuries. Thus, new replacement tools have been developed that include injury descriptors that accurately characterize combat anatomic injury, particularly injury from explosions, and also indicate immediate tactical functional impairment. This Military Combat Injury Scale will enable comparisons to military and civilian legacy databases; will link test, injury, and military crew safety criteria for future military vehicle development; and will incorporate effects of multiple mechanisms of injury to enhance combat trauma outcome prediction. This will add to our understanding of blast-related injury and help quantify the associated risks of morbidity and mortality.

CONCLUSION

Explosion-related blast injuries and numbers of casualties have been constantly increasing. They have devastating consequences and can overwhelm medical resources. The combination of multiple and complex injuries, involvement of multiple body regions, and mass casualty situations are challenging to prehospital personnel, emergency physicians, and surgeons. Knowledge of the mechanisms, clinical aspects, and triage-related issues are of great importance for trauma surgeons and all personnel involved in the management of patients injured by explosive devices.

For the chapter's Suggested Readings list, please visit the book at www.ExpertConsult.inkling.com.

PREHOSPITAL CARE OF BIOLOGIC AGENT–INDUCED INJURIES

Kenneth G. Swan, Charles D. Mabry, and Juan A. Asensio

On a busy Baghdad bridge spanning the great Tigris River coursing through Iraq from north to south, a crowd of people intermingled in their bidirectional flow. Most were hurrying to and from the nearby market on the east side of the river below. Some were carrying parcels, others infant children in their arms or on their backs. Someone shouted something; it was never determined who or what, but those within hearing interpreted the alarm as a warning, presumably of an improvised explosive device (IED) on the bridge. The reaction among the already apprehensive civilians was instant panic and they scattered in all directions. Some attempted to cross to the other side; others tried to retreat from where they were headed, some jumped into the waters below. A herd mentality eliminated all sense of proportion; flight with presumed escape dominated the thought processes of the terrified populace. In the aftermath of the incident, almost 1000 were dead and many more were injured. The causes of death included suffocation, exsanguination from blunt trauma to torso, head injuries, and multiple long-bone fractures. Many drowned. The alleged IED never detonated, nor was it ever identified. The date was August 31, 2005. The inciting event, however, exemplifies two phenomena pertinent to the trauma surgeon.

Acts of civilian terrorism may result from many instruments or have unknown causes. Equally important, if perpetrated in the setting of heightened anxiety or apprehension, they can have devastating consequences of panic, stampede, and resultant blunt trauma. An explosive device need not be the inciting event. Just the threat of one or of any number of alternative hazards to personal safety may have the same result. Such alternatives include the agents of bioterrorism. Ignorance and superstition, primarily the former, cloud rationality when their presence is suspected. Thus, two forms of trauma must be considered by prehospital caregivers under such circumstances: the biohazard itself and the trauma that ensued from the panic that it produced.

Prehospital care is provided by the most medically sophisticated at the scene and en route to a medical treatment facility (MTF). Such caregivers may be emergency medical technicians (EMTs), paramedics, and even physicians. They will be required, by necessity, to perform patient assessment, threat assessment, triage, and first aid until additional help arrives.

Patient assessment proceeds along standardized guidelines established by the American College of Surgeons and its Advanced Trauma Life Support program as modified to complement varying skill levels, such as those relevant to nurses, paramedics, and EMTs (Prehospital Trauma Life Support). Included in the patient assessment is the threat assessment. What caused the panic? Was it explosive, radioactive, chemical, or biologic and does it still pose a threat? Answers to these questions may not be readily apparent, initially; nevertheless, answers will be essential to successful triage, patient resuscitation, stabilization and transport, as well as notification and protection of those not yet exposed to the dangers presented.

Triage is patient-location dependent. Casualties from biologic agent–induced injuries may be encountered in the field or at the scene of agent exposure. At this level the term "field triage," as distinguished from "hospital triage," is appropriate. The word triage is derived from the French verb "trier," which means to sort, and dates back to the 15th century and European marketplaces where fur and fiber were sorted according to quality and price. Any number of triage categories can be designated, but perhaps the simplest arrangement involves three tiers. Most "patients" are apprehensive, bordering on hysteria. They need to be conveniently relocated and comforted by a minimal number of caregivers. This category may comprise the largest percentage of patients at the scene. A small percentage of the remainder are in extremis or agonal. They are termed "expectant," and cannot be helped other than to be allowed to die with a minimum of discomfort and as much dignity as can be provided under the circumstances. The remainder are categorized as "priority," and they all need transport to an MTF. These patients are bleeding, have airway problems, head injuries, burns, chest or abdominal pain, or evidence of spine or long-bone fracture. This latter category may represent only 20% of the casualties, but it is the most important.

Principles of triage that must be understood include the fact that patients are triaged and retriaged, not only at all levels of patient care, but also within levels of patient care. The triage officer does not treat, assuming there is more than one caregiver present. The triage officer only sorts patients according to injury and probable outcome. The latter is dependent upon available resources—time, personnel, and equipment—and their presumed efficient use. Weather, communications, and available transportation will all play critical roles in determining anticipated outcome. Assuming that explosive ordnance, radiation, and chemical threats have been eliminated, but a biologic agent has not, what steps should be taken by the first responder or caregiver present at the scene of an act of civilian terrorism?

The ranking medical caregiver must establish communications, ascertain the risk of additional threat to the immediate area, and in addition to providing first aid to those most in need, attempt to identify the biologic agent responsible for the mass casualties and the probable time of onset of exposure.

At present, there are five specific agents considered likely sources of bioterrorism. They have several general characteristics in common that make them preferable to alternative agents. These characteristics include relative ease of production, packaging, transport, and delivery as well as not only lethality but also morbidity. Agents that kill rapidly may be less inducive of panic and terror than those that cause large numbers to be extremely ill for prolonged periods of time, their condition apparently communicable. The five agents most commonly cited as potential threats are those associated with anthrax, smallpox, botulism, plague, and tularemia. The characteristics of each disease and its agent will be presented with emphasis placed on detection, diagnosis, treatment, precautions, prophylaxis, quarantine, decontamination, and necrology (Tables 1 to 3). Other less likely agents, such as the viruses that cause encephalitis and the Ebola virus, will be mentioned, but only in passing, because of their much lower probability of encounter.

ANTHRAX

Anthrax has a long history as a disease among animals, but is much less commonly encountered in humans. Spores of *Bacillus anthracis*

have been weaponized by the governments of many countries, and individuals have been exposed accidentally in Russia as well as targeted by attacks in Japan and more recently the United States. Although the number of deaths from these exposures is relatively small, the potential is impressive. The World Health Organization (WHO) estimated that aerial release of 50 kg of anthrax spores over an urban population of 5 million, would cause 250,000 casualties, almost half of whom would die without treatment. Similar scenarios have compared an aerosolized attack with anthrax spores to the effects of a hydrogen bomb attack on a large city.

Three forms of exposure to anthrax infectivity occur in humans: inhalation, cutaneous, and gastrointestinal (Fig. 1). Anthrax spores are 1.0 μm, extremely hardy, and when aerosolized, odorless, tasteless, colorless, and invisible (Fig. 2). Obviously, bioterrorists would most likely attempt inhalation exposure via an aerosolized release of spores from an aircraft. A two-stage illness ensues. In the primary phase, which lasts hours to days, the victim experiences fever, dyspnea, cough, headache, nausea, vomiting, chills, weakness, and pain in chest and abdomen within days to weeks of exposure, depending on number and size of spores inhaled. The second phase begins with an abrupt increase in severity of symptoms, which coincides with systemic lymphadenopathy, bacteremia, hypotension, and death, if untreated. The massive hilar lymphadenopathy is seen

TABLE 1: Five Most Frequently Cited Bioterrorism Agents and Associated Diseases: Characteristics, Recognition, and Identification

Disease	Organism	Aerosol	Onset	Symptoms	Distinction	Identification
Anthrax	*Bacillus anthracis*	Spore	2 days	Acute onset, flulike illness	Mediastinal widening	Large gram-positive rods, blood
Smallpox	*Orthopoxvirus variola*	Virus	12–14 days	Severe febrile illness	Rash	Viruses (EM), pustular fluid
Plague	*Yersinia pestis*	Bacterium	1–6 days	Severe pneumonia, sepsis	Hemoptysis	Bipolar ("safety pin") gram-negative coccobacilli, sputum
Botulism	*Clostridium botulinum*	Toxin	Hours-days	Paralysis	No fever	Mouse bioassay, blood
Tularemia	*Francisella tularensis*	Bacterium	3–5 days	Acute onset, febrile illness, nonspecific	Slower progression	Small gram-negative coccobacilli, sputum.

TABLE 2: Five Most Frequently Cited Bioterrorism Agents and Associated Diseases: Treatment, Prevention, Cause of Death, and Necrology

Disease	TREATMENT* Parenteral	Oral	Prevention	Cause of Death	Necrology
Anthrax	Ciprofloxacin 400 mg	Ciprofloxacin 500 mg	Vaccination, 6-dose series, U.S. military	Respiratory failure, sepsis	Burial, cremation
Smallpox	For secondary infections		None available	Sepsis	Cremation
Plague	Streptomycin 1.0 g, gentamicin	Doxycycline 100 mg, ciprofloxacin	None available	Sepsis	Burial
Botulism	For secondary infections		Antitoxin	Respiratory failure	Burial
Tularemia	Streptomycin 1.0 g, gentamicin	Doxycycline 100 mg, ciprofloxacin	None available	Sepsis	Burial

*Antibiotics (q12h).

TABLE 3: Five Most Frequently Cited Bioterrorism Agents and Associated Diseases: Prophylaxis, Infection Control, and Decontamination

Disease	Prophylaxis	Infection Control	Decontamination
Anthrax	Same as for treatment, 60 days	No H-HT, SP	Initial, secondary aerosolization without direct contact, soap and water
Smallpox	Vaccination	Isolation and vaccination of all patients plus their contacts	Spontaneous, 6–24 hours
Plague	Same as for treatment, all contacts plus anyone with fever or cough	RDP until 48 hours ABT	Spontaneous, 1 hour
Botulism	Close observation, antitoxin scarce	SP	Toxin easily destroyed, bleach 1:10 dilution, soap and water
Tularemia	Same as for treatment, any exposed	No H-HT, SP	Short half-life, soap and water, bleach 1:10 dilution, alcohol 70%

ABT, Antibiotic therapy; H-HT, human-to-human transmission; RDP, respiratory droplet precautions (with masks); SP, standard precautions.

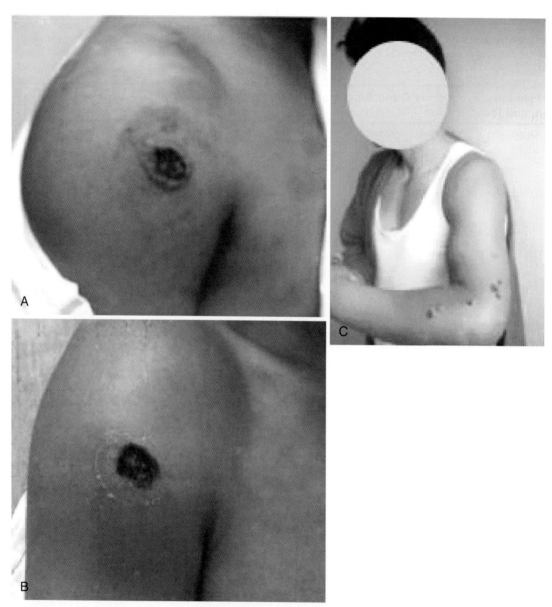

FIGURE 1 Cutaneous lesions of anthrax. **A,** Ulcer with vesicle ring. **B,** Black eschar with surrounding erythema. **C,** Marked edema of extremity secondary to anthrax edema toxin with multiple black eschars. *(Photographs courtesy of the Centers for Disease Control and Prevention, Atlanta, Ga. Available at www.bt.cdc.gov/agent/anthrax/anthraximages/cutaneous. asp. From Dembek ZF: Medical aspects of biological warfare. Washington, D.C., Borden Institute, Walter Reed Army Medical Center, 2007.)*

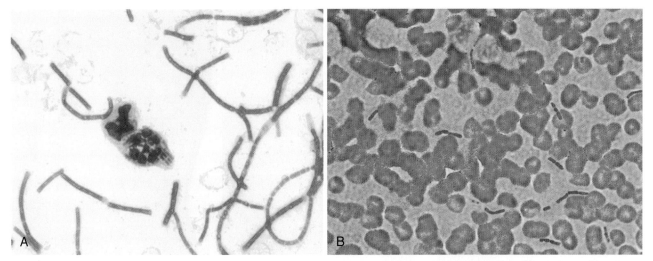

FIGURE 2 **A,** Gram stain of a blood smear from an infected guinea pig demonstrating intracellular bacilli chains within a polymorphonuclear leukocyte. **B,** Gram stain of peripheral blood smear from a nonhuman primate infected with *Bacillus anthracis*, Ames strain. *(Photograph in **A** courtesy of Susan Welkos, PhD, Division of Bacteriology, U.S. Army Medical Research Institute of Infectious Diseases, Fort Detrick, MD; Photograph in **B** courtesy of John Ezzell, PhD, U.S. Army Medical Research Institute of Infectious Diseases, Fort Detrick, MD. From Dembek ZF: Medical aspects of biological warfare. Washington, D.C., Borden Institute, Walter Reed Army Medical Center, 2007.)*

radiographically as a "widened mediastinum." Mediastinitis, meningitis, and cyanosis are common in the second phase. Clues to the diagnosis are the sudden appearance, in large numbers, of previously healthy city dwellers with an overwhelming flulike illness. Differential diagnosis includes pneumonic plague. Treatment includes parenteral antibiotics (penicillin, etc.), assisted ventilation, and pressors if patients can be hospitalized, and if not, oral antibiotics. Blood cultures before antibiotic therapy are confirmatory, but case fatality rates approach 80% and most victims succumb within the first 2 days of symptoms. A potential countermeasure consists of a recently developed human IgG1 monoclonal antibody that interacts directly with the anthrax toxin and neutralizes it. The antibody, raxibacumab, is protective in rabbits and monkeys, but its efficacy in humans has not been tested.

Prophylaxis has consisted of vaccination (six-dose series), which has been administered to all U.S. service personnel. Recent evaluation of a large military cohort, however, revealed that over half of the vaccines had low serum levels of in vitro toxin neutralization capacity.

Because there is no threat of patient-to-patient transmission of anthrax, patient contacts do not require treatment; however, the dead should be cremated because of spore hardiness. Decontamination of all suspected victims of inhalation anthrax is necessary to avoid secondary aerosolization of spores that remain on clothing and other surfaces. Health care workers must wash their hands after contact with anthrax victims for the same reason.

Should first responders and health care providers at the site suspect an anthrax aerosolization as the source of the ensuing scene of fear and panic, several important measures need immediate attention. As in all cases of suspected bioterrorism, appropriate local, state, and federal reporting centers must be notified. Also, local hospitals need also to be alerted and appropriate steps taken to maximize availability of ventilators because those who do sustain inhalation anthrax will likely require endotracheal intubation and respiratory support. Numbers may overwhelm resource availability in such situations. Triage is implemented.

When relatively large numbers of burn victims require triage for resource management, a 50% total body burn is considered sufficiently lethal to designate expectancy under such circumstances. Often there are associated injuries in burn victims; additional trauma is added to the burn percentage. For example, if a person jumped from a burning building and fractured his femur, his burn percentage

(50%) would be increased to 55% (5% is added for each long-bone fracture). Similarly, the trauma patient who was injured while attempting to flee an anthrax attack that exposed him or her to inhalation of the agent more likely might be declared expectant because of an inevitably poor prognosis. The unpredictable timing of disease onset, under this set of circumstances, will challenge the triage officer.

SMALLPOX

Perhaps the most feared of the biologic agents on the top five list for likely agents of bioterrorism is the virus that causes smallpox. It is especially threatening for several reasons. Because global eradication through vaccination was declared almost 30 years ago, vaccination has been terminated. Thus, no one today is protected from a smallpox attack; the only known sources of the virus (*Orthopoxvirus variola*) are in state-controlled laboratories in the United States and Russia. In addition, there is no known treatment for smallpox. Person-to-person contact enables aerosol transmission of body secretions. Contaminated clothing and bedding readily holds as well as transmits the virus from patient to contacts. Only a few viruses are necessary for infection to progress to viremia, which lasts a few days. The hemopoietic and reticuloendothelial systems are inoculated, and a secondary, heavier viremia results within 8 days. Victims exhibit high fever, malaise, headache, prostration, backache, and abdominal pain. A characteristic vesicular skin eruption progresses centrifugally and involves the palms of the hands and soles of the feet, which distinguishes smallpox (variola) from chickenpox (varicella) (Fig. 3). The former lesions conform to a single stage, whereas those of varicella appear in crops and also progress centrifugally.

Treatment of smallpox consists of supportive measures, including antibiotics, but case fatality rate is in excess of 30%. Contacts need vaccination, and this of course includes not only all exposed health care workers, but also all those who have had contact with the victim. Patients must be isolated. They can be confined in a designated hospital, and even their own home when possible. The incubation period is 12 to 14 days, and the subsequent viremia progresses as outlined previously. Because the patients remain heavily infective, even in death, cremation is necessary, as with victims of anthrax.

Although the smallpox virus is perhaps most feared as an agent for bioterrorism, world condemnation of its use for such purposes,

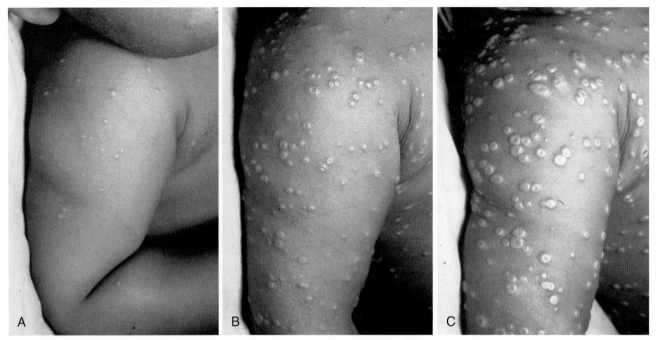

FIGURE 3 This series of photographs illustrates the evolution of skin lesions in an unvaccinated infant with the classic form of variola major. **A,** The third day of rash shows synchronous eruption of skin lesions; some are becoming vesiculated. **B,** On the fifth day of rash, almost all papules are vesicular or pustular. **C,** On the seventh day of rash, many lesions are umbilicated, and all lesions are in the same general stage of development. *(From Fenner F, Henderson DA, Arita I, et al: Smallpox and its eradication. Geneva, Switzerland, World Health Organization, 1988, pp 10–14. Photographs by I. Arita. As printed in Dembek ZF: Medical aspects of biological warfare. Washington, D.C., Borden Institute, Walter Reed Army Medical Center, 2007.)*

coupled with the very difficult, virtually impossible access to sufficient stores of the virus, make its use extremely impractical and unlikely. Nonetheless, because Russia remains somewhat unpredictable, and because Russia and the United States may not be the only repositories for the virus, the threat remains and so must the registration of smallpox in all bioterrorism training programs in the United States and elsewhere.

PLAGUE

Plague has its own history of bioterrorist use, and rivals any other disease due to a biologic agent in terms of numbers killed, certainly as a percentage of world population, including the Great Influenza Epidemic of 1918. Plague is high on the list of choices for current bioterrorists because of ready availability, ease of production, and applicability to aerosolization. It is estimated that 50 kg of *Yersinia pestis*, the causative organism, aerosolized over an urban population of 5 million, would result in pneumonic plague in 150,000, of whom 36,000 would die. The organisms would be expected to survive within the area for 1 hour and remain a threat during that time. Because pneumonic plague can be transmitted from one person to another, panic and flight could readily spread the initial infection. The disease presents as a severe respiratory illness 1 to 6 days following exposure (Fig. 4). Because actual exposure may not be known, the clue to recognition of pneumonic plague is its nearly simultaneous presentation in a relatively large number of previously healthy individuals with negligible risk factors. Historically, plague has been anticipated in the wake of large numbers of dead and dying rats in an urban population, causing the fleas carrying the bacilli to turn to humans as hosts. In a terrorist attack, however, this phase of the life cycle would be obviated.

The disease in humans became known as the "Black Death" from the acral cyanosis associated with digital vasospasm and gangrene associated with septicemic plague, a complication of any form of infection with *Y. pestis*. Others attribute the term to the intense, generalized cyanosis coincident with pneumonic plague and its resultant hypoxemia. Because the prodroma of pneumonic plague include coryza, a sneeze in the 14th century was greeted with "God bless you" by those in attendance, who quickly scurried away because the presumption was that the person who sneezed was about to succumb to the plague, for which there was no treatment and death was a certainty.

Because of its similarity to anthrax, several distinguishing features are mentioned. Hemoptysis is more suggestive of pneumonic plague than the pneumonia caused by anthrax (Fig. 5). Sputum from patients with plague reveals gram-negative coccobacilli that have been likened to "safety pins" in appearance because of their bipolar nuclei (Fig. 6). Treatment is with parenteral antibiotics (tetracycline, gentamicin) preferably; but faced with large numbers of patients and limited hospital space, oral tetracycline, doxycycline, or ciprofloxacin is recommended. A vaccine was developed for prevention of bubonic plague, but it offers little protection against pneumonic plague contracted from aerosolization, and in fact, it is no longer manufactured. Once the organism is identified, health care providers should isolate patients because they remain infective and those in attendance should implement standard respiratory droplet precautions, which include mask and eye screens in addition to gown and gloves. Patients who do not survive can be buried because the organisms will not survive. Environmental precautions are usually not a concern because the organisms have a limited life expectancy following release (1 hour).

BOTULISM

A fourth agent for bioterrorism is *Clostridium botulinum*, a bacterium that produces botulinum toxin, considered the most poisonous

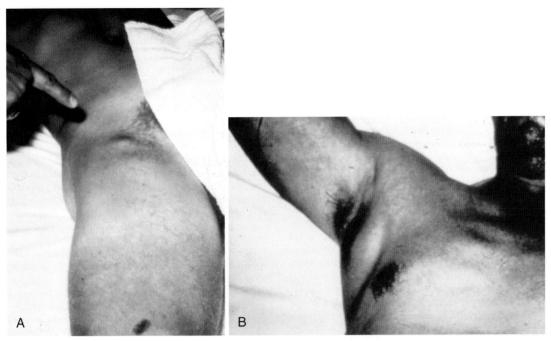

FIGURE 4 A femoral bubo (**A**) the most common site of an erythematous, tender, swollen lymph node in patients with plague. This painful lesion may be aspirated in a sterile fashion to relieve pain and pressure; it should not be incised and drained. The next most common lymph node regions involved are the inguinal, axillary (**B**), and cervical areas. Bubo location is a function of the region of the body in which an infected flea inoculates the plague bacilli. *(Photographs courtesy of Kenneth L. Gage, PhD, Centers for Disease Control and Prevention Laboratory, Fort Collins, Colo. From Dembek ZF: Medical aspects of biological warfare. Washington, D.C., Borden Institute, Walter Reed Army Medical Center, 2007.)*

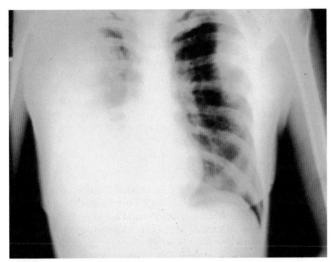

FIGURE 5 This chest roentgenogram shows right middle and lower lobe involvement in a patient with pneumonic plague. *(Photograph courtesy of Kenneth L. Gage, PhD, Centers for Disease Control and Prevention Laboratory, Fort Collins, Colo. From Dembek ZF: Medical aspects of biological warfare. Washington, D.C., Borden Institute, Walter Reed Army Medical Center, 2007.)*

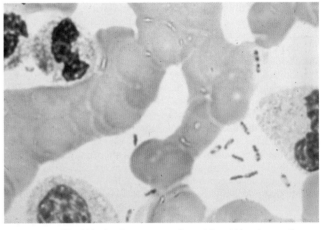

FIGURE 6 This Wright-Giemsa stain of a peripheral blood smear from a patient with septicemic plague demonstrates the bipolar, safety pin appearance of *Yersinia pestis*. Gram and Wayson stains can also demonstrate this pattern. *(Photograph courtesy of Kenneth L. Gage, PhD, Centers for Disease Control and Prevention Laboratory, Fort Collins, Colo. From Dembek ZF: Medical aspects of biological warfare. Washington, D.C., Borden Institute, Walter Reed Army Medical Center, 2007.)*

substance known to humankind. Aerosolization of 1 g of the toxin, if adequately dispersed and inhaled by those exposed, could kill 1 million people. One tenth of 1 µg (0.1 µg), given intravenously, is sufficient to kill an adult. The toxin blocks acetylcholine release at neuromuscular junctions, and it does so by binding irreversibly with cholinergic synapses. The clinical picture is a classic triad of symptoms: (1) symmetrical, descending flaccid paralysis with prominent bulbar palsies, in (2) an afebrile patient, with (3) a clear sensorium. The bulbar palsies are often referred to as "the 4 Ds": diplopia, dysphoria, dysarthria, and dysphagia. Recovery from inhalation botulism requires intensive care and ventilatory and nutritional support, and may take weeks to months because neural regeneration is required to displace the previously blocked synapses at myoneural junctions. For this reason alone, the prolonged disability and delayed recovery of so many victims, the toxin is a highly prized agent for bioterrorism. In fact, prior to the outbreak of the Gulf War in 1991, Iraq is said to have stockpiled and weaponized enough botulinum toxin to kill three times the world's population. The toxin is easily produced and can be readily stored and transported, as well as delivered, to a target.

Recognition of botulism without a history of a terrorist attack will be dependent upon a high index of suspicion. Otherwise healthy individuals, who do not have a history suggestive of alternative forms of the disease, such as food poisoning or wound abscess, but present with the neurologic symptoms mentioned previously, progressing in a descending fashion to involve upper and then lower extremities symmetrically, must be suspect. Appropriate notification must be initiated while confirmatory evidence is sought from serum bioassay in the case of inhalation botulism, and stool samples in the case of intestinal botulism. Because ventilatory support will be required to avoid death from respiratory paralysis, hospital preparedness is critical to successful management of any significant number of victims from such an attack. Large numbers of prolonged, ventilator-dependent patients could exhaust the resources of even a large medical community. Thus, the value of an antitoxin, which can ameliorate the paralysis and shorten the recovery time, has increased. Currently there is such treatment available through the Centers for Disease Control and Prevention (CDC) in Atlanta, Georgia, but supply is limited and the antitoxin is released for clinical use only, on a case-by-case basis.

The outbreak of botulism in Thailand in 2006, from ingestion of bamboo shoots, affected 209 people, 42 of whom developed respiratory failure. Of this group 25 required hospitalization for ventilatory support. Patients who received botulinum antitoxin (anti-BoNT, CDC) on day 4 of their disease recovered faster than those who received the antitoxin on day 6.

What might be expected at the prehospital phase of the bioterrorist attack with aerosolized botulinum toxin? The agent, like anthrax spores, even in large volume and concentration, is colorless, odorless, tasteless, and invisible. Hence, its detection would go unnoticed, at least initially. Symptoms might not appear for an hour and for obvious reasons. Experience with human inhalation botulism is very limited. In its only delivery against civilians, Japanese terrorists failed on three occasions in the early 1990s to injure anyone, presumably for technical reasons. Nonetheless, word of the attacks did terrorize those in attendance. Many who fled the scene sustained injuries, but the final report concluded, "non-toxin casualties were light." Had the population been forewarned of a possible attack or, like the Iraqi civilians on the bridge mentioned earlier, been subjected to potential terror attacks for several years before, the ensuing panic could have been infinitely more injurious to those present. Add to that possibility the likelihood that symptoms occurred more rapidly and that word spread among the crowd that death was imminent unless the victims could reach a major treatment facility. Pandemonium would ensue; nearby hospitals would be inundated and overwhelmed within a matter of minutes. Such examples point to the need for education of the populace and those who care for them in the field and at the MTF. The former need to know that they should avoid panic, await instructions, vacate the area, and listen to the radio and other media for further information and instructions. Similarly, field and hospital staff must be notified of probable patient surge, and the likely agent, and the latest diagnostic, treatment, and reporting algorithms to follow. Prehospital teams, EMTs, paramedics, and first responders should assess the scene for symptomatic victims who need to be transported expeditiously to the MTF.

The toxin is readily decontaminated with a variety of solutions, including soap and water or 0.1% hypochlorite bleach. Without attention, the toxin decays at a rate of 1% per minute in a neutral environment.

TULAREMIA

Francisella tularensis, a small, nonmotile, aerobic, gram-negative coccobacillus, is responsible for tularemia in humans and is one of the most infectious pathogenic bacteria known to humankind. Inoculation or inhalation of as few as 10 organisms is sufficient to cause disease. Because of its extreme infectivity, the ease of its dissemination, and its capacity to cause severe illness and even death, *F. tularensis* is a likely agent for use in bioterrorism. WHO estimated that 50 kg of live organisms, aerosolized over an urban population center of 5 million, would cause 250,000 casualties including 19,000 deaths.

The bacterium is ubiquitous. Its vectors are arthropods and its reservoirs are small mammals. It can be transmitted to humans by insect bite, direct contact with animal carcasses or soil, ingestion of contaminated water or food, and inhalation. The latter would be the method of choice for terrorism. Person-to-person transmission does not occur; hence, human infection would not spread the disease as in smallpox.

The result of an aerosolized release of *F. tularensis* would be a large number of patients with an unusual respiratory disease 3 to 5 days after inhalation. A high index of suspicion is again needed to distinguish tularemia from community-acquired infections such as influenza or atypical pneumonia. If a bioterrorist attack is suspected, the differential diagnosis includes other related diseases such as plague, anthrax, and, yet to be discussed, Q fever. Tularemia generally has a slower progression of symptoms and a lower case fatality rate. Plague progresses to hemoptysis, respiratory failure, sepsis, and shock, which are not usually seen in tularemia. Anthrax has a characteristic radiographic appearance (widened mediastinum), which is not seen in tularemia. Although light microscopy of sputum may reveal the gram-negative coccobacilli, culture from sputum establishes the diagnosis. Treatment consists of parenteral antibiotics, such as streptomycin or gentamicin, under ideal conditions. When mass casualties exceed, numerically, the facilities for parenteral antibiotics, oral doxycycline or ciprofloxacin are substituted. Vaccination is not useful because of the very short incubation period of the organism in humans. Patients need not be isolated because person-to-person transmission does not occur. Standard precautions are all that are necessary for patient care providers. Environmental decontamination is minimally problematic because of the presumed short half-life of the organism when exposed to environmental factors such as desiccation and solar radiation. Alcohol, soap and water, and household bleach (dilute) are decontaminants if there is concern about additional potential contamination of equipment or other materials.

OTHER AGENTS

Other agents are available and the list of possibilities is extensive. We will conclude, as indicated earlier, with a brief presentation of other agents that are often mentioned, but thought less likely to be deployed than "the big five" discussed previously. Agents included here are *Coxiella* (Q fever), *Staphylococcus* (staphylococcal enterotoxin B), the equine encephalitis viruses, and the hemorrhagic fever viruses. Each has a special characteristic that makes it attractive to bioterrorists, but also at least one that makes it less likely to be used than one of the big five.

Q fever is a flulike illness that results from inhalation of the etiologic agent, *Coxiella burnetii*. The latter has been called a *Rickettsia* by some, and a bacterium by others. It is from this conflict that the resultant disease derives its name. "Q" stands for "query," indicating the enigma surrounding its definition. The terrorist appeal relates to the organism's high infectivity. This "asset" is countered by a relatively low lethality and self-limited clinical course. Diagnosis is problematic; a high index of suspicion is necessary. Confirmation requires serologic testing. Treatment, if necessary, is antibiotic (doxycycline).

Staphylococcal enterotoxin B is an exotoxin that can be aerosolized and, when inhaled, results in sepsis. Its appeal is its ability to produce an incapacitating illness that would persist long enough to spread terror, even panic, among a large number (essentially all) of those exposed. Theoretically, the living can more readily dramatize the threat than can the dead because they remain vocal. The "disadvantage" of the agent for bioterrorists is its very low lethality and ease of therapy, which is largely supportive. Diagnosis again depends on a high index of suspicion; identification is based upon serologic confirmation. Of concern is the potential mixture of agents for aerosolization that would cause obvious confusion among caregivers and heighten the terror and panic.

The equine encephalitides are caused by three viruses that have special interest to bioterrorists. These RNA viruses are highly infectious; the Eastern form is especially lethal, but none pose of significant risk for human-to-human transmission. The diagnosis is based on the appearance of a viral illness that progresses to encephalitis. Treatment is supportive, and identification is based on culture of the organism from throat swabs or blood samples.

The hemorrhagic fever viruses include a final agent of probable interest to bioterrorists, the Ebola virus. The latter is the one most often mentioned because of its case fatality rate, which approaches 100%. This group of viruses also includes those responsible for dengue fever and yellow fever. These viruses attack endothelial cells, and for this reason the resultant diseases are characterized by bleeding disorders among other symptoms. Human-to-human transmission

is unlikely, and bioterrorists, apparently, have not yet attempted its use. Most likely all of these agents would be delivered by aerosolization.

SUMMARY

Because victims of bioterrorism may seek different treatment facilities and because onset of symptoms may not always be synchronous, health care deliverers must have surveillance systems in place so that any "flulike illness," unusual in number or presentation, is reported to all regional health care facilities. This practice is essential for early detection of an otherwise silent bioterrorist attack. What else can be done in preparation for such an event? As of this writing, vaccines are available for prevention of anthrax, cholera, plague, Q fever, and smallpox, but there are no licensed vaccines available to prevent botulism or viral encephalitis. Concerns have been raised regarding the ethical, economic, and political considerations as significant factors, currently limiting development of needed vaccines against agents of bioterrorism. Antibiotics are the recommended treatment for exposure to anthrax, plague, and Q fever. Antitoxins and antiviral agents are available for treatment of botulism and smallpox, respectively.

For the chapter's Suggested Readings list, please visit the book at www.ExpertConsult.inkling.com.

WOUND BALLISTICS: WHAT EVERY TRAUMA SURGEON SHOULD KNOW

Laszlo Kiraly, John C. Mayberry, and Donald D. Trunkey

After an earlier period of decline, the incidence of firearm injuries and fatalities in the United States has remained relatively stable in the past decade. Wounds caused by firearms will be encountered not only in urban "high-crime" areas but also rural areas, where hunting accidents occur. Wounds encountered in a military environment have unique characteristics that are clinically important and distinct from those seen in the civilian sector. Operation Iraqi Freedom (OIF) and Operation Enduring Freedom (Afghanistan) (OEF) have provided important observations in the treatment of military projectile injuries. The study of wound ballistics is an essential part of the general and trauma surgeons' training.

BALLISTICS THEORY

Although there are many variables, the muzzle velocity (speed of the bullet as it leaves the barrel) and the bullet characteristics such as mass and deformability are the most important determinants of the wound that a particular weapon will produce (Table 1). The muzzle velocity is determined by the caliber (diameter) of the bullet, the capacity of the casing (amount of powder), and gun barrel length. The bullet's velocity rapidly increases as it travels down the barrel, but gradually slows upon meeting air resistance once it has exited. Handguns generally accept smaller bullets with less powder and have shorter barrels than rifles, and therefore produce projectiles of considerably less velocity (Table 2).

After a projectile strikes its target, two distinct interactions occur between the bullet and the tissue. First, the rapidly traveling bullet creates a path of direct tissue destruction. This destructive interaction is commonly termed the "permanent cavity." Along the tract of the bullet, a "temporary cavity" is also formed. This "temporary cavity" is formed by the lateral displacement of adjacent tissues as the bullet is forced through the body. These forces can affect an area many times greater than the bullet diameter itself. Depending on the site and elasticity of the tissue, the temporary cavity can have varying clinical importance. For example, rapid displacement of tissue in the chest can result in significant pulmonary contusion.

Because of its heavier mass, and therefore its increased energy per given velocity, lead is the principal element of most bullets. Lead, however, is a relatively soft metal that deforms readily during high-velocity flight. "Jacketed" bullets have a lead body covered with metal alloys that prevent deformation during flight, and therefore help the bullet retain speed and accuracy over a long distance. Conventionally jacketed bullets will deform when they strike dense tissue, but bullets with thicker jackets are intended to retain their shape and therefore penetrate deeply into large game animals, such as elephants (Fig. 1). Bullets that deform upon striking the body will cause considerably more collateral tissue damage by direct contact, cavitation, and shock waves than nondeformable bullets. Fragmentation of bullets will also occur when the bullet strikes bone and will add to the damage by shredding surrounding tissue (Fig. 2). Animal models have demonstrated clearly more tissue destruction and larger areas of injury with deformable hollow point bullets. Full jacketed bullets, however, are more likely to exit the victim, thereby not transferring all of the kinetic injury to the body.

According to The Hague Declarations of 1899, military rifle bullets "which expand or flatten easily in the human body, such as bullets with a hard envelope which does not entirely cover the core" are banned. This prohibition was designed to reduce the severity of wounds, and therefore the suffering of soldiers on the battlefield, but does not apply to combatants of noncontracting organizations and does not apply to bullets commonly used for hunting. In fact, "full-metal-jacket" (FMJ) bullets are prohibited for game hunting in many jurisdictions. For this reason, hunting rifle wounds may

TABLE 1: Factors Involved in Wound Ballistics

Bullet Design

Caliber (diameter)

Mass

Shape (profile)

Jacket

Pellets

Powder (amount and type)

Weapon Design

Barrel length

Rifling

Single shot

Automatic

Semiautomatic

Portability (weight and size)

Victim

Position

Distance from weapon

Location of wound

Tissue characteristics (bone, muscle, vessel, organ)

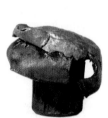
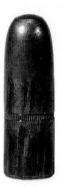
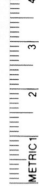

FIGURE 1   Full-metal-jacket 308 caliber rifle bullet that has opened upon impact with a game animal *(left)* compared with same caliber bullet with a thicker jacket that has passed undeformed through the animal *(right)*. Notice the grooves on the base of each bullet caused by the internal rifling of the barrel. (Bullets courtesy of Gerald Warnock, MD, Portland, Ore.)

TABLE 2: Muzzle Velocity by Gun and Bullet Type

Handguns	Velocity (m/sec)
.38 special	290
.44	305
9 mm	315
.44 magnum	420
Rifles	
.22 long	380
30.06	890
.308 (7.62 mm)	860
Military	
.223 (M-16)	950
.30 (AK-47)	720
.50 (Browning)	850

be more severe than those resulting from an equivalent military rifle. The exception to this principle is the assault rifle, which although its bullet is jacketed, can cause severe wounds from the bullet's tendency to tumble in tissue.

■ HANDGUNS

Handguns are commonly used in urban areas because they are lightweight and can be concealed. Fortunately, handguns cannot produce as highly accelerated and accurate a projectile as rifles. The amount of gunpowder packed into a handgun bullet casing must be limited to avoid barrel damage and permit the shooter to fire the weapon supported only by the arms and hands. Experienced sharpshooters can master the handgun under controlled circumstances, but both police and criminals probably strike their target less than half the time in the field. Accuracy is dramatically decreased with distance. The majority of handgun wounds, therefore, are generated from 10 yards or less.

The immediate danger of a handgun wound stems from direct injury to vital organs such as are found in the head, neck, or chest. The probability of proximity injury to vasculature is less with handgun wounds than it is with rifle or automatic weapon injuries, but should still be considered. Because the velocity of a handgun bullet is less as the bullet strikes the tissue, the bullet is less likely to deform or fragment and tissue cavitation may be slight. Jacketed handgun bullets cause even less collateral damage than the nonjacketed and in some cases may penetrate the tissue and subsequently exit the body with much of their destructive potential intact.

Nonetheless, several measures designed to increase the wounding potential or "stopping power" of handguns are available and will be encountered. These include "hollow-point" bullets designed to expand (Fig. 3) and bullets designed to disintegrate into tiny pellets after impact. These bullets are favored by law enforcement and security personnel for immobilizing a human target in a crowded environment such as an airport or an airplane without concern of overpenetration or ricochet into innocent bystanders. "Magnum" handguns have extra powder and longer barrels that will produce a devastating wound at close range. Fortunately, magnum editions are not as commonly seen as regular handguns because they are expensive, heavy, and difficult to master.

Indications for operation of handgun wounds of the neck, chest, and abdomen would include mandatory exploration for zone II neck injuries, selective exploration of the chest based on hemorrhage, and

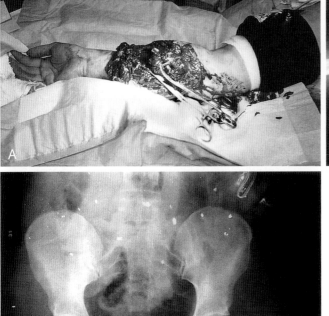

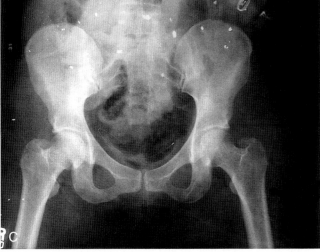

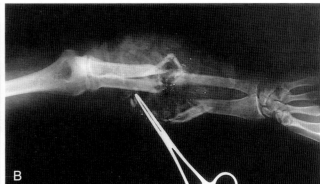

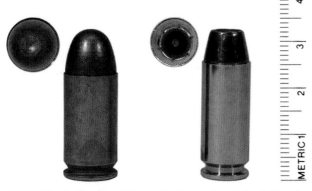

FIGURE 2 **A,** Close range 30-06 hunting rifle wound to the right forearm. **B,** Radiograph of same injury showing extensive bony comminution and bullet fragmentation. **C,** Radiograph of same patient's pelvis demonstrating extensive fragmentation of the bullet. This patient required lower abdominal wall reconstruction.

FIGURE 3 A .45-caliber full-metal-jacket handgun bullet *(left)* and 10-mm "hollow-point," partially jacketed bullet *(right)*. *(Bullets courtesy of Bruce Ham, MD and Gerald Warnock, MD, Portland, Ore.)*

and managed nonoperatively if the bullet clearly injures only the liver. Laparoscopy may be used to evaluate the diaphragm in stable, nontender patients with chest wounds or as an adjunct to nonoperative management of liver penetrations that result in bile leaks.

HUNTING RIFLES

Civilian rifle wounds, such as those resulting from hunting accidents, are among the most destructive injuries seen by surgeons. The increased amount of gunpowder contained in the bullet case and the enhanced length of the barrel that exposes the bullet to the force of the powder blast for a longer distance leads to dramatically more projectile acceleration than is possible with a handgun (Fig. 4). Rifling, the barrel's internal spiraling grooves, causes the bullet to spin and consequently improves distance and accuracy. The average muzzle velocity of a 30-06 hunting rifle is 890 m/sec and may maintain up to 90% of its kinetic energy at 100 m. A rifle wound to an extremity, whether close range or distant, will destroy soft tissue, bone, and vessels, and cause dramatic hemorrhage that may need to be controlled with direct pressure or a tourniquet at the scene (see Fig. 2).

Because of the potential for extensive damage to an extremity struck by a rifle bullet, plain radiographs looking for fractures, operative wound exploration with débridement, and intraoperative angiograms are highly recommended. Even if the overlying skin is uninjured, the soft tissue hidden beneath may be irreversibly damaged. All devascularized tissue and pieces of clothing should be removed. Serial débridements at daily intervals may be necessary to

mandatory exploration of all abdominal penetrations except tangential injuries that do not penetrate the fascia and selective liver injuries. Patients with bullet entrance sites below the nipple on the chest require abdominal exploration if the abdomen is tender, a diagnostic peritoneal lavage is suspicious, or the diaphragm is not well visualized on radiograph. Stable patients with right upper quadrant wounds may be selectively evaluated by computed tomography scan

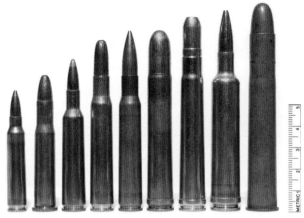

FIGURE 4 Various rifle bullets compared. **Left to right,** .223 caliber FMJ (M-16 assault rifle), 30-30 soft point, 6-mm soft point, 30-06 soft point, .308 caliber military-style FMJ (7.62 mm NATO), .458 caliber FMJ magnum, .375 caliber FMJ magnum, .378 caliber FMJ hollow tip, World War II–era .47 caliber FMJ. FMJ, full metal jacket. *(Bullets courtesy of Bruce Ham, MD and Gerald Warnock, MD, Portland, Ore.)*

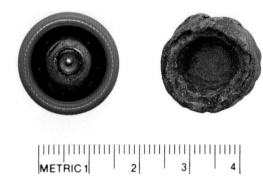

FIGURE 5 Shotgun shell loaded with lead slug instead of pellets *(left)*. Same type of slug removed from game animal. Note deformity of central zone from flight and contact. *(Bullets courtesy of Gerald Warnock, MD, Portland, Ore.)*

identify all nonviable tissue. Abdominal gunshot wounds from hunting rifles are best managed by open abdomen techniques with second-look operations if several organs are simultaneously injured.

ASSAULT RIFLES

The M-16 (United States), AK-47 and AK-74 (Russia), Uzi and Galil (Israel), Fal (Belgium), and their variations are relatively lightweight, short-barreled military rifles that fire rapidly sequential, high-velocity bullets that tumble and yaw shortly after striking tissue. Military actions that rely on these weapons seek to rapidly disable as many combatants as possible. Although these rifles and their ammunition are no longer sold on the civilian market in most Western countries, rifles that the owner possessed prior to 1994 can be legally fired in the United States, such as in target practice. These are the most common assault rifles that will be encountered in military actions; it is estimated that tens of millions of AKs and Uzis have been manufactured and distributed around the world. The caliber of bullet used in assault rifles ranges from the smaller 5.45-mm (0.21-inch) AK-74, to the 0.223-inch M-16, to the 7.62-mm (0.3-inch) AK-47, to the 9-mm (0.35-inch) Uzi.

In general, these bullets will produce severe wounds that will require soft tissue débridement; however, surgeons who have operated on injuries caused by assault rifles have occasionally noted their surprise that more injury is not apparent. This is because both the M-16 and the AK-74 deliver an FMJ bullet not much larger than a 22-caliber small-game rifle. If a single bullet passes cleanly through an extremity, the surrounding tissue damage will not be as dramatic as what a deformable, larger-caliber hunting rifle bullet would cause. The decision to débride additional tissue should thus be at the discretion of the operating surgeon and should not be based on the type of weapon or ammunition alone.

Another characteristic of assault rifles is the difficulty there can be in determining the bullet's trajectory after it strikes the victim. Abdominal wounds may contain several areas of bowel injury as well as solid organ disruptions. Thoracic penetrations need ultrasonic visualization of the pericardial space and esophageal contrast radiography if nonoperative therapy is chosen. Extremity wounds may require operative exploration and débridement and an angiogram is indicated if the ankle-brachial index (ABI) is 0.9 or less.

SHOTGUNS

Shotguns and their shells come in four main sizes: 410 juvenile, 20-gauge, 12-gauge, and 10-gauge. The gauge sizes correspond to the diameter of a lead sphere of a fraction of a pound. For example, a 10-gauge shotgun has a bore enabling a $^1/_{10}$ pound lead ball to enter the barrel. Pellets are of variable sizes and are made of lead or steel. Smaller pellets are referred to as birdshot and have a diameter of less than 0.11 inch (number 6 shot). Birdshot has considerably less range, but more spread in comparison to heavier larger buckshot. Heavier lead pellets scatter less than steel pellets but are illegal for shooting waterfowl. Slugs are also available for shotguns and are commonly used for game hunting in some states, such as New Jersey (Fig. 5). The shotgun, particularly with birdshot, is ineffective against humans at distances greater than 10 or 15 yards (30–45 ft), but close-range (<4 ft) blasts to the chest or abdomen are 85% fatal. Shotguns fire with a relatively low muzzle velocity, but their wounds are extremely morbid and often require several operations and multidisciplinary management. Pellets spread in every direction and strike multiple types of tissue, but fortunately because of their small mass the damage potential of the shot dissipates quickly. Pellets may enter arteries and veins and embolize peripherally or centrally (Fig. 6). A search for the plastic insert or wadding dispelled from the shell and pieces of the patient's clothing hidden in the wound is advised in close-range injuries (Fig. 7). There is no indication to remove all the pellets—lead poisoning does not occur from pellets or bullets left permanently in human tissue.

Thoracic wounds created by close-range shotgun blasts may be challenging to cover if part of the chest wall is lost—diaphragm transposition or emergent muscular flaps have been described. Abdominal wounds are best managed with serial operations and débridement. The blast effect can cause ischemia and injury that may not manifest itself on initial examination. The resultant open abdomen can be managed with a vacuum or other temporary dressing. Extremity shotgun blasts usually require wound exploration and débridement with intraoperative angiograms if indicated.

NONLETHAL AMMUNITION

Nonlethal rounds are increasingly common with law enforcement agencies. These rounds theoretically allow police officers in not immediately life-threatening circumstances to incapacitate subjects with lower risks of mortality or permanent disability. Nonlethal ammunition can take the form of softer lighter bullets. Rubber or plastic bullets have been used extensively in cases of civil unrest by the Israeli and British governments. The wounds produced are not entirely benign and frequently require treatment. Despite their

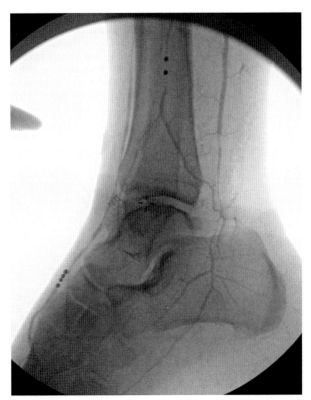

FIGURE 6 Angiogram of patient hit with a shotgun round to the right femur. He suffered a superficial femoral artery injury resulting in emboli of birdshot. Reconstruction of the femoral artery and embolectomy of the anterior tibial artery were performed.

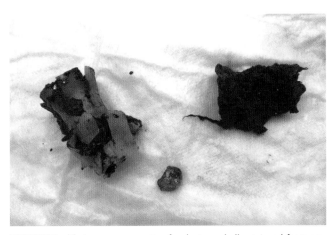

FIGURE 7 Various components of a shotgun shell retrieved from an extremity wound.

design, penetration of the skin does occur and injuries to the face and head have been noted to be fatal.

Beanbag rounds have also been used as nonlethal ammunition. These rounds are composed of light pellets in a cloth shell and are fired from a standard 12-gauge shotgun. These rounds theoretically diffuse the impact over a larger surface and the containing cloth prevents penetration. The injury itself is however dependent on the distance traveled and the site of impact. Severe blunt abdominal injuries as well as penetrating injuries have been described. When treating patients with these injuries, a thorough evaluation is required to rule out deeper injuries.

PROTECTIVE VESTS

There are many varieties of "bullet-proof" vests manufactured with successive layers of synthetic materials such as Kevlar (DuPont), which is a lightweight aramid fiber with extreme tensile strength. These vests are categorized according to their level of protection: Level I will protect the wearer from a .38 handgun at 259 m/sec, Level II from a 9-mm FMJ at 332 m/sec, and Level III from a 9-mm FMJ (assault rifle) at 427 m/sec. Protection from rifle bullets at higher velocities requires the addition of a ceramic plate to the vest. No vest is 100% effective, however. Even if the bullet does not penetrate, chest wall and pulmonary contusions can occur from the blunt force that is dissipated into the vest and onto the chest wall. High-fidelity models have studied the ensuing pressure effects after a bullet strikes body armor. Significant pressure waves affect hollow and solid organs. Care should be taken to rule out injuries despite lack of noticeable entry or exit wounds. Many varieties of "armor-piercing" bullets are manufactured for both handguns and rifles and may be encountered in both military and nonmilitary situations, even though they are illegal for civilian use. These projectiles are jacketed and have a lead inner shell and a hardened steel or tungsten interior core. As the conventional portion of the projectile strikes the vest, it deforms and "softens up" the barrier. The hardened cores of these bullets pass through their softer shells to penetrate body and vehicular armor and even, in some cases, concrete walls.

LANDMINES AND IMPROVISED EXPLOSIVE DEVICES

The improvised explosive device (IED) has gained notoriety during OIF and OEF. IEDs are the leading cause of fatality for U.S. and coalition forces in the current conflicts. These IEDs are highly variable in their sophistication and construction. The devices vary from small conventional explosives to complex powerful shaped charges. The detonation of an IED has the potential to cause instantly fatal injuries. A direct detonation of a concealed explosive device such as a conventional landmine or an IED usually results in the immediate amputation or at least partial amputation of the triggering extremity. Exsanguination from major vessel injury is possible, and therefore a field tourniquet may be necessary. Fragments of metal and debris will also shower the contralateral extremity, perineum, torso, and face. Abdominal injuries often have diffuse injuries requiring an open abdomen for multiple explorations. Additional damage from the blast effect can result in injuries not immediately evident at the time of initial laparotomy. The current military standard for operative management is damage control. Repeated débridements of devascularized tissue and the use of external fixators for bone stability are recommended. In austere settings, vascular injuries can be temporized with the use of shunts. Conventional landmines triggered by the foot will cause an umbrella effect that spares the skin and subcutaneous tissue of the lower leg while destroying underlying muscle and bone (Fig. 8A). The overlying skin will hide significant destruction and contamination beneath (Fig. 8B). Aggressive débridement to prevent infection tracking along the popliteal vessels and neural sheaths is advised. Robin Coupland of the International Red Cross makes an argument, however, to conserve the partially protected gastrocnemius muscle for reconstruction.

WOUND EXPLORATION AND BULLET REMOVAL

Not all gunshot wounds need to be explored or débrided. Frequently these wounds do not have significant tissue destruction or associated fractures. Simple wounds caused by a bullet passing through soft tissue and muscle without vascular injury or significant hematoma can be observed. Wounds should be evaluated and basic irrigation should

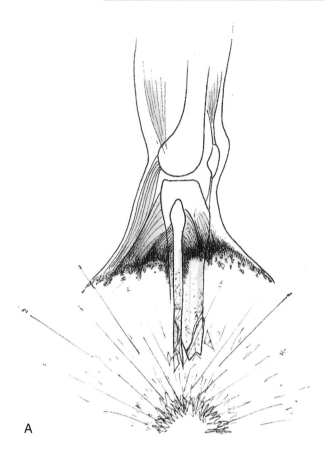

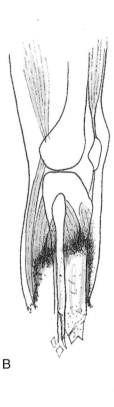

B

FIGURE 8 **A,** "Umbrella" effect of foot-triggered mine on the lower leg. **B,** Severe damage to the compartments of the lower leg may be concealed by overlying skin. *(From Coupland RM: War wounds of limbs: surgical management. Oxford, Butterworth-Heinemann, 1993.)*

A

be performed within 6 hours as the most significant risk factor of infection is delay in treatment. Intravenous antibiotics are unnecessary because the risk of infection is less than 2%. In both simple and complex wounds, the practitioner should address the patient's tetanus status.

Bullet removal is generally unnecessary and ideally would not be used as the only indication for a surgical procedure. An occasional patient is symptomatic enough from an irritating focus to tempt the surgeon to remove the projectile. Many a surgeon, however, has searched subcutaneous tissue in vain looking for a foreign body that seems to be just beneath the skin. Radiographic localization may be necessary.

The only risk of lead poisoning seems to be from bullets in contact with synovial fluid and. by extrapolation, spinal cord fluid. Bullets that pass through colon and subsequently lodge in bone are at risk to cause osteomyelitis. Controversy exists as to the magnitude of the risk, but at our center we favor removal depending on the accessibility of the projectile. The alternative is irrigation of the tract and a minimum of 10 days of broad-spectrum intravenous antibiotics. Other true indications for bullet removal include removing bullet emboli in arteries and veins and bullets lodged in cardiac chambers.

For the chapter's Suggested Readings list, please visit the book at www.ExpertConsult.inkling.com.

COMMON PREHOSPITAL COMPLICATIONS AND PITFALLS IN THE TRAUMA PATIENT

Frank L. Mitchell, Charles M. Richart, and Harry E. Wilkins

The evolution of prehospital care in this country has an interesting and continually evolving record. Although there is recorded history of wagons and carts being used to transport the sick and injured as early as 900 ACE, the term "ambulance" was not used until introduced by Queen Isabella of Spain in the early 15th century. Even at that time, it referred more to military field hospitals and tents for the wounded than to a means of transporting wounded and dead from battlefields. Not until the time of Baron Larrey would the term "ambulance" take up its more current meaning of "a specially equipped motor vehicle, airplane, or ship for carrying sick or injured people, usually to a hospital."

Baron Dominique-Jean Larrey was Napoleon Bonaparte's surgeon and developed what was known as "flying ambulances." Prior to 1792, there was very little organized transportation of the wounded from the battlefield. As is the case with most medical advances, advances in ambulance transportation occurred as a result of military conflict. Throughout the remainder of the 1800s and the conflicts of the early 20th century, ambulances and other means of transporting individuals from the field of battle were employed.

During the 1950s through the 1970s, helicopters were employed to transport the injured from battlefields to MASH (mobile army surgical hospital) units attaining particular effectiveness in the Korean and Vietnam conflicts. Throughout the first several decades of the 20th century, civilian transport for the injured continued to lag behind advances established in the military.

One of the prime factors identified as contributing to the continued reduction in battlefield casualties from 8% in World War I to less than 2% in the Vietnam War was reducing the time from injury to initiation of medical care. On this backdrop, the mid-1960s and early 1970s sought to improve prehospital care, education, equipment, and processes. The early 1960s called for an extension of basic and advanced first aid training to greater numbers of the lay population, and preparation of nationally accepted texts, training aids, and courses of instruction for rescue squad personnel, police, firefighters, and ambulance attendants. Ambulance service in the 1960s was very piecemeal and adequate at best. In a few major cities, there were specially equipped ambulances prepared to care for the injured and sick, and trained professional prehospital personnel were available. However, approximately 50% of the country's ambulance services at that time were provided by over 12,000 morticians mainly because their vehicles were able to accommodate transportation of patients on gurneys or stretchers.

In the mid-1960s, the National Traffic and Motor Safety Act and the Highway Safety Act provided for the establishment of national standards for used motor vehicles, motor vehicle inspections, and emergency services. Communications were also problematic. At a time when the United States had just placed a man on the moon, it was easier in most instances to communicate with that extraterrestrial individual than it was for prehospital providers to communicate with the emergency department where they were headed.

Over the next several decades, the education and provision of specifically equipped vehicles progressed until the mid-1980s when *Injury in America: A Continuing Public Health Problem* was published. Although the report found that there had been significant progress in the credentialing and education of prehospital care providers, more than 2.5 million Americans died from injuries in the 1966–1985 period. This prompted the expenditure of more federal dollars to study the continuing public health problem, as the report noted and called for the institution of more systems of communication and transportation of the injured to facilities specially equipped for managing critically injured patients.

In 1992, the Model of Trauma Care Systems Plan, developed by Health Resources and Services Administration under the Authority of the Trauma Systems Planning and Development Act of 1990, marked the next major step in the evolution of health policy related to trauma care. This plan emphasized the need for a fully inclusive trauma care system that involved not only trauma centers, but also all health care facilities according to availability of trauma resources, including prehospital providers. As a result, the numbers of dedicated trauma centers and state trauma systems increased, although at a still less-than-adequate pace. Trauma centers were charged with becoming resource facilities for emergency medical response agencies. Educational programs such as Prehospital Trauma Life Support, Basic Trauma Life Support, and others were developed with states being empowered to license and credential prehospital providers at various levels.

Today, the initial care of the injured patient continues to reside primarily with trained prehospital providers. Emergency medical technicians, with basic, intermediate, and paramedic levels of instruction, with police and fire departments also being trained in basic life support, as well as increased communication and education with the lay public with regard to cardiac arrest, seat belt usage, wearing of helmets, and other prevention initiatives, are in place to continue to try to combat the unacceptably high level of death and disability in this country from intentional and unintentional injury.

Along with the ever-evolving technologies available to the prehospital provider come the unintended risk of complications associated with the implementation of these devices and processes. This chapter addresses some of the more common prehospital complications.

INCIDENCE

According to the National Highway Traffic Safety Administration, the leading cause of death in the United States in 2002 for people aged 4 to 34 was overwhelmingly motor vehicle traffic crashes (Table 1). In terms of years of life lost, motor vehicle crashes rank third, after malignant neoplasms and heart disease, at 5% of total years of life lost for the entire population.

A total of 37% of trauma deaths are caused by motor vehicle crashes and motorcycle crashes. Other important causes of trauma deaths are gunshot wounds, stabbings, and falls. Today's prehospital provider is in a position to be the first responder to the vast majority of these injuries at or shortly after the time they occur.

The major causes of death in the prehospital period are secondary to severe head injury, respiratory compromise, and exsanguinating hemorrhage. Initial and emergent prehospital treatment focuses on the treatment and prevention of these eventualities.

The foundation of Advanced Trauma Life Support of the American College of Surgeons stresses an ABC (airway, breathing, and circulation) approach. Much of the emphasis on prehospital care and subsequent care involves appropriate management of the airway, providing for ventilation by breathing for the patient, and control of circulation consisting of hemorrhage control and restoration of intravascular volume. Not surprisingly, the most common prehospital complications occur in these three areas.

AIRWAY

Ensuring that the trauma victim has a patent airway is the highest management priority. If manual maneuvers (clearing the airway of foreign bodies, jaw thrust, or chin lift) or basic adjuncts (oropharyngeal or nasopharyngeal airways) are not adequate to maintain the airway, then alternate, more invasive methods are required.

Current prehospital techniques used for airway management and ventilation include (1) bag-valve-mask (BVM), (2) laryngeal mask airways (LMAs), (3) dual lumen tubes (i.e., Combitubes), (4) endotracheal intubation (with or without the use of paralytics), and (5) emergency cricothyroidotomy.

BVM can be a temporizing method for providing adequate oxygenation and ventilation of the injured patient, but can occasionally be problematic related to obtaining an adequate seal at the mouth, potential for aspiration, problems with bleeding from soft tissue injury, patient cooperation, and the lack of satisfactory ventilation and oxygenation depending on the specific clinical situation. Acute gastric dilatation from overzealous ventilation can also lead to ventilatory impairment from increased intraabdominal pressure, and, in extreme cases, gastric rupture.

The prehospital use of LMAs and dual lumen tubes has an advantage over conventional endotracheal intubation related to ease of technique and maintenance of insertion skill. LMAs and dual lumen tubes are beneficial in an unconscious patient who cannot be adequately ventilated with a BVM device or cannot be successfully intubated. However, because the trachea is not completely protected, the use of an LMA may result in aspiration. The use of dual lumen tubes may also result in aspiration if the gag reflex is intact, and there is also potential for damage to the esophagus and the possibility for hypoxia if the wrong lumen is used.

The identification of patients requiring definitive airway management may sometimes be problematic based on the patient's injuries, mental status (secondary to injury, alcohol, or drugs), underlying medical conditions, and the experience of the prehospital provider. Delay of intubation until respiratory arrest increases morbidity and mortality risks and should be avoided if at all possible. Early recognition of

TABLE 1: Deaths, Top 10 Causes by Age Group, United States, 2002*

Rank	Infants under 1	Toddlers 1-3	Young Children 4-7	Children 8-15	Youth 16-20	Young Adults 21-24	OTHER ADULTS 25-34	35-44	45-64	Elderly ≥65	All Ages	Years of Life Lost[†]
1	Perinatal period 14,106	Congenital anomalies 474	MV traffic crashes 495	MV traffic crashes 1,584	MV traffic crashes 6,327	MV traffic crashes 4,446	MV traffic crashes 6,933	Malignant neoplasms 16,085	Malignant neoplasms 143,028	Heart disease 576,301	Heart disease 696,947	Malignant neoplasms 23% (8,686,782)
2	Congenital anomalies 5,623	MV traffic crashes 410	Malignant neoplasms 449	Malignant neoplasms 842	Homicide 2,422	Homicide 2,650	Suicide 5,046	Heart disease 13,688	Heart disease 101,804	Malignant neoplasms 391,001	Malignant neoplasms 557,271	Heart disease 22% (8,140,300)
3	Heart disease 500	Accidental drowning 380	Congenital anomalies 180	Suicide 428	Suicide 1,810	Suicide 2,036	Homicide 4,489	MV traffic crashes 6,883	Stroke 15,952	Stroke 143,293	Stroke 162,672	MV traffic crashes 5% (1,766,854)
4	Homicide 303	Homicide 366	Accidental drowning 171	Homicide 426	Malignant neoplasms 805	Accidental poisoning 974	Malignant neoplasms 3,872	Suicide 6,851	Diabetes 15,518	Chronic lower respiratory disease 108,313	Chronic lower respiratory disease 124,816	Stroke 5% (1,682,465)
5	Septicemia 296	Malignant neoplasms 285	Exposure to smoke/fire 151	Congenital anomalies 345	Accidental poisoning 679	Malignant neoplasms 823	Heart disease 3,165	Accidental poisoning 6,007	Chronic. lower respiratory disease 14,755	Influenza/pneumonia 58,826	Diabetes 73,249	Chronic lower respiratory disease 4% (1,466,004)
6	Influenza/pneumonia 263	Exposure to smoke/fire 163	Homicide 134	Accidental drowning 270	Heart disease 449	Heart disease 518	Accidental poisoning 3,116	HIV infection 5,707	Chronic liver disease 13,313	Alzheimer's disease 58,289	Influenza/pneumonia 65,681	Suicide 3% (1,109,748)
7	Nephritis/nephrosis 173	Heart disease 144	Heart disease 73	Heart disease 258	Accidental drowning 345	Accidental drowning 238	HIV 1,839	Homicide 3,239	Suicide 9,926	Diabetes 54,715	Alzheimer's disease 58,866	Perinatal period 3% (1,099,767)
8	MV traffic crashes 120	Influenza/pneumonia 92	Influenza/pneumonia 41	Exposure to smoke/fire 170	Congenital anomalies 254	Congenital anomalies 186	Diabetes 642	Chronic liver disease 3,154	MV traffic crashes 9,412	Nephritis/nephrosis 34,316	MV traffic crashes 44,065	Diabetes 3% (1,050,798)
9	Stroke 117	MV nontraffic crashes[‡] 69	Septicemia 38	Chronic lower respiratory disease 131	MV nontraffic crashes[‡] 121	Accidental falls 134	Stroke 567	Stroke 2,425	HIV infection 5,821	Septicemia 26,670	Nephritis/nephrosis 40,974	Homicide 2% (822,762)
10	Malignant neoplasms 74	Septicemia 63	Benign neoplasms 36	MV nontraffic crashes[‡] 115	Accidental discharge of firearms 113	HIV infection 130	Congenital anomalies 475	Diabetes 2,164	Accidental poisoning 5,780	Hypertension renal disease 17,345	Septicemia 33,865	Accidental poisoning 2% (675,348)
ALL[§]	28,034	4,079	2,586	6,760	16,239	15,390	41,355	91,140	425,727	1,811,720	2,443,387	All causes 100%

HIV, Human immunodeficiency virus; MV, motor vehicle.

Note: The cause of death classification is based on the National Center for Statistics and Analysis (NCSA) Revised 68 Cause of Death Listing. This listing differs from the one used by the NCHS for its reports on leading causes of death by separating out unintentional injuries into separate causes of death, such as motor vehicle traffic crashes, accidental falls, motor vehicle nontraffic crashes, etc. Accordingly, the rank of some causes of death will differ from those reported by the NCHS. This difference will mostly be observed for minor causes of death in smaller age groupings.

*When ranked by specific ages, MV crashes are the leading cause of death for ages 3 through 33.

[†] Number of years calculated based on remaining life expectancy at time of death; percents calculated as a proportion of total years of life lost due to all causes of death.

[‡] A motor vehicle nontraffic crash is any vehicle crash that occurs (entirely) in any place other than a public highway.

[§] Not a total of top 10 causes of death.

From NHTSA (National Highway Traffic Safety Administration), U.S. Department of Transportation Technical report (DOT HS 809 843), June 2005, National Center for Statistics and Analysis. Available at http://www-nrd.nhtsa.dot.gov/pdf/nrd-30/NCSA/Rpts/2005/809843.pdf. Data from National Center for Health Statistics (NCHS), Centers for Disease Control and Prevention, mortality data, 2002.

the need for intubation is of paramount importance for the prehospital provider.

Late endotracheal intubation may result because of a false sense of security by the provider, the inability to obtain an airway, and lack of recognition of likely deterioration in a patient's ventilatory status (secondary to airway and chest injuries, traumatic brain injury [TBI], alteration in mental status, or the overall complexity of the injuries). Patients with facial burns and maxillofacial trauma may have progression of their underlying injury, and may deteriorate secondary to edema or hematoma formation, causing airway obstruction. Intubation of these patients can be a difficult challenge with the potential for disastrous results if proactive intubation is not accomplished. This is especially true if paralytic agents have been used and the vocal cords cannot be easily visualized. Anticipation of this problem along with early intubation may prevent a catastrophe.

The use of paralytic agents for intubation in the prehospital setting results in a quicker and higher success rate of intubation. However, many prehospital providers do not have access to use these agents. Additionally, if paralytic agents are used, it is critical that adequate analgesia and sedation are also administered, so that the injured patient is not chemically paralyzed, while awake and hurting. At the time of hand-off of the trauma patient from the prehospital provider to the trauma team in the emergency department, it is important that all of the medications that have been administered to the patient prior to arrival are reviewed, so that the emergency physician and trauma surgeon will ensure adequate pain management and sedation, even when the patient is chemically paralyzed.

Successful endotracheal intubation is beneficial for the trauma patient whose airway needs to be secured, but there are potential complications and pitfalls that may occur during the process of intubation, regardless of the expertise of the provider. Prehospital personnel should be aware of these potential complications and how to clinically recognize them if they occur.

Esophageal intubation is a known complication of intubation, and should be quickly recognized by the prehospital provider if it occurs. The difficulty of the intubation and in visualizing the vocal cords should increase concerns of an esophageal intubation, and warrants aggressive evaluation to ensure adequate placement of the endotracheal tube (ETT). The placement of an esophageal ETT should be clinically evident by routine chest auscultation immediately after intubation. The routine use of end-tidal CO_2 detectors ($ETCO_2$) is beneficial in rapidly detecting the presence of CO_2 in the exhaled air. The calorimetric devices have a chemically treated indicator strip that reflects the CO_2 level. If there is a question of the exact location, visualization of the ETT location should be repeated and appropriate location confirmed.

Right mainstem intubation is an occasional complication of intubation that occurs up to 30% of the time in pediatric trauma patients, and should be detected by physical examination at the time of intubation, and with frequent routine clinical reassessments, or urgent reassessment if the patient clinically deteriorates. The distance of the tip of the ETT should be evaluated, relative to the size of the patient and the expected appropriate distance of ETT. Repositioning of the ETT while auscultating the chest helps in determining the appropriate location of the ETT. Other possible traumatic injuries that may lead to similar clinical findings must also be considered in severely injured patients, including a pneumothorax, hemothorax, pulmonary contusion, or ruptured hemidiaphragm.

Surgical airways are occasionally needed when endotracheal intubation cannot be successfully achieved secondary to facial trauma, anatomic difficulties, and soft tissue injuries. Although the use of surgical airways in the prehospital setting is controversial, local protocols should outline the specific indications and circumstances for their use.

Complications of needle cricothyroidotomy include inadequate ventilation resulting in hypoxia and death, esophageal laceration, hematoma formation, posterior tracheal wall perforation, thyroid laceration, and bleeding. Complications of surgical cricothyroidotomy include false passage into the tissues, hemorrhage or hematoma formation, esophageal laceration, vocal cord paralysis, and potential subglottic stenosis/edema. If a surgical airway is needed, a surgical cricothyroidotomy should be performed. A formal tracheostomy should not be performed by prehospital providers because of the difficulty and length of time needed to successfully accomplish the procedure.

BREATHING

A tension pneumothorax is a life-threatening situation as a result of an injury to the lung causing a pneumothorax that results in air leaking into the pleural space, causing increased pressure that results in difficult ventilation and decreased venous return. Typically it is recognized by a variety of signs and symptoms, including tachypnea, dyspnea, decreased breath sounds or unilateral absence of breath sounds, air hunger, respiratory distress, tachycardia, hypotension, tracheal deviation, neck vein distention, and cyanosis (late). Hyperresonant percussion tone and absent breath sounds are typical of a significant pneumothorax. Although there are many signs and symptoms that are associated with a tension pneumothorax, some may be difficult to recognize in the prehospital setting, and some may not be present in all situations. In a patient who has required intubation and positive pressure ventilation, a minimal lung injury may develop into a clinically significant tension pneumothorax, and should be anticipated if a patient in this type of setting suddenly deteriorates.

The management of a tension pneumothorax in the prehospital setting includes the recognition of the presence of a clinically significant pneumothorax, and then prompt needle decompression with a large-bore needle, classically inserted into the pleural space in the second intercostal space, midclavicular line. This location minimizes the risk of injuring underlying internal structures; however, the development of a hematoma or lung laceration is possible. There is also the possibility of the needle not being placed deep enough to reach the pleural cavity, thus not relieving the tension pneumothorax. Placement of the needle in the lateral aspect of the affected chest cavity has also been shown to be of benefit in resolving tension pneumothoraces. Once a pleural cavity has been decompressed with a needle, a definitive chest tube should be placed. The lack of recognition of a tension pneumothorax, and a delay in its management may result in a life-threatening situation. In a patient who is intubated, the location of the ETT should be determined to make sure that it is not in a mainstem bronchus as the cause of absent breath sounds, prior to needle decompression of the chest cavity.

CIRCULATION

One of the most common prehospital complications related to circulation is hemorrhage, and the failure to detect and address ongoing hemorrhage can be dangerous. External hemorrhage is best controlled by applying direct pressure to the bleeding site. Common areas that are sources of external hemorrhage that may be missed include the posterior scalp, axillae, perineum, and posterior trunk. Bulky dressings, particularly applied to the scalp, may be dangerous for a number of reasons. First, they can hide posterior scalp hemorrhage from view of the providers while providing a false sense of security that the bleeding has been controlled. Failure to recognize signs and symptoms of intrathoracic, intraabdominal, and pelvic bleeding can lead to another potential prehospital complication related to circulatory insufficiency.

Prehospital intravenous fluid therapy is an area of continued controversy. A thorough discussion of the types and amount of fluid to be administered in the prehospital setting is beyond the scope of this chapter. In general, there are very few complications in the prehospital setting related to fluid excess. There is also evidence that subsets of patients—particularly trauma patients who have suffered penetrating trauma—may do better with no prehospital fluid or limited prehospital fluid than those who receive prehospital fluid. There is general agreement among providers of trauma care that extra time spent in the field trying to obtain intravenous access is detrimental to efforts to get the patient to definitive care and attempts to obtain access should be limited in most situations. In the case of significant intracavitary bleeding, fluid cannot be administered in adequate amounts in the prehospital setting to restore effective intravascular volume. Therefore, efforts should be directed toward expeditious transfer to definitive care.

Other causes of circulatory insufficiency must be kept in mind. Pericardial tamponade manifested by Beck's triad of hypotension, jugular venous distention, and muffled heart tones may be difficult to discern in the frenetic prehospital setting. A temporizing measure for this rare prehospital occurrence is pericardiocentesis. Complications related to this procedure are significant and include, but are not limited to, inadvertent ventricular laceration/puncture, laceration of the coronary arteries or vein, injury to the thoracic or upper abdominal great vessels, pneumothorax, and injury to the upper abdominal viscera. Prehospital attempts at pericardiocentesis are discouraged except by the most experienced providers and then in only the most dire of circumstances. Restoration of intravascular volume may temporarily offset the negative circulatory effects of pericardial tamponade, but again, rapid transport to definitive care is the best approach in this situation.

DISABILITY

The major goal during the resuscitation of patients with traumatic neurologic injury is to avoid or minimize secondary brain injury and spinal cord damage. Avoiding hypoxemia and shock are also major priorities. Management of ventilation and maintenance of cerebral perfusion pressure can and should be addressed, altered, and optimized in the prehospital setting. Maintaining adequate perfusion and oxygenation in order to prevent secondary brain injury makes a positive difference in morbidity and fatality from TBI. The ABCs are important in the management of TBI in order to prevent secondary brain injury. The goals should be to maintain systolic blood pressure greater than 90 mm Hg and oxygenation saturations of at least 95% and provide ventilation to maintain $ETCO_2$ at 30 to 35 mm Hg.

There are multiple reasons for the development of altered mental status in trauma patients other than TBI (hypoxia, hypotension, alcohol, and other mind-altering drugs). However, in the prehospital setting the patient with an altered mental status and a mechanism of injury consistent with a TBI should be assumed to have suffered a significant brain injury until proved otherwise and treated aggressively in order to prevent secondary brain injury. Severity of the TBI may not be readily apparent in the prehospital setting. A high index of suspicion should be maintained based on the mechanism of injury and the patient's initial neurologic examination findings.

Historically, prehospital intubation has been the highest priority for patients with TBI with an associated coma (Glasgow Coma Scale score ≤ 8), but recent evidence has shown that prehospital intubation may worsen outcomes for patients with TBI. These results appear to be related to the expertise of the prehospital provider and the use of neuromuscular blockade agents (rapid sequence intubation). Intubation with pharmacologic agents is thought to lessen the "struggling" and difficulty in intubation. Without adequate sedation or paralytics, the intubation time may be prolonged, resulting in hypoxia, which may be the reason for the worsened outcomes, versus providers that have full pharmacologic agents available. Additionally, some prehospital providers have more expertise in intubation techniques, based on frequency of intubation. Therefore, it likely depends on the expertise and ease of intubation whether intubation is beneficial or harmful in the prehospital setting for patient outcomes with TBI. Using the BVM technique and maintaining adequate minute ventilation and

oxygenation is preferred compared to a prehospital provider with less proficiency at endotracheal intubation and the potential for the patient to have significant (degree and duration) hypoxemia and hypercarbia while attempting to accomplish endotracheal intubation. The use of intravenous lidocaine (1 mg/kg) may blunt an increase in intracranial pressure (ICP) during intubation.

Mannitol for severe head injuries should only be used for patients with localizing signs or evidence of elevated intracranial hypertension, when the patient is adequately volume resuscitated. Otherwise, the patient's volume status may be worsened, producing hypovolemia, and contribute to secondary brain injury, thus further worsening cerebral perfusion. Patients should be maintained in a euvolemic state.

Controlled hyperventilation—mild therapeutic hyperventilation ($ETCO_2$ of 25 to 30 mm Hg)—may be used in situations with acute neurologic deterioration with signs of herniation or obvious increase in ICP. Hyperventilation should be stopped if the signs of intracranial hypertension resolve (i.e., dilated pupil responds). Prophylactic hyperventilation should not be used in the prehospital management of TBI. Overaggressive hyperventilation produces cerebral vasoconstriction that in turn leads to a decrease in cerebral oxygen delivery. Routine prophylactic hyperventilation has been shown to worsen neurologic outcomes and should not be used.

The use of benzodiazepines for treating seizures should be used with caution (titrated) because of the potential for developing hypotension and ventilatory depression.

Patients with TBI should be taken to the appropriate facility, one that cares for patients with TBI. If the transport time to a facility is prolonged, sedation, analgesia, chemical paralysis, controlled hyperventilation, and treatment with mannitol (osmotherapy) should be utilized as indicated. Prolonged attempts at intubation should be avoided—especially if a short transport time—as an oropharyngeal airway with BVM ventilations is a reasonable alternative.

Patients with suspected TBI should be placed in spinal immobilization, because of the significant incidence of cervical spine fractures. A tight cervical spine collar may impede venous drainage from the head, thereby increasing ICP.

TRANSPORT

Upon arrival at the scene of injury, it is of paramount importance that the prehospital providers have a good understanding of the local resources available in terms of transport times, the transport environment, the transport vehicle, and the receiving facility. It is also very important that information gathered at the time of the initial evaluation be transmitted to the receiving facility in order to facilitate the receiving facility's ability to properly prepare for the patient's arrival. At the scene of a crash or injury incident, the paramedic must make a decision based on his or her resources as to which of the patients (if there are multiple patients) requires the first and most resources. Ideally, the most critically injured patient would be attended to first and sent out of the scene toward definitive care in the most expeditious fashion. Toward this end most health providers who care for the injured patient advocate a rapid transport team rather than spending additional time on the scene employing other modalities of advanced access, advanced airway techniques, or any other attempts at what would be definitive control at the scene. Put another way, there's more of a desire by health care providers for a "scoop-and-run" than a "stay-and-play" approach. Subsequently, prehospital complications surrounding this scene include too much time on the scene allowing for the patient with potential intracavitary bleeding to deteriorate beyond the ability to provide definitive control. Second, there is the tendency to perform too many procedures at the scene that may be provided more effectively in the hospital setting.

Finally, there may be a tendency to employ protocol over what may in fact be better for the patient. An example is forcing patients with massive maxillofacial injury, who may otherwise be stable, into a supine position where they may choke on their own secretions. These patients may need to be transported in the decubitus position with cervical spine control or even transported in the sitting position to allow gravity to help secretions fall away from the airway. Similarly, patients who have potential tracheal injuries may actually do worse with repeated attempts at endotracheal intubation, when in fact their airway may be adequate and patent for transfer. Another delaying factor is intravenous access.

COMORBID CONDITIONS

With advances in medicine and medical care, Americans are living longer with chronic medical illnesses. Failure to recognize the underlying chronic medical condition in the victim of trauma is a common prehospital complication.

With advancement of age of the general population, the use of anticoagulants (warfarin, clopidogrel, aspirin) is becoming more common. Failure to recognize the patient who is fully medically anticoagulated may lead to a delay in recognizing significant intracranial, intrathoracic, or intraabdominal bleeding. Alternatively, recognition of the medically anticoagulated state can lead to a higher index of suspicion on the part of prehospital providers as to the potential for significant injury, despite what might otherwise be considered minor trauma.

Chronic medical conditions that must be considered include those involving the cardiopulmonary, renal, hepatic, and endocrine systems.

Patients with chronic congestive heart failure are often on a number of medications that may blunt their ability to mount a response to trauma. Beta-blocking drugs, for instance, may prevent these patients from mounting a tachycardic response to acute hemorrhage. Chronic diuretic therapy may cause these patients to be chronically intravascularly depleted. These patients are often severely dyspneic, precluding their ability to lay supine on a transport gurney, and finally, their chronic congestive failure may predispose them to easy fluid overload with relatively minimal amounts of intravenous fluid therapy.

Patients with chronic obstructive pulmonary disease (COPD) may be difficult to assess, as they have chronically diminished breath sounds on auscultation. This makes it difficult, if not impossible, to clinically detect a condition such as pneumothorax, hemothorax, and pericardial tamponade. In addition, patients with severe COPD may be dependent on relative hypoxemia to promote respiratory efforts, and too much supplemental oxygen administration may acutely blunt this drive resulting in acute respiratory arrest.

Patients with chronic renal and hepatic insufficiency may manifest diminished clearing of administered intravenous medications used in the prehospital setting. Choice and dosage of these medications such as benzodiazepines and opioids must be made carefully with the patient's estimated hepatic and renal clearances in mind.

Patients with diabetes, adrenal insufficiency, and thyroid disorders may also manifest altered physiologic responses to acute trauma, and the ability to elicit this history from the patient or guardian may be helpful in the acute and subsequent management of these patients. Many of these disorders can be ascertained from a review of the medications that the patient is taking. Eliciting this history from a family member, caregiver, or the patient is extremely useful in helping to manage the patient in the prehospital setting and beyond.

CONCLUSION

The initial management of the trauma victim is a challenging endeavor that lends itself readily to the application of an ordered approach to care. Following the ABCs of care, prioritizing the injuries with which a patient presents, and prioritizing rapid transport to definitive care yield the best possible outcome for the patient. Errors in the prehospital arena, as in others, include those of omission and those of commission. Both types of errors are avoidable with careful attention to defined principles of the approach to the patient.

For the chapter's Suggested Readings list, please visit the book at www.ExpertConsult.Inkling.com.

INITIAL ASSESSMENT AND RESUSCITATION

AIRWAY MANAGEMENT: WHAT EVERY TRAUMA SURGEON SHOULD KNOW, FROM INTUBATION TO CRICOTHYROIDOTOMY

Andrew R. Doben and Ronald I. Gross

The concept of immediate and appropriate airway management spans all disciplines of medicine. Achieving, protecting, and maintaining the airway have been well recognized as the initial steps necessary in resuscitation of the critically ill or injured patient. The basic premise of the *Advanced Trauma Life Support for Doctors Course* (ATLS) is that all resuscitations should follow the mnemonic ABCDE: Airway, Breathing, Circulation, Disability, Exposure. This mnemonic, according to the ATLS, "defines the specific, ordered evaluations and interventions that should be followed in all injured patients."

The optimal airway is one that an awake patient can maintain without assistance; the worst-case scenario is an airway that can be achieved only with surgical intervention—the dreaded "cannot intubate, cannot ventilate" situation. The success or failure to achieve an adequate and protected airway is dependent on many factors. Techniques available to the clinician range from the simple to the complex. The concept of tracheal intubation is by no means a new one. In fact, the first documented report of tracheal intubation dates back to 1543, and actually refers to a tracheostomy. In his atlas *On the Fabric of the Human Body*, the Renaissance anatomist Andreas Vesalius observed, "Life may, in a manner of speaking, be restored. An opening must be attempted in the trunk of the trachea into which a reed or cane should be put; you will then blow into this so that the lung may rise again."

From the clinician's standpoint, the appropriate management of the airway can be the most stressful part of a patient's initial care. This chapter will deal with the anatomic aspects of the head, neck, and respiratory system in which a clinician must be adept to successfully manage the airway. It will also address how these anatomic variations, in association with the clinical situation, will affect the clinician's choice of airway management. The chapter will describe many of the available techniques used to obtain and maintain a secure airway.

AIRWAY ANATOMY

Successful execution of any procedure demands a thorough understanding of the procedure: indications, technical requirements, and necessary equipment to complete the task. In addition, the operator must be cognizant of potential complications and their management. Obtaining an airway, whether by conventional or surgical means, is no different from any other procedure. The anatomy and normal functions of the structures that comprise the upper airway are complex. The surgeon must recognize the essential anatomic structures to effectively manage the airway.

The nose and mouth are the two natural external openings to the airway. The nasal cavity is separated by the nasal septum into two pyramids containing bone, cartilage, and sinus orifices. The roof of the nose is formed by the nasal and frontal bones, the ethmoid cribiform plate, and the body of the sphenoid bone. The floor is formed by the maxilla and palatine bones, and the medial wall by septal cartilage, the vomer, and the perpendicular plane of the ethmoid. Laterally, the wall contains a portion of the ethmoid bone, along with the superior, middle, and inferior turbinate bones. In addition, it contains the openings to the paranasal sinuses and the nasolacrimal duct (Fig. 1). The nerve supply to the nasal cavities is from the olfactory and the trigeminal nerves (cranial nerves I and V, respectively). The blood supply is from the anterior and posterior branches of the ophthalmic artery, as well as branches of the maxillary and facial arteries.

The mouth is defined by the lips and cheeks externally; the gingiva, teeth, and palate superiorly; and mucosa and tongue inferiorly. The palate forms the roof of the mouth and the floor of the nasal cavity. The hard palate forms the anterior four fifths of the palate and is a bony framework covered with a mucous membrane. The soft palate, composing the posterior one fifth of the palate, is a fibromuscular fold that moves posteriorly against the pharyngeal wall to close the oropharyngeal cavity when swallowing or speaking.

Although separated anteriorly by the palate, the mouth and nasal cavities join posteriorly at the end of the soft palate to form the pharynx. The pharynx is separated into the nasopharynx and the oropharynx. The pharynx extends to the inferior border of the cricoid cartilage anteriorly and the inferior border of the body of C6 posteriorly. The wall of the pharynx is composed of two layers of pharyngeal muscles: the external circular layer consists of the constrictor muscles and the internal longitudinal layer consists of muscles that elevate the larynx and pharynx during swallowing and speaking. The nasopharynx follows directly from the nasal cavity at the level of the soft palate, and communicates with the nasal cavities through the nasal choanae and with the tympanic cavity through the eustachian tube. It contains the pharyngeal tonsils in its posterior wall. The oropharynx begins at the soft palate and continues to the tip of the epiglottis (Fig. 2). It contains the palatine tonsils, important landmarks in the Mallampati airway classification.

Pharynx

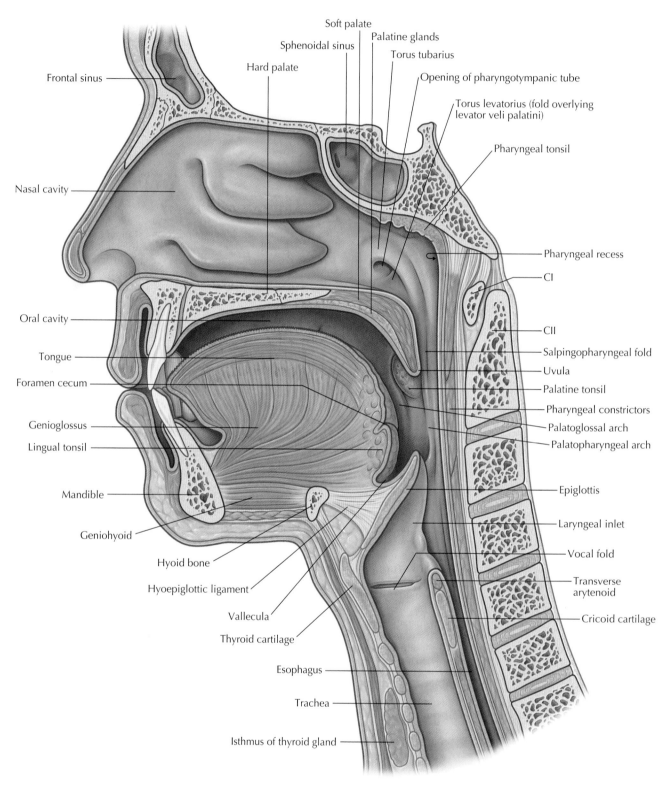

FIGURE 1   Lateral view of the pharynx (nasal, oral, and larynx). *(From Drake RJ, Vogl AW, Mitchell AWM, et al, editors: Gray's atlas of human anatomy. Philadelphia, Churchill Livingstone, 2008.)*

Pharynx

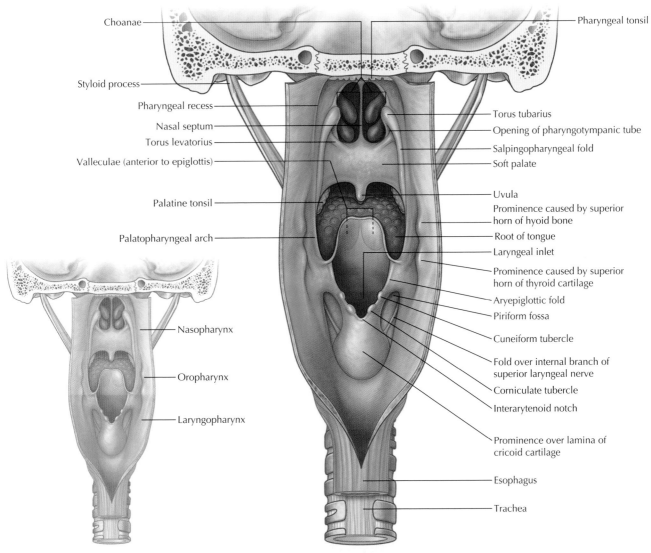

Choanae

Styloid process

Pharyngeal recess

Nasal septum

Torus levatorius

Valleculae (anterior to epiglottis)

Palatine tonsil

Palatopharyngeal arch

Nasopharynx

Oropharynx

Laryngopharynx

Pharyngeal tonsil

Torus tubarius

Opening of pharyngotympanic tube

Salpingopharyngeal fold

Soft palate

Uvula

Prominence caused by superior horn of hyoid bone

Root of tongue

Laryngeal inlet

Prominence caused by superior horn of thyroid cartilage

Aryepiglottic fold

Piriform fossa

Cuneiform tubercle

Fold over internal branch of superior laryngeal nerve

Corniculate tubercle

Interarytenoid notch

Prominence over lamina of cricoid cartilage

Esophagus

Trachea

**Features of the pharynx
(posterior view with the pharyngeal wall opened)**

FIGURE 2 Posterior view of the pharynx (nasal, oral, and larynx). *(From Drake RJ, Vogl AW, Mitchell AWM, et al, editors:* Gray's atlas of human anatomy. *Philadelphia, Churchill Livingstone, 2008.)*

The epiglottis is a spoon-shaped plate of elastic cartilage that lies behind the tongue. It prevents aspiration by covering the glottis—the opening of the larynx—during swallowing. The laryngopharynx/hypopharynx extends from the upper border of the epiglottis to the lower border of the cricoid cartilage. It is separated laterally from the larynx by the arytenoepiglottic folds, which contain the piriform recesses. The piriform sinuses are found at each side of the opening of the larynx, in which the inferior laryngeal nerve lies and swallowed foreign materials may be lodged.

The laryngeal skeleton consists of several cartilages connected by ligaments and muscles: the thyroid, cricoid, epiglottic, and (in pairs) the arytenoid, corniculate, and cuneiform. The larynx serves as a sphincter to prevent the passage of food and drink into the trachea and lungs during swallowing. It also contains the vocal

cords and regulates the flow of air to and from the lungs for phonation. It is through the abducted vocal cords of the larynx that an endotracheal tube is advanced during endotracheal intubation (Fig. 3).

The thyroid cartilage is a large anterior structure that consists of right and left laminae that meet in the midline, forming the thyroid notch and thyroid prominence. The right and left superior projections (horns) of the thyroid cartilage connect to the hyoid bone, and the cricothyroid membrane connects the inferior edge to the cricoid cartilage. This latter anatomic relationship is of particular importance when an emergency surgical airway must be obtained (Fig. 4).

Unlike the thyroid cartilage, which does not project posteriorly, the cricoid cartilage is a complete signet-shaped cartilaginous ring

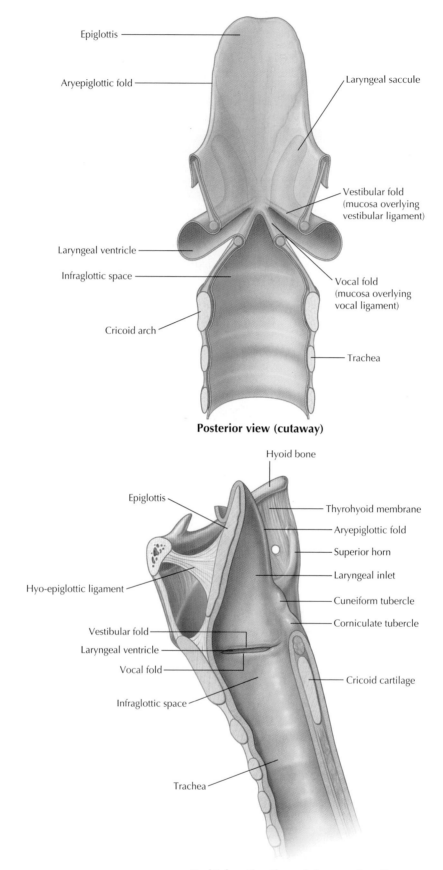

Posterior view (cutaway)

Sagittal section through laryngeal cavity

FIGURE 3   Posterior and lateral views of the laryngeal cavity. *(From Drake RJ, Vogl AW, Mitchell AWM, et al, editors: Gray's atlas of human anatomy. Philadelphia, Churchill Livingstone, 2008.)*

Muscles of the Larynx

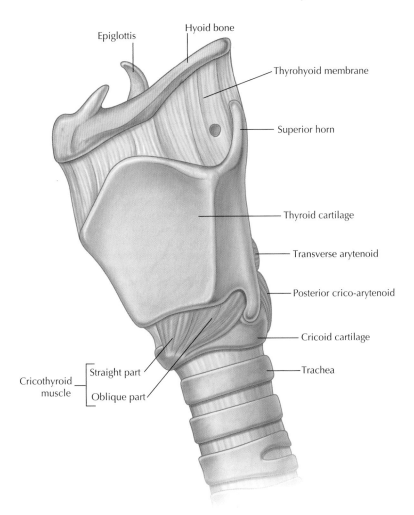

Epiglottis
Hyoid bone
Thyrohyoid membrane
Superior horn
Thyroid cartilage
Transverse arytenoid
Posterior crico-arytenoid
Cricoid cartilage
Trachea
Cricothyroid muscle
Straight part
Oblique part

Lateral view

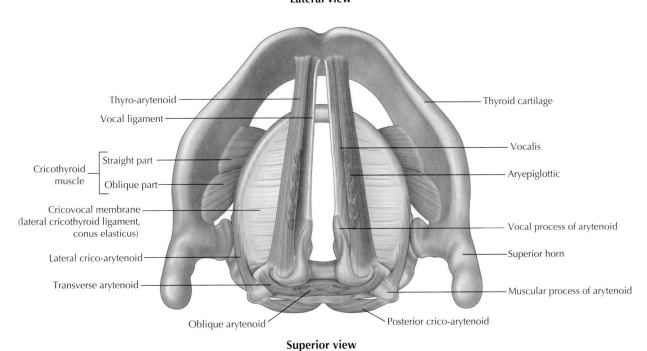

Thyro-arytenoid
Vocal ligament
Cricothyroid muscle
Straight part
Oblique part
Cricovocal membrane
(lateral cricothyroid ligament,
conus elasticus)
Lateral crico-arytenoid
Transverse arytenoid
Oblique arytenoid
Thyroid cartilage
Vocalis
Aryepiglottic
Vocal process of arytenoid
Superior horn
Muscular process of arytenoid
Posterior crico-arytenoid

Superior view

FIGURE 4 Muscular and bony landmarks of the larynx. *(From Drake RJ, Vogl AW, Mitchell AWM, et al, editors: Gray's atlas of human anatomy. Philadelphia, Churchill Livingstone, 2008.)*

connected to both the thyroid cartilage and the first tracheal ring. This anatomic relationship was used by Sellick, who described the prevention of passive regurgitation of gastric contents by posterior pressure on the cricoid cartilage during the induction of general anesthesia, a technique that has since become the accepted standard of care.

The epiglottis is an elastic cartilaginous structure covered by a mucous membrane. The reflection of this mucous membrane forms a slight depression known as the vallecula. It is at this point that the tip of the laryngoscope blade is placed so as to elevate the epiglottis and visualize the vocal cords. The epiglottis is anteriorly attached, superiorly to the hyoid bone by the hypoepiglottic ligament, and inferiorly to the thyroid cartilage by the thyroepiglottic ligament. The quadrangular ligament extends between the lateral aspects of the arytenoid and epiglottic cartilages. Its free inferior edge is the vestibular ligament, and covered with mucosa, it forms the vestibular fold, which lies above the vocal cord (fold) and extends from the thyroid to the arytenoid cartilage. The arytenoids articulate with the superolateral aspect of the cricoid, and each has an anterior vocal cord process that attaches to the vocal cords via the cord ligament. The free superior margin forms the aryepiglottic ligament, and its mucosal covering forms the aryepiglottic fold. It is within the posterior aspects of aryepiglottic folds that the cuneiform and corniculate cartilages can be seen. These cartilages rest on the apex of the arytenoids. Their elastic properties facilitate the return of the arytenoid cartilages to their anatomic position of rest after abduction, and can usually be seen during direct laryngoscopy. They can, therefore, be used as a landmark for the tracheal opening when it is difficult to visualize the vocal cords (Fig. 5).

The glottis is contained within the larynx, and is the narrowest part of the adult airway. It is composed of the vocal cords (or folds) and the space between them is called the rima glottides. Because the true vocal cords are covered by stratified epithelium, they have the characteristic pearly white color when illuminated. The recurrent laryngeal nerves innervate the cords, and the musculature of the larynx receives its innervation from branches of the vagus nerve (cranial nerve X). The larynx is inclusive of the structures noted previously.

The trachea extends from the inferior border of the cricoid cartilage for a variable distance, dividing into the right and left mainstem bronchi at the carina, which anatomically corresponds to the T4-T5 junction posteriorly and the sternal notch anteriorly. Like the thyroid cartilage, the 16 to 20 tracheal cartilages form incomplete C-shaped rings that open posteriorly, allowing for variability in the tracheal diameter needed for normal airway functional changes. The trachea is in direct apposition posteriorly to the esophagus. This may be of significance in patients who have esophageal tumors or mediastinal hematomas (either traumatic or postoperative in origin) or have ingested large foreign bodies. All of these masses can cause upper (tracheal) airway obstruction.

FIGURE 5 Landmarks of the tracheal opening. *(From Putz R, Pabst R, editors: Sobatta atlas of human anatomy, 13th ed. Baltimore, Williams & Wilkins, 2001.)*

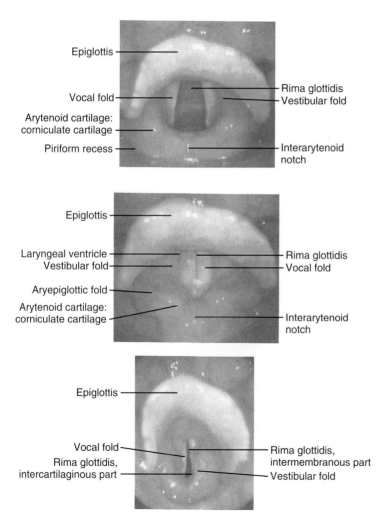

ASSESSING THE AIRWAY

A thorough but rapid initial assessment of the trauma patient begins with the airway and breathing as first priorities. This step must be done with the understanding that, unless the cervical spine has already been "cleared" clinically, every patient has a cervical spine injury until proved otherwise. Breathing and speech are impossible without an intact airway. Simply asking the patient his name is revealing. Lack of response or change in voice because of a compromised airway is immediately apparent and an indication for adjuncts to secure an airway.

Any patients with a Glasgow Coma Scale (GCS) score of 8 or less, regardless of cause, will need to be intubated to protect and secure the airway. Intoxication and use of illicit substances are frequent causes of an altered mental status, as are closed head injuries and hypoxia. One must, therefore, err on the side of caution, and always assume that the depressed GCS score is injury related, and that intubation will be needed to protect the airway. Hoarseness, shortness of breath, carbonaceous sputum, or evidence of external burns to the nares and mouth should alert the clinician that an airway may be in jeopardy even if the patient can respond appropriately. These patients must have careful and frequent interval reevaluations, with a low threshold for intubation. In addition, these patients may pose particularly difficult challenges to intubation, and this situation underscores the need for a rapid and careful assessment of each individual airway.

Patient anatomy, both inherent and as altered by injury, is an important factor that requires careful assessment by the clinician prior to attempting definitive airway management. In the trauma patient, the clinician must always be cognizant of the potential for cervical spine injury. This is particularly important in the patient whose physical examination is compromised by an altered mental status, regardless of the cause. The presence of maxillofacial trauma or injuries of the soft tissues of the neck must also be considered when deciding the best way to secure and protect the airway. In the absence of injury or pathologic conditions, the ability to ventilate and control the supraglottic airway is a function of the size of the airway and the compliance of the supralaryngeal tissues. It should be remembered that under normal conditions, airflow through the nasal cavity is not usually a concern in that this portion of the airway is usually supported by rigid elements in its walls. Conversely, the pharynx does not have a rigid support system, and therefore, it is predisposed to collapse. The most common cause of supralaryngeal obstruction is the tongue in obtunded or comatose patients; usually this problem can initially be dealt with effectively with the use of the oral airway.

A more ominous situation arises when the airway is compromised in the immediate vicinity of the laryngeal inlet because of the size of the base of the tongue or the epiglottis. Airflow in this region will be inversely proportional to the size of these structures, as well as the condition of the perilaryngeal tissues. Restriction of airflow to these areas can come from a number of causes; some of the more common causes are trauma to the neck causing anatomic disruption or tissue edema, prior irradiation to the neck, head and neck tumors, and redundant fatty tissue in the perilaryngeal area secondary to obesity. These conditions may lead to the aforementioned "cannot ventilate, cannot intubate" scenario, a potentially fatal situation for even the most skilled airway personnel.

As with any other medical procedure, it is always prudent to perform a methodical evaluation of the situation, and determine the preferable approach and equipment needed to perform the task efficiently. In addition to factors previously discussed, one must also assess for scarring and fibrosis to the airway and surrounding tissues; injury to the trachea; congenital anomalies; acute inflammatory or neoplastic diseases of the airway; and, finally, gingival, mandibular, and dental anomalies or disease. Short, muscular individuals with very short necks and obese patients tend to be difficult to intubate. Morbidly obese patients can compromise the airway with excessive redundant tissue in the paratonsillar and paraglottic areas, masking visualization and accessibility of the glottis during laryngoscopy. Anatomic factors that should be assessed include mandibular mobility at the temporomandibular joints; mobility of the head at the atlanto-occipital joint (when cervical spine injury has been ruled out); the length, size, and muscularity of the neck; size and configuration of the palate; the proportionate size of the mandible in relation to the face; and the presence of an overbite of the maxillary teeth. Two rapid assessments of these factors can be useful. A thyromental distance of less than 3 fingerbreadths has been shown to be associated with more difficult mask ventilation. Also, the Mallampati score used by anesthesiology in elective cases (see Fig. 1 in "Prehospital Airway Management" located in Part II) has also been shown to be a predictor of difficult direct laryngoscopy.

In order to classify a Mallampati score, the patient is asked to open the mouth as widely as possible and protrude the tongue out as far as possible while seated, with the head in the neutral position, something that is near impossible to accomplish in the trauma setting. However, a clinician familiar with the Mallampati classification can perform a cursory evaluation of the oropharynx using a tongue blade or laryngoscope, which provides the clinician some idea as to the potential for difficulty in intubation. It will also demonstrate the existence of any evidence of injury to the oropharynx and the presence of foreign bodies, blood, or vomitus.

Because one cannot always rely on the anesthesiologist to secure the airway, all clinicians caring for the trauma patient must have the ability to provide immediate and effective airway protection and ventilation. Clinicians must, therefore, be able to recognize limitations to airway access, and must possess techniques to overcome these limitations. Many tools and techniques are available to the anesthesiologist in the elective setting, and although many of them may not be practical in the emergent trauma setting, several can be used, and they will be the focus of the rest of this discussion.

CONTROLLING THE AIRWAY

The best airway is the airway that the patient can safely maintain without any external intervention. The Eastern Association for the Surgery of Trauma has cited the need for emergency tracheal intubation in trauma patients with airway obstruction, hypoventilation, severe hypoxia in spite of supplemental oxygen administration, severe cognitive impairment (GCS score < 8), cardiac arrest, and severe hemorrhagic shock. Once it has been decided that the airway is not adequate, or that the patient is unable to protect the airway, then intubation must be accomplished in a rapid, efficient, and safe manner. It is important to remember that all trauma patients must be intubated with one person maintaining in-line cervical immobilization throughout the procedure to protect the possibly injured cervical spine.

As with all other procedures, a successful outcome depends on the operator's experience and on having immediate access to all of the correct equipment. Most emergency departments have airway carts that contain all of the equipment that will routinely be needed for emergency intubations, as well as specialty carts designed for the "difficult airway." Although the contents of these carts will vary from institution to institution, they will usually be standardized within each hospital.

Once the decision to intubate has been made, all patients should be preoxygenated with 100% oxygen. The jaw thrust and chin lift can be done without endangering the cervical spine, and should be performed in an attempt to open an airway that may be obstructed by the tongue, which tends to fall posteriorly in the obtunded patient. The chin lift technique is accomplished by placing one's fingers under the mandible and gently lifting the mandible upward. The thumb of the same hand is used to depress the lower lip and open the mouth. Care must be taken to prevent hyperextension of the neck while performing the chin lift. The jaw thrust can be performed alone or used in conjunction with bag-valve-mask (BVM) ventilation of the obtunded, but breathing patient, and the respiratory efforts are

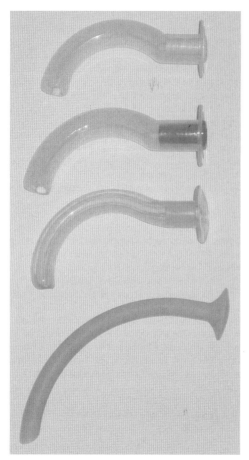

FIGURE 6   Oral airways *(upper three)* and nasal airway.

assisted with compression of the bag. By grasping both mandibular angles and displacing the mandible forward, one is able to simultaneously open the airway and obtain and maintain an effective seal with the mask during assisted bag-mask ventilation. Although this technique is possible to perform with a single operator, it is most effective with two skilled staff members.

Oropharyngeal and nasopharyngeal airways (Fig. 6) are useful, but must be inserted with care, and are contraindicated in severe facial trauma with concern for cribriform plate fractures. Although neither one is well tolerated by the awake patient, the nasopharyngeal airway is better tolerated in the semiresponsive patient, and is less likely to stimulate gagging and vomiting. They can both be used to help maintain a patent upper airway in the obtunded patient. In the adult, the oral airway is inserted with the convexity facing down initially. It must be placed carefully, so that it does not push the tongue posteriorly but, rather, is seated posterior to the tongue, displacing the tongue anteriorly. In children, the oral airway must always be placed with the convex surface facing cephalad initially to avoid injury to the soft tissues of the mouth and pharynx. It is important to remember that in patients with a persistent (intact) upper airway gag reflex, the insertion of the oral airway can precipitate laryngospasm and bronchospasm, as well as coughing, gagging, vomiting, and ultimately, aspiration.

DOCUMENTATION OF PROPER ENDOTRACHEAL TUBE PLACEMENT

Regardless of technique used to secure the airway, it is imperative that proper tube position is confirmed and documented once a definitive airway has been obtained. The best confirmation of proper tube placement is the direct visualization of the tube passing through the vocal cords during laryngoscopy. Because this is not always the case, tube placement can be rapidly but tentatively confirmed by physical examination. Observation and auscultation of the chest is a valuable clinical tool. In the absence of chest wall disruption due to rib fractures, the clinician will see symmetrical chest wall motion upon ventilation with appropriate tube placement.

Auscultation of the chest is done both anteriorly and in the axillae, and is useful when breath sounds are heard bilaterally and are equal. This is not always the case, even with appropriate tube placement, because of the presence of pneumothoraces or hemothoraces seen in the trauma patient population. It is incumbent on the clinician to immediately treat the pneumothorax and hemothorax, and then confirm tube thoracostomy placement by both physical examination and chest radiograph. Auscultation over the left upper quadrant of the abdomen is important; with appropriate placement of the endotracheal tube, there will be no gurgling in the stomach during ventilation.

Cyanosis as an indicator of a fall in oxygen concentration is a late event, and is influenced by factors such as room lighting, anemia, and hemoglobin anomalies. Resolution of hypoxia is a reliable sign of proper tube placement, but minutes may elapse before a patient shows desaturation by pulse oximetry, especially in patients who have been properly preoxygenated. Identification of carbon dioxide (CO_2) in exhaled gas has become the standard for verification of appropriate placement of an endotracheal tube in the elective or emergent setting. This can be accomplished with capnography (the instantaneous display of the CO_2 waveform during ventilation), which is the measurement of CO_2 in the expired gas. Colorimetric CO_2 detectors have become the standard in most institutions due to the ease of use and rapid availability. Colorimetric CO_2 detectors are routinely inserted into the respiratory circuit between the end of the endotracheal tube and the ventilator tubing or Ambu-bag, and will detect the presence of CO_2 as soon as ventilation begins after intubation. A change in color signifies the presence of CO_2 in the exhaled gas. It must be remembered that although useful, the presence of CO_2 is not, by itself, absolute assurance of proper tube placement. The endotracheal tube could be improperly positioned in a mainstem bronchus and one would still detect CO_2. CO_2 will not be detected in patients who are in cardiac arrest. In patients who have been actively ventilated prior to intubation, CO_2 can be detected in gas from the stomach when the endotracheal tube is improperly placed in the esophagus. This will clear with several breaths, however, and indicate to the clinician that the tube is improperly placed.

The cuffed portion of the endotracheal tube should be at least 1 to 2 cm below the cords, and in the average patient, the endotracheal tube will be taped in position at the 21- to 23-cm mark at the teeth. Lastly, a chest radiograph should be performed to confirm proper placement of the endotracheal tube after every intubation. The tip of an appropriately placed endotracheal tube should be visible on chest radiograph approximately 5 cm above the carina in the average adult.

Even with all of the equipment and technical advances available to the clinician, clinical judgment, the physical examination, and attention to detail are essential in management of the airway.

COMBITUBE

The inability to intubate can be a fatal event due to the hypoxia resulting from the inability to ventilate and, therefore, oxygenate the critically ill or injured patient. There are certain "rescue" techniques available, and one such technique involves the use of the dual lumen esophagotracheal tube, known as the Combitube (Tyco Healthcare Group LP, 2001). This tube, which comes in a regular and small adult size, has minimized the problems that had been seen with the use of the esophageal obturator airway as an airway rescue technique. Although Wissler recommends using the laryngoscope for placement of the tube under direct vision, the tube can be inserted blindly through the mouth.

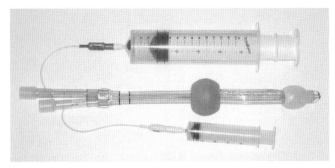

FIGURE 7 Combitube with both balloons inflated. Larger syringe inflates the blue tube (No. 1) balloon.

Although the tip of the tube can end up in the trachea, it will enter the esophagus 99% of the time. Once the tube is successfully placed, the balloons are inflated with air, 100 mL in the pharyngeal balloon to occlude the pharynx, and 15 mL in the distal balloon occluding either the esophagus or the trachea. Ventilation is now begun using tube no. 1. If the tip of the tube is positioned in the esophagus (the preferred position), one will hear breath sounds bilaterally, capnography will be positive for CO_2, and auscultation over the left upper quadrant of the abdomen will be negative for gastric insufflation. At this point, a gastric tube can be placed through tube no. 2 (Fig. 7).

If the tip of the tube is in the trachea, no breath sounds will be heard in the chest, and capnography will be negative for CO_2. Ventilation should immediately be switched to tube no. 2, and the examination repeated to confirm breath sounds by auscultation and CO_2 by capnography.

The Combitube has been shown to be an effective alternative to prehospital cricothyroidotomy after failed rapid-sequence intubation (RSI) attempts in patients with severe maxillofacial trauma. In fact, Blostein et al studied 10 such patients who failed in-field intubation. The Combitube was successfully replaced in hospital by an orotracheal tube in 7 of the 10 patients, and only 3 required a surgical airway. It must be remembered that the Combitube must be replaced with a definitive airway as soon as the clinical situation permits. Furthermore, it should be remembered that contraindications to use of a Combitube include patients who: (1) are younger than 16 years, (2) are responsive with an intact gag reflex, (3) have known esophageal disease, and (4) have a known ingestion of a caustic substance. Although the Combitube remains an important adjunct to endotracheal intubation in the field, the use of the Combitube in the trauma bay remains limited.

ENDOTRACHEAL INTUBATION

In the adult, the placement of a cuffed tube within the tracheal lumen is considered to be a secure airway. This definitive airway can be achieved nasally, orally, or surgically (cricothyroidotomy or tracheostomy). The level of urgency for airway control and the skill set of the clinician will determine the indication for each of these techniques.

Nasal Intubation

Nasal intubation is a well-accepted technique for intubation in the obtunded patient, but the patient must be spontaneously breathing and not in extremis. Most trauma patients have contraindications to nasal intubation. Because injured patients are often in extremis in conjunction with depressed neurologic status and the possibility of occult and as yet unrecognized facial bony fractures, nasal intubation is rarely performed on the multiple-injured trauma patient. Additionally, because most trauma patients have not been fasting, and are at risk for vomiting and aspiration, intubation is most often performed using the RSI technique. This technique renders the patient apneic, and nasal intubation is therefore contraindicated.

Orotracheal Intubation

Orotracheal intubation is the mainstay for definitive airway control in the emergent setting. When performed by an anesthesiologist in the elective setting, orotracheal intubation is completed with the patient's head in extension, the so-called "sniffing position." In the trauma patient with a potential cervical spine injury, extension of the neck is contraindicated. It is important to remember that in the trauma population, orotracheal intubation is a *two-person* procedure, with one person performing the intubation and a second person maintaining constant in-line cervical spine immobilization.

Trauma patients who require intubation often have a variety of anatomic and physiologic derangements that make intubation difficult. These patients frequently have varying degrees of hypoxia, acidosis, and hemodynamic instability. Compromised cardiac or pulmonary function, especially in the elderly patient, further increases the risk of myocardial or cerebral ischemia when attempts at intubation are prolonged. Associated conditions related to the traumatic event, such as intracranial hypertension, myocardial dysfunction, upper airway bleeding, inhalation injury, and vomiting can actually be exacerbated by the physical manipulation of the oropharynx required to intubate the patient. These factors necessitated the development of a standardized approach when emergency intubation is warranted. The advent of RSI has provided this standardized approach to those caring for the critically ill patient.

RSI is the near simultaneous administration of an induction agent (sedative, anxiolytic, amnesic) and a paralyzing dose of a neuromuscular blocking agent (NMBA). The goal of RSI is to obtain a secure airway while avoiding complications such as vomiting and aspiration, cardiac arrhythmias, or the reflex sympathetic response caused by laryngoscopy. Relative contraindications include those situations in which BVM ventilation will most likely be ineffective or impossible. When used appropriately, RSI has been shown to decrease complications associated with intubation while increasing the intubation success rate to 98%. The most commonly used RSI medications include lidocaine, the induction agent midazolam or etomidate, and the NMBA succinylcholine or rocuronium. See Table 1 for a summary of the depolarizing and nondepolarizing neuromuscular paralytic agents.

Lidocaine is commonly used to decrease the hypertensive response and airway reactivity of laryngoscopy, to minimize intracranial hypertension, and to decrease the incidence of cardiac arrhythmias during intubation. To be effective, however, 1.5 mg/kg should be administered intravenously 3 minutes prior to oropharynx manipulation.

Induction agents will facilitate intubation by rapidly rendering the patient unconscious. Both midazolam and etomidate are rapidly effective and have a similar elimination half-life. Given parenterally, midazolam (1–2.5 mg/kg) has a greater propensity to precipitate hypotension and myocardial depression. Conversely, etomidate (0.15–0.3 mg/kg) does not affect blood pressure, and has a cerebral protective effect in that it reduces cerebral blood flow and cerebral oxygen uptake. It is, therefore, favored for use in the trauma patient with hypotension.

Succinylcholine, a depolarizing agent, is the most commonly used NMBA. It has a rapid onset (30–60 seconds) and relatively short duration of effect (5–15 minutes) that will allow for effective return of spontaneous ventilation after 9 to 10 minutes. About 10 to 15 seconds after administration of succinylcholine, fasciculations occur that are associated with brief increase in intracranial, intraocular, and intragastric pressures. However, the potential increase in intracranial pressure is so small that its effects are outweighed and offset by the avoidance of hypoxia seen with an improved success rate of intubation. Succinylcholine cannot be used in patients with penetrating globe injuries, pseudocholinesterase deficiency, any history of myopathy, or muscular dystrophy. In addition, patients who have or are at risk for hyperkalemia, such as patients with thermal (burn) injuries more than 24 hours old, or crush syndromes with myonecrosis/rhabdomyolysis,

TABLE 1: Depolarizing and Nondepolarizing Agents

Agent	Dose
Depolarizing Agents	
Ultrashort (<10–12 minutes)	
Succinylcholine	1.5 mg/kg
Nondepolarizing Agents	
Short acting (15–20 minutes)	
Mivacurium	0.2 mg/kg
Intermediate (20–50 minutes)	
Vecuronium	0.08–0.1 mg/kg
Rocuronium	0.6–1.2 mg/kg
Atracurium	0.5–0.5 mg/kg
Cisatracurium	0.15–0.2 mg/kg
Long acting (>50 minutes)	
Pancuronium	0.06–0.1 mg/kg
Pipecuronium	0.07–0.1 mg/kg
Metocurine	0.2–0.4 mg/kg
Doxacurium	0.05 mg/kg
Gallamine	1 mg/kg (max 100 mg)
Alcuronium	0.2–0.3 mg/kg
Tubocurarine	0.5–0.6 mg/kg

Modified from Miller RD: *Miller's Anesthesia,* 7th ed. Philadelphia, Elsevier, 2010, and consulting editors, Micromedex 2.0 5/2/2012.

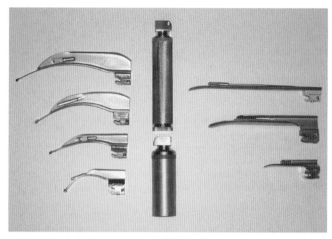

FIGURE 8 *Left,* Macintosh curved blades (from top to bottom, nos. 4, 3, 2, and 1). *Center,* Laryngoscope handles. *Right,* Miller straight blades (from top to bottom nos. 3, 2, and 0).

In the comatose and apneic patient, no medication is needed, and the patient can be intubated upon laryngoscopic visualization of the cords. Several different laryngoscope blades are available (Fig. 8). The appropriate shape and size should be selected for intubation. The laryngoscope is inserted into the mouth with care taken not to injure the lips or teeth. The blade of the laryngoscope is advanced posteriorly, sweeping the tongue upward and to the left. Once the tonsillar pillars are visualized, the tip of the blade is placed into the vallecula, exposing the larynx and the triangular glottic opening, which is formed and bordered by the vocal cords. If the epiglottis is seen to overhang the larynx, the blade is advanced farther into the vallecula, exposing the cords. Once the cords are visualized, the endotracheal tube is gently placed through the cords into the trachea. The use of an endotracheal tube stylette is common, but not mandatory. Endotracheal tubes vary in size, and are sized based on the patient. Historically, children were intubated using uncuffed endotracheal tubes, but according to the new recommendations from PALS for the in-hospital setting, children should have cuffed tubes placed. In the adult, the cuffed tube size will be determined by the size of the opening between the cords. Most adults will tolerate an endotracheal tube with an internal diameter of 7, 7.5, or 8 mm, placed to a depth of about 21 to 24 cm at the lip. In the child, the endotracheal tube should be cuffed, and about the same size as the child's nostril or little (fifth) digit of the hand. Placement should not be any further than 2 cm past the cords. The endotracheal tube should never be forced through the cords, but rather, should be gently guided through the glottis (Fig. 9).

Securing a difficult airway can be a frightening obstacle. Complications related to hemodynamic alterations, as well as difficulties in

or poorly compliant dialysis patients should not receive succinylcholine. Rocuronium, a nondepolarizing NMBA, also has a short onset of action (30–60 seconds) after a dose of 1.0 mg/kg, but a longer recovery time to spontaneous respiration (45–60 minutes) than succinylcholine. It does not have any of the deleterious side effects of succinylcholine, and according to Perry et al, the success of intubation is similar with rocuronium and succinylcholine under all study conditions.

RSI can be used in the pediatric patient, but dosing is different from that recommended in the patient over age 10 years. Pediatric patients have increased vagal tone and a decreased functional residual capacity. Bradycardia during intubation can result from both vagal stimulation and hypoxia. In addition, succinylcholine can cause bradycardia in the pediatric population. It is recommended that each institution develop an RSI protocol for pediatric patients based on the Pediatric Advanced Life Support course (PALS) recommendation and a combination of weight based or Breslow sizing for medication dosing.

Intubation ideally is preceded by preoxygenation with 100% oxygen by mask until the So_2 by pulse oximetry is either at 100% or has reached a maximal level. BVM ventilation can be used to assist the breathing patient, and is used to control the airway in the apneic patient prior to intubation. The direct cricoid pressure known as the Sellick maneuver should be performed whenever possible to reduce the possibility of aspiration. The stomach may be insufflated during BVM ventilation, and an orogastric or nasogastric tube must be inserted immediately after successful intubation.

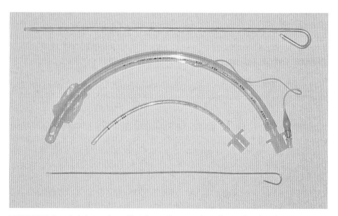

FIGURE 9 Adult and pediatric stylets and endotracheal tubes.

oxygenation and ventilation, have been shown to be significant issues in the patient population requiring emergent intubation outside the elective operating room (OR) setting. One study has shown that difficult intubations requiring more than three attempts account for almost 10% of all out-of-OR intubations, and that airway-related and hemodynamic-related complications were "relatively common." This points to the fact that anyone dealing with the emergent airway must always have a secondary or backup plan. These rescue plans should include the Combitube (discussed earlier), flexible bougies, laryngeal mask airways (LMAs), intubating LMAs, glidescope video laryngoscopy (GVL), and finally, the emergency cricothyroidotomy. In addition, whenever possible, additional assistance by those proficient in intubation must be readily available if one hopes to avoid complications that include death when dealing with the difficult airway.

Adjuncts to Orotracheal Intubation

GVL has become more predominant in the emergent airway over the past several years. This rigid indirect video laryngoscopy has been shown to increase success of orotracheal intubation using laryngoscopy (Fig. 10). Studies have shown that the glidescope has successful intubation rates of 94% to 97% even as a rescue technique for failed direct laryngoscopy. And although studies have not shown increased success rates with intubation in patients with cervical spine immobilization, it does produce favorable laryngoscopic views.

Although the glidescope does allow for a two-hand technique in which the endotracheal tube is placed through the cords, it also allows for a second hand to suction and clear the posterior pharynx. In addition, the speed at which the equipment is set up makes this technique more effective in a trauma scenario than flexible fiberoptic bronchoscopy. Although the glidescope clearly offers superior views and an additional tool in the arsenal of airway techniques, massive facial trauma with significant blood and fluid in the oropharynx is a contraindication to its use because any substance that obscures the camera lens will render this technique ineffective.

Bougies are semirigid, gum-elastic stylette-like devices with a bent tip. They should be a standard piece of equipment on any difficult airway cart, and should be immediately available whenever a difficult airway is anticipated. They are used most often when only the arytenoids or the epiglottis can be visualized. During laryngoscopy or GVL, the bougie is advanced into the larynx, through the cords, and into the trachea. As the bougie moves down the trachea, the tip of the bougie rubs against the tracheal rings. This is transmitted

up the bougie and one can experience what has been referred to as the "washboard effect." Care must be exercised so as not to advance the bougie too far; this has the possibility of creating a bronchial injury. Once in position, the bougie is maintained in position by one clinician as a second clinician advances a lubricated endotracheal tube over the bougie, through the cords, and into position in the trachea under laryngoscopic visualization (whenever possible). The bougie is then removed, and the steps to confirm endotracheal tube placement are performed as mentioned earlier (Fig. 11).

Originally introduced by Brain in 1983, the LMA is now routinely used for airway management in the elective anesthesia setting. The LMA (Laryngeal Mask Company, Ltd.) and the LMA Fastrach are also now becoming valuable additions to the armamentarium of emergency airway management, although less commonly used (Fig. 12).

The LMA is a large-bore tube that is attached to an ovoid or elliptical silicone cuff that, once well lubricated, is inserted blindly into the airway as far as it will go. Once properly positioned, and the cuff is inflated with 20 to 30 mL of air, the leading edge or tip of the cuff will obstruct the esophageal lumen and the cuff provides a low-pressure seal around the entrance to the larynx, allowing for ventilation in an emergent setting. It is important to remember that the LMA will not be well tolerated in any patient with an existing gag reflex, and may precipitate vomiting and aspiration in these patients. The LMA comes in several sizes, and can be used in the pediatric and adult populations. As with endotracheal intubation, successful insertion will require the appropriate size selection. Indications for the emergent placement of the LMA in trauma patients include a GCS score of 3 after rapid-sequence drug administration and attempted orotracheal intubation has failed; once the ventilation has been established, a more definitive airway must be obtained.

Although the LMA has been used to secure the airway in the trauma patient, it is, indeed, more suited for elective airway management situations. The LMA Fastrach (Fig. 13), or intubating LMA, on the other hand, has been shown to be effective when used in the trauma center setting. The pharyngeal orifice of the LMA Fastrach is different from that of the regular LMA (Figs. 13 and 14), and it allows the passage of a specifically designed and compatible endotracheal tube once the LMA Fastrach is appropriately placed. The maximal size endotracheal tube that the LMA Fastrach will allow is an 8-mm internal diameter. As with the LMA, the LMA Fastrach is placed in trauma patients when attempts to place an orotracheal tube with RSI have failed, the patient has a GCS score of 3, and an airway must be controlled immediately. Placement of the intubating

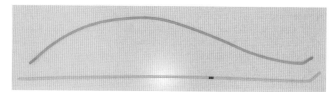

FIGURE 11 Semirigid gum-elastic bougies.

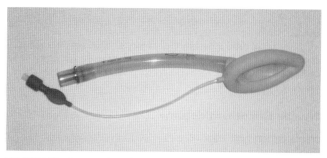

FIGURE 12 Laryngeal mask airway.

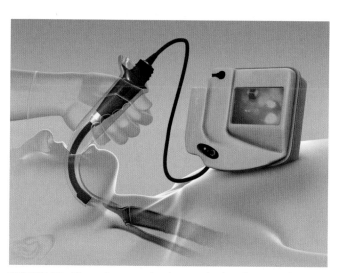

FIGURE 10 Illustrative example of orotracheal intubation with glidescope. *(Used with permission © Verathor Inc.)*

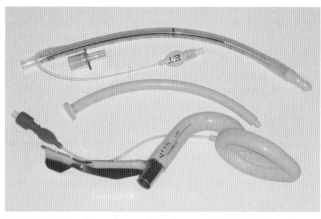

FIGURE 13 Intubating laryngeal mask airway (LMA). LMA-specific endotracheal tube *(top)*, stylet *(middle)*, and intubating LMA with intubating handle *(bottom)*.

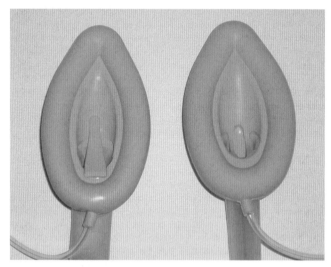

FIGURE 14 Pharyngeal orifices of the intubating laryngeal mask airway (LMA) *(left)* and regular LMA *(right)*.

LMA is done in the same manner as with the LMA, but passage of the endotracheal tube is usually done as a two-person technique, with one person controlling the LMA and a second passing the very well lubricated endotracheal tube. Once placement of the endotracheal tube is confirmed, the LMA can carefully be removed while maintaining the position of the endotracheal tube.

SURGICAL AIRWAY

The preferred method of management of the airway is by the patient with minimal assistance from the physician. The clinician can monitor the flow of air into the airway and observe any difficulty in ventilation. Unfortunately, this is not always possible.

Once any of the aforementioned airway adjuncts have been unsuccessfully attempted and the patient has an unprotected airway and cannot be ventilated, a surgical approach to the airway is indicated.

Needle Cricothyroidotomy

Needle cricothyroidotomy is a rapid, effective, and safe method of gaining access directly into the airway through the cricothyroid membrane. The advantages of this procedure are that it is relatively easy to use and requires minimal equipment. It bypasses obstructions at the level of the cords and allows for direct air entry into the tracheobronchial tree.

The disadvantages are that even a large-caliber needle is insufficient to adequately ventilate the patient for more than a few minutes. This method of airway control is designed to provide some oxygenation for a patient with inability to ventilate until a more formal surgical airway can be obtained.

Unfortunately, even though high-flow oxygen can be delivered through a 14-G or larger needle, there is minimal ability to exhale. Carbon monoxide levels rise and the ability to deliver oxygen to the alveoli is compromised.

Procedure

A syringe with a 14-G needle is obtained. A Y-connector is obtained and oxygen is attached to one branch of the Y. The other branch of the Y can be occluded with a finger to allow oxygen to flow into the trachea. The chest is then observed to rise with inspiration. Removing the occluding finger can effect expiration. The larynx is palpated and the inferior border of the larynx is identified. The cricothyroid cartilage is then identified as the first cartilaginous structure inferior to the larynx. The space between the larynx and the cricothyroid is the cricothyroid membrane (see Fig. 4). This is palpated with a finger and the needle is attached to the syringe with 2 mL of fluid inside and is advanced at a 45-degree angle through the skin, the cricothyroid membrane, and into the lumen of the trachea. As the needle is inserted, gentle retraction on the syringe should occur. As soon as the needle "pops" through the cricothyroid membrane, there should be a gentle bubble of air within the 2 mL of fluid in the syringe. Air should flow easily into the syringe. The needle should then be withdrawn from the sheath and the cannulae secured in place. The oxygen line is then connected with the Y-connector to the barrel of the cannulae. Oxygen can then be delivered through the tubing directly into the trachea. By removing one's finger from one branch of the Y-connector, CO_2 can be vented from the endobronchial tree. Oxygen should be delivered at a high flow rate of 10 to 12 L/minute. Oxygenation and ventilation can occur only for minutes until a more definite, larger gauge airway is secured.

Cricothyroidotomy

A formal cricothyroidotomy has considerable advantages over a needle cricothyroidotomy. A large cannula can be introduced through the cricothyroid membrane and adequate ventilation can then occur. The advantages are similar to the needle cricothyroidotomy in that the anatomy is easy to identify and the procedure is relatively easy to perform. The disadvantages are that this otomy is too superior in the neck to be a long-term airway. For this reason, a cricothyroidotomy is to be used as a temporary measure until a tracheostomy can be performed in a controlled setting.

Procedure

The larynx is identified in the midline and the cricothyroid ring is also identified. The diamond-shaped cricothyroid membrane is palpated between both of these structures. It is essential to stay in the midline, as the midline is avascular. As the operator moves laterally, there is an opportunity to encounter the anterior jugular veins and the major vessels and nerves in the neck. The medial strap muscles are just lateral to the midline. Although it has been written that it is preferable to make a horizontal incision directly over the cricothyroid membrane, in the emergent situation this can lead to significant venous injury and profuse bleeding that can obscure visualization. As such, a vertical incision provides a safer approach and should be the preferred approach for cricothyroidotomy in the emergent situation. The incision should be 1 to 2 cm in length. It is carried through the skin and subcutaneous tissue and the platysma. As soon as the platysma is entered, a finger is introduced and the cricothyroid membrane is identified digitally (see Fig. 4). A transverse incision is made with the scalpel through the cricothyroid membrane and into the trachea. The scalpel blade is used to make a small nick in the cricothyroid membrane in the midline. The handle of the scalpel is then turned perpendicular to the vertical incision and placed into the lumen of the trachea through the tiny defect in the membrane described in the previous step. The handle is then rolled through 90 degrees. Alternatively, a Halsted's mosquito clamp can be used to spread the cricothyroid membrane horizontally and then longitudinally. This provides a generous otomy directly into the trachea. This scalpel handle technique is useful because there is a blood vessel at each lateral aspect of the cricothyroid membrane and it is preferable to perform a blunt dissection of the cricothyroid membrane. A no. 4, and certainly no larger than a no. 6, tracheostomy tube can then be inserted directly through the cricothyroid membrane into the trachea. If no tracheostomy tubes are available, a no. 6 endotracheal tube may be inserted.

If the anatomy is distorted or if there is significant injury with a hematoma to this area, it is wise to pass a Robinson red rubber tube through the cricothyroid membrane into the trachea. The tracheostomy tube can then be advanced over the red rubber catheter. This will avoid creating a false passage or creating trauma to the trachea itself. Once the tracheostomy tube is in the trachea, the patient is then ventilated via the tracheostomy tube. It is imperative to secure this tube with a suture fixation. Confirmation of tube placement should occur as described in the orotracheal intubation section of this chapter.

Emergency Surgical Tracheostomy

This procedure should be reserved for life-threatening situations. It is indicated rarely. One of its indications is the uncommon cricotracheal separation often resulting from clothesline injuries. It is preferable to use any of the aforementioned airway adjuncts to gain control of the airway and adequately oxygenate the patient prior to performing an emergency tracheostomy. A vertical incision should be made for all emergency life-threatening tracheostomies when time is of the essence.

Procedure

The trachea is identified below the thyroid cartilage and cricothyroid cartilage and controlled with one hand. An incision is made and carried down through the skin and platysma. Once the platysma is opened, it is essential that all dissection be performed in the midline. This will avoid the anterior jugular veins and the medial strap muscles. A dissection should be carried down to the trachea under direct vision. It is preferable to use a blunt clamp for dissection and then use the tip of the finger to identify the tracheal rings. If the isthmus of the thyroid is palpated on the surface of the trachea, it should be retracted cephalad and the trachea then identified. The membrane between the tracheal ring should be opened with a cruciate incision for a distance of approximately 1 cm. A 2.0 Prolene suture should be placed in the lateral aspects of the trachea and left as a long retractor suture. The lumen of the trachea should be identified and a red rubber catheter introduced to ensure that there is no false passage. This is particularly important if there is an injury to the trachea and there is blood or mucosal hemorrhage in the trachea. The tracheostomy tube is then

introduced into the tracheostomy and the obturator removed and replaced with the inner cannula. Ventilation should then occur. The tracheostomy tube should then be secured in place and the Prolene sutures should be brought out through the superior aspect of the wound and left in situ. This technique is extremely useful in the event there is dislodgement of the tracheostomy tube.

Management of Airway When Neck Is Lacerated

Lacerations to the anterior and lateral neck may involve the airway. It is essential to obtain a history as to how the laceration occurred. Whether this injury was a knife wound or an impaled object from a motor vehicle crash or a fall has different implications. An impaling object has the ability to create an injury to the cervical spine and spinal cord, and therefore, the neck has to be treated as if there were a potential injury to the spinal column. This requires stabilization of the neck.

In the event of a knife laceration in an assault, it is highly unlikely that there would be injury to the bony elements of the spinal cord and therefore, spinal cord injury is not a major factor.

The wound should be inspected for obvious pulsatile or nonpulsatile hemorrhage. Direct, focused digital pressure should be applied to pulsatile arterial hemorrhage to control the hemorrhage. If the bleeding is nonpulsatile dark venous blood, it is important to remember that major venous injuries can precipitate air embolism by sucking air into the deep venous system and into the heart. This results in air embolism into the main pulmonary artery. An air lock is then created and pulmonary perfusion is significantly compromised.

There are major nerves in association with the vascular structures in the neck, and therefore blindly placing clamps into the wound should be avoided. Hemorrhage control should be either under direct vision or by a noncrushing clamp.

The wound should be palpated for crepitus. Air in the wound is a harbinger of an injury to the airway or the esophagus. Both of these structures would need to be identified and any injury dealt with in the operating room. The airway should be controlled either with an endotracheal tube or with a surgical airway. Once the airway is adequately controlled and the patient is effectively ventilated, then the patient should be transferred to the operating room for definitive control of hemorrhage and an evaluation of the aerodigestive tree through external visualization, endoscopy, or a combination of both in the operating room. The appropriate repair should then be carried out.

SUMMARY

Management of the airway in the trauma patient continues to be the most important lifesaving event in the management of the severely injured and dying patient. It is essential that all surgeons are aware of the noninvasive and invasive methods of managing the airway. Identifying those patients who will not be able to be managed by conventional airway techniques is critical. It is very important to determine when to proceed to a surgical airway and to be aware of the landmarks and potential pitfalls of obtaining an emergent surgical airway. Mastering all of these techniques and procedures will facilitate the emergent management of the severely injured patient's airway.

For the chapter's Suggested Readings list, please visit the book at www.ExpertConsult.inkling.com.

RESUSCITATION FLUIDS

Ron Barbosa, Brandon Tieu, Laszlo Kiraly, Michael Englehart, Martin Schreiber, and Susan Rowell

Fluids have been given intravenously since the 1600s. Slow progress was made after William Harvey provided a modern description of the circulatory system in 1638. William O'Shaughnessy theorized that patients suffering from volume loss secondary to cholera would benefit from restoration of blood to its natural specific gravity by replacing its "deficient saline." This became the first concept of contemporary intravenous (IV) fluid therapy. Thomas Latta was credited with applying O'Shaughnessy's theory and treating victims of cholera in 1832. Later in the 19th century, Sydney Ringer described a physiologic solution with a focus on electrolyte concentrations in his animal models. Hartman modified this solution by the addition of lactate as a buffer. Many of these concepts were criticized and largely forgotten until the 20th century. The advent of modern surgery was associated with increased recognition of the importance of maintaining intravascular volume and led to investigation of the use of IV fluids for that purpose.

World War I provided tremendous experience with resuscitation of hemorrhagic shock. Walter Cannon's work eloquently described the natural history and presentation of shock with primary accounts of battlefield victims. His work suggested that a delay in surgical control of bleeding was accompanied by a large increase in fatality. Furthermore, he indicated that aggressive resuscitation without surgical control could worsen hemorrhagic shock. He also indicated that resuscitation with saline could worsen existing acidosis. In subsequent decades, however, much of his work was forgotten or ignored. Then in World War II and the Korean War, practice shifted to resuscitation with plasma and blood. Blalock supported this based on his dog studies, suggesting that crystalloid fluids were rapidly lost from the intravascular space. In 1963, Shires showed that shock is accompanied by a shift of interstitial fluid into the vasculature. This discovery brought renewed interest in salt solution therapy (Table 1). Subsequent decades have been characterized by further optimization in aggressive resuscitation. Specific gains have been made in the realm of intensive care, monitoring, IV access, and end points of resuscitation. Despite these advances, many controversies and questions remain. Choice of fluid has remained controversial. The study of the mechanism of shock has provided a vast amount of information at the cellular and molecular level, but this has yet to translate into a directly applicable clinical treatment. More importantly, the complications of modern resuscitation are commonly seen in trauma intensive care units (ICUs).

CHOICE OF FLUIDS

The use of crystalloids versus colloids has been an ongoing debate for decades (Fig. 1). In the Vietnam War, isotonic crystalloids were used when laboratory work from the 1960s by Shires and others showed larger volume resuscitation with isotonic crystalloids resulted in the best survival. They noted that extracellular fluid redistributed into both intravascular and intracellular spaces during shock, and rapid correction of this extracellular deficit required an infusion of a 3:1 ratio of crystalloid fluid to blood loss. Using this resuscitation strategy, the overall rate of mortality and the rate of acute renal failure decreased but a new entity of shock lung, now better known as acute respiratory distress syndrome, was encountered.

There are a number of theoretic advantages to the use of colloids for fluid resuscitation. Colloids increase the plasma volume and oncotic pressure immediately after being given. It has been commonly assumed that this effect lasts for a clinically significant amount of time, but recent animal studies have suggested that this effect might be short lived, and that colloid molecules may diffuse into the extravascular space within seconds of administration. It has also been commonly assumed that administration of colloids leads to less tissue edema than with crystalloids. This has never been verified in the clinical setting, and recent clinical trials show that extravascular fluid volume and requirement for mechanical ventilation are equivalent after administration of colloid or crystalloid.

Colloids have been compared to crystalloids in a large number of clinical studies in various patient populations over the last few decades. Many studies are difficult to interpret owing to small number and methodologic flaws. In the last several years, however, several high-quality randomized trials and metaanalyses have been conducted in this area. The Saline versus Albumin Fluid Evaluation (SAFE) study randomized 6997 ICU patients to receive 4% albumin or normal saline (NS). The study population was heterogeneous and included 43% surgical patients and 17.4% trauma patients. Physicians were blinded and were allowed to determine the rate and amount of fluid infusion depending on the clinical circumstances. There were no

TABLE 1: Composition of Balanced Salt Solutions (mEq/L)

Solutions	Glucose (g/L)	Na^+	Cl^-	NCO_3^-	K^+	Ca^{2+}	Mg^{2+}	HPO_4^-	NH_4^+
Extracellular fluid	1000	140	102	27	4.2	5	3	3	0.3
5% dextrose and water	50								
0.21% sodium chloride (0.25 NS)		34	34						
0.45% sodium chloride (0.5 NS)		77	77						
0.9% sodium chloride (NS)		154	154						
3% sodium chloride (HS)		513	513						
7.5% sodium chloride (HS)		1283	1283						
Lactated Ringer's solution		130	109	28*	4	2.7			

HS, hypertonic saline; NS, normal saline.

*Present in solution as lactate, but is metabolized to bicarbonate.

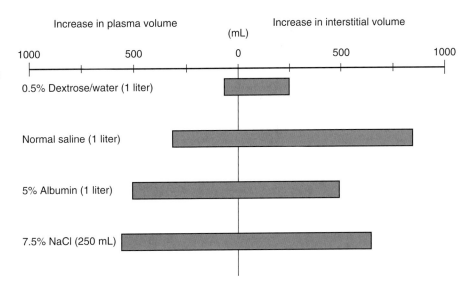

FIGURE 1 The influence of colloid and crystalloid fluids on the volume of the extracellular fluid compartments. *(Data from Imm A, Carlson RW: Fluid resuscitation in circulatory shock. Crit Care Clin 9:313, 1993.)*

significant differences in mortality rate, ICU days, days of mechanical ventilation, or days of renal replacement therapy. The SAFE investigators later performed a post hoc analysis of the patients with traumatic brain injury (TBI) in the original cohort and found that the use of albumin significantly increased mortality rate. Among patients with severe TBI, 41.8% of the patients in the albumin group died versus 22.2% in the saline group. Because there was no difference in resuscitation end points between groups, it was hypothesized that vasogenic or cytotoxic cerebral edema might be exacerbated by albumin.

A recent Cochrane Collaboration metaanalysis examined randomized controlled trials in critically ill patients receiving colloid or crystalloid for resuscitation and found no advantage to the use of colloid. Albumin, hydroxyethyl starch, modified gelatin, and dextran were each examined individually and in each case the relative mortality risk for patients receiving colloid was between 0.91 and 1.24. Other metaanalyses have either shown no benefit to the use of colloids or have suggested that some patient populations may have a worse outcome. Other possible disadvantages are an increased incidence of allergic reactions and renal failure (dextrans), altered platelet function (dextrans, hetastarches), hyperchloremic acidosis (hetastarch), and greater expense. In summary, there is no clinical evidence to support giving colloid products over crystalloid solutions for fluid resuscitation.

The choice of crystalloid has also been a source of controversy over the years. NS has been commonly used for fluid resuscitation in trauma patients. NS is composed of 154 mEq/L of sodium and 154 mEq/L of chloride. It has been chosen by some trauma systems in part because of the concern that lactated Ringer's (LR) solution may lead to clotting of blood filters when given with red blood cell (RBC) transfusions. NS also has higher osmolarity than LR solution and therefore has a potential benefit in patients with severe brain injuries. However, large volume resuscitation with NS can lead to hyperchloremic metabolic acidosis. Studies in elective surgical patients showed that patients receiving NS required more bicarbonate and had lower pH values after surgery than those receiving LR solution.

Ringer's solution was originally developed by Sydney Ringer after laboratory experiments involving isolated frog hearts suspended in sodium chloride became contaminated with inorganic salts, and it was noticed that potassium and calcium increased contractility. The solution was later modified by Hartman by the addition of sodium lactate and is now known as lactated Ringer's solution. Use of LR solution for fluid resuscitation avoids the hyperchloremic metabolic acidosis that can result from NS. Clinical trials in elective surgical patients suggest that use of LR solution may lead to less blood loss compared to NS. Animal models of uncontrolled hemorrhagic

shock show that LR solution resuscitation leads to less blood loss and more favorable effects on extravascular lung water index compared to resuscitation with NS.

LR solution is not approved by the American Association of American Blood Banks for infusion with packed RBCs because of the concern that calcium in the fluid may be chelated by citrate in the blood, leading to clotting of the filters. The clinical significance of this is unclear, and recent studies suggest that simultaneous LR solution resuscitation and rapid RBC infusion does not lead to increased clotting. In the 1980s, LR solution was found to cause neutrophil activation and studies subsequently showed that the D-isomer of lactate, which is not a part of normal human metabolism, was responsible for this activation. It is recommended that LR solutions containing only the L-isomer be used for resuscitation.

Plasma-Lyte is a balanced crystalloid solution that is sold commercially using a variety of different formulations around the world. It was designed to be a balanced solution and most formulations contain sodium, potassium, magnesium, and chloride, but not calcium. Acetate, gluconate, or lactate is present as a bicarbonate precursor. It does not lead to hyperchloremic acidosis and is safe to give with medications or blood products. Most clinical studies have involved use of plasma-Lyte in cardiac surgical or transplant patients, and it has not been well studied in hypovolemic shock. At present, there is no evidence that its theoretic advantages lead to an improvement in outcome in trauma patients compared to other crystalloids.

Hypertonic saline (HS) has been studied extensively over the last few decades as a resuscitation fluid. It raises the serum oncotic pressure, drawing fluid from the interstitial space into the intravascular space, leading to increased blood pressure and improved microcirculatory blood flow. A smaller volume of fluid is required than with isotonic crystalloids. The osmotic effect also reduces intracranial pressure in patients with severe brain injury and may modulate the systemic inflammatory response after injury. Numerous animal studies using 3% or 5% HS have been performed, but clinical data in patients with hemorrhagic shock are lacking. One study showed that hypotensive trauma patients receiving 3% HS had adequate restoration of blood pressure and urine output, and another small study using 5% HS showed a trend toward decreased mortality rate in patients with severe brain injury. Neither solution has been evaluated in recent years in a randomized controlled trial.

Hypertonic saline-dextran (HSD) has been investigated more extensively in clinical trials. It is a mixture of 7.5% NaCl and 6% dextran-70. Dextran was added in an attempt to prolong the hemodynamic effects of hypertonicity. A number of trials of prehospital administration of HSD showed a trend toward increased survival, but statistical significance was not reached. Three metaanalyses by

Wade et al were later conducted. One analysis showed an overall survival benefit in the HSD group and another showed a survival benefit for hypotensive patients with TBI. In 2003, a randomized trial of HSD versus LR solution administered in the prehospital setting to blunt injured patients with hypovolemic shock began patient enrollment. The study was stopped in 2005 after the second interim analysis for futility. It was hypothesized that the lack of improvement in outcome was at least partially explained by enrollment of patients with transient hypotension who were not truly in hemorrhagic shock. A subsequent trial by the Resuscitation Outcomes Consortium randomized patents with either hypovolemic shock or severe TBI to receive 7.5% saline, HSD, or NS in the prehospital setting. Enrollment in the shock cohort was suspended due to futility and a potential safety concern in the hypertonic group. Enrollment in the TBI group was later suspended for futility as well. Currently, HSD has not shown a significant clinical benefit for fluid resuscitation in the civilian trauma setting.

RESUSCITATION STRATEGIES

Traditional resuscitation strategies have been directed toward restoring normal intravascular fluid volumes and arterial blood pressures to maintain perfusion to vital organs. Since the early 1990s, this approach has been reexamined. In delayed resuscitation, fluids are withheld until control of the hemorrhage has been established. This is not a new concept. Cannon stated that early control of hemorrhage was paramount and attempts at fluid resuscitation prior to this would result in increased bleeding and mortality risk. Rapid resuscitation can exacerbate bleeding by dislodging fragile clots, decreasing blood viscosity, and creating compartment syndromes of the cranial vault, abdomen, and extremities. It also exacerbates the "lethal triad" of hypothermia, acidosis, and coagulopathy. In hypotensive resuscitation, fluid is administered at lower rates (or is withheld altogether) with a lower systolic blood pressure (SBP) goal. Tissue injury from regional hypoperfusion is a risk of these strategies. A single accurate method to assess regional hypoperfusion has not been established.

Previous animal studies used controlled hemorrhage models in which hemostasis was achieved early allowing rapid restoration to a normovolemic state. Unfortunately, in the clinical setting the bleeding source may not be immediately known or immediate control is not possible. A number of animal models of uncontrolled hemorrhage have been developed. In a swine aortotomy model, Sondeen noted the average mean arterial pressure (MAP) at which rebleeding occurred following uncontrolled hemorrhagic shock and spontaneous clotting was 64 mm Hg. This was independent of time of resuscitation. Using an aortotomy model in immature swine, Bickell and colleagues showed unfavorable outcomes in those swine resuscitated with LR or HSD compared with no fluid.

This issue has also been examined in clinical studies. In a prospective randomized study, Bickell et al compared immediate and delayed fluid resuscitation in hypotensive patients (SBP < 90 mm Hg) with penetrating injuries to the torso. There was a statistically significant difference in survival between the two groups, 62% versus 70% ($P = .04$), suggesting delayed resuscitation improved outcomes in penetrating injuries to the torso. The study was criticized for its predominantly young, male patient population, and its urban setting with short transfer times. Subsequent subgroup analysis showed survival benefits only in patients with cardiac injuries and no difference in survival when deaths were divided into preoperative, intraoperative, and postoperative time periods. Dutton et al compared fluid resuscitation to a goal SBP of 70 mm Hg versus SBP higher than 100 mm Hg in actively hemorrhaging patients. Resuscitation to a lower SBP did not affect overall mortality rate. Both blunt and penetrating trauma patients were included in this study.

Further randomized controlled trials are needed before a hypotensive resuscitation strategy can be defined. Currently, patients suffering from blunt injuries should be managed with traditional

strategies. Although the ideal target blood pressure remains elusive, in penetrating injuries an SBP of 80 to 90 mm Hg may be adequate. A significant association exists between prehospital hypotension (SBP < 90 mm Hg) and worse outcomes in severe TBI. Attempts to maintain SBP higher than 90 mm Hg may decrease adverse outcomes in head-injured patients, although no class I evidence is available to corroborate this.

The current literature on hypotensive resuscitation cannot be extrapolated to all trauma patients but it emphasizes the importance of rapid diagnosis and treatment. Early identification of bleeding sources and control of hemorrhage will lead to more rapid replacement of intravascular volume and decreased morbidity and mortality risks.

Blood Transfusions

The use of blood transfusions in resuscitation has been an ongoing debate since its initial use in World War I and in World War II, when it became the standard of care. There was an increase in early survival, but many casualties later died of acute renal failure. It is generally accepted that a patient in shock who fails to respond adequately to 2 L of crystalloid is in need of blood transfusions. It is clear in unstable patients with active bleeding and hemorrhagic shock that blood should be given immediately. When larger volumes of crystalloid and RBCs are given, fresh frozen plasma, platelets, or cryoprecipitate may also be needed to reverse the associated dilutional coagulopathy. One must also consider the inherent risks of blood transfusion, such as transfusion reactions, transfusion-related acute lung injury, infection, and immunosuppression. It has been observed that blood transfusions contain proinflammatory mediators that both prime and activate neutrophils. This has been proposed as a key mechanism in the development of multiple organ failure. Stored RBCs also undergo substantial shape changes and impaired deformability by the second week of storage. This decreased deformity can lead to microvascular obstruction, and has been found to be associated with the development of splanchnic ischemia. Malone et al reported that trauma patients who underwent blood transfusions within the first 24 hours of admission, independent of shock severity, were almost three times more likely to die than those who did not receive transfusions.

Early clinical studies concluded that hemoglobin (Hb) levels of 10 g/dL were optimal for shock resuscitation; however, recent consensus panels have suggested that a lower concentration is adequate. A prospective randomized trial showed that ICU patients who received blood transfusion for Hb less than 7.0 g/dL and were maintained at Hb 7.0 to 9.0 g/dL did as well, and possibly better, than patients who were liberally transfused for an Hb level less than 10 g/dL and maintained at 10 to 12 g/dL. All these patients were without ongoing bleeding, acute myocardial infarction, or unstable angina. Subgroup analysis looking at the safety of a restricted RBC transfusion strategy in trauma patients showed there was no statistically significant difference in mortality rate, multiple organ dysfunction, or length of stay, when compared to those managed with the liberal transfusion strategy. Randomized, controlled investigations need to be conducted to provide evidence to help dictate the use of blood in critically ill trauma patients.

Artificial Oxygen-Carrying Blood Substitutes

Although both crystalloids and colloids can replace intravascular volume, neither product restores the oxygen-carrying capacity of the lost RBCs. Artificial Hb products have the potential to improve oxygen-carrying capacity without the storage, availability, immune suppression, transfusion reaction, compatibility, or disease transmission problems associated with standard transfusions. Unfortunately, these products also fail to restore coagulation components, and hemostasis can be hindered with the loss of cellular elements that lower the viscosity of circulating blood. The use of a large volume of artificial oxygen-carrying solutions in severe hemorrhage has not been adequately studied.

Hemoglobin-based oxygen carriers (HBOCs) have been derived from human blood, bovine blood, and recombinant DNA technology dating back to 1933. Carrier solutions need to be stroma-free polymerized or cross-linked Hb tetramers with oxygen-carrying capabilities that remain within the intravascular space for a prolonged period of time. Early Hb substitutes had a greater oxygen affinity because of the loss of 2,3-diphosphoglycerate. However, with pyridoxylation of the Hb tetramer, this problem was addressed. HBOCs can also cause vasoconstriction because tetrameric Hb binds the nitric oxide in the vascular wall and results in unopposed vasoconstriction. Because of this phenomenon, blood pressures may be higher than expected for the level of intravascular volume replacement in hemorrhagic shock patients. Initial studies of these products in humans have been disappointing. A phase III trial of diaspirin cross-linked Hb was prematurely stopped owing to an unexpectedly high mortality rate in the treatment group (46% vs. 17%). PolyHeme, glutaraldehyde-polymerized pyridoxylated human Hb, showed promise in phase I and II trials as a blood substitute. However, in a phase III trial, no survival benefit was seen and there was a trend toward increased adverse events, especially myocardial ischemia. The Food and Drug Administration did not grant approval, and currently PolyHeme is not being actively studied for clinical use.

An alternate blood substitute, HBOC-201, raised MAP more than colloids or crystalloids in an animal model and showed immunomodulatory effects in other preclinical studies. It has been shown to be noninferior to 6% HS in the military setting. However, in a phase III clinical trial in a civilian population, more adverse events were seen in patients receiving HBOC-201 than in those receiving RBC transfusions. It is thought that many of the adverse events resulted from vasoactivity secondary to nitric oxide scavenging by HBOC-201, and basic science efforts to prevent this process are ongoing. Because of this issue, HBOC-201 clinical trials are currently being done.

Perfluorocarbons are chemically and biologically inert liquids that dissolve large amounts of gas. They require dispersion in plasma-like aqueous fluids such as albumin or in physiologic electrolyte solutions to be an adequate oxygen-carrying substitute. They have a lower oxygen-delivering capacity than normal blood and require an F_{IO_2} of greater than 70% to carry physiologically useful concentrations of oxygen. The long-term biologic effects of absorption, distribution, metabolism, and excretion, and the effects on the reticuloendothelial system (RES) require further evaluation. Concern about toxicity to the RES and high F_{IO_2} requirements may limit their use in severe hemorrhage.

■ COMPLICATIONS OF RESUSCITATION

In the 1980s and 1990s, there was a shift toward the use of large volumes of fluid for resuscitation in acutely injured patients. Advances in critical care and the adoption of damage control techniques led to an increasing number of critically ill patients surviving the immediate postinjury period. However, the large volumes of crystalloids used for resuscitation led to an increase in complications of resuscitation, such as acidosis, hypothermia, coagulopathy, and the development of abdominal and extremity compartment syndromes. This can lead to a positive feedback cycle in which the acidosis, hypothermia, and coagulopathy worsen each other (Fig. 2).

Hypothermia

Hypothermia is defined as a core body temperature of less than 35° C. The internal core temperature is a net result of heat production and heat loss. Heat loss is a result of evaporation, radiation, conduction, or

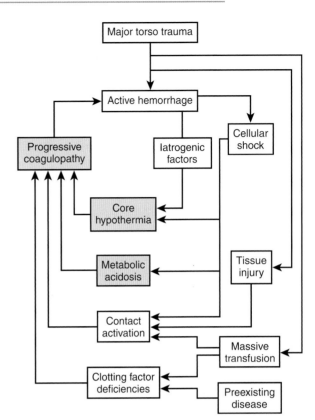

FIGURE 2   The lethal triad. *(Modified from Moore EE: Staged laparotomy for the hypothermia, acidosis, coagulopathy syndrome. Am J Surg 172:405–410, 1996.)*

convection. Heat production largely occurs as a result of cellular metabolism. Acutely injured patients have numerous sources of potential heat loss. Exposure in the field can cause the patient to be hypothermic on admission. Further exposure per Advanced Trauma Life Support (ATLS) protocols causes further heat loss. Operations involving exposure of body cavities cause significant losses through evaporative and conductive means. IV fluids present the highest potential for heat loss. This can be quantified by the following equation:

$$\text{Heat} = \text{mass} \times \text{specific heat} \times \left(T_{\text{body}} - T_{\text{fluid}}\right)$$

Given a specific heat of water of 4.19 kJ/kg/° C, 1 L of 25° C crystalloid infused in a normothermic patient would result in a heat loss of 50.3 kJ. This heat loss exceeds the heat that can be returned to the patient by conventional methods in 1 hour. Blood products are commonly stored at 4° C and administration of large volumes on unwarmed blood products leads to an even greater degree of heat loss. Heat loss can be minimized by the use of blood and fluid warmers. Rewarming is a more gradual process, as it takes approximately 12 L of warmed fluid to raise core temperature by 1° C.

The incidence of hypothermia in trauma patients during resuscitation may be as high as 66%. Although Gregory et al found that only 12% of patients arriving in the emergency department were hypothermic, 46% were hypothermic on arrival to the operating room, and 57% were hypothermic when leaving the operating room. This suggests that the majority of heat loss occurs in the resuscitation bay, and current adjunctive measures are not able to prevent intraoperative heat loss entirely.

Hypothermia in the trauma patient is a poor prognostic indicator and it has been shown to be independently predictive of mortality rate. The mortality rate of victims of accidental exposure with moderate hypothermia is normally about 20%. However, trauma victims studied with similar core temperatures (<32° C) have almost 100%

TABLE 2: Approximate Rate of Heat Transfer with Available Rewarming Methods

Rewarming Technique	Rate of Heat Transfer (kcal/hr)
Airway rewarming	8–12
Overhead radiant warmer	17
Heating blankets	20
Convective warmers	15–26
Body cavity lavage	36
Continuous arteriovenous rewarming	92–139
Cardiopulmonary bypass	710

Modified from Gentilello LM: Practical approaches to hypothermia. In Maull KI, Cleveland HC, Feliciano DV, et al, editors: *Advances in Trauma and Critical Care*, Vol. 9. St. Louis, Mosby, 1994, pp 39–79.

mortality rate. This difference has several explanations. Trauma patients have similar heat losses secondary to exposure; however, they also have further losses secondary to hemorrhage and exposed body cavities. Beyond this, the decreased cardiac output and oxygen consumption secondary to blood loss and shock lead to decreased heat production. Given these mechanisms, the mortality rate documented may be more a manifestation of the severity of injury rather than isolated hypothermia.

Because of the strong association of hypothermia to mortality risk and the other elements of the "lethal triad," rewarming and prevention of ongoing heat loss should be a priority of resuscitation (Table 2). The first step is to obtain an accurate core temperature. Esophageal or bladder temperatures have been shown to be more reliable than rectal or axillary measurements. Given the high rate of heat loss with infusion of room temperature fluids, all resuscitation solutions should be warmed. Operating room temperatures should be

elevated to minimize losses due to conduction and radiation. Once the secondary evaluation is complete, the patient should be covered. Significant heat loss can occur from the scalp, and covering of the head is often overlooked. A Bair Hugger or similar device can be used to actively warm the patient. For profound hypothermia, active internal rewarming can be used. This is done either with lavage of a body cavity (peritoneal or thoracic) or by intravascular rewarming. Options for intravascular rewarming include venovenous rewarming, arteriovenous rewarming, or cardiopulmonary bypass. Continuous arteriovenous rewarming (Fig. 3) has been shown to decrease early fatality in critically injured hypothermic trauma patients.

Coagulopathy

Hemorrhage is a major cause of early trauma deaths. Coagulopathy in trauma patients is common during major resuscitations. The mechanisms are thought to be related to hypothermia, metabolic disturbances, dilution, and disseminated intravascular coagulation. Most of these mechanisms can be traced in some way to resuscitation.

Dilution is a major cause of coagulopathy in resuscitated trauma patients. Intravascular fluid containing coagulation factors is lost and replaced with solutions lacking these factors. The actual degree of coagulopathy is not easily predictable as the plasma shifts are quite complex. Coagulation factors are continually produced and sequestered in the posttrauma setting. Dilutional coagulopathy is not thought to play a significant role until approximately 1 blood volume (70 ml/kg) of replacement fluid is infused into a patient. Therefore, giving prophylactic products without clinical evidence of bleeding or laboratory data is generally not recommended. However, there is increasing evidence that the early administration of coagulation factors is indicated in the presence of hemorrhagic shock.

Hypothermia has a profound effect on coagulation activity. Reed and Rohrer, in different experiments, showed that hypothermia resulted in prolonged partial thromboplastin time (PTT) and prothrombin time independent of the actual level of enzymes. Gubler et al showed that the effect of hemodilution and hypothermia are additive (Fig. 4). In addition to these enzyme effects, fibrinolysis is thought to be increased by hypothermia. Animal studies have

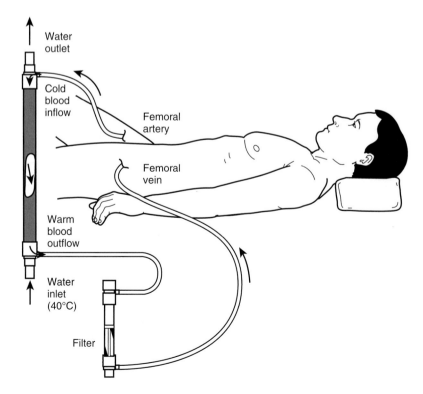

FIGURE 3 Continuous arteriovenous rewarming. *(From Gentilello LM, Jurkovich GJ, Stark MS, et al: Continuous arteriovenous rewarming: rapid reversal of hypothermia in critically ill patients. J Trauma 32:316–327, 1992.)*

Water outlet

Cold blood inflow

Femoral artery

Femoral vein

Warm blood outflow

Water inlet (40°C)

Filter

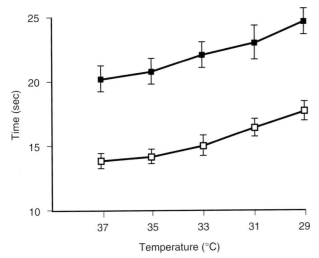

FIGURE 4 The effect of hypothermia and dilution on prothrombin time. Filled squares, diluted specimens; open squares, nondiluted specimens. *(From Gubler KD, Gentilello LM, Hassantash SA, Maier RV: The impact of hypothermia on dilutional coagulopathy. J Trauma 36:847–851, 1994.)*

suggested that platelets are sequestered by the spleen in the presence of hypothermia. Platelet adhesion is also decreased in hypothermic patients. A recent in vitro study suggests that platelet effects cause the majority of hypothermic coagulopathy at temperatures above 33° C, whereas enzymatic dysfunction had a significant effect when the temperature was below 33° C. Clinical studies have shown that acidotic and hypothermic patients with adequate blood, plasma, and platelet replacement still develop significant bleeding.

As with any disease, treatment of coagulopathy begins with recognizing the problem. Any trauma patient with evidence of significant tissue injury or ongoing bleeding should be screened to determine an international normalized ratio (INR), PTT, platelet count, and fibrinogen level. In the setting of active traumatic bleeding, the platelet count should be kept above 50,000/μL, the INR less than 2, the fibrinogen greater than 100 mg/dL, and the PTT less than 1.5 times normal. Again, close monitoring of these parameters is recommended as empiric therapy often yields unpredictable results. In the absence of laboratory results, empiric therapy can be started.

Coagulopathy is also specifically linked to brain injury. The release of thromboplastin from injured brain tissue is thought to cause severe consumptive coagulopathy leading to disseminated intravascular coagulation. More extensive coagulation monitoring is indicated in the setting of head trauma. Thrombelastography (TEG) is currently being investigated for this purpose, because studies have suggested that TEG may detect clinically significant abnormalities in coagulation earlier than standard assays.

Acidosis

Metabolic acidosis is commonly seen in trauma patients with hemorrhagic shock and is postulated to occur secondary to tissue hypoperfusion in the setting of decreased cardiac output and oxygen-carrying capacity. This cascade of events eventually leads to anaerobic metabolism with the production of lactate. Massive resuscitation with crystalloid solutions has been associated with the development of a worsening metabolic acidosis. Following the Stewart model of acid-base equilibrium, the administration of solutions with supraphysiologic levels of chloride relative to sodium results in a decreased strong ion difference (SID) (Na + K + Ca + Mg – Cl – lactate). This decreased SID causes further dissociation of H^+ from H_2O to maintain charge neutrality, resulting in a decreased pH. Crystalloid solutions vary in

their propensity to alter the SID because they have differing concentrations of positive and negative strong ions. LR solution has a higher SID than NS does. Because of this difference, large volumes of LR solution will not cause the same degree of metabolic acidosis that can result from large volumes of NS.

Although the presence of a hyperchloremic acidosis has not been directly associated with increased mortality risk, there are many potential hazards of profound acidosis. Acidosis has a depressant effect on the myocardium and increases ventricular dysrhythmias. The sympathetic-adrenal axis is stimulated in the setting of acidosis; however, the myocardium has decreased responsiveness to circulating catecholamines. The prolonged acidotic state also increases respiratory drive, increases intracranial pressure in head-injured patients, and worsens coagulopathy. A more common danger exists in misinterpreting a hyperchloremic acidosis for continued hypoperfusion and shock leading to unnecessary therapies.

In order to avoid hyperchloremic acidosis, fluids with supraphysiologic concentrations of chloride should be avoided. LR solution contains a more physiologic concentration of chloride (109 mEq/L) compared to NS (154 mEq/L). Several clinical series and animal studies document profound acidosis in the setting of large-volume NS administration. Although less probable, this acidosis can still be seen with LR solution, as its SID is less than the SID of plasma. Careful monitoring of electrolytes with measurement of the anion gap can aid in guiding therapy. A normal or narrowed anion gap should be seen in the setting of an isolated hyperchloremic metabolic acidosis, as opposed to the elevated gap seen in lactic acidosis. Transitioning to fluids with less chloride (LR solution or Plasma-Lyte) or no chloride (sodium acetate) can resolve the hyperchloremic acidosis.

The mechanism of coagulopathy in acidotic patients is a matter of active investigation. In vitro experiments have shown a decrease in the activity of factor VIIa-tissue factor and factor Xa-Va complexes. In vivo animal experiments have shown that acidosis independently decreases fibrinogen and platelet counts, increases PTT, and increases clinical bleeding time. In a study of patients undergoing massive transfusion, a pH less than 7.10 independently predicted coagulopathy.

Compartment Syndromes

Tissue edema is a frequent result of large volume resuscitation in the setting of shock. In most cases, this edema has little immediately obvious harmful effects. However, in restricted body compartments, the resulting increase in pressure can lead to ischemia and subsequent tissue necrosis. The three affected areas are the extremities, abdomen, and cranial vault.

Extremity compartment syndrome most often results secondary to traumatic injury with or without an associated fracture. Although infrequent, compartment syndromes have been described in the absence of injury in the setting of large-volume resuscitation. This entity has been labeled secondary extremity compartment syndrome. This process likely results from reperfusion after a period of severe shock. The subsequent release of inflammatory mediators results in a capillary leak phenomenon. When this is combined with large volumes of blood and fluids, the edema can overwhelm the fascial compartments, leading to limb or muscle ischemia. As with any compartment syndrome, early recognition, diagnosis, and treatment are paramount for limb salvage.

The abdominal compartment syndrome (ACS) has been described over the past century, but was clearly recognized and defined in the early 1990s. It is defined as organ dysfunction secondary to intraabdominal hypertension. ACS was originally described in patients with abdominal operations or abdominal trauma. Since that time, ACS has been further classified as primary ACS, occurring from an insult to the intraabdominal contents, and secondary ACS, occurring as a result of shock and massive resuscitation. Secondary ACS is theorized to occur by several mechanisms. As more IV fluid is given, more interstitial edema develops. Plasma proteins are also further diluted, potentially diminishing intravascular oncotic pressure. The edema that forms increases intraabdominal pressure and decreases splanchnic venous return. This process eventually leads to decreased central venous return, prompting further administration of fluids. This forms another vicious cycle of resuscitation.

Several studies have investigated the risk factors and mortality of secondary ACS. All studies indicate that severe shock and massive resuscitation are predisposing factors. Reviewed case series report a resuscitation volume averaging from 16 to 38 L of crystalloid and 13 to 29 units of blood. Balogh et al concluded that trauma patients undergoing supranormal resuscitation ($Do_2 > 600$) had received significantly more crystalloid and had a significantly higher rate of ACS (16% vs. 8%). The supranormal arm received an average of 13 L of LR solution versus 7 L in the standard resuscitation group. Patients suffering from secondary ACS had mortality rates ranging from 38% to 67%. This suggests that ACS may be prevented with judicious use of fluids and avoiding unnecessary volume overload.

Bladder pressures should be monitored in patients showing clinical signs of ACS or patients in shock who are receiving large resuscitations. A tense abdomen in the setting of low urine output, high airway pressures, and hypotension are diagnostic of ACS. Maxwell's series observed that nonsurvivors of secondary ACS had a time to operating room of 25 hours versus 3 hours for survivors. This indicates that secondary ACS can happen very early in resuscitation. Furthermore, prompt diagnosis and treatment may be beneficial for survival.

Elevated intracranial pressure is a frequent result of TBI and subsequent intracranial hemorrhage. The total volume of the intracranial vault is approximately 1600 mL. This is generally divided into 80% cerebral tissue, 10% blood, and 10% cerebrospinal fluid. Cerebral edema results from direct injury and a capillary leak phenomenon similar to the other compartment syndromes. Resuscitation with too much IV fluid can worsen this process. The use of HS may help minimize cerebral edema, but its role in fluid resuscitation for brain-injured patients remains controversial. Given the composition of the vault contents, medical management offers limited treatment once pathologic intracranial hypertension develops. More invasive methods, such as ventriculostomy or craniectomy, should be considered in a timely fashion when medical therapy fails.

For the chapter's Suggested Readings list, please visit the book at www.ExpertConsult.inkling.com.

RESUSCITATIVE THORACOTOMY

Juan A. Asensio, Patrizio Petrone, Alejandro Perez-Alonso, Wendy Jo Svetanoff, Molly Hartmann, Eric Elster, Gerd Daniel Pust, and Michel Wagner

Emergency department thoracotomy (EDT) remains a formidable tool within the trauma surgeon's armamentarium. Since its introduction during the 1960s, the use of this procedure has ranged from sparing to liberal. At many urban trauma centers, this procedure has found a niche as part of the resuscitative process. Because of improvements in emergency medical services systems, many critically injured patients now arrive in extremis, prompting trauma surgeons to perform this procedure to attempt saving their lives. This technically complex procedure should be performed only by surgeons familiar with the management of penetrating cardiothoracic injuries.

Indications for the use of EDT appearing in the literature range from vague to quite specific. It has been used in a variety of settings including penetrating and blunt thoracic and thoracoabdominal injuries, cardiac injuries, and exsanguinating abdominal vascular injuries. It has also been used rarely in exsanguinating peripheral vascular injuries arriving in cardiopulmonary arrest and also in pediatric trauma. Many studies in the literature have also reported its use in patients presenting in cardiopulmonary arrest secondary to blunt trauma.

HISTORICAL PERSPECTIVE

In 1874, Schiff was first to promote the concept of open cardiac massage. Rehn in 1896 reported the first successful repair of a cardiac injury, a stab wound of the right ventricle. In 1897, Duval described the median sternotomy incision widely used today. Igelsrud in 1901 was the first to report successful resuscitation of a patient sustaining a posttraumatic cardiac arrest with a thoracotomy and open cardiac massage. Spangaro in 1906 described the left anterolateral thoracotomy widely used today for resuscitation as an intercostocondral thoracotomy.

Zoll in 1956 was the first to introduce the concept of external defibrillation, and Kouwenhoven in 1960 described closed cardiopulmonary resuscitation (CPR). Beall et al in 1961 were the first to propose that patients experiencing cessation of cardiac action should undergo immediate resuscitative thoracotomy and cardiac massage, whether in the ED, operating room, or recovery ward, and Beall was first to attempt this procedure. Similarly, in 1966, he advocated the use of immediate cardiorrhaphy in the emergency room and setting up an instrument tray; he was also the first to successfully perform this procedure.

OBJECTIVES

Objectives of the EDT procedure include the following:

- Resuscitation of agonal patients with penetrating cardiothoracic injuries (Figs. 1 through 6)
- Evacuation of pericardial blood and clot to relieve cardiac tamponade (Figs. 7 and 8)
- Control of thoracic hemorrhage
- Repair of cardiac injuries (Figs. 9 through 11)
- Cross-clamp of the descending thoracic aorta (Figs. 12 through 14)

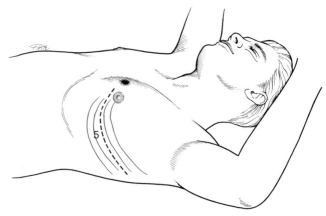

FIGURE 1 Left anterolateral thoracotomy incision.

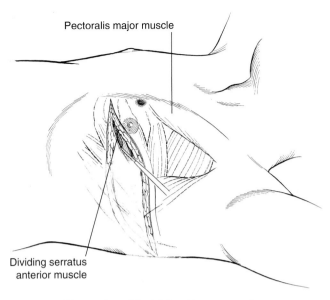

FIGURE 2 Transection of the left hemithorax musculature to access the chest.

Pectoralis major muscle

Dividing serratus anterior muscle

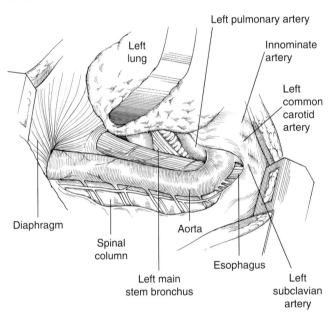

Left lung

Left pulmonary artery

Innominate artery

Left common carotid artery

Diaphragm

Spinal column

Left main stem bronchus

Aorta

Esophagus

Left subclavian artery

FIGURE 3 Anatomy of the left hemithoracic cavity. Notice the relationship between the esophagus, anterior to the descending thoracic aorta.

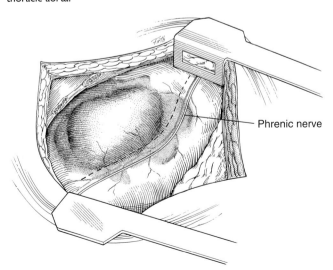

Phrenic nerve

FIGURE 4 Tense hemopericardium. Incision is made anterior to the left phrenic nerve.

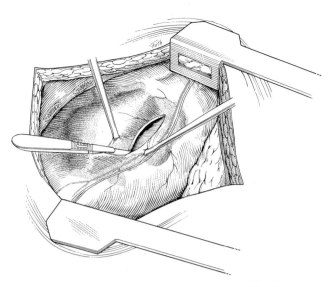

FIGURE 5 The tense pericardium is grasped between Allis clamps and a small incision is made with a scalpel.

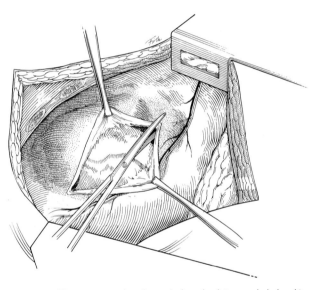

FIGURE 6 The incision is sharply carried out both in a cephalad and in a caudal direction, utilizing Metzenbaum scissors.

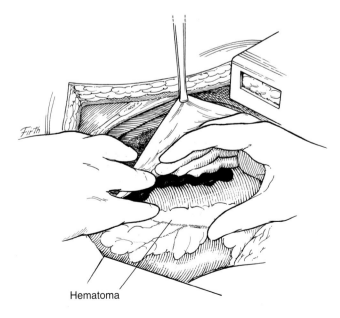

Hematoma

FIGURE 7 The pericardial clot is manually extracted.

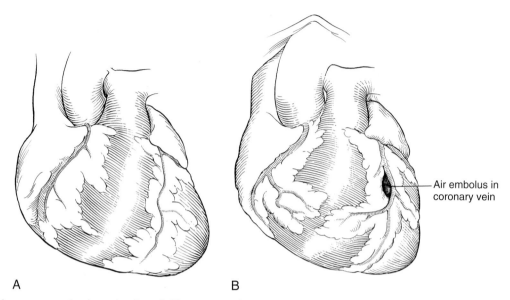

A   B

Air embolus in
coronary vein

FIGURE 8   Findings upon opening the pericardium. **A,** Vasoconstricted coronary vessels due to hypoperfusion. **B,** Air emboli noticed in the coronary veins. Air emboli create a temporary occlusion to flow in coronary arteries but cannot be seen due to the thickness of their wall. When detected, the ventricles should be vented with a needle. Air emboli are strong predictors of poor outcome.

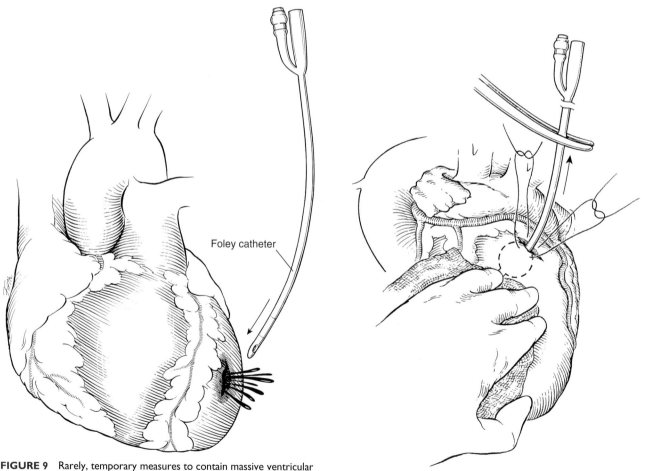

Foley catheter

FIGURE 9   Rarely, temporary measures to contain massive ventricular hemorrhage are necessary.

FIGURE 10   Depicts insertion of a Foley catheter to stop hemorrhage.

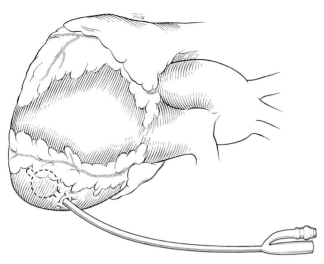

FIGURE 11 Depicts inflated intraventricular Foley catheter balloon.

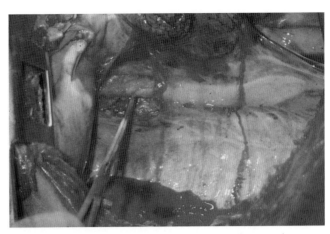

FIGURE 13 The descending aorta when entering the aortic hiatus. The aorta was dissected prior to being clamped. Note the esophagus superiorly.

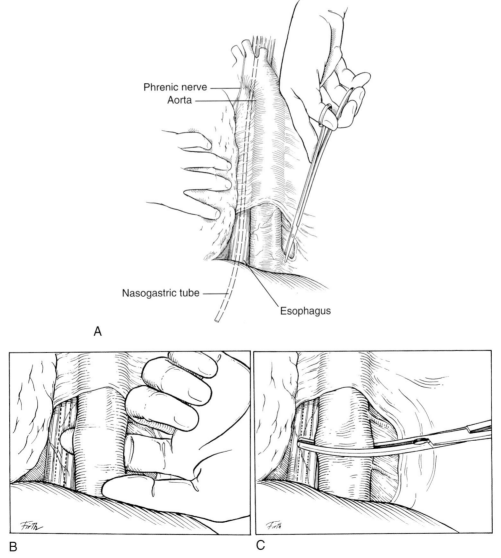

Phrenic nerve

Aorta

Nasogastric tube

Esophagus

A

B

C

FIGURE 12 **A,** Sharp dissection of the descending thoracic aorta. The left lung is displaced anteriorly. Notice the esophagus directly interior to the descending thoracic aorta. **B,** Digital mobilization of the descending thoracic aorta. **C,** Placement of a Crafoord-DeBakey aortic cross-clamp.

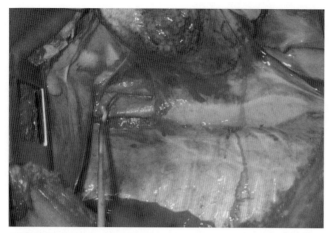

FIGURE 14 Aortic cross-clamp in place. Note the size of the left hemithorax cavity, which can hold the entire patient's blood volume during exsanguinating injuries.

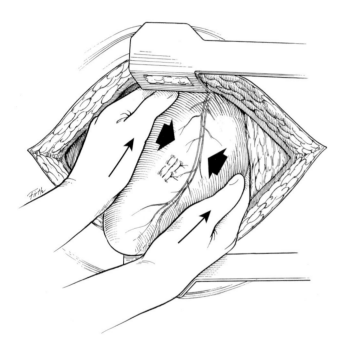

FIGURE 15 After performing ventricular cardiography it is often necessary to perform open cardiopulmonary resuscitation, which is performed with the palms of both hands.

- Performance of open cardiac massage, which can produce up to 60% of the normal ejection fraction (Figs. 15 and 16)
- Cross-clamp of the pulmonary hilum to control pulmonary vessel hemorrhage
- Cross-clamp of the pulmonary hilum and aspiration of both the right and left ventricles to prevent or treat pulmonary embolism

PHYSIOLOGY

The physiologic effects of thoracic aortic cross-clamping include positive and negative effects, yet others are unknown:

Positive Effects

- Preservation and redistribution of remaining blood volume to improve coronary/carotid arterial perfusion

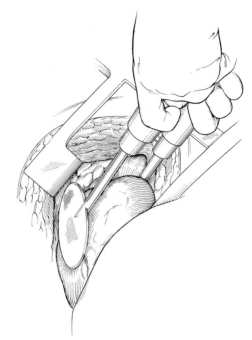

FIGURE 16 If ventricular fibrillation is detected, open defibrillation with 50 J is carried out in addition to pharmacologic manipulation.

- Reduction of subdiaphragmatic blood loss
- Increases left ventricular stroke work index
- Increases myocardial contractility

Negative Effects

- Decreases blood flow to abdominal viscera to approximately 10% of normal
- Decreases renal perfusion to approximately 10% of normal
- Decreases blood flow to the spinal cord to approximately 10%
- Induces anaerobic metabolism
- Induces hypoxia/lactic acidosis
- Imposes a tremendous afterload onto the left ventricle
- Unknown factors
- Prolonged length of safe cross-clamp time
- Incidence of reperfusion injury

INDICATIONS

Indications for EDT can be subdivided into three categories: (1) accepted, (2) selective, and (3) rare.

Accepted Indications

EDT is best applied to patients sustaining penetrating cardiac injuries who arrive in trauma centers after a short scene and transport time with witnessed or objectively measured physiologic parameters (signs of life); pupillary reactivity; spontaneous ventilation, even if agonal; presence of a carotid pulse; measurable or palpable blood pressure; extremity movement; and cardiac electrical activity.

Selective Indications

EDT should be performed selectively in patients sustaining penetrating noncardiac thoracic injuries owing to its very low survival rate. Because it is difficult to ascertain whether injuries are noncardiac thoracic versus cardiac, this procedure may be employed to establish a diagnosis.

EDT should be performed selectively in patients sustaining exsanguinating abdominal vascular injuries owing to its very low survival rate. Meticulous selection of patients should be exercised. This procedure should be used as an adjunct to definitive repair of abdominal vascular injuries.

Rare Indications

EDT should be performed rarely in patients sustaining cardiopulmonary arrest secondary to blunt trauma owing to its very low survival rate and poor neurologic outcomes. Extreme caution should be exercised in selecting patients for this procedure. It should be strictly limited to those who arrive with vital signs at the trauma center and experience a witnessed cardiopulmonary arrest. Most authors would caution against this indication.

TECHNIQUES FOR CARDIAC INJURY REPAIR

Incisions

Two main incisions are used in the management of penetrating cardiac injuries. Trauma surgeons should be aware that injuries caused by missiles can be unpredictable in their trajectory and that a missile injury that penetrates a hemithoracic cavity may not remain confined in the original area of entrance and may produce injury to the contralateral cavity. This will require the trauma surgeon to access the contralateral hemithoracic cavity.

Median sternotomy, described by Duval, is the incision of choice for patients admitted with penetrating precordial injuries who arrive with some degree of hemodynamic instability and may undergo preoperative investigation with either FAST or chest radiograph. It is also the incision of choice for those who are thought to harbor occult cardiac injuries. The left anterolateral thoracotomy is the incision of choice in the management of patients who arrive in extremis. This incision is used in the ED for resuscitative purposes.

The left anterolateral thoracotomy described by Spangaro can also be extended across the sternum as bilateral anterolateral thoracotomies if it is determined during the resuscitative period that the patient's injury extends into the right hemithoracic cavity (Table 1). Extension into bilateral anterolateral thoracotomies is the incision of choice for patients who are hemodynamically unstable after incurring mediastinal traversing injuries. This incision allows full exposure of the anterior mediastinum and pericardium as well as both hemithoracic cavities. It is important to note that upon transection of the sternum, both internal mammary arteries are also transected and must be ligated after restoration of perfusion pressure. Uncontrolled, they can serve as a significant source of blood loss. This is a frequent pitfall during the institution of damage control, as trauma surgeons may forget to ligate these vessels, prompting return to the operating room for a patient who can ill afford it. For patients who sustain thoracoabdominal injuries, the left anterolateral thoracotomy is also the incision of choice if patients deteriorate in the operating room while undergoing a laparotomy.

Adjunct Maneuvers

Trauma surgeons must possess several maneuvers in their armamentarium to deal with penetrating cardiothoracic injuries. The first adjunct maneuver dealing with these injuries was described by Sauerbuch in 1907, as quoted by Brantigan. This maneuver entailed controlling blood flow to the heart by compression of the base. This

TABLE 1: Algorithm for Emergency Department Thoracotomy

Operator	Well-trained surgeon
Initial assessment and resuscitation	Endotracheal intubation Immediate venous access Rapid infusion
Position	Supine with left arm elevated
Incision	Left anterolateral incision Fifth intercostal space from left sternocostal junction to latissimus dorsi muscle
Procedure	Incision as previously mentioned Sharp transection of intercostal muscle Open pleura Place a Finnochietto retractor Open cardiac massage Elevate left lung medially Locate and dissect descending aorta Cross-clamp aorta by Crafoord-Debakey clamp
If cardiac injury (bluish and tense pericardium)	Open pericardium longitudinally with preserving phrenic n. Evacuate blood clot Repair cardiac injury (mattress sutures of Halsted with Prolene 2-0)
If active bleeding at pulmonary hilum	Cross-clamp pulmonary hilum with Crafoord-Debakey clamp
If pulmonary parenchymal laceration	Clamp with Duval clamp
If associated injury in contralateral thoracic cavity	Extend incision to the contralateral side Transect sternum sharply Convert to bilateral anterolateral thoracotomy
If air embolism is suspected (air in coronary vein)	Aspirate left ventricle
Miscellaneous	Ligate internal mammary artery Systemic or intraventricular epinephrine administration Internal defibrillation 10–50 J Temporary pacemaker
Immediately transport to operating room after successful resuscitation	

maneuver is difficult to perform via a left anterolateral thoracotomy, has been abandoned, and is mentioned because of historical interest only.

Total inflow occlusion to the heart is a complex maneuver that entails cross-clamping both the superior vena cava and inferior vena cava (IVC) in their intrapericardial location to arrest total blood flow to the heart. Crafoord-DeBakey cross-clamps are employed, resulting in the immediate emptying of the heart. The trauma surgeon must recognize that cross-clamping the IVC intrapericardially at the space of Gibbons can be quite treacherous, as it is often fused with the posterior aspect of the pericardium. Inexperienced trauma surgeons will often force the cross-clamp in an attempt to rapidly achieve total occlusion, leading to an iatrogenic injury of the intrapericardial IVC. Similarly, circumferentially dissecting this delicate vessel can also lead to iatrogenic injury. The clamp must be placed carefully and sometimes at an angle so as to totally occlude the intrapericardial IVC.

Total inflow occlusion of the heart is indicated for the management of injuries in the lateral most aspect of the right atrium and the superior or inferior atriocaval junction. Total inflow occlusion will lead to immediate emptying of the heart and allow the injury to be visualized and thus repaired. Frequently, this procedure results in cardiopulmonary arrest as tolerance by the injured, acidotic, hypothermic, and ischemic heart is very limited. The safe period for this maneuver is unknown, although a 1- to 3-minute range is often quoted in the literature as the period of time after which clamps must be released. As the clamps are released, venous return fills the right cardiac chambers and forward cardiac pumping motion will begin. More often than not, the heart will fibrillate, requiring immediate direct defibrillation along with pharmacologic manipulation. This may be unsuccessful, particularly if a period of 3 minutes has been exceeded. Restoration of a normal sinus rhythm is often impossible.

Cross-clamping of the pulmonary hilum is another valuable maneuver indicated for the management of associated pulmonary injuries, particularly those that have hilar central hematomas or active bleeding. This maneuver arrests bleeding from the lung and prevents air emboli from reaching the systemic circulation. However, one of its negative effects is responsible for significantly increasing the afterload of the right ventricle, as half of the pulmonary circulation is no longer available for perfusion. We recommend sequential declamping of the hilum to be carried out as expediently as possible, along with a direct approach by stapled pulmonary tractotomy for identification and control of hemorrhaging intraparenchymal pulmonary vessels. This will promptly unload the right ventricle. In the presence of acidosis, hypothermia, and ischemia, the right ventricle may not be able to tolerate this maneuver, leading to fibrillation and arrest.

Grabowski recently described a maneuver to facilitate exposure of posterior cardiac wounds by placing a Satinsky clamp at the right ventricular angle, which is formed at the acute anteroinferior margin of the right ventricle as it reflects on the right diaphragm. Grabowski recommends that the clamp only grasp a small portion of the right ventricle. He recommends this maneuver for elevating the heart out of the pericardium to repair posterior injuries. We have no experience with this maneuver and cannot recommend it. We strongly feel that if used inappropriately, it will lead to the development of significant cardiac dysrhythmias.

Maneuvers such as venting either the right or left ventricle postcardiorrhaphy are recommended to provide an avenue of egress for air emboli trapped in these chambers. This is usually accomplished by placing 16-G intravenous catheters. Theoretically, air should eject out of the repair chambers, thus preventing air emboli. Although the authors have used this maneuver successfully, little has been written in the literature describing its outcome.

At times, a trauma surgeon will need to elevate the heart out of the pericardium in order to repair certain injuries. Rapid and injudicious manipulation of the heart will often result in complex dysrhythmias that might include ventricular fibrillation and even cardiopulmonary arrest. Occasionally, given the degree of exsanguinating hemorrhage, the heart must be extracted rapidly from pericardium in order to perform cardiorrhaphy. The trauma surgeon must communicate with the anesthesiologists whenever this maneuver is performed. If hemorrhage can be digitally controlled, gradual elevation of the heart by placing multiple laparotomy packs will allow better tolerance of this maneuver while decreasing the chances for the development of dysrhythmias.

Recently described mechanical stabilizer systems to the heart have been utilized in the performance of conventional coronary artery bypass grafts, which have traditionally used cardiopulmonary bypass to allow cardiac surgeons to operate on a motionless heart arrested by means of cardioplegic solutions. The deleterious systemic inflammatory effects of circulating blood through the extracorporeal circuit of the cardiopulmonary pump have prompted the development of mechanical stabilizer systems to allow off-pump coronary artery bypass grafting to be performed by cardiothoracic surgeons.

Waterworth recently reported the first case in which the Octopus IV Mechanical Cardiac Stabilizer was used on a 20-year-old patient who sustained a 2-cm stab wound in the right ventricular outflow tract approximately 1 cm below the pulmonary valve. According to the author, this area was difficult to suture without causing further tearing due to tachycardia sustained by the patient and the fragile nature of this area. After control of hemorrhage by direct pressure, the Octopus IV Mechanical Cardiac Stabilizer was placed, which provided for immobility to this area of the heart and thus facilitated repair. In this case report, the author describes the use of this device, suggesting that cardiac stabilization devices with adjustable suction foot blades may be used to control hemorrhage in addition to facilitating repair, particularly in areas difficult or dangerous to handle manually. The recommended positioning parallel to the direction of the wound and approximating the foot plates may result in closure of the wound, providing a clear field for repair. This case report by Waterworth appears to be the first and only case reported in the literature utilizing a mechanical cardiac stabilizer in the management of a penetrating cardiac injury. Whether stabilizers will be routinely used in the management of penetrating cardiac injuries in the future remains to be seen.

Repair of Atrial Injuries

Atrial injuries can usually be controlled by placement of a Satinsky partial occlusion vascular clamp. Control of the wound will allow the trauma surgeon to perform cardiorrhaphy. We recommend utilizing 2-0 or 3-0 polypropylene monofilament sutures on an MH needle in a running or interrupted fashion. It is important to visualize both sides of the atrial injury, particularly those caused by missiles. Missile injuries can usually cause a significant amount of tissue destruction, which might require meticulous débridement prior to closure. Similarly, a portion of the atria may be resected and cardiorrhaphy performed utilizing a running suture of 2-0 or 3-0 polypropylene monofilament suture. The trauma surgeon must be aware that the atria have fairly thin walls and demand gentleness during cardiorrhaphy, as they can easily tear and enlarge the original injury. The use of bioprosthetic materials in the form of Teflon pledgets is not recommended for management of these injuries.

Repair of Ventricular Injuries

Ventricular injuries usually cause significant hemorrhage. They should be occluded digitally and simultaneously repaired by either simple interrupted or horizontal mattress sutures of Halsted. Ventricular cardiorrhaphy can also be accomplished with a running monofilament suture of 2-0 polypropylene on an MH needle. Performing cardiorrhaphy for ventricular for stab wounds is usually less challenging than for gunshot wounds. Missile injuries often produce some degree of blast effect that causes myocardial fibers to retract. Frequently, missile injuries that have been successfully sutured and controlled enlarge, as the damaged myocardium retracts and becomes more friable. Frequently, these injuries require multiple sutures to control significant hemorrhage. In the presence of this scenario, bioprosthetic materials such as Teflon strips or pledgets are often needed to buttress the suture line. This is usually performed by fashioning a Teflon strip that may measure anywhere from 1 to 5 cm (Figs. 17 and 18). This strip is held by two straight Crile clamps held by an assistant. Simultaneously, the trauma surgeon may then place double-armed 2-0 polypropylene monofilament sutures on an MH needle, first through the strip, and then through both sides of the injury. A second strip is then held in a similar fashion so that the trauma surgeon then

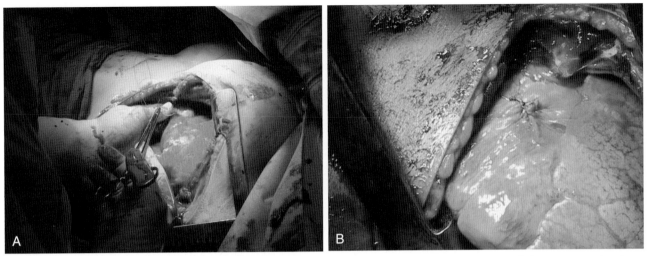

FIGURE 17 **A,** Repairing a stab wound to the heart, after emergency department thoracotomy. **B,** Same patient with the suture completed.

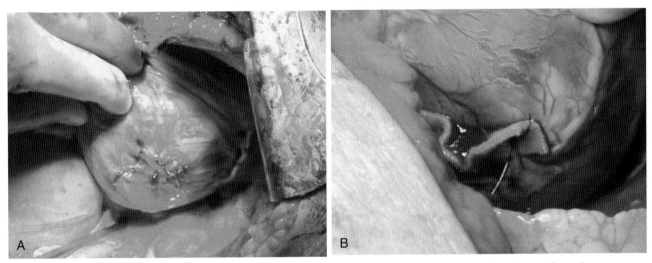

FIGURE 18 **A,** Patient sustained a penetrating injury to the cardiac apex. **B,** Same patient with Teflon patches used to reinforce the sutures.

places both needles thru the second Teflon strip. The sutures are then gently tied against the Teflon strip or pledget, which will buttress and reinforce the suture line. This maneuver must be repeated until total control of ventricular hemorrhage is achieved. The authors have recently used commercially made fibrin sealants to seal complex ventricular injuries.

Coronary Artery Injuries

The repair of ventricular injuries adjacent to coronary arteries can be very challenging. Injudicious or inappropriate placement of sutures during cardiorrhaphy may narrow and occlude a coronary artery or one of its branches. Therefore, it is recommended that sutures be placed underneath the bed of the coronary artery. Coronary arteries are usually divided into three segments: (1) proximal, (2) middle, and (3) distal. Injuries to the proximal segment of a coronary artery will usually require cardiopulmonary bypass for repair, although this is infrequently necessary. Injuries of the middle segment of the coronary artery may also require cardiopulmonary bypass or, if ligated in desperation, may result in immediate myocardial infarction at the operating table. These patients may benefit from the institution of intraaortic balloon counterpulsation followed by aortocoronary bypass. Lacerations of the distal segment of the coronary artery particularly in the distalmost third of the vessel are managed by ligation.

Use of Bioprosthetic and Autogenous Materials

Trauma surgeons are familiar with the use of Teflon pledgets or strips to buttress suture lines on friable myocardial tissue. Mattox provided the first reference in the literature alluding to the use of this material. The authors strongly believe in the necessity to buttress complex suture lines and use Teflon when indicated. However, no studies have been performed to determine if the use of Teflon increases tensile strength of the repair. The use of autogenous materials such as the pericardium to bolster suture lines is also well known. A small flap is developed and excised from the pericardium to be used in a manner similar to use of Teflon pledgets. Inexperienced trauma surgeons will often suture the pericardium to a ventricular injury causing the chamber to be fixated, which leads to dysrhythmias. This is mentioned, as it is a pitfall that should be avoided at all costs.

Complex and Combined Injuries

As trauma surgeons and trauma centers continue to develop greater expertise in the management of penetrating cardiac injuries, and patients are subjected to greater degrees of violence in urban arenas of warfare, a significant number of patients arrive harboring multiple associated injuries in addition to their penetrating cardiac injuries. Complex and combined cardiac injuries can be defined as a penetrating cardiac injury plus associated neck, thoracic, thoracic-vascular, abdominal, abdominal vascular, or peripheral vascular injuries. These injuries are quite challenging to manage. Priority should be given early to the injury causing the greatest blood loss or threatening the patient's life.

Wall and Mattox described 60 patients with complex cardiac injuries, which they defined as those beyond lacerations of the myocardium. These injuries were defined as those with concomitant coronary artery injuries, cardiac valvular injuries, intracardiac fistulas, and other unusual injuries. In this series, the authors described 39 coronary artery injuries; 2 valvular injuries; and 14 intracardiac fistulas including ventriculoseptal defects, atrioseptal defects, and another 10 injuries that they considered unusual ranging from ventricular false aneurysms to coronary sinus injuries and 2 patients who developed missile emboli to the heart. These types of injuries can also be considered complex and combined injuries.

RESULTS

The literature abounds with retrospective series describing the use of EDT. Great difficulties, however, exist in evaluating the results of these series. Close scrutiny reveals several flaws; most series have been retrospective reviews, many from institutions that employ this technique infrequently. Furthermore, many institutions report many overlapping studies that encompass the experience of many years. Whereas many series have selected physiologic parameters as predictors of outcome, none have statistically validated their predictive values. Invariably, these series omit data pertaining to the physiologic status of the patient upon initial presentation. To our knowledge, there is only one prospective study in the literature. As a result, there are still many questions to be answered.

Which patients should be subjected to this procedure?
Are there any prospectively validated physiologic predictors of outcomes that can safely and accurately identify patients who will benefit from the procedure and also safely exclude those who will not?
What are the true survival rates of this procedure?
Of the surviving patients, how many survive with severe neurologic impairment or remain in a persistent vegetative state?
How can we ensure that individuals performing this procedure are qualified?

Well-known physiologic factors predictive of poor outcome include prehospital and ED absence of vital signs, fixed and dilated pupils, absence of cardiac rhythm and motion in the extremities, and agonal breathing. Similarly, the absence of a palpable pulse in the presence of cardiopulmonary arrest is also predictive of poor outcome. These factors have been validated by Asensio and colleagues, who tracked cases in the field, during transport, and upon arrival in the ED in two prospective studies dealing with penetrating cardiac injuries. Interestingly enough, many of these physiologic predictors of outcome, as well as any data describing the physiologic condition of the patient prior to EDT, are often absent in many studies.

Previous work by Buckman et al and Asensio and colleagues applied and validated the cardiovascular respiratory score (CVRS) of the trauma score (TS). The cardiovascular respiratory component of the TS reflects individual elements of blood pressure, respiratory rate, respiratory effort, and capillary refill. The highest possible CVRS is 11, which denotes a systolic blood pressure of greater than 90 mm Hg, respiratory rates that fluctuate between 10 and 24/minute, along with a normal respiratory effort and capillary refill. The lowest possible CVRS score is zero, which reflects an absence of blood pressure and no palpable carotid pulse, along with an absence of breathing, respiratory effort, and capillary refill. This score has been statistically validated and applied to the only three perspective cardiac injury series reported in the literature.

Asensio and colleagues, in the only prospective study on the use of EDT reported in the literature, analyzed parameters measuring the physiologic condition of patients incurring cardiopulmonary arrest in the field, during transport, and upon arrival at the trauma center. The CVRS, injury mechanism, and anatomic site of injury, along with restoration of blood pressure, were tracked prospectively with the objectives of identifying a set of parameters that would reliably predict mortality risk and exclude patients from EDT. This 2-year prospective study had a single inclusion criterion—cardiopulmonary arrest secondary to traumatic injury—as well as a single intervention, EDT for resuscitation. The main outcome of this study was survival at 1 hour and survival to discharge.

A total of 215 patients who sustained cardiopulmonary arrest were studied prospectively. Of this total, 167 (78%) sustained penetrating injuries, including 142 (66%) gunshot wounds, 21 (10%) stab wounds, and 4 (2%) shotgun wounds. In addition, there were 48 (22%) who sustained blunt injuries. The mean revised trauma score was 0.6, the mean injury severity score was 42, and the mean CVRS was 1, denoting a severely injured and physiologically compromised patient population. The mean duration of CPR prior to arrival at the trauma center was 12 minutes.

A total of 162 patients (75%) succumbed in the ED. Fifty-three patients (25%) survived up to 1 hour, after successful ED resuscitation with some restoration of vital signs so that they could be transported immediately to the operating room. Of the 215 patients, only 6 (3%) survived, all of whom sustained cardiac injuries. None of the 48 patients who were injured due to blunt trauma survived. Upon comparing patients succumbing in the ED with those who survived at least 1 hour, all physiologic parameters were predictive of outcome ($p < .001$). When all patients who survived 1 hour were compared with overall survivors, none of the physiologic parameters predicted outcome. Duration of CPR ($p = .04$), penetrating mechanism of injury ($p < .001$), and exsanguination ($p < .006$) were predictors of outcome. The CVRS showed a trend toward the prediction of survival ($p = .07$). When all nonsurvivors were compared with survivors, restoration of blood pressure was a strong predictor of outcome ($p < .001$).

The authors concluded from these data that physiologic parameters plus the CVRS score were predictive of survival for patients undergoing EDT. On the basis of these criteria, the authors estimated that 75% of these patients could be safely excluded from this procedure at a cost savings of over $500,000 at their institution, and recommended that EDT should be limited to patients sustaining penetrating cardiac injuries and should not be applied to patients sustaining cardiopulmonary arrest secondary to blunt trauma.

Precisely because of the lack of uniformity in the reporting process in many of the reports in the literature, Asensio and colleagues in the working group of the Ad Hoc Subcommittee on Outcomes of the American College of Surgeons Committee on Trauma closely scrutinized the literature to generate practice management guidelines for EDT.

In an extensive literature search, studies were classified into three classes. Class I comprises prospective randomized controlled trials and remains the gold standard of all clinical trials. In this category, the studies found were generally poorly designed, had inadequate numbers, or suffered from methodologic inadequacies, rendering them clinically nonsignificant. In this group, no prospective randomized controlled trials were found. Studies in class II included clinical studies in which data were collected prospectively, as well as retrospective analyses based on clearly reliable data. Included here are observational, cohort, prevalence, and case-controlled studies. The authors found 29 studies that qualified for class II, three of which were prospective. Finally, for class III—defined as retrospectively collected data including clinical series, databases or registries, case reviews, case reports, and expert opinion—the authors located 63 studies.

Analysis was conducted by stratifying the series into series dealing with EDT, series reporting neurologic outcomes of patients subjected to EDT, series dealing exclusively with penetrating cardiac injuries, and series dealing with pediatric patients. In the 42 series dealing with EDT (Table 2), there were 7035 EDTs and 551 survivors, for a survival rate of 7.83%. When data were stratified according to mechanism of

TABLE 2: Analysis of 42 Series Dealing with Emergency Department Thoracotomy

Lead Author*	Year	Type of Study	Survivors/ Total EDT	Neurologic Impairment (n)	Survivors/ Penetrating Trauma	Survivors/ Blunt Trauma
Mattox	1974	R	11/106	0	8/87	3/19
McDonald	1978	R	3/28	0	3/26	0/2
Moore	1979	R	12/146	4	11/98	1/48
Baker	1980	R	32/168	2	31/108	1/60
Hamar	1981	R	5/64	0	—	—
Ivatury	1981	R	8/22	1	8/22	—
Flynn	1982	R	4/33	0	4/13	0/20
Bodai	1982	R	0/38	0	—	0/38
Rohman	1983	R	24/91	0	24/91	—
Vij	1983	R	5/63	1	5/57	0/6
Cogbill	1983	R	16/400	4	15/205	1/195
Shimazu	1983	R	6/267	2	4/50	4/217
Danne	1984	R	10/89	1	10/60	0/29
Tavares	1984	R	21/37	0	21/37	—
Washington	1984	R	6/23	0	6/23	0
Washington	1985	R	8/55	0	8/55	—
Brantigan	1985	R	6/32	1	6/32	
Feliciano	1986	R	28/335	1	25/280	3/53
Roberge	1986	R	7/44	0	7/44	—
Schwab	1986	R	14/51	0	14/36	0/15
Moreno	1986	R	4/69	0	4/69	—
Ordog	1987	R	6/80	1	5/64	2/16
Demetriades	1987	R	5/73	0	5/73	—
Baxter	1988	R	29/632	0	22/313	7/319
Clevenger	1988	R	3/72	0	3/41	0/31
Hoyt	1989	R	33/113	0	33/74	0/39
Mandal	1989	R	7/23	0	——	0
Esposito	1991	R	2/112	1	1/24	1/88
Ivatury	1991	R	16/163	0	16/134	0/29
Lewis	1991	R	8/45	0	8/32	0/13
Durham	1992	R	32/389	0	32/318	0/69
Lorenz	1992	R	41/424	4	37/231	3/193
Blake	1992	R	5/22	0	5/22	—
Bond	1992	R	2/28	0	2/11	0/17
Millham	1993	R	13/290	4	13/290	—

Continued

TABLE 2: Analysis of 42 Series Dealing with Emergency Department Thoracotomy—cont'd

Lead Author*	Year	Type of Study	Survivors/ Total EDT	Neurologic Impairment (n)	Survivors/ Penetrating Trauma	Survivors/ Blunt Trauma
Mazzorana	1994	R	10/273	0	10/252	0/21
Velmahos	1995	R	43/855	0	42/679	1/176
Jahangiri	1996	R	1/16	0	1/4	0/12
Brown	1996	R	4/160	0	4/149	0/11
Bleetman	1996	R	8/25	0	8/24	0/1
Branncy	1998	R	41/868	7	33/483	8/385
Asensio	1998	P	6/215	0	6/167	0/48

Modified from Working Group, Ad Hoc Subcommittee on Outcomes, American College of Surgeons, Committee on Trauma: Practice management guidelines for emergency department thoracotomy. *J Am Coll Surg* 193(3):303–309, 2001.
EDT, Emergency department thoracotomy; P, prospective; R, retrospective.
*Studies listed here are cited in Suggested Readings, available online.

injury, there were 4482 thoracotomies for penetrating injuries; of these, 500 patients survived, yielding a survival rate of 11.16%. There were 2193 thoracotomies performed for blunt injuries; only 35 patients survived, for a survival rate of 1.60%.

Of the 14 series reporting neurologic outcomes and their results, a total of 4520 patients were subjected to EDT with 226 survivors, yielding a 5% survival rate. Of these 226 survivors, 34 (15%) survived with neurologic impairment. In the series dealing exclusively with EDTs performed to repair penetrating cardiac injuries (Table 3), in a total of 1165 EDTs, 363 patients survived, yielding a survival rate of 31.1%. Only four series were found that dealt exclusively with pediatric patients (Table 4). There were 142 EDTs performed. Of 57 thoracotomies

performed for penetrating injuries, 7 patients survived, yielding a survival rate of 12.2%. Eighty-five thoracotomies were performed for blunt injuries; 2 patients survived, for a survival rate of 2.3%.

Although EDT does not lend itself to be studied with prospective randomized control trials, the authors have produced the following recommendations:

1. EDT should be performed rarely in patients sustaining cardiopulmonary arrest secondary to blunt trauma because of its very low survival rate and poor neurologic outcomes. It should be limited to those who arrive with vital signs at the trauma center and experience a witnessed cardiopulmonary arrest.

TABLE 3: Emergency Department Thoracotomy for Cardiac Injuries: Analysis of 46 Reports

Lead Author*	Year	Type of Study	Survivors/Total EDT	Survivors/Penetrating Trauma
Boyd	1965	R	0/0	17/25
Beall	1966	R	3/16	42/197
Sauer	1967	R	12/0	12/13
Sugg	1968	R	0/0	63/459
Yao	1968	R	0/0	61/80
Steichen	1971	R	7/21	35/58
Beall	1971	R	29/52	42/66
Borja	1971	R	0/0	24/145
Carrasquilla	1972	R	8/30	20/245
Beall	1972	R	0/0	67/269
Bolanowski	1973	R	0/0	33/44
Trinkle	1974	R	0/0	38/45
Mattox	1974	R	25/37	31/62
Harvey	1975	R	0/0	22/28

TABLE 3: Emergency Department Thoracotomy for Cardiac Injuries: Analysis of 46 Reports—cont'd

Lead Author*	Year	Type of Study	Survivors/Total EDT	Survivors/Penetrating Trauma
Symbas	1976	R	0/0	50/98
Beach	1976	R	0/4	26/34
Asfaw	1977	R	0/0	277/323
Sherman	1978	R	32/41	37/92
Trinkle	1978	R	0/0	89/100
Evans	1979	R	0/4	29/46
Breaux	1979	R	39/44	78/197
Mandal	1979	R	/38	26/55
Gervin	1982	R	4/21	4/21
Demetriades	1983	R	2/16	40/125
Demetriades	1984	R	1/11	45
Tavares	1984	R	21/37	64
Feliciano	1984	R	5/15	3/2
Mattox	1985	R	50/119	204
Demetriades	1986	R	1/18	70
Moreno	1986	R	4/69	100
Ivatury	1987	R	28/91	—
Jebara	1989	R	4/17	—
Attar	1991	R	21/55	—
Knott-Craig	1992	R	5/13	—
Buchman	1992	R	1/2	23
Benyan	1992	R	1/13	—
Macho	1993	R	12/24	—
Mitchell	1993	R	7/47	—
Kaplan	1993	R	2/23	
Henderson	1994	R	6/122	215
Coimbra	1995	R	0/20	
Arreola-Risa	1995	R	11/40	
Karmy-Jones	1997	R	3/6	16
Rhee	1998	R	15/58	41/96
Asensio	1998	P	6/37	6/37
Asensio	1998	P	10/71	10/71

Modified from Working Group, Ad Hoc Subcommittee on Outcomes, American College of Surgeons, Committee on Trauma: Practice management guidelines for emergency department thoracotomy. *J Am Coll Surg* 193(3):303–309, 2001.
Note: There were no survivors of blunt trauma.
EDT, Emergency department thoracotomy; P, prospective; R, retrospective.
*Studies listed here are cited in Suggested Readings, available online.

TABLE 4: Emergency Department Thoracotomy in Children

Lead Author*	Year	Type of Study	Survivors/Total EDT	Survivors, Penetrating Trauma	Survivors, Blunt Trauma
Beaver	1987	R	0/17	0/2	0/15
Powell	1988	R	5/19	4/11	1/8
Rothenberg	1989	R	3/83	2/36	1/47
Sheikh	1993	R	1/23	1/8	0/15

Modified from Working Group, Ad Hoc Subcommittee on Outcomes, American College of Surgeons, Committee on Trauma: Practice management guidelines for emergency department thoracotomy. *J Am Coll Surg* 193(3):303–309, 2001.
EDT, Emergency department thoracotomy; R, retrospective.
*Studies listed here are cited in Suggested Readings, available online.

2. EDT is best applied to patients sustaining penetrating cardiac injuries who arrive at trauma centers after a short scene and transport time with witnessed or objectively measured physiologic parameters (signs of life), such as pupillary response, spontaneous ventilation, presence of carotid pulse, measurable or palpable blood pressure, extremity movement, or cardiac electrical activity.
3. EDT should be performed in patients sustaining penetrating noncardiac thoracic injuries, but these patients generally experience a low survival rate. Because it is difficult to ascertain whether the injuries are noncardiac thoracic versus cardiac, EDT can be used to establish a diagnosis.
4. EDT should be performed in patients sustaining exsanguinating abdominal vascular injuries, but these patients generally experience a low survival rate. Judicious selection of patients should be exercised. This procedure should be used as an adjunct to definitive repair of the abdominal vascular injury.
5. For the pediatric population, guidelines 1 to 4 are applicable.
6. In conclusion, EDT remains a very powerful tool in the trauma surgeons' armamentarium. It should be employed wisely with strict indications, and should be performed only by trauma surgeons and surgeons properly trained. Only by judicious scientific inquiry can we push the envelope, save lives, and advance science.

For the chapter's Suggested Readings list, please visit the book at www.ExpertConsult.inkling.com.

Focused Assessment with Sonography for the Trauma Patient

Andrés M. Rubiano, Glyn Estebanez, and Aurelio Rodríguez

The use of focused assessment with sonography in trauma (FAST) in the management of the trauma patient has become increasingly widespread over the past two decades. Serial improvements in ultrasound technology, its portability, and the quality of the images have facilitated rapid and reliable diagnostic images during the initial resuscitation in the emergency room. Confirmation of the acceptance, and importance, of its use was highlighted by the American College of Surgeon's (ACS) incorporation of FAST into the Advanced Trauma Life Support (ATLS) curriculum in 1997. Presently, multidisciplinary teams perform worldwide FAST, including trauma surgeons, emergency medicine physicians, and prehospital providers. There are several guidelines and evidence-based reviews about FAST in different settings, including operational and tactical scenarios in war zones. Extensions of the classic technique have been promoted and wireless devices have been developed. The aim of this chapter is to describe the technique, the indications, the controversies, and the evolution of the process.

BRIEF HISTORY OF THE ULTRASOUND

In 1917, the first piezoelectric generator was used in the creation of ultrasound. The crystals of the generator also served as a receiver, generating electrical signals upon detection of the reflected mechanical vibrations or sound waves. During World War II the vast potential of ultrasound technology began to be recognized with its use in SONAR (Sound Navigation and Ranging) systems that enabled the detection of submarines and subsequently saved countless lives. In 1959, the use of the Doppler effect during ultrasound examination enabled the flow of peripheral arteries to be detected; however, it was the introduction of the gray scale, in 1971, that marked the beginning of the widespread acceptance of ultrasound as a diagnostic tool.

During the 1980s, the German physicians pioneered the utilization of ultrasound in trauma, introducing standardized ultrasound training programs for its surgical residents in 1988. In 1992, North America recognized the potential role of ultrasound in patient care and began implementing its teaching in the assessment of the trauma patient, as described in seminal papers of Hoffman TSO and Rodriguez. After the publication of several case series demonstrating the successful use of ultrasound in the management of the trauma patient, the ACS incorporated FAST into their algorithm for the management of abdominal trauma in 1995. Initially, the technique was focused to the abdominal region and, in 1996, the term FAST (focused abdominal sonogram for trauma) was described according to papers published by Rodriguez, Rozycki, and others. Later in the same year, the method was included in ATLS training program and the definition of FAST was changed to focused assessment with sonography for the trauma patient. In 1997, when it was included into the ATLS course, FAST became acknowledged as a fundamental and valuable tool in trauma patient care.

FAST TRAINING EVOLUTION

The technique initially was widespread between surgeons and surgical residents. But actually other specialties involved in the trauma care also participate in the training process, including emergency medicine physicians, critical care physicians, and prehospital providers. The aim of the FAST training program is simply to improve the ability to accurately diagnose the presence of free fluid. FAST is a rapid, accurate, noninvasive, and easily repeated method of detecting free fluid that can be performed during the primary survey and also in the unstable patient during the initial resuscitation. Guidelines for appropriated FAST use have been developed in several consensuses, including the following recommendations:

- Evaluation with ultrasound must be available to be performed 24 hours a day at the bedside in the resuscitation room.
- The trauma surgeon performing FAST must be appropriately trained in accurately performing and interpreting the scan.
- Each hospital must train and evaluate its doctors to ensure effective use of the resource, with use of different specialists to help candidates improve their interpretation and decision making.
- Training in FAST must form part of the curriculum for surgical residents (Fig. 1).
- The value of FAST in decision making during the management of the trauma patient is operator dependent; therefore, effective teaching, and continued training, of doctors in the accurate performance and interpretation of the technique are priorities.

PRINCIPLES OF ULTRASOUND

Ultrasonography may be defined as the imaging of deep body structures by recording the echoes of pulses of ultrasonic waves directed into the tissues and reflected by tissue planes where there is a change in density. Audible sound waves have a frequency range between 20 KHz and 15 Hz; infrasound wave frequency is below 15 Hz, and ultrasound waves used in medical imaging range from 1 MHz to 60 MHz. The ultrasound waves used in medical imaging are longitudinal waves that may pass through liquid and soft tissues but are not readily transmitted in the absence of these substances; hence, air-filled structures such as the lungs are poorly visualized by ultrasound. Once an ultrasound wave encounters a material with a different density or acoustic impedance, a fraction of that sound wave is reflected and detected by the transducer. The greater the density of the tissue or structure, the greater the reflection or echo and therefore higher density tissues appear as brighter images upon the display. The transducer acts as both the transmitter and receiver. The ultrasound waves are generated from the mechanical movement or oscillations of crystals that are excited by electrical pulses, the piezoelectric effect. Of those sound waves transmitted into the patient's body, a small percentage is reflected back to the crystals within the transducer and

the reception of these reflected sound waves generates electrical impulses, which are processed to create an image.

The intensity of the electrical pulses that act on the crystals within the transducer allows a period of silence that is sufficient to allow the reception of both, superficial and deep reflected sound waves or echoes, prior to the generation of the next transmitted sound wave. A pulse consists of three phases: (1) the emitting phase, (2) the phase of balance, and (3) the receiving phase. The emitting phase occurs when the ultrasound wave is generated; the receiving phase is the period in which reception of the reflected sound waves occur; and the phase of balance is the period in which there is neither reception nor emission of ultrasound waves.

The majority of ultrasound scanners have a maximum depth of examination of 20 cm and on occasions it is important to analyze the area from different angles so as to obtain the best possible image. Sound waves have a constant speed of 1540 m/second; therefore, if a wave has a reduced duration of "emission and reception" to the transducer, this indicates that the particular soft tissue, which is reflecting the sound wave, is of greater density. When soft tissue does not reflect the sound wave, and no signal is obtained, this often indicates cystic content.

Transducers

Transducers consist of several basic components; the crystal of the transducer is made of a piezoelectric material, typically single-crystal quartz or lead zirconate titanate. The purpose of the crystal is to convert the electrical impulses into transmitted sound waves and vice versa. Insulation material, most commonly rubber, is used for the "nose" of the transducer and increases the focused transmission of the sound waves, thus increasing the axial resolution and depth of the sound wave penetration. An external protector or acoustic insulator is used to envelope the transducer and isolate it from any unwanted sound wave interference. The transducer is connected to the external display via an electronic cable, which allows the transmission of electrical impulses toward and away from the piezoelectric crystals.

Types of Transducers and Their Uses

The suitability of the use of specific transducers is dependent upon the purpose of the scan being performed as well as the depth of view that is required. Frequencies more often used for medical imaging range from 2 to 20 MHz, with higher frequencies being used for the optimal viewing of superficial structures. This is because higher frequencies have smaller wavelengths, which are subject to greater levels of attenuation of the sound waves over shorter distances when compared with lower frequencies. Transducers used for viewing superficial tissues tend to use frequencies ranging from 7 to 12 MHz and have a maximum depth of imaging of 4 cm. Transducers utilizing lower frequencies between 3 to 5 MHz allow transmission of sound waves to

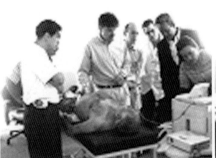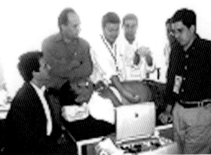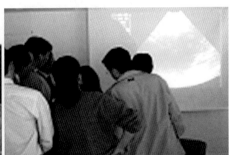

FIGURE 1 Focused assessment with sonography for trauma training session for surgery and emergency medicine residents. The Ultrasound in Trauma and Emergency Room training program is a Pan-American Trauma Society course developed for FAST training in Latin American countries. *(Courtesy Dr. Andres Rubiano [USET instructors group].)*

greater depths and therefore are suitable for use in imaging abdominal and pelvic regions and thus are used in the performance of FAST.

The shape of the transducer "nose" is an important factor in when its use is appropriate. Linear scanners allow the transmission of sound waves that run parallel to each other and remain the same distance regardless of the depth of transmission, and thus, linear scanners are best at visualizing superficial structures and soft tissues. Curved surface scanners transmit ultrasound waves in a fan-shaped manner, thus increasing the width of view perceived. When used in combination with better penetrating lower frequency sound waves, curved scanners provide the most appropriate view with which FAST may be accurately performed (Fig. 2).

Ultrasound Settings

Modern ultrasound machines come with preset optimized combinations of different shaped transducers and wavelength frequencies to be used when scanning different parts of the body (Fig. 3). Therefore, the operator often has to merely select the appropriate viewing settings on the machine and choose the appropriate transducer prior to performing the scan. While performing FAST it may be necessary to make real-time adjustments of the setting of the ultrasound equipment so as to fine-tune the quality of the images obtained.

Detailed knowledge of the various means of improving the quality of the ultrasound picture increases the accuracy of the treatment

decisions made based upon them and therefore potentially avoids errors in diagnosis:

- **Acoustic power/output:** This controls the voltage applied to the piezoelectric crystal, increasing the power output increases the intensity of the sound wave created. Typically, the lowest level of power output is used to obtain suitable images for interpretation.
- **Cineloop:** A sequence of images stored digitally that may be reviewed upon completion of the examination.
- **Depth:** Depth determines the degree of penetration visualized upon the display screen. The maximum depth varies according to the type of transducer used. The greater the frequency, the lesser the depth (>5 MHz $<$ depth), and the lower the frequency, the greater the depth (<5 MHz $>$ depth).
- **Focus:** Focus allows increased clarity of image to be attained at the selected depths of interest during the scan. The point of focus can be varied according to the interest point during the examination.
- **Gain:** Gain regulates the degree of amplification applied to all ultrasound waves returning to the transducer. Too much or too little gain can affect the quality of the images obtained. If the gain is set too high, then the image acquired will become distorted with artifact noise and additionally there will be a loss in the contrast between different structures as all reflecting echoes become progressively brighter. If gain is set too low, the

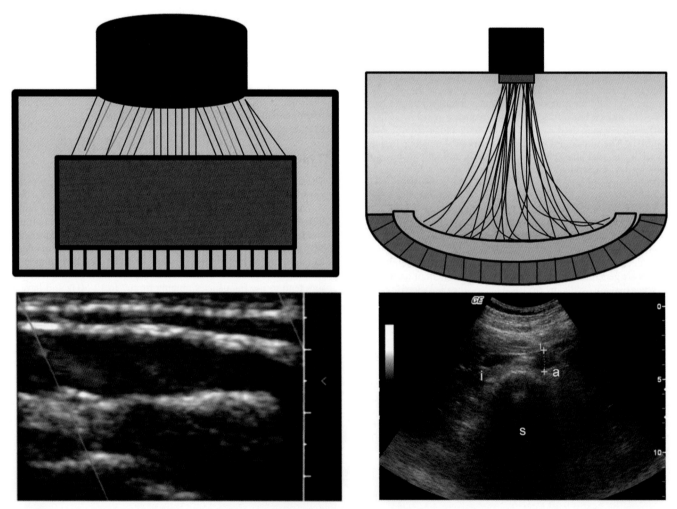

FIGURE 2 The 7.5 MHz linear *(left)* and 3.5 MHz convex *(right)* transducers scheme. The image of the first one is a typical square box used frequently in vascular scan. The trapezoidal view form is characteristic from the convex transducer, used for focused assessment with sonography for trauma.

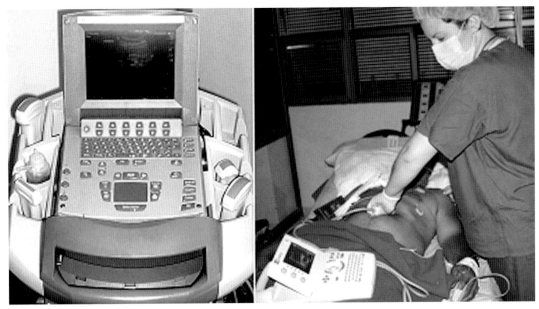

FIGURE 3   Modern portable ultrasound equipment allows performing focused assessment with sonography for trauma procedures at the bedside in short periods of time. Preset transducers normally save time and minimize the operator's error factor.

perception of some real echoes will be lost and thus the quality of the image reduced.

■ **Near gain:** This controls the amplification of the echoes within the superficial field.
■ **Far gain:** This controls the amplification of the echoes in the deep field.
■ **Zoom lens:** The zoom lens allows us to magnify the image to better visualize small structures; however, this magnification can cause some distortion of the image and subsequent loss of image quality.

USING FAST

Artifacts in FAST Imaging

■ **Noise:** Interference of the image caused by the presence of other electrical equipment.
■ **Veiling:** Bands of increased echogenicity viewed at certain depths when several focal zones are used simultaneously. It is recommended to use few focal zones.
■ **Reverberation:** Artifacts that occur in the presence of multiple reflections of the sound waves with the waves being reflected back into the body from the skin-transducer interface.
■ **Mirror imaging:** Duplication of the image of the structure that is being visualized. Revisualization of the point of interest from alternative angles or sites of the body may improve this defect.
■ **Enhancement:** An area of increased brightness underneath fluid that results from the lack of impedance of the sound wave by the fluid compared to the greater reflective tissue behind it. Typically, enhancement may occur during visualization of cystic structures.

Vocabulary Used in FAST

■ **Anechoic:** Structures that do not cause reflection of sound waves and therefore appear black upon the ultrasound image.

■ **Attenuation:** The reduction in amplitude of the sound wave as a function of the distance traveled through the tissue or medium being imaged. Progressive weakness of the sound wave is typically due to absorption by various tissues.
■ **Echogenicity:** The degree to which tissue echoes ultrasonic waves (generally reflected in ultrasound image as degree of brightness).
■ **Hypoechoic:** Less echoic (darker) than surrounding tissue.
■ **Hyperechoic:** More echoic (brighter) than surrounding tissue.
■ **Isoechoic:** Having appearance similar to that of surrounding tissue.

FAST TECHNIQUE

The appeal of FAST is that it provides a rapid, safe, noninvasive, and easily repeatable method of accurately identifying the presence of free fluid within the peritoneum or pericardium. Unlike diagnostic peritoneal lavage (DPL), FAST is a noninvasive investigation that is relatively easy to perform, is without contraindication, and is safe to perform in the pregnant trauma patient.

The four windows or views obtained in the FAST assessment may be remembered as the "four Ps": (1) pericardial, (2) perihepatic, (3) perisplenic, and (4) pelvic. These views enable the evaluation of the sites at which the presence of free fluid is more easily identified. The sequence of views obtained in the FAST examination may be varied. Some groups start by the pericardial view, especially if the patient is hemodynamically unstable, to exclude the presence of a pericardiac tamponade. Most commonly, the sequence starts at the right quadrant, Morison pouch view (perihepatic), because statistically it is the most frequent place to find free fluid (Fig. 4). There are also some groups that start by the pelvic window to obtain an appropriate view of the fluid in the bladder and then retain this image in memory to compare against other views. This technique can be useful when the operators are not well experienced.

An extended version of the classical FAST examination (E-FAST) has been developed, which also incorporates bilateral views of both hemithoraces to identify the presence of pneumothorax or hemothorax. Although this extended examination has the potential

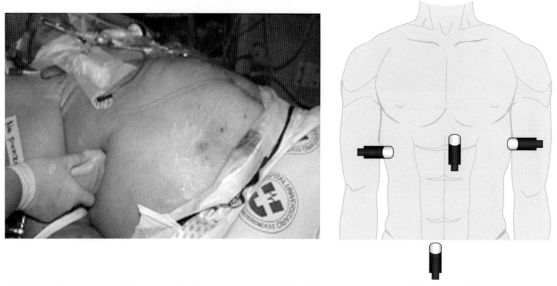

FIGURE 4 The focused assessment with sonography for trauma sequence has different ways to start. The right quadrant is statistically the most frequent area to find free fluid (Morison pouch).

to provide useful additional information, it has not as yet been formally incorporated into the routine ultrasound assessment of the trauma patient. When performed by experienced trauma clinicians, FAST assessment has been shown to positively identify the presence of as little as 250 mL of free intraperitoneal fluid. Unlike computed tomography (CT), however, the sensitivity and specificity of FAST are largely operator dependent and are dependent upon the level of experience in the use of the technique. Several studies have revealed that the accuracy of the FAST at "ruling in" the presence of free intraperitoneal or pericardial blood improves with the increased number of previous scans that the examiner has performed.

The examination is exclusively toward the detection of free fluid and cardiac obstruction. The injuries of solid organs, hollow viscera, and retroperitoneum are of difficult valuation with this technique.

The type of transducers (more in the portable equipment) are those of 2.5 MHz (for obese patients), 3.5 MHz (convex), and 5 MHz (for pediatric patients). Gel is applied in the four areas and then a sequence is followed: right superior quadrant, pericardium, left superior quadrant, and pelvic view:

- **Perihepatic window:** The transducer is positioned in the right midaxillary line, between 11th and 12th ribs. Check for Morison pouch and identify the liver, kidney, and diaphragm. The planes among them are reviewed to check for free fluid. Statistically, this is the most common location of the free fluid (Figs. 5 and 6).
- **Pericardiac window:** The classic position is the subxiphoid approach. The transducer is positioned against the xiphoid process pointing to the left shoulder. The pericardium is

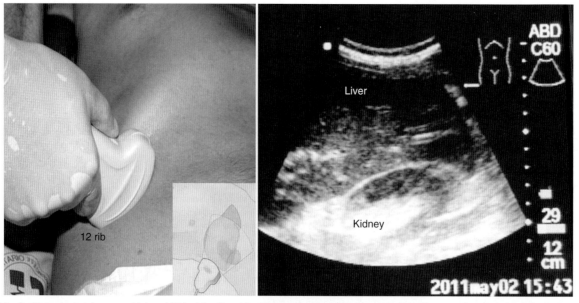

FIGURE 5 Perihepatic view between 11th and 12th right ribs with middle axillary line. The liver and the kidney are identified and there is not free fluid between them. Normal view.

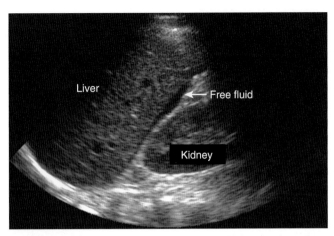

FIGURE 6 Perihepatic view between 11th and 12th right ribs with middle axillary line. The liver and the kidney are identified and there is free fluid between them. Abnormal view. *(Courtesy of M. Perdomo, USET Instructors Group.)*

checked for free fluid. In some patients, especially the obese ones, this approach is difficult. An alternative approach is between the 4th and 5th ribs parallel to the left sternal border. This approach is frequently used by a cardiologist performing echocardiography. Microconvex transducers have advantages over the regular convex transducer when performing this approach (Fig. 7).

■ **Perisplenic window:** The transducer is positioned in the left posterior axillary line, between the 10th and 11th ribs. Check for the renal-spleen fossa and identify the spleen, the kidney, and the diaphragm. The planes among them are reviewed to check for free fluid (Fig. 8).

■ **Pelvic window:** The transducer is positioned approximately 4 cm over the pubic bone. The bladder is easily identified, especially if it is full of urine. If not and a Foley catheter is in position, saline can be injected to fill the bladder. The rectovesical and the rectouterine space (pouch of Douglas) are examined for free fluid. This is the second most frequent location of free fluid in several studies (Figs. 9 and 10).

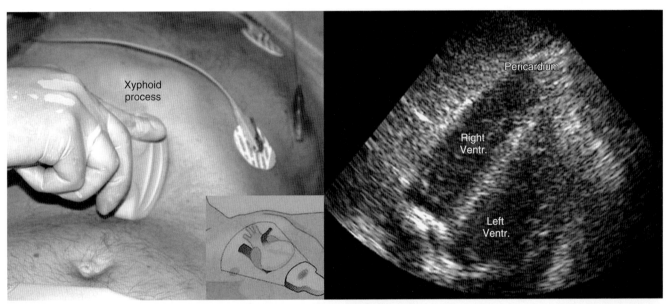

FIGURE 7 Subxiphoid approach for pericardiac window. The ventricles are identified and the surrounding pericardium is free of fluid. Normal view.

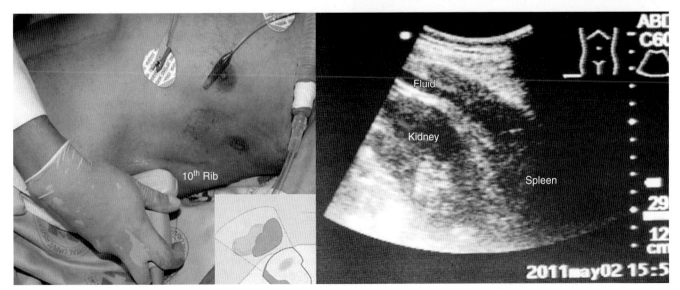

FIGURE 8 Perisplenic window. Under the 10th rib with posterior axillary line, the spleen and the kidney are identified. This patient has a penetrating injury and there is free fluid between the two organs. Abnormal view.

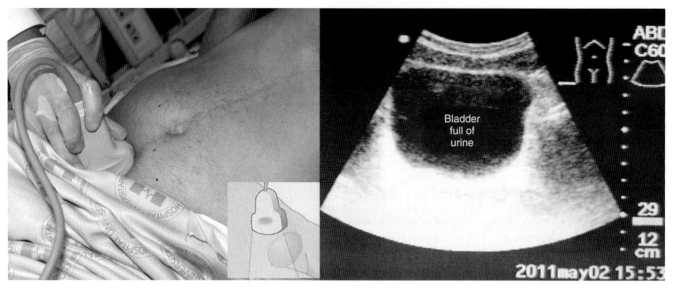

FIGURE 9 Pelvic window: 4 cm above the pubic bone, the bladder is identified. There is not free fluid surrounding the organ. There is hyperechogenic enhancement after the bladder. Normal view with normal artifact (enhancement) due to the lack of impedance of the sound wave by the fluid compared to the greater reflective tissue behind it.

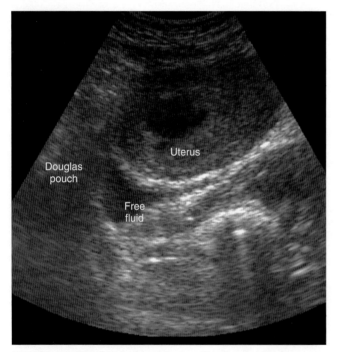

FIGURE 10 Free fluid in the pelvic view. The Douglas pouch (rectouterine space) has free fluid around the uterus. Some free fluid can be normal in this view. *(Courtesy of M. Perdomo, USET Instructors Group.)*

▣ EXTENDED FAST FOR THORACIC TRAUMA ULTRASOUND

Lichtenstein et al were the first to describe the utilization of ultrasound in the diagnosis of pneumothorax in the intensive care unit, and, subsequently, ultrasound was shown to be applicable for this purpose in the emergency department. In 2004, Kirkpatrick et al proposed "extending" FAST to incorporate visualization of the thorax, hence modifying the acronym to E-FAST. Unlike the chest radiograph or CT scan, ultrasound assessment of the thorax for the presence of pneumothorax or hemothorax is a rapid assessment tool that provides an immediate diagnosis at the time of performance, may be performed during the resuscitation of the patient, and does not expose the patient to potentially harmful radiation. Additionally, ultrasound has been shown to have comparable and even superior accuracy in the diagnosis of pneumothorax and hemothorax when compared to current established diagnostic methods. In 1997, Ma and Mateer demonstrated that ultrasound has equivalent accuracy to chest radiograph in the detection of traumatic hemothorax with the additional benefit that the examination may be performed faster. In the detection of traumatic pneumothorax, ultrasound has been shown to have superior sensitivity compared to supine chest radiographs (49% vs. 21%; 98% vs. 75.5%), and also to have comparable accuracy to CT scans.

E-FAST Technique

The technique for identifying pneumothorax with ultrasound involves utilization of a higher frequency transducer (7.5 MHz) due to the reduced depth of visualization involved. With the patient in the supine position, each hemithorax is examined by placing the transducer over the third to fourth intercostal spaces along the mid-axillary line and slowly moving the transducer medially and laterally between the ribs in both sagittal and transverse orientations. The lung pleura is examined to assess for the presence of "pleural sliding" and "comet-tail" artifacts, both of which should be present within the normal hemithorax examination (Fig. 11). To confirm, the motion mode in real time can be used to evaluate the "stratosphere sign." If air is not present, the differences between the soft tissue image (stratosphere lines) and the lung tissue image (beach sand lines) will be identified. If air is present, the entire image will show "stratosphere" pattern without the beach sand lines (Fig. 12).

Pleural sliding describes the presence of a hyperechoic line between visceral and parietal pleura representing the continuous apposition of these layers, throughout the movement of inspiration and expiration. In the presence of a pneumothorax, air separates the layers of the pleura and subsequently prevents the transmission of the ultrasound waves and thus visualization of the visceral pleura is lost, and pleural sliding cannot be seen. Comet-tail artifacts occur when ultrasound waves reverberated in between two closely related tissue layers, resulting in the emergence of multiple reverberations and the formation of a bright vertical line—the "comet tail." In the

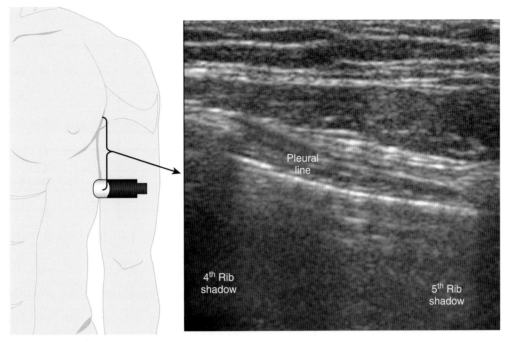

FIGURE 11   E-FAST (extended focused assessment with sonography for trauma). The pleural line is identified between the 4th and 5th ribs. The sliding movement is identified and the "comet-tail" artifact is the normal finding. The photograph shows a normal pleural space. *(Photograph courtesy of M. Perdomo, USET Instructors Group.)*

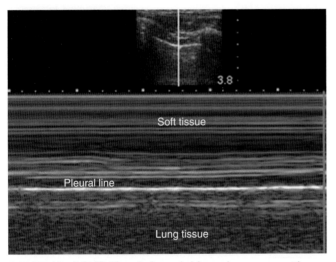

FIGURE 12   E-FAST, M-mode (extended focused assessment with sonography for trauma, using motion mode). The pleural line is identified between the soft tissue (stratosphere lines) and the lung tissue (beach sand lines). Air is not present. If air were present, the entire image will appear as soft tissue. The photograph shows a normal pleural space. *(Courtesy of M. Perdomo, USET Instructors Group.)*

normal hemithorax ultrasound waves are strongly reflected by the lung and thus the hyperechoic tapering comet tail is visualized deep to the visceral pleura. In the presence of a pneumothorax, propagation of the ultrasound waves is hindered by the air within the pleural space and there this artifact is lost.

FAST ALGORITHM

FAST provides a rapid and accurate means of triaging the trauma patient, commonly within the resuscitation room, to the operating theater, the CT scanner, or the angiography suite. The role of FAST is of particular importance in the assessment of patients with blunt abdominal trauma (BAT). In the hemodynamically stable, BAT patients with a finding of free intraperitoneal fluid on FAST should undergo CT to identify the potential source of bleeding. In the hemodynamically unstable BAT patient, the finding of free intraperitoneal fluid on FAST typically denotes the necessity for an emergency laparotomy. Although FAST does not claim to rival the accuracy of CT in the detection of abdominal visceral injuries, for which it is poorly sensitive, it does provide a rapid and accurate means of assessing the unstable patient, a group in whom the use of CT would not be safe or appropriate. The role of FAST as a means of rapidly triaging the trauma patient has been emphasized by several studies, which have shown that the use of FAST is associated with a significantly decreased duration of time from arrival at the emergency department to arrival in the operating theater (Figs. 13 and 14).

FAST SCORING SYSTEMS

Some groups propose scoring FAST systems to identify patients with surgical requirements according to the amount of fluid. Huang et al developed a scoring system, giving 1 point for each area of the abdomen positive for blood, and an additional point for free-floating intestine. Two points were given for a fluid depth of greater than 2 mm in the perihepatic or perisplenic windows (Table 1). They found that 96% of patients with 3 or more points required laparotomy; however, 38% of patients with a score less than 3 still required laparotomy. The sensitivity and specificity for collections greater than 1 L at laparotomy were 84% and 71%, respectively.

McKenney et al developed a second score. This score was defined as the depth in centimeters of the deepest pocket of fluid collection, plus the number of additional spaces where fluid was seen. They found that 85% of patients with a score greater or equal to 3, and only 15% of patients with a score less than 3, required laparotomy. The sensitivity, specificity, and accuracy of this scoring system were 83%, 87%, and 85%, respectively. Both scores are useful but still there is not wide consensus regarding their use.

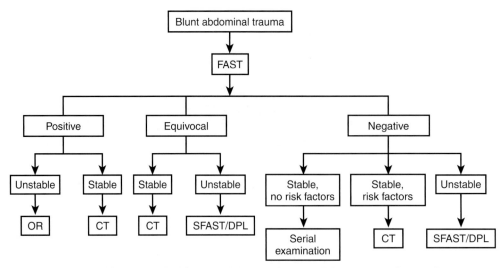

FIGURE 13   Blunt abdominal trauma FAST algorithm. Risk factors include pelvic fracture, rib fracture, spine fracture, hematuria, transient hypotension, abdominal tenderness, head injury, intoxication, and persistent base deficit. CT, Computed tomography; DPL, diagnostic peritoneal lavage; FAST, focused assessment with sonography for trauma; OR, operating room; SFAST, secondary FAST. *(Dunhan M, McKenney M, Shatz D: The role of focused assessment with sonography for trauma: indications, limitations, and controversies. In Asensio JA, Trunkey DD, editors:* Current therapy of trauma and surgical critical care. *St. Louis, Mosby Elsevier, 2008, pp 121–135.)*

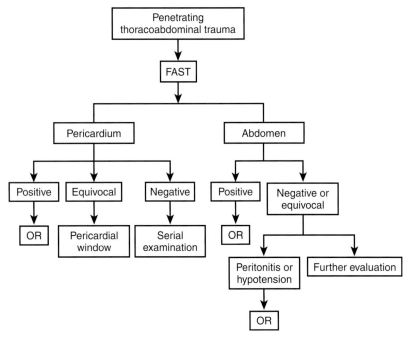

FIGURE 14   Penetrating thoraco abdominal trauma FAST algorithm. FAST, Focused assessment sonography for the trauma patient; OR, operation room. *(Dunhan M, McKenney M, Shatz D: The role of focused assessment with sonography for trauma: indications, limitations, and controversies. In Asensio JA, Trunkey DD, editors:* Current therapy of trauma and surgical critical care. *St. Louis, Mosby Elsevier, 2008, pp 121–135.)*

PEDIATRIC FAST

For more than 20 years, FAST has been routinely used in the examination of pediatric trauma patients in the identification of free intraperitoneal or pericardial fluid, and in the determination, based upon hemodynamic stability, of the need for urgent surgical intervention. The indications for performing FAST in children are identical to those in adults. Techniques used in performing the examination in children are also identical to those used in adult assessment, except that a 5-MHz transducer is often used to improve visualization.

Children are better suited to FAST examination as they have smaller abdominal cavities and the quality of the views obtained are rarely diminished by the presence of fat or morbid obesity, as may be the case in the adult population. FAST is also potentially beneficial for children as it provides a suitable alternative to unnecessary CT scanning and the associated risk of radiation-induced malignancy. One case of fatal radiation-induced malignancy occurs per 500 CT scans in adolescents and potentially 3 cases of nonfatal malignancy may be induced for every 1 case of fatal malignancy.

The accuracy of FAST in the assessment of pediatric BAT is comparable to that of the adult population. One study of 196 pediatric

TABLE 1: Huang's FAST Scoring System

Window	Size	Score*
Morison pouch	>2 mm	2
	<2 mm	1
Douglas pouch	>2 mm	2
	<2 mm	1
Perisplenic view		1
Perihepatic view		1
Free floating intestine		2

Modified from Huang M, Liu M, Wu JK, et al: Ultrasonography for the evaluation of hemoperitoneum during resuscitation: a simple scoring system. *J Trauma* 36:173, 1994.
FAST, Focused assessment with sonography for trauma.
*96% of patients with 3 or more points required laparotomy.

trauma patients found FAST to have a sensitivity of 80% and a specificity of 100%, as well as revealing that FAST was positive in 5.3%. This latter point reflects the reduced incidence of hemoperitoneum in the pediatric population. One study looking at FAST in 224 hemodynamically stable and unstable pediatric patients revealed a sensitivity of 82% and specificity of 95%, as well as finding that 7 of 7 patients who were unstable and had positive FAST were found to have intraperitoneal injury on emergency laparotomy. In the pediatric population, the need for exploratory laparotomy is the exception as opposed to being the rule with the majority of hemodynamically stable patients with positive FAST subsequently undergoing CT scans or being observed expectantly. In the hemodynamically unstable pediatric trauma patient, a positive FAST has been shown to strongly correlate with the need for urgent explorative laparotomy.

FASTER: E-FAST for Pediatrics

In addition to its role in the assessment of intraperitoneal, pericardial, and intrathoracic injuries in the pediatric trauma patient, ultrasound has also been advocated in the detection of extremity fractures. Dulchavsky et al suggested that extremity evaluation for fractures be added to the E-FAST examination, thus creating another acronym, the FASTER examination. Several studies have shown ultrasound to have a specificity of more than 90% in identifying the presence of a long-bone fracture in the pediatric patient, and sensitivities varying ranging from 78% to 97% in the exclusion of fractures. Ultrasound has been used to assist the immediate reduction of grossly displaced long-bone fractures with accompanied vascular compromise. Unlike radiographs or CT scans, ultrasound does not expose pediatric patients to harmful radiation, and, additionally, due to its portable nature, it may be utilized in the prehospital environment to help expedite the emergent treatment of potentially limb-threatening injuries.

FAST: FACTS AND EVIDENCE

Training

The accuracy of FAST is heavily dependent upon the experience and competence of the operator performing the examination. The significance of operator experience upon the sensitivity and specificity of FAST is reflected by the conclusion of one international consensus that recommended that 200 supervised scans be performed before the operator may be credentialed. Conversely, other studies have

concluded that satisfactory levels of accuracy are attained after performing only 10 proctored evaluations. This lack of clarity has highlighted the belief that credentialing of FAST should be based upon the individual's competence in performing the skill and not on the number of times it has been performed. At present, there exists no consensus as to the number of supervised FAST examinations that are needed to be performed before the clinician may be deemed as competent. International consensus ranged between 50 and 200 supervised FAST examinations to reach an appropriate level of expertise. In our own experience training different levels of physicians, including residents and primary and specialized physicians in Latin American countries through the Pan-American Trauma Society Course: Ultrasound in Trauma and Emergency Room (USET) (nearly 600 students in more than 9 countries trained in a 8-hour theoretic-practical program) we recommend 50 supervised examinations before trainees start scanning without a senior expert. We encourage health institutions in developing countries to design appropriate guidelines according to the local resources and appropriate ways for accreditation of the level of training according to local councils or scientific associations based on international consensus. In 1997, the FAST committee of the World Consensus Conference on Ultrasound, an international expert panel of different specialties recommended a 1-day training program including a 4-hour didactic component followed by a 4-hour practical component, and 200 supervised examinations.

An interesting study from Thomas et al shows how the number of studies improve the sensitivity and minimize the time needed to perform the technique (Table 2) (Figs. 15 and 16).

The use of FAST as a rapid triaging tool has been shown to have significant benefits when compared to groups in which FAST was not utilized. Melniker et al found that the use of FAST was associated with reduced duration of time until operative care in patients requiring surgery for traumatic injuries (57 minutes vs. 166 minutes) compared to patients receiving standard trauma care. This study also revealed that patients within the FAST group had a reduced length of hospital stay (6 days vs. 10.2 days), reduced resource use ($10,600 vs. $16,400), and a reduced incidence of CT scan use (53% vs. 85%). A reduction in CT use following FAST examination was also demonstrated by Rose et al, whose randomized control trial of 208 patients revealed that 36% of the FAST group underwent CT, compared to 52% of the standard trauma care group.

In 2008, a Cochrane systematic review analyzing the effect of emergency ultrasound, based algorithms on the diagnosis and management of BAT, revealed a 50% reduction in the use of CT scans in the FAST assessed patient group. Despite this, the overall conclusion of the report was that there was insufficient evidence from

TABLE 2: Accuracy of the FAST Examination in a Cohort of Physicians

Accuracy of the Examination	Hemoperitoneum (%)	Surgical Requirement (%)
Sensitivity	81.0	73.9
Specificity	99.3	99.3
Positive predictive value	89.5	89.5
Predictive value	98.0	97.9
Final accuracy	98.0	97.3

Modified from Thomas B, Falcone RE, Vasquez D, et al: Ultrasound evaluation of blunt abdominal trauma: program implementation, initial experience and learning curve. *J Trauma* 42:384–390, 1997.
FAST, Focused assessment with sonography for trauma.

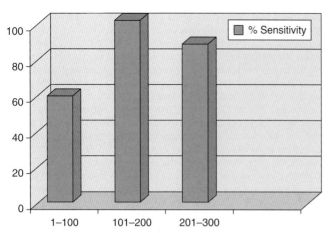

FIGURE 15 Sensitivity curve for focused assessment with sonography for trauma examination according to the number of studies performed. The best sensitivity is acquired after 100 studies and decreases a little bit after 200 examinations. *(Thomas B, Falcone RE, Vasquez D, et al: Ultrasound evaluation of blunt abdominal trauma: program implementation, initial experience and learning curve. J Trauma 42:384–390, 1997.)*

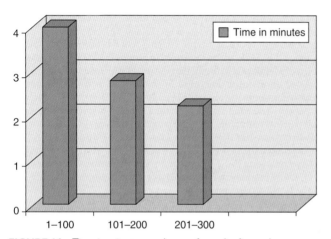

FIGURE 16 Time in minutes used to perform the focused assessment with sonography for trauma examination. The times start to decrease after 100 studies and the best performance is achieved after 200 examinations. *(Thomas B, Falcone RE, Vasquez D, et al: Ultrasound evaluation of blunt abdominal trauma: program implementation, initial experience and learning curve. J Trauma 42:384–390, 1997.)*

randomized clinical trials to justify the promotion of ultrasound based clinical pathways in diagnosing patients with BAT. Thus, at present, despite providing a safe, noninvasive, rapid and easily repeated means of accurately assessing and triaging the trauma patient, there remains a need for more large-scale studies to assess the significance of the role that FAST should play in trauma patient care.

FUTURE OF FAST

Although there is still a lot of controversy regarding the future of the FAST technique, new studies have been structured focused on the advantages of the portable devices for prehospital providers in mass casualty incident's triage, austere environments (war theaters), and in new in-hospital applications (Fig. 17). A recent systematic review of

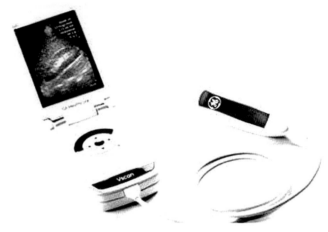

FIGURE 17 General Electric V-scan handheld ultrasound. This small device can be used for focused assessment with sonography for trauma wireless transmission miles away. The resolution of the image is fair for remote assistance. *(Courtesy of General Electric Company.)*

the applications of FAST in prehospital care shows the benefits of the technique but also the lack of studies in this field. Few studies were also performed before taking the handheld and portable devices to the Iraq war scenario. Wireless devices were used by nonmedical prehospital providers who performed the examination and sent the images miles away to emergency medicine doctors, who decided how to triage the scanned patients.

Recently, studies regarding the use of intravenous ultrasound contrast agents to enhance ultrasound imaging in the evaluation of solid organ injury have been published. The diagnostic test performance of contrast-enhanced ultrasound imaging may approach the sensitivity and specificity of abdominal CT scan for solid organ injury in abdominal trauma. If the risks of radiation-induced malignancy from CT scan become unacceptable in the future, implementation of methods to eliminate unnecessary CT scans will become high priority. Research incorporating ultrasound into clinical decision-making rules for abdominal CT scans in pediatric trauma are already in course.

Key Points to Remember in FAST

- The presence of free intraperitoneal fluid may not represent blood. Other sources of free fluid may come from a ruptured ovarian cyst, ascites, or a ruptured bladder. These can be sources of false-positive results of FAST examinations.
- Intraabdominal injury may be present even in the setting of a negative result from the FAST examination. Solid organ, bowel, and diaphragm injuries with minimal bleeding may be undetectable on ultrasound assessment.
- Thoracic ultrasound can detect a pneumothorax (lack of lung sliding) only when it is located directly under the probe. Multiple sites over the chest wall may need to be interrogated, particularly the supraclavicular fossa, to visualize the small pneumothoraces at the lung apices, especially in patients who are sitting upright.
- Fracture detection at the ends of bones or near joints can be difficult because of the curved and irregular contours where diagnostic accuracy is decreased. Comparing with the contralateral normal extremity can help to differentiate normal from abnormal.

For the chapter's Suggested Readings list, please visit the book at www.ExpertConsult.inkling.com.

ROLE OF RADIOLOGY IN INITIAL TRAUMA EVALUATION

Kim M. Caban, Gary H. Danton, Anthony M. Durso, Felipa Munera, and Luis A. Rivas

U se of radiology studies in the trauma setting, including radiography, fluoroscopy, ultrasound (US), computed tomography (CT), and magnetic resonance imaging (MRI), has increased substantially in the emergency room and trauma setting over the last decade. The use of CT, which is most concerning because of expense and radiation dose, increased 330% from 1996 to 2007 such that almost one quarter of all CT scans are performed in the emergency department. The increase in total patients seeking emergency room care during that period increased by only 30%. Substantial costs to the health care system and patient safety issues derive from overutilization of imaging resources. Safety concerns include the theoretical risk of cancer in patients exposed to radiation, the risk for renal failure or allergic reactions from contrast media, and nephrogenic systemic fibrosis from MRI contrast agents. Although these risks are often outweighed by the benefits of diagnosis, radiologists from all across the country report an excessive number of negative findings in examinations performed for questionable indications. Although medical-legal issues are often cited as a reason for imaging, the not too distant future may herald litigation for physicians who overorder radiation-based tests. Despite these concerns, imaging will remain an important tool in the diagnostic armamentarium of trauma physicians. Determining the best study to order for a particular indication requires an understanding of each modality's uses and risks, as well as an understanding of how pretest probability and evidence influence diagnostic decision making.

RADIOGRAPHY

Plain radiography (also termed plain films or "x-rays") uses ionizing radiation (potentially a cause of cancer) to produce an image based on the relative densities of tissues. Metal (most dense) appears most white and air (least dense) appears black, with all other tissues filling in the range of appearances. The spatial resolution of plain radiographs is excellent and with portable units, images are acquired with minimal patient transfer. Before CT came into common use, radiographs were the most reliable assessment for musculoskeletal injuries and evaluation of the chest. It is still commonly used in the trauma setting for a rapid evaluation of the chest, pelvis, and extremities.

The initial radiograph of the chest and pelvis is useful as a quick screening tool to assess extent of traumatic injuries, though sensitivity to detect soft tissue and bony injuries should be considered low or moderate at best if patient position is not optimal. Sensitivity also depends partly on radiograph quality (Fig. 1). Overlying structures, such as backboards and electrocardiographic leads, limit assessment of soft tissues and obscure the lung apices where small pneumothoraces may reside. Because lung volumes are typically low, the heart and mediastinum normally appear wide or enlarged. Subtle findings that suggest aortic injury, such as thickening or obscuration of the paraspinal stripe, are difficult to appreciate. Retrocardiac density may obscure the descending aorta and left diaphragm owing to atelectasis common to the supine patient in the expiratory phase of respiration. Anterolateral rib fractures in particular may be missed.

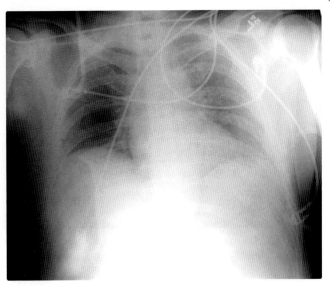

FIGURE 1 Typical chest radiograph in a trauma patient illustrates features that limit sensitivity in evaluating the chest. The chest in this patient was normal other than an old clavicle fracture. The lung volumes are low, which makes the lung appear hazy. This could be taken as a false positive for contusion. The backboard and overlying wires obscure parts of the bones and the chest, altering normal densities. Because of the supine position and low volumes, the heart and mediastinum appear wide, which is normal for this kind of study but could result in a missed mediastinum injury.

The pelvis radiograph may also miss subtle injuries, and evidence of pelvic trauma through physical examination is key to interpreting these films with respect to pretest probabilities (Fig. 2).

Fluoroscopy uses x-rays in a similar fashion as plain radiographs, but the images are viewed in real time, typically with the introduction of contrast agents. The radiation dose administered during a burst of fluoroscopy is typically less than for a conventional radiograph; however, because multiple bursts of fluoroscopy are given during a typical procedure the cumulative radiation dose can increase rapidly. Diagnostic fluoroscopic procedures are useful for evaluating hollow viscus or any structure into which contrast agent can be placed. The image is then a lumenogram, useful for identifying leaks in the bowel (Fig. 3), bladder, or extravasation during angiograms. Fluoroscopy is often used by orthopedic surgeons to set bones. Operators who use fluoroscopy should wear leaded gowns, thyroid shields, and radiation badges.

ULTRASOUND

US uses a transducer to generate sound waves, which pass into the body and bounce off tissues that have features that reflect sound. The reflected sound returns to and is detected by the transducer. By knowing how much sound returned to the transducer and how long it took for the sound wave to make the round trip, the computer calculates the depth and relative brightness of the tissue. Therefore, the image is not a density map; rather, the image is based on the ability of various tissues to reflect sound. For this reason, something that is bright is called echogenic or hyperechoic (many echoes), something that is darker than surrounding tissues is hypoechoic (less echoes), and something completely black is anechoic (no echoes). Because water conducts sound, it appears black because no sound waves are

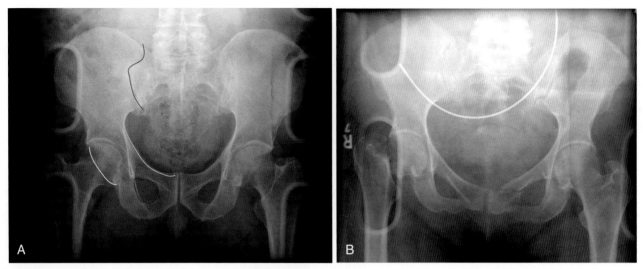

FIGURE 2 Radiographs of a normal (**A**) and a fractured (**B**) pelvis in two different patients. In both radiographs the backboard interferes with image quality, decreasing sensitivity for fracture. In **A**, a dark line along the left iliac bone is an artifact. Physicians should be cautious when reading these limited examinations. At minimum, the following lines should be glanced at to ensure they are smooth and regular: iliopectineal line *(orange)* reflecting the anterior column, sacroiliac joint *(blue)*, obturator ring *(pink)* assesses the pubic rami, teardrop *(green)* reflects the medial acetabular wall and the acetabular notch and anterior portion of the quadrilateral plate, and the posterior rim of the acetabulum *(yellow)*. **B** shows fractures of the right femoral neck, right inferior pubic ramus, left superior, inferior rami, and the left pubic bone. The sacroiliac joint on the left side is slightly widened.

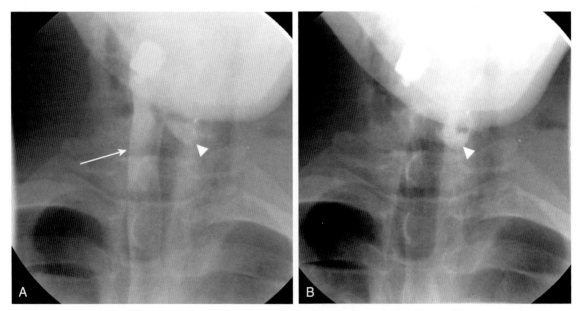

FIGURE 3 Esophagogram during (**A**) and immediately after (**B**) swallowing gastrografin. In **A**, the column of contrast material is seen in the esophagus *(arrow)* and a small outpouching of contrast material begins to form *(arrowhead)*. The contrast material persists after the esophagus is cleared (**B**), indicating that it has leaked. In the setting of a gunshot wound as illustrated by the metallic shrapnel, this is most likely posttraumatic.

reflected. In contrast, air is a strong reflector of sound, so most of the sound is reflected to the transducer. Therefore, air appears as a white line with "dirty shadowing" or an indistinct fuzzy appearance beneath it that obscures features of tissues deeper than the air. Radiology technologists sometimes say that a structure like the pancreas is "gassed out," meaning that gas from bowel is obscuring that structure. If gas is a problem, you can ask the patient to drink water, which fills the stomach and duodenum and allows better images of structures in the upper abdomen. When structures are obscured by gas or bone, it is said that the patient has "poor windows" and giving water can improve those "windows" (Fig. 4).

US has excellent temporal resolution and allows real-time imaging of the body. It is particularly useful for detecting fluid and the characteristics of fluid such as hemoperitoneum in the trauma setting. It is also useful for detecting injuries to solid organs and confirming the patency of vasculature using Doppler techniques. Importantly, because US uses sound waves, there is no ionizing radiation. Because US contrast agents are not typically used in the trauma setting, there is no risk of contrast or allergic reactions, so the safety profile of US is excellent. However, the sensitivity to detect disease such as solid organ injuries is lower than that with other modalities, such as CT.

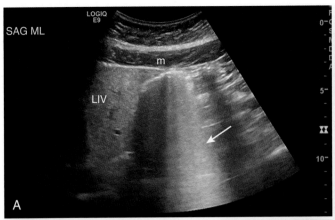

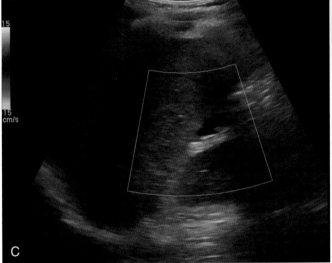

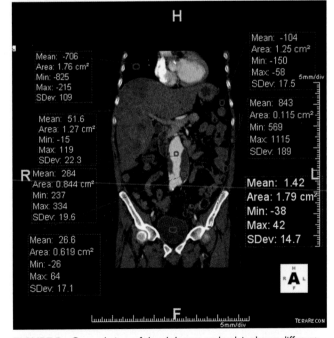

FIGURE 4   A, Ultrasound image of the right upper quadrant shows the liver *(LIV)* and an area of white hazy shadowing *(arrow)*. This is the dirty shadowing created by air within the bowel at the uppermost aspect of the abdomen just beneath the striated muscle *(m)*. B, Longitudinal views of the liver *(LIV)* and right kidney *(RT KID)* shows a small subhepatic anechoic area. To ensure this is not a vascular structure, color Doppler was placed on the area. C, Because it showed no flow, it is confirmed as a small amount of free fluid. Although more obvious cases could have been provided, it is important to realize that small areas of fluid could herald a more significant injury, and trauma surgeons performing a FAST examination should be on the lookout for small areas of free fluid.

COMPUTED TOMOGRAPHY

CT has become the work horse in the trauma setting owing to improved availability and the brief time it takes to acquire images. CT does use x-rays, a potentially cancer-causing form of ionizing radiation. By measuring the attenuation of x-rays of a particular spot in the body using a variety of projections, a computer assigns a value to that area based on the Hounsfield scale, in which water is assigned a value of 0 and air is assigned −1000. All other densities are then assigned HUs reflecting their relative density (Fig. 5). CT has excellent spatial resolution and good contrast resolution. Spatial resolution for CT is the ability to differentiate two lines separated by a very small distance. Spatial resolution allows a viewer to see small structures. Contrast resolution for CT is the ability to differentiate two adjacent tissues of slightly varying density. The ability to see a liver contusion is very dependent on contrast resolution and image noise. A noisy image appears grainy to the viewer and can obscure findings by decreasing contrast resolution. Generally, the more radiation dose used, the less noise and better overall image quality will result. Another way to improve contrast resolution is to use intravenous (IV) CT contrast agent. IV contrast agents for CT are made up of iodinated molecules that attenuate x-rays and appear bright on the image.

IV contrast reflects the vascularity of a tissue or pathologic features within the tissue and the timing of the contrast bolus is important as the different phases of contrast affect what can be seen in the image. This is important to understand because it explains why radiologists have to scan the patient multiple times and why it's important to let the radiologist know exactly what is being looked for before the study is performed. The arterial phase is obtained between 15 and 30 seconds after injection of contrast agent, depending on what part

FIGURE 5   Coronal view of the abdomen and pelvis shows different Hounsfield units (HU) of the circled tissue. Notice that the mean HU value is calculated based on all the pixels in the circled area and as such, the minimum, maximum, and standard deviation are calculated. Mean HU values in this patient are as follows: lung −706, liver 51.6, enhanced aorta 284, aortic thrombus 26.6, fat −104, cortical bone 843, and urine 1.42.

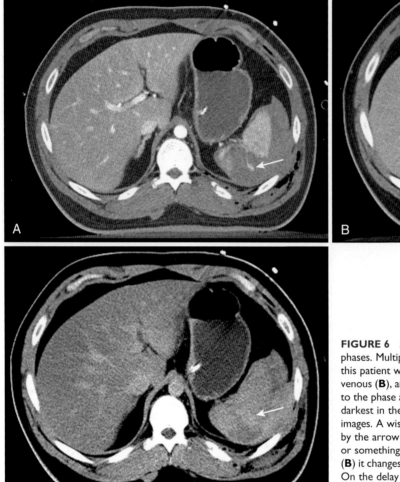

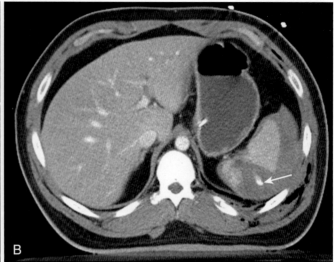

FIGURE 6 Active extravasation and computed tomography (CT) phases. Multiple axial CT images of the abdomen were obtained in this patient with trauma to the left abdomen in arterial (**A**), portal venous (**B**), and 5-minute delayed (**C**) phases. The aorta clues the reader to the phase as it is brightest in arterial, less bright in portal venous, and darkest in the delayed phases. A grade IV liver laceration is seen in all images. A wisp of contrast material on the arterial phase (**A**) marked by the arrow shows what could be either extravasated contrast agent or something dense like a calcification. On the portal venous phase (**B**) it changes shape, indicating the finding is extravasating contrast agent. On the delay phase, the contrast agent is spread out in a blush and is denser than surrounding fluid but similar to vascular structures. This confirms active extravasation.

of the body is being scanned and how fast the CT scanner is. A CT scan obtained in the arterial phase is called a CT angiogram, or CTA. The arterial phase shows only arterial supply and is excellent for seeing extraluminal contrast (active extravasation) against the background of unenhanced tissue (Fig. 6). Unfortunately, it is sometimes difficult to decide if a particular line of contrast seen on the image is part of a small vessel or actually a spurt of extravasated contrast material. For this, a more delayed phase of contrast is required. Splenic parenchyma is also particularly difficult in the arterial phase as the heterogeneous blood supply causes a mixed pattern that can be mistaken for a splenic injury.

The "portal venous" phase is usually acquired between 60 and 75 seconds after injection of contrast agent. During this time, the portal veins and solid organs including the liver, kidneys, pancreas, and spleen should be optimally enhanced for evaluation of the parenchyma. It is ideal for detecting subtle contusions or lacerations. The arteries remain enhanced but because the parenchyma of solid organs is enhanced, extravasation may be difficult to evaluate. Large veins are also enhanced at this phase and venous injuries may be detected. The delayed phase is acquired 5 minutes after contrast injection and is best for evaluating the renal collecting system and urinary bladder as they should be filled with contrast material. Solid organs have lost most of their parenchymal enhancement by 5 minutes. Because arteries are certainly not enhanced during the delayed examination, extravasated contrast will appear as a larger,

more diffuse area of contrast enhancement (a blush) than the focus of extravasated contrast seen on the arterial phase. By comparing the delayed phase or sometimes even the portal venous phase to the arterial phase, active extravasation can be diagnosed. The downside of obtaining multiple phases of contrast is the doubling or tripling of radiation dose. To reduce the chances of obtaining unnecessary scans, the radiologist may view the images before the delay phase and decide then whether or not additional phases are necessary.

CT technology has dramatically changed over the past 15 years. Conventional CT scanners obtained one image (a slice) of a given thickness. After acquiring the image, the table moved the patient to the next position and another image was obtained. This is called step and shoot. For various reasons, reconstructed images were limited and the scans were relatively slow. With helical or spiral CT, the table moves at a constant rate throughout image acquisition as the gantry rotates around the patient. Software reconstructs the images into a volumetric data set that can be reconstructed in any plane. Multidetector computed tomography (MDCT) uses multiple rows of detectors to scan a wider area of the body with each rotation. Because the scan covers a greater area, the table speed can be increased and the total time decreases. This is particularly helpful in the trauma setting as patients with altered mental status may not hold still and motion degrades image quality, making diagnosis difficult. Some of the newest and fastest units have acquired diagnostic images while a child tried to sit up on the CT table during the scan. All new CT units are MDCT and detector rows of 64, 128, and 320 have revolutionized CT imaging.

Computed Tomography Image Processing

With the advent of spiral CT and isotropic data sets (each voxel or part of the image makes up a cube of equal sides), the image can be reconstructed into any plane. By changing the color or brightness that a particular density is assigned, a variety of images can be generated. Three-dimensional (3-D) images are produced by assigning colors to various densities in the volume data set. Maximum intensity projected (MIP) images emphasize high-density structures such as contrast-enhanced vessels and bone. Lower density structures are suppressed. MIP images are very useful for assessing arteries in the trauma patient. These image-processing techniques help show spatial relationships between injuries, anatomy, and foreign bodies (Fig. 7).

MAGNETIC RESONANCE IMAGING

MRI has limited use in the early trauma setting, given its somewhat limited availability due to its overuse by other specialties. It takes a relatively long time to acquire the images, and the patient must be free of metallic foreign bodies. MRI has excellent contrast resolution but spatial resolution of CT is superior. CT is able to make the most of the diagnoses that are important to stabilize the patient. Detailed evaluation of the spinal cord or evaluation of subtle diffuse axonal injury (DAI) lesions may be improved with MRI.

MANAGEMENT OF IODINE ALLERGIES

If the patient has a known severe iodinated contrast allergy then CT may be performed without the administration of IV contrast agent, although it will be significantly limited in evaluation for vascular, solid organ, and hollow viscus injury. Another option would be to premedicate the patient with corticosteroids and diphenhydramine; however, the fastest widely accepted protocol requires a 6-hour preparation time. IV contrast agent administration after premedication should be performed only in patients who report prior minor reactions to IV contrast material, history of moderate to severe asthma, severe reaction to one substance, or multiple known food, medication, or other substance allergies. Contrary to prior beliefs, studies have shown that a history of minor shellfish allergy does not pose a significant risk of reaction to contrast administration. Premedication should not be administered if there is a history of anaphylaxis or bronchospasm after exposure to IV contrast agent. Caution should also be taken in administering contrast agent despite premedication

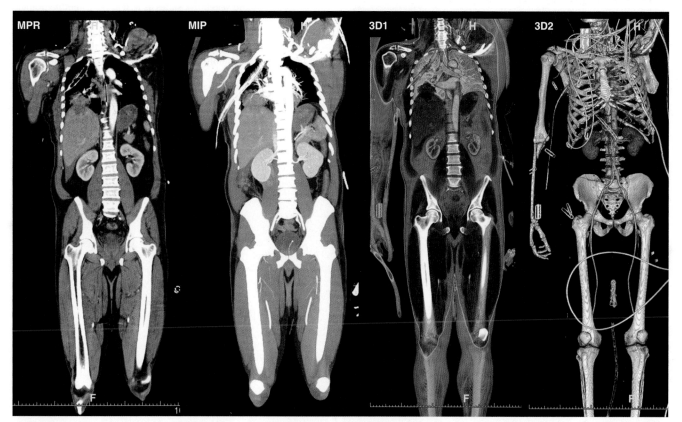

FIGURE 7 Multidetector computed tomography: Coronal images of a trauma patient with a liver laceration after a gunshot wound with diaphragm injury. These images were acquired in the standard axial plane, but because they are isotropic, they were reconstructed into the coronal plane. The multiplanar reformat (MPR) is the typical computed tomography image with a 1.5-mm slice thickness with gray scale displayed on soft tissue windows. The laceration at the liver dome and fluid inferior to the liver border is easily visible. Maximum intensity projection (MIP) image in this example has slice thickness of 90 mm of tissue and displays higher density structures like bone, contrast-enhanced vessels, and the kidneys as brighter than lower density structures. By assigning color instead of gray scale to 90 mm thickness of tissue (3D1) or looking at the entire full thickness of tissue (3D2) the three-dimensional volume rendered display can be created. In 3D2, soft tissue was assigned no color; therefore, those structures are not included on the image.

in patients on chronic corticosteroid therapy, those with severe allergic reaction to any one substance, and those with severe allergies. Keep in mind that even with premedication, a patient may still adversely react to IV contrast material. No set premedication protocol exists. Tables 1 and 2 list widely accepted premedication protocols.

TABLE 1: Standard Premedication Protocol

Drug	Dosage	Delivery
Prednisone or Methylprednisolone or Hydrocortisone	50 mg PO 32 mg PO 200 mg IV	Administer 13 hours, 7 hours, and 1 hour prior to IV contrast agent administration Administer 12 hours and 2 hours prior to IV contrast agent administration Administer 13 hours, 7 hours, and 1 hour before IV contrast agent administration
Diphenhydramine	50 mg PO IV, or IM	administer 1 hour prior to IV contrast agent administration

IM, Intramuscular; IV, intravenous; PO, orally.

TABLE 2: Urgent Premedication Protocol

Drug	Dosage	Delivery
Hydrocortisone	200 mg IV	Administer 6 hours prior to IV contrast agent administration
Diphenhydramine	50 mg IV	Administer 1 hour prior to contrast agent administration

IV, Intravenous.

SKULL AND BRAIN

Traumatic brain injuries (TBIs) lead to significant morbidity and mortality risks in trauma patients. Evaluation with a noncontrast CT of the brain is routine and should be the first step to exclude TBI. Candidates for imaging include those who suffer loss of consciousness, altered mental status, neurologic deficits, intoxication, battle signs, fluid or bloody otorrhea, suspected cerebrospinal fluid leaks, and facial trauma.

Subarachnoid hemorrhage will appear as extraaxial serpiginous areas of high density within the interpeduncular cistern, focal high-density collections in sulci and cerebellar folia, and high density along the interhemispheric fissure or along the tentorium (Fig. 8). Acute subdural hemorrhage usually appears as dense extraaxial crescent-shaped collections, but they may also present as dense thickening of the interhemispheric fissure or blood layering along the tentorium. Acute epidural bleeds present as lentiform or convex-shaped extra-axial dense collections and commonly have an adjacent skull fracture. Hemorrhagic cortical contusions appear as high-density foci within the cerebral cortex. DAIs to the white matter tracts are difficult to diagnose. MRI is more sensitive than CT in identifying these lesions and therefore the preferred imaging choice to identify these lesions. MRI gradient echo sequences and diffusion tensor imaging are the best sequences to identify these lesions. On MRI, 1 to 15 mm foci of edema or hemorrhage may be seen in the white matter tracts. DAIs may present on CT as foci of hemorrhage (high density) at the gray-white matter junction, within the corpus callosum, thalami, cerebral peduncles, and basal ganglia. DAIs are a leading cause of persistent unconsciousness and vegetative states as well as persistent neurologic impairment in the trauma patient. In a patient with persistent coma and negative CT, MRI should be obtained to evaluate for DAIs.

Both penetrating injuries and blunt trauma to the head and neck may result in vascular injury. CTA of the head and neck should be performed if there is concern for vascular occlusion, dissection, transection, vascular extravasation, or carotid cavernous sinus fistula (Fig. 9). CTA should be performed following a noncontrast brain CT as contrast material typically obscures hemorrhage (see Fig. 8B).

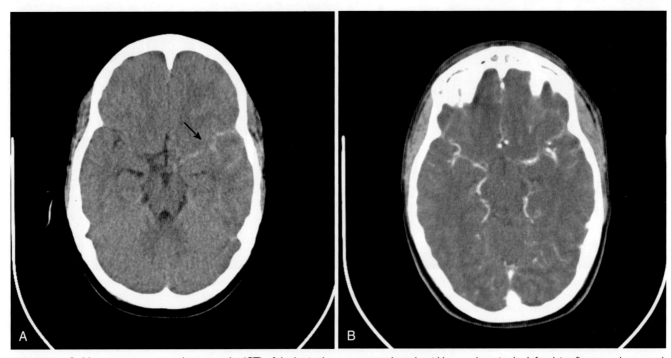

FIGURE 8   A, Noncontrast computed tomography (CT) of the brain demonstrates subarachnoid hemorrhage in the left sylvian fissure and temporal lobe *(arrow).* **B,** CT angiogram of the brain in the same patient. Note how contrast agent can obscure the subarachnoid hemorrhage.

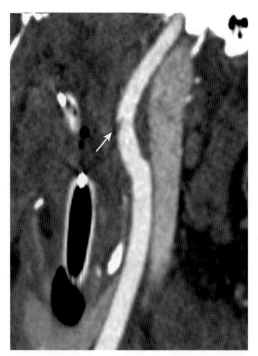

FIGURE 9   Computed tomography angiogram of coronal reconstructed image of the internal carotid artery demonstrating an intimal flap *(arrow)*.

If the patient exhibits signs of skull base injury, then a dedicated temporal bone CT should be performed. Axial 1 to 2 mm thin-section CT images are obtained through the temporal bones. Sagittal and coronal images should be reformatted to aid in the detection of subtle nondisplaced fractures and to evaluate the extent and path of injury.

SPINE

Traditionally, radiographs of the spine were used to evaluate for fractures and ligamentous injuries. With the advent of CT, their use has diminished as the limitations of conventional radiography are better recognized. CT is not only faster but has been proved to be more accurate in the evaluation of spine injuries. The spine is now routinely incorporated in whole-body CT protocols. Sagittal and coronal reformatted images aid in the evaluation of spine injuries (Fig. 10). MRI remains the best modality to evaluate for ligamentous injury, spinal cord injury, and epidural hematomas.

FACE

Any patient with signs of facial trauma, abrasions, swelling, gross deformities, and lacerations should undergo facial CT. Coronal and sagittal reconstructed images of the face aid in the diagnosis of subtle and nondisplaced fractures. 3-D images have also been proved to be useful for surgical planning. Facial CT can identify injuries to the globe, retrobulbar hematomas, extraconal hematomas, muscular entrapment, and presence of foreign bodies.

VASCULAR INJURIES

CTA has taken over DSA (digital subtraction angiography) in identifying vascular injuries (Fig. 11). CT poses minimal risk to the patient and can quickly identify areas of hemorrhage. By utilizing multiphasic imaging, CT can identify not only the location of hemorrhage but also its severity, and can differentiate arterial from venous hemorrhage. CTA therefore serves to guide patient management whether it be observation, transcatheter embolization, other endovascular therapy, or surgical intervention. Research has shown that up to 40% of patients suffering from pelvic fractures have underlying active hemorrhage and 20% will require transcatheter embolization.

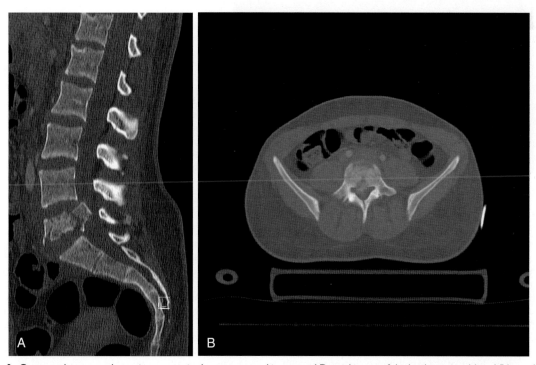

FIGURE 10   A, Computed tomography angiogram, sagittal reconstructed image, and **B,** axial image of the lumbar spine. Note L5 burst fracture with bony retropulsion into the spinal canal.

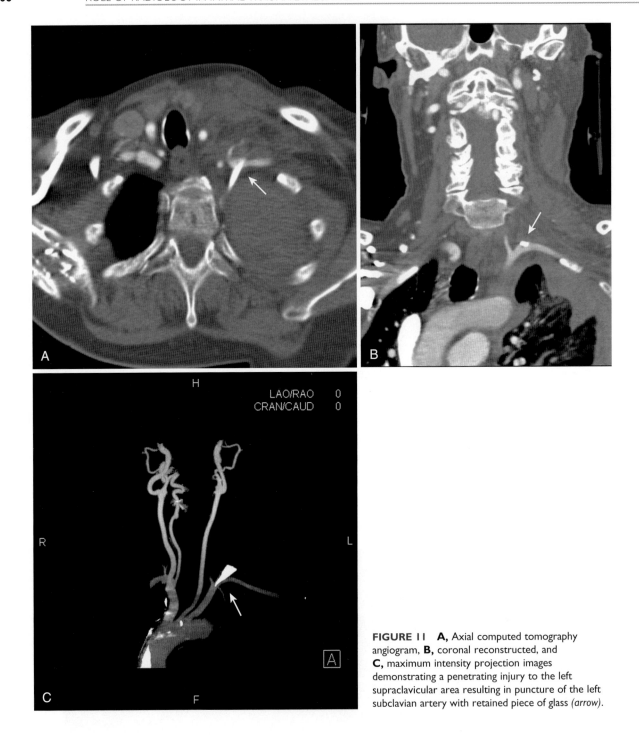

FIGURE 11 A, Axial computed tomography angiogram, **B,** coronal reconstructed, and **C,** maximum intensity projection images demonstrating a penetrating injury to the left supraclavicular area resulting in puncture of the left subclavian artery with retained piece of glass *(arrow).*

Injury to the vessels may result in occlusion, pseudoaneurysm formation, arteriovenous fistula (AVF) formation, intimal injury, dissection, spasm, active bleeding, and transection. Occlusion can result from direct blunt injury, spasm, or emboli. Occlusion presents as abrupt cutoff of a vessel. The vessel may reconstitute via collaterals or branches (Fig. 12). An intimal injury or dissection appears as an eccentric filling defect within the vessel lumen (Fig. 13). AVFs present as early asymmetrical contrast opacification of a vein. Pseudoaneurysm formation occurs when the wall of a vessel is disrupted and blood is contained by the adventitia or adjacent soft tissue. They appear as focal lobulated outpouchings of the vessel lumen that opacify with contrast. The attenuation of the pseudoaneurysm should remain equal to that of the originating vessel on all phases of images (Fig. 14). Delayed CT images can differentiate a pseudoaneurysm from areas of active extravasation as the former will not change in size or shape.

Transection of a vessel can lead to occlusion or active bleeding. Areas of active contrast extravasation consistent with active hemorrhage appear as extraluminal areas of hyperattenuation that usually increase in size during each phase of imaging (Fig. 15). With arterial sources, the attenuation value of these areas are equal to or greater than the aortic attenuation in the early arterial phase of imaging, and are greater than the aortic attenuation in the subsequent portal venous and delayed phases. With venous sources of contrast extravasation, extraluminal contrast blush is identified only on the portal venous or delayed phases of imaging. Occasionally, subtle areas of arterial extravasation or intermittent arterial bleeding can be seen only on the portal venous phase images.

Artifact arising from adjacent metallic foreign bodies, overlying lines and monitoring leads, spinal or orthopedic hardware, prosthesis, contrast-filled urinary bladder, and bone fragments may obscure the identification of or mimic vascular extravasation (Fig. 16). Reviewing CT images in the different phases helps to differentiate bone fragments from areas of contrast extravasation, as no change in size or attenuation occurs with bone fragments. Compression of the vasculature from adjacent soft tissue hematoma or edema may also mimic a vascular injury. Patient and respiratory motion may also limit evaluation of injuries.

On initial chest radiograph, the presence of a widened mediastinum, left pleural collection, indistinct aortic knob, widened left paratracheal stripe, widened left paraspinal line, and left apical capping should prompt further evaluation with a thoracic CTA to exclude injury to the thoracic aorta (Fig. 17). With blunt trauma, the thoracic aorta is most commonly injured at its sites of attachment: aortic root, aortic arch, aortic isthmus (proximal descending thoracic aorta), and aortic diaphragmatic hiatus (Fig. 18). Ninety percent of the injuries seen in clinical practice occur at the aortic isthmus. Most aortic injuries present with periaortic hematomas. CTA will demonstrate aortic intimal flaps/tears, intimal thrombi, pseudoaneurysms, contour abnormalities, transections, and sites of active bleeding. CTA utilizing cardiac gating is recommended in evaluation for proximal aortic injury as this area is limited in evaluation with routine CTA secondary to aortic pulsation. Aortic injuries are commonly associated with emboli to its branches resulting in parenchymal infarctions. CTA also demonstrates injuries to aortic branches. Perivascular hematomas surrounding the great vessels should raise suspicion for vascular injury.

Mediastinal hematomas may result from aortic, internal mammary artery, internal thoracic vein, brachiocephalic artery/vein, carotid artery, subclavian artery, or mediastinal vein injury. Hemopericardium may result from injury to the proximal aorta, pulmonary artery, pulmonary veins, superior vena cava, inferior vena cava (IVC), pericardium, and heart.

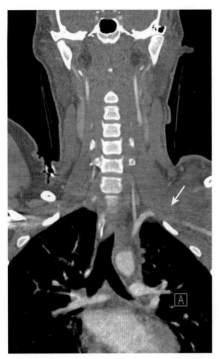

FIGURE 12 Computed tomography angiogram coronal reconstructed image of the left subclavian artery demonstrating segmental occlusion with distal reconstitution *(arrow)* secondary to blunt traumatic injury.

■ NONVASCULAR CHEST/THORAX

An anteroposterior (AP) supine chest radiograph is the standard initial imaging of the trauma patient and serves to quickly diagnose conditions that require immediate attention/treatment. Tension pneumothorax, pleural collection, widened mediastinum, diaphragmatic injuries, and life support line positioning are well demonstrated on chest radiograph. Tension pneumothorax classically presents as contralateral mediastinal shift, hyperinflated ipsilateral lung, and inverted or flattened ipsilateral diaphragm. Pleural collections are suggested when the costophrenic angle becomes blunted, a meniscus sign is present, and when there is asymmetrical increased density of a hemithorax.

CT is used to confirm and evaluate the cause of injuries suggested by the chest radiograph such as lung contusions, lung lacerations, pneumomediastinum, pneumothorax, rib fractures, mediastinal hematoma, aortic injury, pericardial effusion, and differentiated types of pleural collections. Pleural collections are well demonstrated on CT. The CT HU attenuation value of hemothorax (blood) is equal to or greater than 35 HU, and simple pleural fluid is less and 20 or less for simple fluid.

CTA of the thorax is recommended to evaluate the trauma patient. It is best to image the thorax in the arterial phase in order to evaluate the vasculature and heart. Thin section imaging should be performed

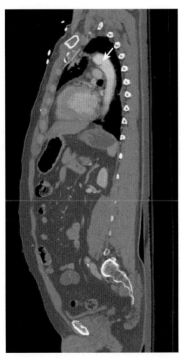

FIGURE 13 Computed tomography angiogram sagittal reconstructed image of the descending thoracic aorta demonstrates an intimal flap at the aortic isthmus *(arrow)*.

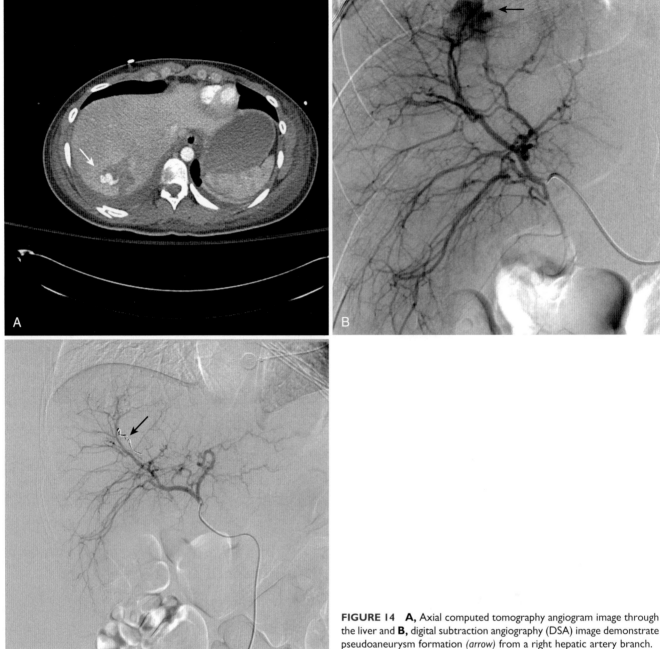

FIGURE 14   A, Axial computed tomography angiogram image through the liver and **B,** digital subtraction angiography (DSA) image demonstrate pseudoaneurysm formation *(arrow)* from a right hepatic artery branch. **C,** Postcoiling DSA image confirms obliteration of the pseudoaneurysm *(arrow).*

in the axial plane so that CTA and multiplanar reformations (in the coronal and sagittal planes) may be obtained.

CT can also identify subtle injuries and occult injuries on chest radiograph. It is important to remember that pneumothoraces tend to accumulate in the anterior, inferior, and medial pleural space when the patient is supine and may therefore be occult on the initial supine AP chest radiograph. There are several signs on a supine chest radiograph that can suggest the presence of a pneumothorax: deep sulcus sign, sharply defined mediastinal contour, sharply defined lung base, and double diaphragm sign.

Parenchymal injury to the lung is common, consisting of pulmonary contusions and lacerations. Contusions are the most common injuries encountered with blunt trauma to the chest. They appear as patchy nonsegmental airspace opacities or consolidations that have ill-defined borders and classically spare the subpleural space (Fig. 19). Within 24 to 48 hours, contusions begin to clear, with complete clearing occurring anywhere from 3 to 10 days. Lacerations appear as cavities within the lung parenchyma that may fill with air or blood. These tears in the lungs may persist for months. Lacerations are graded by mechanism of injury, association with rib fractures, and appearance on CT.

Pneumomediastinum can develop from pneumothorax or esophageal or airway injury. With pneumothorax and alveolar injuries, air can track through the bronchovascular bundles into the mediastinum. Lacerations of the trachea and bronchi may also occur, leading to pneumomediastinum. The "fallen lung sign" (collapsed lung lies in a dependent position, posterolaterally within the hemithorax hanging from the hilum by its vascular pedicle) occurs when there

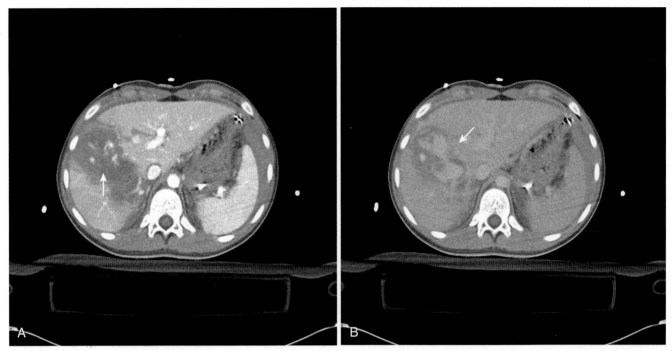

FIGURE 15 Axial computed tomography image through the liver in the arterial phase (**A**) and portal venous phase (**B**). A blush of extraluminal contrast *(arrow)* is seen within the right lobe of the liver during the arterial phase. This area of extraluminal contrast then increases in size *(arrow)* during the portal venous phase, consistent with active arterial contrast extravasation.

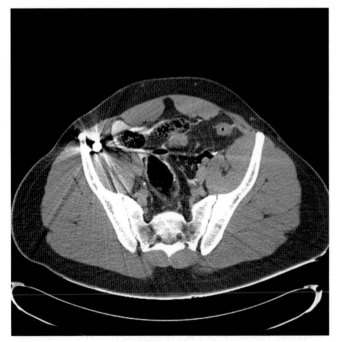

FIGURE 16 Axial computed tomography angiogram image through the pelvis. Note how the bullet results in streak artifact, limiting evaluation of the surrounding structures.

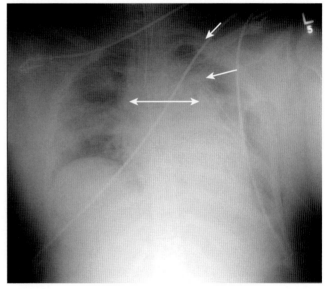

FIGURE 17 Portable anteroposterior chest radiograph demonstrates a widened mediastinum *(double arrow)*, left apical capping *(top arrow)*, left pleural collection *(middle arrow)*, and an indistinct aortic knob. This constellation of findings should raise the suspicion for aortic injury.

has been a complete transection or rupture of a bronchus. Tracheal injuries present with pneumomediastinum, subcutaneous emphysema tracking into the neck, and an overdistended or herniated endotracheal tube balloon projecting outside the confines of the trachea.

The proximal and distal portions of the esophagus are the most commonly injured. Injury to the esophagus is more common after

penetrating injuries and is rarely seen with blunt trauma. Clinically, patients with esophageal injuries present with odynophagia or dysphagia. Blood or hematoma within the esophagus can be seen with endoscopy. If esophageal injury is suspected, oral contrast agent may be administered prior to chest CT. CT findings suggesting esophageal injury consist of pneumomediastinum; periesophageal fluid, gas, or fat stranding; thickened esophageal wall; mediastinitis; extravasated oral contrast material; and hydropneumothorax. An

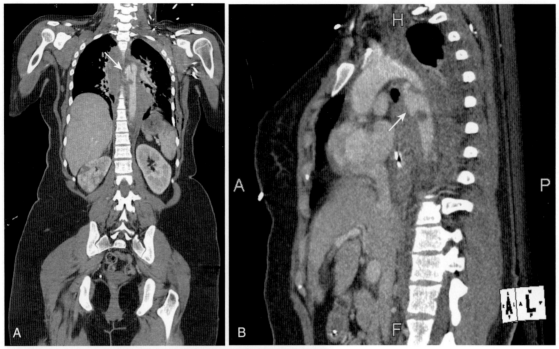

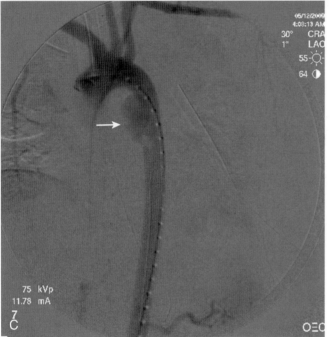

FIGURE 18 Coronal (**A**) and sagittal (**B**) reconstructed computed tomography angiogram and digital subtraction angiography (**C**) images demonstrate a pseudoaneurysm arising from the proximal descending thoracic aorta, surrounding mediastinal hematoma, and accompanying right renal infarcts.

esophagogram utilizing water-soluble contrast agent as well as endoscopy should be performed to evaluate for esophageal injuries if CT cannot exclude or findings are equivocal.

CARDIAC INJURIES

Both US and CT are useful in evaluation of cardiac injuries. Echocardiography can evaluate for pericardial fluid, valve function, wall motion abnormalities, aneurysms, myocardial hematomas, and intraluminal thrombus. Findings on CT suggesting cardiac injury include a displaced heart, hemopericardium, pneumopericardium, myocardial hematoma, intraluminal thrombus, aneurysm, and IV contrast extravasation into the pericardial space or mediastinum.

DIAPHRAGMATIC INJURIES

Penetrating and blunt traumatic injuries may both lead to diaphragmatic injury and subsequent hernia. Penetrating injuries to the diaphragm are more common and tend to result in small defects, making visualization difficult. With blunt trauma, diaphragmatic injury most commonly involves the posterolateral aspect but can occur anywhere along its surface. The left hemidiaphragm is most commonly injured with blunt trauma as the liver is thought to provide reinforcement of the right hemidiaphragm. Diaphragmatic tears can result in herniation of fat and organs into the thorax, putting them at risk for perforation, incarceration, and strangulation. Hernias may present immediately or become apparent years later. The initial AP

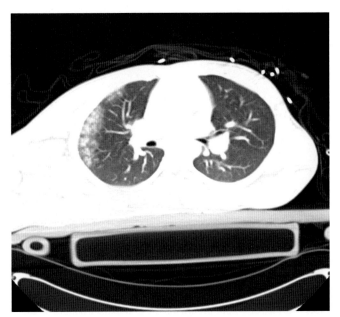

FIGURE 19 Axial computed tomography image through the lungs demonstrates the typical appearance of lung contusions.

supine chest radiograph may demonstrate a masslike opacity of the hemithorax, ill-defined or elevated hemidiaphragm, or even a gastric tube projecting in the hemithorax (Fig. 20). Subsequent injury to the adjacent lung and pleural collections are commonly seen on chest radiograph. MDCT can demonstrate the location and size of the diaphragmatic tear, herniated contents, and their effects on the lung and heart. Many signs have been described on CT with diaphragmatic hernias: "hump sign, collar sign, and dependent viscera sign." With penetrating injuries, if the injury trajectory crosses the diaphragm or if adjacent injuries are noted on both sides of the diaphragm, a diaphragmatic tear should be suspected. Fluid or blood on both sides of the diaphragm should also raise suspicion for possible diaphragmatic injury, keeping in mind that this finding is nonspecific in the setting of multiple penetrating wounds.

FOCUSED ASSESSMENT WITH SONOGRAPHY IN TRAUMA

US, like AP chest and pelvic radiographs, can be used in the initial assessment of the unstable trauma patient. It is quick and without risk in directing the management of the unstable patient. FAST evaluates five spaces for the presence of fluid that could indicate a hollow viscus or solid organ injury. The following five spaces are investigated: (1) pericardial, (2) splenorenal, (3) hepatorenal, (5) both paracolic gutters, and (6) the pouch of Douglas. US can also sometimes differentiate the presence of simple fluid from hemoperitoneum, as blood is usually more echogenic and clots can be seen. US cannot differentiate free fluid from urine and is limited in evaluating the retroperitoneal space.

FREE FLUID

Multiple diagnostic modalities exist to evaluate for the presence and type of free fluid present in the abdomen: DPL, FAST, or CT. Intraperitoneal free fluid should arise suspicion for solid or hollow viscus organ injury. In an MDCT study evaluating bowel and mesenteric

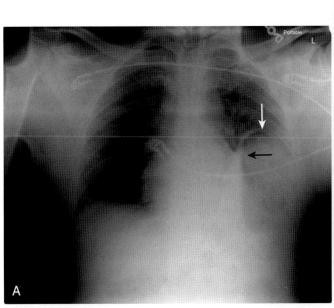
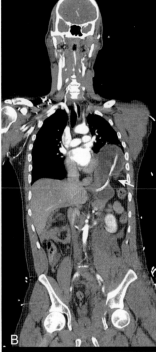

FIGURE 20 Anteroposterior portable chest radiograph (**A**) and reconstructed coronal computed tomography angiogram (CTA) (**B**) images. The chest radiograph demonstrates a masslike opacity in the left lung base containing the nasogastric tube *(arrows)*. CTA image confirms the herniation of the stomach through the diaphragm *(arrow)* into the left hemithorax.

blunt trauma performed by Brofman et al, 50 (93%) of 54 patients with either bowel or mesenteric injury had intraperitoneal fluid. Usually the fluid is located at or near the site of injury but may be seen distant to or diffusely throughout the abdomen and pelvis.

Keep in mind that a small amount of free fluid within the cul de sac is expected in premenopausal females and can be seen in postmenopausal females as well. It has also been suggested that a small amount of simple attenuation free pelvic fluid in a male may be normal. Intraperitoneal and retroperitoneal free fluid can also result from aggressive hydration, but is usually accompanied by other supporting signs, including periportal edema, engorged IVC, engorged hepatic veins, and diffuse bowel wall edema. Also, DPL may result in free air and fluid, making it hard to discern the source of the findings.

FREE AIR

Extraluminal free air is classically seen deep to the anterior abdominal wall parietal peritoneum, in the mesentery, within the mesenteric and portal veins, and in the porta hepatis region. Retroperitoneal free air should raise suspicion for duodenal, ascending, or descending colonic injuries.

There are many causes of free air in a trauma patient that one must keep in mind besides bowel perforation/injury. Intraperitoneal free air can be seen when air from a pneumothorax or pneumomediastinum dissects into the abdomen, after DPL, with barotrauma from mechanical ventilation, in abdominal and chest wall penetrating injuries, and after Foley catheter placement in existing intraperitoneal bladder perforation.

GASTROINTESTINAL TRACT

Both penetrating injuries and blunt trauma may result in hollow visceral organ injury. Bowel may be torn because of deceleration forces, and it may be crushed or ruptured by direct forces. MDCT has been shown to be more specific and sensitive than both FAST and DPL. The use of "triple contrast" is recommended for evaluation of penetrating injuries to the abdomen and pelvis, if the patient is stable. Triple contrast refers to the concomitant IV, oral, and rectal administration of contrast agent for CT. The presence of free air or free fluid suggests peritoneal violation but is not diagnostic for either hollow viscus or solid organ injury. In cases of inconclusive source of free air or fluid on initial CT without oral contrast administration, a repeat CT in 6 to 8 hours may be performed with the administration of just oral contrast.

Injuries to the bowel may present as surrounding free fluid, surrounding fat stranding, mesenteric hematomas, bowel wall thickening, bowel wall discontinuity, free air, discontinuous and irregular avid enhancement of the bowel wall, decreased enhancement of the bowel wall secondary to devascularization, abdominal wall injury, and oral contrast extravasation. The most highly specific signs of bowel injury include disruption of the bowel wall, active oral contrast extravasation, and free air. The only unequivocal sign of a hollow viscus organ injury is the presence of extraluminal gastrointestinal contrast agent (Fig. 21).

Most commonly, the small bowel is injured near fixed/attached sites such as the distal ileum near the ileocecal valve and the proximal jejunum near the ligament of Treitz. Remember that the second, third, and fourth portions of the duodenum are retroperitoneal and therefore free fluid or air in the retroperitoneum should raise suspicion for duodenal injury. Also, free fluid in the right anterior pararenal space should raise suspicion for duodenal injury.

Penetrating injuries are the most common cause of rectal injury. Injuries to the rectum from blunt trauma are rare and are usually the result of straddle injuries or other trauma to the perineum. Patients

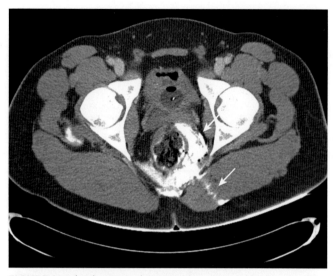

FIGURE 21 Axial computed tomography angiogram triple contrast image through the pelvis after gunshot wound to the left gluteal region. Note that the rectal contrast agent has extravasated from the rectal lumen into the perirectal space and bullet tract (arrows).

with rectal injuries usually present with bright red blood per rectum. CT may demonstrate perirectal fat stranding, perirectal hematoma, perirectal free air, presacral fluid/hematoma, and focal rectal wall thickening.

MESENTERIC INJURIES

It is frequently difficult to separate mesenteric injuries from bowel injuries, as the less specific and sensitive imaging findings may be similar in both cases. Although the imaging findings of bowel and mesenteric injuries may overlap, the presence of a mesenteric hematoma, IV contrast extravasation in the mesentery, occlusion of a mesenteric vessel, and a beaded appearance of the mesenteric vessels are specific to mesenteric injury (Fig. 22). A mesenteric injury may lead to devascularization of an adjacent bowel loop, which can present as bowel wall thickening and irregular enhancement. Other nonspecific findings seen with mesenteric injuries include mesenteric fat stranding, abdominal wall injury, and well-defined mesenteric hematomas.

SOLID ORGAN INJURIES (LIVER, SPLEEN, AND KIDNEYS)

Injuries to the solid organs manifest in similar presentations despite difference in organ whether it be the liver, spleen, kidneys, or pancreas. Beyond the scope of evaluating for periorgan free fluid, hemoperitoneum, or subcapsular hematoma, US is limited in evaluating for solid organ parenchymal injury. On US, focal lacerations, contusions, and hematomas may be seen as hyperechoic, hypoechoic, or heterogeneous diffuse or geographic areas within the organ parenchyma. Lacerations, on US, may also appear as hypoechoic linear and branching areas that are oriented perpendicular to the organ surface.

Solid organ injuries are optimally seen during the portal venous phase of CT imaging. Subtle and less severe injuries may present as varying degrees of periorgan fat stranding or fluid. Subcapsular hematomas typically present as hypodense periorgan fluid collections that conform to the confines of the organ capsule. Subcapsular

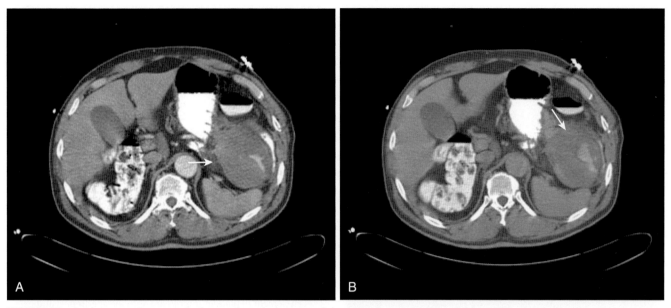

FIGURE 22   Axial computed tomography images through the upper abdomen in the arterial (**A**) and delayed (**B**) phases of imaging. A mesenteric hematoma *(arrow)* is noted in the left upper quadrant in **A**. In **B**, the contrast blush *(arrow)* enlarges on the delayed phase of imaging consistent with active hemorrhage.

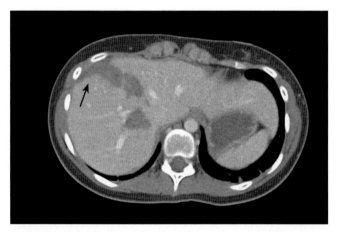

FIGURE 23   Axial computed tomography angiogram image through the liver demonstrates lacerations of the liver and subcapsular hematoma *(arrow)*.

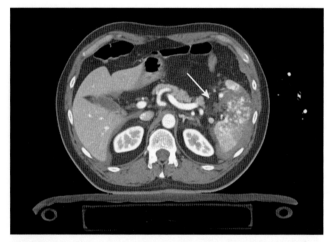

FIGURE 24   Axial computed tomography angiogram image through the spleen demonstrates a shattered spleen with perisplenic hematoma, active arterial contrast extravasation, and multiple small pseudoaneurysms *(arrow)*.

hematomas may be hyperdense and demonstrate areas of IV contrast extravasation consistent with areas of active bleeding, typically when the organ capsule is torn (Fig. 23). Contusions present as hypoattenuating areas or areas of decreased enhancement within the organ parenchyma. Hematomas on noncontrast CT may appear as hyperattenuating parenchymal areas. Lacerations appear as linear nonenhancing, sometimes branching, or even complex appearing, hypoattenuating defects through the parenchyma of the organ (Fig. 24). It is important to identify if the injury involves the organ's hilum. CT also serves to identify solid organ vascular injuries. Infarcts appear as peripheral wedge-shaped hypoattenuating or hypoenhancing areas. Infarcts can occur from vascular injury and may be secondary to thromboembolic disease because of aortic injury.

The American Association for the Surgery of Trauma (AAST) solid organ injury classifications take into account the size of lacerations, size of parenchymal and subcapsular hematomas, and presence

of vascular injury. The AAST grading scale for the kidneys also takes into account injury to the collecting system.

COLLECTING SYSTEM

Renal lacerations can extend into the collecting system (Fig. 25). Hematuria, whether it be gross or microscopic, along with mechanism of injury and signs of shock should prompt evaluation for a renal collecting system injury. Note that hematuria may be absent if the ureteropelvic junction or ureter is completely transected. Delayed CT images, 5 minutes after initial IV contrast agent administration, are important in evaluating for urinary tract injury and urinary extravasation (Fig. 26). Urinary extravasation may be encapsulated or free. Injury

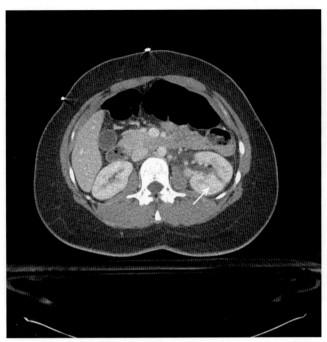

FIGURE 25 Axial portal venous phase computed tomography image through the kidneys demonstrates a left renal laceration *(arrow)* extending into the collecting system with surrounding perinephric fluid (hematoma and urine).

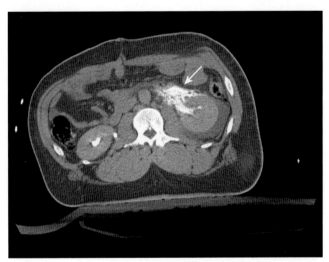

FIGURE 26 Axial delayed phase computed tomography image through the kidneys demonstrates extravasation from the left proximal collecting system and perinephric hematoma *(arrow)*.

to the collecting system may be partial or complete. If contrast material is seen within the collecting system distal to the site of extravasation, then a partial tear can be assumed.

Bladder injury should be suspected with pelvic fractures as well as known posterior urethral injuries. A conventional fluoroscopic or CT cystogram may be performed to identify bladder injury. In major trauma centers, CT has replaced the conventional fluoroscopic cystogram. Via Foley or suprapubic catheter the bladder is instilled with 300 mL of a mixture consisting of 50% saline and 50% IV contrast agent, and then a limited CT of the pelvis is performed. For the

pediatric patient 100 to 150 mL of the saline/contrast mixture should be instilled into the bladder. Bladder integrity is not confirmed until full bladder distention is obtained. CT cystography should be performed last as a contrast-filled bladder or an injured/ruptured bladder can obscure adjacent vascular or gastrointestinal tract contrast extravasation.

Seventy percent of bladder injuries are extraperitoneal and most are associated with pelvic fractures. With extraperitoneal bladder rupture, fluid (urine) or bladder contrast agent will accumulate in the perivesical or prevesical spaces (Fig. 27). The prevesical extraperitoneal space, also known as the space of Retzius, extends from the pubic symphysis to the umbilicus. The extravasated contrast takes on a "flame"-shaped appearance. If the urogenital diaphragm is disrupted, urine or contrast agent will extravasate into the scrotum, thigh, and penis.

Twenty percent of bladder injuries are intraperitoneal. The dome, covered by the peritoneum, is the weakest point of the bladder. In intraperitoneal bladder injury, urine or contrast material will extravasate into the peritoneal space and can be seen surrounding the intraperitoneal bowel and solid organs, in the paracolic gutters, in the pouch of Douglas, and in the subphrenic spaces.

Ten percent of bladder injuries are both intraperitoneal and extraperitoneal and usually result from penetrating injuries.

URETHRA

Injury to the urethra should be suspected with pelvic fractures, if there is a history of penetrating injury near the urethra, or known straddle injury. Patients may present with blood at the meatus, hematuria, or inability to void. The prostate gland may also be high riding on rectal examination. Placing a Foley catheter when a urethral injury exists may exacerbate the injury. If there is suspicion for a urethral injury, then a retrograde urethrogram should be performed prior to Foley catheter placement. The urethrogram can localize the site of injury (anterior vs. posterior urethra) and determine if the injury is complete or incomplete. With posterior urethral injuries, contrast agent will accumulate in the retropubic space. Keep in mind that patients suffering posterior urethral injuries may also have bladder injuries. Anterior urethral injuries will demonstrate contrast extravasation into the corpus cavernosum or spongiosum, and may reflux into the draining veins of the penis. Contrast material may accumulate in the perineum when injuries involve the urogenital diaphragm. Partial filling of the urinary bladder may be seen with partial urethral rupture. Sometimes urethral injuries can be detected on delayed phase CT even with existing Foley catheter.

RETROPERITONEAL INJURIES

Evaluation of retroperitoneal injuries is limited on physical examination and laboratory studies as well as DPL and FAST US.

PANCREAS

Most pancreatic injuries occur because of blunt trauma or deceleration injuries. In motor vehicle accidents, bicycle accidents, and motorcycle collisions the pancreas is injured because of direct impact of the steering wheel or handle bar. Contrast-enhanced CT is the modality of choice in identifying pancreatic injuries. Injury to the pancreas may present as subtle findings such as peripancreatic fat stranding or fluid. Contusions appear as areas of decreased attenuation/enhancement in the parenchyma and may have associated surrounding fat stranding and fluid. Lacerations present as linear

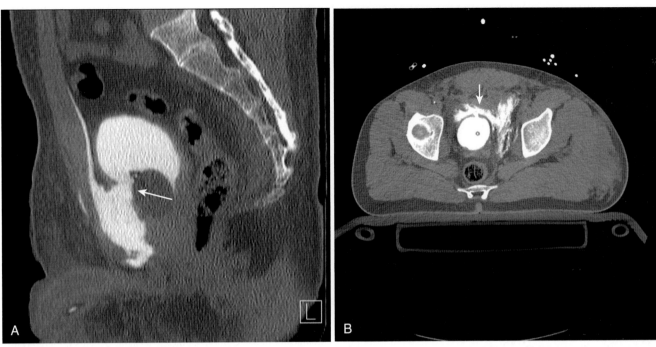

FIGURE 27   Sagittal reconstructed (**A**) and axial (**B**) computed tomography cystogram images. Note the extraperitoneal extravasation of contrast agent through a defect *(arrow)* in the urinary bladder.

hypoattenuating nonenhancing defects through the pancreatic parenchyma. Transections are lacerations that involve greater than 50% of the gland thickness and involve the pancreatic duct. Most transections occur in the pancreatic neck. Magnetic resonance cholangiopancreatography can further evaluate injury to the pancreatic duct. Pancreatic injuries are usually associated with duodenal injuries.

ADRENAL GLANDS

Injury to the adrenals can be readily detected on both contrast and noncontrast CT. Findings range from periadrenal fat stranding to an enlarged hypoattenuating gland (Fig. 28). Hemorrhage can arise from the superior adrenal artery. Adrenal gland injuries are associated with hepatic lacerations and IVC injuries.

BONES OTHER THAN SPINE

MDCT can also demonstrate occult fractures on radiograph and further evaluate the extent of fractures noted on radiograph. Subtle widening of the sacroiliac joints, diastasis of the pubic symphysis, intraarticular fracture extension, intraarticular loose bodies, and subluxation of joints are all well demonstrated on CT (Fig. 29). Fractures that course in the axial plane may be occult on the axial CT images but

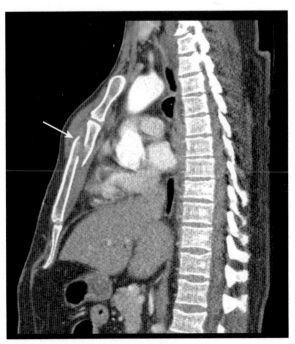

FIGURE 29   Sagittal reconstructed computed tomography angiogram image of the chest demonstrates an oblique sternal fracture *(arrow)* and retrosternal hematoma.

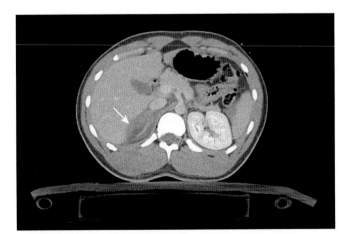

FIGURE 28   Computed tomography angiogram axial image demonstrating a right adrenal gland hematoma *(arrow)*.

usually are well demonstrated on the sagittal and coronal reformatted images.

SHOCK

There are several CT telltale signs of hypovolemic shock: avid adrenal gland and bowel wall enhancement, flattened IVC, small aortic caliber, pancreatic edema, retroperitoneal edema, and diffuse small bowel wall edema/thickening.

RESUSCITATION EFFECTS

CT findings include engorged IVC and hepatic veins, periportal edema, and low attenuation free fluid in the dependent portions of the pelvis and retroperitoneum. Periportal edema on CT appears as tubular low attenuation paralleling both sides of the intrahepatic portal venous branches.

ABDOMINAL COMPARTMENT SYNDROME

CT findings include abdominal distention, compressed IVC by fluid, dense retroperitoneal infiltration, renal compression, inguinal herniation, bowel wall thickening, and avid bowel wall enhancement.

For the chapter's Suggested Readings list, please visit the book at www.ExpertConsult.inkling.com.

INTERVENTIONAL RADIOLOGY: DIAGNOSTIC AND THERAPEUTIC ROLES

David J. Quintana, Jason Salsamendi, and Felipa Munera

One of the most preventable causes of death in abdominal and pelvic trauma is arterial hemorrhage that goes untreated or unrecognized. Over the last decade, radiology has undergone many advances, particularly in noninvasive imaging and interventional angiography, such that critical arterial hemorrhage is both recognized and treated faster, often with life-preserving results. Yet as we will see, interventional radiology extends beyond angiography as computed tomography (CT)-guided percutaneous interventions and other imaging-guided techniques also play a significant role in the acute management of the trauma patient.

The cornerstone of arterial hemostasis is early intervention, whether via a direct approach to injured blood vessel, endovascular techniques, thoracotomy, open laparotomy, or a combination of interventions. Early intervention requires a highly sensitive and specific diagnostic study that can be both performed and interpreted quickly. In the past, arterial injuries were largely identified during diagnostic angiography, which was both time-intensive and invasive. Yet, with technological advancements in CT, CT angiography (CTA) has essentially replaced traditional diagnostic angiography to evaluate vascular injury. Patients who are hemodynamically stable have traditionally forgone laparotomy, are assessed with CTA, and receive nonoperative management (NOM). Angiography has been reserved for these NOM patients, yet with interventional techniques evolving over the last decade, embolization has become integrated in the management of both the nonoperative and operative patient. Further advances in endovascular techniques have allowed tremendous strides in the management of the unstable patient, and in the appropriate clinical setting, many leading trauma centers have utilized arterial embolization as a component of primary resuscitation, especially in pelvic trauma.

In short, interventional radiology plays a major role in the diagnosis, treatment, and management of the trauma patient. The use of interventional radiology requires a multidisciplinary approach in which the trauma surgeon and interventionalist understand both its indications and limitations.

COMPUTED TOMOGRAPHY ANGIOGRAPHY

CTA is typically reserved for those trauma patients who are hemodynamically stable. Hemodynamically unstable patients undergo resuscitation, and once vital signs are stabilized, CTA is performed. Yet, development in CT technology has pushed the envelope, so to speak, and CTA is being performed on less stable patients. This is largely due to advancements in multidetector CT (MDCT) technology which has decreased time of acquisition, and has allowed faster localization of active hemorrhage. State-of-the-art multislice scanners not only provide improved temporal and spatial resolution, but can acquire total body images in less than 1.5 seconds, which is faster than traditional plain chest and pelvic radiographs. MDCT acquires isovolumetric data, enabling the interpreter to reconstruct images in an infinite number of planes. Multiplanar reconstruction and maximum intensity projections aid in confirming suspected vascular lesions and uncover vascular injuries that may be obscured by adjacent hyperattenuating bone or foreign bodies.

In the 1980s, it was well established that between 50% and 70% of all liver and splenic injuries cease bleeding at the time of operation and can be treated conservatively as long as patient hemodynamic status is not compromised. However, vascular injury has become a primary focus in CTA evaluation, as its presence is associated with failure of NOM. Solid organ injuries are also evaluated with CTA and historically have been defined and graded through the American Association for the Surgery of Trauma (AAST) scale. Yet, these grading scales are based on anatomic findings, and have not been shown to accurately select those patients who will fail nonoperative treatment or decompensate from delayed hemorrhage. In fact, Durham compared CT scan results with operative findings and concluded that CT may actually underestimate the degree of liver injury. Subsequently, there have been a number of attempts to define clinically relevant CT imaging findings. Though currently there is no universally accepted standardization, the goal of this section is to define those CT findings considered high risk and which may benefit from early intervention.

Contrast extravasation is one of the most reliable CTA findings of vascular injury, and has a 99% specificity and 80% to 97% sensitivity for identifying patients who will require embolization. In 1993, Shanmuganathan found that active bleeding can be differentiated from clotted blood on CT. Continuous bleeding is hyperattenuated on CT, averaging 130 Hounsfield units (HU), and clotted blood measures between 40 and 70 HU. Therefore, attenuation greater than 100 HU is suspicious for active hemorrhage. With contrast agent administration, a contrast blush can be seen, which often fades into a parenchymal hematoma or peritoneal fluid. The attenuation of extravasated contrast material will often be within 10 HU of the adjacent feeding arterial source. Active extravasation typically has ill-defined margins with either a linear or focal region of hyperattenuation. On delayed CTA imaging, hematoma that has expanded in size or changed attenuation values suggests active hemorrhage. Overall, the key for the diagnosis of active extravasation is a hyperattenuated entity, which changes on delayed imaging.

It is critical to distinguish between active hemorrhage from intraparenchymal hematoma and laceration. If vascular injury is suspected despite no evidence of active extravasation, serial CTA may help monitor patient progression. Delayed bleeding may be seen as a hematoma that has increased in size, rupture of a central solid-organ hematoma, or rupture of a pseudoaneurysm in contact with fluid collection such as biloma or hematoma. Sudden change in clinical status or increase in pain should lead to suspicion of delayed bleeding. Moreover, hepatic lacerations involving more than three liver segments and extension of laceration into the hilum are associated with vascular injury and should prompt early intervention. Care should be taken in lacerations with hilar extent, as these are more likely unstable lesions involving the portal vein or inferior vena cava (IVC) and are better managed surgically.

The location of intraparenchymal hematoma is equally important. Certain locations potentially communicate with larger compartments and are at higher risk of decompression due to the lack of supporting structure for tamponade. Hepatic hematomas involving segment VII may extend to the bare area of the liver, causing decompression into the retroperitoneum. A central hepatic hematoma communicates with the perivascular spaces, and may decompress into the hilum. Finally, hepatic or splenic parenchymal hematoma may extend into the capsule. If the capsule is compromised, hematoma may expand into the peritoneal cavity. In fact, the more quadrants containing free fluid, the more specific CTA is for vascular injury. Patients with free fluid extending into the paracolic gutters and pelvic cul-de-sac more frequently fail NOM, and require embolization, but free fluid contained in Morrison's pouch and perisplenic regions are more likely to pass without embolization. Though hemoperitoneum is not a specific CT finding alone, free fluid in more than three quadrants with contrast extravasation or sentinel clot increases the specificity for vascular injury, requiring early intervention. If hemoperitoneum is found in more than one quadrant, comparison of the fluid attenuation should be made. Blood closest to the injury site has more time to retract, and forms higher density clotted blood; the so-called "sentinel clot sign." This is important for the interventionalist in patients with multiple solid organ injuries, as it may facilitate deciding which selective arteriography should be performed first.

Other signs of vascular injury seen on CT include contrast-contained vascular lesions and intimal injuries. Pseudoaneurysm and arteriovenous fistula (AVF) are classified as contained arterial lesions. Pseudoaneurysms exhibit different characteristics on CT when compared to active extravasation. They commonly exhibit attenuation that is similar to the adjacent feeding artery, yet demonstrate well-defined margins in a round configuration. Pseudoaneurysm is also less apparent on delayed imaging, and if an adjacent hematoma is present, it will not change in size or attenuation. Depending upon the location, pseudoaneurysms may be readily characterized on Doppler ultrasound (Fig. 1). Contained AVF is difficult to diagnose on CT, as CTA requires long intravenous injection times, which nonselectively opacify the vasculature. Finally, traumatic visceral intimal injuries may be detected on CTA and are most commonly found in the renal arteries. Blunt renal artery injuries are considered high-risk lesions owing to the risk of thrombosis, parenchymal dysfunction, and even renal failure.

Diagnostic CTA does have its limitations. It is important to understand that current CTA imaging is only a snapshot in time, and it may not detect all vascular lesions that are present. Furthermore, CTA is unable to accurately predict delayed hemorrhage. As stated earlier, CTA potentially underestimates solid organ injuries, and therefore clinical presentation is most critical. Ultimately, however, CTA is a powerful tool that reliably aids in management decisions of the trauma patient.

TRANSCATHETER ANGIOGRAPHY

Diagnostic Angiography

Angiography confirms 80% to 90% of CTA findings suspicious for arterial injury, yet presents a continuous diagnostic challenge. Active hemorrhage and vascular injury may be subtle, and the appearances of these lesions differ on angiography from CTA. Contrast extravasation is seen as a persistent blush of contrast on angiography that appears earlier than the venous phase, and fails to wash out in the delay phase. Pseudoaneurysm is diagnosed as a contained saccular outpouching, which has equal density to the adjacent vessel and no evidence of extravasation. Abrupt arterial truncation indicates transection and occlusion of the vessel.

When a discrepancy between CTA and angiography manifests, it is important to determine whether it is due to the cessation of arterial bleeding or if vasospasm, the physiologic response to hemodynamic instability, is masking the vascular injury. If active hemorrhage is highly suspected, and diagnostic angiography does not locate the lesion initially, provocative angiography may be warranted to reveal contrast extravasation. The most frequently used medications are nitroglycerin, heparin, or tissue plasminogen activator. Nitroglycerin is the safest in a trauma setting, due to its short half-life of 3 minutes. Its effect allows the interventionalist to identify potential life-threatening hemorrhage yet is brief enough as to typically not cause further hemodynamic demise. If a discrepancy persists after provocative angiography or if there is a high clinical suspicion of hemorrhage in the absence of CTA, prophylactic embolization may be performed. However, it is important to consider spontaneous cessation of arterial hemorrhage or that hemorrhage may be from a venous source.

Arterial access is extremely important prior to performing diagnostic and therapeutic angiography. The most common arterial access site in the trauma setting is the right common femoral artery (CFA), due to its superficial location. If the CFA cannot be accessed, it may be obtained from the contralateral side, or via a brachial approach. CFA is accessed over the lower third of the femoral head, to facilitate compression at the termination of the procedure. After palpation, the micropuncture needle is advanced at a 45-degree angle through the anterior wall of the artery until blood return is noted. If access is gained distal to the bifurcation of the CFA, compression may become difficult. Additionally, iatrogenic arteriovenous fistula (AVF) can complicate CFA access, as the femoral vein lies posterior to the artery at this level. If the CFA cannot be accessed, then the brachial artery can be accessed. Brachial access has an established risk of stroke ($\sim$0.5%) due to the necessity of crossing the vertebral and carotid arteries. Additionally, there is a slight increased risk of hematoma formation, which has potentially adverse consequences in the upper extremity. Compressive hematoma risks medial brachial compartment syndrome and peripheral nerve injury. Finally, the left brachial artery is preferred to the right, as there is only one cerebral vessel crossed with this approach.

Angiographic evaluation will largely depend on preassessment CTA. If CTA has been performed, selective angiography can be performed first to address the known or suspected vascular injuries diagnosed on CTA. After selective angiography, nonselective angiography should always be performed to identify undiagnosed vascular lesions and assure there are no additional sites of active hemorrhage. In unstable patients with pelvic trauma, CTA many times will not be available, and nonselective angiography should be implemented first to provide a roadmap for more selective arteriography.

Nonselective aortography not only offers a roadmap to the visceral vasculature, it may also demonstrate potential anatomic collateral pathways important for embolization. These collateral pathways, though rare, may provide sustained blood flow to active hemorrhage, and thus are important to identify. Additionally, these collateral pathways may be important in the surgical management of the trauma patient in cases that may subsequently end up in the operating room. The arc of Buhler is an embryologic communication of the celiac axis and the superior

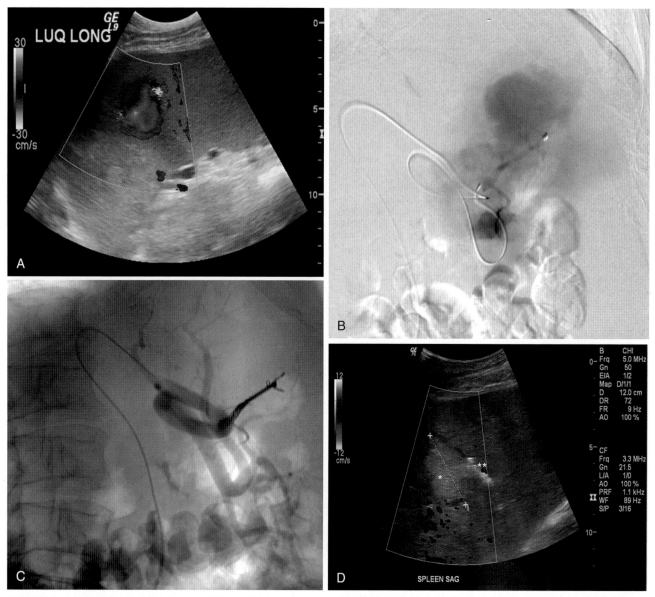

FIGURE 1   Sagittal color Doppler ultrasound (**A**) readily demonstrates a 4.5 cm upper pole splenic pseudoaneurysm confirmed by superselective splenic angiogram (**B**). The psuedoaneurysm extends close to the capsule at the confirmed site of splenic injury seen on prior contrast enhanced CT. Intraparenchymal pseudoaneurysm was treated with super selective embolization with detachable microcoils and liquid embolic (onyx) (**C**). Postembolization Doppler ultrasound demonstrates no flow within the thrombosed pseudoaneurysm *(single asterisk)* as well as echogenic material *(double asterisks)* in the parent splenic artery branch (**D**).

mesenteric artery (SMA), which persists via the dorsal pancreatic artery. The arc of Barkow represents a collateral pathway between the celiac and SMA via the omental arteries. The right and left gastroepiploic arteries, which originate from the gastroduodenal and splenic arteries, respectively, give collateral flow to the greater omentum. Additionally, the posterior epiploic arteries of the transverse pancreatic and the middle colic arteries (from the SMA) supply the greater omentum, and connect with the gastroepiploic arteries, thus forming the arc of Barkow. Though less important in the trauma setting, the arc of Riolan represents communication of the SMA with the inferior mesenteric artery via a central connection from the proximal middle colic artery and proximal left colic artery.

Therapeutic Angiography

When considering vascular injury, a vast array of tools is available, and a good foundation in angiographic techniques is required. The main agents discussed in this chapter are stent grafts, occlusion balloons,

and embolic agents (both liquid and solid). Stent graft may be used to stop arterial bleeding as well as presage native arterial flow to the distal organs and tissues. The successful utilization of a stent graft requires a suitable artery, and therefore cannot be used for every vascular lesion. Vessels should be at least 5 mm or greater and should follow a relative straight course; tortuous vessels are not amenable to stent grafts due to migratory risk. Furthermore, bifurcating vessels are not candidates for stent grafts for similar reasons and risk of branch occlusion; they should also be avoided in young patients due to in-stent stenosis from neointimal hyperplasia. Arteries that are ideal for stent grafts include the external iliac and superficial femoral arteries. Occlusion balloons are typically used as temporizing measures as a bridge to surgery or as definitive endovascular treatment in rapid exsanguination.

Embolization can be performed with coils, vascular plugs, Gelfoam pledgets, particles, liquid embolics, or a combination of these. Coils function as embolic agents by inducing thrombosis, not mechanical occlusion; the thrombogenic effect is enhanced by Dacron wool tails, which are incorporated in the coil. These agents are very effective in

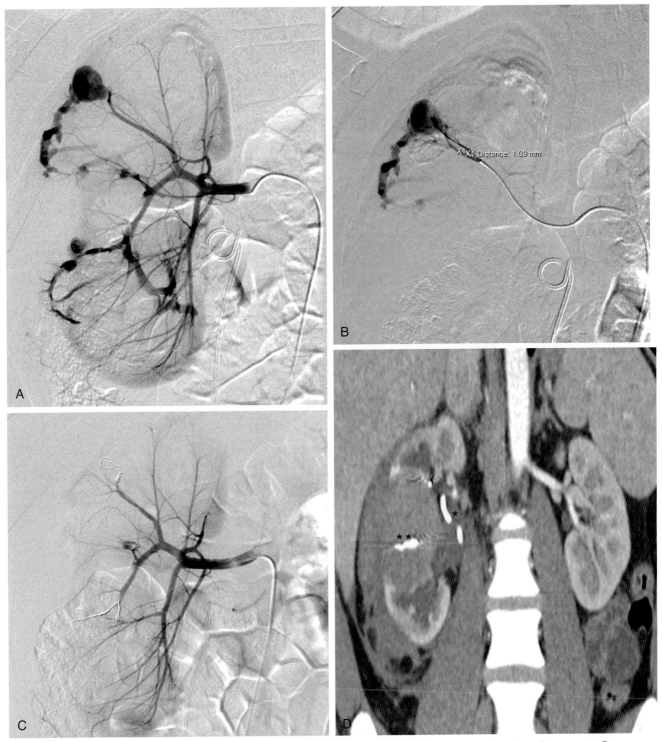

FIGURE 2   A, Selective right renal angiography demonstrates multiple arteriovenous fistula and intraparenhymal pseudoaneurysms. **B,** Superselective interpolar arteriography demonstrates a well defined pseudoaneurysm and communicated arteriovenous fistula. **C,** Right renal angiogram post superselective embolization with detachable microcoils demonstrates resolution of previously noted pseudoaneurysms and arteriovenous fistulas. **D,** Followup contrast CT demonstrates maintained perfusion of the uninvolved renal parenchyma as well as an interpolar intraparenchymal hematoma. Ureteral stent *(single asterisk)* and microils *(double asterisks)* are noted.

proximal embolization, and can also be used in sandwich techniques. The sandwich technique is typically used in regions of potential collateralization, such as hepatic or splenic arterial injury. Situations in which the sandwich technique is useful are discontinuous flow in a ruptured hepatic artery or isolated pseudoaneurysm of the splenic artery. Coils and vascular plugs may also be used in cases of AVF or bleeding refractory to other embolic agents. Detachable microcoils

may allow for accurate pin point embolization, which is key for treating underlying vascular injuries while preserving normal tissue perfusion, especially in the setting of injury to end vessel organs, such as in renal trauma (Fig. 2). The major disadvantage of coil/vascular plug embolization remains that once proximal embolization is performed, distal access to the vessel is blocked, and therefore repeat endovascular intervention is not possible.

Gelfoam is another embolic agent; it is water-soluble and can be prepared rather quickly. It is a temporary embolic agent that is completely absorbed by the body. The arterial vessel typically recanalizes within 2 to 3 weeks. It is effectively used in regions of multiple pseudoaneurysms and extensively used in pelvic trauma, following arterial flow distally to seal active hemorrhage quickly.

Embolic particles are sometimes used in the trauma setting. Particles are available in many different sizes; however, those used in trauma range from 500 to 700 μm and 700 to 900 μm. Though not as frequently used, liquid agents are also very effective embolic materials. *N*-butyl cyanoacrylate, or NBCA, is commonly referred to as liquid adhesive or glue, and polymerizes immediately on contact with ionized fluid such as blood. The glue forms as a result of an exothermic reaction, which destroys the vessel wall, and therefore it is reserved for smaller vessels accessed with a microcatheter. Once the glue is injected, the catheter must be quickly removed from the vessel lumen in order to prevent catheter-vessel wall adherence. Particles and liquid embolics are permanent distal embolizing agents, and there is a potential risk of tissue ischemia, especially if there is occlusion of the capillary bed. In general, liquid and particulate embolic agents should be avoided in the spleen and inferior gluteal artery to reduce the incidence of abscess and sciatic nerve injury, respectively.

PITFALLS FOR THE INTERVENTIONALIST

Pitfalls may arise even for the most experienced interventional radiologist. A sound understanding of potential variations of normal visceral and pelvic vasculature is essential to master and may prevent treatment failure. Traditional anatomy of the celiac trunk is present in only 70% of patients. Although the common hepatic artery arises from the celiac trunk in 95% of patients, the arterial vasculature of the liver is anatomic in only 55% of the population. Though numerous variations exist in visceral and pelvic vasculature, three major anomalies are of most importance when searching for angiographic extravasation (Table 1). First, the dorsal pancreatic

TABLE 1: Visceral Arterial Vasculature

Vessel	Arterial Variant	Frequency
Celiac	Celiac origin of left gastric artery, common hepatic artery, and splenic artery	70%
	Left gastric artery, common hepatic artery, dorsal pancreatic artery, and splenic artery with celiac origin	10%
	Aortic origin of left gastric artery	2%
	Celiac origin of left gastric artery and splenic artery only	3%
Hepatic	Right and left hepatic artery originating from common hepatic artery	55%
	Replaced right hepatic artery	12%
	Accessory right hepatic artery	6%
	Replaced left hepatic artery	11%
	Accessory left hepatic artery	11%
	Right hepatic artery originating from superior mesenteric artery, left hepatic artery originating from left gastric artery	2%

Modified from Kaufman JA: Fundamentals of angiography. In Kaufman JA, Michael JL, editors: *The requisites: vascular and interventional radiology,* Philadelphia, Mosby, 2004, pp 31–66.

artery arises from the celiac trunk in 10% of patients, and should not be mistaken for hemorrhage. Second, 12% of patient's right hepatic lobe is supplied by a replaced right hepatic artery, which arises from the SMA. In this circumstance, selective arteriography of the SMA is required to rule out hemorrhage of the right hepatic lobe. Finally, in pelvic angiography the obturator artery may arise from the common femoral or inferior epigastric arteries in 20% of individuals, requiring selective angiography of the external iliac artery. Initial nonselective angiogram or prior CTA imaging is usually sufficient to diagnose these anomalies.

Angiographic interpretation is also a potential source of problems. In pelvic angiography of the male patient, it is important to distinguish between active extravasation and cavernosal blush. Differences may be subtle, but consequences from penile artery embolization are significant, especially in young patients. Important to understand is that the cavernosal blush is typically midline at or below the pubic symphysis, arises from the internal pudendal artery, and completely washes out, but active extravasation will persist through the delayed phase. Another potential downfall is small vessel arterial truncation from obstructive thrombus. These lesions may also be extremely subtle; however, if the angiogram is not meticulously examined, arterial truncation can be easily missed. Ultimately, it is important to understand the limitations of angiography, and potential false–negative findings that may occur. As mentioned earlier, the hemodynamic status of the patient significantly affects the appearance of diagnostic angiography. Vasospasm may temporarily cease active hemorrhage, and if extravasation is not identified, delayed hemorrhage can result in further demise.

SOLID ORGAN INJURY

Splenic Trauma

The spleen is the most commonly injured abdominal organ in blunt abdominal trauma. In fact, 97% of trauma surgeons consider hemodynamic instability an indication for emergent splenectomy in blunt splenic injury. However, the current standard of care for splenic trauma in hemodynamically stable patients is nonoperative management. Nonoperative management fails in 12% to 15% of splenic trauma, and it has been shown that early embolization reduces these rates. Embolization is additionally advantageous for splenic salvage, with reports demonstrating salvage rates of above 85%. Yet, there is no uniform consensus for indications for angiography or embolization in splenic trauma. Some strongly advocate angiography for all splenic injuries, but others reserve angiography for high-grade solid organ injury, presence of vascular injury on CTA, and large hemoperitoneum.

Splenic embolization can be performed proximally in the splenic artery or distally within intraparenchymal branches, or approached with a combination of both. Proximal embolization is preferable by many interventionalists, though outcomes for both proximal and distal embolization are similar. Proximal techniques execute hemostasis by decreasing the arterial pressure heading to the spleen. It has a decreased risk of infarction due to the preservation of collateral flow; however, there is a concern of the overall function of the spleen after embolization, as the spleen is rendered globally ischemic. The proximal technique is used for multiple vascular injuries or high-grade parenchymal injury. Coils or vascular plugs are typically deployed in the splenic artery distal to the pancreatic vessels. Distal embolization is used in those patients with isolated vascular injury or lower-grade splenic injury. A major advantage of the distal technique is preservation of splenic function. Gelfoam slurries are usually used because theoretically the temporary agent has lower risk of abscess formation than that of permanent embolic agents, such as particles.

Splenic intervention is not without risk, and there is up to a 35% complication rate, combining distal and proximal techniques. Though complications are relatively common, there is no adverse effect on splenic salvage rates. Splenic infarction, defined as devascularization of greater than 25%, is the most common complication, occurs in 20% of patients, and is more frequently seen in distal embolization. The majority of splenic infarction is asymptomatic, and can be managed nonoperatively, resolving without sequelae. The most common major complication is rehemorrhage (11%), which often requires reembolization or surgical splenectomy. Another major complication, which is less common, is abscess formation. If caught early, abscess cavities can be drained percutaneously or may need surgical débridement. Abscess complications are more frequently encountered with combined embolization techniques and with the use of particles. Proximal embolization techniques have unique late sequelae not seen in distal intervention in which hypertrophic short gastric vessels may result in Dieulafoy-type lesions of the gastric mucosa. This is a chronic complication, resulting from collateralization of the splenic artery, and is never seen in the acute setting. Pancreatic and gastric wall infarction is extremely rare as the visceral vasculature is extraordinarily resilient, providing collateral blood flow via the short gastric arteries and surrounding vasculature.

Hepatic Trauma

The liver is the second most commonly injured abdominal organ in blunt trauma. Because of the exocrine function of the liver, and its anatomic complexity, there is a significant risk of complication, as trauma can cause venous, arterial, and even biliary injury. As a result, over 85% of trauma-related liver injuries are treated with some sort of intervention. Most hepatic bleeding is from low-pressure venous hemorrhage, yet arterial and biliary injuries are of most significance to the interventionalist. Asensio et al described the multidisciplinary approach to the management of complex hepatic injuries AAST grades IV and VI as it is well known that AAST-grade injury increases the risk of arterial and biliary injury, and subsequently raises the need for early intervention. Furthermore, high-grade hepatic injury and hemodynamic instability often require a multidisciplinary surgical and endovascular approach with operative management primarily performed and postoperative embolization adjunctively used for remaining arterial hemorrhage.

The morbidity associated with embolization and subsequent liver-related complications is not completely understood, as there is overlap with trauma-related complications. However, the efficacy of embolization for severe hepatic injury has been well established, with success rates of 85% to 100% and a significant mortality rate benefit. Furthermore, recent studies have demonstrated no significant difference in hepatic morbidity with or without embolization. Embolization techniques used in hepatic trauma are similar to those techniques used in splenic trauma. Owing to the rich collateral network of arterial vasculature in the liver, sandwich techniques (see therapeutic angiography) are used more often in hepatic trauma. Coil embolization and liquid embolic agents are also commonly used in the liver.

Complications related to hepatic trauma can be divided into early and late manifestations. Persistent bleeding is the most common early complication, which can occur in up to 9% of conservatively managed patients. It is important to distinguish between active bleeding and delayed bleeding in those patients with follow-up CTA (refer to earlier CTA discussion). Active arterial hemorrhage can be treated with embolization, but delayed hemorrhage may require operative management. Late manifestations of hepatic trauma include biliary fistula, abscess formation, and hemobilia. Biliary injury resulting in bile leak or biloma occurs in up to 14% of patients with high-grade liver injuries. Percutaneous imaging-guided drainage plays a critical role in the management of biliary fistula, and is the primary treatment of choice. Endoscopic retrograde cholangiopancreatography (ERCP) with stenting of the common bile duct is typically reserved for those injuries difficult to access percutaneously or in those patients with a significant bile leak. Ultimately, the goal is to reduce pressure on the adjacent tissues to prevent necrosis and allow adequate bile drainage. Typically, patients require an average of 4 weeks to fully repair the biliary radicals. Output of the drainage catheter should be monitored daily and will generally decrease over the course of a few weeks. Minimal drainage output suggests antegrade flow of bile into the duodenum, and indicates the bile duct has fully healed. The catheter can then be removed. Dual drainage with ERCP should be considered in those patients with prolonged bile

drainage over 6 weeks. Abscess formation may also complicate hepatic trauma. Abscess is thought to represent sequelae from the high pressure of intraparenchymal collections on the surrounding tissue, leading to necrosis, and eventually abscess. Imaging-guided percutaneous drainage is the treatment of choice for abscess formation.

Severe complication with hemobilia typically manifests late in the patient's course. This is a result of deep arterial injury, usually a pseudoaneurysm, which communicates or ruptures into the biliary tree, resulting in extensive clot burden, obstructive cholangitis, and possible exsanguination. The mortality rate of untreated hemobilia reaches 60%, and therefore, urgent angiography and embolization are required. Finally, gallbladder and biliary necrosis is rare in the trauma setting, unlike hepatic arterial embolization in hepatocellular carcinoma (HCC). This is likely due to normal hepatic parenchyma and preserved collateral flow in the majority of the trauma population. The risk of gallbladder necrosis may increase in those trauma patients with a history of cirrhosis or HCC and should be strongly considered.

Renal Trauma

The incidence of renal injury in blunt trauma is approximately 2%, and blunt renal artery injury is even less common, seen in under 1% of blunt trauma patients. Renal injuries are almost never isolated in blunt trauma, and typically the spleen and liver are injured first. Most injuries to the kidney are minor. Over 80% are small hematomas or lacerations with an intact capsule and can be managed conservatively. Of those patients with renal lacerations, 17% extend beyond the capsule, and 7% of these have some sort of communication with the collecting system, which may require intervention. Patients with high-grade injury risk renal dysfunction, renovascular hypertension, or even renal failure. Therefore, though there is no unified consensus for the management of renal injury, higher-grade renal injuries are typically intervened upon. Grade II to IV parenchymal injuries are managed in a multidisciplinary approach with angiography or surgery with an attempt at renal salvage, and grade V parenchymal injuries are by and large managed surgically, many times with nephrectomy.

The renal vasculature differs from that of the liver or spleen, as the kidneys depend on end-arteries for blood supply due to poorly developed collaterals. Although proximal embolization and sandwich techniques are favored in the liver and spleen, alternative approaches are required in the kidney to preserve renal function. Subsequently, peripheral embolization techniques have been developed, selectively embolizing as distally as possible. These techniques typically require a coaxial approach with microcatheters to get as selective as possible and minimize the risk of parenchymal infarction. Microcoils and liquid embolics, like NBCA, are commonly used for these intraparenchymal arterial injury. A recent 10-year review demonstrated an embolization success rate of 94% when used as primary management. Severe complications related to embolization are rare. Renal infarction is a relatively common phenomenon, but adverse sequelae are typically not seen. Renal abscess, from progression of infarction, occurs in less than 5% of postembolization patients.

Traumatic injury to the main renal artery can result in renal artery dissection, intimal flaps, and even acute arterial truncation from thrombosis. Intimal flaps may progress to nonocclusive dissection, which can further progress to occlusive dissection and thrombosis, resulting in parenchymal death. Therefore, renal artery stenting is a reasonable option in those patients with renal artery intimal injury/dissection, especially if there is a pressure gradient or if subsequent renovascular hypertension develops. Typically, covered or bare-metal stents are used with good 1-year primary patency rates. Renal artery truncation suggests arterial transection and occluding thrombosis; these lesions should be left alone as unstable thrombus may potentially dislodge, leading to exsanguination into the retroperitoneum. Although some interventionalists may employ provocative angiography, in our experience these lesions are best managed conservatively. Once the patient's condition stabilizes, surgical nephrectomy may be performed for the infarcted kidney. In certain situations, polytrauma patients or those with high operative risk may require main renal artery embolization, either as definitive treatment or followed by interval nephrectomy once the patient's clinical condition improves.

Finally, active hemorrhage and parenchymal hematoma can cause significant clot burden in the urinary collecting system, which may subsequently cause obstructive uropathy. Foley catheterization and continuous bladder irrigation with or without cystoscopic stent placement is typically required with good success rates. Complicated cases with extensive clot burden in the ureter may require percutaneous nephrostomy placement to decompress the urinary collecting system. Additionally, perinephric hematoma can cause extrinsic renal compression, the so-called perinephric compartment syndrome, which can be treated with percutaneous drainage under ultrasound guidance.

PELVIC TRAUMA

Because of the anatomic constraints of the pelvic girdle and the close approximation to the osseous structures, vascular injury is relatively common in pelvic trauma, and is the cause of the high mortality rate of over 25% in this subset of patients. Hemorrhagic sources in the pelvis are largely due to venous, osseous, and arterial bleeding. Venous and bone hemorrhage can be successfully controlled with pelvic fixation; however, life-threatening arterial hemorrhage cannot be tamponaded due to the high-pressure system. In fact, it has been reported that 10% to 15% of pelvic hemorrhage is due to an arterial injury, and mortality rate is substantially increased once an arterial source is identified. Owing to the potential increase in the pelvic volume, pelvic fracture results in hemodynamic instability in up to 20% of patients.

Pelvic fracture results from lateral compression, anteroposterior (AP) compression, vertical shear, or a combination of mechanisms. AP compression, vertical shear forces, and combination mechanisms demonstrate a higher failure rate to pelvic fixation alone, and typically

require angiography. Furthermore, embolization in pelvic trauma boasts success rates of over 87%. As a result, embolization has advanced to the vanguard of primary hemostasis in pelvic trauma, and has become the standard of care in many institutions. Patients with active extravasation or those with pelvic fracture and hemodynamic instability are candidates for angiographic embolization.

The branches of the internal iliac artery (IIA) are the most frequently injured arterial vessels in pelvic trauma (Fig. 3). The superior gluteal artery, which originates from the posterior division of the IIA, is the most common, followed closely by the internal pudendal artery from the anterior division. Embolization is usually performed with Gelfoam slurry or coils to control hemorrhage. Dehydrated alcohol is typically avoided in the pelvis, due to the risk of nerve damage and mucosal sloughing of the large intestine. In patients with hemodynamic instability, angiographic contrast extravasation can be difficult to identify because of profound vasospasm. If extravasation is not identified and provocative angiography not indicated, prophylactic proximal IIA embolization can be performed. The side of the pelvic fracture is identified and subsequent embolization of the ipsilateral IIA is performed with Gelfoam or coils. Bilateral prophylactic IIA embolization may be indicated in certain clinical scenarios. This effectively treats arterial hemorrhage, and indirectly ceases bleeding from venous and osseous sources in the pelvis. The risk of gluteal claudication and necrosis is significantly increased in this approach, which should only be performed in specific critical situations.

The external iliac artery (EIA) can also be injured in pelvic trauma. The most common types of injury are intimal injury resulting in dissection, and transmural injury resulting in active extravasation. EIA dissection is treated with a bare metal stent. Most critical is ensuring to deploy the stent over both the site of entry and reentry. Stenting on the site of reentry can lead to further dissection and even rupture, as this is where the arterial wall is weakest. EIA hemorrhage can be

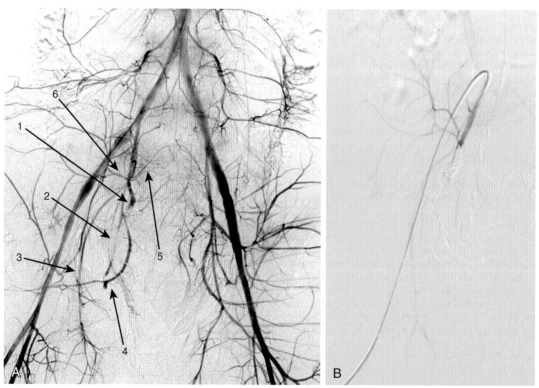

FIGURE 3 **A,** Pelvic angiography demonstrates mainly right-sided pelvic vascular injury (numbered in decreasing incidence of injury): (1) Right superior gluteal (posterior), which is truncated; (2) Right internal pudendal (anterior), which demonstrates truncation and spasm; (3) Right obturator (anterior); (4) Inferior gluteal (anterior) which demonstrates a small pseudoaneurysm; (5) Right lateral sacral (posterior); (6) Right iliolumbar (posterior). **B,** Selective right internal iliac postembolization angiography demonstrates microcoil occlusion of the inferior gluteal, internal pudendal, and superior gluteal arteries and patent obturator, lateral sacral, and iliolumbar arteries.

treated with a covered stent graft if the lesion can be crossed. The 1-year patency rates of EIA stents are well over 90%, and these patients typically follow an uncomplicated course. In specific clinical situations in which the EIA is transected, temporary endovascular ballooning can be a lifesaving procedure prior to surgical revascularization.

Complications of angiographic embolization are generally acceptable, considering the high mortality rates with pelvic trauma; furthermore, just as in the liver, most complications are difficult to distinguish from actual trauma-related complications. Gluteal necrosis though can be seen in unilateral IIA embolization and is more frequently encountered in bilateral embolization of the IIA. Skin ulceration and necrosis are seen in about 10% of pelvic trauma. Recent studies demonstrate no significant difference in skin necrosis, sloughing, or perineal infection rate between embolized and nonembolized patients. Impotence and infertility are also potential risks with embolization of the internal pudendal artery, though there have been no long-term studies to evaluate this. Care must be taken to not mistake caverosal blush for extravasation, as this may increase the risk of impotence and infertility if embolized.

INFERIOR VENA CAVA FILTER PLACEMENT FOR PROPHYLATIC EMBOLIC PROTECTION

Pulmonary embolism (PE) and deep venous thrombosis (DVT) have a high incidence in the trauma population with reports of up to 15%. Virchow's triad of venous stasis, vessel wall injury, and increased coagulability put patients at increased risk of DVT and PE, and the trauma patient epitomizes these characteristic traits. IVC filters have no effect on the treatment of PE, and do not prevent DVT, yet act as venous interruption for recurrent PE. Although IVC filter placement has traditionally been reserved for those patients diagnosed with PE and contraindications to anticoagulation, prophylactic IVC filters are being placed with more and more frequency due to the high association with trauma and DVT/PE. Currently, there are two indications for placement of prophylactic IVC filter: (1) polytrauma patients at high risk of PE; and (2) patients undergoing a major surgical procedure with history of PE/DVT and high postoperative risk of DVT.

IVC filters are typically placed below the lowest renal vein, which is frequently at the L3 vertebral body level. Before placement of the filter, an inferior vena cavogram is usually obtained to ensure patency of the IVC and to screen for anatomic variants. Though rare, venous anomalies, of which the interventionalist must be aware, include circumaortic left renal vein, retroaortic left renal vein, duplicated IVC, left-sided IVC, and mega cava. With scenarios in which a circumaortic left renal vein is encountered, the IVC filter must be placed suprarenally. Retroaortic renal veins usually insert lower on the vena cava, which also influences the placement of filters. A duplicated IVC requires a dual filter placement in each of the IVCs. The left-sided IVC is important, as it appears different angiographically, and may be technically more difficult to place under fluoroscopy. Finally, mega cava, defined as an IVC greater than 30 mm in diameter, requires placement of the larger bird's nest filter; alternatively, filters can be placed in the common iliac veins bilaterally. Through recent advances in ultrasound technology, the ability to perform bedside IVC filters is becoming more feasible via intravascular ultrasound guidance.

Careful consideration should be made for the type of filter placed and future management as IVC filters in and of themselves, are prothrombotic. Trauma patients are only temporarily in a hypercoaguable state, and thromboembolic protection is not needed outside the acute setting. Furthermore, the trauma population is, by and large, a young patient population in which IVC occlusion from clot propagation can result in significant morbidity. Subsequently, retrievable IVC filters are preferred in the trauma setting, with plan of removal within 3 to 6 months to prevent intimal incorporation.

CONCLUDING DISCUSSION

In conclusion, interventional radiology has a pivotal role in the diagnosis, management, and treatment of abdominal and pelvic trauma. The major goal in the evaluation of the trauma patient is rapid identification of potentially life-threatening hemorrhage and early intervention. Interventional techniques are used in nonoperative and operative management schemes—in those patients who are hemodynamically stable and those who are unstable. Angiography and surgery are complimentary in providing hemostasis, often requiring a multidisciplinary approach. In certain clinical scenarios, angiography may even be considered an alternative to surgery.

Given the complexity of many of these traumatic injuries, which are often multiple, it is imperative both to understand the indications for such interventional techniques, and to prepare for the inevitable trauma-related complications that may require further intervention. Within interventional radiology, much emphasis has been placed on the design of newer angiography suites, which are becoming integrated into the emergency room layout for easier access. Furthermore, some leading institutions are combining CT machines with angiography suites to reduce the time delay between diagnosis and intervention. Ultimately, as the field of interventional radiology progresses, research and further investigation on techniques specifically for the trauma population are needed, not only to allow for earlier intervention, but to advance patient care and provide the safest, most effective treatment.

For the chapter's Suggested Readings list, please visit the book at www.ExpertConsult.inkling.com.

ENDPOINTS OF RESUSCITATION

Susan Rowell, Ronald Barbosa, Michael Englehart, Brandon Tieu, and Martin Schreiber

The optimal end point of resuscitation has been debated since the early 20th century when Walter Cannon, MD, proposed his controversial viewpoint of limited volume resuscitation, and it continues to be a topic of discussion and study. The ideal end point of resuscitation should be readily obtainable, easily interpreted, and directly correlated with clinical outcome. The goal is to provide adequate oxygen delivery (DO_2) and tissue perfusion without producing complications of overresuscitation. This is accomplished primarily by increasing cardiac output via increases in preload (volume loading) or vasoactive drugs. Multiple diagnostic measurements have been used to determine both optimal cardiac performance and adequate tissue perfusion. Although no single value can be used exclusively, various measurements do allow uniformity in comparing adequacy of resuscitation. These values provide the ability over time to determine whether a patient is being properly resuscitated. They can be categorized into hemodynamic parameters, metabolic parameters, and regional perfusion end points.

CLINICAL AND HEMODYNAMIC END POINTS

Shock has been defined in a multitude of ways, but can best be described as a lack of adequate tissue perfusion. Oxygen delivery and removal of waste products are impaired. The six basic advanced trauma life support physiologic parameters that have been used to identify shock are heart rate, respiratory rate, blood pressure, urine output, level of consciousness, and pulse pressure. Urine output and level of consciousness are direct correlates of tissue perfusion, and are defined for each class of shock. Renal blood flow correlates with arterial pressure, but can be subject to significant autoregulation during periods of hypoperfusion. Level of consciousness is less reliable when influenced by intoxication, central nervous system injury, and medication. Heart rate and respiratory rate can be notoriously misleading (Table 1). Anxiety, pain, and stress secondary to the emotional impact of trauma can falsely elevate these physiologic parameters. This can confuse the picture and mask the underlying severity of shock. Clinical studies and animal models both show that a degree of disconnection between the systemic circulation and the microcirculation is frequently present. The presence of relatively normal vital signs does not guarantee that regional perfusion is adequate. The diagnosis of shock is best made by observing the body's main compensatory mechanism: redistribution of blood flow.

Due to austere conditions and inability to measure blood pressure, U.S. combat medics in Operation Iraqi Freedom and Operation Enduring Freedom have been trained to resuscitate patients until they are conscious, or when consciousness cannot be assessed, until they have a palpable radial pulse. Current British Army guidelines also include resuscitation to a palpable radial pulse. During World War I, Cannon stated that 75 mm Hg was the critical systolic blood pressure to maintain. However, many have advocated avoiding hypotension in patients with severe brain injury to ensure adequate cerebral perfusion pressure. The presence of hypotension is predictive of worse outcome after head injury. Additionally, patients with previous hypertension may display symptoms of organ hypoperfusion despite a "normal" mean arterial pressure (MAP). Owing to complex interactions of the patients' preexisting disease states and the severity of the injury, there is unfortunately no uniform "goal" MAP to determine adequate resuscitation.

Oxygen delivery is a function of hemoglobin concentration, oxygen saturation, and cardiac output. Hemoglobin concentration and oxygen concentration are relatively easy to manipulate and monitor, but cardiac output can be more problematic. Adequate cardiac performance is largely a function of preload. Multiple methods have been devised to estimate the patient's volume status indirectly by evaluating the venous return to the heart. With the introduction of central venous and pulmonary artery catheters (PACs), central venous pressure (CVP) and pulmonary artery occlusion pressure (PAOP) have been used as measurements of volume status. Although these measurements serve to guide the resuscitation, absolute values should be interpreted with caution. Valvular or global cardiac dysfunction, as well as restrictive pulmonary disease, can dramatically alter these measurements. The use of mechanical ventilation, particularly when pressure settings are high, also make CVP and PAOP more difficult to interpret. Considerable variability can also be introduced between observers due to differences in transducer zeroing or failure to measure the pressures at the same reference points in the respiratory and cardiac cycles.

Newer volumetric or oximetric PACs have the capability for dynamic measurement of additional hemodynamic parameters that were previously unobtainable. Cardiac output can be continuously monitored due to the development of catheters using heated filaments to obtain measurements. Cardiac performance can be evaluated using calculations of ventricular power and end-diastolic volume index. A recent study demonstrated that the right ventricular end-diastolic volume index (RVEDVI) is a more sensitive measurement of preload than CVP or PAOP, particularly in the mechanically ventilated patient. Cheatham et al demonstrated that cardiac index (CI) correlated better with RVEDVI than with PAOP, even at very high levels of positive end-expiratory pressure. In a comparison of RVEDVI with splanchnic perfusion in trauma patients, both Miller et al and Chang et al found that resuscitation to a RVEDVI of greater than 120 mL/m^2 during shock was associated with better outcomes. Other studies have shown similar advantages. However, use of these techniques requires a significant institutional commitment that may be prohibitive given the small number of patients that benefit from this type of monitoring.

Despite the advances in PACs, their effectiveness has been in question since the mid-1990s. Connors et al published an observational study suggesting that PACs were associated with increased mortality rate and increased utilization of resources. Despite the study's limitations, critically ill patients who had a PAC placed had a higher 30-, 60-, and 180-day mortality rate, increased hospital cost, and longer intensive care unit (ICU) stays. A recent metaanalysis including 5051 medical and surgical ICU patients enrolled in 13 randomized controlled trials evaluating PACs showed that the use of PACs did not improve survival or decrease length of stay in the hospital. It did not demonstrate increased mortality risk in the patients who had a PAC placed. Recent studies show that PAC use is declining in the United States in general, and in the trauma population in particular. Overall, these data suggest that PACs should not be used routinely in surgical ICU patients unless effective therapies can be found that improve outcomes when used in conjunction with this diagnostic tool.

Pulse contour–derived CO measurement (PCCO) can also continuously measure cardiac output and correlates well with thermodilution measurements. PCCO requires placement of an arterial catheter and a central venous catheter on opposite sides of the diaphragm. It may be a more accurate indicator of cardiac preload than CVP or PAOP. Unfortunately, rapid changes in hemodynamic status can alter the monitoring and recalibration is necessary.

Many have attempted to define an oxygen consumption/delivery end point itself, but with no clear results. The Fick equation states that Do_2 and Vo_2 are functions of CI, hemoglobin (Hb), and arterial and venous oxygen saturations (Sao_2 and Svo_2, respectively):

$$Do_2 = CI \times 13.4 \times Hb \times Sao_2$$
$$Vo_2 = CI \times 13.4 \times Hb \times (Sao_2 - Svo_2)$$

Unfortunately, Do_2 and Vo_2 are both derived from cardiac output, and the stable plateau described in Figure 1 is virtually impossible to obtain. Goal-directed therapy, aimed at ensuring a CI greater than

TABLE 1: Relationship of Degree of Shock to Pulse Rate (106 Cases)

| Pulse Rate | DEGREES OF SHOCK* | | | |
	None (n = 13)	Slight (n = 24)	Moderate (n = 34)	Severe (n = 35)
Minimum	70	88	80	60
Maximum	140	150	160	144
Average	103 ± 7.2	111 ± 3.4	113 ± 3.6	116 ± 3.3

Modified from The Board for the Study of the Severely Wounded: *The Physiologic Effect of Wounds.* Washington, DC, Office of the Surgeon General, 1952.

*These data were gathered in the North African–Mediterranean Theater during World War II. There was minimal variability observed between groups despite significant differences in the severity of shock. Slight shock = 80% of normal blood volume; moderate shock = 70% of normal blood volume; severe shock = 55% of normal blood volume.

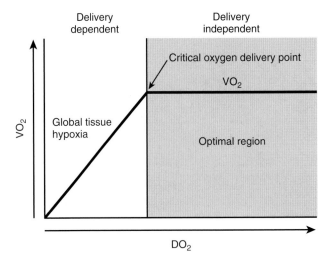

Delivery dependent   Delivery independent

Critical oxygen delivery point

VO_2

Global tissue hypoxia

Optimal region

VO_2

DO_2

FIGURE 1   Relationship between oxygen delivery (Do_2) and oxygen extraction (Vo_2). *(From Bilkovski RN, Rivers EP, Horst HM: Targeted resuscitation strategies after injury.* Curr Opin Crit Care *10:529–538, 2004.)*

4.5 L/minute/m², Do_2 index greater than 600 mL/minute/m², and Vo_2 index greater than 170 mL/minute/m², has been advocated by Shoemaker and others, demonstrating reduced morbidity and mortality rates in critically ill patients. However, Gattinoni in a multicenter randomized controlled trial, and Heyland in a metaanalysis, showed no such benefit. Furthermore, a prospective, randomized controlled trial by Velmahos comparing conventional versus supranormal end points demonstrated that despite all efforts, only 70% of patients were able to reach these end points. They concluded that regardless of the resuscitation strategy, the ability of the patient to achieve "optimal hemodynamic values" significantly affected outcome. Looking at O_2 delivery alone, McKinley et al found that there was no difference in outcome between groups resuscitated to an O_2 delivery goal of 600 mL/minute/m² versus 500 mL/minute/m².

Resuscitation to supranormal end points has been associated with numerous complications. Shoemaker's protocol included volume loading with crystalloids and blood, and enhancement of cardiac output with dobutamine. Improvements in blood pressure and cardiac performance by vasoactive drugs can be negated by reduced tissue perfusion, and can often result in tissue ischemia. Hayes et al found in medical and surgical critically ill patients that the use of dobutamine to augment O_2 delivery may actually increase mortality risk. Overresuscitation with crystalloid solutions can lead to the development of compartment syndromes, coagulopathy, hyperchloremic acidosis, and other iatrogenic complications, such as congestive heart failure, in patients with cardiac disease.

Less invasive techniques for measuring cardiac performance have been developed. Thoracic electrical bioimpedance measures the resistance of the chest to low-voltage currents. It is inversely related to thoracic fluid content, thereby allowing calculation of cardiac output. Several studies have demonstrated that this method correlates well with thermodilution measurements of cardiac output. However, a metaanalysis demonstrated clinical utility in trend analysis but not accuracy for diagnostic interpretation. There can also be significant imprecision with tachycardia or with pathologic fluid collections such as pleural effusions.

Transesophageal echocardiography can assess preload and peak velocity measurements, as well as continuous cardiac output monitoring, and has been validated with thermodilution techniques. In animal models of hemorrhagic shock, it has accurately reflected the magnitude of change on cardiac output. Bedside transthoracic echocardiography (TTE) has also been recently studied by Gunst et al. In this study, trauma surgeons with a modest amount of echocardiogram training were able to obtain estimates of CI that correlated well with those derived from a PAC. However, the utility of TTE is limited by interobserver variability and frequent technical difficulties with obtaining sufficient quality images, especially in the supine position. Ferrada et al have also used TTE to measure inferior vena cava diameter and respiratory variation as a measure of the fluid status of critically ill patients. Though technically feasible, interventions based on these data have yet to demonstrate direct clinical benefit.

Heart rate variability (HRV) has been studied in critically ill patients in an attempt to identify patients at risk for clinical deterioration earlier than standard hemodynamic parameters. HRV is based on the observation that critically ill patients have a degree of autonomic dysfunction that manifests in, among other things, a decreased variability in heart rate, both on a minute-to-minute basis and over a 1-hour period. Clinical studies show that mortality risk increases in trauma patients that manifest a decreased HRV. Heart rate complexity (HRC) has also been studied in the trauma population. HRC is a different method of analyzing heart rate data that analyzes the degree of irregularity and randomness in the signal. In a recent study by Cancio et al, increased HRC was correlated with an increased need for prehospital intubation. Though some authors have suggested that HRV and HRC can potentially be used as a new vital sign for resuscitation, they have not been widely accepted for a number of reasons. First, there is no standard method for measuring or reporting HRV and HRC and most institutions studying these methods have designed their own custom algorithms. Furthermore, the underlying physiologic mechanisms behind the mathematical observations are poorly understood. Additionally, it is unclear whether HRV and HRC can be used as true resuscitation end points (i.e., that restoration of normal HRV or HRC after resuscitation leads to a better outcome).

METABOLIC END POINTS

Measurable metabolic end points allow the clinician to effectively assess the microcirculation. Accumulation of lactate occurs under anaerobic conditions, and therefore, is a marker of inadequate microcirculatory oxygen delivery. Thus, lactate levels can provide a measure of the extent of shock. Although elevated levels indicate a worsening degree of shock, there is no clear cutoff value to determine "satisfactory" resuscitation and adequate oxygen delivery to the tissues. Manikas et al found that initial and peak lactate levels, along with duration of hyperlactatemia, correlated with the development of multiple organ dysfunction syndrome after trauma. Lactate clearance over time is probably more predictive of mortality rate than isolated values. Serial lactate levels in trauma patients have been associated with 0% to 10% mortality rate if cleared (lactate level < 2 mmol/L) within 24 hours, 25% mortality rate if cleared by 24 to 48 hours, and 80% to 86% mortality rate if cleared beyond 48 hours.

Base deficit has been advocated as a useful clinical marker for assessing reduced tissue perfusion and as a convenient marker of elevated lactate levels. It is defined as the amount of base (mmol) required to raise 1 L of whole blood to a normal pH. Davis first classified the base deficit according to severity: mild (2–5 mmol/L), moderate (6–14 mmol/L), or severe (>15 mmol/L). The severity of the deficit directly correlated with the volume of crystalloid and blood replaced within the first 24 hours. It has been shown that serum bicarbonate levels, which may be more readily available, correlate well with base deficits, but they are affected by the patient's ventilatory status. Similar to lactate, the absolute base deficit can estimate the severity of shock, but no single value can be used as an end point. A persistently high or worsening base deficit may be an indicator of complications such as abdominal compartment syndrome or ongoing hemorrhage. Greater severity of base deficit has been demonstrated to predict diminished oxygen consumption, increased risk of multiple organ dysfunction syndrome, and greater mortality risk. However, base deficit secondary to hyperchloremic acidosis is not associated with increased mortality risk or complications as demonstrated by Brill et al (Table 2). The inaccurate interpretation of an elevated base

TABLE 2: Hyperchloremic Group vs. Combined High and Mixed Anion Gap Group

Parameter	Hyperchloremic Group	Combined Group	p Value
Number of patients	37	38	
Mean age	53.9 ± 19.8	54.8 ± 22.9	0.85
Male sex (%)	54	60	0.71
APACHE II	12.2 ± 6.01	15 ± 7.5	0.10
Mean days SICU	7.8 ± 6.9	10.4 ± 9.9	0.19
Mean estimated blood loss (mL)	1088 ± 1835	1343 ± 1930	0.61
Mean resuscitation (mL)	5598 ± 3950	6500 ± 5227	0.41
Mean lactate (mg/dL)	1.5 ± 0.29	3.9 ± 2.2	<0.001
Mean base deficit (mEq/l)	5.3 ± 2.5	7.8 ± 5.4	0.01
Deaths	4	13	0.03

Modified from Brill SA, Stewart TR, Brundage SI, Schreiber MA: Base deficit does not predict mortality when secondary to hyperchloremic acidosis. *Shock* 17:459–462, 2002.
APACHE II, Acute Physiology and Chronic Health Evaluation II; SICU, surgical intensive care unit.
Note: Mortality rate is significantly reduced in surgical intensive care unit patients when acidosis is secondary to hyperchloremic acidosis as opposed to lactic acidosis.

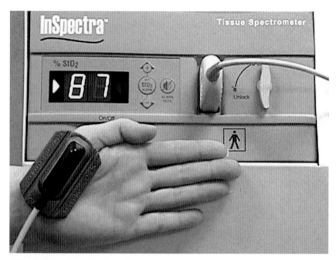

FIGURE 2 Near-infrared spectroscopy measuring tissue oxygen saturation. InSpectra Tissue Spectrometer with thenar shield in place. Shield may also be used on the deltoid muscles.

deficit that is truly related to hyperchloremic acidosis may result in unnecessary interventions such as ongoing fluid resuscitation, blood transfusion, or even operative interventions. As with lactate, the trend of the base deficit over time is more useful in predicting outcomes.

Mixed venous oxygen saturation ($S\bar{v}o_2$) has been used as an end point of resuscitation because it varies directly with changes in Sao_2, cardiac output, and hemoglobin. Decreased values suggest that tissue hypoxia is present. Current Surviving Sepsis Campaign guidelines recommend a goal $S\bar{v}o_2$ 70% or higher. The ideal $S\bar{v}o_2$ for resuscitation in hemorrhagic shock is less clear. Measurement of $S\bar{v}o_2$ also requires placement of a PAC. The use of central venous oxygen saturation ($Scvo_2$) has also been investigated because it only requires placement of a central venous line. Measured $Scvo_2$ values reflect the venous oxygen saturation of the upper body, but are thought to directly correlate with $S\bar{v}o_2$ values. The interchangeability of $S\bar{v}o_2$ and $Scvo_2$ values, however, remains controversial.

REGIONAL PERFUSION END POINTS

A multitude of techniques that directly measure the tissue microcirculation have been developed. They include gastric tonometry, sublingual capnography, and near-infrared spectroscopy (NIRS). Gastric tonometry monitors the gastric intramucosal pH (pHi), by measuring the level of tissue Pco_2. pHi decreases as splanchnic perfusion decreases. For this test to be accurate, gastric feedings need to

be withheld and gastric acid secretion needs to be suppressed. Unfortunately, it correlates poorly with lactate and base deficit, and has a prolonged calibration time. It has been suggested in studies that a lower pHi correlates with the development of multiorgan dysfunction syndrome and increased mortality risk. Sublingual capnography uses the premise that global tissue hypoperfusion causes systemic hypercarbia. It has been shown to correlate with lactate levels, as well as the severity of shock, and has been used as a predictor of mortality.

Finally, NIRS can be used to determine peripheral tissue oxygen saturation (Sto_2) (Fig. 2) based on the absorption of infrared light by hemoglobin. The NIRS technology allows the simultaneous measurement of tissue Po_2, Pco_2, and pH. In animal models of hemorrhagic shock, Sto_2 closely correlated with measured oxygen delivery, and was a superior measurement of shock when compared to lactate, base excess, or $S\bar{v}o_2$. McKinley et al found that Sto_2 correlated with oxygen delivery, base deficit, and lactate levels in severely injured trauma patients. NIRS can also monitor mitochondrial function by monitoring the redox state of cytochrome aa3, which reflects mitochondrial oxygen consumption. Under normal conditions, tissue oxyhemoglobin levels and cytochrome aa3 levels are tightly coupled. In a study of 24 severely injured trauma patients, Cairns et al noted that patients who developed multiple organ failure were more likely to have decoupling. Sto_2 monitoring has been shown to also be technically feasible in the prehospital setting, though its potential role is far from clear. Current Sto_2 devices have not yet been widely used and parameters for resuscitation have not been established.

SUMMARY

In conclusion, the goals of resuscitation should be to optimize preload, cardiac performance, blood pressure, oxygen delivery, and end-organ perfusion. Unfortunately, no single hemodynamic value or laboratory test will be universally helpful. The best method is to incorporate and optimize each of these end points. Given that shock remains a clinical diagnosis, the assessment of resuscitation is best made at the bedside, relying on an accurate assessment of the physical signs and symptoms.

For the chapter's Suggested Readings list, please visit the book at www.ExpertConsult.inkling.com.

TRAUMATIC BRAIN INJURY: PATHOPHYSIOLOGY, CLINICAL DIAGNOSIS, AND PREHOSPITAL AND EMERGENCY CENTER CARE

Aileen Ebadat and Alex B. Valadka

D eath. Long-lasting or even permanent loss of function. Those are the burdens borne by many traumatic brain injury (TBI) patients and their families. Even some patients who initially appeared to have injuries that were mild according to clinical or radiographic criteria can suffer permanent deficits that prevent them from returning to their jobs and to their family roles as husband or wife, parent, breadwinner, etc.

Emergency craniotomies and insertion of intracranial monitors are the most high-profile aspects of management of TBI patients. However, the vulnerability of the injured brain to even mild and transient metabolic derangements underscores the major impact that systemic parameters can have on influencing outcome from TBI. Thus, non-neurosurgeons can influence management in ways that are just as important, and in some cases perhaps more so, than the interventions performed by neurosurgeons.

This chapter will discuss a few principles of the underlying pathophysiology, initial assessment, and prehospital and emergency center management of TBI patients. The following chapter addresses topics relevant to the acute hospital admission. This discussion is weighted toward patients with severe TBI, but many of the basic principles apply to patients with mild or moderate TBI as well.

INCIDENCE

It is frequently stated that, in multiply injured patients, the head is the most commonly injured part of the body. Outcome from polytrauma is more dependent upon the extent of brain injury than on injury to other organ systems. Perhaps a third of the entire cost of trauma, including medical and rehabilitative care, lost income to the patient, and lost productivity to society, is attributable to brain injury.

According to data reported by the Centers for Disease Control in the 1990s, 1.5 million Americans sustain a TBI every year. Of this number, hospitalization and ultimate survival occur in approximately 230,000 patients, but 50,000 will die. Long-term disability will occur in 80,000 to 90,000 patients annually. It has been estimated that more than 5 million men, women, and children in the United States are living with a permanent TBI-related disability.

Motor vehicle crashes are the most common cause of TBI that produces hospitalization, whereas violence is the major cause of TBI-related deaths. Falls predominate as the leading cause of TBI in elderly patients. In 1990, gunshot wounds to the head overtook falls as the most common cause of TBI-related deaths in the United States.

The TBI death rate in the United States is approximately 20 per 100,000 population. In all age groups, the mortality rate is higher in males than in females. The incidence of TBI-related fatality peaks in the late teens and early twenties, subsequently decreasing during the next few decades, until taking off exponentially at about retirement age.

MECHANISM OF INJURY

Although an epidural, subdural, or intraparenchymal hematoma may have a dramatic appearance on a computed tomography (CT) scan, the clinician must remember that these lesions are distinct from the cerebral parenchymal injury that is the true cause of long-term neurologic deficits. TBI is best thought of as a diffuse disturbance of cerebral function, not as a blood clot or contusion. This diffuse disturbance may occur in parallel with, but may also be independent of, those processes that lead to the development of traumatic mass lesions.

Subdural Hematoma

Classically, a subdural hematoma (SDH) (Fig. 1) has been said to develop after tearing of a bridging vein (i.e., a vein passing directly from the cortex to the overlying dura). The mechanical forces of the trauma can cause tearing and bridging of these veins. More recent evidence indicates that at least some of these hematomas actually form from splitting of inner and outer layers of the dura; thus, they may actually be "intradural hematomas." Finally, some SDHs are caused by direct bleeding into the subdural space from parenchymal contusions or hematomas or from injured cortical arteries or veins.

Epidural Hematoma

Epidural hematomas (EDHs) classically arise after a blow to the side of the head results in a fracture of the thin temporal bone immediately overlying the middle meningeal artery. The patient may briefly lose consciousness after the initial impact, but he or she quickly awakens; thus, the brain injury was mild. Unfortunately, the fracturing of the

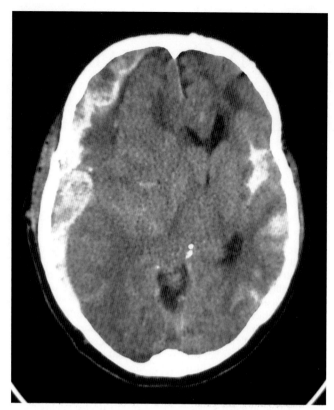

FIGURE 1 Large acute subdural hematoma (SDH) with midline shift. Subarachnoid hemorrhage is evident contralateral to the SDH.

skull lacerated the middle meningeal artery. Continued bleeding from this source produces an enlarging EDH, the presence of which may be signaled by such symptoms as severe and worsening headache, vomiting, and decreasing level of consciousness.

The period between awakening from the initial concussion and subsequent lapsing into a coma has historically been described as a "lucid interval." Importantly, loss of consciousness (LOC) does not always occur after the skull is fractured, and many patients with large EDHs are awake until they begin to lapse into a terminal coma. It must also be mentioned that many EDHs are not associated with meningeal arterial bleeding. In these cases, perhaps the source of the hematoma is oozing from the overlying edges of fractured bone.

Referring again to the classic scenarios, patients with EDHs are said to fare better than patients with similarly sized SDHs. Why should this be so? The answer is that a "pure" EDH essentially represents a skull fracture with no direct parenchymal injury to the brain. On the other hand, the rotational forces that are said to be an important cause of SDHs via tearing of bridging veins may also cause widespread axonal injury, as discussed later. Thus, SDH is said to be associated with a greater burden of parenchymal injury, which explains the worse outcomes. Of course, this explanation refers only to the extreme ends of the spectrum of the pathophysiology of EDHs and SDHs. Many patients with EDHs will do poorly, but SDH patients often recover well from their injuries. Nevertheless, this explanation is a useful way to conceptualize the interactions between mass lesions and diffuse injury.

Subarachnoid Hemorrhage

The most common post-traumatic intracerebral hemorrhage is not a mass lesion, but rather diffuse subarachnoid hemorrhage (SAH) (see Fig. 1). Several retrospective series report that SAH after TBI is independently associated with worse outcomes, but the mechanism that might explain such an association is unclear. In the acute setting,

SAH does not seem to have much effect on patient management, which is driven instead by more immediately pressing concerns.

Parenchymal Lesions

Contusions occur commonly after TBI, especially at the base of the frontal lobes and at the anterior edges of the temporal lobes. The brain in these regions is said to continue moving over or into the skull base after the head suddenly stops moving after a violent blow or rapid rotational movement. Fortunately, most such contusions remain small and surgically insignificant. Emergency surgery may be required, however, for larger lesions or for smaller ones that subsequently enlarge.

Unlike contusions, in which extravasated blood mixes freely with brain tissue, parenchymal hematomas consist of solid blood clots within the brain itself. They occur less commonly than contusions. They tend to be more variable in their distribution.

Ischemia

Diffuse injury may be of several types. Ischemia is a common form of diffuse injury. In some cases, mass effect from a traumatic hematoma may cause elevated intracranial pressure (ICP) and local compression of underlying tissue that can lead, respectively, to global and local reduction of cerebral blood flow (CBF). However, post-traumatic cerebral ischemia may also occur when no mass lesion is present, especially very early after injury. Although the CT scans in these cases may be relatively unimpressive, these patients may be quite vulnerable to the effects of such secondary insults as hypotension or hypoxia. Over the subsequent hours and days, CBF usually increases, but the damage from early ischemia may have already been done long before the increase in CBF (Fig. 2). Some centers have utilized xenon CT or perfusion CT to measure CBF and identify ischemia immediately after injury.

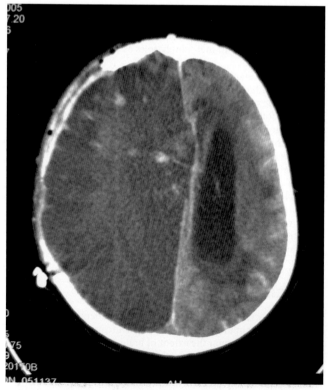

FIGURE 2 Infarction of an entire cerebral hemisphere is evident on the left side of this computed tomography scan.

Diffuse Axonal Injury

Another common type of diffuse injury is diffuse axonal injury (DAI). Although the axonal disconnection that characterizes DAI is commonly thought to occur at the time of injury, such immediate loss of axonal continuity probably occurs only when an injury produces severe cerebral parenchymal disruption. Instead, it appears more likely that the rotational and mechanical forces that are operant during the traumatic event produce a focal impairment of axoplasmic flow which, in turn, culminates in axonal disconnection several hours after injury. This slight delay creates hope that a therapeutic window may exist for the administration of a yet-to-be-developed treatment that would prevent loss of axonal integrity and function.

Of course, axonal disease cannot be visualized on a CT scan. However, DAI frequently occurs in conjunction with small scattered parenchymal hemorrhages commonly described as "shear injuries," probably because they have been postulated to occur as tissues at different depths of the brain undergo rotation at different velocities. The interface between these regions is said to undergo shearing, resulting in the small punctuate hemorrhages. Regardless of whether this explanation is true, the presence of scattered small hemorrhages may serve as a clue that DAI may be present.

Cellular and Molecular Factors

At the cellular level, the abnormalities caused by TBI are numerous and complex. Release of glutamate and other excitatory neurotransmitters may lead to excessive neuronal depolarization and intracellular calcium influx, with activation of proteases and other processes that lead to cell death. Inadequate blood flow can cause a conversion from aerobic to anaerobic metabolism. The lactic acid that is produced lowers local tissue pH, and the consequent acidosis contributes to tissue injury and death. Trauma-induced apoptosis may promote further cell death. These and other biochemical and cellular processes take place against the backdrop of an individual patient's genetic makeup; the presence of specific alleles for various genes may make an individual more or less susceptible to the damaging effects of various pathophysiologic processes.

CLINICAL DIAGNOSIS

Clinical Examination

Ideally, the severity of TBI is determined and classified according to a patient's neurologic examination. The size and appearance of a mass lesion as seen on imaging studies are not as important as the effect that that lesion may be having on a patient's neurologic function and level of alertness.

The single most important question in the evaluation of a potentially head-injured patient is whether or not the patient obeys simple one-step commands. A simple definition of coma is that a person will not do such things as hold up two fingers or stick out his tongue when asked to do so. Failure to obey commands is widely used as an indicator of the presence of severe TBI. Other simple, but important, observations are the type of movement exhibited by the patient (localization of noxious stimuli, withdrawal, flexion, extension, etc.); whether the right and left sides are symmetrical; the type of speech; the presence or absence of eye opening; and pupillary size, reactivity to light, and bilateral symmetry.

Because the nerve fibers that mediate pupillary constriction lie on the surface of the third cranial nerve, compression of this nerve by herniating brain tissue that is being displaced by a large mass lesion may cause inactivation of the pupilloconstricting fibers. The resulting pupil appears large and unable to constrict in response to bright light. This physical finding in a comatose TBI patient suggests that an

TABLE 1: Glasgow Coma Scale

Score	Motor	Verbal	Eye Opening
6	Obeys commands	–	–
5	Localizes stimulus	Oriented	—
4	Withdraws from stimulus	Confused	Spontaneously
3	Flexes arm	Words/phrases	To voice
2	Extends arm	Sounds	To pain
1	No response	No response	Remain closed

immediate CT scan is needed to identify a large acute hematoma. However, fixed and dilated pupils may also be caused by brainstem ischemia or by direct ocular trauma.

Many scales have been developed for the assessment of consciousness or neurologic status after injury, but by far the most widely used is the Glasgow Coma Scale (GCS) (Table 1). In conjunction with such information as the status of pupillary reactivity and the tempo or rate of change of a patient's neurologic condition, the GCS is an extremely useful tool for assessing a patient's baseline condition and subsequent progress.

Serum Markers

There currently exists intense interest in identifying serum markers of brain injury. Applications could include more accurate patient assessment in prehospital or battlefield settings; a more thorough evaluation of apparently mild TBI patients in emergency departments; and serial tracking in intensive care units. Many compounds have been found to be sensitive for revealing the presence of TBI, but their specificity is poor. Given the pressing clinical need for such markers and the potential commercial gain that could result from their identification, it is possible that such testing could see widespread use in the near future.

INITIAL CLINICAL INTERVENTIONS: PREHOSPITAL AND EMERGENCY CENTER CARE

The basic principles of TBI care, which have remained unchanged for decades, are maintenance of normal homeostasis and prevention and prompt treatment of secondary insults. The acutely traumatized brain is much more vulnerable than the uninjured brain to even mild deviations from normal, such as transient episodes of hypotension or hypoxia. Some evidence suggests that events like febrile episodes, seizures, and hyperglycemia may also worsen outcome. Brief insults are usually tolerated well by the normal brain, but they may have a profound detrimental effect on the injured brain.

The basics of TBI care revolve around the ABCs: airway, breathing, and circulation. Although some of the specifics of management of these parameters differ between the prehospital setting and the intensive care unit (ICU), it is important to view management of the ABCs as a continuum with goals that remain constant throughout the acute phase of a patient's illness. Because of this continuity, the following discussion of the ABCs begins with the prehospital setting, but then moves into ICU considerations as well.

Airway

In terms of control of the airway, prehospital endotracheal intubation should be considered in patients with severe TBI or with other problems that may impair movement of air or protection of the airway from aspiration. Recent reports in the trauma literature associate worse outcomes with prehospital intubation of severe TBI patients. One possible explanation of these findings may be the difficulty of performing successful endotracheal intubation in the prehospital setting, especially if prehospital providers do so only infrequently. Patients may suffer severe hypoxia while an inexperienced rescuer makes repeated attempts to place an endotracheal tube successfully. Another explanation may be overly zealous ventilation (with decrease in $Paco_2$ to dangerously low levels) after intubation.

Breathing

In terms of breathing, standard recommendations advocate the lowest Fio_2 capable of maintaining adequate oxygenation. Although the minimum acceptable Pao_2 based on the oxygen-hemoglobin dissociation curve is 60 mm Hg, most practitioners target a minimum of 80 to 100 mm Hg in TBI patients in order to create a bit of a cushion.

Hyperventilation is no longer recommended as a prophylactic measure to prevent intracranial hypertension. Hyperventilation is known to cause constriction of the cerebral vasculature, and the resultant decrease in cerebral blood volume can acutely lower ICP. However, the constriction of cerebral arteries may cause CBF to drop to critical levels. Also, within 24 hours of initiation of hyperventilation, the cerebral arteries probably dilate back to their original diameter. Subsequent attempts to allow the $Paco_2$ to increase can cause the arteries to dilate beyond their original baseline, possibly raising ICP.

Most clinicians aim for the low-normal range of $Paco_2$, targeting a value of approximately 35 to 40 mm Hg. Keeping the $Paco_2$ toward the lower end of the normal range may optimize the ability of the cerebral vasculature to autoregulate.

Hyperventilation should be reserved for acute deterioration accompanied by signs of a mass lesion, such as raised ICP with asymmetrical pupils or asymmetrical motor examination. In such cases, the assumption is that the patient will need emergency surgery to evacuate the lesion. Hyperventilation and other measures, like administration of mannitol, are intended only to buy a few minutes to obtain an emergency CT scan prior to going to surgery. If the scan reveals that no surgical lesion is present, attempts should be made to manage the elevated ICP without hyperventilation by using some of the steps explained in the next chapter (Traumatic Brain Injury: Imaging, Operative and Nonoperative Care, and Complications).

Circulation

The "C" in ABCs stands for circulation. For brain-injured patients, this can be thought of as management of blood pressure and intravenous fluids.

In years past, common practice was to dehydrate patients "to prevent the brain from swelling." In the 1990s, the pendulum swung the other way as TBI patients were aggressively managed with intravenous fluids and pressors in order to artificially elevate their blood pressure. However, subsequent studies showed that patients treated with aggressive elevation of blood pressure through fluids and pressors did not show improved neurologic outcome and, in fact, had a fivefold higher likelihood of developing acute respiratory distress syndrome.

Current management strategies call for maintenance of a normal blood pressure, with aggressive elevation of blood pressure reserved for those patients in whom clinical or physiologic monitoring

suggests a need for such therapy, for example, to treat cerebral hypoxia or to reverse neurologic deterioration.

Direct monitoring of brain tissue oxygen tension ($Pbto_2$) is now possible via small intraparenchymal catheters. Although some clinicians treat low $Pbto_2$ by increasing the Fio_2, we prefer to treat low brain tissue Po_2 initially by raising blood pressure in order to optimize perfusion of the affected tissue. Ischemic thresholds of brain tissue are difficult to identify with precision. A $Pbto_2$ below 15 to 20 mm Hg is generally regarded as low, whereas values below 8 to 10 mm Hg may suggest that further evaluation and intervention might be appropriate.

IMAGING MODALITIES: WHAT, WHEN, AND WHY?

Computed Tomography Scanning

After initial assessment and stabilization of a TBI patient, the next order of business is the procurement of imaging studies. The most important radiologic study for the evaluation of acute TBI is a CT scan. This imaging modality is excellent for revealing acute hemorrhage, cerebral edema, and mass effect, which are the features of greatest interest during the initial assessment. Bone settings can also detect calvarial and skull base fractures. Another advantage is that CT scanning is a quick procedure that is widely available, at least in most developed countries. To overcome difficulties posed by prehospital intubation and the frequent use of sedation in these patients (which complicate accurate clinical assessment), Marshall devised a TBI classification scheme based on CT scan findings (Table 2).

Magnetic Resonance Imaging

Historically, magnetic resonance imaging (MRI) has limited application in the acute setting for several reasons. Obtaining a study requires a fair amount of time; access to the patient is limited during the study;

TABLE 2: Marshall Computed Tomography Classification Scheme

Category	Definition
Diffuse injury I (no visible disease)	No intracranial injury visible on computed tomography scan
Diffuse injury II	Cisterns are present with midline shift 0–5 mm and/or: lesion densities present no high- or mixed-density lesion >25 cm³
Diffuse injury III (swelling)	Cisterns compressed or absent with midline shift 0–5 mm; no high- or mixed-density lesion >25 cm³
Diffuse injury IV (shift)	Midline shift >5 mm, no high- or mixed-density lesion >25 cm³
Evacuated mass lesion	Any lesion surgically evacuated
Nonevacuated mass lesion	High- or mixed-density lesion >25 cm³, not surgically evacuated

and ferromagnetic monitoring and resuscitative equipment must be removed before the patient can enter the magnet. After a patient has stabilized, however, MRI may reveal the presence of subtle parenchymal injuries, which may shed light on the unexplained failure of some patients to improve. There may also be a role for MRI in evaluating mild TBI patients, especially when their symptoms seem disproportionately severe in comparison to the appearance of their CT scans.

Angiography

Angiography continues to have an ambiguous role in the initial evaluation of the brain-injured patient. Prior to the development of CT scanning in the 1970s, neurosurgeons were limited to pneumoencephalography or angiography for detecting midline shift or other types of mass effect. Skull radiography could also indicate displacement of the calcified pineal gland.

Since the advent of CT scanning, cerebral angiography has usually been reserved for cases in which there exists a high index of suspicion for intracranial vascular injury, such as pseudoaneurysm formation or arterial dissection. However, the optimal treatment of any such findings is unclear. Most acutely brain-injured patients should not receive heparin or warfarin, yet interventional radiologic procedures often require that the patient be anticoagulated. Similarly, critically low CBF is present in a sizeable percentage of severe TBI patients. The wisdom of occluding a major artery in a patient who may already be ischemic is questionable.

Continuing advances in CT angiography and MR angiography have made these technologies comparable to conventional angiography for detecting vascular injury in many cases. Thus, angiography will probably continue its historical trend of declining use in the acute assessment of TBI patients.

INJURY GRADING

Glasgow Coma Scale

Many different schemes have been proposed for the grading and classification of brain injury. As discussed earlier, the best-known is the GCS. Introduction of this scale reinforced the need for an accurate neurologic examination as part of the assessment and classification of brain-injured patients. This point is as fundamental today as when the GCS was initially described. Because this scale made possible a more objective assessment of patients, interobserver and intercenter variability could be reduced, thus enabling the creation of multicenter and even multinational studies.

However, accurate determination of the GCS score is often difficult in patients who are intoxicated with alcohol or other drugs or in patients with injuries that cause such extensive periorbital edema that the eyes are swollen shut, making assessment of eye opening impossible. Other factors that complicate the determination of the GCS score reflect changes in prehospital and emergency department practices since the initial description of the GCS over a generation ago. Presently, many patients are endotracheally intubated in the prehospital setting, and paralytics and sedatives are often administered before an accurate and thorough neurologic assessment is performed. These problems have led to the creation of other assessment tools, such as those based on CT findings. Another way of getting around the problem of an inaccurate neurologic examination might be the use of serum markers to identify trauma patients who are likely to have serious central nervous system injury, analogous to the manner in which serum levels of cardiac enzymes are used in the diagnosis of acute myocardial injury. This is an area of rapidly growing interest.

Common practice classifies brain injury as mild, moderate, or severe based on the GCS score. Mild TBI is traditionally equated with

a GCS score of 13 to 15, whereas moderate TBI refers to a GCS score of 9 to 12. Some authorities, however, consider a score of 13 to be more indicative of moderate injury. Severe TBI refers to patients with a GCS score of 8 or less.

It is worth emphasizing that this widely used scheme of classifying TBI is based on functional, not anatomic, criteria. This approach contrasts with that used in much of the general trauma literature, in which anatomic criteria are used as the primary means of classifying injuries.

Marshall Computed Tomography Scale

Marshall and colleagues developed a CT-based classification scheme using data from the Traumatic Coma Data Bank (see Table 2). This system, commonly referred to as the Marshall scale or the TCDB scale, classifies CT scans according to such factors as midline shift and compression of cerebrospinal fluid cisterns. Although this scale is useful in certain circumstances, it should not be considered a substitute for an accurate neurologic examination.

Abbreviated Injury Scale

The Abbreviated Injury Scale (Table 3) for the head assigns a score of 1 for minor scalp injuries such as abrasions, contusions, and lacerations. Longer and deeper lacerations receive a score of 2, whereas scalp injuries accompanied by significant blood loss or characterized by total scalp loss are scored as 3. Cranial nerve injuries are coded as 2.

TABLE 3: Abbreviated Injury Scale for Head Injury

AIS Score	Injury Severity	Head Injury Examples
1	Minor	Minor scalp injuries
2	Moderate	More severe scalp injuries Cranial nerve injuries Simple calvarial fractures LOC <1 hour Post-traumatic amnesia
3	Serious	Worst scalp injuries Cerebral vascular injuries Skull base fractures Comminuted calvarial fractures Small parenchymal contusions Traumatic SAH LOC 1–6 hours
4	Severe	Worse cerebral vascular injuries Worst skull fractures Hematomas LOC 6–24 hours
5	Critical	Worst cerebral vascular injuries Larger hematomas LOC >24 hours
6	Lethal	Massive destruction Crush injuries

AIS, Abbreviated Injury Scale; LOC, loss of consciousness; SAH, subarachnoid hemorrhage.

Injuries to major cerebral vessels are generally coded as 3 or 4 for thrombosis or traumatic aneurysm formation, or as 4 or 5 for laceration.

Scores for fractures of the skull and skull base range from 2 for simple fractures of the vault, to 3 for skull base fractures or comminuted vault fractures, to 4 for the most complex open fractures with exposed brain tissue or for significantly depressed closed fractures.

Scoring for brain parenchymal injuries ranges from 3 to 5. Small single or multiple contusions receive a score of 3, as does SAH, edema, or infarction directly related to trauma. Hematomas are scored as 4 or 5, depending upon their size.

Massive destruction or crush injuries are scored as a 6.

The duration of LOC and presence of associated neurologic deficits may be used to score injury severity if such scores exceed those based on anatomic injuries. Such scores range from 2 to 5.

The American Association for the Surgery of Trauma organ injury scale does not address brain injuries.

Other Classification Schemes

The limitations of the GCS affect clinical research trials as well as patient care. The major agencies of the U.S. government that fund clinical TBI trials have convened workshops of clinical trialists to begin rethinking the ways in which TBI has been classified, especially to facilitate the development of treatments targeted at specific aspects of TBI pathophysiology.

Mild and Moderate Traumatic Brain Injury

This chapter and the following one focus on patients with severe TBI. Those with moderate brain injury, who are commonly described as patients with a GCS score of 9 to 12, often have significant intracranial damage and yet still obey commands. Their management is similar to that of severe TBI patients in the sense that careful observation and prevention of secondary insults are of paramount importance.

However, intracranial monitors may not be needed in many of these patients, and they may not require the same intensity of care for the same amount of time as severe TBI patients.

The vast majority of patients seeking medical attention after a brain injury have mild TBI. They are often diagnosed as having had a concussion. Importantly, the diagnosis of mild TBI (or concussion) does not require that a patient lose consciousness. Some data indicate that the majority of patients with mild TBI never lose consciousness, but they may complain of a variety of symptoms such as headache, post-traumatic amnesia, difficulty concentrating, ringing in the ears, and unsteadiness of gait.

Unlike the situation with severe TBI, the major concern with mild TBI is not whether a patient will live or die or whether a patient will become vegetative or severely disabled. Almost all these patients survive. Instead, the major morbidity relates to disturbances of memory, cognition, attention, emotional stability, and similar areas. The lack of "hard" evidence of neurologic impairment leads many physicians to downplay the significance of these symptoms. However, these patients often go on to lose their jobs, drop out of school, divorce their spouses, or go through other major upheavals in their lives. Eventually, most of them recover, but such a process may take months. Reassurance of the patient and family may be all that is needed, and in fact, may be all that can be offered. Counseling and formal testing may be appropriate if objective documentation of injury is needed or if a physician suspects malingering or symptom magnification for secondary gain.

CONCLUSIONS AND ALGORITHM

Figure 3 summarizes the priorities in assessment and initial management of TBI patients. Accurate neurologic assessment and careful attention to the ABCs are of paramount importance. These goals continue to be emphasized while patients are transported to a hospital, are resuscitated, and are taken to a CT scanner.

For the chapter's Suggested Readings list, please visit the book at www.ExpertConsult.inkling.com.

FIGURE 3 Basic initial assessment and management of traumatic brain injury (TBI) patients. ABCs, Airway, breathing, and circulation; CT, computed tomography.

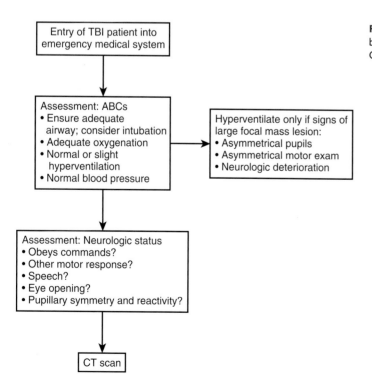

TRAUMATIC BRAIN INJURY: IMAGING, OPERATIVE AND NONOPERATIVE CARE, AND COMPLICATIONS

Aileen Ebadat and Alex B. Valadka

The previous chapter described pathophysiology and initial management of traumatic brain injury (TBI) patients. This chapter provides an overview of selected aspects of surgical management, nonoperative care, complications, and outcome.

SURGICAL MANAGEMENT

The strength and rigidity of the skull, its covering by the highly vascular scalp, and the need to do something with the overlying hair all combine to make it harder to get to the brain than to most other organs. Consequently, the surgeon must prepare carefully prior to any craniotomy, especially in an emergency. Disaster can occur if the original positioning and exposure prove to be inadequate to deal with the known injury, much less with the unexpected contingencies that seem to arise all too frequently during emergency craniotomies. If additional exposure should suddenly become necessary in the middle of a case, the price that might need to be paid to gain this additional access may include considerable blood loss, brain swelling, or other complications.

Positioning

Most traumatic lesions can be accessed by positioning the patient supine, with the head turned to the contralateral side (i.e., to the right for a left-sided craniotomy). A large roll of sheets or other support placed parasagittally under the ipsilateral shoulder blade and upper chest can also facilitate rotation of the head. Rigid fixation of the head via pins is not needed for most trauma craniotomies. Instead, the hospital's usual doughnuts, foam head holders, or other devices are commonly used. In most trauma cases, the goal is to have the midline of the head more or less parallel to the floor.

In patients with rigid cervical collars, this goal may be achieved by varying the positioning described previously so that the patient is placed in the lateral position. Putting a patient into such a position requires more work from all members of the surgical team, but an experienced crew should be able to secure a patient in this position quickly.

The seemingly infinite variety of anatomic lesions that may be found in head-injured patients makes it necessary for the surgeon to know how to gain access to all parts of the brain and skull. Treatment of occipital, posterior temporal and parietal, and posterior fossa trauma may require that the patient be positioned prone. Injuries to the anterior midline skull base, such as depressed frontal sinus fractures, are usually operated on with the head neutral and the neck slightly extended. A detailed discussion of the variety of positionings and approaches that are used in neurosurgery is beyond the scope of this book. The essential message is that flexibility and familiarity with different surgical approaches are key parts of the management of head and brain injury.

Bone Flap

Another general principle of surgery for TBI is to create a large bone flap. This principle is especially true for an acute subdural hematoma (SDH). The blood in these lesions often layers out over much of the cerebral hemisphere. Trying to remove clot from far under the edges of a small bony opening is often frustrating for the surgeon and may be dangerous for the patient. Furthermore, the intradural bleeding that often accompanies SDHs may arise almost anywhere: from draining veins that enter the superior sagittal sinus near the midline, from the floor of the anterior or middle cranial fossa, from inferior or medial to the frontal pole, or from the transverse sinus, to name just a few common areas. A large bone flap is the best way to ensure that as many potential bleeding sites as possible have been made accessible.

Most trauma incisions begin at the posterior root of the zygoma, just anterior to the tragus. They then curve posteriorly, above and behind the ear. In trauma cases, this posterior extension should extend as far as possible. The incision then curves medially and superiorly. It is wise to take the skin incision to the midline to permit access to the superior sagittal sinus in the event that troublesome bleeding arises from the midline.

Although the scalp flap extends near or to the midline, it is wise to keep the medial edge of the bone flap several centimeters off the midline. Attempts to remove bone on or near the midline may produce brisk epidural bleeding from arachnoid granulations or severe dural bleeding from dural venous lakes. Such bleeding is usually controllable with gentle tamponade, but these maneuvers delay and distract attention from the goal of rapid evacuation of the SDH. Similarly, recurrence of this bleeding may go unnoticed while the surgeon is preoccupied with evacuation of the clot. If brisk bleeding originates from underneath the medial edge of the craniotomy opening, the best treatment may be tamponade with absorbable hemostatic agents and placement of numerous closely spaced dural tack-up sutures.

The size of the opening needed to evacuate an epidural hematoma (EDH) may often be smaller than that for an SDH because the tight adherence of the dura to the overlying skull often constrains the spread of these lesions. For this reason, EDHs often appear to be "short and fat" on computed tomography (CT) scans, but SDHs often spread out and appear to be "long and thin" because of the absence of barriers to their spread over the surface of the hemisphere. Care must still be taken, however, not to make the bony opening too small when attempting evacuation of an EDH.

Intraparenchymal lesions such as hematomas and contusions are often amenable to evacuation via smaller openings. In fact, even large parenchymal lesions can be evacuated through very small openings in the cerebral cortex. Careful retraction of the cortical edges is made easier because of the cavity that is left behind as the clot is removed.

Brain Swelling

Rapid brain swelling is a major concern after evacuation of an acute SDH. The speed with which this phenomenon occurs suggests that defective autoregulation may play an important role. A popular current practice is simply to leave the native dura open (but loosely cover the brain with a dural graft) and not replace the bone flap. Some neurosurgeons strongly advocate this practice, and it does seem to be effective in lowering intracranial pressure (ICP); still, its effects on outcome remain unclear. Publications going back several decades report that a persistent vegetative state was commonly seen in survivors. Recent data suggest that decompression for diffuse brain swelling does not improve outcome and may even be deleterious. Other concerns are that decompressive craniectomies may be performed too frequently or for poor or inadequate indications. Often, the bony opening that is left behind is too small, causing swollen brain to strangulate and die, with the resulting edema tracking back intracranially and further aggravating intracranial hypertension.

Although the surgeon sometimes has no choice but to leave the bone flap off, a better strategy is to undertake several steps to minimize the likelihood of being placed in such a situation. Instead of a wide dural opening, slits may be made in the dura in the four different quadrants of the exposure, and the clot carefully aspirated through these slits. Slow, controlled evacuation of the hematoma may prevent sudden massive brain swelling more than immediate removal of the entire clot. If it appears that most of the hematoma has been removed, and no evidence of ongoing intradural bleeding exists, the slits can be closed quickly if the brain begins to swell. However, if continued intradural bleeding persists, a wider dural opening must be created by connecting two or more of the slits in order to identify and control the source of the bleeding. Such a maneuver must be performed as rapidly as possible so that dural closure can be achieved before the brain begins to swell.

Implicit in the preceding discussion is the need to close the dura before brain swelling makes this impossible. As mentioned previously, this goal may seem antiquated in light of the current popularity of simply not replacing the bone flap. However, the authors have rarely encountered problems using this strategy, even when a retractor had to be used to gently depress swelling brain while the dural edges were forcibly pulled together with forceps so that they could be sutured together. This experience is consistent with laboratory data suggesting that decompressive craniectomy may actually promote cerebral edema.

Epidural Hematomas

Surgery for EDHs is usually more straightforward. Occasionally, the surgeon may feel the need to make a small opening in the dura to verify that no subdural blood is present. It is common to see a thin layer of subdural blood when this maneuver is carried out, but this blood can usually be irrigated away without too much difficulty. Another common problem in the epidural space is persistent bleeding, either from dural veins or dural venous sinuses or from underneath the bony edges of the craniotomy. If epidural venous bleeding cannot be stopped with cautery, gentle pressure with any of the various commercially available neurosurgical hemostatic agents is usually effective. In most cases, leaving these bioabsorbable materials in place is better than attempting to remove them. Of note, bleeding from the middle meningeal artery is not encountered as frequently as some books suggest, but when seen, it is usually possible to cauterize the bleeding artery directly.

Intraparenchymal Lesions

Evacuation of intraparenchymal hematomas and contusions can often be performed via a small corticectomy. Fortunately, as soon as one of these lesions is evacuated, the brain becomes much more relaxed. The main difficulties in these cases are ensuring complete lesion evacuation and verifying hemostasis. These goals may be difficult if the hematoma cavity is large. Occasionally, for large contusions or hematomas, a second corticectomy may facilitate lesion evacuation and hemostasis of parts of the lesion that would be inaccessible via the original cortical opening.

Intracranial Pressure Monitoring

The question of whether these patients require postoperative ICP monitoring is often difficult to answer. In general, if a patient is not expected to "wake up" after surgery (i.e., not expected to obey commands or to have a Glasgow Coma Scale [GCS] score > 8), insertion of a monitor should be strongly considered. Ventriculostomies are preferred because they permit therapeutic drainage of

cerebrospinal fluid (CSF) in the event that ICP becomes elevated. Insertion of these devices during the initial craniotomy is usually possible, but some surgeons prefer to wait until the craniotomy has been closed and then insert the ventriculostomy in the operating room or in the intensive care unit (ICU). If the ventricles cannot be cannulated, a parenchymal monitor may be used.

Coagulopathy

If patients appear to be coagulopathic, the blood bank should be given early notification that platelets and fresh frozen plasma are urgently needed in the operating room. Severe diffuse oozing may require the use of recombinant factor VIIa. Laboratory studies can be used during surgery to track the effects of these interventions on coagulation studies and platelet counts, but an easier way to gauge the status of hemostasis is simply to check whether blood that trickles down into the dependent parts of the surgical field is able to form a solid clot.

Summary

In summary, the surgeon can often avoid trouble by thinking ahead about possible setbacks and their avoidance. Planning the exposure to permit adequate clot evacuation is crucial. Elevating the head of the bed slightly may minimize venous bleeding. Major bleeding should be anticipated if depressed fractures overlying major dural venous sinuses are elevated. A controlled dural opening during evacuation of an acute SDH may be helpful for minimizing massive brain swelling.

NONOPERATIVE MANAGEMENT

Location of Care

The complexity of TBI management and the tremendous impact of TBI on long-term outcome suggest that brain-injured patients should initially be admitted to an ICU with physicians and nurses experienced in the care of TBI patients. This specialized experience in TBI may be more important than expertise only in general trauma or critical care. During the first few days after injury, TBI patients may require blood pressure monitoring, frequent checking of hemoglobin concentrations, complex ventilator management, and other interventions that are standard for patients without a brain injury, but in addition to these basic measures, careful assessment and management of the brain injury and integration of general management practices with brain-specific therapies must also occur. Although many general ICUs or trauma ICUs are not comfortable with the nuances of TBI management, most neurosurgical ICUs are quite capable of managing patients with major systemic illnesses.

If a TBI patient improves or remains neurologically stable for a few days, he or she can then be transferred to another ICU, to an intermediate care unit, or to a regular care ward. This approach differs from the commonly advocated view that patients should initially be admitted to a standard trauma unit instead of to a neurosurgical ICU. In many standard surgical ICUs, however, management is based on a patient's systemic parameters, which may not necessarily be optimal for the brain injury. In the real world, these discrepancies are handled differently at each institution according to whatever arrangements have been made among the different parties who care for these patients.

Secondary Insults

The prehospital emphasis on prevention and early treatment of secondary cerebral insults continues during the ICU management of these patients and, in fact, forms the foundation of their management. Special attention should be paid to basic metabolic and physiologic parameters, including blood pressure, oxygenation, hemoglobin concentration, and serum sodium concentration. Surgery for associated injuries that do not absolutely require immediate treatment, such as facial fractures, hand or foot injuries, and even most long-bone fractures, is best deferred while the injured brain is still vulnerable to possible intraoperative metabolic disturbances.

Ventilator Weaning and Tracheostomy

Attempts at weaning and eventual extubation are dictated by the patient's clinical course. Many intensivists advocate very early tracheostomy in these patients. However, if patients appear to be recovering consciousness, there is usually little harm in gradually decreasing the intermittent mandatory ventilation rate or even adding trials of continuous positive airway pressure. In most TBI patients, the indication for continued intubation is the brain injury, not a primary pulmonary problem. Thus, the decision to extubate is based primarily on improvement in mental status. Even if a patient is clearly not going to wake up soon, continued intubation may be necessary because of the potential risk of aggravating intracranial hypertension if a tracheostomy is performed while the patient is still having frequent or continual elevations of ICP.

Sedation

In many ICUs, there exists an automatic reflex among practitioners to sedate patients heavily and to administer pharmacologic paralytics, often via simultaneous intravenous infusions of multiple drugs. Few people seem to ask why the patient receives such extensive medication. If a TBI patient's ICP is not elevated and if he or she is not thrashing about, there is probably little need for heavy sedation beyond reasonable doses of analgesics on an as-needed basis. This philosophy permits accurate assessment of neurologic status and also facilitates more rapid weaning from the ventilator. Partly for this reason, we are less eager than some other institutions to perform immediate tracheostomies on these patients, preferring instead to allow them the opportunity to recover to the point of extubation if they demonstrate early progress toward that goal.

Cerebral Monitoring

Monitoring of cerebral physiologic function can provide important information that may be used to titrate treatment toward the goal of preventing and promptly treating secondary insults.

ICP monitoring has been widely available for decades. Whenever possible, a ventriculostomy catheter is preferred because of its relatively low cost, its ability to act as a therapeutic tool by draining CSF, and the ability to re-zero the monitor as needed. The development of antibiotic-impregnated catheters seems to have lowered the risk of ventriculostomy infection.

Additional cerebral monitoring devices are commercially available. Jugular venous oxygen saturation may be tracked continuously via oximetric catheters inserted in a retrograde manner up the jugular vein and into the jugular bulb. A decrease in the oxygen saturation of the blood in the jugular bulb signals an increase in cerebral oxygen extraction because of ischemia or other pathologic processes.

Intraparenchymal monitors of the oxygen tension of the brain ($Pbto_2$) have generated considerable interest because of the usually good relationship between $Pbto_2$ and cerebral blood flow (CBF). Importantly, interpretation of these data requires knowledge of whether the catheter is measuring normal brain or whether it lies near contused or injured brain. Such positioning dictates whether the catheter is acting as a monitor of global metabolism or a gauge of the regional metabolism of the brain around the probe. Large areas with significantly abnormal regional metabolism may get lost in the background and not be detected if only a global monitor is used. Our preference has been to use local monitors like $Pbto_2$ catheters to target brain tissue around contused or otherwise injured areas.

Other monitors provide methods of tracking CBF, performing cerebral microdialysis, following brain electroencephalographic activity, and measuring other physiologic parameters. These can all provide valuable information that supplements careful neurologic assessments and CT scans. It will be difficult to conduct prospective, randomized, controlled trials to demonstrate the utility—or lack thereof—of these devices. There is growing interest in creation of a large international prospectively created database, including collection of neuropsychological and other prespecified outcome measures, to enable performance of comparative effectiveness studies. Such analyses could provide important data about the value of various interventions, as well as guiding judicious use of monitoring techniques in order to facilitate targeted patient management.

Nutrition

Nutrition should be started as soon as possible, usually via the enteral route. If feedings via this route cannot be initiated despite several days of trying, consideration should be given to parenteral nutrition. The increasing attention being paid to the association between poor outcomes and elevated glucose levels suggests that protocols for frequent monitoring and, if needed, treatment of serum glucose concentration should be considered.

Fluids and Electrolytes

Other basic principles include maintenance of a normal intravascular volume to avoid either dehydration or fluid overload. We aim for a serum sodium level in the normal range and do not deliberately drive the sodium to supranormal levels. However, we have become more concerned that hyponatremia may contribute to cerebral edema and increased ICP. Thus, we have become more liberal about treating serum sodium values (in mEq/L) in the 120s or even low 130s with hypertonic saline to establish a more desirable osmotic gradient between the brain and the vasculature.

Physical, Occupational, and Speech Therapy

Early involvement of physical therapy and occupational therapy can be quite helpful to preserve range of motion of extremities and, later during a patient's recovery, to expedite sitting up and even ambulation. Speech therapy may also be helpful for some patients.

Fever

Hyperthermia is receiving more scrutiny as a contributor to adverse outcomes in patients with neurologic injuries. Various cooling devices might be considered in patients who remain febrile despite antipyretics, external cooling, and treatment of known sources of fever.

Deep Venous Thrombosis

Prevention of deep venous thrombosis (DVT) is important in comatose patients who may be bedridden for a prolonged period. Application of sequential compression devices immediately upon patient arrival in the ICU has been effective in our unit. We have not generally used pharmacologic prophylaxis immediately after injury for fear of aggravating potential coagulopathy and possibly contributing to delayed or recurrent intracranial hemorrhage. Our usual policy is to begin prophylaxis with low-molecular-weight heparin (LMWH) 72 hours after injury. Occasionally, however, we have used shorter intervals in patients who seemed to be at especially high risk. We have also used LMWH to treat DVT when it occurs. We do not routinely place prophylactic inferior vena cava (IVC) filters. Instead, we have generally reserved IVC filters in TBI patients for cases of documented DVT. We are more aggressive with patients who are paralyzed as a result of a spinal cord injury.

Transfusion Thresholds

Transfusion thresholds continue to be a controversial area. Historically, neurosurgeons have advocated that hemoglobin levels be maintained at approximately 10 mg/dL in patients with TBI or aneurysmal subarachnoid hemorrhage. Although the O_2-carrying capacity of blood is decreased at this subnormal value, the nonlinear relationship between O_2-carrying capacity and viscosity causes the viscosity to be reduced much more than the O_2-carrying capacity at this hemoglobin level. Thus, the improvement in flow from the lower viscosity was felt to more than offset the reduction in O_2-carrying capacity. Several studies, however, have demonstrated that blood transfusion increases the risk of fatality and that patients fare better with a "permissive" transfusion strategy of not administering blood until the hemoglobin decreases as low as 7 mg/dL. On the other hand, some data suggest that patients with myocardial ischemia do better when hemoglobin is maintained at 10 mg/dL rather than 7 mg/dL. Debate rages about whether these findings apply to patients with TBI, stroke, and other neurologic diseases. At the present time, we favor the traditional approach of targeting a hemoglobin of approximately 10 mg/dL during the first few days after severe brain injury.

Treatment of Intracranial Hypertension

Many algorithms exist for the treatment of elevated ICP (Fig. 1). These generally begin with safe, noninvasive interventions. If ICP continues to be elevated, progressively more aggressive treatments are applied. The variety of the algorithms that are available reflects the differences with which various centers embrace the individual treatments that make up those algorithms. Of note, use of steroids to treat TBI is not recommended.

Computed Tomography Scanning

Repeat CT scanning should be considered if there is any suspicion that elevated ICP readings may be caused by a delayed or recurrent hematoma, by hydrocephalus or ventriculostomy malfunction, or by a large infarction (Fig. 2).

Sedation and Paralysis

Sedation and analgesics may help to lower ICP, supplemented if needed by neuromuscular blockade.

Cerebrospinal Fluid Drainage

Persistently elevated ICP may respond to CSF drainage if a ventriculostomy has been inserted. The older practice of routinely changing a ventriculostomy catheter every 5 to 7 days to prevent infection does not seem to be justified by more recent studies, and some centers have reported leaving catheters in place for 2 weeks or even longer without an increase in infection rates. The subsequent development of antibiotic-coated ventriculostomy catheters seems to have had a considerable impact on lowering the incidence of ventriculostomy-related infections.

Osmotic Diuretics

Administration of mannitol is often a useful step. Mannitol has an osmotic effect that pulls fluid from the brain into the vascular

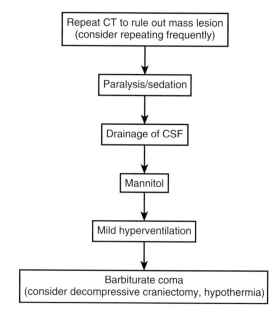

FIGURE 1 Basic algorithm for the management of elevated intracranial pressure. CSF, Cerebrospinal fluid; CT, computed tomography.

compartment. It also decreases blood viscosity, which enables cerebral arteries to constrict (and thereby lower intracerebral blood volume) without decreasing CBF because the decrease in viscosity facilitates adequate flow through the narrower artery. Hypertonic saline is receiving a great deal of interest as a possible surrogate or supplement to mannitol. Its use has become especially widespread among pediatric intensivists. Although preliminary reports are encouraging, more solid data are still pending about the optimal method of administration and about relative indications, contraindications, and adverse events.

Hyperventilation

Continued elevations of ICP may respond to judicious use of mild hyperventilation. Whenever possible, we attempt to use monitors of cerebral oxygenation to make sure that cerebral ischemia does not result from hyperventilation that is more aggressive than the brain can tolerate.

Barbiturate Coma

Persistent intracranial hypertension may respond to pentobarbital-induced coma. This treatment is effective at lowering ICP, but hypotension is a major problem. Prior to administering barbiturates, we have pressors ready for immediate infusion if the blood pressure begins to decrease.

Decompressive Craniectomy

Intracranial hypertension that persists despite initiation of the treatments listed in Figure 1 is a serious problem. Decompressive craniectomy, in which a large part of the skull is temporarily removed so that the injured brain has room to swell, is currently a popular intervention. It seems clear that a large craniectomy can lower ICP, but uncertainty remains about whether it improves patient outcomes. It is possible that many of these operations are performed prematurely or with inadequate removal of bone (Fig. 3). The complications of decompressive craniectomy can also be troubling, including development of contralateral subdural fluid collections and herniation of brain through the craniectomy defect (Fig. 4).

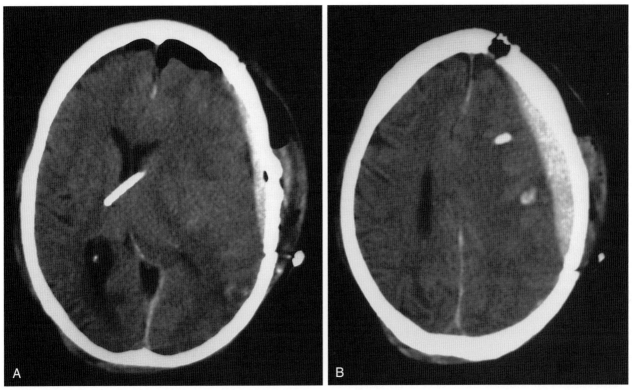

FIGURE 2 Postoperative computed tomography (CT) scans from a patient who had undergone evacuation of an acute subdural hematoma. Intracranial pressure readings remained elevated after surgery. CT scan revealed postoperative epidural hematoma, for which the patient had to be taken back to surgery.

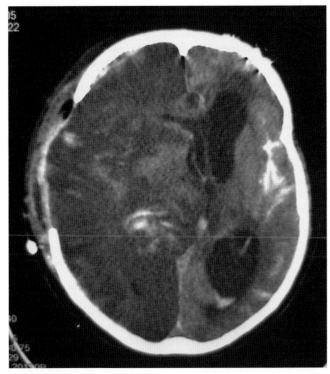

FIGURE 3 Postoperative computed tomography (CT) scan from the patient whose initial CT scan is shown in Figure 1 of the previous chapter (Traumatic Brain Injury: Pathophysiology, Clinical Diagnosis, and Prehospital and Emergency Center Care). Although the bone flap was not replaced, the size of the craniectomy was too small for adequate decompression.

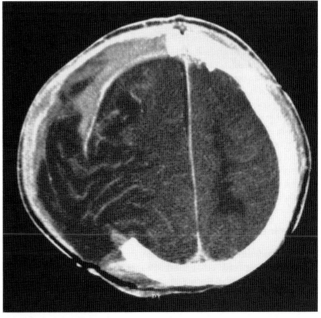

FIGURE 4 Massive herniation of necrotic brain through a craniectomy defect.

Hypothermia

Another potential treatment is hypothermia. The results of the first National Acute Brain Injury Study: Hypothermia (NABIS:H) study demonstrated lack of effect when this treatment was applied indiscriminately to all patients. The same result was seen in the second NABIS:H study, which aimed for more rapid cooling in younger patients. However, like decompressive craniectomy or any other intervention, it is likely that a specific subpopulation of TBI patients can benefit. Also, immediate initiation of a treatment in all patients is different than applying that treatment selectively to those patients with refractory elevations of ICP. The difficulty for investigators and clinicians lies in identifying those patients for whom an intervention has the most optimal benefit/risk ratio.

Individualization of Treatment

Although most algorithms recommend that patients be treated according to the same sequence of interventions, patients are in fact unique. Ideally, treatments would be applied not according to an algorithm that forces all patients into the same pathway, but rather according to a patient's particular metabolic picture. In terms of treating elevated ICP, patients with considerable amounts of cerebral edema might benefit most from osmotic diuretics; those with obstructed CSF flow may need a ventriculostomy; and those with elevated cerebral blood volume might benefit from mild hyperventilation performed early in their course.

It is highly likely that each of these ICP-lowering treatments represents the optimal intervention for a certain type of patient. Our weakness lies in our inability to identify which treatment represents the best intervention for a given patient at that particular time in a patient's course. Part of this weakness is explained by the fact that clinical trials in severe TBI have generally enrolled all severe TBI patients, regardless of their pathophysiologic picture. A treatment that may be beneficial in only certain types of patients might not be proved "effective" in a clinical trial because of the background noise from all the other patients who do not benefit. Targeted trials are more difficult to perform, but there appears to be a large need for the type of information that they can provide.

Failure of Intracranial Pressure Prophylaxis

Another important lesson that has been learned over and over again is that treatments for elevated ICP cannot be applied proactively. Doing so is not beneficial and, in fact, may cause harm in many cases. Our natural inclination as clinicians is to try to prevent ICP from rising by aggressively instituting treatments known to lower ICP; we worry that waiting until ICP rises may subject patients to the risk of harm. However, over the years, prophylactic use of hyperventilation, barbiturate coma, pharmacologic paralysis, hypothermia, or blood pressure elevation has been shown in class I or class II studies to have no benefit and, in many cases, to have significant risks. Thus, the best we can do at this time is to monitor patients carefully, to focus on the ABCs (airway, breathing, and circulation) and on prevention of secondary insults, and to intervene promptly when ICP elevation or another adverse event occurs.

Guidelines

Various guidelines for the management of brain-injured patients have enjoyed widespread circulation. Properly constructed, guidelines summarize a review of the literature with a weighting of that literature based on the quality of the design and execution of the reviewed studies. Methodologically solid studies are given a higher classification than trials that are poorly conceived or carried out. The resulting recommendations are weighted accordingly.

Not surprisingly, most clinical decisions have little in the way of randomized, prospective, controlled trials to support them. At the same time, such well-constructed trials are usually designed to answer a specific question in a specific population, and with specified outcome measures. Generalizability of findings to a larger population is often problematic.

These limitations of guidelines suggest that it is unwise to follow their recommendations blindly. Instead, a much more reasoned approach is to integrate evidence-based guidelines with a particular

physician's judgment and experience, with a particular patient's situation, and with the particular aspects of the environment in which care is being delivered. This approach should avoid unthinking adherence to guidelines while, at the same time, ensuring that they receive serious and appropriate consideration.

Failure of Clinical Trials

Millions of dollars and countless hours of effort have been poured into clinical trials to test drugs and other treatments that were designed to improve outcome after TBI. These have all failed, including hypertonic saline and starches. Analysis of these trials and recommendations for improving the design of future trials have become dynamic fields of inquiry, but such considerations are beyond the scope of this chapter. The lesson learned from these failures is that, for the time being, we must continue to focus on the basics of patient care instead of placing unjustified optimism in the development of a single pharmacologic "cure" for TBI.

MORBIDITY AND COMPLICATIONS

TBI patients are prone to the same complications as any other trauma patients. These complications include infections of the respiratory tract, urinary tract, and other body systems, as well as infections of therapeutic devices such as central and peripheral venous catheters and arterial lines. DVT, decubitus ulcers, myocardial infarction, and loss of lean body mass are just a few of the many other adverse events that may develop during a critically ill patient's prolonged stay in an ICU.

For the most part, these complications are managed just as they would be in a patient without a brain injury. A common temptation is to blame unusual developments on the brain injury by ascribing them to a "central process." However, that conclusion must be a diagnosis of exclusion that is appropriate only after a thorough workup has eliminated more likely sources.

Some complications are unique to the brain-injured patient. Elevated ICP and its management have already been discussed. Excessive and inappropriate sedation not only impairs accurate neurologic assessment of a patient, but may also unnecessarily subject a patient to the risks of sedation and of a lengthened stay in the ICU.

Prophylaxis against seizures is currently recommended for the first week after injury. After that time, anticonvulsants may be discontinued in patients who have not had a seizure. If seizures occur in a patient who is already receiving anticonvulsants, serum levels of the drug should be checked. Options include administering a bolus and increasing the maintenance dose of the drug, or adding a second agent. The optimal duration of seizure treatment in these patients remains unclear, but certainly treatment is reasonable for at least several months and probably longer.

Rebleeding or delayed intracranial bleeding can be catastrophic (see Fig. 2). Some of these events may be caused by suboptimal surgical technique in which inadequate time was spent ensuring that hemostasis was present. Often, however, patients may have a preexisting history of liver disease, and the trauma itself can predispose to a coagulopathic state. Aggressive use of fresh frozen plasma and sometimes platelets may help achieve hemostasis in patients with persistent diffuse oozing. Recent reports describing the successful use of recombinant factor VIIa in such cases have generated considerable interest.

MORTALITY

Many studies in the trauma literature report outcomes in terms of patient mortality rate at hospital discharge. This choice of outcome measure is often driven by the data contained in a hospital's trauma registry. Such an end point is an understandable choice for reports about chest and abdominal injuries, from which patients tend to

TABLE 1: Glasgow Outcome Scale

Score	Category	Description
5	Good recovery	Able to live and work independently despite minor disabilities.
4	Moderate disability	Able to live independently despite disabilities. Can use public transportation, work with assistance/supervision, etc.
3	Severe disability	Conscious but dependent upon others for self-care. Often institutionalized.
2	Persistent vegetative state	Not conscious, but may appear "awake."
1	Death	Self-explanatory.

either recover reasonably well or die soon after admission from their initial injuries or from subsequent complications.

Unfortunately, mortality rate at hospital discharge is a poor outcome measure for TBI. Survival is not considered to be an ideal outcome if a patient will remain in a persistent vegetative state. Most TBI studies have considered death, persistent vegetative state, or severe disability to be a poor outcome, whereas good recovery or moderate disability has been viewed as a good outcome. These outcome categories are based on the Glasgow Outcome Scale (GOS) (Table 1). In addition or instead of the GOS, some studies use more detailed instruments to assess outcome, especially if data are sought about less obvious measures, such as neuropsychological function.

The timing of outcome assessment is important. A patient who begins to recover quickly may have a high level of function upon discharge from the acute care hospital, which may take place just a week or two after injury. Another patient who is transferred early to a long-term care facility or to a rehabilitation hospital may have a low level of function upon leaving the acute care hospital. Yet at six months after injury, both patients may have comparable levels of function if the second patient makes gradual progress. Recovery from brain injury may continue for several years. For practical reasons, most TBI studies collect outcome data at six months.

Some recent studies report quite good outcomes after TBI, with mortality rates of approximately 20% or lower. However, many of these studies did not enroll patients with a GCS score of 3, with fixed and dilated pupils, or with other findings to suggest that they were unlikely to have a good recovery. The Traumatic Coma Data Bank, which enrolled all patients who presented to four academic centers, included 753 patients. Approximate outcomes were as follows: 27% good recovery, 16% moderate disability, 16% severe disability, 5% persistent vegetative state, and 36% fatality. Current experience suggests that these percentages remain valid today. However, these data were collected in the 1980s. Because of subsequent advances in emergency medical services systems and in neurocritical care, it might be interesting to collect such data again to see if these advances have resulted in a noticeable improvement in outcomes.

Penetrating Brain Injury

Most penetrating brain injuries are caused by gunshot wounds to the head. The vast majority of these result in death before the patient ever reaches the hospital, and most studies indicate that the majority of patients who reach the hospital alive proceed to die. On the other hand, among survivors, there is a reasonable likelihood of reaching a good outcome.

Some authors recommend that heroic measures not be instituted in patients with a GCS score of 3 or 4, and perhaps for a score of 5 as well. Others, however, report that good outcomes can occasionally be attained by patients whose initial neurologic examination was quite poor. Thus, they advocate uniformly aggressive resuscitation and stabilization of these patients. The extent of surgical intervention that is necessary varies from extensive craniotomy and reconstruction to simple débridement that can be accomplished at the bedside.

It is important to remember that the possibility of organ donation represents the only good thing that can come from many of these often-tragic cases.

CONCLUSIONS AND ALGORITHM

Figure 5 lists some basic principles and goals in the management of TBI patients. As always, the main goal remains the avoidance of secondary insults. The best monitor is a reliable neurologic examination repeated at regular intervals. Patients who do not obey commands may require monitoring of ICP and other parameters to facilitate prompt detection of adverse metabolic events. Generic algorithms

FIGURE 5 In-hospital management of traumatic brain injury (TBI) patients. ICP, Intracranial pressure; ICU, intensive care unit.

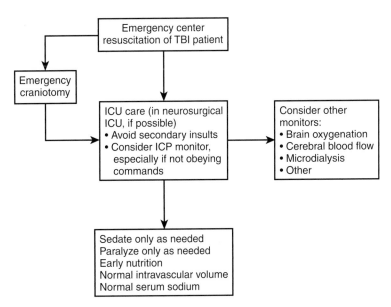

are available for the treatment of intracranial hypertension (see Fig. 1). Patient-specific interventions may supplement or replace these algorithms if monitoring data suggest the existence of particular pathophysiologic patterns in given patients.

Key Points

- Think ahead when positioning for surgery.
- Use a large flap.

- Expect brain swelling during evacuation of a large SDH; consider gradual decompression via dural slits.
- Be compulsive about hemostasis before closing.
- If in doubt, monitor ICP.
- After surgery, continue the focus on preventing secondary insults in the ICU.
- Don't sedate unnecessarily.

For the chapter's Suggested Readings list, please visit the book at www.ExpertConsult.inkling.com.

SPINE: SPINAL CORD INJURY, BLUNT AND PENETRATING, NEUROGENIC AND SPINAL SHOCK

Vartan S. Tashjian, Nestor R. Gonzalez, and Larry T. Khoo

In the acute setting, spinal cord injury (SCI) represents a complex management issue, with optimal patient care depending on the smooth execution of diagnostic and therapeutic interventions, involving several different disciplines within the medical field. These include emergency medical services (EMS) personnel, emergency department (ED) staff, radiologists, orthopedic and neurologic surgeons, intensivists, and physiotherapists. Of these, the immediate interventions employed within hours of injury often dictate the overall prognosis, and provide the patient with the best opportunity to improve long-term functional outcome. For this reason, adequate spinal immobilization, prompt diagnosis, and early consultation of the appropriate surgical service are measures that every ED physician should strive to incorporate into the evaluation of each individual trauma patient. This chapter focuses on the epidemiology, classification, and management of SCI, as well as the complications that are typically encountered in both the acute and chronic spine-injured patient. It is through a healthy understanding of the diagnostic and therapeutic guidelines and recommendations that the morbidity and mortality rates associated with SCI can continue to trend downward, as they have consistently over the past 30 years.

10-year period between 1980 and 1990, the overall proportion of SCI caused by vehicle trauma decreased from 47.2% to 38.1%. In rural centers, falls account for the second highest cause of SCI, whereas in urban centers, violence has rivaled vehicle trauma as the leading cause of SCI. Specifically, gunshot wounds (GSWs) from handguns represent approximately 90% of all SCI resulting from violence in urban centers, with an overrepresentation of minorities in these specific cases. Sports-related injuries continue to play a significant role in the overall incidence of SCI, regardless of the socioeconomic setting. In a study focusing on sports-related SCI out of the University of Alabama, Birmingham, the following sports contributed most to SCI in descending order: diving/surfing, football, winter sports, gymnastics, wrestling, and horseback riding. With the ever-increasing geriatric population, and youth violence on the rise, it is likely that falls and penetrating SCI will represent an increasing proportion of total SCI cases in years to come.

SCI represents a major economic burden on the health care industry for a variety of reasons. At the core of the problem is the fact that SCI patients not only represent an acute management challenge, with the average first year postinjury costs ranging from $123,000 to $417,000 depending on the neurologic level of injury, but they also represent a chronic financial burden when long-term direct and indirect costs are factored in. Whereas direct costs are absorbed as a direct result of the injury, including rehospitalizations, nursing home care, durable equipment, and attendant care, indirect costs are more esoteric and include loss of future wages, fringe benefits, and productivity. Although it is indeed a triumph of modern medicine and critical care that greater than 95% of SCI patients survive their initial hospitalization, with an overall lifespan now approaching that of the average citizen, these factors have only further contributed to the escalating direct and indirect costs associated with the lifelong care for SCI patients. The young average age of SCI patients at the onset of injury contributes further to the economic impact of SCI, with the estimated lifetime direct and indirect costs in excess of $2.5 million for high cervical injury patients (injury between C1 and C4).

INCIDENCE

SCI as a whole most often afflicts young men between the ages of 16 and 30. The mean age is 29.7 years, and there is an 82% male gender bias, likely reflecting the greater tendency of young males to engage in risk-related activities. Injury most often occurs in the warmer summer months, especially during the weekend, with 53% of all SCIs occurring between Friday and Sunday. With regard to specific causes of SCI, results often vary from one trauma center to the next, based largely on the socioeconomic setting of the respective institution. Vehicle trauma is common to both rural and urban health care centers as the leading cause of SCI. Prevention programs, including mandatory seatbelt laws, coupled with evolving innovations in automobile safety have served to drastically reduce the overall proportion of SCI attributable to motor vehicle accidents (MVAs) in recent years. In one

ANATOMY AND BIOMECHANICS

Spinal Anatomy

First described by Denis, the three-column model of spinal anatomy divides the spine into three distinct longitudinally oriented anatomic columns (Fig. 1). The anterior column includes the anterior longitudinal ligament (ALL), the anterior half of the vertebral body, and the intervertebral disk. The middle column consists of the posterior half of the vertebral body/intervertebral disk and posterior longitudinal ligament (PLL). Finally, the posterior column represents all bony/ligamentous elements posterior to the PLL (pedicles, lamina, spinous process, ligamentum flavum, and the interspinous ligament). By definition, SCI resulting in disruption of at least two of these three

FIGURE 1 Schematic representation of the three-column model of the spine. The anterior column consists of the anterior longitudinal ligament (ALL) and the anterior half of the vertebral body/intervertebral disk complex. The middle column is composed of the posterior half of the vertebral body/intervertebral disk complex and the posterior longitudinal ligament (PLL). The posterior column includes the intact vertebral arch and associated ligamentous structures.

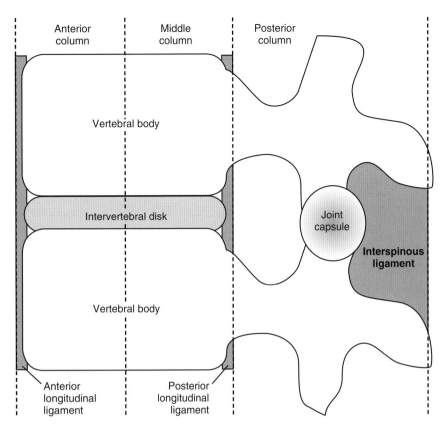

columns is considered an unstable injury. This somewhat simplistic representation of spinal anatomy serves to provide a mental framework for appreciating spine biomechanics and the potential injuries that may result from various blunt and penetrating forces to the spinal column.

Biomechanics of the Spine

Prior to delving into potential mechanisms of SCI, a healthy understanding of the biomechanics of the spine is imperative. As is frequently the case, there is often a certain degree of discrepancy between the actual level of deforming injury to the spine and the resultant radiographic findings and neurologic deficits associated with the injury. Multiple mechanisms are often simultaneously involved in producing SCI. In their simplest forms, the four types of injurious forces that may be imparted to the intact spinal column are: (1) flexion and extension (deflexion) injuries, (2) vertical compression and longitudinal distraction trauma, (3) rotational injuries, and (4) injuries with combined mechanisms.

Regarding flexion-extension injuries, the spinal cord is often damaged by compression, transverse/longitudinal shear, torsion, and rotational forces. These injuries typically involve the cervical spine, often result in disk protrusion, and may include interspinous/anterior column/posterior column ligamentous tears. When an associated disk protrusion or subluxation is present, there is a high incidence of concomitant local cord damage with mainly central cord necrosis and hemorrhage seen. In children under the age of 8, extreme hyperflexion injuries are often associated with complete cord transection, secondary to the physiologic high cervical ligamentous laxity normally found in the pediatric population.

Hyperextension (retroflexion) injuries most often result in damage to the spinal cord at the C5–C6 level, as extension is maximal at this specific level from a biomechanical perspective. These injuries

are often associated with bony dislocation, ventral fracture-dislocation, avulsion of articular processes, disruption/displacement of the intervertebral disks, and disruption of the ALL/PLL, all of which result in significant compromise of the anteroposterior diameter of the spinal canal and subsequent central cord lesions.

Compression and longitudinal distraction injuries are most often seen in the setting of vertical stress to the spinal column secondary to the falls on the head, buttocks, or neck. They also often occur with an acute increase in axial load forces during an MVA. Radiographically, these injuries are typically characterized by vertebral body flattening, end-plate fractures, and acute disk herniations. Often, there is associated retropulsion of bony fragments/disk material into the spinal canal, and varying degrees of resultant cord compression. When the mechanism of injury involves a fall, the majority of these injuries occur at the thoracolumbar junction, the most mobile segment of the spinal column. Conversely, the lower cervical spine is more often involved in cases in which a vertical axial load is imparted the spinal column.

Similar to compression/longitudinal distraction injuries, rotational injuries of the spine most often involve the thoracolumbar junction and upper lumbar spine. By definition, they may involve all parts of the vertebral body, including the pedicles, articulating facets, and ligamentous complex. These injuries often result in unilateral or bilateral dislocation or stable/unstable fracture dislocation due to interlocking of the vertebral bodies and distraction of the intervertebral disks.

MECHANISM OF INJURY

Spinal cord trauma is a broad term describing an injurious event that results in disruption of the functional or anatomic integrity of the spinal cord at a particular level(s). Although isolated lumbar spine injuries represent a significant proportion of SCIs, the majority of debilitating SCIs involve trauma to the cervical and thoracic spine. It is for this reason that the focus of this discussion will be injury of the spine from the cervical spine down to the thoracolumbar junction. With respect to the general mechanism of injury, all SCIs can be categorized in one of three subgroups: (1) direct (penetrating) SCI, (2) indirect (blunt) SCI, or (3) combined direct/indirect SCI. Depending on the underlying mechanism of injury involved, the pathogenesis of SCI can be further subclassified. Primary traumatic lesions are due to direct mechanical disruption of the cord parenchyma, typically occurring at the time of the original injury. Secondary traumatic (reactive) lesions do not develop directly from the injurious stimulus, but instead evolve as a consequence of injury-related factors, including the development of edema, ischemia, improper immobilization with secondary mechanical injury, and other biochemical disorders. Finally, common to both primary and secondary traumatic lesions is the potential for delayed neurologic sequelae, including scar formation, secondary degeneration, or regenerative phenomena.

Penetrating Spinal Cord Injury

Historically, the management of penetrating spinal cord injury (PSI) was a task relegated mainly to military physicians, as the majority of these injuries occurred in the setting of active combat. Unfortunately, the emergence of violence as a leading cause of SCI in many urban centers over the past 20 years has served to underscore the importance of emergency room physician familiarity with the acute management of these injuries in civilian practice. In general, PSI can be classified as either GSW–related or lacerating (non-GSW) PSI. Both types of PSI most commonly involve the thoracic spine, and seldom involve more than one vertebral segment. Depending on the series, 52% to 57% of all PSI results in complete neurologic deficit (no sacral motor/sensory sparing), although lacerating PSI often results in incomplete neurologic injury. Although by definition, PSI implies direct dural/parenchymal disruption, in some cases the pathogenesis of PSI resembles that of a concussive model. This has been demonstrated in numerous military-based studies in which normal-appearing dura was encountered at the time of laminectomy in many cases.

Blunt Spinal Cord Injury

In clinical practice, closed injuries of the spine are typically the most frequent type of SCI encountered. They often occur in the setting of MVA, industrial accidents, falls, and sport-related activities. In these cases, underlying injury to the spinal cord may occur in the presence/absence of concomitant soft tissue injuries, including fracture dislocation and subluxation of the spine. Biomechanics and mechanism of injury play a central role in the type and extent of SCI incurred. A thorough understanding of the potential types of mechanical forces distributed throughout the spine at the time of injury is paramount in order to be able to anticipate the evolution of secondary reactive lesions following the initial insult. In general, closed SCI can be distilled down into two broad categories. The first involves indirect cord injury arising from blunt trauma without space-occupying or penetrating lesions within the spinal canal. This type of injury is frequently observed in cases in which the mechanism of injury involves longitudinal shearing/distraction, flexion, rotation, rotation-flexion, or posteroanterior acceleration. The second type of closed SCI involves direct cord injury secondary to blunt or penetrating forces resulting in canal compromise from a variety of space-occupying lesions. These include bony/ligamentous damage, fracture dislocation, or subluxation. It is important to note that SCI is rarely confined to the anatomic point of impact. In approximately 15% of SCI cases, lesions are observed at multiple levels due to both primary and secondary traumatic changes.

SEVERITY/GRADING OF SPINAL CORD INJURIES

The neurologic level of injury (NLI) is a specific term that refers to the most caudal spinal cord level at which normal motor/sensory function persists following SCI. Although some degree of correlation often exists between the anatomic and neurologic levels of injury, this relationship is not always consistent. Several factors, including the spinal segment involved and the underlying mechanism of injury, contribute to the ultimate NLI, once secondary traumatic lesions have manifested. Overall, according to the American Spine Injury Association (ASIA) database, approximately 53% of SCI patients are tetraplegic, 46% are paraplegic, and the remaining 1% experience complete recovery by the time they are discharged from the hospital. The classification of SCI can be further categorized as complete or incomplete injury, referring to the absence/presence of sacral motor/sensory sparing, respectively. The most common neurologic category is incomplete tetraplegia (31.2%), followed by complete paraplegia (26%), complete tetraplegia (21.9%), and incomplete paraplegia (20%).

Neurologic and Functional Outcome Scales

Numerous classification schemes have been devised to describe patients with SCI over the years. Generally speaking, two types of assessment scales exist: (1) neurologic examination scales and (2) functional outcome scales. It is now generally accepted that the most meaningful description of SCI in the acute setting occurs when a neurologic assessment tool is applied in conjunction with a functional outcome assessment scheme, in order to provide perspective on the significance of any neurologic recovery on the day-to-day life of SCI patients. The first standardized neurologic assessment scale for SCI was proposed by Frankel and associates in 1969. In this scheme, a five-grade scale (A to E) is employed to discriminate SCI patients on the basis of differing degrees of motor/sensory function preserved after their injury. Frankel grade A patients are those with complete motor and sensory lesions. Grade B patients have sensory-only functions below the level of injury. Grade C patients have some degree of motor and sensory function below the level of injury, but their retained/recovered motor function is useless. Grade D patients have useful, but abnormal, motor function below the level of injury, and grade E patients are fortunate enough to experience complete motor/sensory recovery prior to discharge from the hospital. The main deficiencies involving the Frankel scale proved to be the difficulty involved in discerning grade C from grade D patients, as well as the relatively poor interobserver reliability with practical application of the scale. Despite these shortcomings, the Frankel scale provided an important classification framework from which several contemporary classification schemes have been derived. In fact, the ASIA impairment scale, largely regarded as the most studied and useful of the SCI neurologic classification schemes, is essentially a permutation of the original Frankel scale, in which objective parameters are provided to better assess the significance of retained motor function between grade C and grade D patients.

Analogous to the Frankel scale as a neurologic examination tool in SCI is the Functional Independence Measure (FIM) as a functional outcome scale. The FIM is an 18-item, 7-level scale designed to assess the severity of patient disability, estimate the burden of care, and prognosticate on medical rehabilitation and overall functional outcome. Specifically, the FIM complements neurologic assessment by providing scores for activities of grooming, bathing, eating, dressing the upper body, dressing the lower body, and toileting.

Concomitant assessment of both the neurologic and functional deficits in acute SCI is imperative in assessing the impact of injury on the patient as a whole. Additionally, linkage of these independent scales allows clinicians to specifically evaluate whether therapeutic interventions resulting in improvement of the gross neurologic assessment score also result in enhanced functional recovery for the patient. It is on the basis of functional outcome that the overall significance of various therapeutic interventions can be truly assessed. Omission of such functional outcome assessment in the National Acute Spinal Cord Injury Study (NASCIS) I and II clinical trials assessing the benefit of acute methylprednisolone (MP) therapy in acute SCI patients is often cited as a critical shortcoming of the design study, rendering the interpretation of improved neurologic outcome scores essentially impossible. A recent meta-analysis of the current literature regarding classification schemes for SCI prompted the Section on Disorders of the Spine and Peripheral Nerves of the American Association of Neurological Surgeons (AANS) and the Congress of Neurological Surgeons (CNS) to recommend the ASIA standards for neurologic and functional classification of SCI as the preferred neurologic examination for clinicians involved in the evaluation and management of acute SCI. This recommendation was based largely on the finding that the ASIA scale provided the greatest discrimination in grouping subjects with SCI into mixed-injured categories, with a relatively high degree of interobserver reliability. Similar to the other SCI classification schemes, the ASIA scale has undergone several revisions since its inception in 1984. Currently, the scale now consists of several components, including the ASIA impairment scale, the ASIA motor index score, the ASIA sensory score, and the FIM (Fig. 2).

Spinal Cord Syndromes

Several spinal cord syndromes have been described in the setting of acute SCI. Central cord syndrome typically occurs with a cervical region injury leading to greater weakness in the upper limbs than the lower limbs, associated with sacral sparing. Brown-Séquard syndrome is classically seen in the setting of penetrating SCI resulting in a hemisection lesion of the cord. It is typically associated with a relatively greater ipsilateral proprioceptive and motor loss, with contralateral loss of sensitivity to pain and temperature below the NLI. Conversely, anterior cord syndrome is associated with a lesion causing variable loss of motor function and sensitivity to pain and temperature, while posterior tracts including proprioception are spared. Conus medullaris syndrome is associated with injury to the sacral cord and lumbar nerve roots, leading to areflexic bladder, bowel, and lower extremity, while sacral segments may occasionally demonstrate preserved reflexes. Finally, cauda equine syndrome is due to injury involving the lumbosacral nerve roots within the spinal canal, resulting in areflexic bladder, bowel, and lower extremities. Similar to the various brainstem vascular syndromes (e.g., Wallenberg syndrome), spinal cord syndromes often do not present with the classic textbook constellation of signs and symptoms. However, as is the case with brainstem vascular syndromes, an understanding of the

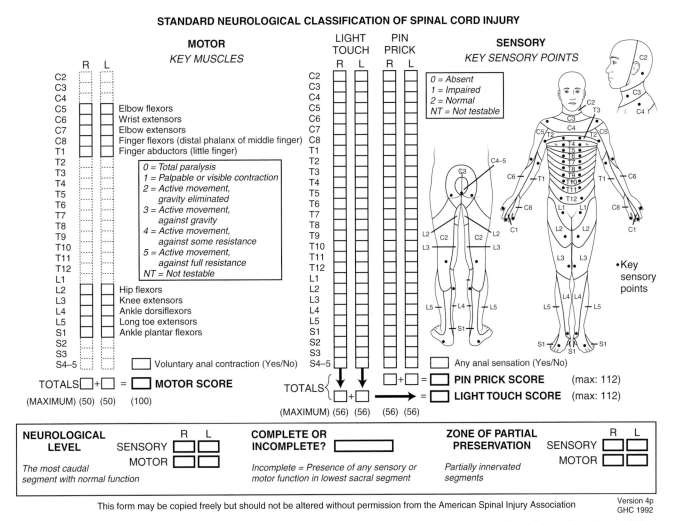

FIGURE 2 The American Spinal Injury Association (ASIA) Impairment Scale and ASIA neurologic classification scheme for spinal cord injury (SCI). The Impairment Scale is a permutation of the original Frankel Scale for SCI. The actual ASIA classification scheme includes the ASIA Impairment Scale and ASIA motor/sensory indices, as well as the Functional Independence Measure, which is not pictured. (*Courtesy of The American Spinal Cord Injury Association and The International Medical Society of Paraplegia.*)

various spinal cord syndromes serves to provide a rough neuroanatomic framework regarding the complex structural organization intrinsic to the spinal cord.

DIAGNOSIS

The organization of the central nervous system provides the physician with the opportunity to localize traumatic lesions to the spinal cord with a relatively high degree of accuracy, based on careful neurologic examination alone. However, adequate presurgical care, as well as optimal surgical planning, are both heavily dependent upon accurate imaging of the spine. For decades, plain roentgenograms of the spine have been an invaluable localization tool in SCI for several reasons. First, unlike other more sophisticated imaging modalities, the technology and resources required are not typically a limiting factor. Second, the portability of x-ray technology and the relative ease of acquisition provide the physician the opportunity to rapidly attain important anatomic information, even under the most hectic conditions. Lastly, plain films of the spine can provide a whole host of information regarding underlying SCI, including the presence/absence of fractures, subluxation/dislocation, and spinal canal patency (Fig. 3). Although soft tissue structures are not well visualized with standard x-ray technology, malalignment/angulation of the spine detected on a plain film may hint to underlying acute ligamentous or disk injury.

Since 2000, the increased availability of computed tomography (CT) in most trauma centers has served to revolutionize the diagnosis of SCI in the acute setting. In many centers, CT has supplanted the plain x-ray study as the acute imaging modality of choice for the evaluation of the spine in trauma patients, largely because of the improved accessibility of this technology. CT is superior to plain x-ray studies in many respects. It provides an outstanding view of the osseous structures, unparalleled by any other imaging modality. Additionally, the

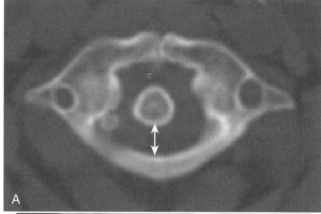

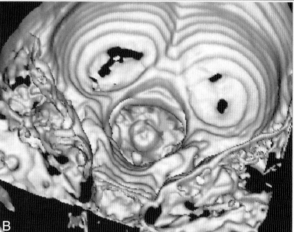

FIGURE 4 An example of post-traumatic atlantoaxial subluxation in a 35-year-old patient with Down syndrome. **A,** Note the generous atlanto-dens interval, as well as the marked reduction in the anteroposterior canal diameter *(double-headed arrow)*, appreciated more readily on the three-dimensional reconstruction (**B**).

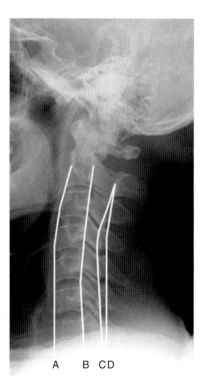

FIGURE 3 Lateral radiograph of the nonpathologic cervical spine, demonstrating normal alignment of the anterior vertebral bodies (**A**), the posterior vertebral bodies (**B**), the laminar-facet line (**C**), and the spinolaminar line (**D**).

recent advent of three-dimensional reconstruction software now provides the added benefit of viewing the relevant anatomy in the axial, coronal, and sagittal planes (Fig. 4). For these reasons, CT is generally considered to be able to detect vertebral fractures with greater sensitivity/specificity than plain x-ray study alone. Although far inferior to magnetic resonance imaging (MRI) technology with regard to the associated soft tissue anatomy, CT can provide some resolution of soft tissue, including the presence of paraspinous hematoma, which further raises the likelihood of underlying unstable ligamentous injury. Combined with myelography, CT technology can provide a view of intracanal anatomy that approaches MRI specificity in diagnosing space-occupying lesions of the spinal canal. Unfortunately, the technical burden and logistics involved with myelography on polytrauma patients has limited its applications for assessment of the acute spine-injured patient.

Since its inception as a medically applicable imaging modality by Raymond Damadian in 1971, MRI technology has continuously evolved into the diagnostic tool that it is today. This evolution in technology has been mirrored by a concomitant increase in its availability. Although inferior to CT technology in terms of resolution of bony architecture, MRI undoubtedly provides the most information regarding injury to soft tissue structures, particularly the spinal cord itself. In particular, T2 sequencing provides valuable information regarding the actual NLI, once secondary traumatic lesions, such as cord edema, have manifested (Fig. 5). Most importantly, active

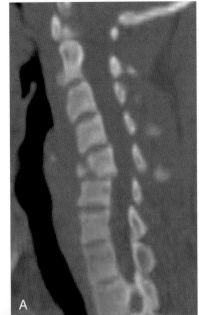

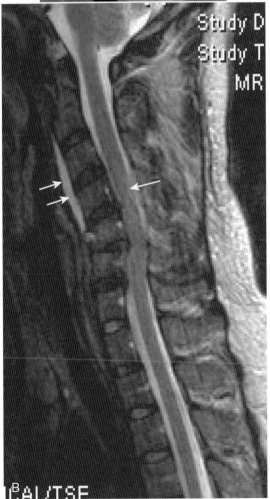

FIGURE 5 The use of both computed tomography (CT) and magnetic resonance imaging (MRI) technology to evaluate spinal cord injury can provide complementary pieces of information. Whereas CT (**A**) provides a superb view of the C5 anterior teardrop fracture and focal kyphotic deformity present in this specific example, MRI technology (**B**) provides a greater resolution of the associated spinal cord edema (*single arrow*) and prevertebral hematoma *(double arrows)*.

mechanical compression of the spinal cord and direct spinal cord parenchymal injury can be directly ascertained by MRI, thus guiding the overall time table for surgical decompression/stabilization.

MANAGEMENT OF ACUTE SPINAL CORD INJURY

The optimal management of acute SCI represents a daunting task, requiring a well-executed multidisciplinary effort in order to provide patients with the greatest chance for meaningful neurologic recovery. In the broadest sense, the management of acute SCI can be fractionated into several important phases, beginning with care rendered by EMS personnel in the field, and culminating with intensive spinal cord rehabilitation following the acute hospitalization. In between, careful orchestration of patient care between ED personnel, radiologists, surgeons, intensivists, and physiotherapists is key, as all play equally important roles in the overall prognosis and outcome of SCI patients. In general, the phases of management in SCI include: (1) prehospital care, (2) acute ED evaluation/care, (3) postacute care, and (4) posthospital care/rehabilitation. Certain aspects of care rendered during a particular phase of treatment may overlap with subsequent phases of management. For instance, pharmacotherapy initiated during acute evaluation in the ED often continues into the postacute phase of care. Additionally, certain treatment options, such as surgery, may be offered at different points of care (e.g., acute vs. subacute surgical intervention).

Prehospital Care

The main tenet of prehospital care of SCI has remained rapid and effective spinal immobilization in order to prevent further neurologic deterioration secondary to pathologic motion of the unstable spine. It is estimated that approximately 3% to 25% of SCIs occur after the initial traumatic insult, either during transport or early in the course of management. For this reason, it is recommended that complete spine immobilization utilizing a rigid cervical spine collar with supportive blocks on a rigid backboard with straps be performed on all trauma patients in which the underlying mechanism of injury suggests potential underlying SCI. The judicious use of spine immobilizers must be tempered with their rapid discontinuation once definitive evaluation and treatment have been rendered, given concern over immobilization device–associated morbidity. Specifically, elevated intracranial pressure, development of pressure sores, significant patient discomfort/distress, falls, and increased risk of aspiration have all been associated with spinal immobilization devices. Once a patient is safely extricated and immobilized, timely transport to a regional medical center capable of evaluating and treating acute SCI is paramount.

Acute Emergency Department Evaluation/ Management

Once the patient has made it to the ED, the onus then falls on the evaluating physician to expeditiously perform the patient workup. Early in the evaluation of a trauma patient, an important responsibility of the ED physician is to ensure that appropriate spine precautions have been implemented in the field, and to closely adhere to these precautions during the primary and secondary surveys. Care must be taken to adequately palpate the spinal column in its entirety, to assess for potential bony separation malalignment and associated soft tissue swelling/injury. A thorough neurologic examination and physical palpation should be performed in conjunction with the primary survey, and any overt neurologic deficit should prompt early consultation of the appropriate surgical service (neurosurgery or orthopedic surgery), if available. Next, rapid acquisition of the appropriate radiographic studies should be obtained, as well as interpreted by the staff radiologist. Any radiographic structural abnormality potentially representing acute spinal injury should further prompt surgical consultation.

If neurosurgery or orthopedic surgery services are not available at a given institution, then transfer of the patient to the closest ED with appropriate surgical coverage is warranted at the earliest sign of neurologic impairment or radiographic abnormality. Transfer should be delayed only in cases in which the patient is hemodynamically unstable, requiring additional resuscitation prior to transport.

Depending on the institution, evaluation of acute SCI lies within the realm of either neurologic or orthopedic surgery. In many regards, the most important aspect of the surgeon's involvement actually begins in the setting of the ED. It is the surgeon's responsibility to rapidly process several diverse pieces of information including the neurologic examination findings, radiographic findings, and the presence of other detracting injuries, in order to arrive at the major branch point in the early management of the spine-injured patient: acute surgical intervention versus conservative management with the potential for delayed surgical intervention. The decision to intervene surgically is typically made on a case-by-case basis, as each case represents a unique set of circumstances to consider and diagnostic/therapeutic obstacles to overcome. Generally speaking, the decision to operate in the acute setting is heavily influenced by the specific type of injury radiographically present, the patient's neurologic examination findings, and the overall stability of the patient vis-à-vis other potentially immediately life-threatening traumatic injuries. Polytrauma in the SCI patient is common, with the following injuries occurring with decreasing frequency: fractures of the trunk (17.2%), long-bone fractures (13.9%), head and facial trauma (13.8%), pneumothorax and chest injury (8.8%), and abdominal injury (8.6%). In these cases, surgery should be delayed until the patient is first adequately resuscitated, including treatment of immediately life-threatening injuries, maintenance of adequate blood pressure parameters, and the employment of cervical traction and corticosteroid therapy, if deemed appropriate.

Surgical Intervention

Regarding surgical intervention in SCI, the Section on Disorders of the Spine and Peripheral Nerves of the AANS and CNS recently undertook the herculean task of reviewing the pertinent literature in order to provide recommendations on surgical management of various types of cervical spine injury. The surgical options advanced in this section are a reflection of their recommendations, albeit in a more condensed format.

Traumatic atlanto-occipital (C1-occipital) dislocation injuries may be best treated with internal fixation and arthrodesis utilizing any variety of craniocervical fusion techniques. Although traction and external immobilization have been used to successfully treat a subset of these injuries, transient or permanent neurologic worsening, or delayed instability, has been observed more often in these cases than in cases with surgical stabilization. Occipital condyle fractures may be optimally treated with external cervical immobilization. Management of isolated fractures of the atlas (C1) is typically dictated by the specific atlas fracture present. It is recommended that all isolated atlas fractures with preservation of the transverse ligament be treated with immobilization alone. Isolated atlas fractures occurring in the context of transverse ligament disruption may be treated with either external cervical immobilization alone or with surgical fixation. The rule of Spence states that in the setting of atlas fractures, when the sum of the displacement of the lateral masses of C1 on C2 exceeds 8 mm on plain open-mouth x-ray film, the likelihood of underlying transverse ligament disruption is especially high, and may require an MRI for further assessment.

Management of fractures of the axis (C2) similarly depends on the type of fracture present. Type I (tip of dens), type II (base of dens), and type III (involvement of dens with extension into the body of C2) odontoid fractures may all be initially managed conservatively with external immobilization (Fig. 6). However, surgical fixation should be entertained in cases of type II/III odontoid fractures in which the dens is displaced greater than 5 mm, there is comminution of the dens fracture (type IIA), or fracture alignment is difficult to maintain with external immobilization alone. Additionally, initial surgical fixation should be considered in patients over age 50 with type II odontoid fractures, given the relatively high rate of nonunion in this subset of patients. Hangman's fractures of C2 (traumatic spondylolisthesis of the axis) may also be managed with external immobilization in most cases, although it is important to balance these considerations with the morbidities associated with halo vest use. Surgical stabilization should be considered in cases of severe C2–C3 angulation, disruption of the C2–C3 disk space, or inability to maintain alignment with external immobilization. Isolated fractures of the axis body should be treated with external immobilization alone. The management of combination fractures of the atlas and axis should be based primarily on the specific characteristics of the underlying axis fracture. The majority of C1–C2 combination fractures may be treated with external immobilization, with the exception of C1-type II odontoid combination fractures with an atlanto-dens

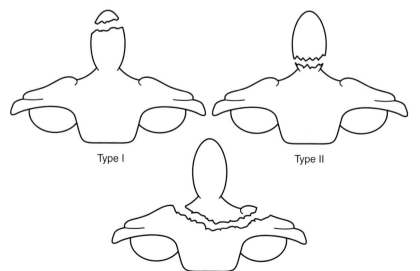

FIGURE 6 Schematic representation of odontoid fracture types. Type I fractures involve the tip of the dens. Type II fractures involve the base of the dens. Type III fractures involve the base of the dens with extension into the vertebral body of C2.

Type I

Type II

Type III

interval of 5 mm or more, and C1-hangman's combination fracture with C2–C3 angulation of 11 degrees or more. The surgical technique employed must be modified to accommodate for any loss of integrity of the ring of the atlas.

Management of subaxial cervical facet dislocation and fracture/dislocation injuries may be treated with either closed or open reduction, followed by rigid external immobilization, anterior arthrodesis with plate fixation, or posterior arthrodesis with plate, rod, or interlaminal clamp fixation.

Thoracolumbar Fractures

The three-column model of spine anatomy is particularly helpful in evaluating injuries to the thoracic and lumbar spine. In general, there are four main types of blunt injury that can be imparted to the thoracolumbar spine: (1) compression fractures, (2) burst fractures, (3) flexion distractions, and (4) fracture dislocations. Compression fractures are characterized by intact middle/posterior columns, with compression and loss of height of the anterior column. Conversely, burst fractures typically involve both the anterior and middle columns, and are most often generated by pure axial load injuries. They most commonly occur between T10 and L2 and, by definition, are associated with retropulsion of bone/ligament complex into the spinal canal, often resulting in significant cord compression (Fig. 7). Flexion distraction injuries typically involve horizontal fractures that can extend exclusively through bone (type I), through bone and ligament (type II), and through the disk, facet capsule, and the interspinous ligament (type III). These injuries may be missed by conventional axial CT because of the horizontal orientation of the fractures. Fracture dislocations are typically caused by shear forces, are highly unstable injuries, and are often associated with significant canal compromise (Fig. 8).

Optimal Timing of Surgical Intervention in Spinal Cord Injuries

The role of surgical decompression in acute SCI remains a topic of considerable debate. Whereas experimental data involving early surgical decompression in animal models has consistently demonstrated enhanced neurologic recovery, these results have proved difficult to extrapolate back to actual SCI patients, mainly due to the lack of clinical trials needed to demonstrate definitive and unequivocal benefit of acute surgical decompression in SCI. The majority of studies on surgical decompression in the literature represent retrospective case series with historical control subjects. Generally speaking, most studies comparing decompressive surgery with conservative management actually fail to definitively demonstrate improved outcome with surgery. Interestingly, in a recent meta-analysis by La Rosa et al, early surgical decompression performed within 24 hours of injury resulted in statistically significant neurologic improvement when compared to both delayed surgical intervention (more than 24 hours postinjury) and conservative management, particularly in patients with initial incomplete injury. Despite the lack of irrefutable supportive evidence, early surgical decompression remains the recommended treatment option in patients with acute cord compression.

Penetrating Spinal Cord Injuries

Similar to early surgical intervention for blunt (nonpenetrating) SCI, the value of early surgical intervention in PSI remains debatable. Retrospective analyses of PSI typically do not demonstrate any improved outcome with early surgical intervention. Additionally, the rate of complication tends to be higher in PSI patients who have been treated with laminectomy in the acute setting. For this reason, early surgical intervention in the setting of acute PSI is recommended as a treatment option only in cases associated with progressive neurologic deterioration. However, open wounds or wounds with suspicion of cerebrospinal fluid (CSF) leakage may require surgical débridement/exploration and dural repair.

Nonoperative Acute Interventions

Concomitant with the assessment for potential acute surgical intervention, several other interventions may be implemented during the acute phase of SCI, while the patient is still in the ED. These measures include closed reduction of cervical spine dislocation injuries, pharmacotherapeutic intervention, and correction/prevention of hypotension. Awake patients with isolated cervical fracture dislocation injuries should undergo early closed reduction with craniocervical traction in order to restore the anatomic alignment of the spine. The overall rates of transient and permanent neurologic complication associated with closed reduction are 2% to 4% and 1%, respectively. If the patient is alert and can be examined, then the risk of reduction/traction without a prior MRI is low. Therefore, external cervical reduction should be performed as soon as possible after the diagnosis has been made radiographically. Prereduction MRI examination is recommended only in cases when the patient cannot be examined during the reduction. The presence of a significant disk herniation under these conditions represents a relative indication for open ventral decompression prior to reduction. Additionally, MRI is recommended for patients who fail initial attempts at closed reduction. An algorithm for the clearance of the cervical spine in a trauma patient is presented in Figure 9.

Pharmacotherapy and Spinal Cord Injury

Unlike the case of closed reduction for cervical dislocation injuries, the role of pharmacotherapy in the treatment of acute SCI has been less definitive. Of the various agents available for treatment of acute SCI, MP has, by far, been the most extensively studied. After initial enthusiasm over the potential benefit of early corticosteroid (MP) therapy in acute SCI, recent studies and intense scrutiny of the study parameters and data interpretation employed in the original NASCIS clinical trials have served to weaken the argument that MP therapy is associated with a meaningful improvement in functional outcome of SCI patients. The main criticisms of the NASCIS trials have been related to the determination of optimal timing of therapy, the method of motor assessment, and the apparent lack of correlation between motor recovery scores and functional outcome measures. These shortcomings, coupled with the inability to demonstrate any clear therapeutic benefit of MP therapy on outcome of SCI in several independent studies, have prompted the AANS and CNS to recommend MP therapy as a treatment option only, which should only be undertaken with the knowledge that evidence suggesting harmful side effects is more consistent than any suggestion of clinical benefit. Harmful side effects of MP therapy include pneumonia, sepsis, hyperglycemia, gastrointestinal ulcers/bleeding, and avascular necrosis of the femoral head, all of which have been observed to occur at significantly higher rates in NASCIS II/III protocol MP-treated SCI patients. GM1 ganglioside has similarly been implicated in enhancement of neurologic recovery in acute SCI. However, available medical evidence does not support such a benefit, and thus, the administration of GM1 ganglioside in the setting of acute SCI is recommended only as a potential treatment option at this time. Nimodipine, naloxone, and tirilazad mesylate have also been implicated as potential neuroprotectants following SCI, and are currently the focus of ongoing clinical trials.

Institution of Blood Pressure Parameters

Yet another intervention that should be implemented in acute SCI patients relatively early in their course is the maintenance of adequate blood pressure parameters. Hypotension is commonly encountered in the setting of acute SCI and is often due to associated traumatic injuries with resultant hypovolemia and spinal/neurogenic shock. Whatever the underlying mechanism at play, hypotension should be avoided in the setting of acute SCI, owing to the potential for cord

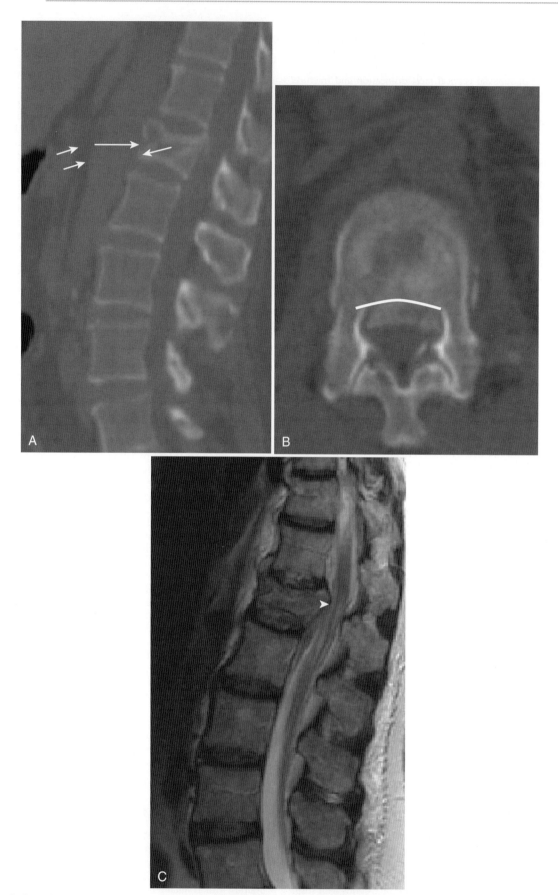

FIGURE 7   A, Sagittal computed tomography reconstruction demonstrating an L1 burst fracture *(arrows)*, with marked canal compromise secondary to retropulsion of bony elements noted on the axial views (**B**). In **B,** the white line represents the normal posterior boundary of the vertebral body. **C,** Magnetic resonance imaging scan demonstrates significant compression of the conus medullaris secondary to the retropulsed fragments *(arrowhead).*

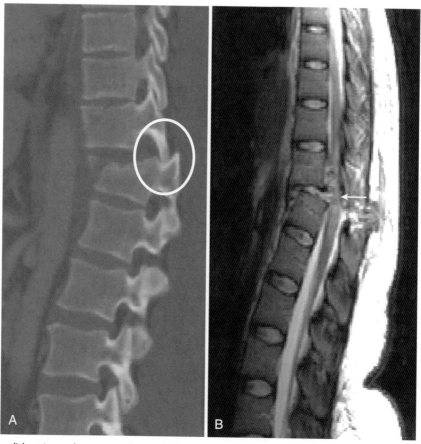

FIGURE 8 T12–L1 fracture dislocation as demonstrated on sagittally reconstructed computed tomography (**A**), with complete facet dislocation *(circle)*, and on magnetic resonance imaging (**B**), with significant compression of and T2 signal changes within the conus *(arrow)*.

FIGURE 9 Algorithm for the clearance of the cervical spine in a trauma patient. AP, Anteroposterior; CT, computed tomography; lat, lateral; MRI, magnetic resonance imaging.

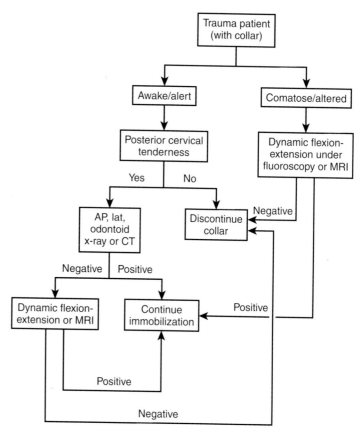

hypoperfusion, ischemia, and exacerbation of secondary traumatic lesions. Because of associated ethical concerns, only retrospective (class III) evidence is available in the literature on neurologic outcome in SCI patients with hypotensive episodes early in their hospital course. Based on the available data, the prevailing recommendation by the AANS and CNS is to avoid systolic blood pressure less than 90 mm Hg in acute spine-injured patients, with the goal of maintaining mean arterial pressure (MAP) greater than 85 mm Hg for the first 7 days after injury. This often entails placement of a central venous catheter and use of intravenous pressor agents.

Subacute Management of Spinal Cord Injury

Following initial resuscitation and acute surgical intervention, SCI patients then enter the subacute phase of their initial hospitalization. Review of the literature suggests that severe SCI patients are susceptible to life-threatening cardiovascular instability and respiratory insufficiency in the first 7 to 14 days after injury. This is particularly true for severe cervical SCI patients. For this reason, it is strongly recommended that patients with severe cervical level SCI be managed in an intensive care unit (ICU) setting, and that cardiac, hemodynamic, and respiratory monitoring devices be employed in their care to detect any cardiopulmonary dysfunction. Even in otherwise stable patients, maintenance of MAP parameters with continuous infusion of pressor agents often necessitates ICU nursing care. While in the ICU, as well as afterward on the wards, SCI patients benefit from prompt evaluation by physical and occupational therapy services and early participation in associated rehabilitation activities. Care should be taken to prevent the development of pressure ulcers and extremity contractures, as these factors negatively impact neurologic recovery potential, as well as outcome in general. Once the patient has been transferred out of the ICU setting, priority should be placed on timely transfer to a qualified rehabilitation center, in order to provide SCI patients with the greatest opportunity to regain neurologic function and improve their overall functional outcome.

MORBIDITY AND COMPLICATIONS MANAGEMENT IN SPINAL CORD INJURY

In discussing the various complications associated with SCI, it is helpful to classify these events by their typical timeline to presentation following the initial injury. Acute complications tend to occur within the first hours to weeks following acute SCI, often occurring during the acute hospitalization. These complications include hemodynamic instability, cardiopulmonary events, pneumonia, urinary tract infection (UTI), sepsis, and thromboembolic phenomena. Conversely, chronic complications tend to occur weeks to years following the initial insult and include respiratory, genitourinary, psychiatric, thromboembolic, musculoskeletal, gastrointestinal, infectious, and skin care issues. Many of the complications encountered during the acute management of SCI, including pulmonary complications, genitourinary issues, and thromboembolism, require the employment of aggressive preventive/prophylactic measures in order to reduce risk of occurrence in the chronic setting.

Neurogenic Shock

Of the potential complications commonly encountered in the context of acute SCI, those implicated in development of hemodynamic compromise are associated with a significant proportion of morbidity and mortality in the early management of these patients. Neurogenic shock is classically associated with the triad of hypotension, bradycardia, and core hypothermia, in the setting of acute SCI with the NLI localized to T6 and above. The loss of thoracic sympathetic outflow produces a state of unopposed predominant vagotonia, with resultant end-organ effects including decreased peripheral vascular resistance, impaired thermoregulation, and bradycardia. The diminished vascular tone, in combination with diminished cardiac output secondary to bradycardia, often results in profound hypotension that may be refractory to crystalloid/colloid resuscitation. Untreated, systemic hypotension can contribute to cord ischemia, facilitating the progression and severity of secondary traumatic lesions. It is this premise that has underscored the rationale of maintaining MAP goals in the acute SCI patient. Typically this is achieved through fluid/colloid resuscitation, the use of pressor agents, or a combination of the two. Pressors with intrinsic β_1-agonist chronotropic activity, including dobutamine and dopamine, are of particular usefulness, as they address both the vasomotor and cardiogenic aspects of neurogenic shock. Persistent bradycardia may be treated with intermittent atropine, with the knowledge that atropine may exacerbate pulmonary dysfunction by thickening secretions. In general, sympathetic tone begins to return in 3 to 7 days. However, during this period, the SCI patient is at greatest risk for developing a cardiopulmonary complication, and thus continued ICU monitoring of these patients during the first 1 to 2 weeks after injury is strongly recommended.

Spinal Shock

Unlike neurogenic shock, spinal shock is a state of transient physiologic reflex depression of cord function below the level of injury, with an associated loss of all sensory/motor functions. Hypertension due to an initial release of catecholamines may be encountered, typically followed by profound hypotension. Flaccid paralysis, including of the bowel and bladder, is the hallmark feature of spinal shock. In many instances, sustained priapism is also observed. These findings typically last from hours to days following the injury, until the reflex arc below the level of injury resumes function. The bulbocavernosus reflex refers to anal sphincter contraction in response to squeezing the glans penis or tugging on the Foley catheter. The reflex involves the S1, S2, and S3 nerve roots and is a spinal cord–mediated reflex arc. Following spinal cord trauma, the presence or absence of this reflex carries prognostic significance. Specifically, in cases of cervical or thoracic cord injury, absence of this reflex documents continuation of spinal shock, or spinal injury at the level of the reflex arc itself. The period of spinal shock usually resolves within 48 hours, and return of the bulbocavernosus reflex signals termination of spinal shock. Complete absence of distal motor or sensory function or perirectal sensation, together with recovery of the bulbocavernosus reflex, indicates a complete cord injury, and in such cases it is highly unlikely that significant neurologic function will ever return. Therefore, if no motor or sensory recovery below the level of injury is present, the patient has a complete SCI and no further distal recovery of motor function can be expected. On the other hand, any spared motor or sensory function below the level of injury is considered an incomplete injury. In the acute setting, the type of shock present may be difficult to discern given the presence of other detracting injuries. Therefore, invasive monitoring of pulmonary artery pressures may be necessary to differentiate among neurogenic, hypovolemic, and cardiogenic shock.

Pulmonary Complications

Pulmonary complications represent a significant source of morbidity and fatality in SCI patients, in both the acute as well as the chronic setting. Injury to the cervical and midthoracic cord often results in underlying respiratory dysfunction, which, in turn, increases susceptibility to pulmonary infections. SCI above C4 often compromises phrenic nerve function, resulting in subsequent diaphragmatic dysfunction. The majority of patients with a high cervical injury thus require prolonged mechanical ventilation, often necessitating tracheostomy to avoid laryngotracheomalacia associated with prolonged intubation. Injury at lower cervical and upper thoracic levels can impair innervation to accessory muscles of respiration, including the intercostal muscles, resulting in a progressive loss of vital capacity, tidal volume, and negative inspiratory pressure. This serves to effectively reduce lung volume, create ventilation-perfusion mismatches with intrapulmonary shunting, and decrease the arterial oxygen saturation. Loss of the ability to produce an adequate cough and the normal sigh mechanism, leads to the accumulation of uncleared secretions, and plugging/collapsing of the terminal pulmonary segments. This serves to promote an optimal intra-alveolar environment for the development of repetitive and in many cases fatal pneumonias. The excessive use of analgesia and sedatives can further depress respiratory function. In order to decrease the risk of pulmonary complications, it is imperative that an aggressive pulmonary toilet regimen be instituted immediately, consisting of aerosol treatments, chest physiotherapy, intermittent positive-pressure breathing, and frequent suction in mechanically ventilated patients. Bronchoscopy has been a valuable tool for retrieval of tenacious mucus plugs in chronically debilitated patients. Additionally, early mobilization, if possible, also serves to improve overall pulmonary function.

Thromboembolism

Thromboembolic phenomena, including deep venous thrombosis (DVT) and pulmonary embolism (PE), represent a significant, and potentially fatal, complication in the SCI patient population. DeVivo and colleagues have documented a 500-fold increased risk of dying from a PE in the first month following SCI when compared against both age- and gender-matched control subjects. Although the risk of DVT and PE appears to decline proportionately with time from injury, SCI patients, especially those with complete injury, are perpetually at an elevated risk for thromboembolism due to immobility. For this reason, prophylaxis for at least 3 months following injury has been advanced as a standard of care in SCI patients. A variety of methods have been used to achieve this end, including the use of low-molecular-weight heparins, caval filters, rotating beds, adjusted-dose heparin, low-dose warfarin, pressure stockings, pneumatic compression stockings, and electrical stimulation. Of these, low-dose heparin, in combination with pneumatic compression stockings, represents the prophylactic regimen of choice in most centers, despite the lack of any direct evidence of synergy. Use of a prophylactic regimen has been observed to reduce the risk of DVT in SCI from 27.3% to 10.3%. In the event of a documented DVT or PE, a 4- to 6-month course of full anticoagulation therapy is warranted. Caval filters are recommended for SCI patients who experience refractory thromboembolic events despite anticoagulation, and in patients in whom anticoagulation is contraindicated (e.g., recent or impending surgery). The diagnosis of DVT can be accomplished with duplex Doppler ultrasound with a sensitivity of approximately 90%. More invasive diagnostic techniques such as venography should be reserved for cases in which the index of suspicion for DVT remains high, despite a negative Doppler study. Similarly, invasive diagnostic modalities for PE, such as transfemoral pulmonary angiogram, should be reserved only for cases in which suspicion of PE remains high, despite a negative ventilation-perfusion or spiral pulmonary CT angiogram study.

Genitourinary Complications

Urinary complications due to elevated bladder pressure, infections, and bladder/renal calculi remain a significant source of morbidity in SCI patients. Alteration of detrusor motor function and bladder sensation, along with compromised sphincter activity, all play a role in incomplete bladder emptying, which, in turn, leads to elevated bladder pressures and secondary genitourinary insult. Chronically elevated bladder pressures can lead to the serious sequelae of hydroureteronephrosis and vesicoureteral reflux. Additionally, urinary stasis increases the risk of UTI, as well as urosepsis, the leading cause of morbidity in SCI. In order to limit these complications, a strict bladder regimen is recommended. The use of indwelling bladder catheters should be limited to the ICU course. Should urinary retention/incontinence prove to be an issue, intermittent clean catheterization every 4 to 6 hours should be employed, with the goal of maintenance of bladder volume under 500 mL at all times. Prophylactic antibiotics are not recommended. However, any indication of possible UTI should be diagnosed and treated promptly.

Gastrointestinal Complications

In the acute setting, SCI patients are at risk of developing stress ulcers of the upper gastrointestinal tract, likely related to gastric capillary bed ischemia, resulting in a diminished resistance of the gastric-enteric mucosa to the normal digestive secretions of the stomach. The utilization of high-dose MP therapy in the treatment of acute SCI also places these patients at higher risk of developing stress ulcers. In recent years, the incidence of bleeding gastric ulcers has gradually decreased in the SCI population, thought to be due, in large part, to the implementation of stress ulcer prophylaxis with histamine receptor type 2 blockers, sucralfate, or proton-pump inhibitors. With neurologic injury, institution of a bowel care regimen is of importance given the likelihood of associated adynamic ileus. A healthy bowel regimen often includes a combination of stool softeners, high-fiber diet, digital stimulation, suppositories, enemas, and manual disimpaction.

Skin Care

In the setting of neurologic injury, the development of pressure ulcers is a significant source of discomfort, and these ulcers represent yet another potential route of infection. The sacral prominence, femoral greater trochanters, ischial tuberosities, and heels are particularly vulnerable to ulcer formation. The incidence of pressure necrosis requiring surgical débridement within 2 years of SCI is approximately 4%. Prevention is paramount, and typically involves early patient mobilization, air mattresses, limited use of braces/orthotics, and aggressive skin inspection and wound care.

Posttraumatic Syringomyelia

Typically occurring on a more chronic timetable, post-traumatic syringomyelia (PTS) has been encountered with increasing frequency in SCI over the past 20 years, likely due to a combination of factors including increased life expectancy in SCI patients, as well as the emergence of MRI technology as a highly sensitive diagnostic tool. By definition, PTS is a central cavitation of the spinal cord, typically occurring months to years after the initial injury. Although presenting symptoms vary based on the location and severity of the syrinx, persistent local or radicular pain, motor weakness, spasticity, dissociated sensory loss, autonomic dysreflexia, sphincter loss, sexual dysfunction, Horner's syndrome, and respiratory dysfunction have all been described. Extension of cervical syrinx cavities into the medulla, termed syringobulbia, has also been described, and typically manifests with corticobulbar dysfunction. Although the exact pathognomonic mechanism involved in syrinx formation has not been definitively elucidated, the prevailing hypothesis favors a progression of posttraumatic cystic myelopathy. Alteration in spinal subarachnoid CSF flow dynamics secondary to posttraumatic arachnoiditis may also play a role. The incidence of PTS ranges from 1.1% to greater than 50%, with the duration of time of injury to diagnosis of syrinx ranging from 2 months to 33 years. Development of symptomatic syringomyelia is a poor prognostic sign. Although several surgical procedures have been employed in the treatment of PTS, including placement of cystoperitoneal and cystopleural shunts, the overall success of these interventions is generally poor.

MORTALITY

Despite significant advances made in first responder management of SCI, approximately 10% to 20% of acute SCI patients do not survive to reach hospitalization, and another 3% of patients die during their acute hospitalization. For those patients who survive the acute hospitalization, the major cause of death is pneumonia and other respiratory complications, followed by heart disease, subsequent trauma, and septicemia. The leading causes of death among incomplete paraplegics are cancer and suicide. Suicide is also the leading cause of death in complete paraplegics, followed by heart disease. In general, the suicide rate is higher among the SCI population under the age of 25 years. In terms of life expectancy, individuals aged 20 years at the time of their injury have life expectancies of approximately 33 years as tetraplegics, 39 years as low tetraplegics, and 44 years as paraplegics.

CONCLUSION

Thanks in large part to marked improvements made in the first-responder and ED management of acute SCI, overall morbidity and mortality rates in this patient population have substantially decreased over the past 30 years. Similarly, the implementation of aggressive prophylactic/preventive measures against many of the common complications of SCI, including thromboembolism, UTIs, pulmonary infections, and pressure ulcers, have served to further improve the quality of life for these patients. With the average life span of SCI patients approaching that of the general public, the economic burden associated with lifelong treatment of these patients will undoubtedly continue to increase in the years to come. Timely diagnosis, in conjunction with the application of appropriate treatment guidelines/recommendations in the acute setting, provides patients with the best opportunity to improve functional neurologic outcome. Whereas certain interventions, including spinal immobilization, closed reduction of cervical dislocation injuries, and maintenance of blood pressure parameters, have gained universal acceptance in the management of SCI, others, including the role of MP therapy and acute surgical decompression, are more widely debated and open for interpretation.

For the chapter's Suggested Readings list, please visit the book at www.ExpertConsult.inkling.com.

MAXILLOFACIAL AND OCULAR INJURIES

MAXILLOFACIAL TRAUMA

Urmen Desai, Rosaine Roeder, Benjamin T. Lemelman, and Seth R. Thaller

Maxillofacial trauma is frequently encountered by both trauma and plastic surgeons but infrequently results in fatality. Maxillofacial trauma is readily apparent when the patient first arrives at the emergency room. Such injuries should not be a distraction to the surgeon during initial evaluation and resuscitation. The exception is the patient who requires a surgical airway. *Advanced Trauma Life Support* directives should be closely followed as a standard procedure.

AIRWAY AND BREATHING

In trauma, the first priority is securing the upper airway, followed by ensuring adequate ventilation and prevention of aspiration. Injury to the maxillofacial region can compromise the airway in several ways including tissue displacement, edema, and hemorrhage. Multiple fractures to the mandible, nasal bones, or maxilla can also lead to loss of the airway. Anatomically, the tongue is secured in the oral cavity by the mandible. Any compromise of this relationship may cause the tongue to descend into the oropharynx, thus obstructing the airway. Surrounding tissue edema and local hematoma due to injury may also narrow the airway. Additionally, blood, emesis, avulsed teeth or dentures, and foreign objects can obstruct the airway. Physical signs of airway obstruction include stridor, cyanosis, and drooling. Patients may also lack a protective gag reflex, owing to alcohol or drug intoxication or concomitant traumatic brain injury. In these cases, endotracheal intubation or cricoidthyrotomy is indicated. Nasotracheal intubation is technically more difficult, as it causes more complications and requires a patent nasal passage.

CIRCULATION AND CONTROL OF HEMORRHAGE

Arterial supply to the face is derived from multiple branches of the external carotid artery. Extensive anastomosis creates a rich vascular network. Many arteries reside superficially in the maxillofacial skeleton and as a result are vulnerable to traumatic injury. Most superficial arterial bleeding can, however, be controlled with pressure and rarely requires vessel repair. Also, because of the rich anastomotic network, ligation of superficial vessels should not compromise blood supply to adjacent facial structures. Arterial repair should be undertaken in the operating room only when a large-caliber artery is damaged.

Veins are more likely to be injured in facial trauma because they are more superficial to arteries and are valveless, and therefore are prone to profuse bleeding. This is managed by pressure and vessel ligation.

Treatment of airway obstruction secondary to hemorrhage is a priority, as bleeding can potentially impede the view of the upper aerodigestive tract. Often, an inadequate view of the vocal cords makes orotracheal intubation difficult. A surgical airway should be considered in such instances. Bleeding from soft tissue lacerations may be addressed after patients are stabilized. The surgical management of soft tissue lacerations is reviewed later in this chapter. Hemorrhage from facial fractures is generally managed with fracture reduction.

Epistaxis

Epistaxis is commonly encountered after facial trauma and is often self-limited. It may be associated with nasal fracture. Bleeding can be from the anterior or posterior nasal cavities. Identification is important for definitive management. Nasal bleeding is frequently controlled with direct pressure for a minimum of 30 minutes. If bleeding persists, the nasal cavity should be packed. Ribbon gauze impregnated with petroleum jelly is generally employed. For anterior bleeding, a nasal speculum is used to visualize and open the nasal cavity. The gauze is then introduced into the nasal cavity layer by layer with the aid of bayonet forceps. Adequate packing should be performed by firmly pressing down after each layer, only tight enough to stop bleeding without causing mucosal or septal necrosis. Direct cautery with silver nitrate is also effective when a localized point of bleeding is easily identifiable.

Posterior nasal bleeding can be controlled by posterior nasal packing. This is accomplished with the aid of a catheter that introduces the packing though the nares into the nasopharynx and can be passed through the oral cavity. Use of a nasal balloon catheter may be simpler. If nasal balloons are not available, a 10 Fr to 14 Fr Foley catheter with a balloon can be used to control posterior bleeding. It is passed into the oropharynx, inflated to 10 cc, and then carefully pulled anteriorly toward the nasal cavity until bleeding ceases. Hyperinflation of the balloon must be avoided so that pressure necrosis does not occur. Cautery, in the form of bipolar diathermy, electrocautery, or chemical cautery, can also be used when the site of bleeding is visible.

HISTORY AND PHYSICAL EXAMINATION

Once the primary survey is complete, the secondary survey is initiated, followed by a brief history and comprehensive physical examination. The acronym AMPLE is used to remember the pertinent history in the trauma patient: Allergies, Medications, Past medical history, Last meal, and Events of the injury. In patients with evident facial trauma, the mechanism of injury is extremely important. This information may assist the clinician in predicting the extent and magnitude of injury, as well as raise suspicion to the possibility of associated occult injury. A history of motor vehicle crash or gunshot wound suggests possible panfacial fractures. Sports injuries often result in an isolated upper midfacial fracture. History of assault is often associated with a unilateral mandible fracture. Facial trauma as a result of gunshot wound or motor vehicle accident is often more severe than trauma resulting from assault, fall, or athletic injury.

The physical examination must be conducted in an orderly fashion from head to toe in order to avoid missing any injuries. It is necessary to document any asymmetry or gross facial deformities. Starting from the scalp downwards, assess for soft tissue swelling, lacerations, abrasions, and contusions. Evaluate the mandible and maxilla for any missing or broken teeth as well as malocclusion. When palpating the bony regions of the face, note any crepitus, step-off points, or areas of tenderness. Normally, jaw excursion is about 4 to 5 cm when measured from the edges of the incisors. Lateral jaw movement is normally about 1 cm and must also be documented. Otoscopic examination, in addition to visualization of the nares and oral cavity, is required to evaluate for additional sites of occult injury. Examination of the cranial nerves is necessary to ascertain any localized deficits.

Reevaluation of the patient is crucial. Many causes of morbidity and subsequent fatality may not be seen on the initial examination. For example, the patient may vomit at any given time and this will place him at risk for aspiration; bleeding or edema may accumulate over time, resulting in eventual respiratory distress.

RADIOGRAPHS

Facial trauma is best evaluated with computed tomography (CT) imaging supplemented with pantomogram (Panorex) films to evaluate status of dentition and the presence of any possible mandibular fractures. On CT scan, axial, coronal, and sagittal sections using 1- to 2-mm cuts are used to visualize the facial anatomy and demonstrate potential fractures and dislocations. Panfacial fractures and bone loss can be further assessed using three-dimensional reconstruction. Pantomogram visualizes the anatomy of the maxilla and mandible, providing the best evaluation of any potential associated odontogenic injury. Plain radiographs may be used in emergency departments today, yet they have no role in the definitive evaluation of facial trauma.

SOFT TISSUE INJURIES

Evaluation and diagnosis of facial soft tissue injuries are an integral aspect of the overall examination of the trauma patient upon arrival to the treatment facility. However, as most soft tissue injuries are not life threatening, initial treatment should be directed toward cleansing wounds, removing foreign bodies, surgical débridement, and controlling bleeding. Once the patient is stabilized, major facial injury should be appropriately repaired in the operating room.

Local Anesthesia

Facial lacerations can be repaired under local anesthesia, with or without intravenous sedation. Lidocaine and bupivacaine are the most commonly used agents. When using 1% solution of lidocaine, a dose of 4.5 mg/kg is advised, and 7 mg/kg if using lidocaine with epinephrine. Effects of lidocaine last approximately 30 to 60 minutes. Bupivacaine is a longer acting drug than lidocaine, lasting about 2 to 4 hours. The addition of epinephrine to local anesthetic is beneficial, allowing the use of more anesthetic and contributing to vasoconstriction. Topical anesthetic creams, such as EMLA (containing prilocaine and lidocaine), can be used, especially in children, to minimize pain from lacerations as well as from injection of local anesthetic.

Antibiotics

First-generation cephalosporins can be administered to patients within 30 minutes of initiating surgical repair. If a patient is allergic to penicillins, clindamycin can be used. For intraoral lesions, the addition of anaerobic coverage is frequently warranted. If animal bites are suspected, more extensive coverage is needed to cover for both gram–negative organisms and anaerobes. Tetanus prophylaxis should be given to all patients.

Abrasions

All abrasions should be washed with mild soap, foreign bodies removed, and clean sterile dressing placed. These patients should be followed daily for onset of possible infection or delayed healing.

General Concepts for Laceration Repair

All repairs should be done in a sterile environment with appropriate lighting and equipment. Ideally, lacerations should be closed within 6 to 8 hours; however, they can be closed within 24 hours and followed closely for signs of infection. Antibiotic coverage is also initiated. All lacerations should be closed in layers; however, for simple superficial lacerations tissue adhesives can be safely used for closure.

Scalp Laceration

Scalp lacerations can bleed profusely. These wounds should be copiously irrigated and any foreign objects removed. Staples can be applied to quickly control bleeding. Cautery can also be used if available. Formal repair should be performed in layers.

Intraoral Injury

Dental injuries have a high occurrence in facial trauma. Dental-alveolar trauma should be addressed with removal of any loose teeth. Mucosal or gingival lacerations can be treated with pressure or sutured with fine absorbable chromic gut suture. Oral chlorhexidine or peroxide mouth rinse should be used by patients to maintain oral hygiene. Fractures associated with intraoral trauma are discussed later in this chapter.

Tongue Laceration

Minor lacerations generally heal without intervention. However, deep lacerations may involve the lingual artery and result in airway obstruction. Suction is applied to clear blood and oral cavity secretions to identify the source of bleeding. If the lingual artery is transected, it should be repaired in a timely fashion once major injuries are treated.

Lip Laceration

The challenge of repairing a lacerated lip is correlated to the amount of swelling in the affected area. Therefore, repair should be done by aligning the vermilion border anteriorly and suturing the laceration with interrupted sutures in layers posteriorly toward the intraoral mucosa. Absorbable braided suture should be used for muscle, while absorbable chromic gut is used for the vermilion and any mucosal surfaces. Skin can be closed with nonabsorbable suture. Frequently, nerve blocks should be used to avoid distorting vital anatomic landmarks. Surgical margins should be tattooed prior to the outset of repair to meticulously align these structures appropriately.

Nasal Laceration

Simple lacerations of the nose can be repaired with fine interrupted nylon suture or tissue adhesive. However, if cartilage or nasal mucosa is lacerated, specialty consultation should be obtained. Cartilage and mucosal surfaces should be repaired with fine fast-absorbing chromic gut suture.

Ear Laceration

Injuries to the auricle should be repaired within 12 hours of injury. Copious irrigation of the injury to remove any debris or foreign body is vital. Repair should be accomplished with fast-absorbing chromic gut suture. Cartilage can be reapproximated, but does not need to be repaired in all cases. Bolsters are used to maintain support to the repaired auricle. These are made from petroleum impregnated gauze. Avulsion injuries of the auricle should be treated with reconstructive repair and reimplantation. Composite grafts and local flaps are the procedures of choice for partial avulsions, but multistage reconstruction is usually needed for total avulsions.

Orbital Laceration

Injuries involving the eye require a complete ophthalmologic consultation. Before any repair is undertaken, a full ophthalmologic examination should be documented in the medical chart. Major injury to the globe must be ruled out. Initially, irrigation of the periocular region should be performed. Simple lacerations involving the brow and lids can be repaired with tissue adhesives or fine interrupted sutures. Complex laceration should be repaired in layers. Special attention is given to alignment of the lid margin while repair is done. Lacrimal ducts may also be damaged in orbital trauma, especially when the medial canthus is involved. Sequelae from this injury can lead to epiphora. Repair is usually performed late when symptoms persist.

Parotid Gland Injury

Injuries to the parotid gland are rare but can result in significant morbidity. Identification and prompt diagnosis are vital. Lewkowicz and colleagues proposed an algorithm for addressing suspected parotid gland injury. First, the parotid gland should be cannulated and either saline or methylene blue dye injected to assess for injury. If this is negative, the cannula should be left in place for 1 week and the facial laceration should be closed. If it is positive, then the extent of injury needs to be determined by identifying both ends of the duct. If both are identified, primary repair should ensue, followed by 48 hours of external pressure, 1 week of intraoral drainage, and maintaining the catheter in the duct for 14 days.

Facial Nerve Injury

The facial nerve branches lie on the deep surface of the facial muscles and are unlikely to be injured in minor trauma. However, in the case of suspected facial nerve injury, careful examination with loupe magnification is necessary. If the facial nerve is visibly injured or suspected to be injured, wound exploration in the operating room equipped with a microscope should be performed and the nerve should be acutely repaired.

FACIAL FRACTURES

Nasal Bone Fractures

The bony nasal vault is composed of paired nasal bones and the frontal process of the maxilla is shaped in a pyramidal structure. On the inner surface of the nose, the nasal bones fuse with the perpendicular plate of the ethmoid to provide additional support of the nasal pyramid. Owing to the prominent projection as well as fragile structure of the nasal pyramid, the nose is the most vulnerable facial structure. Therefore, it is the most common facial bone to be fractured. Details regarding the events surrounding the injury are vital to elicit in order to determine the type and severity of injury. Athletic activity, motor vehicle injury, assault, and falling from standing position are the most common mechanisms of nasal injury. Several variables such as direction of force, speed of impact, nature of object causing injury, and age are just a few of the factors that further influence the degree of nasal trauma. Injuries from lateral impact are more common. They have a better prognosis as compared to front-on forces of impact. Nasal trauma in males occurs at twice the rate as those which occur in females, most often in the second or third decade of life. Older adults tend to suffer more comminution due to the brittle and osteopenic changes to their bones. Younger adults suffer more dislocation of the major segments of bone. In contrast, children are found to have more greenstick fractures because of the greater cartilaginous makeup and incomplete ossification of their nasal bones. Additionally, fractures caused by lateral impaction of force are more common and result in better prognosis. Fractures may be classified as being unilateral, bilateral, comminuted, depressed, telescoped, impacted, or greenstick. Additionally, fractures may extend to the surrounding bony anatomy including the maxilla, lacrimal bone, ethmoids, or frontal sinus.

Patients who present with fracture of the nasal bones characteristically show a nasal deformity, internal and external nasal edema, and epistaxis, as well as periorbital ecchymosis. A detailed history outlining functional changes in nasal breathing, changes in olfaction, epistaxis, clear watery drainage, or a sweet-salty taste must be obtained to rule out possible cerebrospinal fluid (CSF) leak. The provider should also elicit the medical history of the patient as to any previous nasal injury, nasal fracture, allergies, or sinus disease.

Diagnosis of a nasal fracture is made solely by detailed history and physical examination. Presence of deviation and asymmetry of the nasal dorsum may indicate traumatic injury. Additionally, other findings such as epistaxis, periorbital ecchymosis, and internal nasal edema also support the presence of nasal injury. An external, as well as internal, nasal examination should be performed. This will identify deviation of the nasal pyramid, medial collapse of the nasal bones, medial collapse of the upper lateral cartilages, or broadening of the nasal dorsum. Septal hematomas identified during examination should be drained emergently. Failure to recognize and treat a septal hematoma results in septal necrosis, septal perforation, and possibly an eventual saddle-nose deformity. There is no role for plain films or CT imaging for the diagnosis of a nasal fracture. It is also difficult to distinguish old fractures from new fractures. Imaging also does not identify cartilaginous injury, which is more commonly seen in pediatric injuries.

Appropriate timing is essential to obtaining an ideal reduction and satisfactory postoperative results. Two windows exist for ideal surgical management of nasal fractures. The first window lies within the first 3 hours of injury. This is prior to the onset of soft tissue edema, which often obscures the underlying anatomy. The second window lies between 3 to 10 days, after the majority of swelling has resolved. After this period, fibrous connective tissue begins to develop within the fracture line and may limit an adequate reduction. For straightforward injuries such as isolated unilateral nasal fractures, a closed approach is often used. In contrast, more severe traumatic injuries or old fractures greater than 4 weeks require an open approach to reduce the nasal bones.

Nasal injuries are not life threatening. If not adequately reduced, they can result in significant long-term changes to the nasal profile, including decreased nasal projection and saddle nose deformity, as well as persistent nasal airway obstruction. Additionally, nasal fractures in the pediatric population may potentially result in maldevelopment of the nasal pyramid and bony midface structures.

Zygomatic Fractures

Anterior projection of the zygomatic arch provides important aesthetic facial aspects of facial contour. Because of its convexity, its position makes it susceptible to traumatic injury and fracture. Posteriorly, the zygoma provides attachment of the masseter muscle where the zygoma meets the temporal bone. Medially, the zygoma provides structural support for the lateral and inferior orbital rims as well as the inferolateral orbital walls. Inferior and medial extension of the zygoma forms the lateral buttress of the midface where the zygoma is in contact with the maxilla. The zygoma acts as the primary buttress between the maxilla and the cranium, as well as forming the lateral buttress of the midface skeleton. Fracture of all four suture lines of the zygoma (zygomaticofrontal, zygomaticotemporal, zygomaticomaxillary, and zygomaticosphenoid) is termed a tetrapod fracture or zygomaticomaxillary complex (ZMC) fracture. Bones that articulate with the zygoma often absorb the strong impact and result in a fracture. As a result, the orbital floor is often fractured and collapses into the maxillay sinus. The zygomatic arch often fractures at the midpoint in a single location, or in two areas resulting in a central loose fragment. As seen in other fractures of the maxilla, the degree of displacement is directly related to the severity of injury. This determines the complexity of the fracture repair. Patients with ZMC fractures often have a palpable step-off at the zygoma or orbital rim. Additionally, they may have malar flattening secondary to medial displacement of the arch. These findings may not be apparent on initial examination, as they tend to present themselves with resolution of edema of the overlying soft tissue several days after the injury. Patients often experience trismus from compression of the coronoid process and the temporalis muscle by the depressed ZMC. Patients may also experience hypoesthesia or anesthesia due to injury to the infraorbital nerve.

The gold standard for radiologic evaluation and diagnosis of ZMC fractures is axial CT imaging. Patients who are being worked up after trauma often already have had imaging of the brain to rule out an intracranial process. Inferior views through the upper and middle thirds of the face should be included to further evaluate for a ZMC fracture. Such imaging is vital to assist in surgical planning. Both the degree of displacement as well as comminution determine the complexity of the injury and extent of surgical repair.

Surgical repair of the horizontal portion of the arch results in restoration of the anterior and lateral projection of the cheek. Restoration of the vertical portion of the arch restores the height of the malar eminence in relation to the middle third of the face. Also of importance is the inferolateral displaced fracture of the ZMC. This fracture is often associated with fractures of the orbit, which results in increases in orbital volume. It may potentially result in herniation of fat into the maxillary or ethmoid sinuses. It is necessary to also consider these concomitant orbital fractures. This is vital in order to restore the volume of the orbit in conjunction with restoration of the orbital rim. Intraoperatively, the surgeon should remove any bony fragments that may be impinging on important neuromuscualar

structures. After the zygoma has been repositioned, the stabilized framework can be used to repair any corresponding orbital wall fractures.

The most common complication in the surgical management of ZMC fractures is the failure to achieve an ideal reduction. This may result in malocclusion, malunion, or nonunion, which results in motion at the fracture line, facial asymmetry, and possibly osteomyelitis. Malposition may result in enophthalmos or hypophthalmos. Multiple soft tissue complications can also occur and include scarring or lower lid malposition (ectropion).

Orbital Fractures

A thorough understanding of the bony and soft tissue anatomy is vital in the management of orbital trauma. The position of the globe is determined by the extensive ligaments that suspend it, as well as the integrity of the orbital walls. The orbits are a complex set of bony structures that contain structural contributions from a number of facial bones. An orbit is concave along the central floor, and posteriorly slopes upward into the medial orbital wall. The optic canal resides posteromedially behind the medial wall. It is protected from all but the most severe orbital injuries. Forces of impact are transmitted medially through the orbital process to the inferior orbital rim and floor of the orbit. As a result, damage to the anterior maxillary wall and inferior orbital rim frequently results in comminuted injury of multiple fragments lying between the zygomaticomaxillary suture line and the lacrimal fossa. Severity of the strength of impact force almost always correlates to the degree of injury. The concave central portion of the orbit is often involved. High-velocity periorbital forces of impact from objects such as a tennis ball or a baseball may be transmitted to the convex posterior floor and even to the medial orbital wall. This results in significant bony displacement. Although the globe rests anterior to this region of posterior convexity, it is vital to consider this region in the initial evaluation and surgical reconstruction. Injuries that push one or more of the orbital walls outward increase the orbital volume. This also causes damage to the vast network of suspensory ligaments, leading to posterior recession of the globe (enopthalmos) and depression of the globe (hypothalmos). As a result, there is displacement of the orbital soft tissues due to gravitation forces, and simultaneous fibrous scar contracture is initiated.

A complete ophthalmologic examination should be performed on every patient with maxillofacial trauma to the upper third of the face. This examination should include a test of visual acuity, pupillary function, and ocular motility; inspection of the anterior chamber for hyphema; and thorough funduscopic examination. Visual status must be evaluated as soon as possible upon initial evaluation. Progressive loss of vision often indicates increasing intraorbital pressure or optic nerve injury. Early intervention is mandatory. Chemosis and subconjunctival hemorrhage, as well as periorbital ecchymosis, are strong clinical signs of orbital injury. Patients with orbital fractures may have a palpable step-off along the infraorbital rim. This may be less prominent and more difficult to discern with increasing swelling and edema of the overlying soft tissues. Additionally, patients may experience a degree of hypoesthesia due to injury of the surrounding infraorbital nerve (cranial nerve V_2). A thorough evaluation of the extraocular movements should be made. Limitation of upward gaze on command and subjective diplopia may help identify entrapment of the inferior rectus muscle. Manual forced duction testing may identify entrapment of all of the extraocular muscles. Finally, globe position should be evaluated in both its horizontal as well as vertical direction. Documentation of any degree of enophthalmos or hypophthalmos must be made.

A detailed preoperative CT scan should be used to formulate a treatment plan prior to any surgical reconstruction. Axial and coronal CT is considered the gold standard imaging modality to evaluate any type of orbital wall fracture. Sagittal cuts can also provide useful information for surgical decision making (Figs. 1 through 4).

Although axial imaging provides a substantial amount of information regarding the medial and lateral walls of the orbit, coronal imaging is useful to evaluate the orbital floor. This is particularly true for the convex posterior floor. The term blowout fracture implies that the orbital rims are intact with one or more of the walls of the orbit having been fractured. This term also implies the mechanism of injury whereby a force is transmitted by blunt impact to the globe and onto the surrounding walls. Such floor fractures can injure the infraorbital nerve, which runs along the floor of the orbit.

Fractures of the maxillofacial skeleton, which provides support for the globe, orbit, and soft tissues of the cheek, must be thoroughly evaluated and treated aggressively. Reduction and fixation of each

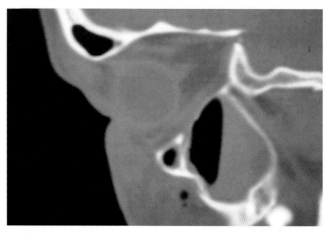

FIGURE 3 Sagittal computed tomography image demonstrating a right infraorbital rim fracture with involvement of the orbital floor and blood in the right maxillary sinus. *(Courtesy of Seth Thaller, MD, DMD, FACS.)*

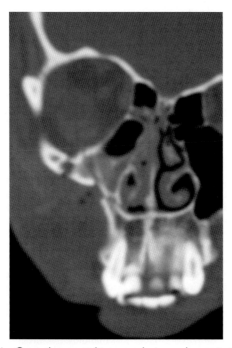

FIGURE 1 Coronal computed tomography image demonstrating a right infraorbital rim fracture with continuity through the infraorbital foramen. *(Courtesy of Seth Thaller, MD, DMD, FACS.)*

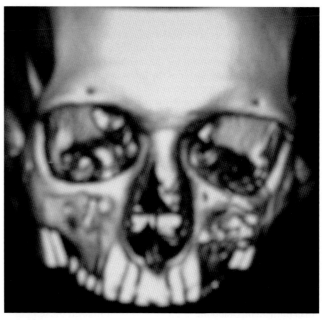

FIGURE 4 Three-dimensional reconstruction image demonstrating a right infraorbital rim fracture with continuity through the infraorbital foramen. *(Courtesy of Seth Thaller, MD, DMD, FACS.)*

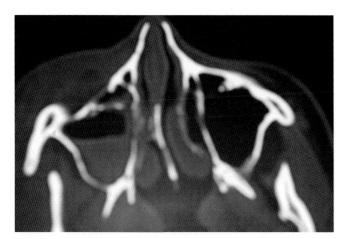

FIGURE 2 Axial computed tomography image demonstrating a right infraorbital rim fracture with blood in the right maxillary sinus and soft tissue edema anterior to the site of fracture. *(Courtesy of Seth Thaller, MD, DMD, FACS.)*

fracture line should be approached in a stepwise fashion in order to consider the orbit as a single unit. Reconstruction of the anterior concave orbital floor can be accomplished with a variety of alloplastic or autogenous material. The orbital floor should be completely exposed in order to allow for two opposing quadrants of the defect to support the implant. Many alloplastic implants are readily available, have minimal migration, and are easily molded and custom trimmed to allow an ideal fit. Calvarial bone has also been used with success.

One of the most common complications is diplopia. This type of visual deficit is usually gaze-evoked with extreme upward or lateral gaze. This often results in entrapment, neuropraxia, or contusion of one of the extraocular muscles. Ectropion, or outward lower lid scarring, results in scarring of the anterior lamella after a subciliary incision. This may manifest to increased scleral show or drying of the cornea, leading to corneal ulceration. Entropion, or inward lower lid scarring, results in scarring of the posterior lamella. It is often associated with a transconjunctival approach to repair. This may lead to a corneal abrasion due to lower eyelashes turned in, as well as corneal exposure. Enophthalmos is also a known complication due to inadequate reconstruction of the orbital floor and medial wall. Another complication is postoperative enophthalmos resulting from an incomplete repair of a defect in the convex posterior aspect of the floor or a failure to properly recognize and repair the medial orbital wall. Finally, plate-related complications may result in soft tissue irritation, cold intolerance, and plate exposure. This may necessitate removal of the plate once the fracture line has properly healed.

For information on orbital compartment syndrome and lateral canthotomy, see the next chapter, Trauma to the Eye and Orbit.

Mandibular Fractures

The workup and management of mandibular fractures are often challenging. The keystone of management is restoration of accurate interdigitation of upper teeth with lower teeth. This makes the surgical management unique. Nonetheless, the same general principles of fracture reduction, rigid fixation, and bone healing are identical to those for long-bone fractures. The mandible is an arch-shaped structure containing both horizontal and vertical landmarks. A dense outer and inner layer consists of cortical bone. Cancellous bone exists along the inner layer. A rich neurovascular bundle and lymphatic drainage system provides nourishment for the mandible and teeth. An important anatomic structure includes the inferior alveolar artery (branch of the internal maxillary artery), which enters through the lingual aspect of the mandible through the mandibular foramen. Also running parallel to the inferior alveolar artery is the inferior alveolar nerve (branch of cranial nerve V_3), which branches to the mental nerve and exits through the anterior aspect of the mandible through the mental foramen. There are a total of 16 teeth in the fully developed mandible. The horizontal portion of the mandible is divided into two primary regions. The superior, or alveolar, portion consists of spongy bone that surrounds and supports the roots of the teeth. The interior, or basal, aspect of the mandible is where the neurovascular bundle courses. The most anterior and central aspect of the mandible is called the symphysis and lateral to this is the parasymphysis. Proximal to the parasymphysis is an area of the mandible called the body. This horizontal aspect of the mandible joins a more vertical component called the ramus. As the ramus ascends and transitions into the condylar neck and coronoid process, it slightly narrows. The condylar neck widens and forms the condyle, which articulates with the glenoid fossa of the temporal bone at the base of skull to form the temporomandibular joint (Fig. 5). This joint contains a fibrocartilaginous structure, which makes up the meniscus of the joint, which is a diarthrodial or ginglymoarthrodial joint. This joint is able to hinge and rotate as well as provide gliding movements. Although the mandible is able to bear an immense amount of force upon impact, there are several areas of inherent weakness. The subcondylar region down to the angle is an area thought to be susceptible to fracture. Interestingly, the presence of a third molar tooth makes this region even weaker. A narrow condylar neck is also frequently involved in injury as forces from the symphysis are transmitted to the neck. This overcomes the compressive strength of the condylar neck, eventually leading to fracture. Similar to the angle region, the presence of a canine tooth root and the location of the mental foramen also make the parasymphysis often involved in a fracture during mandibular trauma. Therefore, owing to the structural properties of the mandible, the most common areas of mandible fracture are found in the subcondylar, angle, and parasymphyseal regions.

Most fractures of the mandible occur as a result of blunt trauma, assault, falls, and motor vehicle accidents. These constitute a majority

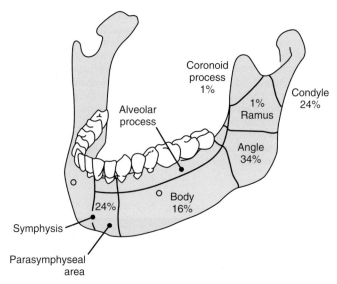

FIGURE 5 Incidence of mandibular fractures by location. *(Modified from Garza JR: Mandible fractures. In Papel I, editor: Facial plastic and reconstructive surgery, 3rd ed. New York, Thieme Medical Publishers, 2009, Chap. 72, p. 1001.)*

of the causes of such fractures. In adults, as opposed to the pediatric population, the mandible is the most projected region in the head and neck, making it more susceptible to injury. When a fracture occurs through the mandible, displaced portions are kept out of alignment because of the unopposed pull of a particular muscle group of jaw elevators (masseter, temporalis, and medial pterygoid) or depressors (suprahyoid musculature and lateral pterygoid muscles).

As discussed previously, fractures of the mandible can also be classified similar to long-bone fractures as being open, closed, simple, complex, or comminuted. Fractures of the mandible are considered open when they extend through the periodontal membrane surrounding the tooth root and communicate with the oral cavity. A further classification exists that divides mandible fractures into favorable and unfavorable. Muscular forces that act on the fractured segments can either favorably reduce the fracture line into a position that is favorable to healing or displace the fracture segments and separate the two fracture segments into a position that impedes adequate healing. Generally speaking, fractures that are inferiorly and posteriorly angled are classified as being more horizontally unfavorable. Fractures that are inferiorly and anteriorly angled are considered horizontally favorable.

The diagnosis of a mandible fracture can often be made by clinical examination. Signs and symptoms include pain, edema, trismus, malocclusion, intraoral bleeding, and deviation of the jaw upon opening. A bony step-off with associated pain may be appreciated upon palpation of the site of fracture. Open fractures may reveal ecchymosis and a mucosal laceration of the floor of mouth in the region of the fracture. A mandibular stress test can be performed, which involves placing the volar aspect of the thumbs on the lingual aspects of the mandibular body and pushing outward. Pain and subtle motion can help confirm the presence of a fracture.

Radiologic tests can confirm the exact location as well as pattern of fracture. A panorex is a panoramic radiograph that can examine the entire aspect of the complex three-dimensional structure of the mandible in a two-dimensional view. A mandible series of imaging can also help with further evaluation of the condylar regions, which may be missed on panoramic imaging. CT imaging is also a modality frequently used to confirm the presence of a mandible fracture. Such imaging can also assist with surgical planning as well as help evaluate other associated facial fractures in the midface.

All open fractures of the mandible should initially be managed with the administration of systemic antibiotics. The earlier a fracture can be surgically managed, the less risk of postoperative complications as well as greater ease in an adequate reduction and fixation. Several principles of the management of mandible fractures must be considered and include the establishment of the premorbid dental occlusion, anatomic reduction of fractures, and an adequate duration of stabilization until the fracture has completely healed. This can be addressed with open reduction and internal fixation techniques using rigid plate and screw fixation. Stabilization of the newly reduced fracture can be achieved by placing external fixation devices that have been developed for comminuted fractures of the mandible. Much controversy continues regarding the total duration of stabilization in intermaxillary wires as well as management of teeth lying within the fracture line.

Complications associated with mandible fractures are often associated with improper surgical technique, poor patient compliance, or healing principles of bone. Infection of the fracture site is often seen due to damaged or infected tooth roots within the fracture line, poor oral hygiene, or a poor surgical reduction leading to significant motion. Additional contributions to motion after surgical reduction include poor plate size selection, improper placement of the plate, and an inadequate number of screws, which lead to excessive motion at the fracture site. This may result in plate failure, place rejection, and nonunion. The latter results in bony necrosis at the fracture site, with fibrous tissue filling the gap rather than newly formed bone. A malunion can also occur when bone heals poorly after an inadequate bony reduction. Damage to surrounding nerves and vessels must also be considered. Inferior alveolar nerve is easily stretched, contused, or even accidentally transected during fracture exposure and plating.

Le Fort Fractures

The maxilla houses two large air-filled sinus cavities. They are known to fracture with far less force than adjacent areas of the facial skeleton. The complex and intricate architecture of the midface is arranged in horizontal beams and vertical buttresses that facilitate the transfer and distribution of forces to other areas of the maxillofacial region and skull base. It is believed that humans evolved this sophisticated architecture in order to absorb the impact of forces to avoid injury to the orbital and cranial contents. Thus, such forces to the midface often result in fractures with significantly less injury than what impact kinetics would predict.

In 1901, René Le Fort originally described a series of classic fracture patterns produced from experimental cadaveric skulls dropped from varying heights (Fig. 6). Although an isolated and pure Le Fort

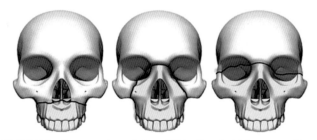

FIGURE 6 Patterns of type I, II, and III Le Fort facial fractures. *(From Orloff G: Management of facial fractures. In Thaller S, Garri JI, Bradley JP, editors: Craniofacial surgery. New York, Informa Healthcare USA, 2007, p 305.)*

fracture is clinically quite rare, his work helped describe fracture patterns that assist in determining the level and severity of injury. A Le Fort I fracture pattern consists of a low horizontal pattern of fracture extending from the maxilla and the palate, lying above the maxillary dentition, separating the teeth from the rest of the craniofacial skeleton. It crosses the nasal septum and posteriorly crosses the posterior maxillary wall and the pterygoid plates. This type of fracture pattern occurs in approximately 30% of all Le Fort fractures. It is usually the result of direct anterior-posterior impacts low on the midface, producing fractures of the vertical and horizontal buttresses of the midface.

A Le Fort II fracture pattern often occurs as a result of either direct horizontal forces to the midface, or alternatively from force transmitted from the anterior mandible to the midface. This fracture often begins at the nasal bones and crosses the frontal process of the maxilla and lacrimal bones. It then descends through the floor of the orbit, infraorbital rim, and lateral maxillary sinus wall, extending posteriorly through the pterygoid plates. The resulting fracture creates a pyramidal fracture of the inferior facial segment, which is separated from the remaining craniofacial skeleton. Similarly, as seen in Le Fort I fractures, the fracture traverses the nasal septum, posterior maxillary walls, and pterygoid plates. This fracture pattern is the most common pattern of fracture, occurring in almost 60% of all cases.

Le Fort III fractures occur at the level of the skull base, where the fracture line separates the zygoma from the temporal bone and frontal bone, crosses the lateral and medial orbits, and reaches the midline at the nasofrontal junction. As with Le Fort I and Le Fort II fracture patterns, there is also fracture through the nasal septum, posterior maxillary walls, and the pterygoid plates. This pattern results in complete craniofacial separation. Such a fracture pattern is often caused by oblique forces to the vertical buttress and is the most rare of all three fracture patterns. It is commonly seen in high-velocity impact and associated with significant comminution and intracranial injury. Although many fractures do not actually follow this strict classification scheme, it does prove a useful tool in assisting with communicating the patient workup and surgical management. Most fractures of the midface are more complex. Often they demonstrate characteristics of several Le Fort injuries on opposing sides of the bony facial skeleton.

Of all facial fractures, Le Fort fractures are seen in approximately 10% to 20% of patients. This pattern of facial fracture is most commonly seen after motor vehicle accident, interpersonal violence, or falls from height. The most frequent demographic group is males in their fifth decade. With an expanding elderly population, there is an expected increase in the number of Le Fort facial fractures in the older population. In contrast, the pediatric population seldom suffer from Le Fort fractures. They generally have a proportionately larger mandible and frontal bone, combined with more flexible facial bones, undeveloped maxillary sinuses, and dentition that has not yet erupted, all of which prevent children from such fracture patterns. Le Fort fractures are often associated with other types of head and neck injuries, including intracranial, ophthalmologic, and neck injuries. Therefore, it is vital that the intial workup and diagnostic tests evaluate all aspects of the head and neck if a Le Fort fracture is identified.

Although it is often difficult in the trauma setting, the surgeon or emergency room physician must perform a thorough evaluation of facial injury after adequate life resuscitating measures have been performed. Bleeding is often found to complicate the evaluation of midface injuries. Often bleeding is secondary to mucosal tear of the septal, nasal, or sinus mucosa. Once stable, premorbid dental occlusion and previous history of dental trauma are important to ascertain. A detailed ophthalmologic history is also vital to evaluation for any acute changes in vision. Examination should also include inspection and palpation of the entire facial skeleton, evaluating for mobility of facial structures. Midface trauma is often associated with a significant degree of soft tissue edema, which may distort facial appearance and potentially mask an underlying depressed fracture. Malocclusion is often seen in which a displaced maxilla may lead to premature contact or an open bite deformity. Often forces of midface trauma cause a posterior displacement of the maxilla along the skull base. This creates a flat and elongated facial appearance. If the injury has extended to the bony orbit, ecchymosis or an abnormal globe position may be encountered. Midface instability is seen with all Le Fort fractures. This can be evaluated by using the thumb and forefinger to grasp the premaxilla while the other hand stabilizes the infraorbital rims. In a Le Fort I fracture, only the premaxilla will show motion, but in a Le Fort II, separation of the infraorbital rims will move with the maxilla. In a Le Fort III, the premaxilla, malar bones, and remainder of the facial bones are mobile at the nasofrontal and zygomaticofrontal sutures. Subcutaneous emphysema and step-off deformities of the orbital rims and cranial nerve V_2 parasthesia may be found in Le Fort II fractures.

CT is the imaging modality of choice when evaluating a trauma patient for a Le Fort fracture pattern. Special attention should be made on imaging through the orbits and the base of skull, as intracranial injury may alter the surgical algorithm.

Surgical management of Le Fort fractures is focused on restoration of function as well as aesthetic aspects of facial symmetry. Reestablishment of facial height and facial projection and reconstitution of premorbid dental occlusion are the primary goals of surgical repair. It was previously believed that repair of Le Fort fractures should wait for resolution of soft tissue edema, allowing a better evaluation of surgical landmarks and a better postoperative reduction. However, it is now felt that early surgical intervention with open reduction and internal fixation allows for a more precise repair before there is any bony resorption or fibrous ingrowth, which is often seen with a delayed repair. Some authors report earlier return to function, decreased infection rate, decreased scarring, and fewer postoperative complications with an immediate repair. Midfacial bones can be exposed by way of concealed surgical incision through a combination of intraoral, transconjunctival, bicoronal, or midface degloving in order to reduce all of the fractured buttresses. Choice of incision is determined by the location and extent of the fracture sites. Once the fractures are adequately reduced, rigid fixation using a combination of low- and high-profile titanium plating systems can be implemented. Patients are also placed into intermaxillary fixation with arch bars with interdental wiring in order to limit the degree of motion and compression on the reduced fracture line.

Complications of midface fractures are often divided into bony and soft tissue defects, which may result in either functional or aesthetic challenges. Bony complications include malocclusion secondary to a combination of delayed union, malunion, nonunion, or fibrous union. When a true nonunion or fibrous union results, all the nonviable bone and fibrous tissue must be débrided and replaced by autologous bone graft. In contrast, soft tissue complications are more easily addressed, such as wound infections, parasthesias or hypoesthesia, hollowing of the malar or temporal area, and eyelid malposition.

Frontal Sinus Fractures

Frontal sinuses are often absent at birth. They begin to develop at the age of 6, and reach their adult size at age 15. The floor of the frontal sinus forms the medial portion of the orbital roof, and the posterior table forms the anterior wall of the anterior cranial fossa. Although the adult frontal sinus is highly variable in size and shape, the frontal sinus is often bilateral and divided by an intersinus septum. Nasofrontal recess resides along the floor of the frontal sinus, which functions as the outflow tract of the frontal sinus. This drains into the nasal cavity. It has been well established that

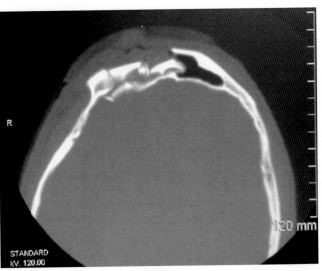

FIGURE 7 Axial computed tomography image demonstrating a bilateral frontal sinus fracture involving both the anterior and posterior tables without pneumocephalus.

the anterior and posterior walls of the frontal sinus are resistant to significant forces of impact. Thick cortical bone, which is characteristic of the frontal sinus, protects the frontal bone, making it the strongest of the bones that make up the facial skeleton. As a result of this inherent property, frontal sinus fractures are quite rare and account for only 5% to 15% of maxillofacial injuries. Such injuries are most often associated with motor vehicle accidents, athletic events, and assault.

An accurate diagnosis of frontal sinus fracture is key to rapid workup and surgical management. Patients with frontal sinus fractures often complain of forehead pain and headache. A detailed history of the mechanism of injury should be made, as well as other clinical attributes such as presence of clear rhinorrhea or salty taste in the oral cavity in order to evaluate for a CSF leak. If, in fact, a CSF leak is suspected, the fluid should be sent for β_2-transferrin testing. On examination, soft tissue edema and erythema in the area overlying the frontal sinus is quite evident. Additional clinical findings include parathesias in the distribution of the supraorbital and supratrochlear nerves, diplopia, and epistaxis.

Diagnosis of frontal sinus fractures requires CT imaging. Anterior table injury, posterior table injury, and pneumocephalus can be evaluated on axial imaging (Fig. 7). The floor of the frontal sinus and the roof of the bony orbit can be evaluated by coronal imaging.

Several surgical goals exist, including protection of the intracranial contents in posterior table fractures, treatment and prevention of CSF leak, prevention of mucocele or mucopyocele, restoration of aesthetic contour of the forehead, and normal function of the frontal sinus. A well-designed treatment algorithm is based on location of fracture (anterior table, posterior table, both anterior and posterior tables), width of fracture, comminution of fracture, injury to the nasofrontal duct, and persistent CSF leak (Fig. 8). Treatment options include observation, open reduction and internal fixation, endoscopic fracture reduction, sinus obliteration, sinus exenteration, and sinus cranialization.

Complications are often attributed to improper surgical management and can result in aesthetic deformities, chronic sinusitis, pneumocephalus, mucopyocele, meningitis, and brain abscess. Mucoceles are known to form when sinus mucosa is disrupted or injured, which can slowly develop and grow over a number of years after the original injury when many trauma patients have not had long-term follow-up care.

FRONTAL SINUS FRACTURE

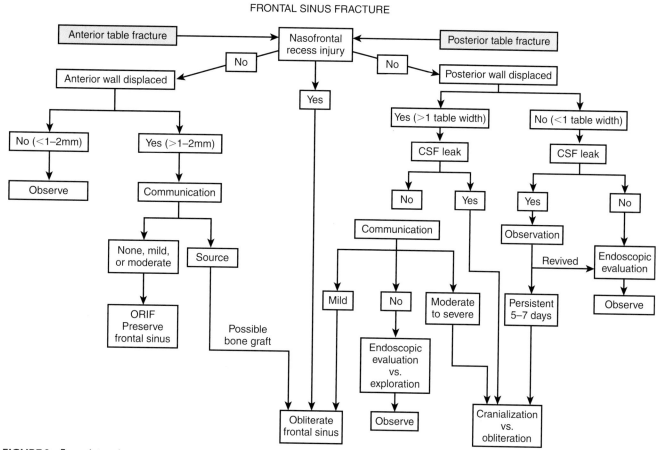

FIGURE 8   Frontal sinus fracture treatment algorithm. CSF, Cerebrospinal fluid; ORIF, open reduction with internal fixation.   *(From Strong BE: Frontal sinus and naso-orbital-ethmoid complex fractures. In Papel I, editor: Facial plastic and reconstructive surgery, 3rd ed, New York, 2009, Thieme Medical Publishers, p 980.)*

Naso-Orbital-Ethmoid Fractures

The naso-orbital-ethmoid (NOE) complex is an intricate anatomic region comprising vital structures including the nasal, lacrimal, ethmoid, maxillary, and frontal bones. Nasal bones can be found attached to the frontal process of the maxilla laterally, and to the frontal bones superiorly. The ethmoid sinuses are located posterior to the paired nasal bones, and separate the orbits from the nasal cavity. The primary horizontal buttresses are the supraorbital rims, and the primary vertical buttress is the frontal process of the maxillary bone. If disruption of either of these paired buttresses occurs, comminution of the entire complex may result.

Medial canthal tendon is the focal point for the NOE complex as it maintains the normal intercanthal distance. A normal intercanthal distance is 30 to 35 mm, which equates to one half of the interpupillary distance or is equal to the alar base of the nose. It arises from the anterior and posterior lacrimal crests and the frontal process of the maxilla.

Fractures of the NOE complex can be diagnosed clinically. Integrity of the medial canthal tendon should be examined by applying lateral tension to each lower lid. A medial canthal tendon that does not have much tensile force, or is the presence of significant medial wall motion, is consistent with a NOE complex fracture. Other clinical findings can be evaluated such as telecanthus, enophthalmos, midface retrusion, pupillary response, and extraocular motion.

Thin-cut CT imaging as well as three-dimensional reconstructions are helpful in defining the pattern of injury as well as providing a useful tool in surgical planning. Areas to focus on during imaging include the cribriform plate, frontal recess, orbit, degree of comminution of the NOE complex, and any other associated facial fractures.

A classification scheme was designed to further describe the degree of bony injury after NOE complex fracture. Such a system is useful in describing the type of injury to the NOE complex. It also helps in the surgical planning of the repair (Fig. 9). The central fragment of bone to which the medial canthal tendon inserts is the anatomic focal point in NOE complex reconstruction. Type I fractures occur when a large central fragment of bone containing the medial canthal ligament is isolated from the surrounding bone. A type II fracture entails significant comminution of that fragment containing the medial canthal ligament. In type III, there is significant comminution, as in type II, but the tendon is detached from that fragment of comminuted bone. Such fractures are extremely uncommon.

It is agreed upon by most experts that the surgical repair of NOE complex fractures are among the most challenging to repair of all fractures of the facial skeleton. An unsatisfactory repair will result in poor surgical exposure, imprecise reduction of fractures, or a poor repair of the medial canthal tendon. Ideal surgical exposure can be achieved through a coronal, midface degloving, glabella, or open sky incision. Once the fracture lines are adequately exposed, a combination of transnasal wires and microplates can be used, depending on the degree of comminution.

Blindness, telecanthus, enophthalmos, CSF leak, and anosmia are all potential complications of injury to the NOE complex. Additionally, more benign complications may also arise including sinusitis, epiphora, and a long-term nasal deformity.

Type I Fracture

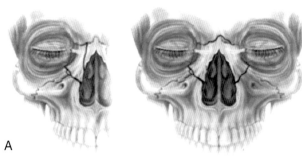

A

Type II Fracture

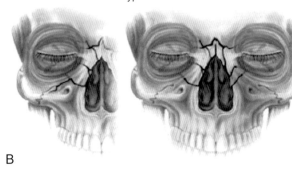

B

Type III Fracture

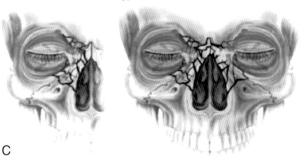

C

FIGURE 9   Patterns of type I (**A**), II (**B**), and III (**C**) naso-orbital-ethmoid fractures. *(From Strong BE: Frontal sinus and naso-orbital-ethmoid complex fractures. In Papel I, editor:* Facial plastic and reconstructive surgery, *3rd ed, New York, 2009, Thieme Medical Publishers, p 989.)*

CONCLUSIONS

Traumatic injury to the maxillofacial skeleton is an injury that requires the clinician to have an extensive knowledge of the three-dimensional anatomy of the face. Once this has been mastered, a systematic approach must be followed in the assessment of the facial trauma patient, and a specific management algorithm must be followed. The principles of bone healing are an important part in the management of maxillofacial trauma. With such knowledge, the use of plating systems for open reduction and internal fixation has been shown to provide superior functional and improved aesthetic results. The ultimate goal in the workup and repair is to restore premorbid function as well as achieve an acceptable aesthetic result. Nonetheless, facial trauma often occurs in the setting of other life-threatening injuries, which should not be overlooked. Facial injuries, although often traumatic, are rarely life threatening. Early initial evaluation and management are extremely important to avoiding significant patient morbidity.

For the chapter's Suggested Readings list, please visit the book at www.ExpertConsult.inkling.com.

TRAUMA TO THE EYE AND ORBIT

Mario A. Meallet and Bibiana J. Reiser

Trauma centers and emergency physicians are frequently confronted with evaluating and managing severe eye injuries, most of which will require immediate consultation and referral to an ophthalmologist. We hope to describe the types of ocular emergencies that can be managed by the emergency and trauma physician, and clearly illustrate the techniques employed. When facial fractures are limited to the orbital bones, an ophthalmology evaluation is sufficient to develop a management plan. In more extensive fractures involving the nasopharynx, skull, maxilla, and mandible, a more collaborative approach with the aid of plastic surgery, ophthalmology, head and neck, and oral-maxillofacial surgery may be needed. The decision for appropriate triage is made within the emergency department and we hope to provide useful guidelines to aid in decision making (Fig. 1).

Direct injury to the eye requires the immediate involvement of eye care providers. Severely injured patients are often unable to cooperate with extensive ocular examination, and management decisions will be based on objective eye findings. In obvious open

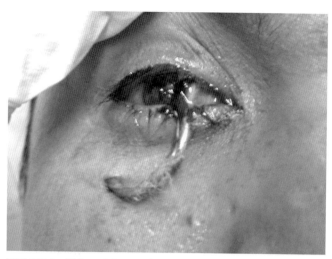

FIGURE 1   Nail gun injury to the eye.

globe injuries, the emergency physician and the trauma surgeon can aid in obtaining a clear history of the injury and making the prompt decision for radiologic evaluation. When an intraocular foreign body (IOFB) is suspected, or a thorough history cannot be elicited, an immediate orbital computed tomography (CT) scan should be obtained. A Fox shield should be placed over the eye for protection and the remainder of the evaluation and management should be deferred to an ophthalmologist. In particular, the emergency medical physician should defer performing a slit-lamp examination and absolutely avoid measurement of intraocular pressure. The patient should also be asked to avoid maneuvers that may cause intraocular hemorrhage, such as coughing or Valsalva maneuver, and be urged to rest quietly until the wound has been repaired.

When an open globe is not clearly obvious, a full ocular examination is carried out in a methodical and rational fashion, beginning with gross external inspection and visual acuity measurement in each eye, independently. Optic nerve function is assessed by testing for a relative afferent pupillary defect (APD), and if appropriate, intraocular pressure is measured and a careful slit-lamp examination is performed. Dilated funduscopic examination can only be performed by trained personnel and can be left to the ophthalmologist. If the combination of clinical findings and ancillary testing is not clearly indicative of an open globe injury, but the suspicion remains high, then formal exploration under anesthesia is recommended. Photo-documentation is recommended whenever feasible. Prompt management by the initial emergency and trauma surgeons can have a profound impact on the ultimate visual function of these patients, and familiarity with the various types of urgent eye injuries will promote a system of ideal triage (Fig. 2).

INCIDENCE

Ocular trauma in the United States occurs at an estimated rate of 2 million eye injuries per year (7 per 1000 population). Data gathered by McGwin et al from national ambulatory care surveys and hospital discharge records reveal that most eye injuries in the United States are treated in emergency departments (50.7%), followed by private physicians' offices (38.7%), and outpatient (8.1%) and inpatient (2.5%) facilities. Demographic analysis of the highest-risk groups reveals that eye injury rates are highest among males in their 20s, with no clear difference among ethnic groups.

The rate of eye injury begins to climb later in childhood, with peak incidence in the third decade, followed by a slow decline. A second peak occurs with very advanced age. This bimodal incidence in younger and older adults, as well as higher rates in males, is a reflection of the types of high-risk activities younger males engage in and the

FIGURE 2   Anatomy of the eye. *(Artistic rendering by Narina Sokolova.)*

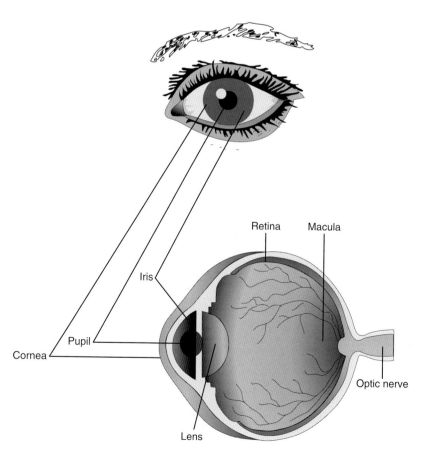

propensity for injuries and falls seen in older adults. These trends apply to injuries in these groups in general.

The setting in which an injury occurs has a marked impact on the severity and the prognosis for visual recovery. A study on the rate of eye injuries in the workplace reported that open globe injuries were the most common (46%), followed by injury to the surrounding ocular adnexal structures (20%), orbital fractures (11%), and traumatic hyphemas (11%). Interestingly, the vast majority (approximately 90%) of eye injuries occur in settings in which protective eyewear can have a major impact (e.g., workplace, sports activities, such as baseball, paintball, and airlift gun play). In fact, in many of these settings, eyewear is mandated but is not being worn at the time of injury. Thus, it is estimated that up to 90% of eye injuries could be prevented if protective eyewear were worn in these settings.

Of the small number of eye injuries related to motor vehicle accidents (estimated at 1.8% of all eye injuries in the United States), very few present as open globe injuries. The mandated use of seatbelts has resulted in a twofold decrease in the number of eye injuries. Curiously, this reduction has been offset by a twofold increase in eye injuries in accidents in which airbags have been deployed. The most frequent injury mechanism related to motor vehicle accidents is impact with the windshield, followed by the airbag, steering wheel, and flying glass. However, these statistics must be viewed in the context of the decreased number of fatalities with the advent of airbag and seatbelt use.

Overall, only a small percentage (2.3%) of eye injuries encountered in the emergency setting present as lacerations and punctures (Table 1 and Fig. 3). The most common causes of eye injuries in this

TABLE 2: Key Mechanisms of Eye Injury in Emergency Setting

Mechanism of Eye Injury	Frequency (%)
Foreign body	44.6
Blunt trauma	33.0
Fire/burn	12.0
Machinery	3.1
Motor vehicle accident	2.3
Fall	1.8
Firearm	< 1.0

Modified from McGwin G Jr, Owsley C: Incidence of emergency department-treated eye injury in the United States. *Arch Ophthalmol* 123:662–666, 2005.

setting are foreign bodies (44.6%) and blunt trauma (33.0%) (Table 2 and Fig. 4). In the subgroup of patients with blunt trauma, many of these injuries represent ruptures of the sclera that may not be clearly obvious to the examiner. In these cases, the examiner must rely on the key clinical findings associated with occult scleral rupture, as outlined in the later section on diagnosis. Werner et al reported on these occult scleral ruptures and found that they can represent up to 25% of all potential ruptured globes that present to physicians. Of these suspected cases of occult rupture, roughly one third were actually found to have eye ruptures at the time of surgical exploration.

There is a significant association of orbital fractures found in patients presenting with head trauma. In a large study of 4426 U.S. Army soldiers with facial and orbital fractures, orbital floor fractures were found in 26%. Within this group, there was also a 30% incidence of injury to the globe and a 70% incidence of concomitant bodily injury. Fractures of the orbital floor and medial wall make up the majority of fractures, with the lateral wall being the third most likely site of fracture and a smaller number of fractures occurring in the orbital roof (Fig. 5). The floor is most susceptible just medial to the infraorbital groove, whereas the medial wall is most likely to rupture at the lamina papyracea, a paper-thin bony septum.

TABLE 1: Posttraumatic Eye Findings in Emergency Setting

Type of Eye Injury	Frequency (%)
Contusion/abrasion	44.6
Foreign body	30.8
Conjunctivitis	10.2
Hemorrhage	9.9
Laceration	1.8
Puncture	0.5

Modified from McGwin G Jr, Owsley C: Incidence of emergency department-treated eye injury in the United States. *Arch Ophthalmol* 123:662–666, 2005.

FIGURE 3   Posttraumatic eye findings in the emergency setting (see Table 1). *(Data from McGwin G Jr, Owsley C: Incidence of emergency department-treated eye injury in the United States.* Arch Ophthalmol *123:662–666, 2005.)*

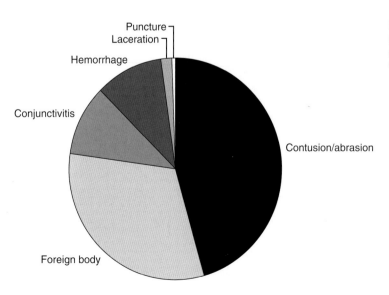

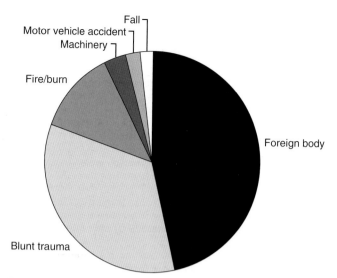

FIGURE 4   Key mechanisms of eye injury in the emergency setting (see Table 2). *(Data from McGwin G Jr, Owsley C: Incidence of emergency department-treated eye injury in the United States. Arch Ophthalmol 123:662–666, 2005.)*

MECHANISM OF INJURY

The mechanisms of injury to the eye and surrounding structures are largely associated with foreign bodies, blunt trauma, and thermal and chemical burns. Machinery, motor vehicle, and firearms are among the less common causes (see Table 2 and Fig. 4). There is often appreciable overlap, and the physician must consider the impact of these mechanisms in combination and treat each injury individually. For example, a ruptured globe from blunt trauma may require a short course of systemic steroids for traumatic optic neuropathy if an APD is noted. Blunt force on an eye can also be described as coup–contrecoup, or compressive force in a manner similar to brain injury. Examples of coup injuries are corneal abrasions, subconjunctival hemorrhages, choroidal hemorrhages, and retinal necrosis. Another example of a coup injury is hyphemas resulting from iridodialysis (shearing off of the iris root) or iris injury from impact from paintball and airsoft gun pellets (Fig. 6). The best example of a contrecoup injury is commotio retinae, with anterior forces being transmitted to the retina and causing shearing of the retinal layers. Compression of the globe usually causes scleral rupture. These open globe injuries are described later.

Orbital fractures can be caused by blunt forces with an increase of intraorbital pressure resulting in blowout fractures of the medial wall and floor, or caused by direct injury to the bones of the face resulting in fracture of any of the four walls. Because the lateral wall and roof are the most resistant to fracture, injury of these bones is an indicator of significant force to the face and eyes, and concomitant injury to the globe should be carefully evaluated. Foreign body penetration of the orbit can involve the eye directly or any of the surrounding structures.

Chemical and thermal injuries to the eyelids and adnexa must be evaluated over the long term, well beyond the healing period for the superficial tissues. Burns to the eyelids and skin lead to scarring and contraction of the eyelids, which place these patients at risk for eyelid retraction and exposure damage to the cornea and ocular surface. Thus, long-term follow-up is important in this patient group, particularly if they are in a critical care setting. They must be treated with aggressive lubrication to the eyes until they demonstrate an ability to blink voluntarily and protect the eye. It is urged that all intensive care units and trauma wards have written eye care protocols for the management of these patients.

Open globe injuries are classically divided into penetrating and nonpenetrating injuries. The latter group is caused by blunt trauma that causes a forceful compression of the eye and results in the physical rupture of the eye wall. The location of the rupture is typically in the areas where the eye wall is the thinnest, namely, the corneoscleral junction (the limbus), at the muscle insertion sites, and at the posterior attachment of the optic nerve. Ruptures posterior to the limbus may be difficult to identify and the clinician must be familiar with the signs of occult rupture, which are described in the section on diagnosis.

FIGURE 5   Diagram of orbital bones with incidence of orbital fractures. *(From Yanoff M, Duker JS: Ophthalmology, 2nd ed. St. Louis, Mosby, 2004, fig. 83-1; Data from Shere JL, Boole JR, Holtel MR, Amoroso PJ: An analysis of 3599 midfacial and 1141 orbital blowout fractures among 4426 United States Army soldiers, 1980–2000. Otolaryngol Head Neck Surg 130:164–170, 2004.)*

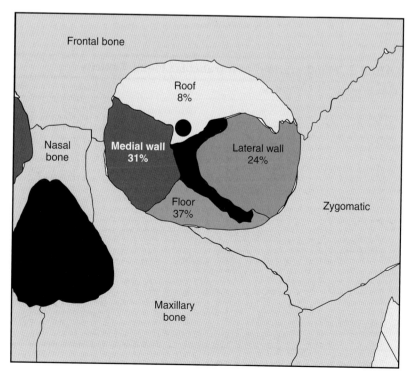

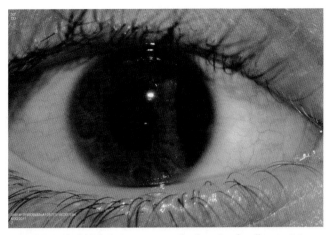

FIGURE 6 Iridodialysis in a young male after airsoft pellet gun injury to the right eye. On presentation, a dense hyphema prevented visualization of the iris.

When the mechanism of injury involves penetration of the globe, the site of entry is usually visible and the decision for surgical intervention is straightforward. The three variables to consider when an entry wound is identified are: (1) whether the penetrating object has exited the eye, (2) whether a foreign body is within the eye, or (3) whether it has passed through the entire eye (perforation), in which case a posterior exit wound should be suspected and the foreign body may be located within the orbit.

If there is evidence of an intraocular or intraorbital foreign body, the type of material may also have implications in toxicity to the eye and the risk of infection to the orbit and the eye (Table 3). When the history of the type of injury is unclear, an orbital CT should be requested immediately and a shield placed over the eye. Even if the foreign body is easily accessible and protruding from the eye or surrounding structures, the emergency or trauma surgeon should make no attempt to remove the object. A shield should be carefully placed over the eye and no manipulation attempted. The extent of injury can be assessed at the time of surgical repair.

DIAGNOSIS

Orbital Trauma

The key clinical features that aid in the decision for urgent management in cases of orbital trauma involve (1) significant limitation of ocular motility, (2) the presence of an APD, (3) the presence of proptosis (abnormal anterior bulging of the eye), and (4) the presence of enophthalmos (abnormal posterior displacement of the eye). Any of these features requires an immediate orbital CT scan, ophthalmologic evaluation, and consideration of surgical intervention. In a study by Lee et al on the role of CT in orbital trauma, of those patients who suffered visual loss secondary to orbital trauma, the causes in order of decreasing frequency were retrobulbar hemorrhage, optic nerve thickening presumably secondary to edema, intraorbital emphysema, optic nerve impingement, retinal detachment, and ruptured globe. In addition to assessing the findings described previously the clinician should palpate the orbital rim for fractures (step-offs) and assess for hypoesthesia just below the eye in the distribution of the infraorbital nerve, and note the presence of hypoglobus (inferior displacement of the eye). Presence of hypoesthesia is indicative of a blowout fracture involving the infraorbital canal and nerve, but it has no urgent significance in itself.

Evaluation of ocular motility involves assessing for limitation of eye movement and eliciting symptoms consistent with decreased motility. The patient will often complain of double vision that disappears with the occlusion of one eye. Defining the orientation of the diplopia (horizontal, vertical, or oblique) can also help focus the examination. During the acute inflammatory period, ocular motility is often affected because of orbital congestion or muscle contusion, and supplementary tests can help distinguish between muscle palsy and muscle restriction or entrapment. Forced duction testing, when the eye is physically displaced using forceps to grasp the eye, can help discern the presence of mechanical restriction. A drop of anesthetic is placed on the eye and the patient is asked to look in the direction of the limited movement. The eye is then physically displaced in that direction to assess for a "tethering" effect (Fig. 7). If significant resistance is encountered, entrapment must be suspected and an orbital CT should be obtained immediately. Clinical signs of entrapment supported by radiologic evidence require immediate surgical intervention to prevent muscle ischemia and necrosis.

TABLE 3: Manifestations of Intraocular Metal Toxicity

Type of Metal	Cornea	Iris	Lens	Vitreous	Retina	Signs/Symptoms
Iron (siderosis)	Rust-colored corneal stromal staining	Anisocoria/ heterochromia	Flower-shaped cataract	Brownish opacities	Diffuse retinal pigmentation	Night blindness, visual field loss
Copper (<85%) (chronic chalcosis)	Fleischer ring	Greenish discoloration	Sunflower cataract	Brownish red opacities	Metallic flecks on vessels and macula	Progressive vision and field loss
Copper (>85%) (acute chalcosis)	Severe inflammation	Greenish discoloration	Sunflower cataract	Diffuse vitritis	Metallic flecks on vessels	Fulminant inflammation/ loss of eye
Gold	—	—	Anterior capsule deposits	—	—	—
Aluminum/zinc	Minimal inflammation	—	—	—	—	—

Data from Yanoff M, Duker JS: *Ophthalmology*, 2nd ed, St. Louis, 2004, Mosby.

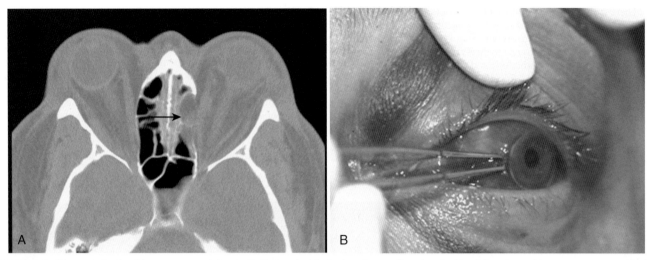

FIGURE 7   Young male after blunt trauma to left eye. **A,** Patient had limited ocular motility when looking left and possible entrapment on orbital computed tomography *(arrow)*. **B,** Forced duction testing revealed full abduction, and entrapment was ruled out.

The finding of posttraumatic proptosis requires immediate measurement of eye pressures to assess for retrobulbar hemorrhage. Proptosis and elevated intraocular pressures are indicative of an orbital compartment syndrome and an axial and coronal orbital CT should be obtained immediately (Fig. 8). The findings on further examination are resistance to retropulsion, diffuse subconjunctival hemorrhage, tight eyelids and orbit, vision loss, an APD, and decreased color vision. Medical therapy should be initiated immediately with pressure-lowering agents as described in the management section in this chapter, and intraocular pressure should be measured frequently to ensure the efficacy of the medical therapy. If the pressures are very high (>30 mm Hg) or if there is no response to medical therapy, a lateral canthotomy and cantholysis should be performed (described under Medical and Surgical Management). This procedure can be performed prior to obtaining an orbital CT if pressures are significantly elevated and there is evidence of an APD.

The presence of an APD should prompt an immediate orbital CT to rule out the presence of bone fragments or a foreign body within the orbit impinging on the optic nerve. With evidence of this type of compression, immediate surgery must be performed to relieve the pressure on the nerve. In the absence of impingement on the optic nerve and absence of obvious lesions of the anterior visual pathway, an APD is highly suggestive of traumatic optic neuropathy and a 3-day course of intravenous (IV) steroids should be instituted.

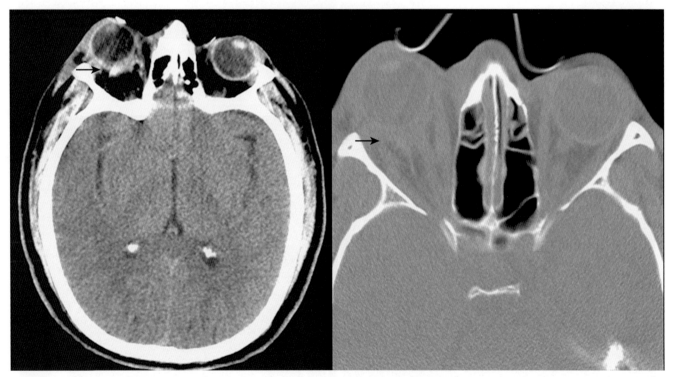

FIGURE 8   Male victim of blunt trauma to the right eye with significant proptosis and radiodensity posterior to the right eye on computed tomography scan (retrobulbar hemorrhage indicated by *arrows*). His intraocular pressure was measured to be 40 mm Hg and was rapidly lowered to 20 mm Hg with a lateral canthotomy and cantholysis.

There is a wide variety of imaging modalities that can be used to visualize the orbit and surrounding bony architecture. The standard head CT consisting of 4-mm sections that is obtained in the emergency setting is often inadequate to assess orbital trauma. The subtle findings of trauma to the orbit, eye, and visual pathway require evaluation with 2-mm axial and coronal sections extending from the eyelids to the optic chiasm. However, signs on the routine head CT that are suggestive of orbital fracture include opacification of the paranasal sinuses, periorbital subcutaneous emphysema, and surrounding soft tissue edema. Presence of these features should prompt the attainment of a full orbital series. The key features of a variety of important CT findings are highlighted in Figures 9 through 11.

Ocular Trauma

The most crucial aspect in evaluating direct trauma to the eye is in determining the presence of an open globe injury. With penetrating injuries, the site of rupture is usually obvious at examination and darkly pigmented uveal structures (iris and choroid) can be seen protruding through the wound (Fig. 12). This can usually be seen at the bedside with the use of a penlight. With a reliable history that the penetrating object was removed from the eye intact, radiologic studies can be deferred. Given a history of a foreign body entering the eye, an orbital CT consisting of 2-mm axial and coronal sections should be obtained immediately. In this scenario, magnetic resonance

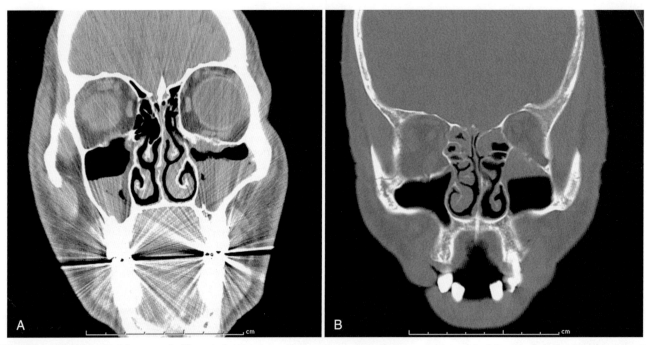

FIGURE 9 Bilateral orbital fractures. **A,** Note air-fluid levels in maxillary sinuses and soft tissue prolapse of the left orbit. **B,** Left orbital fracture with orbital fat prolapse.

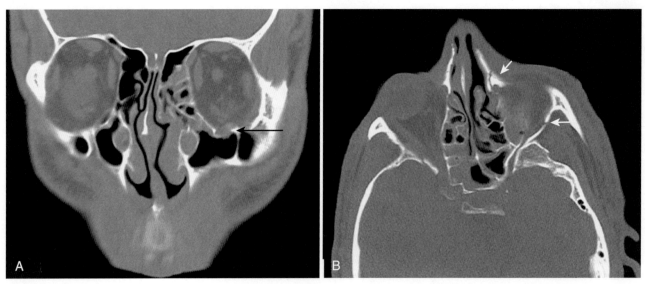

FIGURE 10 Left orbital fracture with muscle entrapment. **A,** The radiopaque muscle can be seen protruding into the "trapdoor" of the fracture *(arrow)*. **B,** Fracture of nasal bone and lateral orbital wall *(arrows)*. The eye was intact in this case.

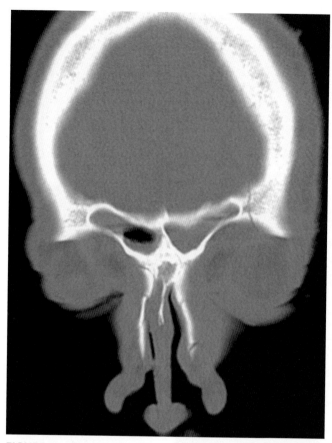

FIGURE 11 Coronal view of fracture through roof of the left orbit.

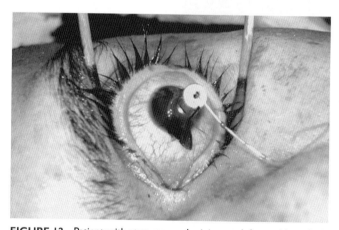

FIGURE 12 Patient with stun-gun probe injury to left eye. Note dark uveal tissue protruding from the cornea. This patient's eye was immediately covered with a cup and he was sent to the eye clinic for further management.

imaging (MRI) is contraindicated as it may cause movement of a metallic object. The eye should be covered with a shield immediately and the remainder of the examination performed by an ophthalmologist, possibly under general anesthesia at the time of surgical repair. The diagnosis of a ruptured globe should not be made by CT alone, although the status of the eye can often be assessed based on its appearance on CT scan (Fig. 13). There is a proven decrease in the rate of infection with prompt diagnosis and repair. The risk of posttraumatic sympathetic ophthalmia must be considered in all ruptured globes. This condition, in which the injured "inciting" eye stimulates the formation of antibodies that can then attack the noninjured

"sympathizing" eye and cause a severe sight-threatening inflammation in the healthy eye, is estimated to be as high as 1 in 500 following an open globe injury.

The most likely areas of rupture from blunt trauma to the eye are the sites where the eye wall is thinnest, namely at the corneoscleral junction (the limbus), at the rectus muscle insertions, and at the attachment of the optic nerve to the eye (Fig. 14). However, the sclera may rupture posterior to the limbus in a manner that is not clearly obvious by standard slit-lamp examination. In these difficult cases, the examiner must rely on the cardinal features of occult scleral rupture to determine the need for surgical exploration of the eye. Werner et al studied 49 eyes with suspected scleral rupture and found that the factors most indicative of true rupture, as determined by surgical exploration, were visual acuity worse than 20/400, lower intraocular pressure in the traumatized eye, the presence of hyphema, an APD, and vitreous hemorrhage. In using these criteria, 17 of 49 patients were found to have true ruptures at surgical exploration. The presence of hemorrhagic chemosis and a peaked pupil has also been found to be sensitive in determining the presence of occult scleral rupture. These data are similar to those of Kylstra et al. The clinical finding of vitreous hemorrhage can only be confirmed by the trained ophthalmologist, often requiring ultrasound examination. This finding is important in the development of proliferative vitreoretinopathy, a fibrous proliferation within the vitreous that causes traction on the retina and predisposes to complicated retinal detachment, as established by Cleary and Ryan. When taken in combination, these findings are very useful in guiding the decision for exploration and repair of a suspected scleral rupture. Figures 15 and 16 illustrate three of these key findings. Their sensitivities and specificities are summarized in Table 4.

Two particularly important subgroups of open eye injuries are those involving IOFBs and the infected open eye. The presence of a foreign body places the patient at greater risk of infection and toxicity, and often requires emergent vitreoretinal surgery to salvage the eye. The materials can range from metals to wood and other organic objects. Orbital CT is very sensitive in detecting metallic foreign bodies (Fig. 17); however, ultrasound examination should be performed on all eyes with suspected IOFB. With an obvious corneal laceration and a history of a small solid projectile to the eye, the anterior chamber angle must be carefully inspected with gonioscopic techniques.

If there is evidence of wound contamination at the time of examination (e.g., injury with plant matter), the concern for infection becomes very acute and must be managed aggressively. Posttraumatic endophthalmitis has been reported to occur in approximately 4% to 8% of open globe injuries and in up to 30% of injuries in a rural setting. The classic finding of hypopyon in an infected eye is not commonly seen in the context of a ruptured globe, as the anterior segment is often distorted and obscured by blood. The role of the trauma and emergency physician in this setting is, as with all other open globes, to obtain in immediate ophthalmology consult and obtain an urgent orbital CT. Further management requires the expertise of eye care providers.

One of the most useful modalities in evaluating globe rupture is ultrasound. Marked lid swelling and patient discomfort often make evaluating ocular trauma very difficult, and the examiner must take the utmost care not to further disturb the open eye. Skilled use of the ultrasound can yield sufficient information on the status of the intraocular contents and on the presence of IOFBs. The eye can be examined from the cornea to the optic nerve, through closed eyelids with virtually no pressure exerted on the globe. In the presence of hyphema or vitreous hemorrhage, the posterior pole of the eye may be difficult to view, in which case an ultrasound examination may allow thorough evaluation. Posterior scleral rupture usually presents with marked hemorrhagic chemosis and vitreous hemorrhage (Figs. 18 and 19). These cases are typically occult with no external signs of rupture and normal intraocular pressure. A clue to the trajectory and ultimate location of an IOFB is the presence

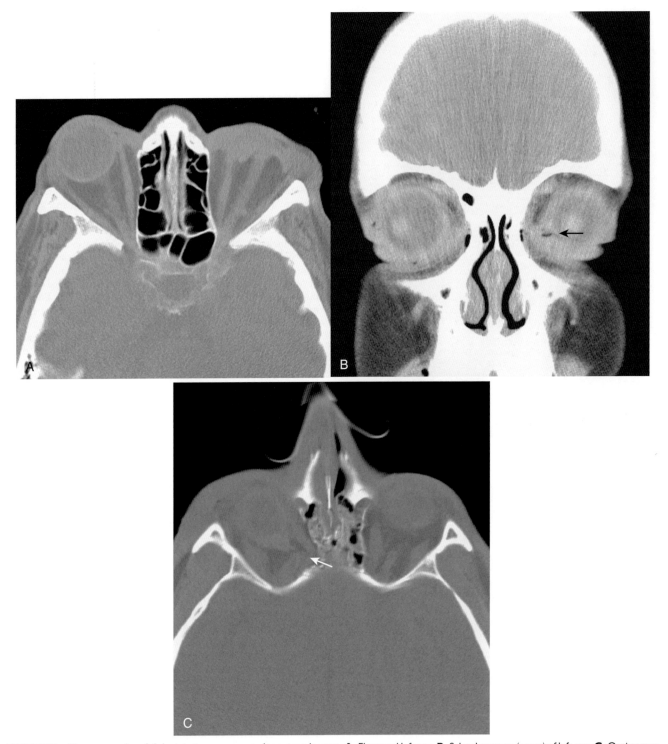

FIGURE 13 Three examples of globe injuries on computed tomography scan. **A,** Flattened left eye. **B,** Scleral rupture *(arrow)* of left eye. **C,** Optic nerve avulsion *(arrow)* of right eye.

of a hemorrhagic tract as seen on ultrasound. By following this tract, the foreign body and its path of destruction can be tracked and defined (Fig. 20). Ultrasound examination should be performed on all forms of IOFBs, even if the foreign body has been previously localized on orbital CT (see Fig. 20). Ultrasound has the advantage of more precisely localizing the position of a foreign body, in assessing the intraocular contents, and in detecting foreign bodies that are not readily visible on CT scan, such as wood, glass, and plastic. Moreover, with a foreign body that is adjacent to the scleral wall,

ultrasound is able to determine whether it lies just inside or outside the globe.

Chemical and thermal burns are often associated with open eye injuries or can occur in isolation. The mainstay of treatment is copious irrigation and treatment with topical steroids and antibiotics. However, in the presence of an open globe, repair of the rupture is of primary importance and should then be followed by management of the chemical and thermal injury. The pH of the ocular surface should be tested with litmus paper and irrigation initiated promptly

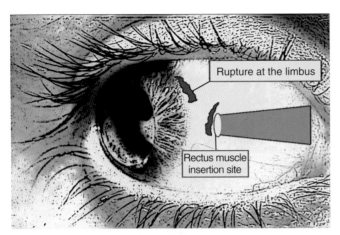

FIGURE 14   The most likely areas of rupture from blunt trauma to the eye. *(Artistic rendering by Narina Sokolova.)*

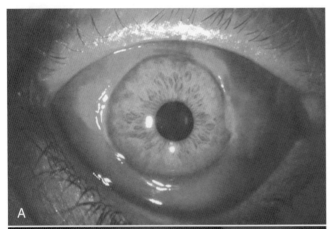

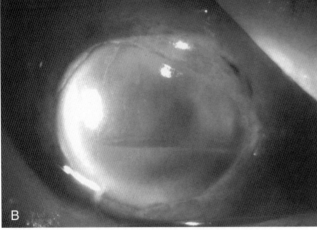

FIGURE 15   A, Hemorrhagic chemosis. Note that the conjunctiva is elevated and boggy, not flat as seen with subconjunctival hemorrhage, a benign condition. **B,** Hyphema of 45% elevation. These are both indicators of occult scleral rupture.

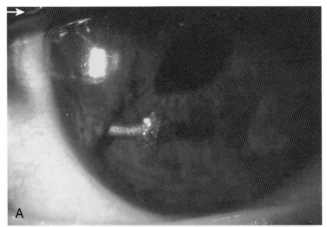

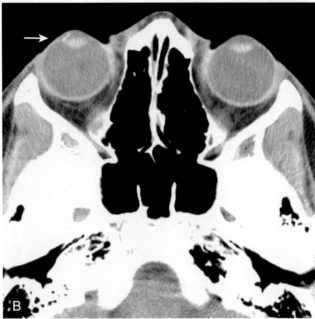

FIGURE 16   A and **B,** Patient with pencil lead penetration into globe (note the "peaked" pupil). Orbital computed tomography scan reveals that foreign body does not extend beyond the anterior chamber *(arrows).*

TABLE 4: Sensitivity and Specificity of Specific Signs in Detecting Eye Rupture

Finding	Sensitivity (%)	Specificity (%)
Vision worse than 20/400	88	47
Intraocular pressure in nontraumatized eye > intraocular pressure in traumatized eye	71	61
Hyphema	69	55
Afferent pupillary defect	80	56
Vitreous hemorrhage	93	38

Modified from Werner MS, Dana MR, Viana MA, Shapiro M: Predictors of occult scleral rupture. *Ophthalmology* 101:1941–1944, 1994.

with a Morgan lens. Between each liter of irrigation, the pH should be reassessed and irrigation continued until the pH becomes neutral. The upper and lower fornices should be swept with a cotton swab for crystallized particles if the pH does not neutralize and lid eversion may be required to remove the particles.

Acids and bases have very distinct effects on the ocular surface. Acids tend to cause denaturation and precipitation of proteins within

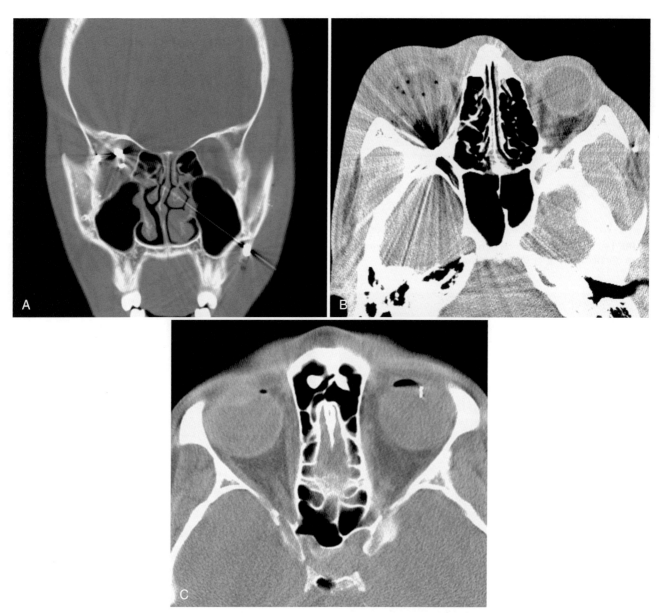

FIGURE 17 **A** and **B,** Shotgun pellets in right eye. **C,** Metallic foreign body and air in anterior chamber of left eye.

the cornea and sclera, and a proteinaceous barrier is formed that prevents the further penetration of acids into the deeper layers. Acidic compounds rarely penetrate into the anterior chamber to cause further damage. On the other hand, bases have the capacity to saponify the superficial lipophilic layers of the cornea and readily penetrate the deeper tissues, frequently causing damage to the intraocular structures and leading to glaucoma and cataract. The eye can appear unusually quiet and the severity of the burn is overlooked. The rule of thumb in these cases is that the quieter the appearance after a chemical burn, the worse the prognosis. This is due to the fact that the vasculature of the ocular surface has been obliterated and the eye will be deceptively blanched in appearance. Over time, the ocular surface becomes inflamed and scarred (Fig. 21). These cases require extensive ocular surface reconstruction, glaucoma surgery, and transplantation of the cornea to regain visual function. Aggressive irrigation within the first few minutes and hours has the most profound impact on the final outcome. Treatment with topical antibiotics and steroids in the first few days is of paramount importance. This is often initiated in the emergency/trauma setting and can be done well before the patient is seen by an eye care provider.

ANATOMIC LOCATION OF INJURY AND INJURY GRADING—OCULAR TRAUMA CLASSIFICATION GROUP

In 1996, the Ocular Trauma Classification Group established a classification of ocular trauma to standardize the definitions for physicians and researchers. One of the goals of this process was to promote the use of trauma-specific terminology in describing eye injuries. This classification applies to both closed and open globe injuries (Table 5). Pieramici et al studied the prognostic significance of this system for classifying mechanical injuries of the eye. The four specific variables in the classification system include: (1) the mechanism of injury, (2) the visual acuity in the injured eye at initial examination, (3) the presence or absence of an APD in the injured eye, and (4) the location of the eye-wall opening. These variables were chosen because they have been shown to be prognostic of visual outcome, and they can be assessed clinically on initial examination or during the initial surgical procedure. The location of the eye-wall opening and the presence of an APD had the strongest prognostic value. The

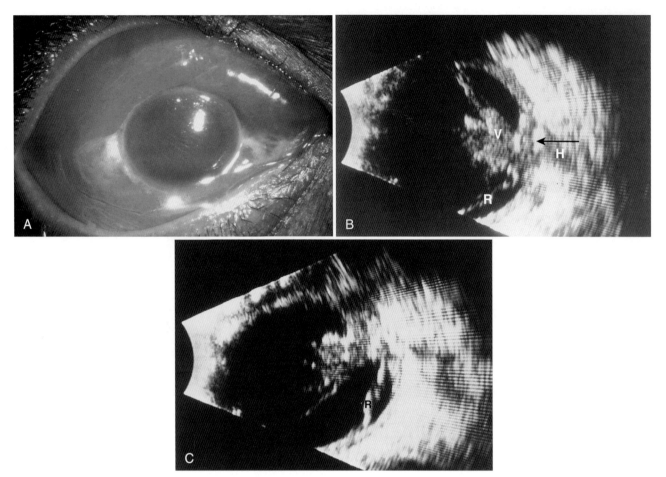

FIGURE 18   Scleral rupture following blunt trauma. **A,** External photograph showing anterior chamber hyphema and hemorrhagic chemosis.
B, Longitudinal B-scan displays vitreous hemorrhage (V), incarceration of vitreous into scleral rupture *(arrow),* and inferior RD (R). **C,** Transverse B-scan
view through area of scleral rupture shows vitreous incarcerated into scleral wound and retinal detachment (R). H, Orbital hemorrhage.   *(From Byrne SF,
Green RL: Ultrasound of the eye and orbit, 2nd ed. St. Louis, 2002, Mosby.)*

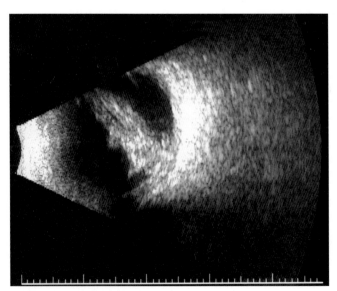

FIGURE 19   Hemorrhagic tract in patient following removal of stun-gun
probe from the eye (see Fig. 11).

key recommendations for the trauma and emergency physician are to
assess for visual acuity and the presence of an APD. However, as previously mentioned, with an obvious rupture, the trauma surgeons and
emergency physicians are urged to cover the eye with a Fox shield and
allow the trained ophthalmologist to perform the remainder of the
examination. With a keen understanding of the findings of closed
and open globe injuries, the trauma surgeons and emergency physicians should be able to appropriately categorize these eye injuries and
aid the eye care provider in making effective medical and surgical
management decisions.

MEDICAL AND SURGICAL MANAGEMENT

Trauma to the Orbit

Conservative medical management of orbital fractures consists of
broad-spectrum oral antibiotics and nasal decongestants, particularly
with CT evidence of disease of the paranasal sinuses or evidence of
foreign body penetration into the orbit. If the patient has no complaints of diplopia and very little restriction of ocular motility, surgical
intervention is not indicated and the patient can be observed weekly.

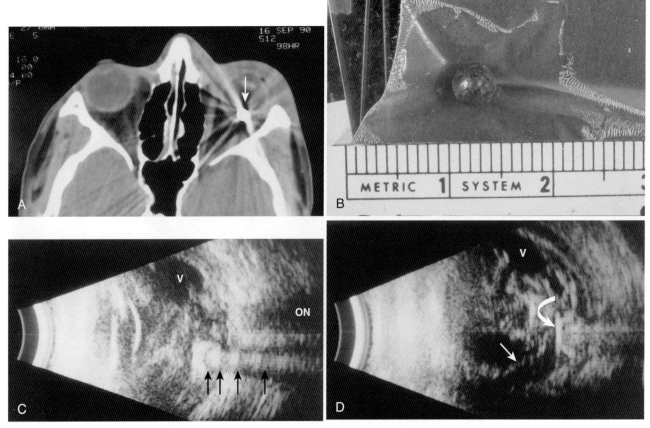

FIGURE 20 Intraocular subretinal BB (gunshot). **A,** Axial computed tomography scan shows spherical foreign body *(straight white arrow)* in vicinity of posterior ocular wall. **B,** Spherical BB removed from eye in A. **C,** Axial B-scan view at high gain shows dense vitreous hemorrhage (V) and large, echo-dense signal from BB. Note the characteristic chain of multiple signals *(comet tail artifact)* produced by BB *(small black arrows)*. **D,** Transverse B-scan at reduced gain shows RD *(straight white arrow)* and underlying BB *(curved white arrow)*. *(From Byrne SF, Green RL: Ultrasound of the eye and orbit, 2nd ed. St. Louis, 2002, Mosby.)*

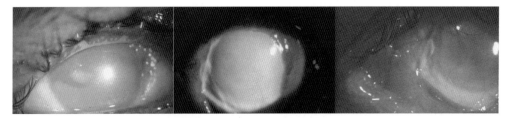

FIGURE 21 Patient with severe alkali burn. Note the white and quiet nature of the eye. The patient has a total corneal epithelial defect as seen with fluorescein stain and cobalt blue light. Despite aggressive management, the patient has a total burn of the ocular surface with extensive inflammation and obliteration of the fornices.

TABLE 5: New Standard Classification of Ocular Trauma Terminology

Term	Definition
Eye wall	Sclera and cornea
Closed-globe injury	Eye wall does not have full-thickness corneal wound
Open-globe injury	Eye wall has full-thickness corneal wound
Rupture	Full-thickness eye wall wound caused by a blunt object; impact results in momentary increase of intraocular pressure and an inside-out injury mechanism
Laceration	Full-thickness wound of eye wall, usually caused by a sharp object; wound occurs at impact site by outside-in mechanism
Penetrating injury	Single laceration of eye wall, usually caused by sharp object
Intraocular foreign body	Retained foreign object(s) causing entrance laceration(s)
Perforating injury	Two full-thickness lacerations (entrance plus exit) of eye wall, usually caused by sharp object or missile

From Ryan S: *Retina*, Vol. 3, 4th ed, St. Louis, 2004, Mosby, p 2380, Table 140-1.

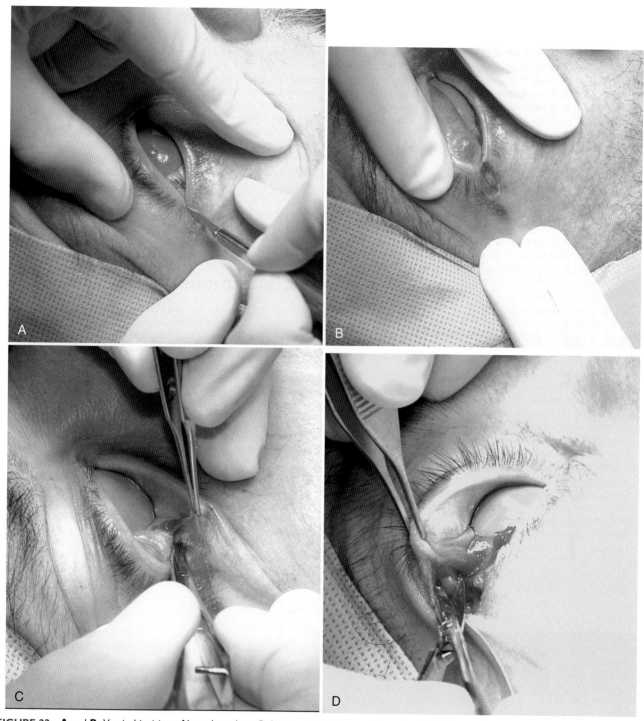

FIGURE 22 **A** and **B,** Vertical incision of lateral canthus. **C,** Incision of inferior canthal tendon. **D,** Incision of superior canthal tendon.

The findings that require immediate repair (within 24 hours) are the white-eyed blowout fracture (normal appearing eye with marked restriction of motility) and fractures with evidence of entrapment clinically and on CT that are associated with nonresolving bradycardia, heart block, nausea, vomiting, or syncope (the oculocardiac reflex). Fractures of the orbital roof, fractures associated with cerebrospinal fluid rhinorrhea, and orbital fractures associated with intracranial hemorrhage require neurosurgical evaluation, and often are repaired collaboratively by neurosurgery and ophthalmology.

Retrobulbar hemorrhage is diagnosed by the presence of significant proptosis and elevated intraocular pressure in the presence of

a tight orbit (very tense eyelids) and evidence of retrobulbar bleeding on orbital CT. If the clinical suspicion is high, a lateral canthotomy and cantholysis can be performed primarily and the orbital CT can be obtained afterward. Performing a lateral canthotomy and cantholysis requires application of local anesthetic and the use of toothed forceps and straight scissors. The lateral orbital rim is palpated and the tissue extending from the lateral canthal angle to the orbital rim is cut in a vertical fashion, splitting the upper and lower connection of the eyelids. The lower lid is grasped with the forceps and tension is placed on the canthal tendon. The tendon can be identified by strumming with scissors and the tendon is cut as close to the orbital rim as possible (Fig. 22). The same approach is taken to locating and incising the upper canthal tendon. Many physicians take a step-wise approach to performing this procedure by cutting the lower canthal tendon and remeasuring the intraocular pressure. If the pressure normalizes by this step alone, cutting the upper canthal tendon can be deferred. Intraocular pressure–lowering agents consisting of IV or oral carbonic anhydrase inhibitors, topical beta blockers, and hyperosmotic agents should be initiated. On completion of this procedure, there is often a release of blood from the retrobulbar space and the eye becomes even more proptotic. However, the result should be the lowering of intraocular pressure and reestablishment of normal blood flow to the eye.

The treatable causes of an APD in cases of trauma include orbital compartment syndrome, mechanical optic nerve compression (by a bone fragment or foreign body), or traumatic optic neuropathy. Central retinal artery occlusion, optic nerve avulsion, and damage to the nerve within the optic canal (fracture or compression within the canal) are less amenable to medical or surgical intervention. Traumatic optic neuropathy is the diagnosis of exclusion once the other causes have been ruled out. If traumatic optic neuropathy is suspected, the recommended treatment involves IV Solu-Medrol, 5.4 mg/kg every 6 hours over 3 days in 12 divided doses. No oral steroid taper is necessary with this regimen. This treatment has been extrapolated from the results of the spinal cord treatment trial, which showed limited benefit for recovery of function in patients who sustained spinal cord injuries when treated with systemic steroids. Studies published in the ophthalmic literature do not conclusively show a benefit of systemic steroids in treating traumatic optic neuropathy, but this approach is widely accepted. Because of the questionable benefit and significant side effect profile, this treatment is used with the utmost caution in young children, the elderly, patients with brittle diabetes, and patients predisposed to infection.

An additional consideration in patients with orbital trauma is the presence of lacerations to the eyelids and surrounding soft tissues. Emergency physicians and trauma surgeons are capable of suturing the majority of these lacerations. Exceptions include lacerations involving the eyelid margin and the lacrimal drainage system (punctum and canaliculus) associated with ptosis (droopy eyelid) and with exposed orbital fat. Repair of these injuries must often be done in the operating room and are often associated with trauma to the eye. Consider tetanus prophylaxis and systemic antibiotics if contamination is suspected (e.g., animal bite). Fast-absorbing suture should be used for the deep aspect of the wound, and slow-absorbing suture for the superficial aspect (e.g., 6-0 Vicryl), particularly if removal after 7 to 10 days proves to be difficult (e.g., children or patients when follow-up may be questionable).

The immediate medical and surgical management of injury to the eye will be directed by the eye care provider. The initial examination by the emergency physicians and trauma surgeons should lead to the rapid decision to obtain an urgent eye consult and to obtain the necessary ancillary tests. Data that will be important to the anesthesiologist are the overall hemodynamic and electrolyte status, pulmonary and neurologic status, and time since last food intake. Also important to the anesthesiologist is to avoid the administration of succinylcholine in the operating room if a ruptured globe is suspected. Depolarizing paralytic agents cause constriction of the extraocular muscles, which may result in the expulsion of the intraocular contents. The repair of lacerations to the eye wall are performed by an ophthalmologist and consists of careful reapproximation of the eye wall in a manner that minimizes the degree of postoperative astigmatism and distortion of the globe and will allow further vitreoretinal surgery if indicated (Fig. 23).

CONCLUSIONS AND ALGORITHM

Although the advanced management of eye injuries requires the experience and training of an ophthalmologist, emergency physicians and trauma surgeons often make the most important decisions in the care of these patients. Following are concise summaries of these key concepts described in this chapter for quick reference. By using this step-wise approach, the critical factors of trauma to the orbit and eye can be documented, and rapid decisions for further management can be made.

The key components of a thorough orbital and ocular examination in the trauma setting are as follows:

1. The initial examination involves the assessment of visual acuity and the presence of an APD. The presence of an APD (even if visual acuity is not severely affected) is a reflection of optic nerve compromise. The potentially treatable causes are retrobulbar hemorrhage with elevated intraocular pressures (orbital compartment syndrome), mechanical compression by a bone fragment or foreign body within the orbit, and traumatic optic neuropathy (nerve contusion). The first two can be diagnosed within the emergency room by the trauma specialist, and the third cause is a diagnosis of exclusion with very few findings on imaging studies. The decision to obtain an orbital CT with 2-mm axial and coronal sections is straightforward in these

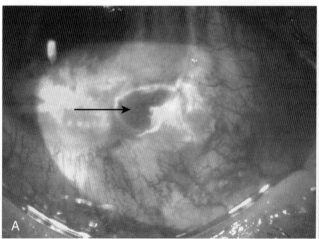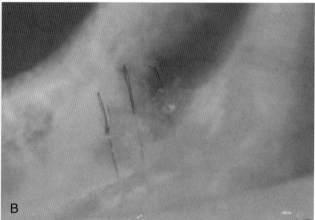

FIGURE 23   A and **B,** Patient shot with blank bullet and suspected plastic shell injury to left eye. Fluorescein stain shows evidence of leak of aqueous at the limbus *(arrow)* with wound extending onto cornea. No extension onto sclera was found on surgical exploration and wound was easily closed with three 10-0 nylon sutures.

cases. If the clinical suspicion for orbital compartment syndrome is high (significant proptosis and elevated intraocular pressure), a lateral canthotomy and cantholysis can be performed prior to obtaining imaging studies and is relatively easy to repair once the condition has been treated. Other causes of an APD that must be ruled out are central retinal artery occlusion, ischemic optic neuropathy, and retinal detachment. These entities are diagnosed only with full examination of the eye.

2. The next step of the examination is to assess for an open globe injury. If rupture or perforation is seen, further examination should be deferred, and the eye should be covered with a shield. An ophthalmologic consult should be obtained immediately and the patient should be started on systemic antibiotics. The patient should be advised to avoid coughing and Valsalva-type maneuvers. Assess for signs of occult rupture: lower intraocular pressure, hyphema, APD, vitreous hemorrhage, hemorrhagic chemosis, and peaked pupil. If rupture is not evident and intraocular pressures are normal, further ocular examination can be safely performed by the trauma physician or the ophthalmologist. Traumatic hyphema is managed with topical steroids and topical atropine 1% for 5 days. The highest rate of rebleeding in cases of traumatic hyphema occurs in the first 5 days and the patient must be seen daily during this time. Intraocular pressure must be monitored closely and the patient is kept on low-dose topical steroids until the hyphema resolves.

3. Evaluation of ocular motility is performed by asking the patient to look in the four main directions of gaze (up, down, left, right) and the eyes are observed for any limitation of movement. The patient should also be asked about double vision either when looking straight or in either direction (the double vision disappears if one eye is covered). If limitation is observed, forced duction testing can be done after placing a drop of topical anesthetic on the eye and asking the patient to look in the same direction of limitation. The physician then attempts to move the eye in the same direction with a forceps. With moderate suspicion of limitation, an immediate orbital CT should be obtained to rule out entrapment of the muscle or orbital fat. Ominous signs of entrapment include bradycardia, nausea, vomiting, and syncope. Also, the quiet appearing eye with significant limitation of movement (the white-eyed blowout) is concerning in children. Oral antibiotics and nasal decongestants are recommended if there is significant disease of the paranasal sinuses (mucosal thickening) on orbital CT.

4. History and presentation consistent with an IOFB require an immediate orbital CT scan consisting of 2-mm axial and coronal sections. An IOFB on CT should prompt an immediate ocular ultrasound to better localize the foreign body and to assess the extent of intraocular injury. Wood, glass, and organic foreign matter is better visualized on ultrasound than orbital CT (i.e., the absence of an obvious IOFB on CT scan does not rule out wood, glass, or organic matter). The ultrasound must be performed by experienced personnel as this must be done with the utmost care so as not to further disrupt the open eye. An immediate eye consult must be obtained and the patient should be started on systemic antibiotics and must remain NPO (nothing by mouth) for anticipated surgery.

5. Evidence of chemical burn requires the measurement of the pH of the ocular surface and initiation of irrigation if an abnormal pH is detected. The physician must be aware that a white, quiet eye following a chemical burn is an ominous sign and must be managed urgently. Continuous irrigation with lactated Ringer's or balanced saline solution is initiated and continued until the repeat pH is normal. Thermal burns must be assessed for direct burn to the eye and managed with antibiotics and lubrication as needed. Burns involving only the eyelids must be monitored until the skin is healed, as contracture may occur and the eye can become exposed. In this setting, lubrication is the mainstay of treatment.

6. The presence of enophthalmos (posterior displacement of the eye) is an indicator of a large fracture of the orbital walls and will require early surgical repair. With a fracture involving more than 50% of the floor, it is assumed that enophthalmos will develop and these patients are scheduled for surgery within 1 to 2 weeks of injury. The other signs of orbital fracture should be thoroughly assessed (hypoesthesia of the cheek below the eye, bony "step-off" of the orbital rim, and limitation of eye movements).

7. A special word of caution with children. If there is a limited examination of the orbit due to inability to cooperate, instead of allowing valuable time to lapse and placing undue pressure on the eye during the examination, do an examination under anesthesia with possible concomitant rupture globe repair.

The points described in this chapter will serve as useful guidelines in assessing the majority of eye trauma cases that present in the emergency room or to trauma surgeons. Additional considerations in the trauma setting involve that of nonaccidental trauma in children (shaken-baby syndrome), Horner syndrome associated with intracranial and neck injury, aneurysmal compressions affecting the cranial nerves to the eye, and the occasional case of carotid-cavernous fistula that can occur in relation to trauma. Although saving the sight of a severely injured patient may seem of secondary concern in the acute setting, it becomes of primary importance once the patient has recovered and is trying to regain normal activity and function.

For the chapter's Suggested Readings list, please visit the book at www.ExpertConsult.inkling.com.

Penetrating Neck Injuries: Diagnosis and Current Management

Leonard J. Weireter, Jr. and L.D. Britt

The neck has been a source of tremendous interest in the trauma surgical literature for several hundred years. Its anatomic compactness places vital anatomic structures in close proximity to each other, making the patient prone to multisystem injuries as the result of a single traumatic event. The debate about the proper treatment of neck trauma has persisted since the 16th century when Ambroise Paré reportedly attended to a victim of a laceration to the common carotid artery and internal jugular vein sustained in a duel. Although Paré's patient survived, he was rendered hemiplegic and aphasic. Complications still highlight discussions today regarding the appropriateness of aggressive surgical management of penetrating cervical injuries.

ANATOMY OF THE NECK

The neck contains a number of vital structures all in close proximity. The carotid artery and the internal jugular vein are juxtaposed immediately deep to the sternocleidomastoid muscle. The pharynx and its junction with the esophagus at the level of the cricopharyngeus musculature are immediately deep to the larynx and the trachea. The thyroid gland and the associated parathyroids are located in the anterior neck overlying the upper trachea. The thoracic duct is well protected as it traverses the neck and enters the jugular-subclavian system in the left side of the neck deep to the sternocleidomastoid muscle. The cervical vertebra and the spinal cord are the most posterior structures, except for the long cervical musculature.

The neck is conventionally divided into a series of triangles. Most surgical discussions center on the anatomy of the anterior triangles that encompass the area between the sternocleidomastoid muscles. Functionally, the neck is divided into three zones (Fig. 1). The boundaries for zone I include the cricoid cartilage (superiorly), the thoracic inlet (inferiorly), and the sternocleidomastoid (laterally). Its surgical significance is the fact that this zone encompasses the major cervicothoracic vasculature, along with components of the aerodigestive tract. Zone III is the horizontal region of the neck cephalad to the angle of the mandible, which superior border is the base of skull. It is important to note that the internal carotid artery, which is cephalad

to the angle of the mandible, is not readily accessible surgically, necessitating special maneuvers to achieve vascular control (e.g., surgical dislocation of the mandible). However, zone II (the area between the cricoid cartilage and the angle of the mandible) is readily accessible with the most direct surgical approach being achieved with an incision along the anterior border of the sternocleidomastoid muscle (Fig. 2).

INITIAL EVALUATION

The initial evaluation of the patient suffering neck injury should be dictated by the Advanced Trauma Life Support guidelines. Such guidelines provide a management framework to expeditiously identify life-threatening injuries and appropriately prioritize treatment. Presentations that warrant urgent surgical intervention, usually referred to as "hard signs" (Table 1) of neck injury, include subcutaneous emphysema, expanding or pulsatile hematoma, or brisk bleeding from the wound. All are overt findings suggestive of a major vascular or aerodigestive tract injury. Diagnostic studies are not essential for these presentations. Optimal airway management is always the first priority.

Without the "hard signs" of injury and, consequently, a need for immediate surgical intervention, a more selective or expectant approach can be initiated. The armamentarium of this selective approach includes multidetector computed tomography (CT) with or without angiography, esophagoscopy, esophagography, laryngoscopy/tracheoscopy, or arteriography. Although subtle findings (so-called soft signs; see Table 1) such as difficulty speaking or change in voice tone could prompt such a selective evaluation, the major controversy centers around whether patients with zone II injury and no "hard findings" should undergo selective management or just observation (expectant management).

A detailed neurologic examination is required for all cervical injuries. Penetrating wounds should never be explored locally. This maneuver should only be done in the operating theater as part of a formal neck exploration. In order to limit patient gagging and coughing, insertion of nasogastric tubes or nasal tracheal suctioning should be withheld, if possible, until the induction of anesthesia in the operating theater.

AERODIGESTIVE INJURY

Simultaneous injuries of the airway and digestive tract are common owing to the close proximity of the trachea and esophagus in the neck. According to Asensio and associates, aerodigestive tract injuries are seen in 10% of penetrating injuries. As highlighted previously, optimal airway management is the top priority.

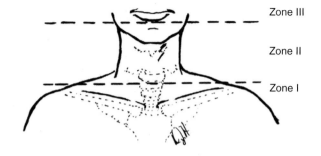

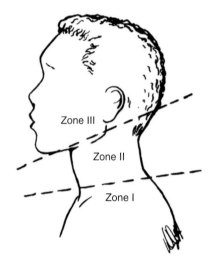

FIGURE 1   Zones of the neck for injury stratification. *(Drawing by Doris Holloman.)*

TABLE 1: Signs of Penetrating Neck Injury

Hard Signs	Soft Signs
Active bleeding	Dysphagia
Expanding or pulsatile hematoma	Voice change
Subcutaneous emphysema or air bubbling from wound	Hemoptysis Wide mediastinum

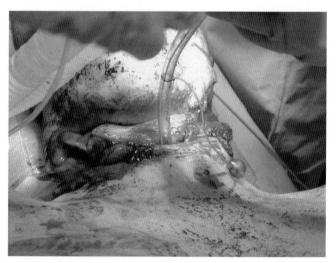

FIGURE 3   Neck wound sustained during an altercation. Note that the airway is established by direct intubation of the lacerated trachea through the wound. Maintaining the patient in the sitting position until intubation is accomplished facilitates airway exposure and minimizes the risk of drowning in secretions.

In a patient who requires urgent airway management, the translaryngeal endotracheal approach is still the best option, particularly when it is performed by skilled practitioners. A surgical airway should always be considered when approaching any patient who might have a difficult airway. Someone who is an expert with airway management should make an attempt at rapid translaryngeal endotracheal intubation. The surgical airway of choice in a true emergency setting is a cricothyroidotomy. A tracheostomy should be considered only in the adult when there is an urgent need for an airway in a patient who you suspect might have a partial laryngotracheal separation.

Even in that setting, an attempt should be made, if possible, by an airway expert to perform a careful translaryngeal endotracheal intubation (Fig. 3).

If a selective management approach is chosen, the available modalities include flexible fiberoptic laryngoscopy, flexible esophagoscopy, flexible bronchoscopy, and contrast esophagography. Using a water-soluble contrast agent and multiple views of the esophagus,

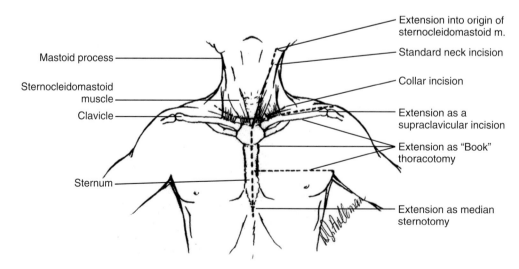

FIGURE 2   Incisions for operative exposure of penetrating neck injuries. *(Drawing by Doris Holloman.)*

extravasation can be safely excluded. The 85% sensitivity and specificity of this study can be increased to near 100% by the addition of esophagoscopy. With increased experience with flexible fiberoptic scopes and enhanced technology, dependence on the use of contrast studies has lessened. Visualization of the proximal 3 to 5 cm of the cervical esophagus immediately inferior to the cricopharyngeal constrictor is critical, for this area can be easily missed during scope insertion and withdrawal. This area has to be specifically inspected.

Although direct laryngoscopy should be used to determine if there is a laryngeal injury, fiberoptic bronchoscopy is used for detection of a tracheal or bronchial injury. Alternatively, CT scan of the neck may identify injuries that require further investigation or operative intervention.

If a tracheal injury is found, it should be repaired by interrupted absorbable suture reapproximating the lacerated trachea after appropriate débridement of devitalized tissue. An accompanying tracheostomy is often not needed unless there is a complex injury.

For suspected laryngeal injuries, fiberoptic endoscopy is the diagnostic procedure of choice and can be combined with surgical exploration depending on the preference of the evaluating team and the suspicion for more severe injury. Laryngeal injury, including the thyroid cartilage, vocal cords, and the arytenoid processes, may require specialized reconstruction. The grading system (Table 2) advocated by Bent et al details their retrospective experience over an 18-year period with laryngeal injuries. The emphasis is on securing an adequate airway and addressing all associated life-threatening injuries. With laryngeal injuries, airway control is best obtained by performing a tracheostomy. Treatment delay in laryngeal injuries beyond 48 hours can lead to inferior results. However, the delay often reflects the fact that the patient is severely injured and is unable to undergo definitive management. Mucosal coaptation and fracture reduction should be performed at the time of initial exploration.

Injury to the cervical esophagus can be difficult to diagnose and may result in the development of a fulminant mediastinitis. Weigelt and associates reported only 7 of 10 injured patients with signs or symptoms of the esophageal injury. The authors noted that there is a false-negative rate of approximately 20% for either endoscopy or esophagography. When the two procedures were combined in evaluation, the false-negative rate decreased to 0%. Armstrong et al reported a retrospective series of 23 patients with penetrating cervical esophageal injury. Contrast esophagograms were only 62% sensitive, but rigid esophagoscopy was 100% sensitive. With advanced fiberoptic technology and greater operative experience, flexible endoscopy has essentially supplanted rigid esophagoscopy.

Most esophageal injuries respond to basic surgical principles. Minimal débridement precedes primary closure, which should be done in two layers. An inner absorbable layer is followed by an outer nonabsorbable suture layer. For concomitant tracheal and esophageal wounds, interposition of viable endogenous tissues, such as muscle flaps, is essential. Complications of treatment, such as esophageal stenosis, tracheoesophageal fistula, and infection are frequent.

Injury to the pharynx, often subtle, requires simple primary repair and drainage.

SOFT TISSUE INJURY

Care of soft tissue follows the same principles of débridement of devitalized skin. Although primary closure can be done, constructing a flap or free tissue graft may be required in order to provide adequate soft tissue coverage, especially in large, open wounds. Penetrating wounds to the thyroid are best controlled by suture ligature, although lobectomy may be warranted depending on the degree of hemorrhage, devascularization, and tissue destruction. Identified injuries to major nerves of the neck or brachial plexus should be tagged for future repair.

THORACIC DUCT INJURY

Injury at the base of the left side of the neck risks laceration of the thoracic duct. Soft tissue injury and bleeding make identifying this injury difficult. Therefore, the classic chylous drainage may not be readily apparent at the time of initial surgical exploration.

VASCULAR INJURY IN THE NECK

In the early 20th century during U.S. military campaigns, major vascular injuries of the neck had very poor outcomes. A 30% neurologic deficit rate was reported after World War I when carotid injuries were treated by ligation. It was not until the 1950s and the military experience in Korea with vascular repair that carotid injury repairs became popular. The superior results were quickly appreciated, and a more aggressive management approach focusing on diagnosis and repair of vascular injuries was established. The first civilian report of carotid injuries appeared in 1956 when Fogelman and Stewart concluded that operative intervention was necessary and that mortality rate increased the longer surgery was delayed. This report was the basis for mandatory exploration of the neck as the standard of care for the next two decades.

Reports challenging the mandatory exploration for penetrating central neck injuries began being widely published in the mid-1970s. Sheely and colleagues reported a series of 632 cases of penetrating neck injuries that still supported mandatory exploration but acknowledged that selected patients might be observed safely, provided they are treated by experienced personnel. Contrary opinion was presented by Saletta et al, who reported a series of 246 patients who underwent mandatory neck exploration. Although the negative exploration rate was high at 63%, morbidity rate was low and there were no fatalities. Although they had negative clinical evaluations, 13 patients had findings at exploration of major injury. Mandatory exploration was thought to be justified. Concurring with this logic, Bishara et al reported a series in which 53% of the patients underwent mandatory exploration and had normal operative findings. However, 23% of the patients had injuries that were not suspected on preoperative clinical evaluation. These were most often isolated venous injuries or isolated pharyngoesophageal injuries. Surgical exploration for a zone II injury was felt to be safe and appropriate. Nevertheless, the high negative exploration rates noted with mandatory neck exploration prompted several institutions to question this approach. Elerding and coworkers reported a series with a 56% negative exploration rate on the basis of a mandatory exploration policy. All the patients with injuries were noted to have clinical signs suggestive of injury preoperatively. Selective exploration was felt to be a legitimate option in the evaluation and management of these patients.

TABLE 2: Laryngeal Injury Classification

Group 1	Minor endolaryngeal hematoma or laceration without detectable fracture
Group 2	Edema, hematoma, minor mucosal disruption without exposed cartilage, nondisplaced fractures noted on computed tomography scan
Group 3	Massive edema, mucosal tears, exposed cartilage, cord immobility, displaced fractures
Group 4	Same as group 3 with more than two fracture lines or massive trauma to laryngeal mucosa
Group 5	Complete laryngotracheal separation

From Bent JP, Silver JR, Porubsky ES: Acute laryngeal trauma: a review of 77 patients. *Otolaryngol Head Neck Surg* 109:441–449, 1993.

Jurkovich et al reported that the diagnostic yield of combined angiographic and fluorographic studies of the vascular and aerodigestive anatomy was 23%. Only 9% of patients benefited from such studies. Using the zone of injury to determine the management approach, Jurkovich and colleagues advocated aggressive use of angiography, chest radiographs and esophagography for zone I injury and angiography for zone III. It was emphasized that zone II injuries could be safely observed, if the patients were asymptomatic. Additional support for a more selective approach to the management of these injuries was published by Obeid and associates who, in a retrospective review, concluded that mandatory exploration should be supplanted by a selective management policy. The rationale behind this support was predicated on several findings, including the fact that missed injuries still occurred with mandatory explorations and that there was morbidity associated with negative exploration and considerable number of hospital days. Obeid et al felt that patients with "hard signs" of injury needed operative intervention, and that those patients with negative physical examinations could be observed. Patients with equivocal findings on physical examination or with changing findings needed ancillary diagnostic studies to determine whether any clinically significant injuries exist. Additional support for a selective exploration policy was published by Belinke et al. In this study, 44 patients were treated with a selective exploration policy, based on physical findings. Twenty-two patients underwent immediate exploration with a negative exploration rate of 23%. In the group of patients observed, there were no delayed operations or complications. If all the patients had been subject to immediate exploration, the negative exploration rate would have been 60%, prompting the authors to advocate a selective approach to penetrating zone II injuries.

Metzdorff and colleagues reported 83 patients with a 56% negative exploration rate. When clinical signs of injury were noted preoperatively, an injury was found in 82% of the patients. If the preoperative physical examination was negative, there were no injuries found in 80% of the patients.

In 1987, Meyer and associates reported a prospective trial of 120 patients with penetrating neck wounds. Seven patients underwent emergency exploration for hemorrhage. The remaining patients underwent arteriography, upper aerodigestive endoscopy, and esophagography plus surgical exploration. Five patients were found to have six major vascular injuries that were not expected preoperatively. The authors concluded that selective management missed too many major vascular injuries and that mandatory exploration was a more prudent approach.

Wood and colleagues advocated selective management based on presenting physical findings. Equivocal findings required diagnostic studies to clarify the need for surgical exploration. In a similar argument, Narrod and Moore confirmed the safety and efficacy of selective management of these patients. Mansour et al endorsed selective nonoperative management when it was determined that only one patient in a cohort of 119 patients required a delayed operation for an occult injury.

Beitsch et al reported a retrospective review of penetrating wounds to the neck. A negative physical examination ruled out 99% of the vascular injuries. Seventy-one angiograms were performed. Only one patient required operative repair. In the light of a normal physical examination, mandatory exploration and the role of angiographic evaluation were questioned.

Scalfani and colleagues reported on a study of proximity angiograms, and noted that physical examination had a sensitivity of 61% and a specificity of 80%. The authors argued that not incorporating proximity angiography in the evaluation of penetrating neck injuries was premature. However, Menawat et al reported that in a series of 110 patients with penetrating neck injuries, only one patient had an injury not predicted by physical examination findings. Nine arterial injuries were treated nonoperatively without sequelae. Atteberry and coworkers reported on a prospective study of 66 patients that highlighted that in the absence of definitive or "hard signs" of vascular injury, these patients could be safely watched. Sekharan et al reported a

missed injury rate of 0.7% with physical examination alone. Jarvik et al reported that physical examination was sensitive and specific enough for detecting clinically significant vascular injuries. Physical examination had a sensitivity of 93.7%. Azuaje and associates' series of penetrating neck injuries demonstrated a sensitivity and negative predictive value of 100% for physical examination in detecting surgically significant vascular injuries. When considering injuries detected by angiography, physical examination showed a sensitivity of 93% and a negative predictive value of 97%. No patient in this series with a negative physical examination required a vascular repair, regardless of the zone of injury.

Referring specifically to zone III wounds, Ferguson et al reports a series of 72 patients with penetrating wounds. The absence of "hard signs" reliably excluded surgically significant injuries. Sixty percent of the patients with "hard signs" of injury were explored. Only one patient in this group had no identifiable injury. The remainder of the patients with "hard signs" of injury underwent emergent angiography with endovascular angiographic treatment. The authors recommended that zone III injuries with "hard signs" of vascular injury should undergo angiography, as they may be amenable to endovascular intervention.

A variety of complementary diagnostic modalities have been proposed as adjuncts to the evaluation of penetrating neck injuries. Ginzburg et al demonstrated, in a prospective double-blind evaluation of angiography and duplex scanning in stable patients with zone I, II, or III penetrating wounds, that duplex scans had 100% sensitivity and 85% specificity.

Newer imaging modalities have emerged. Munera and colleagues prospectively studied 60 patients, and reported that helical CT had a sensitivity of 90%, a specificity of 100%, a positive predictive value of 100%, and a negative predictive value of 98%. The authors concluded that helical CT was an excellent diagnostic study in the evaluation of neck injuries. Mazolewski et al performed a prospective evaluation of 14 stable patients with penetrating zone II injuries. All patients underwent thorough physical examination, infusion CT scan, and operative exploration. Three of the 14 patients had five injuries. Those patients had a high probability for injury based on the CT scan findings. Although a small sample size, results indicated that the CT scan had a sensitivity of 100%, specificity of 91%, positive predictive value of 75%, and negative predictive value of 100%. The authors felt that the CT scan should play a pivotal role in the evaluation of neck injuries. Gracias and coworkers conducted a retrospective series of 23 patients evaluated by CT scan for penetrating neck trauma that spanned all three zones. All the patients lacked "hard signs" of vascular or aerodigestive injury. Thirteen patients had the trajectory of injury remote from important structures identified and no further evaluation carried out. There were no adverse events. Gonzalez et al reported on a prospective study of CT in patients with zone II penetrating wounds without "hard signs" of injury necessitating immediate exploration. The authors concluded that CT added little to the information obtained by physical examination with zone II injuries.

Hollingsworth et al conducted a meta-analysis of computed tomographic angiography (CTA) for detection of carotid and vertebral lesions of either atherosclerotic or traumatic origin. It was concluded there were insufficient high-quality data to comment on the sensitivity or specificity of CTA for trauma.

Woo and colleagues studied patients with zone II penetrating wounds who underwent CTA as a diagnostic test. They reported that with increased utilization of CTA and enhanced staff experience, there was an associated decrease in the number of negative neck explorations. The authors highlighted that with this imaging, wound tracts could be visualized. This finding could assist in determining if other diagnostic studies would be needed. For example, the CT could show that the injury tract was away from any major structure, thus obviating any further investigation. Alternatively, an injury may be demonstrated and surgical exploration or conventional angiography for endovascular intervention could be performed. Finally, an indeterminate study may prompt other investigations depending on the finding in question.

Angiography has been advocated for zone I injuries at the base of the neck because injury in the thoracic outlet would be difficult to diagnose and control. Eddy et al conducted a multi-institutional retrospective study surveying patients over a 10-year period. A total of 138 patients were studied and 28 arterial injuries were found. However, the group concluded that in the presence of a normal physical examination and a normal chest radiograph, angiographic study may not be needed.

Gasparri and associates confirmed this finding after conducting a retrospective review of 100 patients. All patients with "hard signs" of vascular injury were taken for expeditious surgical exploration. Eighty-one patients without "hard signs" of injury underwent angiography, and 11 occult injuries were discovered. When a normal physical examination and a normal chest radiograph are combined, they have a sensitivity of 100%, a specificity of 80%, a positive predictive value of 40%, and a negative predictive value of 100%. The group concluded that proximity alone does not mandate angiography.

A prospective trial by Demetriades et al evaluating the role of physical examination in penetrating neck wounds demonstrated that the lack of hard clinical signs of vascular or aerodigestive injury had a negative predictive value of 100% and reliably excluded all such wounds needing operative repair. The algorithm used by this group specifically looked for physical examination information regarding vascular and aerodigestive injury. Asymptomatic patients were observed safely.

Our own approach is outlined in the algorithm in Figure 4. Patients presenting with "hard signs" of vascular or aerodigestive injury go immediately to the operating room for neck exploration. If the wound is in zone I or II, esophogoscopy and bronchoscopy can be part of the exploration in the operating room. The surgical approach is at the discretion of the attending surgeon. Patients with "soft signs" undergo multislice helical CT/angiography (MHCT). If the wound tract is obviously away from major structures of concern, no specific therapy is initiated. Proximity is a wound tract that passes within 5 mm of a vascular or aerodigestive structure of interest. A study demonstrating such proximity, or that is equivocal due to artifact scatter from retained metallic particles or debris, should prompt further investigation. How this is conducted is at the discretion of the attending trauma surgeon but may entail esophagoscopy, bronchoscopy, angiography, or an appropriate combination of these modalities.

From our own experience, Figure 5 demonstrates air in the soft tissues of the neck and the artifact produced by the retained missile.

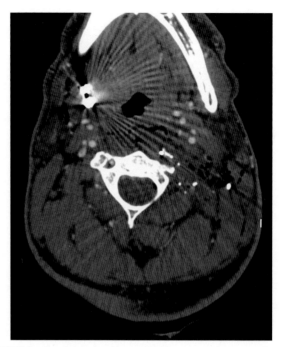

FIGURE 5 Gunshot wound to neck with computed tomography demonstrating subcutaneous air in the soft tissue planes.

The patient lacks hard or soft signs of injury. The uncertainty posed and the proximity to major vascular structures should prompt a CTA. Figure 6 is a lateral view of a similar patient with air in the soft tissues but no hard or soft signs of injury. Figure 7 is a view of a normal CTA of the carotid artery of the patient demonstrated in Figure 6. Figure 8 demonstrates an injury to the internal carotid artery after suffering a zone III gunshot wound. This injury was stented.

A discussion of the evolving role of MHCT is in order. Virtually every body region and organ system has been studied this way and in many ways this has become the de facto standard imaging modality. The wide availability, speed of image acquisition, image quality, lack of dependence on special teams that require mobilization on call, and ability to reconstruct images in multiple planes for specific study all

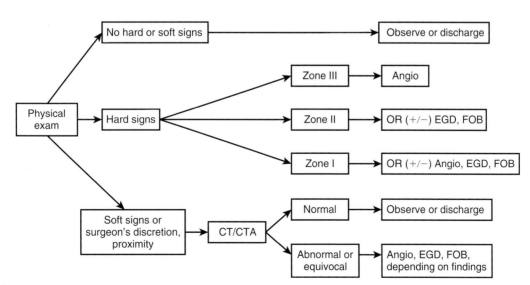

FIGURE 4 Algorithm for evaluation of penetrating neck wounds. Angio, Angiography; CT, computed tomography; CTA, computed tomographic angiography; EGD, esophagogastroduodenoscopy; FOB, fiberoptic bronchoscopy; OR, operating room.

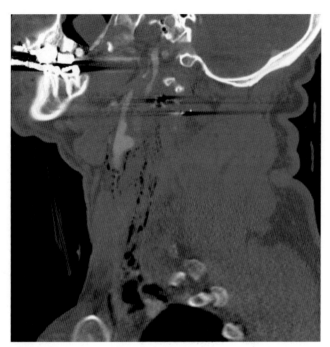

FIGURE 6 Lateral computed tomography demonstrating air in the soft tissue.

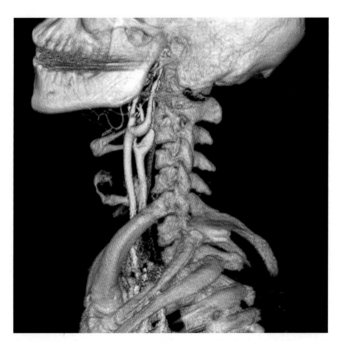

FIGURE 7 Computed tomographic angiography demonstrating normal carotid and vertebral anatomy without injury.

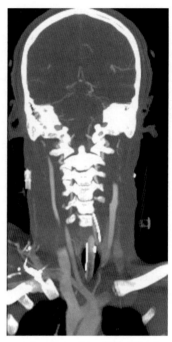

FIGURE 8 Computed tomographic angiography demonstrating interruption of flow in the left internal carotid secondary to a gunshot wound.

contribute to this evolution. The application of this technology to penetrating neck wounds not needing immediate surgical exploration is reasonable.

Inaba and associates in a prospective evaluation of MHCT for penetrating neck wounds not needing immediate surgical exploration note that essentially no injuries were missed by CT imaging. The problem with this conclusion is that the follow-up is short (mean of 33 days) and incomplete (84% of the evaluated population). Studies noted previously and commented on by Inaba all support the premise that MHCT is a highly sensitive and specific screening test that can minimize, if not eliminate, the need for additional diagnostic testing in this patient population. The use of MHCT appears to be a very safe and reliable screening test for penetrating neck injuries that do not require immediate exploration in the operating room.

What is clear is that a policy of mandatory surgical exploration of the neck for penetrating zone II wounds will result in a high negative exploration rate. Routine use of ancillary diagnostic procedures (selective approach) will result in a large expenditure of time and effort and appears to offer no advantage over *experienced* expectant management only. The presence of "hard signs" of vascular or aerodigestive injuries requires surgical exploration. Less overt signs of vascular or aerodigestive injury can be evaluated at the discretion of the surgical team. Astute physical examination directed at signs of vascular injury will detect the overwhelming majority of patients needing surgical exploration and repair. The role of MHCT has evolved to where it may be considered the screening test of choice if evaluation beyond physical examination is contemplated.

An excellent review of imaging options for penetrating neck injuries has been written by Steenburg and associates. This is written from the perspective of the radiologist but makes the same points that the surgical literature does. The ability to delineate a missile tract and see the proximity to major vascular or aerodigestive structures of interest allows planning of additional diagnostic or therapeutic maneuvers. In the absence of such suspicion being raised, no further interventions are necessary.

TREATMENT OF CAROTID ARTERY INJURIES

The surgical approach to the cervical vasculature is predicated on the zone of injury. Zone II injuries are best approached via an incision along the anterior border of the sternocleidomastoid muscle with the head turned to the opposite side. Placement of a towel roll under the patient's shoulders is very helpful. Dissection along this line will encounter the common facial vein, which can be sacrificed, and will allow complete visualization of the common carotid artery, carotid bulb, proximal internal carotid and external carotid arteries, and internal jugular vein. Carotid arterial injuries are best treated by surgical repair. The use of a vein patch taken from adjacent facial vein or Gortex is an alternative to direct suture repair. Shunts are not routinely used in these circumstances. When to repair versus ligate is complicated by the poor ability to discriminate between severe ischemia and evolving infarction. Patients with fixed neurologic deficits do poorly with revascularization. Injuries distal in the internal carotid may require special maneuvers to gain access for repair. Disarticulation of the temporomandibular joint allowing forward displacement of the mandible will allow access to the internal carotid cephalad to the angle of the mandible. The skull base is not surgically accessible and may require interventional techniques to control. Prograde flow in the carotid at the time of surgical exploration is a good indication for repair. In the absence of prograde flow, ligation may be preferable. Ligation of the injured carotid should be reserved only for those patients with devastating neurologic injuries. Liekweg and Greenfield's review of the literature demonstrated lower morbidity and mortality rates in the revascularization group compared to the ligation group. Unger et al and Brown et al in separate reports confirm this recommendation for revascularization over ligation.

Lacerations of the internal jugular are best treated by lateral venography, although ligation is a reasonable alternative, especially when dealing with injuries that nearly completely transect the vein or will result in narrowing greater than 50% of the luminal diameter. Injuries that extend proximally into the thoracic outlet are amenable to surgical exposure by extending the anterior sternocleidomastoid incision as a median sternotomy or a thoracic trapdoor incision. This allows in continuity access to the aortic arch and the take-off of the carotid and subclavian vessels if needed. Likewise, the supraclavicular fossa can be explored by an extension of the anterior neck incision laterally. This may facilitate exposure of the subclavian vessels or vertebral take-off, if necessary.

An extended collar incision, as used for thyroid or parathyroid procedures, can be used for bilateral neck explorations. Transcervical gunshot wounds with the potential for bilateral vascular injury might be better approached through this incision as bilateral control is easy to obtain from one position. This incision may need to be moved cephalad in the neck to facilitate exposure on occasions.

The role of endovascular therapy for penetrating cervical wounds involving the subclavian, carotid, and vertebral vessels is evolving. Experience gained in the treatment of atherosclerotic diseases will, undoubtedly, spill over into injury care, but currently there is insufficient experience to broadly endorse its application. Also, the use of endoluminal stents requires lifelong patient follow-up.

CONCLUSION

Penetrating neck wounds still present serious challenges in diagnosis and management. Astute physical examination with attention to the overt findings of vascular and aerodigestive injury "hard signs" appears to be the most efficient approach to evaluation of penetrating neck injuries. Surgical therapy is usually straightforward, although endovascular approaches are evolving. In the absence of the "hard signs" of injury, careful observation with or without additional diagnostic studies can be a very successful strategy. MHCT appears to be the diagnostic screening test of choice for the patient not requiring immediate surgical exploration.

For the chapter's Suggested Readings list, please visit the book at www.ExpertConsult.inkling.com.

BLUNT CEREBROVASCULAR INJURIES

Clay Cothren Burlew and Ernest E. Moore

O ver the past decade, a wealth of studies has provided the scientific rationale to warrant the early screening and preemptive treatment of blunt cerebrovascular injuries (BCVIs). Initially, BCVIs were thought to have unavoidable, devastating neurologic outcomes, but several reports suggested anticoagulation improves neurologic outcome in patients suffering ischemic neurologic events (INEs). If untreated, carotid artery injuries (CAIs) have a stroke rate up to 50% depending on injury grade, with increasing stroke rates correlating with increasing grades of injury; vertebral artery injuries (VAIs) have a stroke rate of 20% to 25%. Screening protocols, based on patient injury patterns and mechanism of injury, have been instituted to identify these injuries in asymptomatic patients and to initiate treatment prior to neurologic sequelae. Current studies suggest that early antithrombotic therapy in patients with BCVI reduces stroke rate and prevents neurologic morbidity.

SIGNS AND SYMPTOMS

BCVIs were first reported over 30 years ago in patients who presented with stroke following injury. The patient's symptom of cerebral ischemia or the distribution of the symptoms usually indicates the underlying cerebrovascular lesion. CAIs generally result in contralateral sensorimotor deficit, which is generally defined as a stroke. Aphasia occurs when the dominant hemisphere is involved, but nondominant hemisphere strokes may result in hemineglect. VAIs typically manifest as more vague symptomatology, including ataxia, dizziness, vomiting, facial or body analgesia, and visual field defects. Symptoms of carotid-cavernous fistulas include orbital pain, exophthalmos, chemosis, and conjunctival hyperemia.

Although some patients may present with symptoms of BCVI-related ischemia within an hour of injury, the majority exhibit a latent period. This asymptomatic phase has been inferred, based upon the time to onset of symptoms, in patients with defined injuries who did not receive antithrombotic therapy. This time frame appears to range from hours up to 14 years, but the majority seems to develop symptoms within 10 to 72 hours. The goal, then, is diagnosing BCVI during this "silent period" prior to the onset of stroke. Existing data affirm that if you diagnose these injuries during the asymptomatic period, you can effectively treat the patient to prevent stroke. Screening for BCVI during the asymptomatic period was initially suggested in the mid-1990s after the recognition that specific patterns of injuries were associated with BCVI. Although optimal screening criteria have yet to be defined, current screening algorithms include patients considered at high risk based on their injury pattern.

MECHANISM AND PATTERNS OF INJURY

Crissey and Bernstein originally postulated three fundamental mechanisms of injury resulting in BCVI. The first is a direct blow to the neck. This mechanism is often seen with patients in motor vehicle collisions with inappropriately fitting seatbelts, indicated by a seatbelt sign across the neck; it can also be seen in recreational sports with

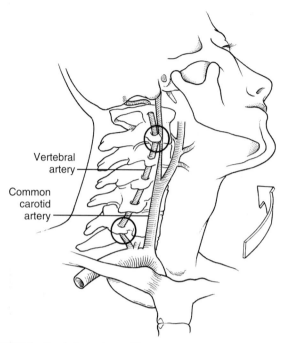

FIGURE 1 Cervical rotation and hyperextension result in a stretch injury of the carotid and vertebral vasculature. *(Modified from Biffl WL, Moore EE, Elliot JP, et al: Blunt cerebrovascular injuries.* Curr Prob Surg *36:505, 1999.)*

TABLE 1: Denver Screening Criteria for Blunt Cerebrovascular Injuries

Signs/symptoms of BCVI	Arterial hemorrhage
	Cervical bruit in patient >50 years of age
	Expanding cervical hematoma
	Focal neurologic deficit
	Neurologic examination incongruous with head CT scan findings
	Stroke on secondary CT scan
Risk factors for BCVI	High energy transfer mechanism associated with:
	Displaced mid-face fracture (LeFort II or III)
	Mandible fracture
	Complex skull fracture/basilar skull fracture/ occipital condyle fracture
	Severe TBI with GCS <6
	Cervical spine fracture, subluxation, or ligamentous injury at any level
	Near hanging with anoxic brain injury
	Clothesline type injury or seat belt abrasion with significant swelling, pain, or altered MS
	TBI with thoracic injuries
	Scalp degloving
	Thoracic vascular injuries
	Blunt cardiac rupture
	Upper rib fractures

Courtesy of Denver Health Medical Center.
BCVI, Blunt cerebrovascular injury; CT, computed tomography; TBI, traumatic brain injury.

a direct blow to the neck. The second proposed mechanism is hyperextension with contralateral rotation of the head. This is the most common mechanism causing CAI with the hyperextension resulting in a stretching of the carotid artery over the lateral articular processes of C1–C3 (Fig. 1). VAI may also be due to a hyperextension-stretch injury due to the tethering of the vertebral artery within the lateral masses of the cervical spine. The third mechanism of injury is a direct laceration of the artery by adjacent fractures involving the sphenoid or petrous bones. Although originally described as the mechanism in association with CAI, this may also be the cause of VAI. With a fracture of the bony elements composing the vertebral foramen, the foramen transversarium, it is not surprising that the vertebral artery can also be injured directly. Regardless of the type of injury mechanism, there is intimal disruption of the carotid or vertebral artery. This intimal tear becomes a nidus for platelet aggregation that may lead to emboli or vessel occlusion, and subsequent stroke.

Although the mechanism of injury is important for determining patients at high risk for BCVI, the patient's associated injuries are also critical to determine which asymptomatic patients need screening for BCVI. Aggressive screening for BCVI was initially suggested after recognition that specific patterns of injuries were associative. Current screening algorithms include patients with signs or symptoms, as well as those considered at high risk by injury pattern (Table 1). With the availability of noninvasive diagnosis using computed tomographic angiography (CTA), and the recognition that historical protocols missed 20% of BCVI, broadening BCVI screening guidelines has been suggested. Injury patterns not originally included that are now potential triggers for diagnostic imaging include mandible fracture, complex skull fracture, traumatic brain injury with thoracic injuries, scalp degloving, thoracic vascular injuries, and clothesline type injury/seatbelt abrasion with significant swelling, pain, or altered mental status. Additionally, original screening protocols included all patients with cervical spine fractures to rule out BCVI. Although some advocate screening all patients with spine fractures, others advocate narrowed criteria based upon mechanism and fracture pattern (cervical spine subluxation, fractures involving the transverse foramen, and upper cervical spine fracture of C1–C3).

DIAGNOSTIC IMAGING

Using defined screening protocols, high-risk patients undergo imaging to identify BCVI. Historically, four-vessel arteriography has been the gold standard to diagnose BCVI. However, many clinicians appropriately questioned the need for subjecting patients to angiography. Angiography is labor intensive, costly, and not without risks; if not available at smaller hospitals, angiography requires emergent transfer of a patient for definitive evaluation.

CTA is an attractive alternative to catheter-based diagnostic imaging. In addition to being a noninvasive imaging modality, the majority of patients undergoing screening for BCVI have indications for CT scanning of other regions. Hence, imaging can often be accomplished with only one "road trip" or via whole-body multidetector CT. Due to its ready availability, CTA can reduce the time to BCVI identification and permits earlier treatment than historical angiography.

Although the accuracy of early-generation 1- to 4-slice CTA was relatively poor for diagnosing BCVI (sensitivity 47% to 68% and specificity of 67%), identification of injuries improved with the introduction of multidetector-row CTA. Five published studies and an additional report have evaluated the accuracy of 16-slice CTA compared with arteriography. Eastman and colleagues evaluated 162 patients with CTA, of whom 146 agreed to angiography. With a screening yield of 28%, they reported 100% sensitivity of 16-slice CTA for CAI, and 96% sensitivity for VAI, with one false-negative CTA of a grade I injury. The Harborview study illustrates the importance of experience in identifying BCVI on a CTA; they performed arteriography on 82 patients who had had a normal screening CTA, and found that CTA missed 7 BCVIs, for a negative predictive value of 92%. However, retrospective review of the CTA images found that the injuries were evident in 6 of the 7 patients, and that the seventh patient's abnormality was most likely not traumatic in origin. Moreover, all missed injuries occurred in the first half of the study period. A very similar finding was noted by the Medical College of Virginia group; they screened 119 patients with 92 undergoing confirmatory angiography. They reported a 43% false-positive rate and 9% false-negative rate for CTA, but all of the missed BCVIs occurred in the first half of the study period. In the second half of the study, the sensitivity and negative predictive value of CTA was 100%. Each of these studies recognize that injuries in the region of the skull base appear to be the most difficult to identify, underlining the importance of carefully examining this high-risk region. The final study to evaluate angiography versus CTA for BCVI diagnosis reported the worst results for high-resolution CTA, with a reported sensitivity of 29% for 16-slice CTA and 54% for 64-slice CTA. Without quality control it is difficult to understand how best to interpret this study's impact on screening options for BCVI. Conversely, a preliminary report by Fakhry et al indicates CTA may be oversensitive in diagnosing BCVI. The most recent evaluation by the Memphis group suggests angiography should continue to be used for the diagnosis of BCVI because of missed injuries by CTA.

All patients with indications for screening, and no contraindications to antithrombotic therapy, should undergo imaging as soon as possible. Patients with documented BCVI should undergo repeat imaging 7 to 10 days after their initial diagnostic study. The importance of routine follow-up imaging is particularly salient in patients with grade I and II injuries; over half of grade I injuries completely heal, allowing cessation of antithrombotic therapy. Conversely, less than 10% of all grade II, III, and IV injuries heal, with injury progression rates of approximately 12% for all treated BCVI. Patients with carotid or vertebral artery occlusions are not as critical to reimage, as over 80% display no change on follow-up imaging. On the other hand, some authors have advocated an endovascular approach to pseudoaneurysms, hence supporting the use of repeat imaging to reassess grade II and III injuries. The optimal timing for reimaging, however, remains to be established as the 7- to 10-day delay is based on the risk of repeat angiography within the first 5 days after injury.

INJURY GRADING SCALE

The identification of disparate outcomes associated with varied luminal irregularities comprising BCVI (dissection, occlusion, transection, and pseudoaneurysms) prompted us to propose a grading scale to facilitate multi-institutional evaluation of the management of these potentially devastating lesions. An injury grading scale was developed to provide not only an accurate description of the injury but also to define the stroke risk by injury grade (Figs. 2 and 3, and Table 2). Untreated injuries have an overall stroke rate of approximately 20%; CAIs have increasing stroke rate by increasing grade, but VAIs tend to have a more consistent stroke rate of approximately 20% for all grades of injury (Table 3).

INCIDENCE OF BLUNT CEREBROVASCULAR INJURIES

Originally thought to be a rare injury, BCVIs are currently diagnosed in 1% of all blunt trauma admissions. Previously, BCVI-related strokes were often attributed to a patient's primary head injury, rather than as a sequelae of cervical arterial injury with subsequent embolic stroke. Therefore, BCVIs were felt to be rare with an incidence reported less than 0.1% among trauma admissions, and with blunt CAI accounting for less than 3% of all traumatic carotid injuries. Once the patient's neurologic changes were recognized as a vascular source, and appropriate imaging was instituted to identify the injured artery, the incidence of BCVI identified tripled. In the first multicenter review of BCVI, performed by the Western Trauma Association, only 49 patients with CAIs were identified at 11 major trauma centers over a 6-year period. With the recognition of BCVI as a specific injury

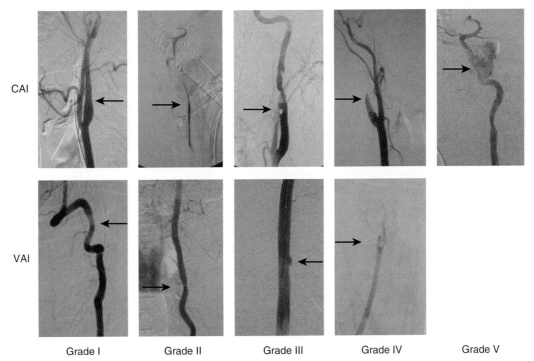

FIGURE 2   Representative angiographic images of blunt cerebrovascular injury by grade. *Arrows* indicate area of injury. CAI, Carotid artery injury; VAI, vertebral artery injury.

FIGURE 3 Representative computed tomography angiographic images of blunt cerebrovascular injury by grade. *Arrows* indicate area of injury. CAI, Carotid artery injury; VAI, vertebral artery injury.

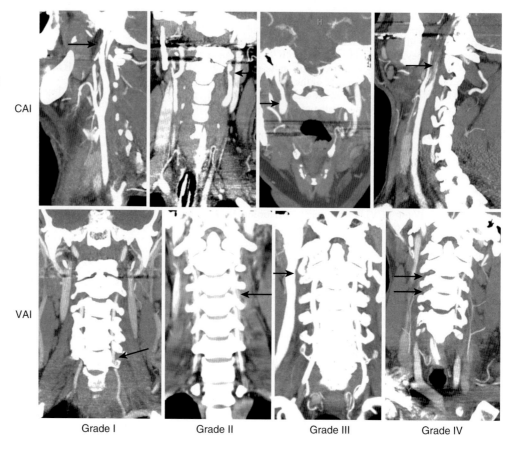

Grade I   Grade II   Grade III   Grade IV

TABLE 2: Denver Grading Scale for Blunt Cerebrovascular Injuries

Grade I	Irregularity of the vessel wall or a dissection/intramural hematoma with less than 25% luminal stenosis
Grade II	Intraluminal thrombus or raised intimal flap is visualized, or dissection/intramural hematoma with 25% or more luminal narrowing
Grade III	Pseudoaneurysm
Grade IV	Vessel occlusion
Grade V	Vessel transection

Courtesy of Denver Health Medical Center.

TABLE 3: Stroke Rate by Blunt Cerebrovascular Injury Grade

Injury	Grade of Injury	Stroke Rate (%)
Carotid artery injury	I	3
	II	14
	III	26
	IV	50
	V	100
Vertebral artery injury	I	6
	II	38
	III	27
	IV	28
	V	100

causing significant stroke-related morbidity and mortality, was the identification of an associated silent period. Specifically, half of patients become symptomatic greater than 12 hours after injury. Consequently, it became evident that there is a therapeutic window of opportunity. With the advent of widespread injury screening in asymptomatic high-risk patients, there has been a veritable epidemic of BCVIs. Currently, in centers with a comprehensive screening approach, the screening yield is over 30% in high-risk populations. In our recent institutional review over an 8½-year period, 0.1% of blunt injury patients presented with neurologic symptoms and 4% underwent screening, with a 34% screening yield for diagnosing BCVI and an overall incidence of 1.5% in all blunt trauma admissions.

ANTITHROMBOTIC TREATMENT

Following the recognition that BCVIs were responsible for patients' adverse neurologic events, treatment modalities were debated. If the injury occurs in a surgically accessible area of the carotid artery, particularly the common carotid artery, operative management is preferred (Fig. 4). The vast majority of BCVI lesions, however, occur

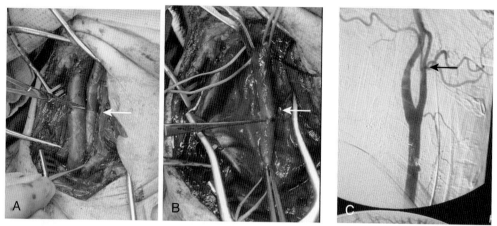

FIGURE 4 Operative approach to a common carotid pseudoaneurysm following angiographic (**A**) diagnosis; identification of the injury (**B**) is followed by primary end-to-end repair (**C**).

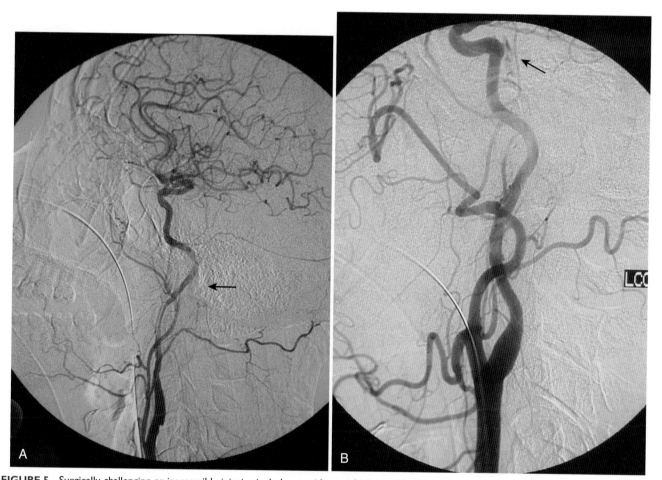

FIGURE 5 Surgically challenging or inaccessible injuries include carotid arterial injury at the base of the skull (**A** and **B**).

(Continued)

in surgically challenging or inaccessible areas of the blood vessels, either high within the carotid canal at the base of the skull or within the foramen transversarium (Fig. 5). Such a location makes the standard vascular repair approaches, including reconstruction or thrombectomy, challenging if not impossible. Heparin was initially the treatment of choice for BCVI, with the assumption that this promoted

clot stabilization if present and clot resolution through intrinsic fibrinolytic mechanisms, and prevented further thrombosis. Treatment with anticoagulation was shown to improve neurologic outcome in patients sustaining BCVI-related INEs. Initial reports, including a multicenter study by the Western Trauma Association, indicated that patients who were treated with anticoagulation had an improved

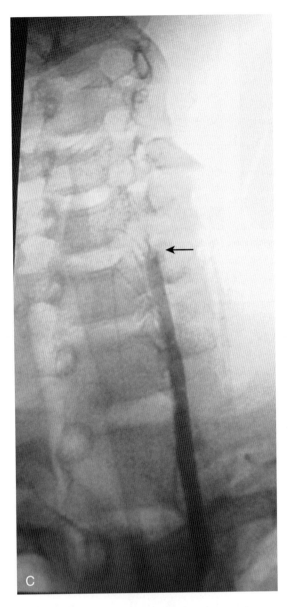

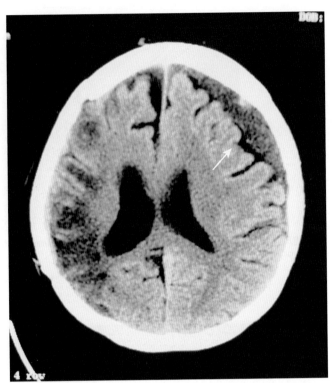

FIGURE 6   Example of intracranial bleeding *(arrow)* complication associated with heparinization of a patient for blunt cerebrovascular injury.

FIGURE 5, CONT'D   C, Vertebral arterial injury within the transverse foramen.

outcome compared to those who were either not treated or had a contraindication to anticoagulation due to associated head injuries. In these studies, up to 45% of patients achieved good neurologic status, and anticoagulation therapy was independently associated with survival and improvement in neurologic outcome.

Subsequently, intravenous heparin was thought to be the treatment of choice for those asymptomatic patients with blunt injuries. Initially, standard heparinization protocols were used, but because of a moderate risk of bleeding in multisystem trauma patients the protocol was modified (Fig. 6). Currently, anticoagulation with systemic heparin is initiated using a continuous infusion of heparin at 15 U/kg/hour, without a loading dose; heparin drips are titrated to achieve a partial thromboplastin time of 40 to 50 seconds. With this adjustment in the BCVI heparin protocol, less than 1% of patients have had bleeding complications necessitating transfusion in our experience. For patients with a contraindication to heparin, antiplatelet agents (currently aspirin 325 mg/day) have been administered. Antithrombotic therapy is not started in patients with closed head injury or intraparenchymal hemorrhage without agreement from the neurosurgery service. Antithrombotic therapy in patients with significant solid organ injuries or a complex pelvic fracture with associated retroperitoneal hematoma is typically not started until at least 24 hours of physiologic stability without transfusion requirements.

Currently there is controversy regarding the ideal antithrombotic therapy for any type of arterial disease—anticoagulation versus antiplatelet agents. A retrospective study by Chimowitz et al indicated that warfarin is superior in patients with vertebrobasilar occlusive disease, but a more recent prospective double-blind comparison by the same authors demonstrated that aspirin is the therapy of choice for patients with symptomatic intracranial atherosclerotic arterial stenosis, due to equivalent stroke prevention rates as warfarin, but decreased hemorrhagic complications. A recent review of vertebrobasilar disease supported the use of antiplatelet agents in patients with arterial stenosis but warfarin in patients with severe, flow-limiting lesions or dissections. Because of the ease of administration, the use of antiplatelet agents has gained favor for the treatment of BCVI. Although the optimal regimen remains unanswered, there appears to be equivalence between anticoagulation and antiplatelet medications in both prevention of stroke as well as healing/progression rates of individual injuries. Our group advocates use of intravenous heparin in the acutely injured patient with transition to antiplatelet agents at discharge owing to easier reversal with fresh frozen plasma should a bleeding complication occur. Which therapeutic agent is utilized, and whether the choice of antithrombotic should be determined by the patient's injury grade, must continue to be evaluated in prospective studies. Future application of thromboelastography (TEG) may help determine the optimal treatment regimen for these patients. Because of variable platelet response to antiplatelet therapy, modified TEG and platelet mapping may become an effective test to assess treatment.

Most importantly, patients who are diagnosed with BCVI early and are treated with antithrombotics almost universally avoid INE. The Memphis group showed a reduction in stroke rate for CAI from 64% in untreated patients to 6.8% in patients treated with antithrombotics (either anticoagulation or antiplatelet agents), and for VAI a reduction from 54% to 2.6% in treated patients. Our group's most recent evaluation demonstrated a stroke rate of 0.3% in 282 patients with BCVI treated with antithrombotics, and untreated patients had an overall stroke rate of 21%. Although the optimal regimen remains unanswered, there appears to be equivalence between the two therapies (anticoagulation and antiplatelet agents) with regard to stroke rate.

Following initiation of antithrombotics, treatment is empirically continued for 6 months based on the assumption of re-endothelialization. Although complete healing of grade I injuries on repeat imaging at 7 to 10 days has been documented in more than half of affected patients, the vast majority of grades II, III, and IV injuries persist. Comprehensive long-term follow-up beyond the acute hospitalization has not been reported in the literature, as is true in most trauma population studies. Therefore, whether these injuries heal or persist at 3 to 6 months is unknown.

ROLE OF ENDOVASCULAR STENTS

Since the turn of the century, there has been an explosion in the use of percutaneous transluminal arterial interventions for both traumatic injuries and atherosclerotic lesions. Although the role of carotid stents for atherosclerotic disease is being explored with randomized, well-controlled trials, the indication for percutaneous intervention for traumatic injuries is less well defined. Carotid stents have been used in patients with blunt injury with persistent pseudoaneurysms because of the concern for subsequent embolization or rupture. In theory, the uncovered carotid stent acts as a filter to trap any thrombus within the pseudoaneurysm, thereby preventing embolization and stroke. The stent may also decrease flow into the pseudoaneurysm by increasing laminar flow within the stented portion of the carotid lumen itself. Decreasing flow into the aneurysmal sac may then reduce any egress of blood from the sac, which in turn may reduce turbulence within the lumen. There are anecdotal reports of carotid pseudoaneurysm rupture, particularly in the petrous portion of the canal leading to epistaxis, but we have not observed this event. However, aside from isolated cases, few other reports of late events are evident in the literature. Thus, it is difficult to confidently state either the true healing rate of these injuries or the risk of rupture or delayed embolic stroke.

Several reports advocate the use of percutaneous angioplasty and stenting of carotid injuries. Although the majority appears to have patency of the stented carotid artery documented in follow-up radiographic evaluation, several cases of carotid artery occlusion following stent placement have been reported. An early evaluation of the use of endovascular techniques, prior to the routine use of cerebral protection devices and the recommendation for antiplatelet treatment following stent placement indicated a significant stroke and carotid occlusion rate associated with carotid stents placed in acutely injured vessels. Without long-term follow-up of patients with traumatic pseudoaneurysms treated solely with antithrombotics it is difficult to determine which treatment modality, stenting versus medical management, is optimal. Our most recent evaluation of the use of endovascular therapy versus antithombotic treatment indicates antithrombotic treatment for BCVI is effective for stroke prevention. Routine stenting entails increased costs and potential risk for stroke and does not appear to add benefit. In our practice, intravascular stents are reserved for the rare patient with symptomatology due to narrowing or a markedly enlarging pseudoaneurysm.

LONG-TERM FOLLOW-UP AND OUTCOME

Following initiation of antithrombotics, treatment is continued for 6 months empirically. Repeat evaluation of the patient's injury and a determination of antithrombotic therapy should be considered at 6 months. Although no long-term studies have been performed to date, we currently recommend multislice CTA for long-term follow-up. Patients with persistent injuries on repeat imaging are often treated with lifelong aspirin, although, as is true for any long-term therapy, the risks of treatment should be discussed with the patient.

The morbidity and mortality rates of BCVI-related INEs are well documented. Historically, BCVI stroke-related permanent neurologic morbidity was greater than 80% with associated mortality rates of 40%. Modern series report lower rates of morbidity but the mortality rate due to BCVI is significant, with CAI patients having a 13% to 21% stroke-related mortality rate and patients with VAI-related strokes a 4% to 18% mortality rate. A less studied variable is the impact of neurologic morbidity on the need for prolonged acute patient care. Our evaluation points to a greater overall rate of discharge to rehabilitation services in patients suffering BCVI-related INEs. Such prolonged acute patient care increases costs to the patient, insurance companies, and ultimately to society. Performing a cost analysis of direct BCVI-related costs is difficult in these multisystem trauma patients; however, a cost analysis of patient life is even more problematic. In our series, overall mortality rate in patients sustaining CAI was 7% for those without neurologic event versus 32% for those with neurologic event; in patients with VAI, those without neurologic event had a mortality rate of 7% and those with a neurologic event had a mortality rate of 18%. The impact on mortality rate due to BCVI-related strokes appears independent of a patient's associated injuries, as the Injury Severity Score was not significantly different between those with and those without INE.

CONCLUSIONS

Diagnosis and treatment of BCVI have evolved over the past three decades, but have moved rapidly since the 1980s. Originally thought to be a rare occurrence, BCVIs are now diagnosed in approximately 1% of blunt trauma admissions. The recognition of a clinically silent period allows for screening for injuries based on mechanism of trauma and the patient's constellation of injuries. Currently, protocols exist for screening, hence limiting imaging to those with the highest risk of injury (Fig. 7). Comprehensive evaluation of patients has resulted in the early diagnosis of BCVI during the asymptomatic phase, thus allowing prompt initiation of treatment. Although the ideal regimen of antithrombotic therapy has yet to be determined, treatment with either antiplatelet agents or anticoagulation reduces the BCVI-related stroke rate. BCVI is a rare but potentially devastating injury; appropriate screening in high-risk patients should be performed and prompt treatment initiated to prevent INEs.

For the chapter's Suggested Readings list, please visit the book at www.ExpertConsult.inkling.com.

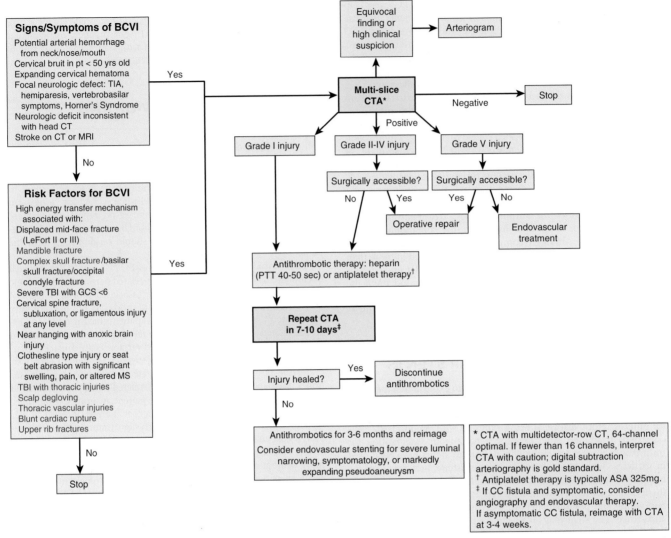

FIGURE 7 Denver Health Medical Center's current BCVI screening algorithm. BCVI, Blunt cerebrovascular injury; CHI, closed head injury; CT, computed tomography; CTA, computed tomographic angiography; DAI, diffuse axonal injury; GCS, Glasgow Coma Scale; MRI, magnetic resonance imaging; MS, mental status; TBI, traumatic brain injury, TIA, transient ischemic attack; PTT, partial thromboplastin time. *(Courtesy of Denver Health Medical Center.)*

TRACHEAL, LARYNGEAL, AND OROPHARYNGEAL INJURIES

Luis G. Fernández, Scott H. Norwood, and John D. Berne

Structural mobility and elasticity are characteristics of the upper airway that make injury to these structures infrequent. Skeletal protection is also provided anteriorly by the mandible and sternum and posteriorly by the bony spinal column (Fig. 1). Upper airway injuries are identified in only 0.03% of patients admitted to major trauma centers. These injuries are frequently lethal, which explains

their higher reported occurrence in autopsy series. Penetrating mechanisms of injury are more common than blunt mechanisms of injury, the true incidence of which is unknown. Twenty-one percent of patients with upper airway injuries die within the first 2 hours after hospitalization. The diagnosis is often delayed in patients without immediate life-threatening upper airway trauma. Such delays often result in serious late complications. Limited experience in nonoperative and operative management of airway injuries has led to a wide variety of recommendations that may be considered under various clinical scenarios. For unstable, immediate life-threatening upper airway injuries, rapid airway control by any available means is essential for patient survival. Most authors agree that tracheal intubation through an open wound that communicates with the tracheobronchial tree is appropriate. Stable patients may benefit from bronchoscopic-guided tracheal intubation distal to the injury site, and blind endotracheal tube placement is almost always a poor choice for airway control. Airway injuries are always challenging to even the most experienced surgeon because traditional approaches to airway control are often contraindicated.

ANATOMY OF UPPER AIRWAY

Oral Cavity

The oral cavity is designed for the articulation of speech and mastication. It also provides an alternate pathway (to the nasopharynx) for the upper airway system.

Boundaries

Anterior—lips
Posterior—anterior tonsillar pillars
Roof—hard and soft palate
Floor—mucosa overlying sublingual and submandibular glands
Walls—buccal mucosa

Contents

Alveolar processes and teeth
Anterior tongue to circumvallate papilla
Orifice of parotid gland (Stenson duct) in buccal mucosa opposite upper second molars
Orifice of submandibular duct (Wharton duct) in anterior floor of mouth
Orifices of sublingual glands

Pharynx

Surgical Anatomy

The pharynx consists of the following elements:

Nasopharynx: Extends from posterior choanae of the nose to the soft palate. It is related posteriorly to the base of the skull. The nasopharynx contains adenoid tissue and the orifices of the eustachian tubes. This area is not accessible to direct inspection and must be examined by mirrors or optical instruments.
Oropharynx: Portion that is visible via the mouth. The oropharynx extends from the soft palate superiorly to the vallecula inferiorly. The posterior and lateral walls of the oropharynx are formed by the superior and middle pharyngeal constrictors.
Palatine tonsils: Lymphoid aggregates between the mucosal folds created by the palatoglossus and palatopharyngeus muscles. The palatine tonsils are covered by stratified squamous epithelium, which continues down into deep crypts. Tonsils vary widely in size and may be sessile or pedunculated.
Hypopharynx: Portion of the pharynx that lies inferior to the tip of the epiglottis. The posterior and lateral walls are formed by middle and inferior pharyngeal constrictors. The hypopharynx extends inferiorly to the cricopharyngeus muscle, where the pharynx empties into the cervical esophagus. Anteriorly, it extends from the vallecula and contains the epiglottis and the larynx. Lateral to the larynx are the pyriform sinuses, two mucosal pouches whose medial borders are the lateral walls of the larynx. The posterior aspect of the hypopharynx contains the posterior pharyngeal wall and postcricoid mucosa (Figs. 2 to 4).

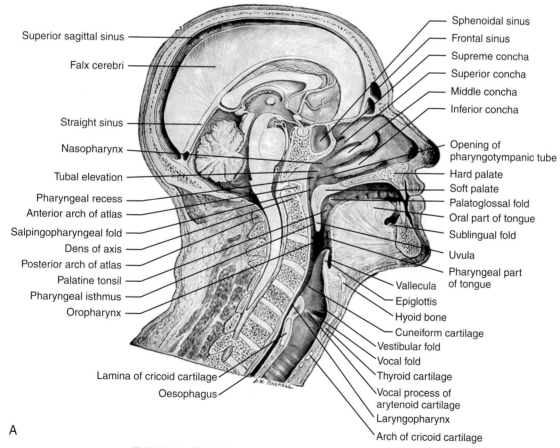

FIGURE I   A, Median sagittal section through the head and neck.

(Continued)

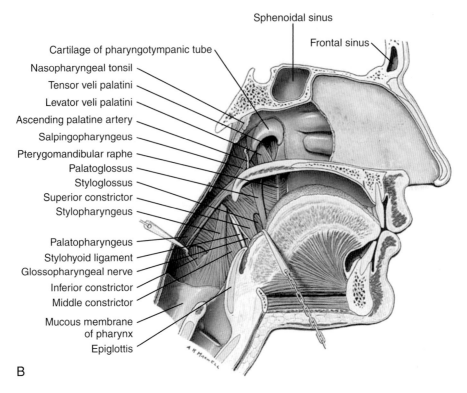

Sphenoidal sinus
Frontal sinus
Cartilage of pharyngotympanic tube
Nasopharyngeal tonsil
Tensor veli palatini
Levator veli palatini
Ascending palatine artery
Salpingopharyngeus
Pterygomandibular raphe
Palatoglossus
Styloglossus
Superior constrictor
Stylopharyngeus
Palatopharyngeus
Stylohyoid ligament
Glossopharyngeal nerve
Inferior constrictor
Middle constrictor
Mucous membrane of pharynx
Epiglottis

B

FIGURE 1, CONT'D   B, Median sagittal section of the head, showing a dissection of the interior of the pharynx, after the removal of the mucous membrane. *(From Gray's anatomy, 39th ed. St. Louis, 2004, Churchill Livingstone, Figs. 35.1 and 35.3.)*

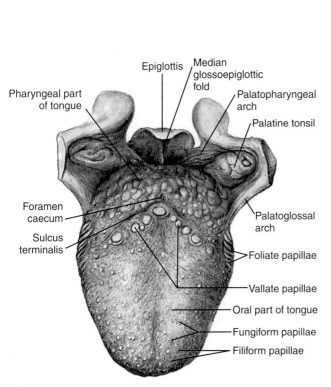

Epiglottis
Median glossoepiglottic fold
Pharyngeal part of tongue
Palatopharyngeal arch
Palatine tonsil
Foramen caecum
Palatoglossal arch
Sulcus terminalis
Foliate papillae
Vallate papillae
Oral part of tongue
Fungiform papillae
Filiform papillae

FIGURE 2   Contents of the oropharynx. *(From Gray's anatomy, 39th ed. St. Louis, 2004, Churchill Livingstone, Fig. 33.4.)*

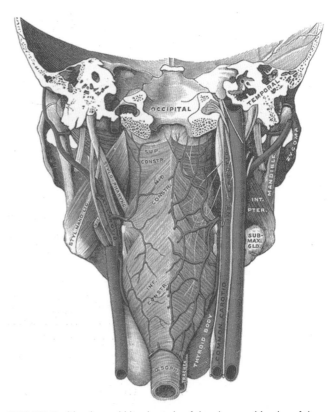

FIGURE 3   Muscles and blood supply of the pharynx. Muscles of the pharynx, viewed from behind, together with the associated vessels and nerves. *(Modified from Gray H: Anatomy of the human body. Philadelphia, 1918, Lea & Febiger. Available at www.bartleby.com/107/.)*

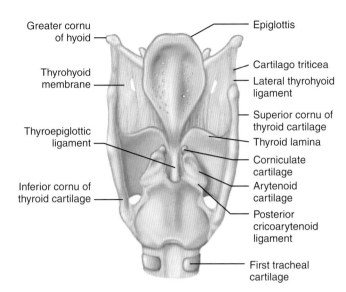

Greater cornu of hyoid

Thyrohyoid membrane

Thyroepiglottic ligament

Inferior cornu of thyroid cartilage

Epiglottis

Cartilago triticea

Lateral thyrohyoid ligament

Superior cornu of thyroid cartilage

Thyroid lamina

Corniculate cartilage

Arytenoid cartilage

Posterior cricoarytenoid ligament

First tracheal cartilage

FIGURE 4 Posterior view of the laryngeal cartilages and ligaments. *(From Gray's anatomy, 39th ed. St. Louis, 2004, Churchill Livingstone, Fig. 36.3.)*

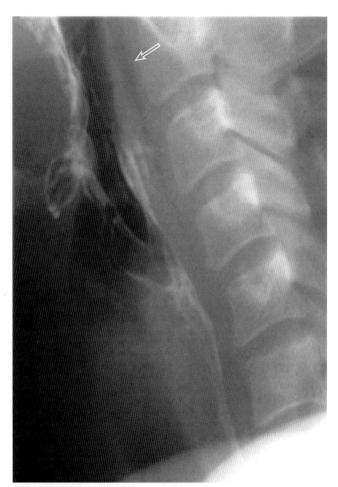

FIGURE 5 Retropharyngeal air *(arrow)* as seen on a lateral cervical spine radiograph/esophagogram.

PHARYNGEAL INJURY

Incidence

Isolated blunt pharyngeal injury is exceedingly rare. It is more often associated with concomitant cervical facial trauma. Penetrating pharyngeal injury occurs more commonly in the pediatric population from lacerations caused by intraoral foreign bodies.

Mechanism of Injury

Pharyngeal trauma may occur from foreign body ingestion, blunt or penetrating trauma, or following laryngoscopy or other endoscopic procedures.

Diagnosis

The initial clinical scenario varies. Patients with nonlethal injuries commonly present with dysphagia and odynophagia. Patients with more severe injuries may present with aphonia, dyspnea, hemoptysis, and severe acute respiratory failure that may rapidly lead to asphyxia if not treated. Injuries to the esophagus and pharynx are difficult to diagnose and may be missed during the management of other immediate life-threatening injuries. Oral bleeding, drooling, and subcutaneous emphysema all suggest upper digestive tract or airway injury. When possible, careful examination of the oropharynx and hypopharynx should be performed at the bedside.

Lateral views of the neck and cervical computed tomography (CT) scan may identify soft tissue air (Figs. 5 and 6). A nonionic contrast-enhanced esophagogram or esophagoscopy is indicated if injury is clinically suspected. Contrast material leak may be revealed on esophagogram (see Fig. 5).

LARYNX

Surgical Anatomy

The larynx is a functional "valve" separating the trachea from the upper aerodigestive tract. It is primarily an organ of communication (the

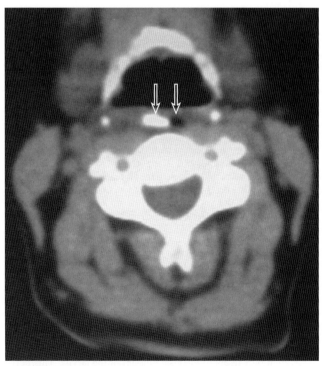

FIGURE 6 Retropharyngeal air as seen on a noncontrast computed tomography scan of the neck.

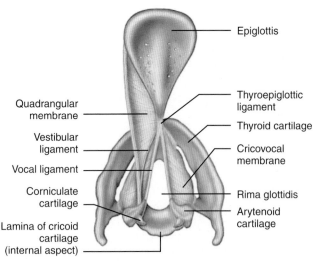

FIGURE 7 Superior view of laryngeal cartilages together with cricothyroid, quadrangular, and related ligaments and membranes. (*From Gray's anatomy, 39th ed, St. Louis, 2004, Churchill Livingstone, Fig. 36.7.*)

voice box), but also serves as an important regulator of respiration. The larynx is necessary for effective coughing and for creating Valsalva maneuvers. The larynx also prevents aspiration during swallowing.

The larynx is composed of the following elements:

Skeleton (Fig. 7)
  Hyoid bone: Attaches to epiglottis and strap muscles.
  Thyroid cartilage: Anterior attachment of vocal folds. Posterior articulation with cricoid cartilage.
  Cricoid cartilage: Complete ring. Articulates with thyroid and arytenoid cartilages.
  Arytenoids: Two cartilages that glide along the posterior cricoid and attach to posterior ends of vocal folds.
Divisions
  Supraglottis: Usually covered with respiratory epithelium containing mucous glands.
  Epiglottis: Leaf-shaped mucosal-covered cartilage, which projects over larynx.
  Aryepiglottic folds: Extend from the lateral epiglottis to the arytenoids.
  False vocal cords: Mucosal folds superior to the true glottis. Separated from true vocal folds by the ventricle.
  Ventricle: Mucosa-lined sac, variable in size, which separates the supraglottis from the glottis.
  Glottis: The true vocal folds attach to the thyroid cartilage at the anterior commissure. The posterior commissure is mobile, as the vocal folds attach to the arytenoids. Motion of the arytenoids effects abduction or adduction of the larynx. The bulk of the vocal fold is made up of muscle covered by mucosa. The free edge is characterized by stratified squamous epithelium. The vocal folds abduct for inspiration and adduct for phonation, cough, and Valsalva manuever.
  Subglottis: Below the vocal folds, extending to the inferior border of the cricoid cartilage.
Innervation—branches of the vagus nerve
  Superior laryngeal nerve: Sensation of the glottis and supraglottis. Motor fibers to the cricothyroid muscle, which tenses the vocal folds. This nerve leaves the vagus high in the neck.
  Recurrent laryngeal nerve: Sensation of the subglottis and motor fibers to intrinsic muscles of the larynx. This nerve branches from the vagus in the mediastinum, then turns back up into the neck. On the right, it travels inferior to the subclavian artery and on the left, the aorta.

Laryngeal Injury

Incidence

Laryngeal and cervical tracheal injuries are difficult and rare injuries and without appropriate diagnosis and management can result in significant morbidity and fatality. These injuries account for less than 1% of trauma cases seen in most major trauma centers and for only 1 in 30,000 emergency department visits. These injuries are rare compared to the total number of injuries that occur to the head and neck, and experience in managing laryngeal injures is limited because of the small number of cases. The rare nature of laryngeal injuries is a consequence of multiple factors including protection by the mandible and sternum, delayed or missed diagnosis of minor laryngeal injuries in major multitrauma victims, and patient fatality at the scene from airway loss and asphyxiation.

Although rare, initial management of laryngeal injuries affects the immediate probability of patient survival and long-term quality of life. The larynx is a well-protected structure that is both anatomically and functionally complex. Blunt and penetrating laryngeal injuries may cause chronic problems with aspiration, phonation, and respiration.

Mechanism of Injury

The mechanisms of laryngeal injury can be divided into blunt trauma (including crushing, clothesline, and strangulation injuries) and penetrating trauma. The degree and location of blunt laryngotracheal trauma are multifactorial. Sheely et al found that 88% of injuries occurred above the fourth tracheal ring. Penetrating injury can occur at any level of the cervical trachea.

Diagnosis

Adherence to the essential principles of initial assessment delineated in the *Advanced Trauma Life Support (ATLS) Manual* is recommended. The ABCs (airway, breathing, circulation), concomitant resuscitation of the trauma victim, and a thorough secondary survey are essential for optimal management of airway injuries. Early recognition of these injuries requires a high index of suspicion based on mechanism of injury and findings identified during cervical and chest examination. Clinical signs and symptoms may include stridor, acute respiratory distress, cervical tenderness, subcutaneous emphysema, and cervical hematoma when associated with major vascular injury. Hemoptysis suggests that an intralaryngeal laceration may be present. This is more common with penetrating injury, but also occurs from blunt laryngeal trauma with an associated laryngeal cartilage fracture. Diagnostic procedures such as direct laryngoscopy, fiberoptic bronchoscopy, and cervical helical, contrast-enhanced multidetector (16 slices minimum, 64 slices preferred) CT with angiography are all beneficial if the patient's clinical condition permits performing these tests. A sample algorithm for the evaluation of patients with laryngeal injuries is described in Figure 8.

Treatment

A recent series of 12 patients with laryngeal facture reported 6 (50%) that were managed nonoperatively. They were all patients with nondisplaced laryngeal factures who were treated with a soft diet, observation in hospital, and intravenous dexamethasone 10 mg every 8 hours for 24 hours. All patients had return to normal voice function after healing. Comminuted or displaced fractures require surgical intervention, and early reduction will usually result in better functional outcome compared to delayed repair. Severity of laryngeal injury can be classified according to the Schaefer-Fuhrman laryngeal injury classification[NR1,NR2] and may be helpful in determining subsequent treatment (Table 1).

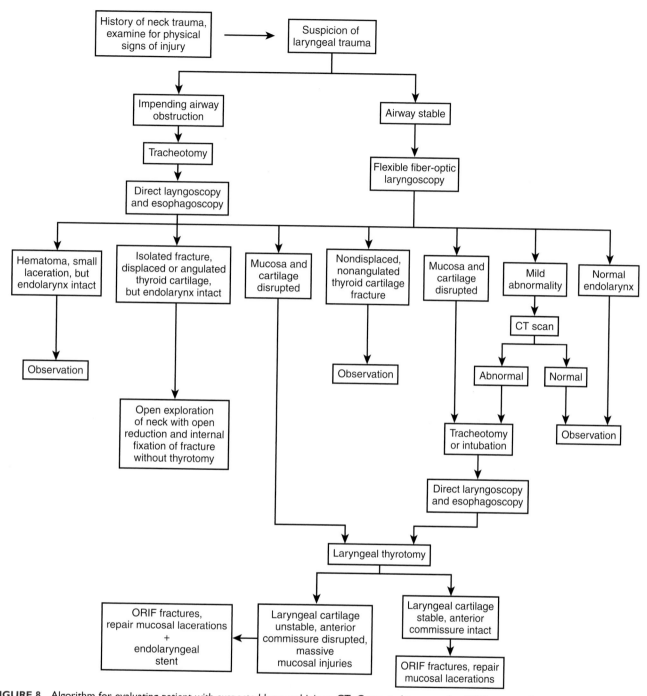

FIGURE 8 Algorithm for evaluating patient with suspected laryngeal injury. CT, Computed tomography; ORIF, open reduction with internal fixation. *(Modified from Pancholi SS: Fractures, laryngeal. Louisa, KY, Three Rivers Medical Center, Department of Otolaryngology, November 3, 2005. Available at http://www.emedicine.com/ent/topic488.htm.)*

TABLE I: Schaefer-Fuhrman Laryngeal Injury Classification[NT1,NT2]

Group	Injury
I	Minor endolaryngeal hematoma without detectable fracture
II	Edema, hematoma, minor mucosal disruption without exposed cartilage, nondisplaced fractures
III	Massive edema, mucosal disruption, exposed cartilage, vocal fold immobility, displaced fracture
IV	Group III with two or more fracture lines or massive trauma to laryngeal mucosa
V	Complete laryngotracheal separation

TRACHEA

Surgical Anatomy

The trachea is a cartilaginous and membranous tube. It extends from the lower part of the larynx, at the level of the sixth cervical vertebra, to the upper border of the fifth thoracic vertebra. There it divides into the two main bronchi. The trachea is an ellipsoid cylinder that is flattened posteriorly. The average adult trachea measures about 11 cm in length with a diameter that ranges from 2 to 2.5 cm. The pediatric trachea is smaller, more deeply placed, and more mobile. Half of the trachea lies within the neck and half is intrathoracic. The anterior two thirds of the trachea are composed of 18 to 22 U-shaped cartilages. The membranous posterior wall of the trachea is in apposition with the anterior wall of the esophagus. The bifurcation of the main bronchi forms the carina at approximately the fourth to fifth thoracic vertebrae. The trachea is supplied with blood by the inferior thyroid arteries. Similarly named veins form the thyroid venous plexus. Tracheal innervation is derived from the vagus nerves, the recurrent laryngeal nerves, and the sympathetic chain. The recurrent laryngeal nerve lies within the tracheoesophageal groove formed by the close proximity of the lateral aspects of the trachea and the esophagus (Figs. 9 to 11).

Tracheal Injury

Incidence

Disruption of the tracheobronchial tree is a rare occurrence and most surgeons' experience is limited. On average, one such case is seen per year in large trauma centers. Bertelsen and Howitz reviewed 1178 postmortem reports of trauma deaths and found 33 (2.8%) with tracheal or bronchial disruptions. Of these 33 cases, 27 were dead at the scene.

Complete cervical transection is rarer still. The true incidence of cervical transection (and tracheobronchial injuries in general) is unknown. There have been a number of case reports and small series described in the literature; however, the extant surgical experience remains limited.

Knowledge of emergency airway management is essential. Loss of the airway in this clinical circumstance can rapidly lead to serious complications and the patient's demise.

Fatality in those patients who do not have complete airway loss at the time of injury is due to the severity of associated injuries. Those patients who arrive alive to a trauma center with isolated tracheobronchial injuries, including complete transection, have a reasonable chance for survival if the trauma surgeon has mastered the skills required for managing a difficult airway.

FIGURE 9 Schematic representation of the anatomy of the larynx: anterior, posterior, midsagittal, and sagittal views. *(From Miller RD, et al: Anesthesia for eye, ear, nose, and throat surgery. Miller's Anesthesia, ed 7, chapter 75, Philadelphia, 2010, Churchill Livingstone.)*

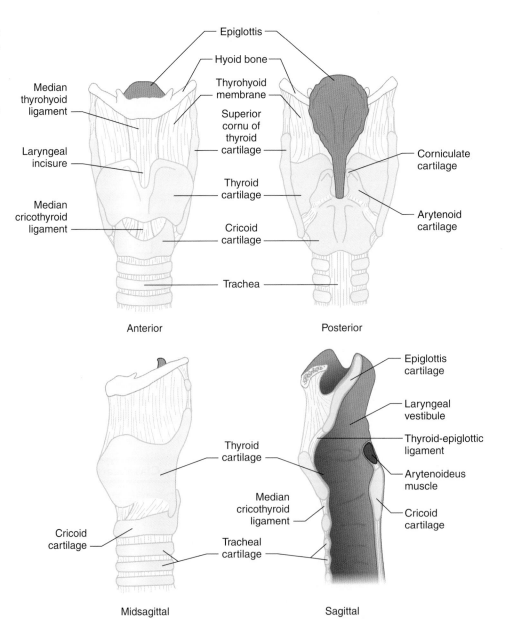

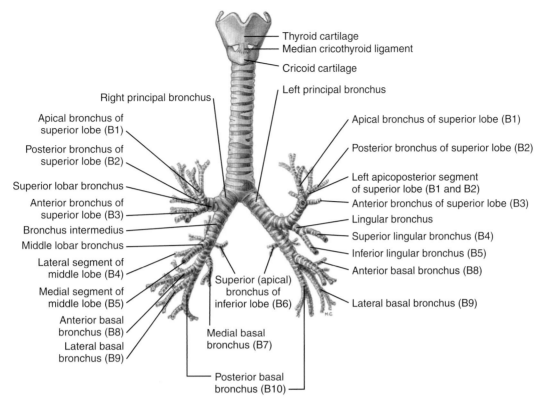

Right principal bronchus

Apical bronchus of
superior lobe (B1)

Posterior bronchus of
superior lobe (B2)

Superior lobar bronchus

Anterior bronchus of
superior lobe (B3)

Bronchus intermedius

Middle lobar bronchus

Lateral segment of
middle lobe (B4)

Medial segment of
middle lobe (B5)

Anterior basal
bronchus (B8)

Lateral basal
bronchus (B9)

Medial basal
bronchus (B7)

Superior (apical)
bronchus of
inferior lobe (B6)

Posterior basal
bronchus (B10)

Thyroid cartilage

Median cricothyroid ligament

Cricoid cartilage

Left principal bronchus

Apical bronchus of superior lobe (B1)

Posterior bronchus of superior lobe (B2)

Left apicoposterior segment
of superior lobe (B1 and B2)

Anterior bronchus of superior lobe (B3)

Lingular bronchus

Superior lingular bronchus (B4)

Inferior lingular bronchus (B5)

Anterior basal bronchus (B8)

Lateral basal bronchus (B9)

FIGURE 10   The cartilages of the larynx, trachea, and bronchi: anterior aspect. *(From* Gray's anatomy, *39th ed, St. Louis, 2004, Churchill Livingstone, Fig. 63.12.)*

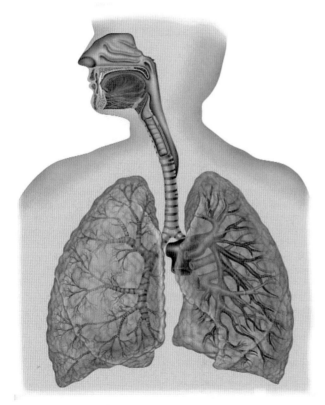

FIGURE 11   The respiratory tract. Those parts of the tract in the head and upper neck are shown in sagittal section, in the lower neck turned anteriorly and, in the remainder of the tract, from the anterior aspect. The right lung shows the bronchial tree in detail whereas the left lung shows the pulmonary vasculature. *(From* Gray's anatomy, *39th ed, St. Louis, 2004, Churchill Livingstone, Fig. 63.1.)*

Beskin reported the first successful repair of a complete cervical transection after blunt trauma in 1957. In 1959, Hood and Sloan collected 18 cases of tracheobronchial injury in the world literature. Complete tracheal transection was "rarely found." In a more recent series, Ecker et al reported a total of 105 tracheobronchial injuries, of which 75 were from penetrating trauma and 30 from blunt trauma. Of these, only 24 patients survived the transfer from the scene of the accident to the trauma center. Of the 30 blunt trauma victims reported in this series, 18 were dead on arrival at the emergency department. The majority of those who arrived alive, regardless of the mechanism of injury, had no other associated injuries (15 of 24 [63%]), and the remainder had only one other associated injury, including esophageal injuries (9 of 24 [37%]). In the same series, the most commonly injured segment of the tracheobronchial tree in survivors was the cervical trachea (37%). The total number of complete tracheal transections in Ecker and associates' series is unknown.

Kelly et al reviewed 106 patients with tracheobronchial injuries of which only 6 had a blunt mechanism of injury. They concluded that a surgeon must adopt a rapid, aggressive surgical approach to these patients in order to prevent fatal outcomes.

Mechanism of Injury

Cervical Trachea

Injuries to the cervical trachea may be caused by blunt or penetrating trauma. Penetrating injury is relatively straightforward. With the exception of shrapnel wounds, this injury consists of a traumatic defect created by the trajectory of a knife or bullet. Knife wounds more commonly occur in the cervical trachea, but gunshot wound injuries may occur at any point along the course of the tracheobronchial tree.

In one review, blunt injury to the cervical tracheal was reported to occur in less than 1% of all 1248 blunt trauma patients admitted over the study period. In this anatomic region, blunt injuries to the larynx are the most frequent. They usually result from motor vehicle accidents or sports injuries and direct blows to this area (e.g., "clothesline injury").

Intrathoracic Tracheal Injury

Injuries in this region are more commonly caused by blunt trauma, but may also result from penetrating injuries. In the former, the exact mechanism is unknown. Several theories have been advanced. This injury is often associated with sudden and forceful compression of the thorax. It is postulated that a rapid anteroposterior compression of the trachea in combination with a closed glottis causes markedly increased tracheal intraluminal pressure. When shearing forces are added to the tracheobronchial tree between the relatively stationary cricoid cartilage and carina (encountered during rapid deceleration), bronchial rupture may occur. Intrathoracic tracheal disruption usually occurs at the junction of the membranous and cartilaginous trachea within 2 cm of the carina. Vertical lesions are rare. When they do occur, they are more commonly located posteriorly where the cartilage is less evident. Bronchial injuries more commonly involve the main bronchi. They tend to occur within 2.5 cm of the carina.

Gunshot wounds are the most frequent penetrating injuries. The incidence of thoracic tracheobronchial injury increases with transmediastinal gunshot wounds. Injuries to the heart, great vessels, and esophagus are common in these cases, and are major contributors to morbidity and fatality.

Diagnosis

A thorough physical examination and knowledge of the mechanism of injury are the first and most important steps in diagnosing a tracheobronchial injury. Clinical findings suggesting airway injury vary according to the mechanism of injury. Cicala et al reviewed nine patients following stab wounds. A laceration directly communicating with the airway was present in five cases. Subcutaneous emphysema was apparent on physical examination and on lateral cervical spine radiograph in three cases. Only one patient had no obvious clinical or radiographic findings to suggest an airway injury. This patient had a small puncture laceration of the cricotracheal membrane, which was diagnosed by bronchoscopy. The majority of patients presenting with gunshot wounds to the trachea will show physical or radiographic findings that suggest airway injury on a plain radiograph of the neck or chest. In the study by Cicala and colleagues, two patients with gunshot wounds to the cervicothoracic trachea developed tension pneumothorax with massive air leak during resuscitation. Two others had fractures of the thyroid cartilage without any airway compromise. One was diagnosed by direct palpation on physical examination. The other patient was diagnosed by cervical CT scan. Hemoptysis, in addition to other findings, was noted in two of the gunshot wound victims.

Blunt trauma patients who survive to the emergency department may present with a wide spectrum of clinical signs and symptoms dependant on the severity and location of the injury to the cervical thoracic trachea. Blunt cervical tracheal injury may create severe respiratory compromise leading to rapid acute respiratory failure and asphyxia. Alternatively, patients with less severe injuries may present with stridor, hoarseness, hemoptysis, and subcutaneous emphysema.

Plain radiographs of the neck and chest may be diagnostic. Subcutaneous emphysema in the neck and chest wall on plain radiographs or CT scan should prompt further evaluation if clinical suspicion favors a major airway injury. Fiberoptic bronchoscopy is the first step in confirming a tracheal injury. Indications for bronchoscopy include a large pneumomediastinum, persistent pneumothorax, or a large, persistent air leak after placement of a functional thoracostomy tube; persistent atelectasis; and expanding severe subcutaneous emphysema. Bronchoscopy is the most accurate and reliable means to establish the diagnosis, determine the site, and define the extent of the injury. Debate remains as to whether rigid or flexible bronchoscopy is superior in this setting. Disadvantages of rigid bronchoscopy include the need for a general anesthetic and a stable cervical spine. Flexible bronchoscopy does not require a general anesthetic and may be used in patients whose cervical spine may be injured. Fiberoptic bronchoscopy is not only diagnostic, but may also be useful in establishing an airway with bronchoscopically guided endotracheal tube placement.

Preoperative assessment of the vocal cords in this setting is strongly recommended. Direct laryngoscopy may be necessary to evaluate the function of the vocal cords. The presence of a recurrent laryngeal nerve injury causing vocal cord paralysis may assist the operating surgeon in determining whether tracheostomy is needed regardless of the location or extent of airway injury.

SURGICAL MANAGEMENT

Surgical management includes appropriate nonoperative observation (by a trauma surgeon) as well as operative intervention. Initial airway management must be approached with caution. Patients who are spontaneously breathing and maintaining adequate oxygenation and ventilation should not be intubated unless their clinical condition deteriorates. Patients intubated prior to arrival in the emergency department should undergo flexible bronchoscopy as soon as possible. Careful intubation over a bronchoscope, performed by an experienced bronchoscopist, is the optimal approach for those patients who require early airway control for clinical deterioration or for treatment of other life-threatening injuries. Intubation is ideally performed in the operating room where emergent cricothyroidotomy or tracheostomy can be performed if necessary. The trauma surgeon must be prepared to extend the tracheostomy incision to a median sternotomy if the distal trachea retracts into the mediastinum. Clinical deterioration may still occur as positive-pressure ventilation is applied if the injury is distal to the tracheostomy. High-frequency ventilation or low tidal volume ventilation with additional tube thoracostomies may be necessary.

Nonoperative Management

Small iatrogenic injuries from endotracheal intubation or from minimal blunt trauma can often be safely observed. Most injuries from high-energy blunt force trauma and all penetrating injuries are not generally considered for nonoperative management.

Gomez-Caro et al reported the successful management of 17 patients with iatrogenic tracheobronchial injuries between 1993 and 2003. Many of these lesions were as large as 4 cm in length. The authors reported no complications or deaths directly caused by nonoperative management. Clinical and endoscopic follow-up in 14 of 17 patients was uneventful. Guidelines for nonoperative management include vital signs stability, no associated esophageal injury, no issues with mechanical ventilation or intubation (if necessary), no development of severe subcutaneous emphysema or mediastinal emphysema, and no signs of sepsis. Additional requirements for nonoperative management have been published and include only small tracheobronchial lacerations, such as those with less than one third of the circumference of the trachea, well-opposed edges, no significant tissue loss, no associated injuries, and no need for positive-pressure ventilation. Intubation, as well as tracheostomy, should ideally be avoided. When necessary, endotracheal intubation with placement of the endotracheal tube balloon distal to the tear has been proposed by Marquette et al. This technique has been successfully used on three occasions by one of the authors. Nonoperative management includes administering prophylactic antibiotics and proton pump inhibitors, very close observation, and close bronchoscopic follow-up. A sample algorithm is provided in Figure 12.

Nonoperative Case Presentation

- The patient is a 43-year-old woman who was injured in a high-speed motor vehicle collision.
- She had suffered significant blunt chest trauma and had diffuse pulmonary contusions and significant hypoxemia resulting in severe acute respiratory distress syndrome. See Figures 13 and 14.
- Because of the severity of the pulmonary injury, operative intervention was not considered an option.

TRACHEOBRONCHIAL INJURY CONFIRMED
- Lesion <one third of tracheal circumference
- Lesion <4 cm in length
- Wound edges well opposed
- No significant tracheal tissue loss

Criteria met   Criteria not met

Nonoperative management ← Yes — Nonoperative risk less than operative risk?

No

Mechanical ventilation required — Yes

Operative management

No

- Humidified O_2
- Voice rest
- Antibiotics
- Proton pump inhibitor or H_2 blocker
- Close observation
- Follow-up bronchoscopy

- Consider high-frequency ventilation
- Consider very low tidal volume ventilation and permissive hypercapnia

FIGURE 12 Algorithm for nonoperative management of tracheobronchial injuries.

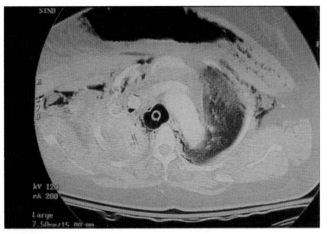

FIGURE 14 Distal tracheal tear from blunt trauma.

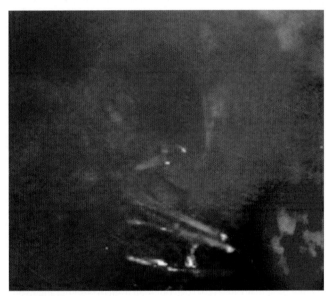

FIGURE 15 A 4-cm distal tear from blunt trauma.

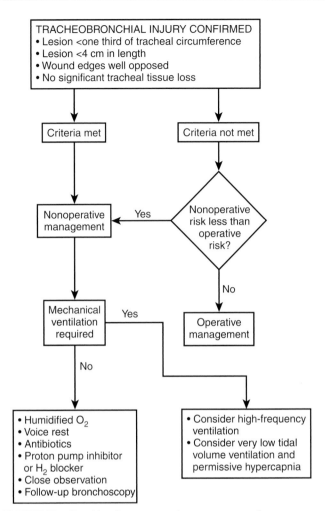

FIGURE 13 Distal tracheal tear from blunt trauma.

- Bronchoscopy revealed a 4-cm tear in the right posterolateral distal trachea extending into the right main bronchus (Fig. 15).
- The patient was treated with daily bronchoscopy, low tidal volume ventilation with permissive hypercapnia (350 mL tidal volume), and controlled mechanical ventilation with 15 cm H_2O positive end-expiratory pressure.
- The laceration closed in 7 days.
- The patient survived hospitalization with return to normal function.

Operative Management

Patients diagnosed with a major tracheobronchial injury should always undergo surgery unless medical instability or severe associated injuries are significantly prohibitive. In those situations, all efforts are made to support and stabilize the patient while maintaining adequate oxygenation and ventilation. High-frequency ventilation may be helpful. Permissive hypercapnia using very low tidal volumes (less than 5 mL/kg) has also been successfully used.

The majority of patients are optimally managed with early surgery. The site of injury dictates the operative approach. These injuries are often challenging to even the most experienced surgeon, and appropriate consultation with an otolaryngologist for high cervical injuries or a thoracic surgeon for more distal intrathoracic injuries may be helpful.

Most cervical injuries are approached through a transverse collar incision (Fig. 16). This incision can be extended cephalad along the anterior border of either sternocleidomastoid muscle, depending on the location of the primary and any associated injuries. Penetrating cervical injuries can often be approached directly, incorporating the wound into the incision. This may be necessary to achieve early airway control.

Blunt cervical tracheal injuries are also approached through a transverse collar incision 2 cm above the sternal notch. The chest

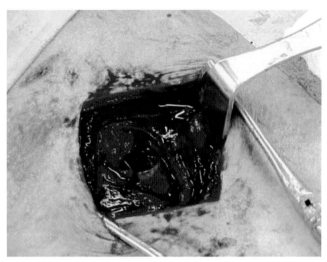

FIGURE 16 Cervical tracheal tear from blunt trauma exposed via a collar incision.

should always be prepped for median sternotomy. An upper median sternotomy is immediately performed if the distal trachea retracts into the chest. Do not necessarily expect to find the trachea in its usual midline position. We have experienced one case in which the distal trachea, upon entry into the chest, retracted 10 cm below the sternal notch and 10 cm to the left of midline.

Most blunt intrathoracic tracheobronchial injuries occur within 2 to 3 cm of the carina. A right posterolateral thoracotomy through the fourth or fifth intercostal space provides the best exposure unless the injury is on the left more than 2 to 3 cm distal to the carina. In this situation, a left posterolateral thoracotomy through the fifth intercostal space is preferred.

Prior consultation with the anesthesiologist is crucial. A variety of endotracheal tubes, connectors, and ventilator tubing should be available on the operative table prior to opening the chest. Intubation over a bronchoscope in the operating room is best for optimal tube placement. Double-lumen tubes are beneficial for providing single-lung ventilation. However, their larger size may cause further damage and hinder the operative repair. Positioning the patient for thoracotomy and opening the chest may cause rapid deterioration from hypoxemia and hypoventilation. Opening the chest quickly with direct intubation of a major bronchus through the operative field may be necessary. The surgeon may also be able to direct the orotracheal tube from the upper trachea into the uninjured bronchus to provide single-lung ventilation. If the anatomy of the injury is not completely known, two ventilators should be available in the operating room so that bilateral single-lung ventilation can be provided if needed. The Univent endobronchial blocker may also be helpful if there is active bleeding from one of the main or segmental bronchi. This device incorporates an endotracheal tube with a maneuverable device that can be directed into and occlude a main bronchus, an intermediate trunk, or a lobar bronchus.

Repair of the trachea and bronchi requires optimal débridement of all devitalized tissue and primary end-to-end anastomosis. Either permanent or absorbable monofilament sutures are preferred. The authors prefer a running monofilament absorbable suture. All knots are tied external to the lumen to reduce the risk of granuloma formation. Management "pearls" are provided in Table 2.

MORBIDITY

Early Complications

In the early postinjury period following tracheal or laryngeal injury, *loss of airway* represents the greatest immediate threat. The need for

TABLE 2: Management Pearls for Acute Laryngotracheal Trauma

Avoid searching for recurrent laryngeal nerves
Avoid tracheostomy through the repair
Conserve viable trachea
Make thorough evaluation of associated injuries
Flex neck postoperatively to reduce tension on tracheal repair
Ensure proper airway management
Separate tracheal and esophageal suture lines

Modified from Mathisen DJ, Grillo H: Laryngotracheal trauma. *Ann Thorac Surg* 43:254–262, 1987.

definitive airway control is dictated by clinical signs of respiratory insufficiency such as dyspnea, tachypnea, hypoxemia, or massive hemoptysis. When laryngeal injury is suspected, care should be taken when passing the tube through the area of injury as partial tears can be converted into complete tears. Tension pneumothorax and massive subcutaneous emphysema may lead to mechanical ventilatory failure from mechanical constraints limiting pulmonary expansion. Endotracheal intubation can be attempted with extreme caution. When advancing the tube past the vocal cords, care should be taken if tracheal injury is present or suspected. Nasotracheal intubation with a no. 7 or smaller cuffed endotracheal tube over a flexible bronchoscope has been proposed as one option in the stable patient. This procedure should ideally be performed in the operating room or where conditions for performing an immediate surgical airway are optimal. Identification of the injury and strategically guided tube placement may be possible while minimizing iatrogenic trauma during intubation. This technique may be particularly useful in cases of near-complete or complete tracheal transection when suspected preoperatively to advance the tube into the distal tracheal segment. This maneuver must be performed by an experienced bronchoscopist. Even in cases when complete tracheal transection has occurred, adequate ventilation and oxygenation may be achieved with intubation of only the proximal tracheal remnant provided that the paratracheal tissues of the neck and superior mediastinum are still intact. Caution should be taken in this setting at the time of operation or attempted surgical airway control when entering this space from a cervical incision; rapid ventilatory failure and cardiopulmonary collapse can occur when this air space is entered and this distal tracheal segment has not been secured with an airway. The distal tracheal segment may retract back into the superior mediastinum and be difficult to access from a cervical incision. This may be prevented by performing a sternotomy prior to entering the pretracheal space when complete tracheal transection is suspected preoperatively.

Tension pneumothorax can lead to rapid cardiopulmonary collapse if not quickly recognized and treated. Although temporary improvement may be achieved, needle thoracostomy should be reserved for patients with impending cardiopulmonary collapse in the prehospital or emergency department setting. Immediate placement of one or more tube thoracostomies is the ideal treatment and may be lifesaving. Patients with tracheobronchial injuries may develop a large air leak following pleural space drainage. In addition to increasing the negative pressure suction applied to the pleural space, advanced ventilatory strategies may be required to improve gas exchange. Low tidal volume ventilation, high-frequency jet ventilation, and high-frequency oscillatory ventilation have all been used with success to reduce peak airway pressure, increase mean airway pressure, reduce air leak, and promote healing at the site of injury.

Pneumomediastinum may occur following tracheobronchial injury. Although hemodynamic compromise has been reported from air under pressure in the mediastinum, this appears to be unusual. Treatment is directed toward the underlying injury and resolution following injury repair, and recovery is the rule.

Subcutaneous emphysema can be massive, spreading to all areas of the body very quickly. Although treatment with multiple incisions or drains has been advocated, the emphysema itself has no direct adverse sequelae and is usually self-limiting.

Massive bleeding into the airways suggests an associated major vascular injury. Initial treatment should be directed at identification and control of hemorrhage from this injury. Large volumes of blood shed into the airway can lead to airway obstruction and profound hypoxemia from impaired gas exchange. Following definitive airway control, the endotracheal cuff should be advanced beyond the site of bleeding into the airway, if possible. Bronchoscopic lavage of retained blood and clots may be of further benefit in clearing retained hemorrhage and improving hypoxemia.

Associated injuries are common and account for a substantial portion of early morbidity. A high index of suspicion for these injuries is maintained throughout early evaluation. Patient management based on ATLS guidelines will minimize associated morbidity.

Late Complications

Late complications following tracheal injury are often related to the integrity of the area of injury or site of surgical repair.

The incidence of tracheobronchial stenosis following injury is 3.8% to 9.3% following surgical repair. Stenosis may also occur when nonoperative management of a tracheal or bronchial tear is attempted. Initial measures to reduce inflammation include corticosteroid therapy and proton pump inhibitors or H_2 blockers to reduce aspiration of acidic gastric contents. Steroid therapy is controversial. The risks of immunosuppression and compromised wound healing must be compared to the benefits of reduced scarring and stenosis. Steroids may be beneficial during nonoperative management to reduce stenosis from hypertrophic granulation tissue, but there are currently no large studies to refute or support this therapy. Factors associated with a higher incidence of tracheal stenosis include degree of tracheal injury and increased time to operative repair. Others have not found increased stenosis rates when operative repair is delayed. Timing of operative repair is determined by associated injuries and overall physiologic status. Surgical repair should proceed as soon as possible to reduce this potential complication. Good surgical technique can reduce postoperative tracheal stenosis. Complete débridement of devitalized tissue, wide mobilization to reduce anastomotic tension, and possibly the use of absorbable sutures are principles that may reduce inflammation and enhance normal healing in the repair site. Vascularized pedicles of muscle, usually the sternocleidomastoid or the strap muscles, sewn as a buttress to the anastomotic site have been shown to reduce the rate of anastomotic dehiscence, leak, and subsequent fistula formation. Tracheal stenosis is suspected when stridor, dyspnea, or air hunger develop following tracheal repair or injury. Usually, the history is one of worsening progression over several days to weeks. Voice changes may occur simultaneously. Other symptoms may include postobstructive atelectasis or pulmonary sepsis, particularly following bronchial or distal segment repairs.

Flexible or rigid bronchoscopy provides an accurate diagnosis and an opportunity for simultaneous treatment. Modern multidetector CT scanners are also highly sensitive and specific for diagnosing tracheobronchial injury. Anatomic detail with three-dimensional reconstruction is very useful in planning operative or interventional repair. Treatment options include: (1) endoscopic dilatation with steroid therapy; (2) silicone, metal, or Teflon stent placement; (3) Nd-YAG laser ablation of scar tissue; or (4) open surgical repair. All of these treatments have been individually successful, and the therapeutic approach in any given patient must be individualized based on the extent of stenosis, severity of comorbid conditions, and the experience and resources of each surgeon and facility. Many different open surgical techniques have been described, but general principles should include resection and débridement of tracheal scar with tracheal mobilization and primary end-to-end anastomosis with absorbable suture.

Tracheoesophageal fistula may occur following a delay in diagnosis or treatment of esophageal and tracheal injuries. A high index of suspicion for esophageal or tracheal injury must be maintained whenever the other is identified, and thorough evaluation with bronchoscopy, esophagoscopy, or esophagography is usually required. Careful and thorough intraoperative evaluation at surgery is mandatory. Full mobilization of the cervical esophagus and intraluminal instillation of methylene blue have been advocated to avoid missing a subtle esophageal tear. Following identification of a late tracheoesophageal fistula, delayed repair is planned following medical stabilization, treatment of aspiration pneumonitis or pneumonia, and gastrostomy tube placement. Repair consists of wide esophageal and tracheal mobilization, débridement to healthy tissue, and primary end-to-end anastomosis. Transposition of a vascularized pedicle of muscle between the areas of repair to be dictated by the anatomic location of the fistula is mandatory to reduce anastomotic dehiscence and recurrent fistula formation.

Voice changes such as dysphonia and laryngeal stenosis can occur following laryngeal injury when architectural relationships within the voice box are altered by healing. Poor outcomes are associated with injuries that create significant mucosal disruption, arytenoid dislocation, or exposed cartilage. One series reported an association between delays in operative repair beyond 24 hours and increased rates of airway stenosis ranging from 13% to 31%. Laryngeal stenting, particularly when one or both vocal cords are mobile, helps preserve the voice by normalizing the shape of the anterior commissure. Stents should be removed as soon as possible (usually 10–14 days) because of the risk of compromised mucosal perfusion with prolonged usage.

Vocal cord paralysis from recurrent laryngeal nerve injury may be unilateral or bilateral following tracheal or laryngeal injuries. Cricotracheal separation carries a 60% risk of recurrent nerve injury, which is often bilateral. Resolution of neuropraxia and nerve regeneration may occur up to 1 year following injury, resulting in resolution of vocal cord paralysis in some cases.

Laryngeal webs, granulomas, and hypertrophic granulation can develop several months following laryngeal trauma. Follow-up endoscopy with laser ablation can prevent chronic problems from these less serious complications.

Other Potentially Life-Threatening Complications

Pharyngeal injuries can lead to serious complications, particularly when the diagnosis is delayed. Retropharyngeal abscess is uncommon but potentially life threatening if upper airway obstruction or mediastinitis develops. A short course of prophylactic antibiotics may reduce the risk of this complication. The diagnosis is usually apparent upon inspection of the oropharynx and palatine tonsils. Retropharyngeal air may be present on lateral cervical radiograph. If present, further evaluation should include cervical and mediastinal CT scan. Surgical drainage of the abscess and broad-spectrum intravenous antibiotics are indicated. Surgical intensive care unit admission and possible intubation may be necessary in severe cases.

Injury to the internal carotid artery should also be considered whenever an impalement injury of the posterior pharynx is diagnosed. Asymptomatic dissection of the internal carotid artery followed by arterial occlusion or embolization to the cerebral vasculature may develop over several hours to days resulting in severe neurologic deficits. Therefore, a high index of suspicion and screening with angiography should be performed when clinical presentation suggests this possibility. CT angiography (CTA) has improved in recent years with multidetector scanners. Experience suggests that CTA may be a good screening tool to identify these injuries.

Anticoagulation to prevent propagation and occlusion of the dissection is standard therapy, but experience with carotid stents is growing. Carotid stenting may be an alternative in selected cases. Surgical repair of the internal carotid artery is usually impossible because of the distal location of most lesions.

MORTALITY

The mortality rate for tracheobronchial injuries in most modern series is less than 30%. A large literature review pooled all patients with blunt tracheobronchial injury reported between 1873 and 1996 and found a 9% mortality rate since 1970 for patients who arrived alive at the hospital. Left-sided injuries, high-speed deceleration, and crush mechanisms are associated with the poorest outcomes. Autopsy series suggest that 80% of patients with tracheobronchial injuries die at the scene. Early fatality results from associated injuries and loss of airway.

Mortality rate from laryngeal injuries has been reported as high as 40% and is primarily attributable to asphyxiation from airway compromise. Penetrating laryngeal injuries appear to have a lower mortality rate (20%). Death from penetrating injuries is more attributable to associated injuries, particularly esophageal and major vascular injuries.

Attributable mortality risk from pharyngeal injuries is difficult to determine because these injuries are rarely life threatening. Death is usually attributable to the internal carotid artery thrombosis, cervical infection, or mediastinitis. When present, the outcome for each of these complications is dependent on early diagnosis and treatment.

For the chapter's Suggested Readings list, please visit the book at www.ExpertConsult.inkling.com.

THORACIC INJURIES

PERTINENT SURGICAL ANATOMY OF THE THORAX AND MEDIASTINUM

Brandon Tieu, Paul Schipper, Mithran Sukumar, and John C. Mayberry

The thorax consists of the chest wall comprising the sternum, ribs, and thoracic vertebrae; the mediastinum containing the pericardium, heart, esophagus, trachea, great vessels, thoracic duct, and thymus; and the paired pleural cavities containing the lungs. This chapter will discuss the anatomy of these structures and spaces, as pertinent to trauma surgery and the surgical intensive care unit.

CHEST WALL

The muscular, tendinous, and bony structures of the chest serve several functions. The chest wall must be rigid enough to protect the thoracic viscera and serve as a fixation point against which the muscles of the upper extremity and abdomen can work yet flexible enough to expand and contract with vigorous respirations.

With gentle respirations, the chest wall is a cylinder with the diaphragm as its piston. With inspiration, the diaphragm contracts, its dome is flattened, and like a piston, it descends in the chest. This motion increases the volume of the thorax, and actively expands the lungs by drawing in air through the trachea. The lungs are very elastic and tend to collapse without outward forces keeping them expanded. With exhalation, the diaphragm relaxes, the elasticity of the lungs causes lung volume to decrease, and air is expelled. Ultimately, the tendency of the lung to collapse is countered by the outward force/rigidity of the chest wall. With vigorous respirations, the intercostal muscles, scalenes, and other accessory muscles of respiration elevate the ribs and increase the thoracic volume much more than usual. With vigorous respirations, the chest wall and diaphragm act in concert like a bellows increasing thoracic volume and then relaxing and allowing the elasticity of the lung to decrease thoracic volume.

The bony structures of the chest wall include 12 ribs, 12 thoracic vertebrae, and the sternum. All ribs articulate posteriorly with the transverse processes and vertebral bodies of their respective

thoracic vertebrae and the vertebral body directly superior (Fig. 1). Ribs 1 through 7 are called true ribs because they articulate anteriorly directly with the sternum through their own costal cartilage. Ribs 8, 9, and 10 are called false ribs because they articulate anteriorly to the costal cartilage of the rib above. This creates a construct of stair-stepping costal cartilages, which ultimately articulates with the sternum and creates the costal arch or costal margin. Ribs 11 and 12 are called floating ribs because they do not articulate with any structure anteriorly (Fig. 2). Rather, they attach to the abdominal wall musculature, primarily the internal oblique muscle.

Because ribs 1 through 10 are fixed anteriorly and posteriorly, they function much like a bucket handle (Fig. 3A). When performing a tube thoracostomy, as you approach the sternum anteriorly and the transverse processes posteriorly, the size of the interspace becomes fixed and narrow. Laterally, away from these points of attachment, the ribs separate and the interspace opens. The widest portion of the interspaces can be found at the lateral apogee or "keystone" of the rib. Tube thoracostomies placed laterally will be easier to place through the interspace and more comfortable for the patient (Fig. 3B). Also, when creating a thoracotomy, division of the intercostal muscles far anterior and posterior will create a larger working space without tearing the intercostal muscle or fracturing a rib with placement of the rib spreader. The skin need only be divided over the working space, not over the entire intercostal incision.

The sternum has three parts, the manubrium, the body, and the xiphoid process. The manubrium is thick and broad, articulating with the clavicle, first rib, and sharing the second rib articulation with the body of the sternum. The sternoclavicular articulation is the only bony articulation of the thorax to the shoulder girdle (see Fig. 2). Understanding the angle of the clavicle, manubrium, and first rib is important in safe placement of central venous catheters into the subclavian vein. The subclavian vein and artery leave the arm and enter the thoracic inlet over the top of the first rib and under the clavicle. Once under the clavicle, a needle directed parallel to the clavicle and first rib will not enter the chest and cause a pneumothorax before finding the subclavian vein. A needle directed too steeply in its approach will quickly enter and exit the triangle where the subclavian vein is found, penetrate the intercostal space, and puncture the lung (Fig. 4).

The second rib inserts into the sternomanubrial junction, also called the angle of Louis. This can be easily palpated in most people as a horizontal ridge in the sternum where the two planes that make up the sternum intersect (Fig. 5). The interspace immediately below the angle of Louis is the second interspace. The angle of Louis serves as a landmark to rapidly locate the second rib and second interspace for placement of a catheter to decompress a tension pneumothorax.

The first rib is short, broad, and flat, and arches sharply from posterior to anterior (Fig. 6). The second rib is longer than but very

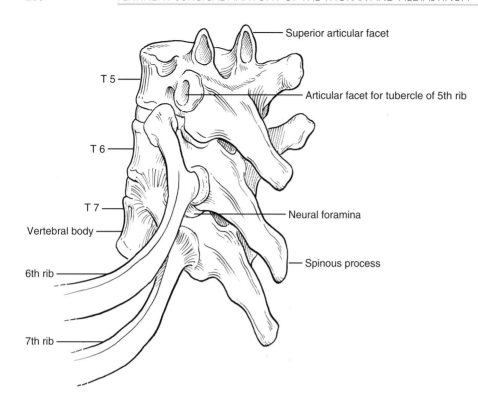

Superior articular facet

T 5

Articular facet for tubercle of 5th rib

T 6

T 7

Neural foramina

Vertebral body

Spinous process

6th rib

7th rib

FIGURE 1 Costovertebral junction. Lateral view showing two left ribs and three vertebrae. Note that ribs articulate with the transverse process and body of one vertebrae and body of vertebra above. *(Modified from Agur AMR, Dalley AF, editors: Grant's atlas of anatomy, 11th ed. Philadelphia, Lippincott Williams & Wilkins, 2005, Figs. 1.13–1.14, pp 14–15.)*

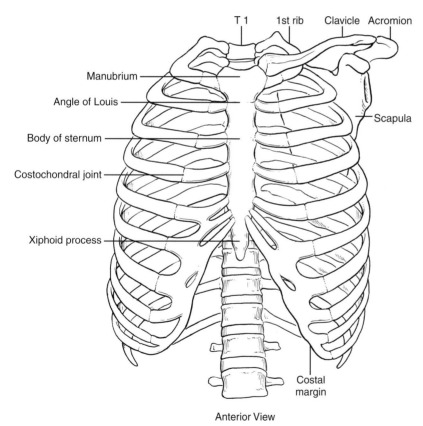

T 1   1st rib   Clavicle   Acromion

Manubrium

Angle of Louis

Body of sternum

Scapula

Costochondral joint

Xiphoid process

Costal margin

Anterior View

FIGURE 2 Bony chest wall. Anterior view. *(Modified from Agur AMR, Dalley AF, editors: Grant's atlas of anatomy, 11th ed. Philadelphia, Lippincott Williams & Wilkins, 2004, Fig. 1.8, p 9.)*

similar to the first rib (Fig. 7). The first slip of the serratus anterior muscle attaches to the second rib approximately one third of the arc from posterior to anterior—this slip also attaches to the inferior aspect of the first rib. Posterior to this attachment, the scalenus posterior muscle attaches to the second rib.

When performing a thoracotomy, counting ribs can identify the correct interspace. Once the latissimus dorsi muscle has been divided and the serratus anterior muscle divided or swept anterior, the scapula is elevated. Thin fibrous attachments hold the undersurface of the scapula to the chest wall. A hand placed deep to the scapula, posterior

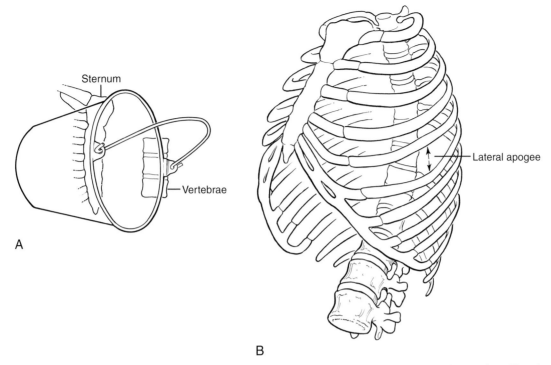

FIGURE 3 **A** and **B,** Bucket handle motion of ribs. Ribs are fixed anteriorly at the sternum and posteriorly at the vertebrae. The ribs will move like a "bucket handle." The widest space between the ribs will be at the lateral apogee or "keystone." *(Modified from Pearson FG, editor: Thoracic surgery, 2nd ed. Philadelphia, Churchill Livingstone, 2002, Fig. 48-3, p 1327.)*

near the spine, and apically can palpate ribs. The first rib is identified by its conspicuously broad and flat contour. Inferior to this, the second rib can be identified by the attachment of the scalenus posterior muscle. This muscle body is palpable by sweeping the finger from posterior to anterior along the second rib (Fig. 8). Less distinct will be the third rib, which seems to "turn the corner" from the apex of the chest to the lateral chest wall (Fig. 9). In a lateral decubitus position, the tip of the scapula overlies the sixth interspace. In a male, the nipple overlies the fourth interspace.

MUSCLES OF THE CHEST WALL

Integral to safe thoracentesis, placement of a tube thoracostomy, or a thoracotomy is understanding the layers of the chest wall and the anatomy of the interspace.

The paired pectoralis major muscles cover the majority of the anterior chest wall. The pectoralis major muscle originates from the clavicle and anterior aspects of ribs 1 through 6 inserting on the proximal humerus. Its origin from the chest wall is broad and an anterior thoracotomy will divide or separate its fibers. Inferiorly, the rectus abdominus muscle inserts onto the costal cartilages of ribs 5 through 7 and the xiphoid process. Lateral to this, the muscle fibers of the external oblique insert onto ribs 5 through 12. The external oblique muscle interdigitates with the serratus anterior muscle as it inserts on ribs 1 through 8 (Fig. 10). Most thoracotomies do not traverse the interspaces guarded by the rectus abdominis and external oblique. These muscles will be encountered with thoracoabdominal incisions crossing the costal margin.

Laterally and posteriorly, two musculofascial layers guard the ribs. The more superficial layer contains the latissimus dorsi muscle laterally. Posteriorly, at the auscultatory triangle, or posterior border of the latissimus dorsi, this layer becomes a thin but tough layer of fascia, which more posteriorly envelopes the trapezius muscle. The second musculofascial layer contains the serratus anterior muscle laterally,

becoming a broader sheet of thin but tough fibrous tissue posteriorly and then becoming the rhomboid major muscle and then the rhomboid minor muscle posteriorly and superiorly (Fig. 11). A tube thoracostomy will traverse these muscle layers to reach the ribs and interspaces. Knowing where you are in these layers allows precious time to be saved in traversing them and getting to where you need to be to complete the procedure.

A typical tube thoracostomy is placed in the fifth interspace at the anterior axillary line. The muscle bodies traversed are thinner here. From superficial to deep, the surgeon will separate skin, subcutaneous adipose tissue, the latissimus dorsi/trapezius musculofascial layer, and then the serratus anterior musculofascial layer. At this depth, the shiny surface of the periosteum of the ribs and the oblique fibers of the external intercostal muscle can be seen. As discussed later, tube thoracostomies are performed over the superior aspect of the rib. It is much easier to locate the superior aspect of the rib when you do not have intervening layers of muscle and fascia.

A thoracotomy can be fashioned to divide or spare these muscles as needed in order to gain access to the rib cage. A full thoracotomy will divide the latissimus dorsi laterally and the trapezius posteriorly. The incision sweeps from horizontal across the lateral chest to vertical and parallel to the spine posteriorly (Fig. 12). Deep to this layer, the serratus anterior can be swept anterior or divided. Posteriorly, the fascial layer coming off the serratus anterior is divided and then the rhomboid major and rhomboid minor muscles are divided. The innervation of the trapezius muscle and rhomboid muscles runs from medial to lateral. The more muscle body that is left medially, the more muscle function will be retained. Enough muscle needs to be left attached to the scapula to allow suture repair of the muscle, and the muscle should not be stripped from the scapula. The posterior and vertical aspect of this incision where the trapezius and rhomboids are divided is done to elevate the scapula off the chest wall, to access the interspaces underneath.

A thoracotomy can be extended anteriorly, dividing the pectoralis major muscle overlying the interspace of interest. The sternum can be

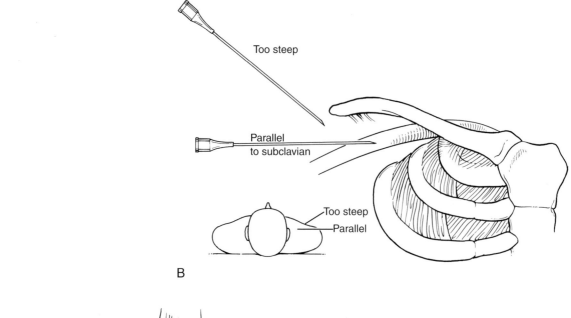

B

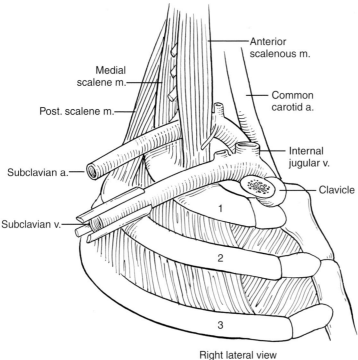

Right lateral view

A

FIGURE 4   Central venous cannulation of subclavian vein. **A,** The clavicle and rib cage form a triangle through which the subclavian vein courses. The vein runs roughly parallel to both the clavicle and the rib cage. **B,** A needle, once passed under the clavicle, directed parallel to the rib cage and clavicle will have a far greater chance of finding the vein. A needle directed too steeply will enter and exit this triangle, penetrate the intercostal space, and puncture the lung. *(Modified from Agur AMR, Dalley AF, editors: Grant's atlas of anatomy, 11th ed. Philadelphia, Lippincott Williams & Wilkins, 2004, Figs. 1.8, 6.29, pp 9, 379.)*

split transversely, and a thoracotomy continued on the contralateral side. This is termed a "clam shell" thoracotomy. The left and right mammary artery will be found 1 cm lateral to and on either side of the sternum, deep to the ribs and intercostal muscles, but superficial to the pleura. These vessels can be cauterized if speed is needed, but are prone to spasm and late bleeding, and should be sought and ligated when possible. Frequently as perfusion is restored they will begin to bleed and should then be ligated.

INTERCOSTAL SPACE

Each intercostal space, from superficial to deep, has two layers of muscle; an artery, a vein, and a nerve; and a diminutive inner layer of muscle. The external intercostal muscles run obliquely with fibers in the same orientation as the external oblique muscle of the abdomen (fingers in pockets). Deep are the internal intercostal muscles running in the opposite direction. The intercostal artery, vein, and nerve run

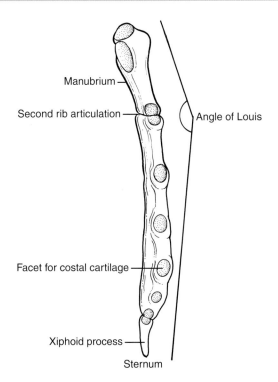

FIGURE 5   Sternum, lateral view. Angle of Louis can be palpated in the midline as a raised horizontal ridge or as the point where the plane of the manubrium and body intersect. The second rib articulates directly lateral to the angle of Louis. *(Modified from Standring S, editor: Gray's anatomy: the anatomical basis of clinical practice, 39th ed. Edinburgh, Churchill Livingstone, 2004, Fig. 57.5, p 954.)*

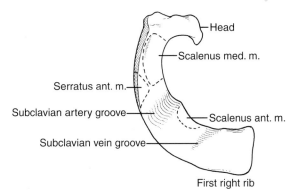

FIGURE 6   Right first rib. *(Modified from Gray H, editor: Gray's anatomy, 20th ed. Lea & Febiger, 1918, Plate 124.)*

along the inferior aspect of each rib, occasionally running underneath a ledge in the costal groove. To avoid injury to these three structures, tube thoracostomies and thoracotomies are directed over the superior aspect of each rib or through the middle of the interspace, but not the inferior aspect of the rib (Fig. 13). The innermost intercostal muscles are located deep to the neurovascular bundle and run in the same direction as the internal intercostal muscles. Although mentioned in anatomy texts, surgically, the innermost intercostal muscles do not need to be considered separately from the internal intercostal muscle (Fig. 14). The intercostal arteries originate as segmental branches off the descending aorta. The intercostal space, including the underlying pleura, can be harvested as a posteriorly based pedicled muscle flap (Fig. 15). This flap is useful for reinforcing bronchial or esophageal repairs.

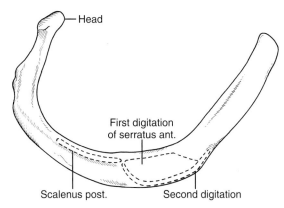

Second right rib

FIGURE 7   Right second rib. *(Modified from Gray H, editor: Gray's anatomy, 20th ed. Lea & Febiger, 1918, Plate 125.)*

The internal mammary artery originates from the subclavian arteries bilaterally, and descends on the inside of the chest wall, approximately 1 cm lateral to the sternum bilaterally (Fig. 16).

PLEURAL SPACE

Normally the lung is coupled to the chest wall by the vacuum that exists between the visceral and parietal pleura. With penetration of the chest wall air is allowed into the pleural space from the outside, or more commonly, penetration of the lung allows air to escape from air spaces within the lung (alveoli, bronchioles, bronchi) into the pleural space. The coupling of the visceral and parietal pleura is broken and the potential space, which is the pleural space, becomes a real space. The elasticity of the lung causes it to collapse and a pneumothorax is formed. The pleural space extends superiorly to where it rises above the circumference of the first rib to inferiorly where the diaphragm inserts on the costal margin and the 12th rib. Lung may or may not be present between the diaphragm and ribs in the lowermost recesses of the pleural space. Anterior to the pericardium and posterior to the sternum, the two pleural cavities can abut but rarely communicate.

DIAPHRAGM

The diaphragm is the movable dome-shaped muscle that separates the thoracic and abdominal cavities. With full exhalation, the dome of the diaphragm can rise to the level of the fourth interspace anteriorly (nipple level). With full inhalation, the diaphragm flattens, bringing the thoracic cavity down to the level of the costal margin anteriorly and the 12th rib posteriorly. The muscle fibers of the diaphragm originate from the sternum, the ribs, and the vertebral column. All three groups insert on a tough, fibrous central tendon. Fibers of the sternal portion are short, arising as small slips from the back of the xiphoid process. Laterally on either side of the xiphoid, fibers originate from the inner surface of the lower six costal cartilages (costal margin). Posteriorly, fibers originate from a thick band arching over the quadratus lumborum (lateral arcuate ligament) and the psoas major (medial arcuate ligament). The paired lateral arcuate ligaments extend from the tip and lower margin of the 12th ribs and arch over the quadratus lumborum muscle to the transverse processes of L1. The paired medial arcuate ligaments complete the journey, arching over the psoas major from the tip of the transverse process of the first lumbar vertebrae to the tendinous portion of each diaphragmatic crus (Fig. 17).

The posterior medial portion of the diaphragm is composed of two crura—an anatomic right crus originating from the upper three

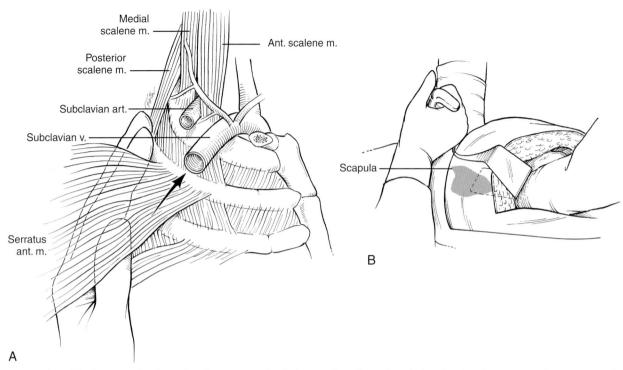

A

B

FIGURE 8   A and **B,** Counting ribs. Once the rib cage is visualized, the scapula is elevated, and a hand is placed posterior and superior to palpate and count ribs. Note that the first rib is broad, short, and flat; the second rib has the insertion of the scalenus posterior; and the third rib "turns the corner" from apex to lateral chest wall.

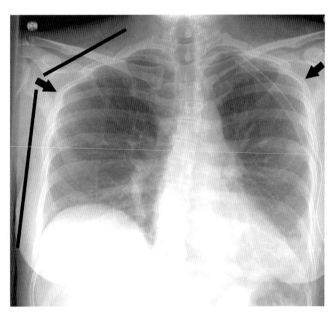

FIGURE 9   Third rib "turns the corner." Anteroposterior chest radiograph illustrating how the rib cage forms a loose box with the third rib at a corner. *Arrows* denote third rib.

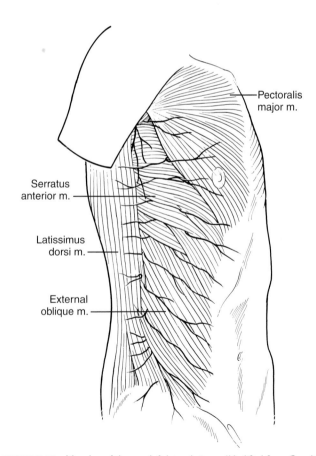

FIGURE 10   Muscles of thorax: left lateral view. *(Modified from Gray H, editor:* Gray's anatomy, *20th ed. Lea & Febiger, 1918, Plate 392.)*

lumbar vertebral bodies and an anatomic left crus originating from the upper two lumbar vertebral bodies. Anterior to the aorta, the medial margins of the two crura form a poorly defined arch called the median arcuate ligament. Anterior to this arch, either the anatomic right crus (64%) or the anatomic left crus (2%) or both (34%) form the esophageal hiatus. Although anatomists name the crura left or right by their origin from the left or right side of the vertebral bodies, surgeons name the crura left or right by their relationship to the esophagus. In the abdomen, visualization of the esophagus

FIGURE 11 Muscles of the thorax. **A,** Superficial layer containing latissimus dorsi muscle and trapezius muscle. **B,** Deep layer containing serratus anterior muscle, rhomboid major muscle, and rhomboid minor muscle. SCM, Sternocleidomastoid muscle. *(Modified from Agur AMR, Dalley AF, editors:* Grant's atlas of anatomy, *11th ed. Philadelphia, Lippincott Williams & Wilkins, 2004, Figs. 4.47, 4.48, 6.13, pp 233, 234, 367.)*

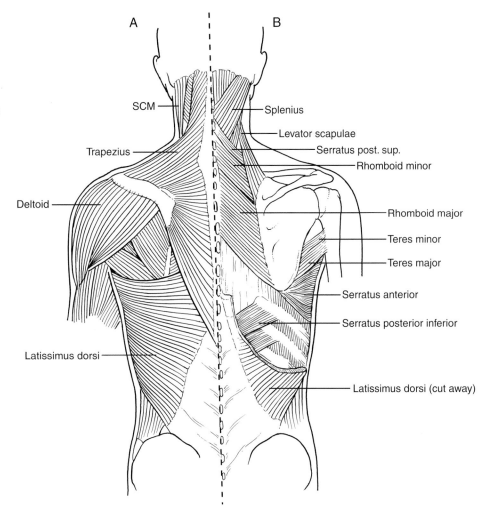

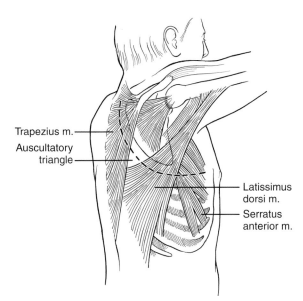

FIGURE 12 Full posterolateral thoracotomy. *(Modified from Agur AMR, Dalley AF, editors:* Grant's atlas of anatomy, *11th ed. Philadelphia, Lippincott Williams & Wilkins, 2004, Figs. 4.47, 4.48, 6.13, pp 233, 234, 367.)*

and division of the crus running to the left of the esophagus will expose the distal thoracic aorta above the level of the celiac artery and renal arteries. A clamp can be applied here to obtain vascular control. Alternatively, the Conn aortic root compressor or a small Richardson retractor wrapped with a laparotomy pad can be used in this position to occlude the aorta by compressing it against the posteriorly located vertebral body (Fig. 18).

The phrenic nerve and twigs from the lower intercostal nerves innervate the diaphragm. The phrenic nerve originates primarily from the C4 nerve root, but receives innervation from C3 and C5 (C3, C4, and C5 keep the body alive). In the neck, the phrenic nerve originates lateral to the scalenus anterior muscle and descends from lateral to medial on the superficial surface of this muscle, deep to the sternocleidomastoid muscle. It enters the thoracic inlet and is found on the medial aspect of the mediastinum just deep to the pleura bilaterally. Superiorly, it is very anterior in the chest and vulnerable to injury, especially with a median sternotomy and dissection of the great vessels, where it is often not readily visible in the wound, but very close to the dissection. On the left, it descends outside the pericardium, deep to the pleura, passing over the arch of the aorta, anterior to the hilum of the lung, and anterior to the inferior pulmonary ligament. As it nears the diaphragm, it is often invested in a veil of pericardial fat, hanging like a curtain between the pericardium and the diaphragm. The nerve reaches the diaphragm just lateral to the left border of the heart and in a plane slightly more anterior than the right phrenic nerve (see Fig. 33). The right phrenic nerve descends along the right lateral border of the superior vena cava and passes anterior to the hilum of the lung, anterior to the inferior pulmonary

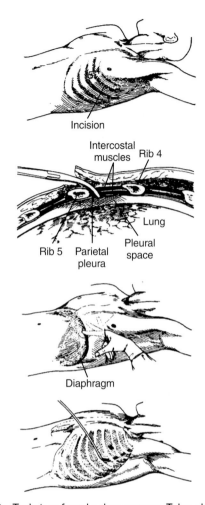

FIGURE 13 Technique for tube thoracostomy. Tubes placed emergently for trauma are placed along the anterior axillary line, fourth or fifth interspace. The intercostal space is entered on the superior aspect of the rib. Finger palpation confirms entrance into the pleural cavity and avoids inadvertent subscapular or intraabdominal placement of tubes as well as injury to adhesed lung. *(From Moore FA, Moore EE: Trauma resuscitation. In Wilmore DN, Brennan MF, Harken AH, et al, editors. Care of the surgical patient. New York, Scientific American, 1989.)*

ligament. It is also invested in a veil of pericardial fat as it approaches the diaphragm. The right phrenic nerve enters the diaphragm just lateral to the inferior vena cava (see Fig. 32).

Both left and right phrenic nerves immediately trifurcate into three muscular branches after entering the hemidiaphragm. One is directed anteromedially toward the sternum, one anterolaterally, and a third posteriorly. The posterior branch bifurcates into a branch directed toward the 12th rib and one toward the crus. Safe incisions in the diaphragm are fashioned to avoid cutting major branches of the phrenic nerve (Fig. 19). A peripheral and circumferential incision will avoid all but distal twigs of the phrenic nerve. Radial incisions can be placed but must be done with care to avoid major branches of the phrenic nerve.

Because the primary innervation of the diaphragm, the phrenic nerve, enters centrally and spreads centrifugally, the diaphragm can be transposed to higher or lower origins from the thoracic cage while maintaining its innervation. This is occasionally required in repair of a diaphragmatic rupture when surface area of the diaphragm is lost or the chest wall has lost its rigidity and can no longer subserve its cylinder function. Care should be taken to maintain a dome shape to the diaphragm. A diaphragm that is flattened at rest will pull the walls of

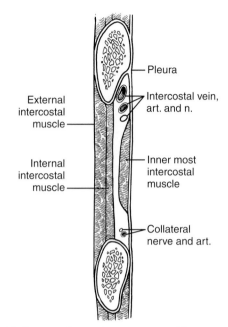

FIGURE 14 Intercostal space in cross section. Note main intercostal bundle along the inferior aspect of the rib. The collateral nerve and artery, although present, are diminutive. *(Modified from Crafts RC: A textbook of human anatomy, 3rd ed. New York, John Wiley, 1985.)*

the thorax closer together when contracting. With contraction, instead of increasing intrathoracic volume, the diaphragm will now decrease intrathoracic volume and become a muscle of expiration (Fig. 20).

PERICARDIUM

The pericardial space is considerably smaller than the pleural space and a small increase in the volume of fluid in this space can have a dramatic impact on cardiac function. The parietal pericardium is a thick, fibrous sac with an inner serosal surface containing the heart, the proximal ascending aorta, the distal superior vena cava, the distal inferior vena cava, the pulmonary trunk and bifurcation, proximal left and right main pulmonary arteries, and a short segment of all four distal pulmonary veins. From this description, it can be visualized that all vessels flowing into and out of the heart have short segments contained in the pericardial sac (Fig. 21). Also, these vascular structures fix the heart in the pericardial sac. If the heart is allowed to rotate, these structures will be twisted or kinked, impeding venous return. Because they are the lowest pressure conduits, the superior vena cava and inferior vena cava are the most vulnerable to kinking and impedance of flow. With decreased blood flow into the heart, there is decreased blood flow out of the heart, and systemic blood pressure falls. This is the physiology of hypotension associated with tension pneumothorax and with cardiac herniation.

There are two sinuses behind the heart. The oblique pericardial sinus is a cul-de-sac behind the heart bounded by pericardial attachments to the inferior vena cava and the four pulmonary veins. Because of the oblique sinus, with a median sternotomy, a hand can be placed around the apex of the heart and the apex gently elevated into the wound. This allows visualization of the lateral and posterior walls of the left ventricle, including the vascular distribution of the diagonal, circumflex, and obtuse marginal coronary arteries. This maneuver is generally poorly tolerated without opening the right pericardium vertically, parallel to the phrenic nerve. This allows the right side of the heart to fall into the right pleural space and maintain filling as the heart is lifted. In addition, severe Trendelenburg position and an apically placed suction retraction device will aid exposure and improve hemodynamics. Internal defibrillating paddles should be

FIGURE 15 **A,** Intercostal muscle flap. Based on intercostal artery with pedicle posterior. **B,** Transverse view of this flap.

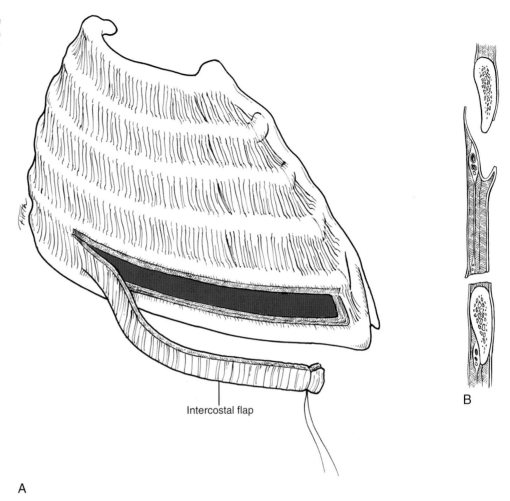

Intercostal flap

A

B

open and ready prior to performing this maneuver, as ventricular fibrillation is not uncommon.

The transverse pericardial sinus allows a finger or clamp to be placed along the right side of the ascending aorta, behind the aorta and pulmonary trunk, and be visualized to the left of the pulmonary trunk and superior to the left superior pulmonary vein in the vicinity of the left atrial appendage (see Fig. 21).

The pericardium can be drained through a median sternotomy, left or right thoracotomy via a subxiphoid approach, or laparotomy. From a left or right thoracotomy, an incision is made anterior or posterior to and parallel to the phrenic nerve. From the left side of the chest the left ventricle and from the right side of the chest the right atrium will be encountered in the pericardial space behind these incisions (Fig. 22).

From a laparotomy, a modification of the subxiphoid approach can be used to enter the pericardium. Alternatively, the central portion of the diaphragm makes up the inferior fibrous parietal pericardial sac. An incision in the diaphragm in this location will enter the pericardial sac, visualizing the inferior wall of the heart.

Subxiphoid Space

The subxiphoid space is a favored access to the pericardium for diagnosis and treatment of pericardial effusions. Both the linea alba and the diaphragm attach to the xiphoid. The peritoneum on the diaphragm is continuous with the peritoneum on the deep surface of the posterior fasciae of the anterior abdominal wall. An incision from

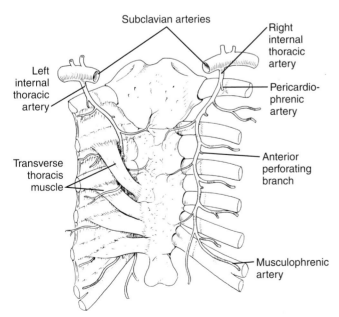

Subclavian arteries

Right internal thoracic artery

Left internal thoracic artery

Pericardio-phrenic artery

Anterior perforating branch

Transverse thoracis muscle

Musculophrenic artery

FIGURE 16 Internal mammary arteries as viewed from inside the chest. *(From Pearson FG, editor:* Thoracic surgery, *2nd ed. Philadelphia, Churchill Livingstone, 2002, Fig. 48-8, p 1330.)*

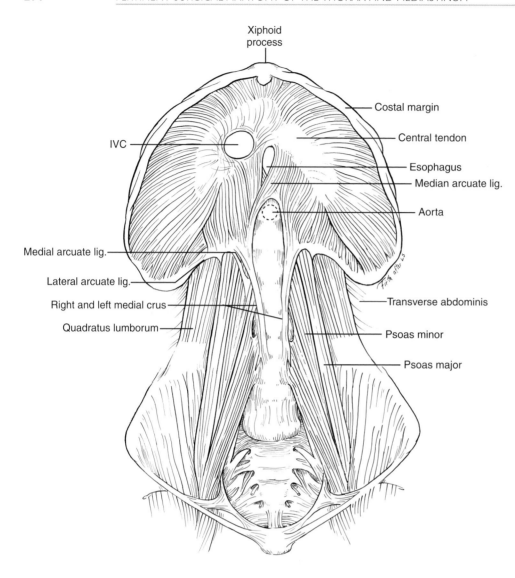

Xiphoid process

Costal margin

Central tendon

IVC

Esophagus

Median arcuate lig.

Aorta

Medial arcuate lig.

Lateral arcuate lig.

Right and left medial crus

Quadratus lumborum

Transverse abdominis

Psoas minor

Psoas major

FIGURE 17 Diaphragm as viewed from the abdomen. The diaphragm originates bilaterally from the xiphoid process, costal margin, lateral arcuate ligament, and medial arcuate ligament, and inserts into the central tendon. The left and right crura originate from the lumbar vertebral bodies and insert into the central tendon. IVC, Inferior vena cava. *(Modified from Langley LL, Telford IR, Christensen JB: Dynamic anatomy and physiology, 5th ed. New York, McGraw-Hill, 1980.)*

above the xiphoid process to 4 cm below will pass through skin, fat, and linea alba. Incising the linea alba will reveal the xiphoid superiorly and the peritoneum inferiorly. The diaphragmatic attachments to the xiphoid can be divided flush with the xiphoid and the xiphoid resected to the level of the sternal body/costal margin. A large vein is routinely encountered at the angle between the xiphoid, costal margin, and sternal body. Posterior retraction of the diaphragm and superior retraction of the sternum will reveal the pericardial reflection on the diaphragm, which is often covered with fat, which must be bluntly dissected with a Kittner dissector sponge stick to reveal the underlying pericardium. Incising the pericardium will enter the pericardial space. The acute margin of the right ventricle will be visible through this incision (Fig. 23). Because this incision is at the corner where two perpendicular planes meet, fluid can be aspirated in two directions. First, straight posterior, parallel to the diaphragm, along the inferior border of the heart, and second, superior, parallel to the sternal body, anterior to the anterior surface of the heart (Fig. 24).

HEART

The heart occupies the central and left portion of the thorax and is the primary content of the middle mediastinum. It is bounded on all sides by the parietal pericardium. Outside this pericardium, it is bounded anteriorly by the sternum and posteriorly by the esophagus, vertebral column, and descending aorta. On the right, mediastinal pleura and

lung are present with the phrenic nerve running just anterior to the hilum of the lung. On the left, the same structures are present but the phrenic nerve runs more anteriorly. Extra care is required to protect this nerve when the heart is approached from the left.

Body Surface Markings for the Heart

The surface projection of the superior border of the heart is a line joining a point 2 cm lateral to the sternum in the left second intercostal space to a point just to the right of the sternum in the same space. This marks the line of the main pulmonary arteries. The right border extends inferiorly to the sixth costal cartilage adjacent to the sternum. This is formed by the right atrium. The inferior border extends from the right sixth costal cartilage to the point of maximum cardiac impulse, which is usually in the left fifth intercostal space just medial to the midclavicular line. The right ventricle forms the inferior border. The left border extends superiorly to the second intercostal space 2 cm lateral to the sternal edge. The left ventricle forms the left border (Fig. 25).

External Features

The heart consists of four chambers divided by three grooves. The atrioventricular groove contains the coronary sinus, which is the largest vein of the heart and lies posteriorly opening into the right atrium.

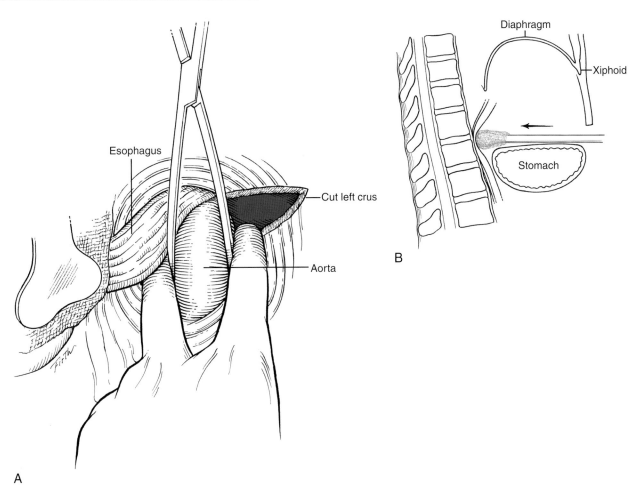

A

FIGURE 18 Cross-clamping of distal descending thoracic aorta from abdomen. **A,** Left crus divided and thoracic aorta found deep. **B,** Lateral view, aorta occluded by compression against vertebral body.

FIGURE 19 Diaphragmatic incisions and branches of the phrenic nerve. Incisions are fashioned to avoid denervating large portions of the diaphragm. Ao, Aorta; IVC, inferior vena cava. *(From Meredino KA, Johnson RS, Skinner HH, et al: The intradiaphragmatic distribution of the phrenic nerve with particular reference to the placement of diaphragmatic incisions and controlled segmental paralysis. Surgery 39:189, 1956.)*

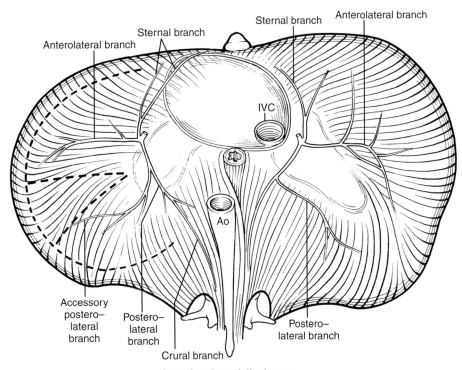

Superior view of diaphragm

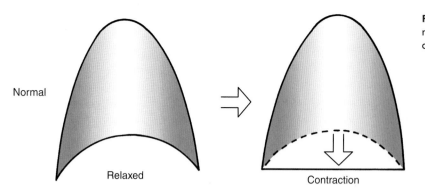

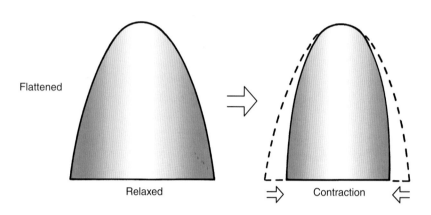

FIGURE 20 A hemidiaphragm is flattened when relaxed; when contracting, it draws the rib cage in and causes expiration, not inspiration.

Normal

Relaxed

Contraction

Flattened

Relaxed

Contraction

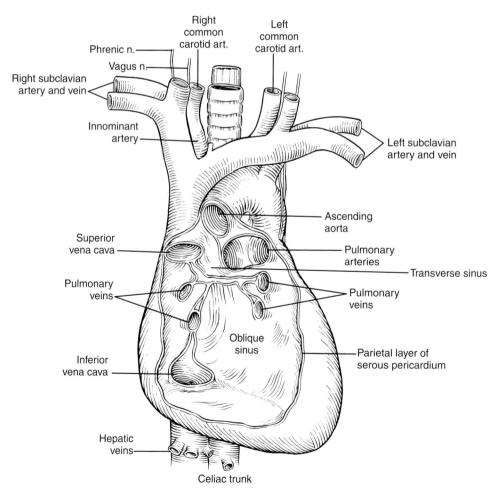

Right common carotid art.

Left common carotid art.

Phrenic n.

Vagus n.

Right subclavian artery and vein

Innominant artery

Left subclavian artery and vein

Superior vena cava

Ascending aorta

Pulmonary arteries

Transverse sinus

Pulmonary veins

Pulmonary veins

Oblique sinus

Inferior vena cava

Parietal layer of serous pericardium

Hepatic veins

Celiac trunk

FIGURE 21 Pericardial sac, posterior and lateral aspects. Anterior pericardial sac has been removed. Heart has been removed. *(Modified from Agur AMR, Dalley AF, editors: Grant's atlas of anatomy, 11th ed. Philadelphia, Lippincott Williams & Wilkins, 2004, Fig. 1.61, p 55.)*

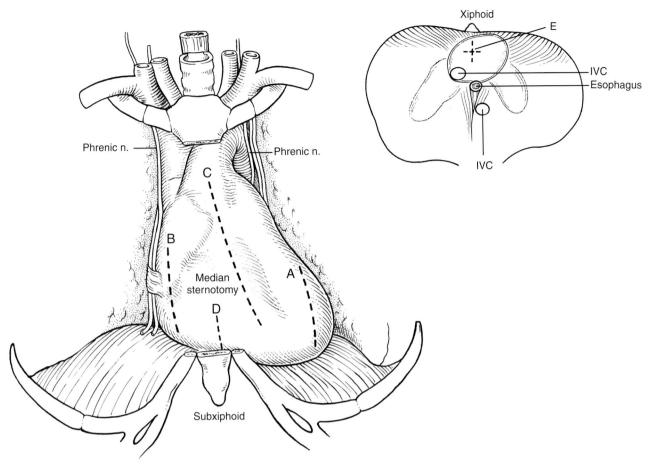

FIGURE 22 Approaches to a pericardial window. The pericardium can be opened from left thoracotomy (**A**), right thoracotomy (**B**), median sternotomy (**C**), subxiphoid (**D**), or abdominal (**E**) approach. IVC, Inferior vena cava. *(Modified from Agur AMR, Dalley AF, editors: Grant's atlas of anatomy, 11th ed. Philadelphia, Lippincott Williams & Wilkins, 2004, Fig. 1.49.)*

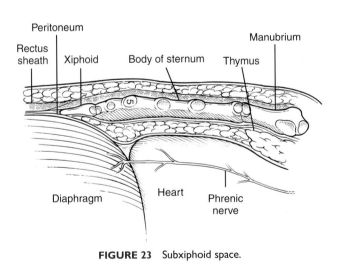

FIGURE 23 Subxiphoid space.

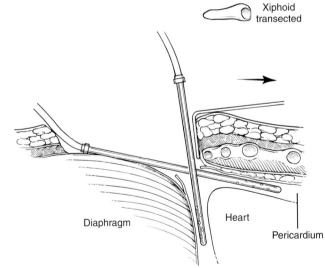

FIGURE 24 Subxiphoid pericardial window.

The interatrial groove is covered anteriorly by the ascending aorta and the main pulmonary artery. The interatrial groove is visible to the right of the heart as a fatty line between the superior vena cava and right superior pulmonary vein. The interventricular groove runs anteriorly toward the apex and contains the great cardiac vein. Posteriorly, it continues along the inferior surface of the heart toward the right margin and contains the middle cardiac vein.

The heart has five surfaces: anterior, posterior, inferior, right lateral, and left lateral. The anterior surface is formed primarily by the right ventricle and the right atrium, and is therefore at risk from any frontal injury. Two thirds of the right atrium and ventricle face anteriorly. The posterior surface or the base of the heart is formed by the left and right atria. The two pulmonary veins on either side, inferior and superior, open into the left atrium at this posterior location.

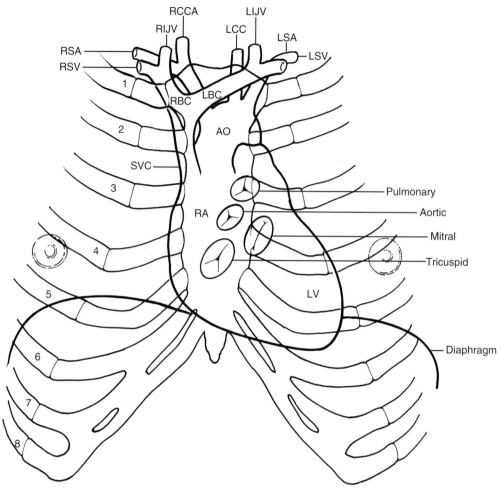

FIGURE 25   Surface projections of heart and lungs. AO, Aorta; LBC, left brachiocephalic; LCC, left common carotid; LIJV, left internal jugular vein; LSA, left subclavian artery; LSV, left subclavian vein; LV, left ventricle; RA, right atrium; RBC, right brachiocephalic; RCCA, right common carotid artery; RIJV, right internal jugular vein; RSA, right subclavian artery; RSV, right subclavian vein; SVC, superior vena cava. *(Modified from Gray H, editor: Gray's anatomy, 20th ed. Lea & Febiger, 1918, Plates 1216, 1218.)*

The superior and inferior vena cava open into the right atrium. The posterior surface of the heart is related to the sixth through the ninth thoracic vertebrae, being separated from them only by the pericardium, right pulmonary veins, esophagus, and aorta (from right to left). One third of the right ventricle and two thirds of the left ventricle form the inferior or diaphragmatic surface of the heart. This part of the heart is in contact with the central portion of the diaphragm. The right atrium and the right ventricle form the right lateral surface of the heart. They are related to the pericardium, the right lung, and the right phrenic nerve just anterior to the hilum. The left ventricle and the left atrium form the left lateral surface. They are related to the same structures as on the right but the phrenic nerve runs across the middle of the surface (Fig. 26).

Coronary Arteries and Veins

Right and left coronary arteries arise from the ascending aorta. The right coronary artery supplies the right atrium, the right ventricle, the posterior one third of the interventricular septum, and the inferior portion of the septum. The left coronary artery supplies the left atrium, the left ventricle, and the anterior two thirds of the interventricular septum. Collateral circulation in the heart is minimal, and therefore, occlusion of a coronary artery results in a specific area of myocardial infarction and dysfunction (Fig. 27).

The named coronary arteries travel just under the epicardium, superficial to the myocardium. Lacerations close to a coronary artery, but not including the artery, can be repaired with unpledgeted horizontal mattress sutures of Halsted. Alternatively, pledgeted horizontal mattress sutures may also be used, placed under the coronary bed, effectively repairing the myocardium but not occluding the coronary artery (Fig. 28). Care should be taken in placing and tying the suture so as not to kink the coronary artery by incorporating too much myocardium. If the left anterior descending artery is the adjacent vessel being avoided, it is possible with this suture to occlude a major septal perforator diving deep to the vessel.

The venous system of the heart is centered on the coronary sinus, which receives the tributaries from the different areas of the heart and drains into the posterior aspect of the right atrium just superior to the tricuspid valve (see Fig. 26B).

Conduction System

The sinoatrial node is the pacemaker of the heart and is located just to the right and anterior to the opening of the superior vena cava. The impulses are transmitted to the atrioventricular node through the wall of the atrium. The atrioventricular node is situated in the posteroinferior portion of the interatrial septum just superior to the opening of

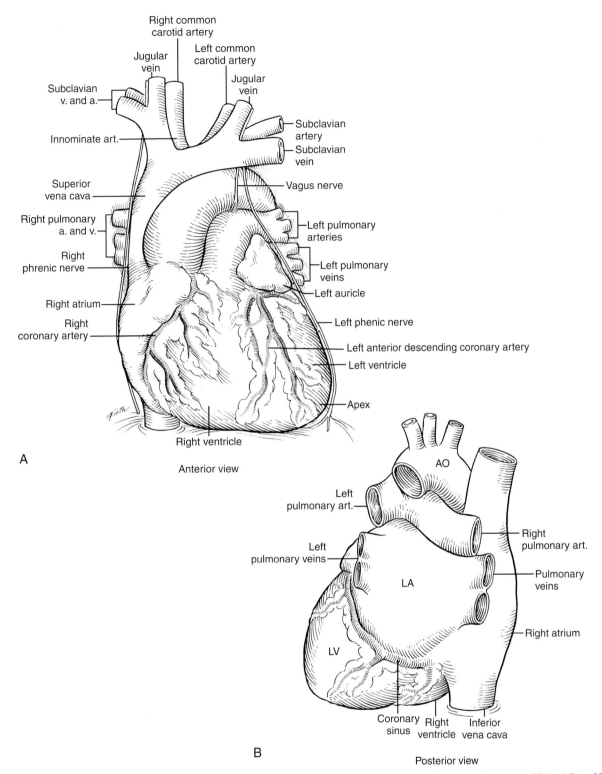

FIGURE 26   Heart. **A,** Anterior. **B,** Posterior. AO, Aorta; LA, left auricle; LV, left ventricle. *(Modified from Gray's anatomy, 39th ed. Plate 970, and Fig. 60.2.)*

the coronary sinus. From here the impulses travel through the bundle of His (atrioventricular bundle) along the posterosuperior edge of the muscular interventricular septum to the right and left bundle branches. These run through the interventricular septum to the papillary muscles in the left and right ventricle and then form a subendocardial network (Purkinje fibers) (Fig. 29).

Internal Features of Heart Chambers

The right atrium has a smooth-walled posterior aspect onto which the vena cava and the coronary sinus open. Anteriorly, the wall is trabeculated muscle. Posteromedially is the interatrial septum with a depression called the fossa ovalis, which marks the previous foramen

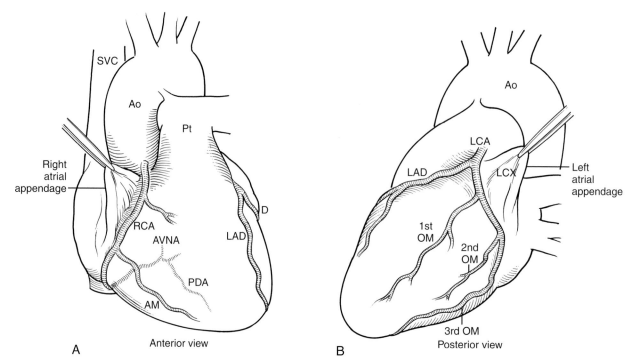

FIGURE 27 Coronary arteries. **A,** Anterior view. **B,** Posterior view. AM, Acute marginal branch of right coronary artery; Ao, aorta; AVNA, atrioventricular nodal artery; D, diagonal branch of LAD; LAD, left anterior descending artery; LCA, left coronary artery; LCX, left circumflex artery; OM, obtuse marginal branch of LCX; PDA, posterior descending coronary artery; Pt, pulmonary trunk; RCA, right coronary artery; SVC, superior vena cava.

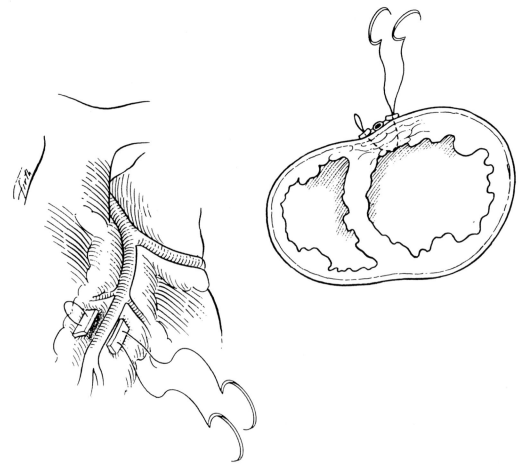

FIGURE 28 Repair of a cardiac laceration near a coronary artery.

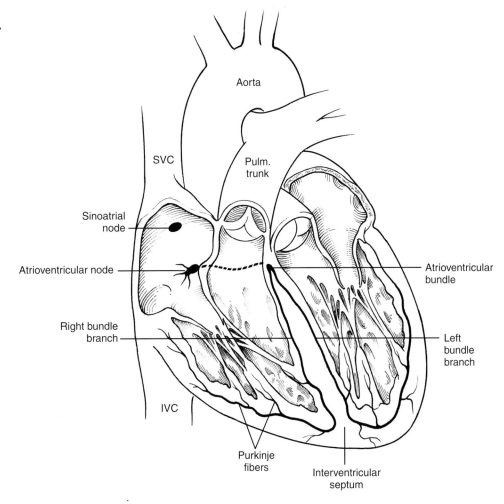

FIGURE 29 Cardiac conduction system. IVC, Inferior vena cava; SVC, superior vena cava. (*Modified from Gray H, editor: Gray's anatomy, 20th ed. Lea & Febiger, 1918, Plate 501.*)

ovale or communication between the atria that existed in utero. Anteroinferiorly is the orifice of the tricuspid valve opening into the right ventricle.

The right ventricle is triangular and muscular with an inflow area from the tricuspid valve and an outflow area, which is smooth, leading to the pulmonary valve.

The ventricular wall gives rise to three (anterior, posterior, septal) conical projections of the papillary muscles. Tendinous structures arise from the apex of each of these to attach to cusps of the tricuspid valve. Injury to any portion of the valve apparatus can give rise to incompetence of the valve. Placed medially and obliquely is the interventricular septum separating the two ventricles.

The left atrium is quadrangular and has smooth walls. The left atrial appendage projects to the left and is the only portion of the atrium that can be seen anteriorly. The openings of the veins lie posteriorly on the left and right. The interatrial septum lies to the right and slopes posteriorly making the left atrium lie behind the right atrium. The mitral valve orifice lies in the anteroinferior part of the atrium (Fig. 30).

The left ventricle is muscular and has an inflow area from the mitral orifice and an outflow area to the aortic root. The ventricular wall gives rise to anterior and posterior papillary muscles that have chordae tendineae that attach to the anterior and posterior mitral valve leaflets (cusps). The anterior leaflet separates the inflow of the mitral valve orifice from the outflow of the aortic root. The aortic orifice is therefore positioned anterior to the mitral orifice. The interventricular septum is present to the right and anteriorly (see Fig. 30).

Pulmonary Artery and Swan-Ganz Catheter Placement

A pulmonary artery catheter is usually introduced via the subclavian or internal jugular vein but the femoral vein can also be used. The catheter passes through these veins into the superior or inferior vena cava and then into the right atrium. The flow of blood carries the tip through the tricuspid valve orifice into the right ventricle and then through the right ventricular outflow tract and the pulmonary valve into the main pulmonary artery. Due to the orientation of the right main pulmonary artery to the pulmonary trunk the catheter tends to pass to the right preferentially and lodge in the distal pulmonary artery.

Occasionally the catheter may pass into the inferior vena cava or the coronary sinus while traversing the right atrium. Entry into the coronary sinus can be recognized by loss of right atrial tracing soon after it appears. Persistence of this tracing after considerable length of the catheter has been introduced suggests coiling within the atrium or passage into the inferior vena cava.

Traditional instruction on pulmonary artery catheter placement includes orienting the coil of the catheter such that it enters the atrium from the superior vena cava and is directed toward the tricuspid valve. The coil of the catheter is oriented on a coronal plane with the tricuspid valve perceived to be a hole in a sagittal plane (Fig. 31A). The tricuspid valve, however, truly exists on a plane rotated 40 to 50 degrees off the sagittal plane (Fig. 31B). In a patient lying supine, blood flows from a right posterior position in the right atrium, through the tricuspid valve diagonally anterior and to the left. The coil of the catheter

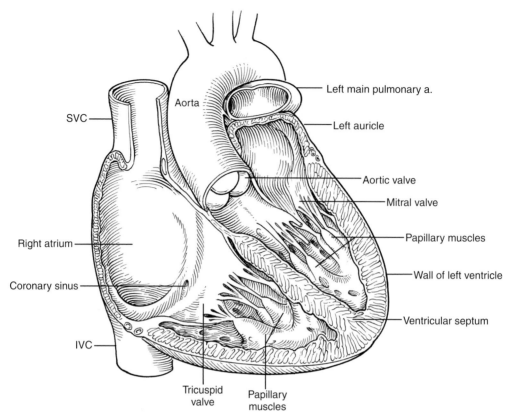

FIGURE 30   Left and right heart chamber anatomy. IVC, Inferior vena cava; SVC, superior vena cava. *(Modified from Gray H, editor: Gray's anatomy, 20th ed. Lea & Febiger, 1918, Plate 498.)*

should therefore have its tip directed 40 to 50 degrees toward the ceiling rather than straight toward the left wall. The right ventricular outflow tract, however, is in the sagittal plane. Once the pressure tracing indicates the tip of the catheter is in the right ventricle, it should be rotated counterclockwise such that the coil is directed toward the left wall.

HILUM OF THE LUNG

The hilum of the lung is the point where the airway and pulmonary artery enter the lung and the pulmonary veins leave. It represents a fixed point where the relatively mobile lung is tethered to the mediastinum. The reflection of the visceral onto parietal pleura occurs at the hilum, adding additional support.

Much thoracic surgery is done through exposures retracting the lung anterior or posterior or looking directly at the anterior or posterior surface of the hilum. Bilaterally, the respective phrenic nerves run anterior to the hilum. On the right (Fig. 32), the esophagus, vagus nerve, thoracic duct, and azygous veins are posterior. On the left (Fig. 33), the descending aorta, esophagus, and vagus nerve are posterior.

Right Hilum

The inferior pulmonary ligament is a reflection of the visceral pleura of the medial aspect of the right lower lobe. This ligament attaches the lung to the mediastinum. Dividing this ligament will bring the right lower lobe into view for inspection or repair through a standard fifth interspace thoracotomy. The ligament should be divided as close to

the lung as possible without injuring lung parenchyma to avoid injury to the underlying thoracic duct, esophagus, and vagus nerve. The superiormost aspect of the inferior pulmonary ligament is the inferior pulmonary vein. This can be visualized as a reflection of the pericardium into the lung. A lymph node will often guard the inferior pulmonary vein at the top of this ligament.

At the superior aspect of the right hilum is the azygous vein coursing posterior to anterior to join the posterior of the superior vena cava. Deep to the azygous vein the trachea bifurcates. Traveling under or medial to the azygous vein is anteriorly the right main bronchus and posteriorly the esophagus. The right main pulmonary artery enters the right side of the chest underneath the superior vena cava just inferior to the azygous vein and anterior to the trachea and right main bronchus. The right main pulmonary artery travels further than the left main pulmonary artery before reaching the pleural space and before branching. After entering the right chest, the pulmonary artery takes an abrupt turn inferior into the deepest part of the horizontal and oblique fissures. It gives off branches to the right upper lobe, right middle lobe, and right lower lobe, respectively. It should be remembered that the pulmonary artery branches distally into the lung like a deciduous tree. Larger vessels will be found close to the hilum and in the horizontal and oblique fissures. Progressively smaller vessels will be found as you approach the outer surface of the lung (Fig. 34). The first branch of the right main pulmonary artery goes to the right upper lobe. This branch may come off the pulmonary artery very proximal and course under the superior vena cava separate from the main pulmonary artery. This branch is often located just anterior to the right upper lobe bronchus and just inferior to the azygous vein as it arches over the hilum. In this location, it is very susceptible to iatrogenic traction injury by too vigorously pulling the lung inferior.

Proximal vascular control of the right pulmonary artery can be obtained as it courses under the superior vena cava either by

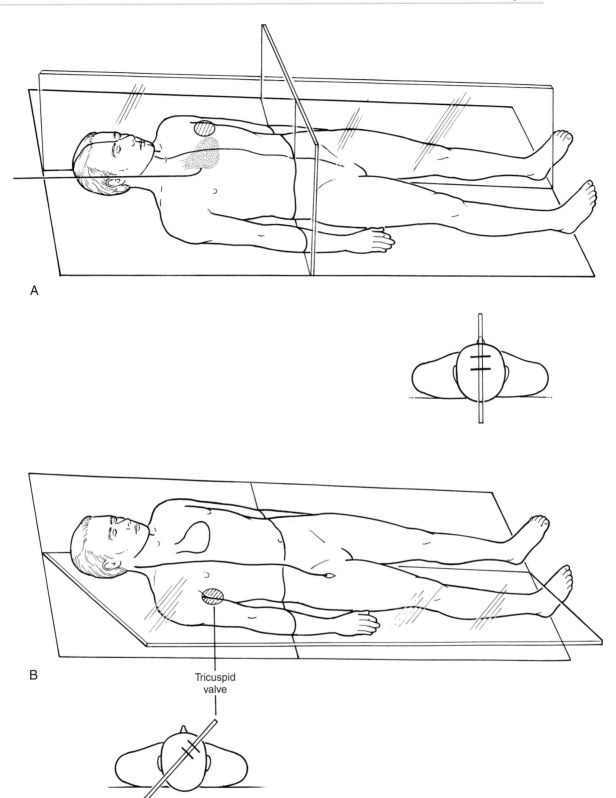

FIGURE 31   Placement of pulmonary artery catheter. **A,** Traditional placement of coil is directed toward the wall to the patient's left on a coronal plane, perceiving the tricuspid valve as an opening on a sagittal plane. **B,** Tricuspid valve is actually an opening on a plane 40 to 50 degrees off the sagittal plane, and correct orientation will direct the catheter 40 to 50 degrees more toward the ceiling.

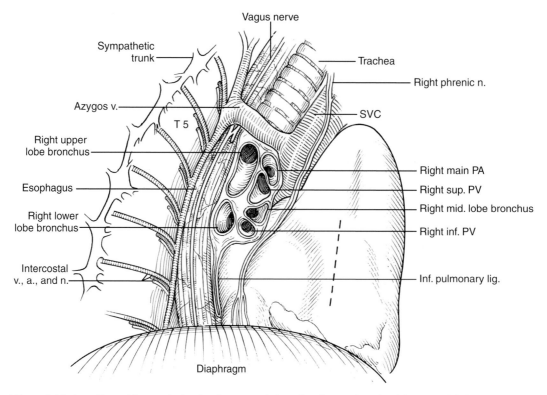

FIGURE 32 Hilum of right lung. Dotted line marks incision for pericardial window from right side of the chest. PA, Pulmonary artery; PV, pulmonary vein; SVC, superior vena cava. *(Modified from Agur AMR, Dalley AF, editors:* Grant's atlas of anatomy, *11th ed. Philadelphia, Lippincott Williams & Wilkins, 2004, Fig. 1.43, p 40.)*

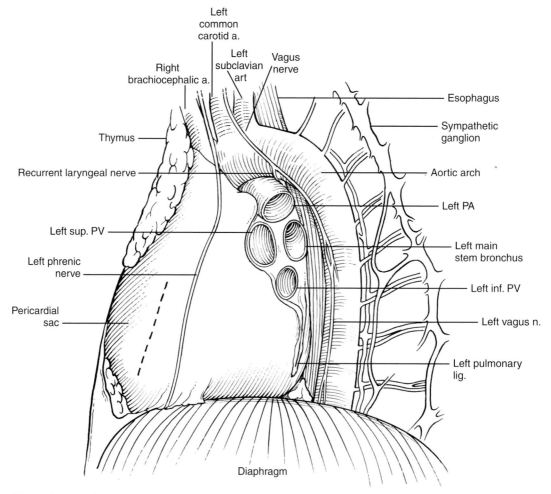

FIGURE 33 Hilum of left lung. Dotted line marks incision for pericardial window. PA, Pulmonary artery; PV, pulmonary vein. *(Modified from Agur AMR, Dalley AF, editors:* Grant's atlas of anatomy, *11th ed. Philadelphia, Lippincott Williams & Wilkins, 2004, Fig. 1.44, p 44.)*

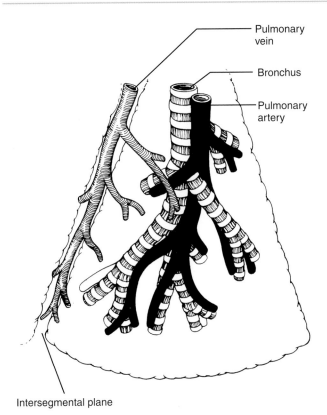

FIGURE 34 *Generic bronchopulmonary segment. (From Pearson FG, editor: Thoracic surgery, 2nd ed. Philadelphia, Churchill Livingstone, 2002, Fig. 20-1, p 428.)*

this allows time and visualization to obtain vascular control of a large hemorrhage such as from a main or branch pulmonary artery. Once the hemorrhage is contained, blood should be allowed to return to the heart before performing a definitive repair. Cardioversion will be necessary if the heart has fibrillated and should be anticipated.

The remaining vascular structure making up the hilum of the right lung is the superior pulmonary vein. This vein is seen anteriorly, sending a superior branch to the upper lobe, which crosses anterior to the pulmonary artery traveling in the horizontal fissure and variable branches to the right middle lobe.

The right main bronchus can be visualized on the posterior superior right hilum. It bifurcates from the carina and travels underneath the azygous vein. While visualizing the bronchus from the posterior hilum, the delicate membranous airway is seen, with the bases of the arching bronchial cartilages visible and palpable on either side.

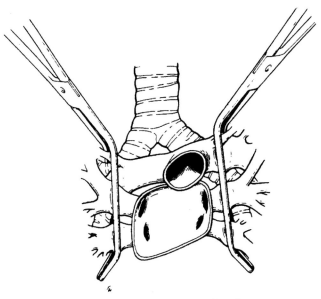

FIGURE 36 "Dirty" clamping of the left or right pulmonary hilum. *(From Pearson FG, editor: Thoracic surgery, 2nd ed. Philadelphia, Churchill Livingstone, 2002, Fig. 68-3, p 1837.)*

encircling the vessel with a vessel loop, careful vascular clamping (Fig. 35), or if needed, applying a nonselective clamp across the entire hilum (Fig. 36). A nonselective clamp is sometimes referred to as "dirty" clamping because the immediate need is control of hemorrhage, and structures other than the offending vessel initially may be included in the clamp.

From the right side of the chest or a median sternotomy, the superior vena cava and inferior vena cava can be clamped in an intrapericardial location. This is termed inflow occlusion or the Shumacker maneuver and will cause cardiac standstill that can be tolerated no more than 3 to 5 minutes. In desperate circumstances,

FIGURE 35 Clamping the right main pulmonary artery (PA) as it courses under the superior vena cava (SVC). PV, Pulmonary vein.

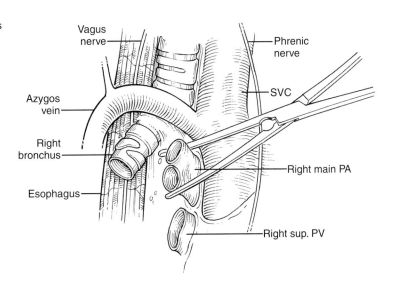

Left Hilum

As with the right lung, the left inferior lobe is tethered to the mediastinum by the left inferior pulmonary ligament. The superiormost aspect of this ligament is the left inferior pulmonary vein, often with a lymph node in the ligament, just inferior to the vein. The superior aspect of the left hilum has the arch of the aorta crossing from the right to the left and from anterior to posterior. The superiormost structure in the hilum proper is the left main pulmonary artery. The left main pulmonary artery is shorter than the right main pulmonary artery. Its first branch is to the left upper lobe and is often buried in the medial substance of the lung parenchyma. This branch is also vulnerable to injury during inferior retraction of the lung. The vagus nerve descends in the left side of the chest anterior to the left subclavian artery, crossing the lateral surface of the arch of the aorta and diving anterior to the descending aorta to join and travel next to the more medially placed esophagus. The vagus nerve gives off the left recurrent laryngeal nerve just below the arch of the aorta. The left recurrent laryngeal nerve will dive around the ligamentum arteriosum and also join the esophagus, but travel superiorly in the tracheoesophageal groove back into the neck to innervate the larynx. The ligamentum arteriosum is the vestigial ductus arteriosus. It is fibrous, possibly calcified, and connects the top of the bifurcation of the pulmonary trunk to the arch of the aorta. It is visible in the left side of the chest and emphasizes the proximity of the bifurcation of the pulmonary trunk to the left hilum of the lung. Minimizing the use of electrocautery in this region and keeping dissections close to the pulmonary artery and away from the aorta and ligamentum arteriosum can avoid injury to the recurrent laryngeal nerve. Proximal control of the left pulmonary artery can be obtained by encircling the pulmonary artery, by application of vascular clamps, or by hilar clamping. Because the left pulmonary artery is so short, it is sometimes necessary to incise the pericardium anterior to the left main pulmonary artery, taking care not to injure the phrenic nerve. The pulmonary trunk and intrapericardial course of the left main pulmonary artery can then be visualized and the left main pulmonary artery clamped. Immediate vascular collapse after placement of this clamp may mean blood flow to the right pulmonary artery was occluded as well and the clamp should be reapplied. The left atrial appendage will be present in this location. It is mobile and often an unwelcome companion. It is susceptible to injury, hemorrhage, and air embolism by clamping and retraction and should be treated with respect.

The left main pulmonary artery turns sharply after entering the chest and descends in the deepest part of the oblique fissure. Like the right superior pulmonary vein, the left superior pulmonary vein is only visible anteriorly. It can be seen inferior to the pulmonary artery as a fold of pericardium entering the lung. The left main bronchus, although long, is hidden by the arch of the aorta and main pulmonary artery. It is often not visible at all without incising the reflection of the parietal and visceral pleura posteriorly and developing the plane between the membranous portion of the left main bronchus and the esophagus.

The left hilum can also be nonselectively clamped to obtain vascular control (see Fig. 36).

LUNG ANATOMY

The right lung has three lobes, the right upper, right middle, and right lower. The left lung has two lobes, the left upper and left lower. The lingula of the left upper lobe is analogous to the middle lobe on the right. Fissures of the lung are usually present, but variably complete. On the right, the horizontal fissure, usually incomplete, divides the right upper lobe from the right middle lobe. The horizontal fissure joins the oblique fissure posteriorly. The oblique fissure divides the right upper lobe from the superior segment of the right lower lobe and the right middle lobe from the right lower lobe. The right lower lobe rests on the diaphragm posteriorly. The right

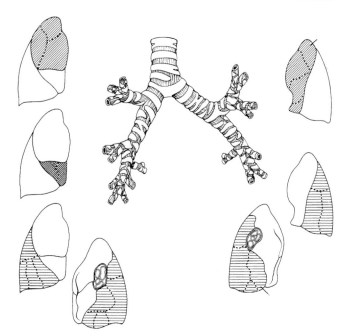

FIGURE 37   Segmental anatomy of the lung. *(From Pearson FG, editor: Thoracic surgery, 2nd ed. Philadelphia, Churchill Livingstone, 2002, Fig. 20-2, p 428.)*

middle lobe will often rest on the diaphragm anteriorly and is mistaken for the right lower lobe in this position. On the left, the oblique fissure divides the left upper lobe from the left lower lobe. The left lower lobe rests on the diaphragm posteriorly. The lingula of the left upper lobe can extend down to the diaphragm anteriorly.

Figure 37 shows the lung segments. Pulmonary arteries and the airway will enter the middle of their respective lung segment and bifurcate toward the periphery. Pulmonary veins travel in the border zones between lung segments and along the walls of the horizontal and oblique fissures (see Fig. 34).

AORTA, TRACHEA, ESOPHAGUS, AND THORACIC DUCT

Posterior to the heart, outside the pericardium, several tubular structures travel parallel to each other. They are the aorta, trachea, esophagus, and thoracic duct (Fig. 38).

Aorta

The thoracic aorta originates from the fibrous trigone of the heart at the aortic valve. The coronary arteries originate immediately distal to the valve from the aortic sinuses of Valsalva. The left coronary artery commonly originates from the left sinus, which is located posteriorly and toward the pulmonary valve. The right coronary artery originates from the right sinus of Valsalva, which is anterior and to the right. The right coronary may be seen coursing from left to right across the anterior wall of the right ventricle from its origin at the aorta. The ascending aorta is short, ending in the aortic arch. The aorta arches mostly from anterior to posterior with some movement from the midline to the left to come to lie just to the left of the vertebral column in the left side of the chest. The great vessels originate at the top of this arch. From proximal to distal and anterior to posterior, they are the right brachiocephalic artery, the left carotid artery, and the left subclavian artery. The right brachiocephalic artery will have the right vagus nerve crossing anteriorly with the right recurrent nerve branching posteriorly from the right vagus just after

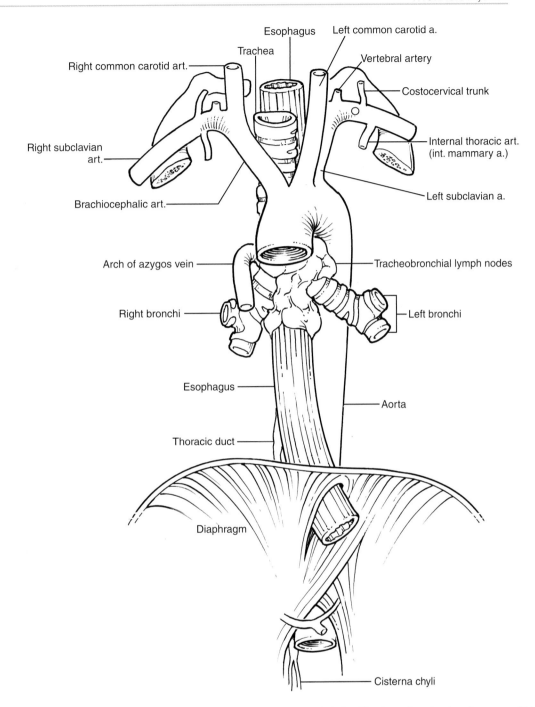

FIGURE 38   Aorta, trachea, esophagus, and thoracic duct. *(Modified from Agur AMR, Dalley AF, editors:* Grant's atlas of anatomy, *11th ed. Philadelphia, Lippincott Williams & Wilkins, 2004, Fig. 1.78, p 68.)*

crossing this vessel. The right recurrent nerve travels to the right tracheoesophageal groove and then superiorly back into the neck. On the underside of the aortic arch, the ligamentum arteriosum attaches the aorta to the pulmonary trunk. The combination of the great vessels and ligamentum arteriosum fix the aortic arch in the chest. The descending thoracic aorta is relatively mobile. The aorta just distal to the left subclavian artery is in the transition zone between fixed and mobile and is a common site for aortic injury in acceleration/deceleration injuries. The descending thoracic aorta gives off segmental branches to the chest wall as intercostal arteries as well as branches to the esophagus, trachea, carina, and proximal bronchi. The aorta enters the abdomen through the aortic hiatus of the diaphragm from T11 to T12. Between T8 and L2, but usually near L2

is the origin of the artery of Adamkiewicz. This is a large segmental artery, most commonly left sided, which anastomosis with the anterior spinal artery and supplies up to two thirds of spinal cord blood flow. Occluding the aorta proximal to this vessel may cause spinal cord ischemia.

Trachea

The trachea begins in the neck at the cricoid cartilage and enters the thorax anterior to the esophagus and posterior to the great vessels, including posterior to the arch and ascending aorta and the pulmonary arteries. Distally, near the carina, the arch of the aorta crosses to

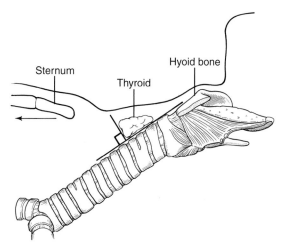

FIGURE 39 Trachea travels diagonally posterior as it leaves the neck and enters the chest. The shortest distance between a point and a line is perpendicular to that line through the point.

the left of the trachea. The trachea bifurcates into the right and left main bronchi at the carina. The carina is at the level of the angle of Louis anteriorly and T4-T5 posteriorly. The average adult trachea is 11 cm in length and varies according to the height of the person. In a young person, hyperextension of the neck can bring 50% of the trachea out of the chest and into the neck. Conversely, in a kyphotic elderly patient, the cricoid cartilage can be at the level of the sternal notch. In the neck, the trachea is anterior and subcutaneous. As it enters the chest, it travels obliquely posterior to the posterior mediastinum. The shortest distance from a point to a line is a perpendicular from that line, intersecting the point. If the trachea is a line, obliquely posterior, the shortest distance from a point on the skin to the trachea will be in a trajectory slightly superior. Visualizing this relationship aids in selecting tracheostomy and cricothyroidotomy incisions (Fig. 39). The trachea is composed anteriorly of cartilaginous arches with fibrous tissue in between. The posterior wall of the trachea is membranous. The blood supply to the trachea is segmental, superiorly primarily from the inferior thyroidal arteries and inferiorly from the bronchial arteries. The subclavian artery, highest intercostal artery, internal thoracic arteries, and innominate artery also supply it. These vessels also supply the esophagus. The blood supply enters the trachea laterally at 3 and 9 o'clock.

Esophagus

The esophagus travels through the posterior mediastinum anterior to the vertebral bodies, to the right of the descending aorta, and to the left of the azygous vein (see Fig. 38). Its blood supply is from segmental branches of the descending aorta, draining into intercostal veins. Above the level of the carina, the esophagus is posterior to the trachea and immediately abuts the membranous trachea. Above the level of the ligamentum arteriosum, the recurrent laryngeal nerve travels in the left tracheoesophageal groove. Above the level of the right brachiocephalic artery the right recurrent laryngeal nerve travels in the right tracheoesophageal groove. Below the carina, the esophagus directly abuts the posterior pericardium. To its left and right from superior to inferior are the superior pulmonary veins, the inferior pulmonary veins, and the inferior pulmonary ligaments. The esophagus enters the diaphragm through the esophageal hiatus at the level of T10 or T11. The area to the left and right of the esophagus at and below the inferior pulmonary ligament and before entering the diaphragm

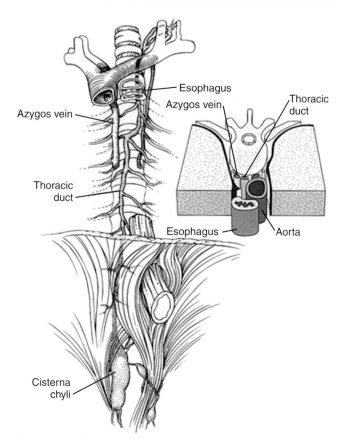

FIGURE 40 Thoracic duct. *(From Pearson FG, editor: Thoracic surgery, 2nd ed. Philadelphia, Churchill Livingstone, 2002, Fig. 20-7, p 431.)*

represents an anatomic weak spot. The wall of the esophagus is not buttressed by other firm mediastinal structures and is exposed to the negative pressure of the pleural space. It is for this reason that increased intraesophageal pressure causing a perforation of the esophagus most commonly occurs here (Boerhaave syndrome).

Thoracic Duct

The thoracic duct originates from the cisterna chyli (Fig. 40). The cisterna chyli is located in the abdomen, at the level of the celiac axis, anterior to the vertebral body and to the right of the aorta. The thoracic duct travels superiorly, entering the thorax through the aortic hiatus of the diaphragm. It ascends in the posterior mediastinum between the aorta and the azygous vein. Above the arch of the aorta, it travels posterior to the esophagus and arches behind the internal jugular vein to join the venous system at the junction of the internal jugular vein and subclavian vein. The thoracic duct is thin walled and often invisible to the naked eye if not distended with lymph. Injury to the duct is visible as a pooling of lymph in the vicinity of the leak. Fat delivered to the small bowel will within 10 to 20 minutes turn this lymph milky white, enhancing visualization. Ligation of the thoracic duct is accomplished by ligating all fatty material and lymphatics bounded by four walls, consisting of the azygous vein, the parietal pleura, the esophagus, and the aorta below the level of the suspected leak.

For the chapter's Suggested Readings list, please visit the book at www.ExpertConsult.inkling.com.

Thoracic Wall Injuries: Ribs, Sternal, and Scapular Fractures; Hemothoraces and Pneumothoraces

David H. Livingston, Carl Hauser, Noelle Salliant, and Devashish J. Anjaria

Though many chest injuries are potentially lethal, early man sustained and survived blunt and penetrating chest trauma with Neanderthal skeletons showing evidence of a healed penetrating trauma and blunt rib fractures. The Edwin Smith Papyrus, written circa 3000 BC, gave explicit instructions for the management of chest injuries, including soft tissue and bony injuries (Breasted). In fact, 8 of the 43 cases discussed concerned chest injuries, suggesting that even at that time, chest injuries accounted for 20% to 25% of all trauma.

Trauma to the chest wall and the underlying lung parenchyma either in isolation or as part of multisystem trauma remains exceedingly common, and such injuries are a frequent source of trauma fatality and morbidity. Hemothoraces and pneumothoraces, although technically not injuries to the thoracic wall, occur commonly in conjunction with such injuries and will be considered here as well. Flail chest and its accompanying pulmonary contusion are mentioned only briefly here and are more completely discussed elsewhere (Pulmonary Contusion and Flail Chest).

INCIDENCE

Thoracic injuries remain common and are directly attributable for 20% to 25% of all trauma deaths. Chest injuries commonly accompany other injuries and contribute to organ failure in patients who have multiple injuries. Rib fractures are among the most commonly encountered injuries. In a review of over 7000 patients seen in a Level I trauma center, 10% had rib fractures; of these, 94% had associated injuries, with a 12% mortality rate. Half of patients with rib fractures required operation or intensive care unit (ICU) admission, one third developed complications, and one third ultimately required extended care in an outpatient facility.

Pneumothorax is found in over 20% of patients arriving to a trauma center. Hemothoraces are encountered with similar frequency. The incidence of both hemothoraces and pneumothoraces is underestimated by plain films, as these injuries are much better visualized by computed tomography (CT) of the chest than the traditional supine anteroposterior (AP) chest radiograph.

Fractures to the bony thorax other than the ribs most commonly occur in the clavicles, which constitute 5% to 10% of all fractures. Fractures of the sternum and scapula are much less common (0.5% to 4% and 0.8% to 3%, respectively) and are more likely to occur in association with other injuries than clavicular fractures. Again, the more liberal use of chest CT has resulted in an increase in the identification of nondisplaced scapula and sternal fractures. Complete scapulothoracic dissociation is a rare but dramatic injury with severe associated neurovascular injury.

MECHANISM OF INJURY

Injuries of the chest wall vary enormously in severity. In routine emergency room settings, chest trauma may be incurred as a result of a low-energy impact and be relatively minor. Conversely, chest injuries sustained by patients treated in trauma centers following high-energy trauma from motor vehicle collisions (MVCs) are potentially severe and often life threatening. The most common causes of chest wall injuries and rib fractures in adults are motor vehicle crashes, followed by falls and direct blows to the chest with blunt objects. It is important to recall that rib fractures in infants and younger children occur almost exclusively in the setting of child abuse. In older populations, falls and motor vehicles versus pedestrian accidents become the predominant mechanism of injury.

Rib fractures are normally the hallmark of significant blunt chest trauma, and increasing numbers of rib fractures are related to increasing morbidity and mortality rates. The presence of greater than three rib fractures on plain chest radiograph in adults is a marker for associated solid visceral trauma and mortality risk, and thus has been used as a marker for trauma center transfer. In hemodynamically stable patients, the presence of blunt chest trauma has also been shown to double the rate of intraabdominal injuries detected by abdominal CT. Rib fractures are less common in children owing to the resilience of their bony chest wall. Thus, children may suffer major intrathoracic injury without rib fractures, and the presence of any rib fracture in a child should be considered a marker for severe injury. The presence of acute rib fractures in a young child whose mechanism of injury is unclear or the finding of rib fractures of varying ages should also serve as an indicator for potential child abuse. Conversely, elderly patients with brittle bones will occasionally have little in the way of intrathoracic injury despite extensive rib fractures.

The different mechanisms of injury provide somewhat different patterns of injury. Penetrating injury causes parenchymal lacerations with hemopneumothoraces. Blunt injury to the lung is most often due to displaced rib fractures, and can result in hemopneumothoraces or pulmonary contusions. Pneumothoraces after blunt trauma occur through (1) alveolar rupture with resultant air leak due to a sudden increase in intrathoracic pressure; (2) laceration of the lung due to displaced rib fractures; (3) tearing of the lung in a deceleration injury; and (4) direct crush injury from a blow to the chest.

DIAGNOSIS

Physical Examination

Expeditious inspection and palpation of the chest will provide much information regarding the patient's injuries (Fig. 1). Auscultation and percussion tend to be less reliable against the high ambient noise of the trauma emergency department (ED). Hypotension, tachycardia, pallor, or cyanosis suggests shock. In the presence of a known or suspected thoracic injury, shock must be assumed to be from an intrathoracic source. Inspection of the chest itself should include assessment of use of the accessory muscles suggestive of airway obstruction, the symmetry of the chest wall, number and location of wounds, presence of open chest wounds, subcutaneous emphysema, and the presence of "flail" segments. Although tracheal deviation in the neck is also frequently cited as a sign of tension pneumothorax, in reality it is rarely if ever seen, even in patients with gross mediastinal deviation on chest radiograph. Palpation can reveal mobile segments of chest wall and further allows appreciation of the symmetry of chest wall motion and of crepitance. Auscultation in trauma has a high specificity but very poor sensitivity, so focus should be placed only on the presence and symmetry of air entry. Heart sounds (such as the muffled heartbeat in Beck triad or the

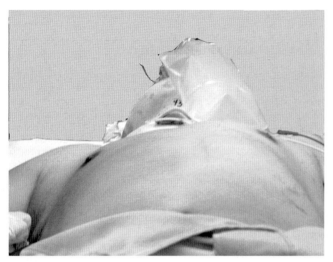

FIGURE 1 Physical examination of the chest in a driver of a motor vehicle discloses marked asymmetry of the right and left hemithoraces.

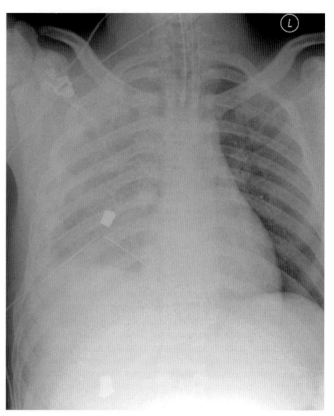

FIGURE 2 Supine chest radiograph demonstrating the overall hazy appearance, which is diagnostic of a right hemothorax (in this case incompletely drained by a tube thoracostomy). Note the difference between the right and left sides.

"mediastinal crunch" of Hamman sign) are also difficult to obtain clearly in the trauma bay. The absence or asymmetry of breath sounds, however, is very suggestive of significant trauma; in the unstable patient, this is an indication for intervention on clinical grounds and a contraindication for imaging studies. Thoracic percussion, even more than auscultation, is difficult to interpret in the trauma setting and is rarely useful.

Physical examination often, but not always, reveals the presence of a hemopneumothorax. It may be suspected in hemodynamically unstable patients by physical examination. In the patient with greatly diminished or absent breath sounds on the affected side, the diagnosis is quickly made on clinical grounds. Breath sounds can be well transmitted from the contralateral lung, further obscuring the results of auscultation. The finding of any subcutaneous emphysema following blunt trauma or at some distance from a penetrating wound is ample evidence of a pneumothorax that requires treatment. An open pneumothorax, of course, is readily appreciated on examination. Confirmation of the hemothorax or pneumothorax occurs with the placement of a chest tube with evacuation of blood or air.

Radiographic Studies

The supine AP chest radiograph is the initial and sometimes most important study in the management of chest trauma. The trauma surgeon must be comfortable interpreting these films, which are often suboptimal owing to the patient's body habitus, supine position, the presence of a spine board, and the use of portable x-ray machines. Still, the portable AP chest radiograph has a high positive predictive value (e.g., findings that are present on the film are usually of great significance and can diagnose or exclude a number of life-threatening injuries). The film must be obtained and reviewed before the patient is transported for any other imaging or procedures.

Interpretation of the chest radiograph should begin with review of the lung parenchyma and pleura. Lung expansion, pulmonary infiltrates or contusions, the position of the endotracheal tube (if present), and the presence of hemothoraces or pneumothoraces should be noted. The mediastinum should be evaluated for evidence of great vessel injury, which is suggested by mediastinal widening, blunting of the aortic knob, apical capping, or a medial displacement of the left main bronchus or of the nasogastric tube. Diaphragmatic elevation or injury should also be noted. Finally, any fractures of the bony thorax—ribs, clavicles, scapulae—should be sought. Alignment of the thoracic vertebrae can be appreciated on chest radiograph, but full imaging of the spine as well as specific radiographs of the bony

thoracic structures should be deferred until the patient's airway, respiratory, and cardiovascular status has been stabilized.

Radiographic imaging is extremely useful in the diagnosis of a hemothorax or pneumothorax. Indeed, in a hemodynamically stable patient, the diagnosis is often made on the portable AP chest radiograph obtained for the secondary survey. In the supine position the AP chest radiograph will reveal hemothorax only when at least 200 to 300 mL of blood is present in the pleural space and is suggested by an overall opacification or haziness compared to the contralateral hemithorax as the fluid will layer posteriorly (Fig. 2). False "negative" appearing chest radiograph may occur in the setting of bilateral hemothoraces (no difference between the two sides) or when there is a simultaneous anterior pneumothorax (decreasing the relative density to be more similar to the other side). In the patient with penetrating chest trauma, the chest radiograph is best taken with the patient upright, which increases the sensitivity for both hemothoraces and pneumothoraces. Chest ultrasound may help to identify the presence of pleural fluid, but its sensitivity and specificity for this purpose have not been well defined.

As routine truncal (chest, abdomen, and pelvis) CT scanning has become more prevalent, many patients with blunt trauma have been found to have significant anterior pneumothoraces not seen on plain chest radiograph. The incidence of missed pneumothoraces on supine AP chest radiograph has been estimated to be between 20% and 35%. A patient with a relatively minor pneumothorax on chest radiograph who nonetheless develops dyspnea and hypoxia may thus in fact have a significant pneumothorax that is better visualized by chest CT. In stable patients, CT scanning also will reveal pleural fluid collections and help to distinguish them from parenchymal injury such as pulmonary contusion.

The appropriate management of the patient with "CT-only" pneumothorax is a matter of some controversy (Fig. 3). The reported

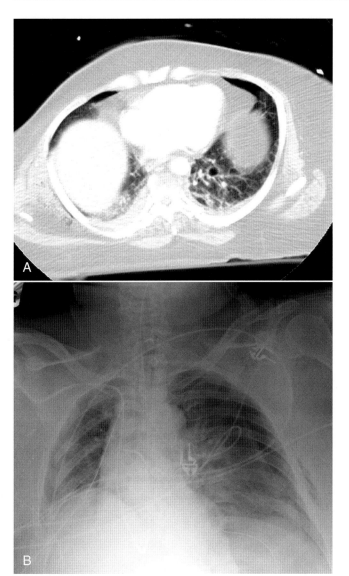

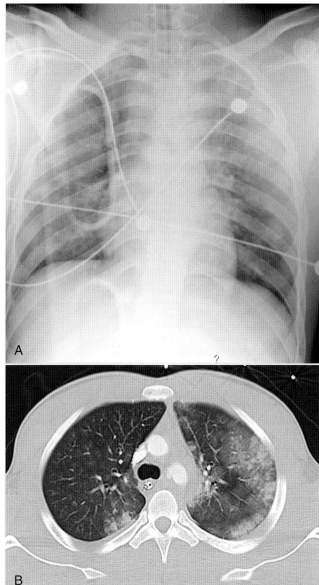

FIGURE 3 Computed tomography (CT) scan (**A**) demonstrating small bilateral "CT-only" pneumothoraces. Chest radiograph of the same patient (**B**), following mechanical ventilation. Note the large left pneumothorax, demonstrating the somewhat unpredictable outcome of these small pneumothoraces. The patient never developed a pneumothorax on the right side.

FIGURE 4 Chest radiograph of a patient ejected from a motor vehicle at a high rate of speed (**A**). The lung fields are essentially clear, although the mediastinal contour is abnormal. Computed tomography scan (**B**) of the same patient demonstrated significant pulmonary contusions, which helped explain the patient's clinical hypoxemia. In addition, an injury to the descending aorta is also visualized.

incidence of these pneumothoraces in blunt trauma patients is 2% to 8%. The available literature suggests that 20% of these patients will require tube thoracostomy. The decision to place a chest tube, however, should be dictated by the patient's overall status. Those patients who have multiple injuries, are in hemorrhagic shock, or have sustained a traumatic brain injury will not tolerate progression of even a small pneumothorax (see Fig. 3). These patients would benefit from tube thoracostomy. In those patients in whom the clinical picture appears stable, observation can be undertaken, with serial radiographs taken at 6 and 24 hours after diagnosis.

CT of the chest has become increasingly accepted in the early management of trauma. CT can reveal injuries not seen on initial chest radiograph in about two thirds of major trauma patients and can lead to therapeutic changes in 5% to 30% of cases (Fig. 4). Specifically for rib fractures, chest radiography has been shown to miss over half of rib fractures seen on CT of the chest. For patients with rib fractures seen on initial chest radiograph, CT scan usually identifies a mean of two additional rib fractures. Despite the increased sensitivity of detecting rib fractures as well as lung contusions, pulmonary morbidity (pneumonia, respiratory failure) and mortality risk is only affected by rib fractures and pulmonary contusions that are visible on chest radiograph, indicating that increased sensitivity is not necessarily related to clinical significance.

In addition, CT scanning may reveal additional findings that are only suggested by an abnormal chest radiograph (Fig. 5). In a number of specific situations chest CT contributes significantly to trauma management. CT of the thoracic spine is the "gold standard" imaging modality for assessing vertebral body as well as posterior element fractures, and is also helpful in imaging the spine at the cervicothoracic junction. In patients with the nonspecific finding of a widened mediastinum on chest radiograph, use of CT can help to limit the

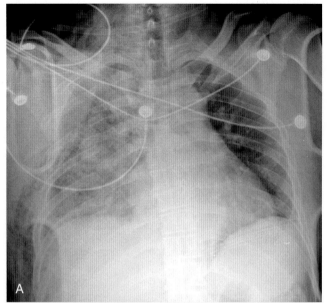

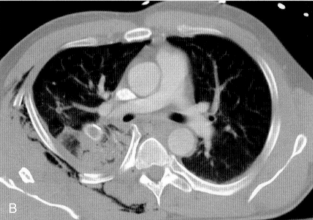

FIGURE 5 The impact of computed tomography (CT) scanning with more obvious severe chest trauma following a motor vehicle collision. Physical examination demonstrated no paradoxical motion in the upper right hemithorax. **A,** Plain radiograph of the chest. There are multiple (seven) rib fractures, a haziness over the entire right hemithorax, and subcutaneous emphysema but no obvious pneumothorax. **B,** CT scan of the same patient shows a chest tube, which was inserted based upon the marked subcutaneous emphysema present on physical examination, drained no air on insertion and minimal amount of blood. The haziness turned out to be only a modest pulmonary contusion with a minimal hemothorax. The scan also revealed a total of 18 distinct rib fractures with considerable more displacement than was noted on the plain radiograph. The reason for the lack of paradoxical motion is explained by the posterior nature of the flail segments. In addition, a nondisplaced scapula fracture and six thoracic transverse process fractures were identified.

use of aortography to assess aortic injuries. As CT technology improves and as further studies become available, the role of CT in chest trauma will become better defined.

Ultrasonography has become important in the assessment of intraabdominal hemorrhage and pericardial fluid collections in the trauma patient. Recent reports also suggest that it might be useful to assess the pleural spaces for pneumothoraces and hemothoraces. The pleural space is interrogated by placing the ultrasound probe between the ribs and looking for the characteristic signs of pneumothorax.

AMERICAN ASSOCIATION FOR THE SURGERY OF TRAUMA—ORGAN INJURY SCALE GRADING

The American Association for the Surgery of Trauma—Organ Injury Scale (AAST-OIS) grading scales for chest wall and lung injury developed by Moore et al are given in Tables 1 and 2.

TABLE 1: Chest Wall Injury Scale

Grade	Injury Type	Description of Injury
I	Contusion Laceration Fracture	Any size Skin and subcutaneous tissue <3 ribs, closed Nondisplaced clavicle, closed
II	Laceration Fracture	Skin, subcutaneous tissue, and muscle ≥3 adjacent ribs, closed Open or displaced clavicle Nondisplaced sternum, closed Scapular body, open or closed
III	Laceration Fracture	Full thickness including pleural penetration Open or displaced sternum Flail sternum Unilateral flail segment (<3 ribs)
IV	Laceration Fracture	Avulsion of chest wall tissues with underlying rib Fractures Unilateral flail chest (≥3 ribs)
V	Fracture	Bilateral flail chest (≥3 ribs on both sides)

Modified from Moore EE, Cogbill TH, Malangoni MA, et al: Organ injury scaling. *Surg Clin North Am* 75:293–303, 1995.

TABLE 2: Lung Injury Scale

Grade	Injury Type	Description of Injury
I	Contusion	Unilateral, <1 lobe
II	Contusion Laceration	Unilateral, single lobe Simple pneumothorax
III	Contusion Laceration Hematoma	Unilateral, >1 lobe Persistent (>72 hours) air leak from distal airway Nonexpanding intraparenchymal
IV	Laceration Hematoma Vascular	Major (segmental or lobar) air leak Expanding intraparenchymal Primary branch intrapulmonary vessel disruption
V	Vascular	Hilar vessel disruption
VI	Vascular	Total uncontained transaction of pulmonary hilum

Modified from Moore EE, Cogbill TH, Malangoni MA, et al: Organ injury scaling. *Surg Clin North Am* 75:293–303, 1995.

MANAGEMENT OF SPECIFIC INJURIES OF THE CHEST WALL

Chest Wall Defects

Chest wall defects create open pneumothoraces and are potentially rapidly fatal. Large sucking chest wounds can allow rapid equilibration of pleural and atmospheric pressure, preventing lung inflation and alveolar ventilation and causing death by asphyxia. As a result, patients sustaining chest wall defects with significant tissue loss rarely survive long enough to be seen in the trauma bay. Patients who do come to medical attention are usually found to have penetrating injuries such as close shotgun blasts or impalements.

The field approach to the relatively small chest wall defect is placement of an occlusive dressing taped on three sides to allow gas to exit from, but not to enter, the thorax. Subsequent treatment consists of tube thoracostomy through clean nontraumatized skin, after which the primary wound may be temporarily closed or dressed with an occlusive dressing. Definitive wound closure is then performed in the operating room.

In large chest wall defects, the occlusive dressing is of no value. These patients must be endotracheally intubated with positive-pressure ventilation. Operative management then focuses on control of hemorrhage from the chest wall and from any associated injuries. Chest wall hemorrhage in these cases may be life threatening and may mandate emergent thoracotomy. "Damage control" with packing may be the optimal initial management of these patients. The chest defect can be temporarily closed with skin or prosthetic material. The definitive closure of these defects, which may require tissue-transfer procedures, is best deferred until the patient is fully resuscitated and physiologically sound and can tolerate a lengthy operation.

Rib Fractures and Flail Chest

Rib fractures can result in chest wall pain, chest wall hemorrhage, and less commonly chest wall instability. A flail chest is said to exist when three or more adjacent ribs are segmentally fractured. The resultant chest wall instability combined with underlying pulmonary contusion is responsible for the respiratory insufficiency that develops in patients with this injury. The pathophysiology and treatment of flail chest injuries are covered in greater detail in another chapter (Pulmonary Contusion and Flail Chest).

Failure to provide sufficient analgesia in the setting of chest wall injuries has been shown to result in hypoventilation, retained secretions, increased atalectasis and lobar collapse, pneumonia, and respiratory failure. Persistence of pain may perpetuate the stress response to injury and may have a negative impact on posttraumatic immune function. Poor pain control will hamper the ability of mechanically ventilated patients to be weaned and extubated. The pharmacologic approach to pain management in chest injury has consisted of the use of narcotics with or without regional anesthesia. The addition of nonsteroidal anti-inflammatory drugs (NSAIDs) such as ketorolac have also proved effective in relieving pain from mild to moderate injuries.

Narcotics

Narcotics are the mainstay for pain control in the majority of trauma patients. Narcotic preparations can be given orally, intramuscularly, or intravenously. But whereas intramuscular administration has been the standard for decades, we strongly advise against this route of administration because it is both painful to the patient and results in unreliable absorption of the narcotic. With the exception of meperidine (Demerol), however, the choice of narcotic is far less important than ensuring adequate dosing for pain control. The amount of narcotic required for pain control may vary greatly depending upon previous or current narcotic use, age, and other factors that may alter the patient's perception of pain.

The use of pain scales in combination with performance on incentive spirometry can be very effective in determining the adequacy of pain control. Our current approach is to begin most awake patients on a patient-controlled analgesia (PCA) regimen using morphine or fentanyl. Later, patients are transitioned to long-acting narcotic preparations such as OxyContin or MS-contin with the use of oxycodone for breakthrough pain. The addition of an NSAID may reduce inflammation and augment the effect of the oral narcotics. It is also important to avoid narcotic-induced constipation, which can result in severe abdominal pain, nausea, and vomiting in patients requiring long-term opioids.

Regional Anesthesia

Rib blocks can be accomplished using a mixture of 1% to 2% lidocaine with 0.25% bipuvicaine to decrease the pain of rib fractures. This simple technique involves the administration 2 to 3 mL of the anesthetic mixture to the inferior rib margin several centimeters posterior to the site of the rib fracture. Optimal analgesia requires blocking at least one rib above and one rib below the fracture. The limitations of the technique are that the pain control is short lived and that it can only be used for patients with mid or lower rib fractures. Last, in our experience the results vary widely and the risks of pneumothorax in patients without a chest tube are real.

Epidural analgesia/anesthesia is the delivery mode that has been shown to have the greatest impact on pulmonary mechanics following moderate to severe chest trauma, especially in those patients with bilateral injuries. Various combinations of local anesthetics and narcotics have been employed. In our institution, the most common combination is fentanyl with bupivacaine. Combination therapy can be advantageous because it works via two different mechanisms of action. Opioids modulate pre- and postsysnaptic nerve transmission in dorsal horn neurons by effects on their specific receptors. Local anesthetics work by blocking sodium channels. Thus, the analgesic effects of the two classes of drug are synergistic. Moreover, the potential for side effects is lessened in combination therapy because the doses of each drug used can be lower than the amount needed if either were administered alone.

Epidural analgesia has significant practical problems including ileus, pruritus, and urinary retention as well as transient hypotension. The use of epidural analgesia requires that the spine be documented to be free of injury, which may be difficult to accomplish for several days in severely injured patients. Also, the concomitant use of low-molecular-weight heparin (LMWH) in patients with an epidural catheter has been implicated in the development of spinal epidural hematomas with resultant neurologic deficits. Finally, epidural catheters can only be left in place safely for 7 to 10 days because of the possibility of epidural abscess formation. Thus, it is strongly recommended that epidural catheters not be placed in mechanically ventilated patients until they are ready to be weaned.

The data supporting the use of epidural analgesia are strong. Mackersie et al demonstrated that the use of epidural fentanyl was associated with significant improvements pulmonary mechanics with 85% of the patients requiring no additional parenteral narcotics. Intravenous (IV) narcotics were associated with increases in Pa_{CO_2} and decreases in Pa_{O_2} that were not observed in the epidural group. In a randomized prospective trial, Bulger et al reported epidural analgesia was associated with half the number of ventilator days compared to patients in the opioid group. They also point out that the technique was limited in trauma patients owing to the presence of exclusion criteria in over 50%. Despite these limitations the use epidural analgesia, when feasible, is of considerable benefit to patients following severe chest injury, as it has been strongly associated with a decrease in the rate of nosocomial pneumonia and a shorter duration of mechanical ventilation.

An alternate method for providing regional analgesia is via thoracic paravertebral catheter providing continuous bupivacaine infusion. This catheter can be an epidural catheter placed in the paravertebral space or a dedicated system such as the On-Q for ease of placement and bupivacaine infusion. Prospective study has shown equivalent pain control to epidural anesthetics with similar rates of pulmonary complications and ICU length of stay. However, the paravertebral infusion was associated with decreased incidence of hypotension. Paravertebral infusion blocks have the potential advantages of being able to be used in patients with spine fractures, being able to be used with heparin products as there is no risk of epidural hematoma, and eliminating the risk of CNS infection or spinal abscess.

Operative Fixation of Ribs

Operative fixation of rib fractures is not a new concept. Initial descriptions of both internal and external fixation were reported in the 1940s and 1950s as a method for treatment of flail chest. This approach was largely abandoned because of the availability of positive-pressure ventilation and lack of effective prosthetic devices to stabilize the ribs, which allowed for pain control while ensuring adequate oxygenation and ventilation. At this point, rib fixation was limited to patients with severe chest wall deformity or patients who required thoracotomy for other reasons in whom fixation was completed "on the way out."

Interest in rib fixation has redeveloped in the past 15 years, initially in Europe and now in the United States. Despite the increased interest, there is not a consensus on indications. In patients with flail chest, studies have shown operative rib fixation in selected patients on mechanical ventilation to result in decreased ventilator days and decreased ICU length of stay. Although rib fixation may improve pain control, in patients with underlying parenchymal disease (lung contusion, pneumonia, etc.) rib fixation is unlikely to change the course of respiratory failure and vent dependence. In studies that advocate rib fixation for flail chest, there is no consensus on timing, although the later the fixation, the greater the potential for decreased benefit in time to liberation from mechanical ventilation.

Patients with open chest wounds or significant chest wall deformity may also benefit from rib fixation, although the reported literature consists of small case series with no consensus on patient selection, timing, and benefit. In addition, there are reports of patients having rib fixation during thoracotomy for other indications (i.e., retained hemothorax) when fixation is performed as part of closure of the chest wall. Conditions that have been reported in the literature but remain controversial as to whether they are appropriate indications include acute pain syndromes and chronic nonunions with pain.

Many techniques have been described for fixation of the ribs. If no commercial hardware is available, fixation can be performed with wire cerclage. The difficulty of this technique is that the fixation is sometimes unstable and risks further rib fracture if the surgeon is not careful. Anterior plates can be used from a generic hand or facial fixation set with anterior screws and wire if a dedicated rib fixation system is not available. Both of these techniques are usually done with the chest open during thoracotomy. Multiple dedicated rib fixation systems are available, allowing for improved bony fixation as well as the ability to perform the fixation without entry into the pleural cavity. These systems include anterior plating with bicortical screws (some with contoured plates to follow the natural curve of each individual rib), intramedullary splints, Judet struts with bendable struts that grasp the superior and inferior edge of the rib without screw fixation, and U-plating systems that eliminate the issue of relatively soft ribs by providing anterior and posterior plating with interlocking screws. In addition, absorbable versions of some of these systems, made of polylactide polymers, are being introduced. This technology has been used successfully in fixation of maxillofacial fractures. It provides the potential advantage of providing an alternative for open chest wounds with contamination, in addition to never having to

be removed, which is a small chance with all metal hardware. Despite the increased interest in operative management of rib fractures and the multiple commercial products to achieve rib fracture fixation, there is still insufficient evidence to definitively identify which patients will benefit most.

Pneumothorax and Hemothorax

Rib fractures can also cause injury to the underlying lung parenchyma, with resultant hemothoraces or pneumothoraces, both of which can also occur without evidence of rib fractures. The severity of pneumothorax ranges from clinically insignificant to life threatening. Pneumothoraces can be categorized as simple, open, and tension. A simple pneumothorax is a collection of air arising from leakage of air from an injured lung into the pleural space. An open pneumothorax arises when air enters the thoracic cavity from an open chest wound, with equalization of pressure between the thorax and the atmosphere. A tension pneumothorax occurs from a "ball-and-valve" effect in which air enters but does not exit the thoracic cavity, causing intrapleural pressure to exceed atmospheric pressure. The resultant pressure can cause the heart and great vessels to shift away from the side of injury and result in progressive circulatory compromise (see Fig. 3).

Hemothorax, the presence of blood in the pleural space, can arise from either thoracic or abdominal sources. Bleeding from thoracic sources can occur from injured lung parenchyma, lacerated intercostal or internal mammary arteries, or the heart and great vessels. Hemothorax from an abdominal source occurs in the setting of diaphragmatic injury with associated abdominal injury, most commonly the liver or spleen.

Treatment of pneumothorax depends upon the type. Small simple pneumothoraces can generally be observed, though larger ones require tube thoracostomy. If the patient is stable and a simple pneumothorax is suspected, a chest radiograph is obtained prior to any intervention. This (1) confirms the diagnosis and prevents unnecessary chest tube placement, (2) helps to exclude unexpected injury such as a diaphragmatic rupture, and (3) may demonstrate other findings (such as a large hemothorax or chest wall hematoma) that would affect the size or location of chest tube placement. Patients with small pneumothoraces who are stable from the hemodynamic and respiratory standpoints may be observed with serial radiographs. Supplemental oxygen may be administered to enhance reabsorption of the pneumothorax. Patients with larger pneumothoraces may be treated either with standard tube thoracostomy or in select patients a "pigtail" catheter.

Open and tension pneumothoraces require urgent treatment. The treatment of open pneumothoraces requires temporary closure of the defect and tube thoracostomy, followed by definitive operative closure of the chest wall defect. Tension pneumothorax is treated with needle decompression followed by tube thoracostomy. If a tension pneumothorax is suspected and the patient manifests any respiratory distress or hemodynamic instability, decompression should be performed without awaiting radiologic imaging. Emergent chest decompression is performed by inserting a 14-G IV catheter in the second or third intercostal space (approximately 2 fingerbreadths below the clavicle) in the midclavicular line. A large chest tube is then placed (see following discussion).

The treatment goal for hemothoraces, as for pneumothoraces, is evacuation of the pleural space and reexpansion of the lung. This is accomplished initially through tube thoracostomy. Apposition of the visceral and parietal pleurae generally provides definitive control of hemorrhage, and thoracotomy is required in less than 10% of all chest trauma patients. Patients may occasionally present to the trauma bay several hours after injury with a large amount of initial drainage from the chest tube. This usually represents the slow accumulation of blood rather than rapid active bleeding, particularly in the patient who remains hemodynamically stable. If the hemothorax

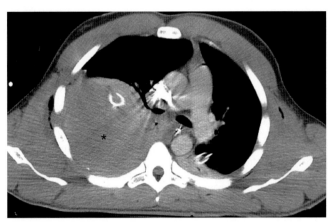

FIGURE 6 Computed tomography scan of the patient shown in Figure 2. The large right retained hemothorax *(asterisk)* is easily seen and can be easily differentiated from the lung parenchyma. The clotted hemothorax was successfully evacuated by video-assisted thoracoscopic surgery.

cannot be adequately drained by one chest tube, another one may need to be placed. Chest radiograph should be obtained immediately after tube thoracostomy to demonstrate successful drainage of the pleural space and lung reexpansion. If residual blood in the pleural space is still suspected and the patient is stable, CT of the chest may help to resolve the issue. If an acute hemothorax cannot be adequately drained because the chest tube is clotted, operative drainage may be necessary as continued bleeding cannot be assessed (Fig. 6). Operative treatment can be accomplished either through thoracotomy or, in selected stable patients, through video-assisted thoracoscopic surgery (VATS).

The chest tube output from any moderate-sized to large acute hemothorax should be collected and autotransfused. Collection systems should be readily available in the trauma ED, as the largest amount of blood loss occurs immediately upon placement of the chest tube. Autotransfusion in our experience appears to diminish the coagulopathy and inflammatory response to injury in these patients.

For patients with hemopneumothoraces, admission to a monitored setting and observation are appropriate for patients who remain hemodynamically stable, have little or no further hemorrhage from the chest tube, demonstrate evacuation of the pleural space on chest radiograph, and have no other emergent operative indications. Rapid active bleeding or persistent brisk bleeding suggests a significant lung injury. The need for emergent thoracotomy is strongly suggested when more than 1 L of blood is immediately evacuated on placement of a chest tube. In patients in whom a lower initial volume is drained, continued chest tube output of 200 mL/hour for 4 hours constitutes an indication for thoracotomy. Observation of patients in this latter group should include a repeat chest radiograph to ensure that the slowing of chest tube output is not due to a clotted hemothorax.

Tube Thoracostomy: Technique and Management

Once the decision is made to place a chest tube, the patient should be positioned to allow easy access to the midaxillary line in the fifth or sixth intercostal space. This location is preferred because it is usually safely above the diaphragm and because the chest wall musculature is thinnest in this area, thus facilitating the procedure. The chest should be cleansed with an antiseptic solution and anesthetized with 10 mL 1% lidocaine in all layers of the chest wall down to the pleura. To provide longer analgesia and increase patient comfort following insertion we suggest mixing the lidocaine with and equal volume of 0.25% bupivacane. Conscious sedation may be administered if the patient's hemodynamic and respiratory status permits. A 2-cm skin incision

is made over the rib immediately below the interspace selected for tube insertion. Sharp dissection proceeds directly to the rib, and the pleural space is entered at its superior margin, care being taken to avoid the intercostal neurovascular bundle at the inferior border of the adjacent superior rib. Although a clamp is commonly used to penetrate through the pleural space, we advocate continuing with the scalpel as it is both easier and less painful to the patient. Once the pleural space is entered, digital exploration will confirm entry into the thorax rather than the lung or abdominal cavity. The presence or absence of adhesions should be noted as well. Digital exploration is particularly important in the patient who may have a diaphragmatic rupture or who has a history of thoracic surgery or pulmonary infection. If no adhesions, diaphragmatic injury, or pulmonary pathology is encountered, the chest tube can be safely placed. The blind placement of chest tubes with trocars is ill advised and not recommended.

Chest tubes, like most medical devices, have markings to aid in placement. Unfortunately, in our experience these markings are too often ignored by residents placing the tube in the heat of battle, with the result that tubes that may be poorly positioned. One of the most common mistakes is to insert the tube too far to ensure that it won't "fall out." The tube will often bend at the last hole which will prevent adequate drainage (see Fig. 2). To prevent this type of malposition the mark at the skin should be evaluated. If the tube is placed in the midaxillary line at the fifth interspace, the mark at the skin level in most patients should be between 10 and 12. A tube placed deeper is likely to be kinked. In addition, once the tube is positioned it should be rotated 360 degrees prior to securing it in place. A tube that cannot be rotated freely should be presumed to be kinked or otherwise malpositioned.

Once inserted, the chest tube is connected to suction with an underwater seal at a negative pressure of 20 cm H_2O. A chest radiograph should be obtained after tube placement to confirm placement, evacuation of air or fluid, and proper reexpansion of the lung. If intrapleural air or fluid remains, a second chest tube should be placed. Complete evacuation of the pleural space with full pulmonary reexpansion will help to decrease bleeding and air leaks, as well as the risk of a posttraumatic empyema. Early surgical intervention is indicated for retained blood in the pleural space.

Chest radiographs should be obtained daily to confirm resolution of the hemopneumothorax. It is not our practice to use prophylactic antibiotics with tube thoracostomies, though opinion in the literature is divided on this issue. The chest tube can subsequently be removed when there is no air leak and when there is less than 100 to 150 mL of drainage over 24 hours, although no data exist to validate this volume of output. A prospective study has shown that a 6- to 8-hour trial of water seal decreases the incidence of recurrent pneumothorax when compared to chest tube removal with no water seal.

Should a new air leak be discovered or the lung fail to reexpand, several potential causes should be investigated. The connections between chest tube, canisters, and wall suction should be inspected for leaks. The chest tube must be checked to ensure that the last hole has not migrated out of the chest wall. If the chest tube is noted to be "out" immediately after placement, it can be repreppped and advanced a small distance; if detection is delayed, however, the chest tube should be removed and replaced at a different site. Placement of the tube into the major fissure may result in inadequate reexpansion, and parenchymal tube placement will result in continuing and ongoing air leaks. These tubes will also require removal and replacement. It is not uncommon for pleural space to become loculated or the chest tube occluded some time following injury, and a tension pneumothorax is always a possibility in a patient on mechanical ventilation, even in the presence of a chest tube.

Sternal Fractures

Sternal fractures are relatively uncommon and occur most often following blunt trauma. The usual mechanism of injury involves an unrestrained driver who strikes the sternum against the steering column of an automobile in a deceleration crash. A fall or other direct impact to the chest may also cause a sternal fracture. Most sternal fractures occur in the upper or midportion of the sternum. As with scapular fractures, the presence of a sternal fracture should be regarded as a marker of potential severe multiple trauma, including rib fractures (40%), long-bone fractures (25%), and head injuries (18%).

The fracture itself often needs no treatment acutely, and more than 95% of patients are treated nonoperatively. Although a baseline electrocardiogram (ECG) should be obtained, particularly in patients over 40 years of age, the need for continuous cardiac monitoring is determined by the associated injuries and the patient's cardiac status rather than by the presence of the sternal fracture itself. Most patients will be found to have a transient right ventricular dysfunction. The patient with an isolated sternal fracture and otherwise normal ED evaluation may be discharged. Similar to rib fractures, the management of sternal fractures is symptomatic and consists of analgesic administration and the avoidance of motion. Patients who have grossly displaced fractures or who have persistent pain due to nonunion may require operative reduction and internal fixation (ORIF). Sternal repair can be accomplished through various techniques utilizing wires or small plates.

Scapular Fractures

Fractures of the scapula are uncommon, occurring with an incidence of 1% to 3% in blunt trauma. Because of its location and structure, the scapula requires considerable direct force to fracture. As a result, associated injuries are common (80% to 98%), and a patient with a scapular fracture should be considered to have sustained a severe chest trauma. Careful examination for thoracic, neurologic, vascular, and abdominal injuries, as well as other orthopedic injuries, should be undertaken. Findings on physical examination include local pain or tenderness, swelling, and crepitus. Though most scapular fractures will be seen on initial chest radiograph, they may be obscured or overlooked. Many scapular fractures may have hitherto gone undetected, with increasing detection of nondisplaced fractures with the increasing use of modern CT technology (see Fig. 5). CT of the shoulder may be necessary to evaluate the fracture and to look for extension into the shoulder joint.

Management of scapular fractures in the vast majority of cases consists of analgesic administration and immobilization initially, followed by progressive physical therapy. Surgical intervention is rarely required and is undertaken primarily for those fractures that will likely cause significant disability. Minimally displaced fractures of the scapular body, neck, coracoid, acromion, and scapular spine are treated nonoperatively and typically result in healing with normal or near-normal function. Glenoid fracture-dislocations, unstable fractures of the neck, and significantly displaced fractures of the coracoid, acromion, and scapular spine, on the other hand, will require operative fixation for restoration of function. Other indications for operative treatment of scapular fractures include intraarticular fractures with step-off of greater than 5 mm or with instability; angulation of greater than 40 degrees of the glenoid neck; displacement of greater than 1 to 2 cm; or disruption of the superior suspensory complex of the shoulder.

Scapulothoracic Dissociation

Scapulothoracic dissociation is due to severe blunt trauma with traction to the shoulder girdle causing the scapula, humerus, musculature of the shoulder, and neurovascular structures to be pulled away from the body. Although this injury is relatively rare, it can be dramatic, not only involving the structures of the shoulder girdle, but also being associated with thoracic, craniocerebral, and spinal injuries. Damschen, in a review of 58 cases, reported complete brachial plexus injury in 81% of patients and partial injury in 13%; subclavian or axillary artery disruption was found in 88%. Because these patients almost universally have severe neurologic deficits in the affected limb, the likelihood of a good functional outcome is low. This should be borne in mind before extensive reconstruction to salvage an essentially defunctionalized limb is undertaken.

Clavicular Fractures

Clavicular fractures, unlike scapular or sternal fractures often occur in isolation. They also occur in association with thoracic and extrathoracic trauma. The clavicle is most commonly fractured in the middle third (80%) after a fall or lateral blow to the shoulder. Clinical findings include local tenderness, crepitus, and deformity. If the fracture is displaced, the shoulder may be found to be positioned inferiorly and medially. Most of these fractures are readily appreciated on AP chest radiograph. The majority (85%) of midshaft clavicular fractures will heal without intervention, and initial management consists of immobilization with a figure-of-eight dressing or shoulder immobilizer.

Traditionally, operative reduction and fixation of the clavicle are indicated in open fractures, displaced fractures with tenting of the overlying skin, and those associated with neurologic or vascular injury. Fractures with greater than 2 cm of shortening, widely displaced fragments with associated chest injuries, a floating shoulder (combined clavicular and scapular fractures), and nonunion are relative indications for operative intervention. Operative treatment consists of either intramedullary fixation or placement of fixation plates.

Recently, the nonoperative approach with sling immobilization has been called into question. The reported nonunion rates are up to 15% after conservative management with suggestion of inferior functional outcomes compared to operative therapy especially in cases of nonunion. One prospective randomized study showed improved functional outcome at 3 months following open reduction and internal fixation with no difference at 6 and 12 months compared to conservative therapy. Another prospective study showed improved functional outcome and lower nonunion rates after operative fixation. Despite these studies, two Cochrane reviews from 2009 on the management of midshaft clavicular fractures were not able to demonstrate superiority of either method of treatment of clavicle fractures. Despite the lack of conclusive evidence, operative fixation of clavicular fracture has gained popularity among the orthopedic community. The Clavicle Trial, a prospective randomized trial, is being undertaken in the United Kingdom. This study aims to enroll 300 adult patients to better answer the question of nonunion rates and functional outcome after operative versus nonoperative treatment of clavicle fractures.

COMPLICATIONS OF HEMOPNEUMOTHORAX

Empyema

Empyema has been reported to have an incidence of between 0% and 18%. At least some of the culture-negative "empyemas" in blunt trauma patients are probably sterile pleural collections that, being rich in inflammatory mediators, produce systemic effects clinically indistinguishable from true empyema collections. The true empyema rate in major trauma patients is probably closer to 5%, though, with the increasing survival of severely injured patients, the incidence of this complication may be increasing. Risk factors for the development of empyema include an inadequately drained pleural collection, mechanism of injury, location and number of chest tubes, presence of pulmonary contusion, and pneumonia.

The clinical presentation of empyema includes unexplained fever, elevated white blood cell count, and respiratory failure. Most patients in whom an empyema is suspected are critically ill. AP chest radiograph in this group may be of little or no help, and liberal use of CT scanning can more easily identify damage that is not evident on plain films

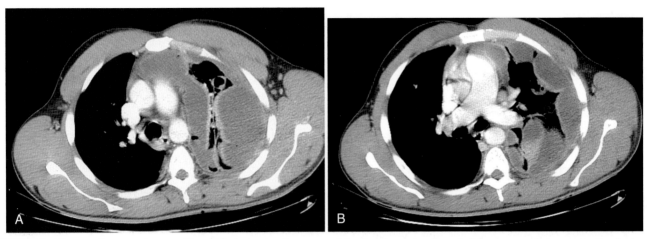

FIGURE 7 Computed tomography scans (**A** and **B**) of a loculated empyema of the chest in a patient 2 weeks following a gunshot wound to the chest and evacuation of a hemothorax. Note the enhancement around the collections. Patient was successfully treated with a thoracotomy and decortication.

(Fig. 7). Early use of CT can prevent the diagnostic delay that may result in the need for more extensive surgical procedures.

Treatment includes (1) drainage via chest tube or CT-guided catheter; (2) chest tube drainage with intrapleural fibrinolytic therapy; (3) VATS; and (4) thoracotomy and decortication. As the empyema progresses from an exudative effusion to a loculated effusion and then to an organized empyema, the pleural fluid becomes increasingly more viscous, and the intervention required becomes more invasive. Early diagnosis and treatment is thus important.

In those patients undergoing decortication, the initial postoperative chest radiograph may look worse rather than better initially. The patient, however, will begin to improve even though the chest radiograph does not. Vigorous pulmonary toilet, suctioning, and culture-specific antibiotics should be administered to all patients.

Pneumatocele

A posttraumatic cyst or pneumatocele can occur after chest trauma. This is usually an air collection within the lung that arises after airway disruption without connection to the pleural space. Most such lesions require no specific treatment and resolve after weaning from the ventilator. If the lesion is large, continues to enlarge, or becomes infected, CT-guided percutaneous drainage is an effective treatment.

Persistent Air Leaks and Bronchopleural Fistula

Air leaks are not uncommon after chest trauma and typically resolve with tube thoracostomy. A large air leak, however, requires workup for a tracheobronchial injury. If such injury is excluded, then complete lung expansion is the cornerstone of therapy. Air leaks may persist for days or even weeks in patients requiring mechanical ventilation with high positive end-expiratory pressure (PEEP); only with weaning from the ventilator will air leaks begin to seal. Tracheostomy can, by decreasing the anatomic dead space, help to lower the peak airway pressures and thus at least slow the air leak. VATS can also help in hemodynamically stable patients with prolonged air leaks.

Complications of Bony Injuries

Complications of bony injuries to the chest are most commonly related to pain. Sternal fractures in isolation or with only mild associated injury appear to have a relatively low incidence of postinjury sequelae; in one study, only 3% of patients at a 6-week follow-up had complaints requiring further intervention, including surgical intervention for a displaced fracture. Twenty-one percent of patients

in that same study reported pain at 6 weeks but required no further intervention.

Scapular fractures are rarely associated with nonunion, but can cause chronic pain. Pain and disability are particularly associated with the degree of glenoid angulation and displacement if the fracture is treated nonoperatively.

Clavicular fractures, by contrast, do carry an incidence of nonunion, though that number is somewhat in dispute. Early studies of nonoperative treatment of clavicle fractures revealed a nonunion rate as low as 0.1%. The nonunion rate has in more recent studies been reported to be much higher, with a rate of 15% for conservative treatment of displaced middle third fractures. Even with operative fixation, some nonunion occurs. An analysis of 8 studies and 14 case series of midshaft clavicle fractures revealed an overall nonunion rate of 4.2%. Nonoperative treatment resulted in a nonunion rate of 5.9%. When results for displaced fractures were identified, a nonunion rate of 4.8% was noted with intramedullary fixation, and displaced fractures treated nonoperatively had a nonunion rate of 15.1%.

Other long-term sequelae of clavicular fractures include pain, cosmetic deformity, and thoracic outlet compression. For these patients, later operative fixation may successfully manage severe symptoms.

Scapulothoracic dissociation, as would be expected, has significant long-term sequelae. A retrospective cohort study with a mean follow-up over 12 years revealed that patients with a complete brachial plexus avulsion had significant physical and mental impairments as measured by the standard SF-36 questionnaire. Primary amputation of the affected limb, though a difficult decision, should be considered to avoid a defunctionalized limb when complete brachial avulsion has occurred.

CONCLUSIONS

Chest wall injuries and concomitant hemopneumothoraces occur frequently following blunt and penetrating trauma and are a significant cause of trauma fatality and morbidity. As the spectrum of thoracic injury is great and occurs in isolation as well as in part of multisystem trauma, providers need to understand the pathophysiology and impact of these injuries on overall patient care. Although most thoracic injuries may be managed nonoperatively, vigilance is required to detect injuries that are potentially life threatening and require urgent intervention. More important, these injuries often result in respiratory failure, ventilator usage, and increased ICU length of stay and thus have a tremendous impact on overall trauma outcome.

For the chapter's Suggested Readings list, please visit the book at www.ExpertConsult.inkling.com.

DIAGNOSTIC AND THERAPEUTIC ROLES OF BRONCHOSCOPY AND VIDEO-ASSISTED THORACOSCOPY IN THE MANAGEMENT OF THORACIC TRAUMA

Ajai K. Malhotra, Michel B. Aboutanos, and Therese M. Duane

Direct injury to the chest and pulmonary complications after any major trauma account for a significant proportion of trauma-related morbidity and fatality. In the past the role of thoracic endoscopy was limited to bronchoscopic diagnosis of major airway injury and assistance with pulmonary toilet. Major injuries to the tracheobronchial tree, significant hemorrhage within the chest, failure of nonoperative management of chest injuries, and major pulmonary complications invariably required thoracotomy with its high morbidity and mortality rates. Technical advances in fiberoptics and videoscopic imaging have led to rapid advances in the field of minimally invasive surgery. In the thoracic region this has led to the advent of video-assisted thoracoscopic surgery (VATS) and the broadening of the role of bronchoscopy, both in terms of diagnosis and therapy. These minimally invasive endoscopic techniques have significantly lower morbidity and mortality rates. This chapter focuses on the evolving role of thoracic endoscopy (thoracoscopy and bronchoscopy) following chest trauma and major pulmonary complications after any trauma.

INCIDENCE

Thoracic trauma accounts for a significant burden of disease in terms of morbidity and mortality. Twenty percent of trauma-associated deaths involve chest injury, and chest trauma is second only to head and spinal cord injuries as a cause of death following trauma. Death as a result of chest trauma in the acute setting is related to either airway injury, direct trauma to the heart, or massive bleeding within the chest cavity. In addition to the acute deaths that are a direct result of chest trauma, pulmonary complications following chest trauma or any trauma add to the mortality and morbidity rates attributable to injuries to the chest.

The majority of chest trauma comprises abrasions, rib fractures, and simple pneumothoraces that are easily diagnosed with chest radiographs and computed tomography (CT) and can be treated with simple measures—pulmonary toilet, pain management, and tube thoracostomy. The indications for open thoracotomy in the acute setting are principally major airway disruption and massive bleeding in the chest or airway. Approximately 1% of all trauma admissions require open thoracotomy in the acute setting. Open thoracotomy in this setting is associated with very high morbidity and mortality rates. Bronchoscopic control of bleeding within the airway and stenting of major airway injury can offer a lower risk alternative to open surgery in selected patients. Similarly, VATS

offers a lower risk alternative for managing hemorrhage within the chest cavity. In the nonacute setting, trauma patients with or without direct injury to the chest have a high incidence of pulmonary complications including pneumonia, retained hemothorax, fibrothorax, empyema, and acute respiratory distress syndrome (ARDS) posing diagnostic and therapeutic challenges. Thoracic endoscopy in this setting is playing an increasingly important role in early diagnosis and therapy for these complications, and possibly improving outcome.

DIAGNOSTIC AND THERAPEUTIC ROLES OF VIDEO-ASSISTED THORACOSCOPIC SURGERY

Indications and Patient Selection

The first diagnostic and therapeutic application of thoracoscopy for the management of thoracic conditions such as pleural effusions, pleural adhesions, empyemas, and thoracic malignancy, was recorded by Hans Christian Jacobaeus at the University of Stockholm in 1922. Thoracoscopy for the treatment of traumatic injuries was first described in 1946 by Branco for the management of hemothorax in penetrating chest injuries. In this century, the advent of minimally invasive access to the thoracic cavity combined with video-assisted technology and selective lung ventilation has revolutionized the diagnosis and the treatment of thoracic injuries with improved use and outcomes.

Patient selection is very important for the application of VATS in thoracoabdominal trauma. The current indications are both diagnostic and therapeutic and include mainly the evaluation of a structural injury (the diaphragm, the pericardium, lung parenchyma, the thoracic duct, etc.) or the drainage of a pleural collection and repair of any structural damage. Aside from the usual bleeding disorders, the main contraindications of VATS include an unstable patient, or a patient with underlying lungs and cardiac trauma that preclude the use of single-lung ventilation. Table 1 lists the current indications and contraindications for the use of VATS.

TABLE 1: Indications and Contraindications of Video-Assisted Thoracoscopic Surgery in Trauma

Indications	Contraindications
Persistent pneumothorax	Hemodynamic instability
Retained collections	Poor lung and cardiac functions with
Hemothorax	inability to tolerate single-lung
Chylothorax	ventilation (chronic obstructive
Bilothorax	pulmonary disease [COPD], heart
Pleural effusion	failure)
Empyema	Contraindication to lateral decubitus
Detection of intrathoracic	position
organ injury	History of bleeding diatheses
(diaphragm, lung,	Massive hemothorax (>1.5 L
thoracic duct,	initially or 200 mL/hour over
pericardium)	3–4 hours)
Intrathoracic foreign body	Obliterated pleural cavity (infection,
Acute hemorrhage in	pleuritis, previous surgery)
stable patients	Suspected cardiac injury
	Indication for laparotomy

Diaphragmatic Injuries

The incidence of blunt diaphragmatic injuries has been reported as low as 0.8% and as high as 7%. Blunt trauma accounts for 10% to 30% of traumatic diaphragmatic ruptures (TDRs) in North American series from urban trauma centers. The incidence of diaphragmatic injuries has been reported to be as high as 67% in penetrating thoracoabdominal trauma.

Diaphragmatic injuries are particularly difficult to diagnose with the use of radiographic imaging such as chest radiograph or conventional CT and can be missed in up to 30% of patients. The advent of multidetector row CT (MDCT) in most urban trauma centers has significantly improved the accuracy of diagnosing diaphragm injury with the use of high-resolution axial, coronal, and sagittal reformatted images. A study from R. Adams Cowley Shock Trauma Center by Stein et al., using a 4- or 16-slice MDCT scanner, improved the sensitivity and specificity up to 94% and 96%, respectively, for the exclusion of a diaphragmatic injury due to penetrating trauma. However, the authors warned that additional diagnostic evaluation is still required to definitively exclude diaphragm injury in patients with equivocal CT findings defined as thickening of the diaphragm, artifact secondary to ballistic fragments, injury in the proximity of the diaphragm, and wound tracts outlined by air, blood, bullet, or bone fragment extending up to the diaphragm.

Together with laparoscopy, thoracoscopy is still considered the diagnostic tool of choice for diaphragmatic injuries when compared to other nonoperative modalities.

Thoracoscopy is particularly useful when laparoscopy may not be optimal or feasible. It is useful for evaluation of right-sided diaphragmatic injuries and posterior wounds from the posterior axillary line to the spine. It is also useful for avoidance of abdominal procedures, particularly in patients with previous laparotomies and expected presence of extensive adhesions.

The therapeutic role of VATS in the treatment of diaphragmatic injuries is well documented. In a report of 24 patients who underwent VATS for thoracic injuries, 9 of 10 patients were successfully diagnosed with diaphragmatic injuries. VATS was used for repair of the diaphragm in 4 patients. Martinez et al evaluated 52 patients with penetrating thoracoabdominal trauma admitted to General Hospital for Accidents in Guatemala City. VATS was used to diagnose 35 patients with diaphragmatic injuries. All 35 diaphragmatic injuries were successfully repaired thoracoscopically. Even though successful thoracoscopic repair of diaphragm injuries is reported as feasible, safe, and expeditious; currently no long-term outcome results are available.

In areas where other abdominal injuries are suspected, a laparoscopic or open surgical approach is preferable depending on the surgical expertise present. A combined thoracic and abdominal cavitary endoscopy can also be useful. Figure 1 shows the thoracoscopic evaluation of a right diaphragm injury from an impaled object in the chest of a patient evaluated in our trauma center. This was followed by the thoracoscopic repair of the diaphragm after the laparoscopic confirmation of a nonbleeding liver laceration and no other associated abdominal injuries. In all cases in which a diaphragm injury is found, an exploratory laparoscopy or laparotomy should be strongly considered to rule out associated intraabdominal injuries.

Retained Thoracic Collection

The evacuation of a retained hemothorax is one of the main indications for VATS. Inadequate evacuation of blood from the pleural space and prolonged thoracostomy tube drainage puts the patient at risk for developing empyema and fibrothorax with prolonged hospital stays and increasing costs. The incidence of a retained hemothorax and empyema after tube thoracostomy placement ranges from 4% to 20% and from 4% to 10%, respectively. A prospective randomized study of 39 patients from Parkland Memorial Hospital with thoracic trauma and retained hemothoraces showed that early evacuation with VATS compared to conventional therapy of a secondary chest tube placement led to a significantly shorter duration of tube drainage (2.5 days), shorter hospital stay (2.7 days), and reduced hospital costs ($6,000). These advantages of VATS were attributed to rapid and complete evacuation of the pleural space, optimal video-assisted positioning of the thoracostomy tubes, and identification and treatment of the sources of the bleeding and of other associated intrathoracic injuries.

It is important to note that these advantages rest on the early use (days 4–7 after injury) of VATS for the evacuation of the hemothorax. A study by Morales et al. to determine the best timing for thoracoscopic evacuation of retained posttraumatic hemothorax noted that the longer the thoracoscopic drainage is delayed, the lower the probability of success, with the best result (>80% success rate) obtained when drainage was performed before the fifth postadmission day. The relative risk of conversion to open thoracotomy or of

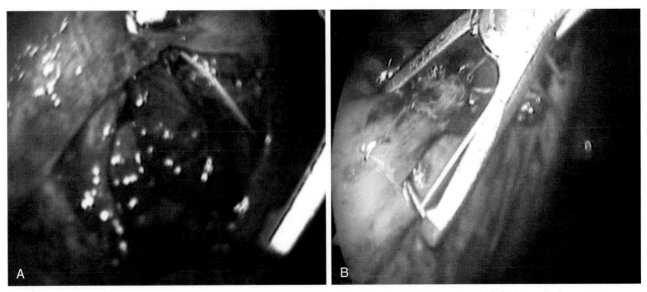

FIGURE 1 This 48-year-old construction worker was impaled with a 4 × 4 wooden object. **A,** Large 5-cm full-thickness diaphragm injury was noted with underlying liver laceration. **B,** The diaphragm was repaired thoracoscopically.

reintervention increased twofold after day 5. Multiple earlier studies from the University of Louisville noted similar success rate (>75%). Failure of VATS correlated with time interval from injury to operation, and with the type of fluid collection (hemothorax vs. empyema). A more recent large study from the same institution confirmed the advantage of early intervention (VATS within 5 days of admission) with significant decrease in conversions to open thoracotomy (8% vs. 29.4%, $P < .05$) and shorter lengths of hospital stay (11 days $\pm$ 6 vs. 16 ± 8, $P < .05$). VATS performed 5 days after admission was more likely to show a diagnosis of empyema (29.4 % vs. 10%, $P < .0001$).

The application of VATS for traumatic empyema is dependent on the phase of the empyema. For the acute/exudative empyema occurring between 1 and 5 days, VATS is uniformly effective. The success rate for the transitional/fibrinopurulent stage (days 6–14) is around 75% to 85% with a sharp drop to around 50% in the organized/chronic phase (>2 weeks). Recent studies confirm the diagnosis of empyema carries a statistically higher conversion rate and increased hospital length of stay (LOS) as compared to retained hemothorax or persistent air leak.

Persistent Hemorrhage

VATS is also useful for patients with persistent but slow hemorrhage, with no hemodynamic instability. Unstable patients with suspected thoracic bleed require open thoracotomy. Smith et al performed VATS on five hemodynamically stable patients for persistent hemorrhage from intercostal vessels. In three patients, the bleeding was successfully controlled with diathermy. Other techniques including endoclips or argon beam coagulators for hemorrhage control can be used. Intracorporeal stitch placement around the rib was used successfully in our center for control of a persistent intercostal bleed not amenable to endoclip placement. The success rate for the thoracoscopic control of a non–hemodynamically compromising hemorrhage is around 80% with a thoracotomy conversion rate of 15% to 20%.

Persistent Pneumothorax

The incidence of persistent air leak and lung reexpansion 72 hours after thoracostomy tube placement ranges from 4% to 23%. Conservative management with continuous pleural suction leads to prolonged chest tube drainage, prolonged hospital LOS, and increased hospital costs. VATS has been shown to be safe and effective in the treatment of persistent pneumothorax with decreased number of chest tube days, hospital LOS, and cost. In a recent report by Smith et al., 8 (10%) of 83 patients underwent VATS for persistent air leak with failed lung reexpansion for greater than 72 hours. All were successfully treated with thoracoscopic surgery without conversion thoracotomy. It is important to note that only in about 50% of patients was the source of the air leak identified. However, all were successfully treated with VATS pleurodesis. In our trauma center, Endo GIA staplers are routinely employed to staple off the affected lung parenchyma. The use of a topical synthetic nonreactive surgical sealant (Coseal; Baxter, Freemont, Calif.) for the creation of an elastic watertight seal has also been reported. Chemical pleurodesis or pleural scarification by electrocoagulation remains a viable option, especially in recurrences after VATS. Carillo et al. reported the successful use of VATS in 10 out of 11 patients with persistent pneumothorax posttraumatic injuries. The 11th patient was successfully treated with chemical pleurodesis. The inflammatory reaction that occurs with chemical pleurodesis, however, is often associated with increased pleural edema, drainage, and postoperative pain. Prior to committing a patient to VATS, it is important to aggressively evaluate the cause of the air leak and rule out a malfunctioning or a malpositioned chest tube, the presence of a foreign body, or a deeply penetrating rib fragment. The patient should be evaluated thoroughly with chest tomography and bronchoscopy to evaluate the tracheobronchial tree, the distal parenchyma, and the pleural cavity.

Other Indications and Applications

Other indications for use of VATS in chest trauma include diagnosis of bronchopleural fistulas, removal of retained foreign bodies, ligation of injured thoracic duct, drainage of chylothorax, and assessment of cardiac and mediastinal structures. Although pericardioscopy for suspected penetrating cardiac injury has been reported as feasible and safe in the hemodynamically stable patient, it remains very controversial, with potential for iatrogenic life-threatening injuries. In a stable patient, the gold standard approach for suspected cardiac injury remains the use of echocardiography or subxiphoid pericardial window followed by immediate sternotomy or left thoracotomy for evacuation of hemopericardium and repair of cardiac injury.

Surgical Approach

The operation is performed under general endotracheal intubation with a dual lumen endotracheal tube. The position of the tube is confirmed bronchoscopically. The patient is positioned in the lateral decubitus position and flexed at the hip to open the rib spaces. The initial port is 10 mm placed at the site of the existing chest tube or in the midaxillary line in the fifth intercostal space. This port is used to introduce a camera with a 30- or 45-degree scope into the pleural cavity and to aid in the placement of additional 5-mm working ports. A maximum of two working ports are most often used, along with a 5-mm 30-degree scope to allow complete inspection of the lung and pleural spaces. Insufflation is not required, but it can be helpful when full lung collapse is not achieved. At the end of the procedure, chest tubes are placed under direct observation through existing port sites. The lung is then inflated under direct vision. Patient-controlled anesthesia along with local intercostal nerve block is used for optimal postoperative pain management.

Morbidity and Complication Management

The reported complication rates for thoracoscopy are less than 10% and the missed injury rates are less than 1%. The perioperative complications include intrathoracic bleed (parietal, intercostal, or parenchymal), recurrent pneumothorax, and hemothorax. Other complications include intercostal neuritis and iatrogenic lung laceration. Conversion to open thoracotomy is reported to be less than 8% and is usually due to inadequate thoracoscopic visibility, dense pleural adhesions with failure to deflate the lung, or uncontrollable bleed. This underscores the importance of the timing of the procedures, within 5 to 7 days—early enough to avoid pleural adhesions and fibrosis and late enough to assure adequate hemostasis. Persistent air leak in the postoperative period is attributed to underlying lung disease, such as emphysema or apical bleb disease. Late complications are rare and include the development of pneumonia, pleural edema, and empyema. Airway complications from malpositioned dual lumen endotracheal tubes or the development of tension pneumothorax during single-lung ventilation have also been reported.

DIAGNOSTIC AND THERAPEUTIC ROLE OF BRONCHOSCOPY

Attempts to directly visualize the interior of the airway date as far back as the time of Hippocrates. However, the first recorded bronchoscopy was performed by Gustav Killian of Freiburg, Germany, in 1887. The only available instrument at that time was a rigid bronchoscope. The principal indications were therapeutic, the commonest being removal of inhaled foreign objects. The field was advanced by Chevalier Jackson, the father of American bronchoesophagology, who designed modern rigid bronchoscopes. In 1963, Dr.

Shigeto Ikeda introduced the flexible fiberoptic bronchoscope, primarily as a diagnostic instrument. Flexible bronchoscopes were much easier to use and flexible bronchoscopy became a diagnostic tool with wide application. The only therapeutic indication that persisted was removal of foreign bodies from within the tracheobronchial tree. Recent technical advances in the instrument itself and in the availability of other therapeutic tools such as stents, electrocautery, and lasers are allowing bronchoscopy to regain a role in therapy and also broadening its well-established diagnostic role. Although in some very limited situations, rigid bronchoscopy may offer some advantages, the ease of use and the greater experience in the use of flexible bronchoscopes have led to rigid bronchoscopy being used rarely in trauma settings.

Basic Technique of Flexible Fiberoptic Bronchoscopy

Almost all bronchoscopies for trauma patients, whether performed in the acute setting soon after trauma or later for pulmonary complications, are performed on patients who have endotracheal tubes in place and are mechanically ventilated.

Preparation

The patient should be administered 100% oxygen, and the ventilator rate set at 10 to 12 breaths per minute. Adequate sedation is essential to avoid inducing stress. This is especially important in head-injured patients as an acute rise in intracranial pressure (ICP) is well documented during bronchoscopy. In our unit we utilize a benzodiazepine (Ativan or Versed 2–4 mg intravenously) and a narcotic analgesic (morphine 4–8 mg or equivalent, intravenously). Although bronchoscopy can be performed without paralysis, we have found that to be able to perform it comfortably, temporary paralysis, using vecuronium (10 mg intravenously) is very helpful. Adequate time should be given to allow the patient to get preoxygenated and the medications to take effect before starting the procedure. The commonly used flexible bronchoscopes have a uniplaner direction control. To be able to manipulate the scope in the other planes the whole scope needs to be rotated along its longitudinal axis. To achieve this, the outside end of the scope is rotated. The rotational movements will not be transmitted to the tip unless the scope is straight, and hence the height of the bed should be so adjusted to keep the scope as straight as possible.

Technique

The basic technique of bronchoscopy is the same irrespective of the indication. However, there are minor variations and adjunctive procedures that are used for different indications. After the height of the bed has been adjusted, the patient preoxygenated, and adequate sedation and paralysis achieved, a lubricated scope is inserted thought a right-angled adaptor that allows some ventilation to continue while the scope is within the endotracheal tube. Once the tip of the scope is beyond the end of the tube, and the carina is visualized, the two main bronchi can be identified by (1) position of the tracheal rings—deficient posteriorly, (2) length of the bronchus—left being longer, and (3) angle of takeoff—right being more straight. A basic knowledge of the lobar anatomy on the two sides and the bronchopleural segments in each of the lobes is essential for successful bronchoscopy. Depending on the patient body habitus, the scope can be inserted into III/IV order bronchioles. It is important to understand that while suctioning and clearing the airway of secretions is an important part of bronchoscopy, it does lead to derecruitment by collapsing alveoli, and hence, like any other medical procedure the risks and benefits should be carefully weighed before embarking on a bronchoscopy and also in deciding how much should be done at one sitting.

Monitoring

The patient undergoing bronchoscopy under sedation and paralysis needs to be carefully monitored for adequate sedation, and also for any cardiorespiratory compromise that may occur during the procedure. The monitoring is best left to another person who should record vital signs continuously. The most important signs to be monitored are (1) heart rate, (2) blood pressure, (3) arterial oxygen saturation by pulse oximetry, and (4) ICP, if the patient has a monitor in place. If the patient is experiencing stress, the heart rate and blood pressure will increase. The procedure should be stopped and adequate sedation achieved before continuing. If the pulse oximeter shows a decline below 90%, except in very rare situations, the scope should be removed so that the patient can be adequately ventilated and oxygenated. Finally, it is possible for the patient to maintain adequate oxygen saturation yet develop arrhythmia, usually bradyarrhythmia, and even cardiac arrest. This happens because even though oxygenation is maintained by high alveolar oxygen content achieved by preoxygenation, ventilation during the procedure is severely compromised leading to an acute rise in $PaCO_2$ and severe respiratory acidosis. This becomes particularly important in patients with head injury as it can lead to an acute and severe rise in ICP with possible deleterious effects on the injured brain. If the patient develops any arrhythmia, the scope should be removed immediately, and adequate ventilation ensured. Resuscitative drugs should be immediately available to treat any arrhythmia that does not resolve spontaneously. A reevaluation of the risks and benefits of the bronchoscopy should occur before proceeding with the procedure.

Complications of Bronchoscopy

A large number of complications have been described after flexible fiberoptic bronchoscopy (Table 2). The incidence of complications is higher the longer the procedure, the sicker the patient, and when the bronchoscopy is performed for therapeutic indications rather than diagnostic purposes. However, in experienced hands when the preceding precautions of technique and monitoring are observed, fiberoptic flexible bronchoscopy is a fairly safe procedure.

Diagnostic Role of Flexible Fiberoptic Bronchoscopy

Acute Trauma

Tracheobronchial Injury

Tracheobronchial injury following trauma is very rare, but the consequences of missed injuries can be significant. Although some injuries can be managed nonoperatively and will heal, if an injury does require repair, delaying the repair significantly increases the chances of failure. Fiberoptic bronchoscopy should be performed early in any patient who may potentially have a tracheobronchial injury. In some instances, if the patient is not acutely hypoxic and tracheobronchial

TABLE 2: Complications of Bronchoscopy

Hypoxemia	Hypercapnia
Barotrauma	Hypotension
Hypertension	Hemorrhage
Aspiration	Intracranial hypertension
Infection	Laryngospasm
Damage to scope	Cardiac arrhythmias

injury is suspected, in addition to its diagnostic role, bronchoscopy can be an invaluable aid to intubation and correct placement of tube. In such situations bronchoscopy should be performed by an experienced bronchoscopist with the endotracheal tube prepositioned over the scope. There is a role for rigid bronchoscopy in patients with injury to the cervical trachea in which the rigid scope can identify the distal ruptured end and align it with the proximal end, allowing the patient to be intubated and the balloon of the tube passed beyond the site of injury. Once an injury has been diagnosed, the bronchoscopic findings are useful in planning appropriate therapy—nonoperative management, open surgery, or bronchoscopic placement of stent. In a report by Lin et al., bronchoscopy was useful in management decisions in one third of the cases.

Acute or Late Onset Bleeding Within the Tracheobronchial Tree

Bleeding within the tracheobronchial tree following trauma is usually caused by pulmonary contusion and rarely by injury to the tree. In later stages, hemoptysis may be caused by pulmonary embolism, infections, tracheobronchial erosions, or tracheo-innominate fistula. Fiberoptic bronchoscopy is useful for diagnosing the cause of the bleeding and to localize the site. It may help temporarily control the hemorrhage, isolate the site to avoid flooding the nonbleeding areas of the lung, and in selected cases, provide definitive control of the bleeding (see later discussion).

Inhalational Injury

Fiberoptic bronchoscopy plays an invaluable role in the diagnosis and management of patients suspected of inhalational injury. Any patient suspected of having suffered inhalational burns to the tracheobronchial tree should undergo early diagnostic evaluation. If signs of impeding loss of airway are present and the patient does not have an endotrachel tube, the bronchoscope may be used as a guide for safe intubation. The bronchoscopic signs of inhalational injury are observed within a few hours of the injury and may be classified as acute, subacute, or chronic. In the acute stage the most prominent finding is airway edema with soot deposition within the mucosa. As the injury progresses to the subacute phase, necrosis of the lining mucosa, and hemorrhagic tracheobronchitis are prominent. The subacute phase may last from several hours to days and in this stage the patient may demonstrate massive bronchorrhea. Repeated bronchoscopic toileting may be necessary to maintain airway patency. Finally, in the chronic phase formation of granulation tissue with stenosis, scarring, and obliterative bronchiolitis are observed. The initial bronchoscopic appearance is poorly correlated with the need and duration of mechanical ventilatory requirements and with the final outcome. In situations when the clinical course does not correlate with the bronchoscopic appearance, repeat examination may be considered to accurately plan therapy.

Ventilator-Associated Pneumonia

Ventilator-associated pneumonia (VAP) is one of the most common nosocomial infections in the modern intensive care unit (ICU). It is associated with high morbidity and mortality rates, and each incidence of VAP significantly increases the cost of care. Early appropriate antimicrobial therapy has been shown to improve outcomes. Despite its relative frequency, the diagnosis of VAP can be challenging especially in the trauma patient. The reasons for this difficulty are primarily the diagnostic criteria for pneumonia (fever with productive cough and leukocytosis, new or changing infiltrate on chest radiograph, and sputum culture demonstrating predominant growth of one organism), which are either nonspecific or falsely positive because of tracheobronchial colonization in the ICU. Quantitative examination of a lower respiratory specimen (lavage or brush) has been suggested as one method of accurately differentiating between nonpathogenic tracheobronchial colonization and VAP. Bronchoalveolar lavage (BAL) specimen from the lower respiratory tree can be obtained easily through the bronchoscope. This method has been proved to be safe, and has been accurate not only in diagnosing VAP but also in ruling it out so that patients are spared unnecessary antimicrobial therapy. A simple scheme practiced at the authors' institution is outlined in Figure 2. Institution of this scheme, in which bronchoscopy plays a central role has significantly reduced the use of antimicrobial agents and as a result has reduced microbial resistance within our ICU.

The technique of obtaining BAL specimen through a flexible bronchoscope is simple. The scope is passed into a tertiary level bronchiole and wedged in it. Suction is avoided while insertion to maintain

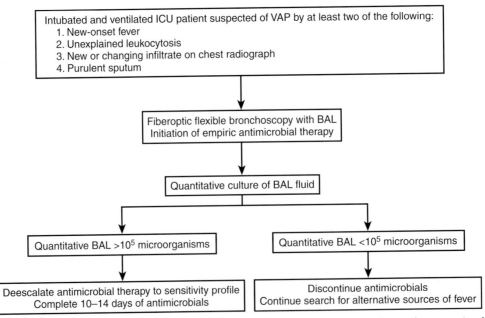

FIGURE 2   A simplified algorithm for evaluating a patient with new-onset fever suspected of being caused by ventilator-associated pneumonia (VAP). BAL, Bronchoalveolar lavage; ICU, intensive care unit.

sterility of the working channel of the scope. The site is selected by using one or more of the following criteria: (1) site of new infiltrate on chest radiograph; (2) site of maximum purulence as observed through the scope; and (3) commonest site of VAP—right lower lobe. Once the scope has been wedged in the selected bronchiole, 5 aliquots of 20 mL sterile nonbacteriostatic saline are instilled through the working port and immediately aspirated. A good specimen is indicated by aspirating 50% or more of the instilled saline and observing floating froth (evidence of surfactant) in the aspirate. This specimen is then sent to the laboratory for quantitative culture and empiric antimicrobials are initiated based on the prevailing flora in the ICU. When the final quantitative culture results are available (usually in 48–72 hours) the antimicrobial therapy is tailored to the culture and sensitivity profile. In our ICU a threshold of more than 10^5 colony-forming units/mL (CFU/mL) of BAL is used for the diagnosis of VAP. Other investigators use a lesser number. An alternative to lavage is the protected specimen brush in which a special brush-tipped catheter is passed through the scope and used to scrape the lining of the bronchiole. A diagnostic threshold of 10 CFU/mL is often used for specimens obtained with the brush. Although non-bronchoscopic methods of obtaining the lower respiratory specimen are available, no comparative trials have been performed to compare the bronchoscopic and nonbronchoscopic methods.

Stricture

The majority of the causes of stricture within the tracheobronchial tree are related to neoplasia. In the trauma setting strictures maybe caused by prolonged intubation, scarring at the site of previous injury, or inhalational injury. Bronchoscopy has both a diagnostic and therapeutic role in the management of strictures. Initially bronchoscopy can confirm the presence of the stricture and localize its site. In addition, the bronchoscopic features in terms of site, length, and character of the tissue can help with the planning of appropriate treatment. Bronchoscopy can help with management of the atelectasis of the pulmonary segments beyond the stricture and can be used to treat the infections in these atelectatic segments.

Therapeutic Role of Flexible Fiberoptic Bronchoscopy

Control of Acute or Late-Onset Hemoptysis

Massive hemoptysis is defined as a volume of blood in the tracheobronchial tree that leads to a life-threatening situation by causing airway obstruction. Bronchoscopy has been used to not only diagnose the source of hemorrhage but also to remove the blood, thereby overcoming the airway obstruction. In some selected cases bronchsocopic techniques can provide temporary control of hemorrhage until preparations for definitive control, by surgery or bronchial artery embolization, are made. In some selected patients bronchoscopic techniques can even provide definitive therapy. The therapeutic tools to control hemorrhage include ice cold saline lavage, injection of 1:200,000 epinephrine, instillation of fibrin glue or other topical hemostatics, balloon tamponade, electrocautery, and laser coagulation. Although most reports about the use of such techniques are from the medical literature, the same techniques are being used for acute hemorrhage following trauma or late-onset hemoptysis in the surgical ICU patient.

Stent Repair of Acute Airway Trauma

Major disruptions of the tracheobronchial tree are rare but life threatening. In the past the only available treatment was major surgery. Recently, covered expandable metallic stents have been developed that can be deployed under bronchoscopic control. This approach offers a low-risk alternative for repairing these potentially devastating

injuries. When injury to the tracheobronchial tree is suspected, early evaluation by bronchoscopy is very helpful in diagnosing or ruling out the injury and then planning therapy. Bronchoscopy can define the site of injury and help with safe placement of the endotracheal tube. Once the patient's airway is secured, a careful assessment should be made of the characteristics of the injury, especially the site in relation to branches, and the size of the injury. Although open repair has been the traditional method of therapy, consideration should be given for stent repair if the injury is so amenable and especially if the patient's other injuries make him/her a poor surgical candidate. If none of the shelf stents are available, customized stents can be ordered to suit the anatomy of the specific injury.

A case at the authors' institution exemplified this point. An 18-year-old man presented after a high-speed motor vehicle collision with the chest CT demonstrating aortic transection. In addition to his massive pneumothorax and persistent high-volume air leak through the chest tube, airway injury was suspected and confirmed at the distal trachea by bronchoscopy. A custom-made stent was placed via the bronchoscope and the air leak stopped. A few days later the patient underwent successful repair of his aortic injury via a thoracotomy. Subsequent bronchoscopies revealed that the tracheal injury had healed with formation of granulation tissue around the stent. The stent was removed intact after 8 weeks, and 2 weeks following removal mucosa was found to be covering the injury site.

Removal of Foreign Body

Prior to the availability of bronchoscopy foreign body removal from the tracheobronchial tree carried high morbidity and mortality rates. Availability of bronchoscopy revolutionized the care of such patients as it offered a very low-risk alternative to major surgery. Although the first removals were performed using a rigid scope, currently the large majority of such cases are performed with flexible scopes that can be inserted into more distal airways and that have a working channel through which instruments can be passed. When inhalation of a foreign body is suspected and the patient has survived the acute obstruction, careful planning should go into any further intervention as poor planning can lead to airway obstruction and death. The procedure should be performed by an experienced endoscopist with the availability and facility with both rigid and flexible scopes. Although the procedure can be performed with the patient awake, often general anesthesia is required. Careful consultation between the endoscopist and the anesthesiologist as to how the airway shall be safely managed is essential. Once the airway plan is determined, endoscopy is carried out. Besides the availability of the two types of scopes, accessory instruments are very helpful in safely removing various bodies that may have gotten embedded into the mucosa. These instruments include balloon catheters, special grasping forceps, and wire baskets. In addition, other adjunctive techniques have been developed to safely remove the foreign body. These techniques include the cryoprobe that can cause the body to adhere to the end of the instrument or neodymium-ytterium-aluminum-garnet (Nd:YAG) laser to break up the foreign body, vaporize the surrounding granulation tissue to dislodge it, and blunt the sharp edges for safe removal.

Toilet for Pulmonary Collapse, Massive Secretions, and Aspiration

Flexible bronchoscopy has become an invaluable tool for managing atelectasis and complete or partial pulmonary collapse due to tenacious mucoid secretions. There is an immediate benefit observed in patients with tenacious mucoid secretions obstructing central airways. In such patients bronchoscopic suctioning for whole lung collapse or lobar atelectasis has been shown to improve oxygenation. In other patients, however, the benefits of bronchoscopic clearing of airways over traditional chest percussion therapy is less clear. In trauma patients, though, because of other injuries, at times it may not be possible to provide good percussion therapy and bronchoscopy may be the only effective method of clearing secretions. For patients who have suffered large volume aspiration of gastric contents, early bronchoscopy and lavage of the airways can help clear the airways and possibly limit the chemical damage. Although bronchoscopy in such settings is often utilized for this aim, no studies have conclusively shown benefit. Based on anecdotal evidence a reasonable approach may be to perform bronchoscopy and lavage on patients suspected of large volume aspiration if they are already intubated or require intubation immediately after the episode. If the patient does not require intubation, he/she should be carefully monitored and managed with aggressive percussion therapy and other measures to encourage pulmonary toilet. As with all procedures it is necessary to balance potential harm with benefit. Extensive suctioning within the airways during bronchoscopy leads to derecruitment of alveoli that can lead to problems with oxygenation and extensive washing within the airways can cause diffusion problems further worsening oxygenation (see complications earlier).

Percutaneous Tracheostomy

Percutaneous tracheostomy has gained in popularity as an alternative to open tracheostomy that can be performed in the ICU at lower cost. Although it is possible to perform the procedure without bronchoscopy, many believe that the addition of bronchoscopic control adds to the safety of the procedure. Over the years the procedure has been refined from a sequence of dilations to one dilation prior to placement of the tracheostomy, resulting in shorter duration of the procedure with equivalent results.

The procedure consists of placing a needle within the trachea, and passing a guidewire through the needle under direct visualization. Once a guidewire has been placed the tract from the skin to the trachea is dilated with a 28 F smooth catheter that is tapered at the end. This step is followed by an 8 Shiley tracheostomy tube, preloaded over a 24 F dilator and passed into the trachea via the established tract. When the procedure is performed under bronchoscopic control, it is possible to ensure that the needle, guidewire, and the dilators are indeed passing into the trachea, as they are supposed to, and not into a false passage within the soft tissues of the neck.

Indications of percutaneous tracheostomy are the same as for open tracheostomy. Skin infection, unstable cervical spine, and elevated ICP are absolute contraindications to the procedure and obesity, high ventilatory requirements, coagulopathy, and any anatomic abnormality in the area are relative contraindications. A recent study reporting on 1000 bedside percutaneous tracheostomies performed in a surgical ICU, showed the procedure can be performed in almost all patients with a low complication rate of 1.4% overall that rises to 1.7% in high-risk patients. Reported complications include mucosal tears, submucosal placement of tube, perforation of the posterior tracheal wall with formation of a tracheoesophageal fistula, paratracheal placement, barotraumas, and damage to the endotracheal tube and bronchoscope. Like the open procedure there is an incidence of late tracheo-innominate fistula and subglottic stenosis.

Management of Bronchopleural Fistula

Bronchopleural fistulas present as a persistent air leak from a thoracostomy tube. When conservative measures, including maintaining continuous negative pleural pressure and chemical pleurodesis, fail to close the fistula by 1 to 3 weeks, surgical correction may be necessary. Bronchoscopy can be useful in identifying the offending segment from which the fistula emanates. Passing the scope into different bronchopleural segments of the lung with the suspected fistula and observing for telltale granulation tissue through which bubbles are emanating is fairly accurate in diagnosing the site of the fistula. After identification a balloon-tipped catheter can be passed with the help of the bronchoscope and the balloon inflated to occlude

the site. If this results in cessation of the air leak, the diagnosis and site are confirmed. Once the diagnosis is confirmed and site identified, a number of substances including fibrin glue, Gelfoam, and lead-shot plugs have been used to temporarily seal the site prior to surgery and, in selected cases, even offer permanent control, obviating the need of major surgery. Fresh autologous blood clot delivered to the site by pasting it onto the balloon of a balloon-tipped catheter has also been used. When blood clot is used an antifibrolytic agent (e.g., epsilon-aminocaproic acid) or tetracycline or doxycycline instillation can enhance the success rate.

Dilatation/Laser Therapy of Tracheobronchial Strictures

Tracheobronchial strictures in trauma patients are usually related to prolonged intubation. However, they can also be caused by granulation tissue due to infections, and after surgical or stent repairs of airway injuries. Although surgical excision and repair of the strictured area have a high success rate, bronchoscopic dilatation, with or without laser vaporization, of the stricture is a lower risk alternative that can offer temporary relief until surgical repair can be carried out or in some cases may even lead to permanent cure. The technical details of the procedure are beyond the scope of this text, but careful consideration has to be given to plan optimal therapy in each individual situation. The important considerations include the anatomy of the stricture—site, length, and type of tissue—and, if laser therapy is opted for, the type of laser to be used—Nd:YAG, CO_2, or potassium-titanyl-phosphate (KTP). In addition, the local expertise and experience are important considerations. Adjunctive techniques that can be used along with laser vaporization include balloon dilatation, placement of a stent, and instillation of mitomycin C to reduce the recurrence rate following laser therapy. No comparative trials have been performed comparing surgical resection with laser therapy, and a multidisciplinary approach to the management of each individual patient is the best way to achieve optimal results.

Drainage of Lung Abscess

Lung abscess is a serious complication following chest trauma or pneumonia following any trauma. It has a high rate of morbidity and fatality. Traditional methods of treatment include adequate early antibiotic therapy and postural drainage. Failing this, surgical drainage was the only available option, but it also carried high morbidity and mortality rates. Interventional radiologic techniques have allowed drainage of the abscess without high-risk surgery. However, radiologically placing drainage catheters deep within the lung in proximity of major airways runs the risk of developing persistent bronchopleural fistulas. Transbronchial approach via the bronchoscope is an additional technique for aspirating such abscesses, and leaving a drainage catheter allows for irrigation of the cavity and continuous drainage. Good results have been reported, but care should be exercised to minimize spillage of pus into the airways.

CONCLUSION

Endoscopic techniques including VATS and fiberoptic bronchoscopy are increasingly useful diagnostic and therapeutic tools in patients with chest trauma or pulmonary complications following any trauma. In carefully selected patients these techniques can offer a lower risk alternative to open surgery both in the acute and nonacute setting. As technical advances improve instrumentation, both bronchoscopy and VATS are likely to play a greater role in the management of chest trauma and pulmonary complications following any trauma.

For the chapter's Suggested Readings list, please visit the book at www.ExpertConsult.inkling.com.

PULMONARY CONTUSION AND FLAIL CHEST

Carl Hauser, Noelle Salliant, and David H. Livingston

Pulmonary contusion and flail chest are the two most common anatomic complications of major blunt chest trauma. Each will directly alter pulmonary physiology in a specific and unique fashion, and thus contribute to pulmonary dysfunction and failure after trauma. Pulmonary contusion was probably first described by Morgagni in the 18th century, but Laurent's description in *The Lancet* in 1883 appears to be the first to recognize the possibility that plasticity of the chest wall, most notably in the young, can allow injury to the underlying lungs without disruption of the bony thorax. Conversely, flail chest is predominantly a disease of the elderly, with most patients being in the sixth decade of life and beyond and older patients having the worst outcomes. Pulmonary contusion and flail chest variably coexist; however, their effects on pulmonary pathophysiology are distinct. Confusion between these two clinical entities can lead to misapplication of studies aimed at one entity or the other and potentially lead to inappropriate treatment.

INCIDENCE

Pulmonary hemorrhage and contusion were first noted at autopsy of patients dying from battlefield and blast injuries during World War I. Similar findings were noted in World War II, and the term "pulmonary concussion" appears to have been coined by Hadfield describing civilian injuries from bomb blasts sustained during the Battle of Britain. In modern military engagement, blast-associated lung injury continues to represent 3% of the overall injury in Iraq and Afghanistan, and its incidence has been rising secondary to increased utilization of explosive devices.

The incidence of pulmonary contusion in the civilian population varies significantly between studies. Initially described in the 1960s in motor vehicular trauma, rates in early reports were quoted to be 10% of thoracic injuries. A recent review of the Department of Transportation's Crash Injury Research and Engineering Network (CIREN) reviewed 2187 passengers involved in frontal and near-side lateral collisions who were evaluated at one of eight participating Level I trauma centers. Just over half (52%) of these passengers sustained blunt chest trauma. Of those, 32% had pulmonary contusion (mean Injury Severity Score [ISS] of 17).

The reported rates of "pulmonary contusion," however, vary markedly because of multiple factors. For one, modern imaging techniques have doubled the rate of detection of small lung volume contusions compared to radiography. Second, the age of the "denominator" patient population examined will clearly affect the disease incidence reported in administrative databases. Younger patients, and specifically pediatric patients, have a compliant chest wall compared to older individuals. Trauma to the young chest transmits more energy to the lung parenchyma, rather than distributing the force to the ribs. Occupants younger than age 25 were 50% more likely to sustain a pulmonary contusion than older occupants, whereas older individuals had almost double the risk of rib fracture.

The relative frequency of flail chest as compared with pulmonary contusion will also vary depending upon the studied population. Pediatric thoracic trauma presents with pulmonary contusions whereas flail chest is very rare, even when multiple fractures are present. One rare exception to this is infants with osteogenesis imperfecta who may manifest their disease with flail chest. Adults, in contrast, have a much higher rate of flail segments. In a large contemporary descriptive series examining adult blunt chest trauma, flail chest was diagnosed in 5% to 13% of chest wall injuries and in 50% of patients with significant pulmonary contusions. Increasing brittleness of the thoracic cage predisposes the frail elderly to a flail chest with relatively minor chest trauma and little or no associated pulmonary contusion.

MECHANISMS OF INJURY

Physical Mechanisms of Injury

All blunt injuries result from the physical transfer of energy to the patient, but because of the rigidity of the bony thorax, most pulmonary contusions and most flail chest injuries are high-energy injuries, with the primary exception being chest wall injuries in the elderly. The overwhelming majority of significant blunt chest trauma in civilian life occurs as a result of motor vehicle crashes and motor vehicle versus pedestrian injuries. Classically, the scenario of injury involves unrestrained drivers striking the steering column. Falls are another common cause of pulmonary contusion and flail chest. Thoracic compression injuries are not as common as vehicular trauma and falls. Although they may produce similar syndromes, the slower speed of impact makes contusion less likely in these injuries than in flail chest. Typically, these patients manifest with traumatic asphyxia. Interpersonal violence, blows with blunt objects, and kicking are occasional causes of pulmonary contusion. Flail chest, however, is rare owing to the younger patient demographic involved in such injuries, and second, because biomechanically they are unlikely to result in segmental injuries of multiple contiguous ribs. The physician should be especially alert to rib fractures in infants and small children as they most commonly occur as a result of child abuse. Any rib fracture in a child is a marker for severe trauma. On rare occasions, tangential gunshot injuries will cause contusions of the underlying pulmonary parenchyma without actually entering the pleural space and lacerating the lung. These injuries are usually very limited in their extent and cause little or no physiologic effect.

As military strategy evolves from conventional engagement to counterinsurgency, improvised explosive devices (IEDs) have become the most common source of injury for American military forces. Blast injuries have four mechanisms of energy transference. Primary blast injuries are directly attributed to the shock wave itself and may occur in the absence of obvious external injury from shrapnel (secondary injury), blunt impact (tertiary injury), or other blast byproducts (quaternary injury). The density interface between air-filled body cavities and the tissue parenchyma predisposes to "spallation," whereby the high-density material transfers its kinetic energy to lower density surfaces, with the excess energy causing implosion of gas bubbles. "Short–duration" blast injuries such as those from IEDs are generally localized pulmonary injuries. Presumably this is based on shearing of the alveolar surfaces due to resistive differences of the tissue and air interface. "Long-duration" blast injuries transfer a compressive, high momentum force to the pulmonary parenchyma and are characteristic of larger bombs such as aircraft delivered bombs and vehicle-borne IEDS. The use of ballistic protective vests and body armor increases pulmonary blast tolerance substantially. These injuries are now also seen in civilians as a consequence of terrorism.

Pathophysiology

The transfer of energy to the chest cavity leads directly to edema and hemorrhage of the lung. A shearing force from the inertial differences

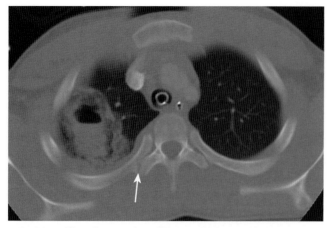

FIGURE 1 The admitting chest CT scan of 14-year-old patient in a high-speed crash. Contusion with pulmonary laceration is evident. There was no significant pneumothorax or hemothorax. No rib fractures were found, but the transverse processes of T4–T7 on the right were fractured *(arrow)*. In our experience, costovertebral joint separations like this are not uncommon on CT, and are the biomechanical equivalents of posterior rib fractures. CT, Computed tomography.

of the hilum and the lung parenchyma can lead to pulmonary lacerations. Although an uncommon occurrence, lacerations to the lung (Fig. 1) have been diagnosed with increasing frequency with the use of routine computed tomography (CT) imaging. Another potential mechanism of pulmonary dysfunction after trauma is the activation of pulmonary vascular endothelium by percussive cellular deformation. This phenomenon is better documented in cerebrovascular endothelial beds, but it is likely to exist in the pulmonary bed as well (see Fig. 1).

Studies from World War I initially proposed that blast injury predominantly resulted in pulmonary hemorrhage and that pulmonary failure reflected blood filling the air spaces. Whereas this effect undoubtedly contributes to the increased pulmonary shunting (Qs/Qt) seen after injury, many other pathophysiologic processes are at work.

It is most convenient to divide the various pathophysiologic influences on pulmonary function into two categories:

1. Those that result in hypoxemia from increased shunt (Qs/Qt)
2. Injuries that mechanically alter the work of breathing and can lead to ventilatory failure with eventual CO_2 retention and respiratory acidosis

These two physiologic insults often overlap, thus compounding the consequences of pulmonary injury. Furthermore, injury may impact mechanical function of the chest wall, pulmonary aeration, and cardiac performance as it relates to lung perfusion, although these considerations are outside the scope of this review.

Shunting and Hypoxemia

Injured, hemorrhagic lung is not the only factor that contributes to $\dot{V}/\dot{Q}$ mismatch in the acutely injured chest. Progressive atelectatic shunting often results from splinting from inadequately treated pain, in addition to the chest injury itself. Systemic shock and ischemia/reperfusion (I/R) are well-known activators of immune system attacks on the lung. This is perhaps most clearly evident in lung transplantation, but is also seen in systemic I/R as well as intestinal I/R. All will activate the innate immune system and cause systemic inflammatory response syndrome (SIRS), which contributes to acute lung injury (ALI) and pulmonary dysfunction after chest trauma.

The use of mechanical ventilation, although necessary, can also result in ventilator-induced lung injury (VILI) through a number of mechanisms. Immunologic injury can be induced by leukocytes in the presence of activating cytokines, resulting in increased lung water and decreased diffusion capacity of the lung (D_L). Finally, secondary immune attack on the "primed" lung can be initiated by pneumonia, shock, injudicious ventilation strategies, or the release of cytokines or damage-associated molecular patterns (DAMPs) into the circulation, as may happen in long-bone fixation.

Increased Work of Breathing and Ventilatory Failure

Ventilatory failure, hypercarbia, and respiratory acidosis after injury are most commonly the result of increased work of breathing. Such increases in work of breathing are typically multifactorial. Chest wall injuries can lead to decreased compliance of the chest wall as well as deficits in neuromuscular chest wall function. The pain and splinting associated with chest wall injuries will lead to decreased tidal volume and a relative increase in anatomic dead space (V_D/V_T). Thus, patients with chest injuries need to increase minute ventilation simply to achieve normal alveolar ventilation. This can be difficult or impossible to achieve in the presence of musculoskeletal chest wall dysfunction and pain.

In the presence of a flail chest, "CO_2 retention" has commonly been attributed to the "pendelluft" phenomenon, where to-and-fro flow of gas has been postulated to exist between the two hemithoraces in the presence of a unilateral flail segment. This concept is intuitively appealing, and the rebreathing of airway gas would indeed create a pathologic dead space. Yet direct application of this concept to clinical chest injury is simplistic. In practice, elevated shunt fractions and hypoxemia are more common in flail chest than is hypercarbia. Moreover, pendelluft occurs in ALI even without chest wall instability. This is a result of the heterogeneous viscoelastic properties of the injured lung, which lead to gas movement between lung segments of differing compliance. Clearly, though, flail segments do make ventilation both painful and increasingly inefficient.

Last, in any major trauma with secondary ALI, the same immune attack on the pulmonary parenchyma that leads to ALI-ARDS (acute respiratory distress syndrome) and hypoxemia will also lead to "stiff" lungs and increased work of breathing. Such decreases in pulmonary compliance may persist even after the chest wall has resumed normal configuration and biomechanics. An extrapulmonary cause of decreased pulmonary compliance that should always be sought in acute situations is abdominal compartmental hypertension. This condition may be difficult to diagnose and should always be suspected when bladder pressures exceed 20 to 25 mm Hg.

Inflammatory Lung Injury

Deteriorating pulmonary function after chest trauma is commonly related to systemic inflammation after injury. ALI and ARDS are terms widely used to reflect the increasing severity of secondary lung injury after trauma. Such injury is widely believed to result from polymorphonuclear neutrophil (PMN)–endothelial cell (EC) interactions that activate pulmonary capillary endothelial membranes, increasing endothelial permeability, causing interstitial and alveolar edema and finally resulting in diminished compliance and gas diffusion. We have recently demonstrated that the interactions of PMNs and ECs are specifically initiated by the circulation of mitochondrial DAMPs after injury. ALI/ARDS is usually defined as a diagnosis of exclusion when hypoxemia exists in the absence of other discrete causes of pulmonary failure such as pneumonia or congestive heart failure. In fact, ALI/ARDS probably exists in all major chest trauma to some extent. Although management of ALI/ARDS is to date supportive, improved understanding of its pathogenesis is critical. The lung is "primed" for secondary insults after chest trauma and at risk for marked deterioration in the event of secondary insults such as shock, pneumonia, and sepsis. There is increased risk of pneumonia after chest trauma, and pneumonia, of course, can act both as a primary cause of pulmonary dysfunction and as a trigger for "second-hit" organ failure. A special problem is that chest trauma is often accompanied by long-bone fractures, and patients with chest injuries are clearly at special risk for pulmonary deterioration after long-bone fracture fixation. Fractures are reservoirs for inflammatory mediators in the early postinjury period that can be mobilized to the bloodstream by operation and potentially contribute to ALI/ARDS. Intracellular DAMPs such as mitochondrial peptides and DNA are generated in high concentration when marrow cavities are reamed and will activate leukocytes as well as endothelial cells. Prospective studies will be needed to determine whether osteosynthetic techniques in these patients should be tailored to the protection of lung function or whether pharmacologic therapies can be developed to protect patients against fracture-related lung injury.

Extravascular Lung Water

Before routine clinical use of pulmonary artery (PA) catheters, it was widely believed that fluid overload and subsequent increases in extravascular lung water were the primary cause of pulmonary dysfunction after trauma. Modern concepts challenge this view and emphasize that hypovolemia, hypoperfusion, and reperfusion can all lead to inflammatory lung injury. Additionally, impaired right-to-left blood flow leads to preferential perfusion of the dependent (West Zone III) lung segments that are poorly ventilated, thus also increasing shunt.

Chest injury may be associated with myocardial dysfunction, but this is typically transient, right ventricular dysfunction that resolves quickly. Shock and resuscitation do expand extravascular water, but pulmonary lymphatics have remarkable reserve to protect the lung from interstitial overload. We therefore stress maintaining euvolemia and circulatory adequacy in patients with chest injuries and ALI. Hypertonic saline (HTS) has been suggested as the resuscitative fluid of choice in lung injury. There is no strong evidence in human subjects to support that recommendation. Limited data have supported the early administration of HTS. Furthermore, HTS has been shown to decrease neutrophil activation that leads to systemic inflammatory response in shock and ALI. In patients with underlying cardiac, renal, or hepatic disease, however, extravascular lung-water accumulation may be a significant issue. These patients may require inotropes, diuretics, or oncotic support. Excellent prospective evidence exists that patients with ALI who require diuresis benefit markedly by plasma volume support using hyperoncotic (25%) albumin.

DIAGNOSIS

Physical Examination

The diagnosis of flail chest is made by visual inspection or often better yet, by palpation of asymmetrical chest wall movement in the spontaneously breathing patient. Radiography and even CT diagnoses of a "flail chest" or a "flail chest segment" (i.e., at least three contiguous ribs fractured in two places) cannot account for the viscoelastic properties of the chest wall. Heavily muscled areas of the chest, whether due to normal anatomy or simply that seen in younger, fitter individuals, are less likely to sustain flail injuries. Such areas tend to remain mechanically stable despite the presence of fractures. Also, true paradoxical motion should not be required to make the diagnoses of a flail chest. Rather, asymmetrical or delayed rise of the affected chest wall segment is the rule.

The area of maximal chest wall weakness is often found at a 60-degree rotation from the sternum, where the ribs are flatter and less supported. Ribs subjected to lateral or anteroposterior (AP) compression will commonly fracture in two places: once at approximately 60 degrees and again posteriorly. AP compression also can create a costochondral disruption, resulting in a sternal flail. If the line of fractures crosses the axillary lines, a flail of the entire anterior chest wall may occur en cuirasse (i.e., like a shield) (Fig. 2).

Finally, it is not uncommon in our experience, especially in the elderly who have been struck by a steering wheel or an airbag anteriorly, to see hinging of the anterior chest wall segment at the

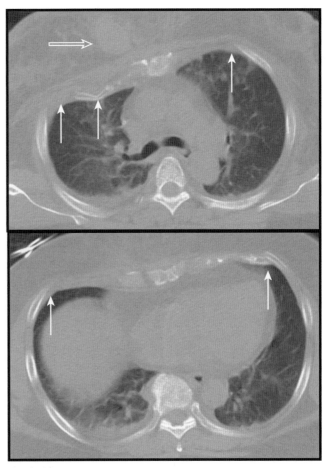

FIGURE 2 Computed tomography scan of an elderly obese woman with steering wheel injury and an anterior chest wall flail en cuirasse. Note that multiple rib fractures (solid arrows) in both anterior axillary lines in this case involved every rib. There is atelectasis and a small amount of pleural fluid, but considering the degree of rib injury this patient has little pulmonary contusion. There is an arterial hematoma in the anterior chest wall (open arrow). This patient was easily managed with pain medication and had no clinical pulmonary dysfunction.

manubrium. This will result in an "anterior flail segment" where the xiphoid depresses as the manubrium rises. Early in the postinjury period, muscular splinting of the chest can mask flail segments, again mandating a careful physical examination and often making palpation the more sensitive test. It is rapid and informative but is often overlooked. Spontaneously breathing patients are often best examined by placing both hands on the two hemithoraces and palpating the symmetry of chest wall motion. Crepitance is also a common finding and point tenderness over the costochondral junctions may point to dislocations or cartilaginous fractures that are not visible on radiographs. Clinical flail chest is associated with worse outcomes and greater need for intubation than pulmonary contusion alone. Auscultation of the chest is usually suboptimal in trauma, and will play little role in the diagnosis of pulmonary contusion and flail chest except to diminish concern in the first few moments in the trauma bay for lesions (such as hemothoraces and pneumothoraces) that may deteriorate acutely.

Chest Radiographs

Chest radiography and CT of the chest play key roles in the diagnosis of chest trauma. The initial AP/supine chest radiographs that are typically done in seriously injured patients may show pulmonary contusion or suggest flail chest (Fig. 3). Injuries diagnosed by AP radiographs

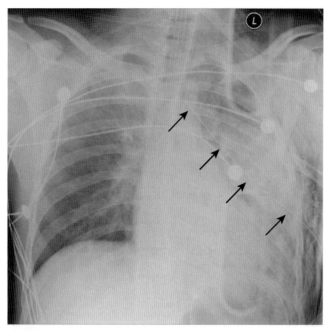

FIGURE 3   Chest radiography done after empirical chest tube placement in a patient with subcutaneous emphysema and arterial desaturation. Note the left lower-lobe pulmonary contusion, the apparently ideal placement of the chest tube (arrows), and the absence of a visible residual pneumothorax. Fractures of the left ribs four, five, and six were visible laterally.

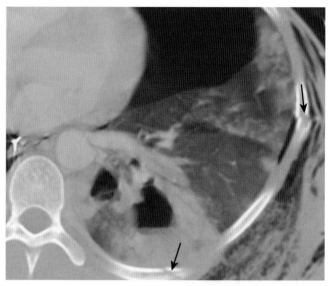

FIGURE 4   Initial chest computed tomography of same patient shown in Figure 3. Multiple segmental rib fractures (arrows) were not seen on chest radiograph. A posterior contusion-laceration and an anterior pneumothorax are present despite the chest tube laterally and the apparent expansion of the lung on chest radiograph. This reflects the superimposition of air and fluid densities.

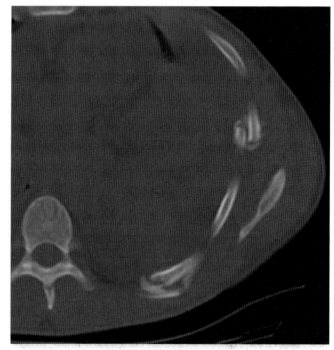

FIGURE 5   Noncontrast computed tomography demonstrating fractures extending over more than three contiguous rib segments. In this location (underneath the fractured scapula) such injuries are rarely found on clinical examination and are unlikely to manifest as chest wall instability.

are almost always clinically significant. Pulmonary contusions identified by radiographs are associated with a statistically significant increased risk of ventilatory support (odds ratio [OR] of 2.05 [95% confidence interval (CI), 1.01–4.14]) and interventions to the chest (OR of 4.01 [95% CI, 1.92–8.37]) compared with those diagnosed by CT alone. However, chest radiographs are of low sensitivity and will miss many very important intrathoracic lesions. Pape et al reported that with radiographs alone only 47% of pulmonary contusions are detected at the time of admission, whereas 92% are seen 24 hours after injury. Although rib fractures may also be apparent, plain radiographs typically show many fewer fractures than CT scans.

Thus, in addition to underestimating pain and disability, chest radiographs only rarely suggest whether rib fracture patterns are likely to be mechanically unstable. So, although the initial chest radiograph remains crucial in the early diagnosis of immediately life-threatening lesions, it often fails to diagnose pulmonary contusions, hemothoraces, pneumothoraces, and lung lacerations that may require specific interventions. This is especially true when anterior pneumothoraces and posterior fluid collections coexist (Fig. 4).

Chest Computed Tomography

Chest CT typically reveals many more rib fractures and pulmonary contusions than chest radiography (Fig. 5). Miller showed that chest CT could often diagnose pulmonary contusions when less than 18% of the pulmonary parenchyma was involved. Furthermore, the authors suggested that the volume of lung involved suggested the likelihood of severe respiratory dysfunction; 82% of patients with a contusion greater than 20% of lung volume developed ARDS versus only 22% of patients with a contusion less than 20%.

Significant flail segments most commonly occur in the setting of segmental fractures of three or more contiguous ribs. CT scans will sometimes demonstrate contiguous rib fractures in a pattern that suggests geographic instability or a dysfunctional area of the chest wall where physical examination is unrevealing, but this does not mean

that all areas where CT shows three adjacent rib fractures necessarily represents a flail segment.

Contusions are often seen as infiltrative lesions that may underlie fractures but are "nonanatomic" in their distribution on chest CT. Dependent infiltrates on the CT after injury may reflect processes, such as aspiration, atelectasis, and later, pneumonia, that can be difficult to distinguish from contusions. In contrast, nonanatomic and antidependent distributions of infiltrative lung lesions on a chest CT may be pathognomonic for pulmonary contusion (Fig. 6). A pleural-based "blast-wave" pattern seen on CT is pathognomonic (Fig. 7). Early chest CT can also aid in the evaluation of pulmonary contusions by determining their extent and allowing prediction of respiratory deterioration.

Physiologic Studies

Radiologic imaging is often of little importance from a functional point of view because multiple nonanatomic and physiologic causes

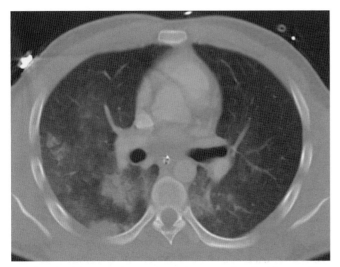

FIGURE 6 Admitting chest computed tomography of a 19-year-old patient after high-speed car crash with severe pulmonary contusions. The only thoracic bony injury was a fractured clavicle. The patient developed severe acute lung injury/acute respiratory distress syndrome 3 days later.

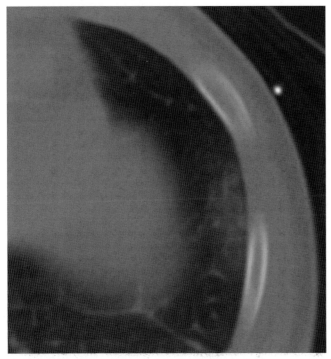

FIGURE 7 Subclinical "computed tomography–only" pulmonary contusion.

of lung injury tend to coexist. The functional and physiologic diagnosis of pulmonary contusion and flail chest will rely on analysis of vital signs, arterial blood gases, and hemodynamic and bedside pulmonary function studies.

The physiologic hallmark of pulmonary contusion is hypoxemia, which results from perfusion of poorly ventilated lung. Hypoxemia can be defined as decreased arterial saturation on a stable F_{IO_2} or by an increasing need for inspired oxygen support to maintain saturation. This is often expressed as a decreasing Pao_2/F_{IO_2} (P/F) ratio. In ventilated patients, increasing positive end-expiratory pressure (PEEP), plateau pressures, or reversed inspiratory/expiratory (I/E) ratios may all indicate a high Qs/Qt. Also, pulmonary parenchymal injury often results in decreased compliance. This can manifest as decreased tidal volume and tachypnea in spontaneously ventilating patients or patients treated with pressure ventilation modes, or it can manifest as increased peak airway pressures in ventilated patients on volume-controlled ventilator settings.

In truly isolated flail chest injuries, there is little initial hypoxemia. Rather, these patients present early with rapid shallow respiration and normal blood gases despite increased minute ventilation and work of breathing (WOB). They commonly develop hypercarbia and hypoxia only as ventilation fails. Often, though, they do have some element of pulmonary contusion initially, and may develop hypoxemia over time because of atelectasis, poor clearance of secretions, or immunologic injury. Ventilated patients may show little pulmonary dysfunction resulting from the flail chest component of their injury as long as their pressure or volume support is sufficient to splint the chest wall and cause it to move in synchrony.

ANATOMIC LOCATION OF INJURY AND INJURY GRADING

The American Association for the Surgery of Trauma Organ Injury Scale (AAST-OIS) for chest trauma as reviewed by Moore and colleagues is shown in Tables 1 and 2. It should be noted that the scores for chest wall and pulmonary injury are separate, but injuries may overlap and interact. For instance, the association of a flail chest with pulmonary contusion results in greater need for intubation and worse outcomes than pulmonary contusion only. Conversely, many of the small pulmonary contusions now found on CT scan alone may be of little prognostic value, or their significance may be limited to situations in which patients are expected to undergo long-bone fixation. Thus, these scales must clearly be considered to be in evolution with respect to the CT diagnosis of intrathoracic injury (see Tables 1 and 2).

MANAGEMENT

Pulmonary contusion/flail chest can be viewed as leading to four common and important sequelae: (1) pain, (2) mechanical chest wall instability, (3) direct lung injury, and (4) secondary (immune) lung injury. To differing extents, these all contribute directly or indirectly to pulmonary gas exchange dysfunction and thus can be important contributors to the morbidity and mortality risks of multisystem injuries.

Immediate Management

Before the early 1980s, the major controversy in early management of pulmonary contusion/flail chest was whether early endotracheal intubation should be emphasized or whether attempts should be made to avoid intubation. This controversy reflected the early perception that patients who were intubated had a worse prognosis. Richardson and colleagues were the first to show that, rather than being a causal relationship, this difference in outcomes reflected worse overall injuries in the intubated than the nonintubated group. Over time, the established

TABLE 1: Chest Wall Injury Scale*

Grade	Injury Type	Description of Injury	ICD-9	AIS-90
I	Contusion	Any size	911.0/922.1	1
	Laceration	Skin and subcutaneous	875.0	1
	Fracture	<3 ribs, closed Nondisplaced clavicle, closed	807.01 807/02 810.00/810.03	1–2 2
II	Laceration	Skin, subcutaneous, and muscle	875.1	1
	Fracture	>3 adjacent ribs, closed Open or displaced clavicle Nondisplaced sternum, closed Scapular body, open or closed	807.03/807.09 810.10/810.13 807.2 811.00/811.18	2–3 2 2 2
III	Laceration	Full thickness including pleural penetration	862.29	2
	Fracture	Open or displaced sternum Flail sternum Unilateral flail segment (<3 ribs)	807.2 807.3 807.4	2 3–4
IV	Laceration	Avulsion of chest wall tissues with underlying rib fractures	807.10/807.19	4
	Fracture	Unilateral flail chest (>3 ribs)	807.4	3–4
V	Fracture	Bilateral flail chest (>3 ribs on both sides)	807.4	5

Modified from Moore EE, Cogbill TH, Malangoni MA, et al: Organ injury scaling. *Surg Clin North Am* 75:293–303, 1995.
AIS, Abbreviated Injury Scale.
*This scale is confined to the chest wall alone and does not reflect associated internal or abdominal injuries. Therefore, further delineation of upper versus lower or anterior versus posterior chest wall was not considered, and a grade VI was warranted. Specifically, thoracic crush was not used as a descriptive term; instead, the geography and extent of fractures and soft tissue injury were used to define the grade.

TABLE 2: Lung Injury Scale

Grade*	Injury Type	Description of Injury	ICD-9	AIS-90
I	Contusion	Unilateral, <1 lobe	861.12 861.31	3
II	Contusion	Unilateral, single lobe	861.20 861.30	3
	Laceration	Simple pneumothorax	860.0/1	3
III	Contusion	Unilateral, >1 lobe	861.20 861.30	3
	Laceration	Persistent (>72 hours) air leak from distal airway	860.0/1 860.4/5 862.0	3–4
	Hematoma	Nonexpanding intraparenchymal	861.30	
IV	Laceration	Major (segmental or lobar) air leak	862.21 861.31	4–5
	Hematoma	Expanding intraparenchymal		
	Vascular	Primary branch intrapulmonary vessel disruption	901.40	3–5
V	Vascular	Hilar vessel disruption	901.41 901.42	4
VI	Vascular	Total uncontained transection of pulmonary hilum	901.41 901.42	4

Modified from Moore EE, Cogbill TH, Malangoni MA, et al: Organ injury scaling. *Surg Clin North Am* 75:293–303, 1995.
AIS, Abbreviated Injury Scale.
*Advance one grade for bilateral injuries up to grade III. Hemothorax is scored under thoracic vascular injury scale.

approach (as reflected in Advanced Trauma Life Support [ATLS] and other algorithms) became early elective use of endotracheal intubation in patients presenting with any hypoxemia. Flail chest injuries in particular are associated with a tendency to early failure of ventilation requiring emergency intubation as the result of unrecognized high work of breathing. This approach is controversial, however, and other works have suggested aggressive attempts to avoid intubation. Analysis of the available data, however, suggests that there are no true prospective series available comparing early intubation to "intubation on demand" in equivalent groups, and that in all reports the intubated patients were simply sicker. In our judgment, arguments that elective intubations lead to worse outcome are unsupported. Our approach has been the use of early rapid-sequence intubation and ventilation to facilitate diagnosis and management wherever there are severe injuries, with early extubation of patients who show that they will tolerate it. Patients who have progressive deterioration of respiratory function despite intubation will require prolonged ventilation and intensive care unit (ICU) management.

Intensive Care Unit Management

Pulmonary contusion decreases parenchymal compliance and increases Qs/Qt. Flail chest causes chest wall dysfunction, pain, and inefficient ventilation. These two injuries contribute synergistically to hypoventilation and ventilatory failure. Pain and impaired coughing contribute to atelectasis and mucus plugging, and decreased chest wall expansion under flail segments decreases functional residual capacity (FRC). Associated systemic injury, shock, and pulmonary infections contribute to secondary pulmonary parenchymal injury. All will contribute to shunting and hypoxemia. Thus, treatment of flail chest/pulmonary contusion is one of the most important and challenging aspects of intensive care in trauma.

The management of flail chest/pulmonary contusion is directed both at minimizing shunt fraction and at limiting the mechanical disadvantage of a deformed chest cavity. Strategies to this aim have included the following:

  Minimizing atelectatic and compressed lung via both noninvasive and invasive positive-pressure ventilation and ventilator recruitment maneuvers
  Preferential conduction of gas exchange to uninjured lung via positioning of patient and strategies to preferentially aerate a noninjured lung with single-lung ventilation
  Strategies to minimize the potential for pneumonia development

In the case of minor injuries, supplemental oxygen can be given by mask as needed. Trunkey was the first to advocate restraint in the use of mechanical intubation. He also emphasized analgesia as a potent supplemental therapy in the clinical management of pulmonary injury.

General Principles of Ventilator Management

True continuous positive airway pressure (CPAP) delivered by a tight-fitting mask has been used to improve oxygenation and support the FRC. Antonelli first supported the efficacy of noninvasive ventilation in a randomized controlled trial in patients with all-cause acute respiratory failure. Gundez examined the same question in a randomized controlled study evaluating CPAP in highly selected, young patients (average age, 40) who presented with flail chest. Respiratory distress was defined as respiratory rate 25 breaths per minute; SpO_2 less than 90% while breathing 10 L/minute O_2, and P/F ratio of 300 while receiving FiO_2 higher than 0.5 in the ICU. Nosocomial infection and survival appeared to be improved in the CPAP group over the intubated group. Despite randomization, bias toward a non-intubated experimental group being healthier is difficult to exclude. Also, the natural history of significant flail chest/pulmonary contusion is a gradual worsening of pulmonary function over the first few days. Thus, in our experience, use of CPAP (and the related nasal form, BiPAP) in chest trauma is often simply a marker for later need for emergent intubation with its attendant risks. Moreover, CPAP predisposes to gastric distention and thus to aspiration. Thus, we have found that using CPAP as a bridge to delay intubation in major chest trauma is often unwise and may risk significant complications. Endotracheal intubation is often required in patients with significant injuries and should be performed before deterioration. As the common medical adage suggests, intubation is usually warranted if it is being considered.

Ventilatory Support

Ventilating chest trauma patients can be different from ventilating other patients. Intubated patients with lesser injuries may require some support for air exchange, but generally should be allowed to spontaneously ventilate to whatever degree is possible. Pressure support ventilation (PSV) mode is very satisfactory for spontaneously breathing patients, but care should be taken when using PSV in the presence of significant flails. In these cases, the negative pressures that trigger the ventilator may destabilize the chest wall and should be minimized. Such motion may be painful and delay stabilization. We often prefer to begin treatment using a volume mode like synchronized intermittent mandatory ventilation (SIMV), keeping minute ventilation high enough to raise arterial pH slightly above 7.4, thus suppressing spontaneous ventilation without undue sedation. The flail segments are allowed to stabilize over about a week, with thicker chest walls often stabilizing more quickly. Patients are then ventilated using PSV and are weaned progressively.

Recent attention has been focused on airway pressure release ventilation (APRV) as a potential ventilator strategy for trauma patients at risk of developing ALI/ARDS. APRV is a pressure-limited, time-cycled ventilation mode that consists of a high-pressure setting that is transiently released to a low-pressure setting to create a deep expiration. Spontaneous breathing is permitted at any time throughout the respiratory cycle to support the patient effort during CPAP breathing. In retrospective data, APRV significantly improved oxygenation by alveolar recruitment, allowed for a reduction in peak airway pressures, and potentially decreased the risk for ventilator-associated pneumonia.

Chest trauma, pulmonary contusion, and ARDS can lower ventilatory compliance. Higher airway pressures are needed to achieve the same tidal volumes that are in the uninjured lung. The ARDSNet data have shown that high airway pressures (35 cm H_2O) should be avoided when possible, and using lower tidal volumes (6–8 mL/g) will decrease peak airway pressures. Limiting airway pressures is especially important in cases of bronchopleural fistulas. "Normal" $PaCO_2$ values are not needed in sedated patients, and "permissive" hypercapnia is often useful in the treatment of hypoxemia after chest trauma. Prospective data showed that hypercapnia is safe in ARDS and blast lung patients, and in some studies there was a significant mortality rate advantage observed. Permissive hypercapnia can require prolonged deep sedation though, and it is important to recall that improved survival has never been demonstrated with a randomized controlled trial. Furthermore, it is important to note that this technique emphasizes control of alveolar pressure, rather than focusing on the numerical PCO_2.

Oxygenation Support

Patients with significant chest trauma all manifest some degree of hypoxemia. This may be managed initially by increasing FiO_2, but prolonged high FiO_2 can be harmful in itself. The longer-term management of hypoxemia therefore entails measures to increase mean airway pressure to maintain and improve oxygenation. This may include PEEP or reversed I/E times that can be delivered by any of several ventilator strategies. These interventions can recruit alveoli and diminish alveolar and interstitial water. The reversal of I/E time is limited by the need to excrete CO_2 and stacking or auto-PEEP at high I/E ratios. Traditional high tidal volume ventilation (10–15 mL/kg) does not contribute to pulmonary expansion, nor does it improve oxygenation in the majority of cases. Rather, it has been known for many years to lead to unequal ventilation, alveolar over distention, and VILI. We began using low tidal volume ventilation in the early 1990s (we called it "the kinder, gentler vent breath"). Since that time, low tidal volume ventilation has been shown to improve the survival of general ICU patients in prospective studies, and we extend these principles to chest trauma in most cases.

Limited data regarding the appropriate use of PEEP have been discussed in the trauma literature. Extrapolating from a meta-analysis of 2299 ALI and ARDS patients, treatment with higher PEEP and recruitment breaths appears to be safe, and perhaps confers a survival benefit in ARDS patients (>12 cm H_2O). Schreiter published a small series that specifically looked at 17 trauma patients with ARDS from pulmonary contusion. Recruitment breaths ranging from 50 to 80 cm H_2O improved their oxygenation and decreased the amount of collapsed lung demonstrated by CT scans of the lung. The impact on patient outcomes was not studied. An alternative approach to improve oxygenation in patients with pulmonary contusion and poor oxygenation is high-frequency oscillatory ventilation (HFOV). Small tidal volumes at a high frequency maintain a mean constant airway pressure, thus minimizing barotraumas and maintaining alveolar recruitment. Small retrospective studies have been performed in surgical patients with improvements in oxygenation. Further study with randomized prospective trials needs to be performed before conclusions regarding the safety and efficacy can be made.

Many other therapies with little or no evidentiary support are in common use as salvage therapies in refractory hypoxemic patients. These include rotating or oscillating beds, differential lung ventilation, inhaled nitric oxide, partial liquid ventilation, HTS, red blood cell transfusions, inotropic support to raise mixed venous oxygen saturation, and other modalities. All may have some effect in individual patients and may on occasion "buy some time" for the primary process to abate. None has been prospectively validated. Extracorporeal membrane oxygenation support or life support (ECMO/ECLS), however, is emerging as a useful adjunct in the care of advanced posttraumatic ARDS, even in the setting of recently controlled bleeding.

Tracheobronchial toilet in the intubated chest trauma patient should have a high priority because of the frequent coexistence of early particulate aspiration, blood casts, or lobar collapse resulting from retained secretions. Both macroaspiration at the time of injury and the continued microaspiration that accompanies endotracheal intubation can increase secretions and allow airway colonization by oropharyngeal flora. Excessive secretions may also predispose to lobar collapse, shunting and hypoxemia, diminished compliance, and postobstructive airway infections. Blood may accumulate in the airway after pulmonary contusion and form bronchial casts. Intubated patients cannot cough and are completely dependent upon suctioning for airway toilet. *N*-acetylcysteine may be used as a mucolytic if secretions are thick, but it causes bronchospasm and should be used with bronchodilators. Also, prolonged *N*-acetylcysteine therapy can cause bronchorrhea. Chest physiotherapy is helpful, but the percussion of injured ribs is often painful. Thus, removal of secretions or particulates frequently requires bronchoscopy. The removal of particulate debris or blood and mucus casts may require retrieval with snares or morcellation (Fig. 8).

Pain Management

The control of chest wall pain is a key consideration in management of chest injuries. Immobility of the chest wall due to splinting resulting from pain is often thought a major contributor to the development of pneumonia after rib fractures. This has never been proved and recent studies suggest that pneumonia in trauma patients, in fact, reflects suppression of immunity. Nonetheless, good pain control is an important contribution to patient care in general, and probably

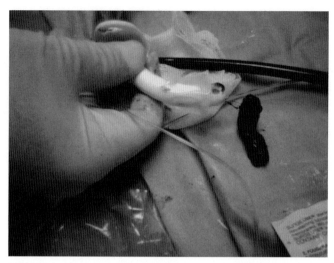

FIGURE 8   Airway cast due to endobronchial bleeding. The cast was too hard to be morcellated. When snared bronchoscopically it was larger than the tracheostomy and could not be removed without first removing and replacing the tracheostomy.

improves pulmonary toilet. Chest wall pain can be treated with appropriate systemic analgesic regimens or with intercostal, intrapleural, subpleural, or paravertebral blocks. At this time, epidural blocks are probably the optimal form of analgesia when possible and not contraindicated. There is no scientific support at all for the historical practice of using chest taping or strapping to relieve pain.

Steroids

As noted previously, all blunt chest injuries will have some element of ALI/ARDS, and as yet no intervention or pharmaceutical agent has been proved to be of significant value in treating posttraumatic ARDS. Some small series, however, have suggested that the late fibroproliferative stage of ARDS may respond in some measure to systemic corticosteroids. Nonetheless, considering the well-established dangers of steroid use, we await prospective data before using them routinely in late ARDS.

Tracheostomy

As with endotracheal intubation, it is often apparent early in patients with severe injuries that tracheostomy will be critical. Also, later deterioration often makes tracheostomy hazardous. Thus, experienced clinicians will often look for an early "window of opportunity" to move airway access from the endotracheal tube to a tracheostomy in sicker patients. Early tracheostomy (generally defined as at <7 days) improves access to the tracheobronchial tree for toilet and allows for better oropharyngeal hygiene. Although controversy persists, this approach has been suggested to result in fewer episodes of pneumonia and more rapid weaning from mechanical ventilation. Last, current studies have shown convincingly that low-volume/low-pressure ventilation is less injurious to the lung than higher ventilator volumes and pressures. Tracheostomy diminishes the anatomic dead space and reliably lowers peak airway pressures at equivalent levels of alveolar ventilation. This is especially helpful in patients with refractory pulmonary failure who require aggressive ventilator settings to support oxygenation.

Operative Stabilization of Flail Chest

Most physiologically significant flail chest injuries are satisfactorily managed by analgesia, selective intubation, and mechanical ventilation. Suggested relative indications for operative therapy include prolonged ventilation, severe mechanical deformity of the chest wall, and thoracotomy for other indications. Theoretically, restoration of the chest wall's three-dimensional silhouette should help correct respiratory impairments caused by flail injuries.

Numerous strategies have been used to stabilize the chest wall. Metal plates, absorbable polymer plates, intermedullary fixation, Judet struts, and U plates have all been employed as potential options without any comparative studies to determine the best intervention.

Anatomically, the limited cortex of each individual rib, the close approximation of the inferior neurovascular bundle, and the tendency for comminuted and oblique fractures can make operative reduction and internal fixation (ORIF) technically challenging. Furthermore, the implantation of foreign material in the chest wall with concomitant chest tubes, respiratory floral contamination, and environmental contamination from the trauma itself also complicates the operation.

The management guidelines for flail chest released by the Eastern Association for the Surgery of Trauma (EAST) considered operative fixation of severe unilateral chest deformity and flail chest requiring ventilation and thoracotomy to be a class III recommendation. The majority of the data, however, is based primarily on nonrandomized, observational studies, without matched control groups.

Two randomized studies, however, have been performed and are worth mentioning. The first, by Tanaka et al, is a prospective randomized study that matched 37 patients by age, ISS, number of ribs broken, severity of pulmonary contusion, and P/F ratio at admission. The study group received Judet strut fixation of ribs T4 through T10 on the fifth postinjury day. The control group was managed with identical respiratory strategies via internal pneumatic stabilization with PEEP, SIMV, and pressure support. A statistically significant advantage was demonstrated in the surgical stabilization group with 8 fewer days of mechanical ventilation, 10 fewer days in ICU, and a 50% reduction in the incidence of pneumonia. Overall cost of care was also diminished in the surgically managed group ($13,455 vs. $23,423, $P < .05$). When the EAST committee reviewed this study it was given a Level 3 designation due to the low number of patients randomized, and failure to compare surgical fixation with "modern" nonoperative treatments such as epidural analgesia and chest physiotherapy. A second randomized trial by Granetzny has since been published that suggested a benefit to surgical fixation of the flail chest. A total of 40 patients were randomized to either surgical wire fixation of the chest wall 24 to 36 hours after injury versus conservative treatment using "strapping and packing" of flail segments with elastic bandages. The study determined that chest wall deformity, described as "stove-in chest" and "rib crowding," was significantly improved in surgically treated patients (1/20 surgical patients versus 9/20 control subjects). Furthermore, pulmonary function tests 2 months after injury showed an improvement of forced vital capacity (FVC), total lung capacity (TLC), and FEF_{75} (forced expiratory flow) in patients with fixation. But the clinical implication of the anatomic "outcomes" chosen as well as the small differences in FVC, TLC, and FEF_{75} found are unclear. In the few patients who were intubated (only 35% control subjects and 45% of surgical patients, or a total of 16 patients) the mean duration of mechanical ventilation was significantly reduced from 12 days to 2 days in favor of surgical repair. Finally, pneumonia was also reduced in the surgical group (10% vs. 50%), although pneumonia was poorly defined. Again, this randomized controlled trial only included small numbers of patients. The biomechanics of chest wall injury were not studied. And critically, we would consider the practice of strapping flail segments itself as done in the control group to be deleterious. Ventilator strategy and analgesic management were not controlled and the role of pulmonary contusion was unstudied.

The implication of pulmonary contusion was discussed by Voggenreiter et al, who studied 42 patients with flail chest. There were no significant differences in age, severity of injury, or extent of injury among the groups. They specifically examined the effects of chest fixation in the presence and absence of pulmonary contusion. Only patients with respiratory failure in the absence of lung contusion benefited from ORIF, likely because they were afforded an earlier extubation and patients with pulmonary contusion did not benefit from ORIF. In summary, operative fixation of a flail chest is clearly not indicated in the vast majority of patients with flail chest.

Evidence is slowly emerging, however, that selected patient populations with respiratory failure related to unstable flail segments may exist, likely those with relatively spared lung parenchyma, in which there may be benefit from early intervention. Furthermore, patients who must already undergo a thoracotomy for related injuries may also benefit. Multicenter study is clearly needed to power adequately controlled clinical trials of surgical fixation versus current ventilator and pain management before consensus can be reached. A better classification of flail chest and future related improvements in operative management would need to be based on the biomechanics of the injury. Current assessments based upon standard chest CT scans may be inadequate. We would suggest that noncontrast dynamic CT scans (similar to those currently done in tracheobronchomalacia) might improve our understanding of which injuries may benefit most. Defining the pathoanatomy of the fracture complex will also allow identification of "hinges" and areas of maximal mobility. Using this information to plan reconstruction could improve postoperative stability while decreasing the extent of operation.

MORTALITY

Most deaths after pulmonary contusion/flail chest result from associated injuries such as head trauma, but major chest wall trauma is still an important independent cause of death. In these instances, death is usually due to ARDS, respiratory failure, sepsis, and multiple organ failure (MOF). Thus, outcomes are covariant with other conditions that predispose to SIRS, respiratory failure, and MOF. These include associated injuries, increasing ISS or Acute Physiology and Chronic Health Evaluation (APACHE) scores, and increasing numbers of blood transfusions. When pulmonary contusions are visible on the admitting chest radiograph of a patient with a flail chest, the need for mechanical ventilation is far greater and mortality rate is more than doubled when compared with either condition alone. Livingston et al specifically looked at the prognostication of CT imaging and determined a stepwise mortality rate increase from 2% in patients with fewer than five rib fractures to 9% for those with five to eight rib fractures and again to 27% for those with greater than nine rib fractures. Similarly, the mortality rate of flail chest increases with age: beyond the age of 55, the likelihood of death related to flail chest increases 132% for every 10-year increase in age and 30% for each unit increase in ISS. Ventilator-associated pneumonia is also an independent risk factor for death in chest trauma, though pneumonia itself may simply be a marker for greater systemic trauma.

Finally, patients sustaining blast injuries of the lung typically have higher energy systemic injuries than those with motor vehicle or pedestrian trauma and so have a higher overall mortality rate. A recent review of the Joint Theatre Trauma Registry reports an initial mortality rate of blast lung injury as 66% prior to reaching a medical facility, with an additional 24% mortality rate in early survivors who eventually succumb to their associated injuries and pulmonary sequelae.

In summary, flail chest and pulmonary contusion are highly morbid and may contribute significantly to fatality in multisystem trauma or in patients with underlying comorbid conditions. Nonetheless, with modern ICU management, death from flail chest and pulmonary contusion alone should be fairly uncommon.

CONCLUSIONS

- Pulmonary contusion and flail chest are common and life-threatening sequelae of blunt chest trauma.
- Pulmonary contusion and flail chest commonly coexist.
- Isolated flail chest tends to occur in older patients with brittle ribs.

- Isolated pulmonary contusions tend to occur in younger patients with flexible ribs.
- Pulmonary contusion and flail chest are each associated with pulmonary dysfunction resulting from shock, SIRS, and inflammatory ALI.
- Impairment of oxygenation in pulmonary contusion and flail chest usually reflects the contributions of contusion and ALI to intrapulmonary shunting (Qs/Qt).
- Impairment of ventilation in pulmonary contusion/flail chest usually reflects the effects of chest wall injury and pain on ventilatory mechanics and on the work of breathing.

- The management of significant pulmonary contusion and flail chest often entails mechanical ventilator support for 5 to 10 days.
- Selected minor injuries can be managed without endotracheal intubation.
- Selected major injuries should be considered for early tracheostomy.

For the chapter's Suggested Readings list, please visit the book at www.ExpertConsult.inkling.com.

OPERATIVE TREATMENT OF CHEST WALL INJURY

R. Stephen Smith and Juan A. Asensio

Thoracic injury is a significant cause of morbidity and death. Rib fractures, one of the most common manifestations of thoracic injury, are frequently encountered in victims of trauma. For example, 94% of severely or fatally injured seatbelt wearers have rib fractures. Approximately 25% of all deaths due to trauma result from injury to the thorax. Despite this, most thoracic injuries are treated with simple interventions such as supplemental oxygen, mechanical ventilation, and tube thoracostomy. The vast majority of thoracic injuries do not require major operative procedures. The basic pathophysiology of thoracic injury involves hypoxia, hypercarbia, and both metabolic and respiratory acidosis. Flail chest is associated with all of these pathophysiologic states.

Approximately 10% of all patients admitted to trauma centers have rib fractures. Most of these patients require only analgesia, pulmonary toilet, and symptomatic care. Approximately 10% of patients admitted with rib fractures have a flail chest. Flail chest results from significant kinetic energy transmitted to the thorax. The classic definition of flail chest is the fracture of three or more consecutive ribs in at least two locations. Patients with multiple consecutive rib fractures may exhibit the same respiratory compromise and pulmonary dysfunction classically associated with flail chest. Mechanical ventilation may be required in more than 50% of patients with flail chest even when optimal support, analgesia, and pulmonary toilet are provided. A key component in the successful treatment of flail chest is adequate analgesia. Failure to provide adequate analgesia in the nonventilated patient results in severe pain, which produces hypoventilation, retention of secretions, progressive atelectasis, lobar collapse, pneumonia, and respiratory failure. The most effective method of providing analgesia for patients with flail chest is thoracic epidural analgesia. This intervention should be initiated as soon as possible to prevent progressive pulmonary insufficiency. All too often, this therapy is delayed past the initial 24 hours following injury. Alternatively, intercostal nerve blocks may be used if long-acting local anesthetics are available. The percutaneous placement of long catheters that permit the continuous installation of local anesthetic adjacent to the site of rib fractures and intercostal nerves may be useful, but is an unproven technique. External patches or dressings containing long-acting local anesthetic agents do not appear to be useful in patients with rib fractures and flail chest. The mortality rate for patients with flail chest is high, ranging from 10% to 36%. This high mortality rate is primarily due to associated injuries.

INDICATIONS FOR OPERATIVE THERAPY

The majority of patients with flail chest are not operative candidates. In most cases, underlying pulmonary contusion is the primary cause of hypoxia and the reason that these patients require mechanical ventilation. Patients with significant hypoxia due to pulmonary contusion should not undergo elective operations until hypoxia has resolved. In some patients, the biomechanical effects of multiple rib fractures and flail chest prevent adequate ventilation. This inadequate ventilation can produce respiratory failure independent of underlying pulmonary contusion.

The indications for surgical stabilization of rib fractures and flail chest are evolving. Indications are different for patients with acute respiratory failure as compared to patients with nonunion of rib fractures producing chronic pain and disability. In the acute setting, potential indications for operative fixation of severely displaced rib fractures and flail chest include patients who must undergo thoracotomy for associated intrathoracic injuries. Hemodynamically stable patients who require thoracotomy may be considered for simultaneous repair of rib fractures. Another group of candidates for operative fixation are patients who do not initially require intubation and mechanical ventilation but have progressive deterioration of pulmonary function despite aggressive nonoperative treatment that includes adequate analgesia, aggressive pulmonary toilet, and the subsequent requirement for mechanical ventilation. Other patients who initially require ventilatory support for pulmonary contusion may become candidates for operative fixation if they remain ventilator dependent after the pulmonary contusion has resolved. Patients with extensive, displaced rib fractures or anterolateral flail chest with progressive dislocation of the fractured ribs are candidates for operative fixation. Operative fixation in this group of patients can prevent unacceptable chest wall deformity and, more importantly, prevent chronic pain by eliminating the development of pseudoarthroses. In these patients, intercostal neuralgia may play a significant role in chronic pain. The use of gabapentin should be considered as a standard component of therapy for chronic pain associated with displaced rib fractures and pseudoarthroses. An algorithm to determine the applicability of operative treatment of acute flail chest injury is represented in Figure 1.

Anatomy and Incisions

The exposure of rib fractures for operative fixation requires knowledge of chest wall anatomy. Major muscle groups of the chest include the trapezius, the rhomboids, the pectoralis major and minor, the latissimus dorsi, the serratus anterior, and the erector spinae muscles. Approaches that are useful for exposure of rib fractures include the apical axillary thoracotomy incision, the curved axillary incision, the horizontal muscle sparing thoracotomy incision, and the posterior lateral thoracotomy incision. Approximately 90% of procedures for operative fixation are performed through a posterolateral incision.

FIGURE 1 Algorithm for operative treatment of acute flail chest.

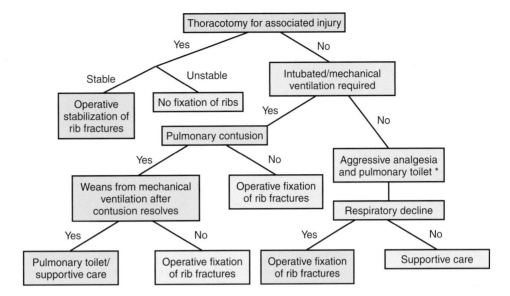

Thoracotomy for associated injury

Yes → Stable → **Operative stabilization of rib fractures**

Yes → Unstable → **No fixation of ribs**

No → **Intubated/mechanical ventilation required**

Yes → **Pulmonary contusion**

Yes → **Weans from mechanical ventilation after contusion resolves**

Yes → **Pulmonary toilet/supportive care**

No → **Operative fixation of rib fractures**

No → **Operative fixation of rib fractures**

No → **Aggressive analgesia and pulmonary toilet ***

Respiratory decline

Yes → **Operative fixation of rib fractures**

No → **Supportive care**

In many cases, it is not necessary to enter the pleural cavity to accomplish rib fixation. The majority of cases for operative repair involved the third through the ninth ribs. Surgical access to the first and second ribs is limited. Ribs 10 through 12 rarely require operative treatment to restore chest wall mechanics. In patients with flail chest, associated injury to chest wall musculature and intercostal nerves is frequently encountered. Injuries to these structures are responsible for altered chest wall mechanics during breathing and can contribute to chronic pain.

Operative Technique

Over the past several decades multiple techniques for surgical stabilization of flail chest have been described in the literature. Today, no stabilization technique has been proved superior. Surgical options for chest wall stabilization include the use of plates (Judet struts), intramedullary devices (Kirschner wires), vertical bridging prostheses including metallic plates and prosthetic mesh, and sternal wires. Improved systems for operative fixation of rib fractures have been introduced recently and are commercially available. These technological advances include a U-shaped fixation plate (Acute Innovations) and a system utilizing curved plates and intramedullary stents (Synthes) specifically engineered for rib fractures. Both of these systems have been used with success in the operative fixation of rib fractures (Figs. 2 and 3). Operative treatment for pseudoarthrosis is more difficult and frequently requires extensive dissection and osteotomy.

Radiographic evaluation of the thorax is essential in patients being considered for operative fixation. In addition to conventional chest radiographs, computed tomography (CT) scanning of the chest provides excellent visualization of the extent of chest wall injury. Three-dimensional reconstructions of CT images are particularly useful for demonstrating the degree of chest wall deformity and the severity of fracture overlap and are essential for operative planning. In patients with chronic pain following rib fractures, CT imaging is particularly useful to demonstrate and localize pseudoarthroses (Fig. 4).

OUTCOMES

The scientific literature regarding surgical stabilization of flail chest is abundant. Unfortunately, the majority of this literature consists of nonrandomized and retrospective studies as well as case reports. The literature is consistent in identifying several advantages of operative fixation of flail segments. These advantages include a decreased

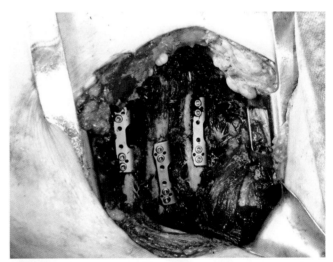

FIGURE 2 Operative treatment of flail chest with U-shaped fixation device specifically designed for the treatment of rib fractures.

length of mechanical ventilation, a shorter intensive care unit (ICU) length of stay, decreased rates of pneumonia, and decreased mortality rate. Disadvantages of operative fixation include the requirement for general anesthesia and extensive incisions, as well as occasional reports of postoperative chronic pain associated with implants. In some cases, this has necessitated removal of the implant. Ahmed and Mohyuddin described a 10-year retrospective review of chest wall injury involving 426 patients. Sixty-four of these patients had flail chest. In patients with flail chest, 26 of these patients received operative repair. The operative group was compared to 38 patients who received continued nonsurgical management. The operatively treated group had a lower mortality rate (8% versus 29%), faster weaning from mechanical ventilation, and decreased rates of tracheostomy, ICU length of stay, and pulmonary infections. Balci et al described 64 patients with flail chest who required mechanical ventilation. In this nonrandomized, retrospective study covering 9 years, operative treatment was performed in 27 patients. Compared to the group treated nonoperatively, the operative group had decreased days of mechanical ventilation, decreased length of stay, and decreased morbidity and mortality rates. Tanaka et al, performed a randomized prospective trial on patients with flail chest who required mechanical ventilation. Both surgical and nonsurgical groups were treated with

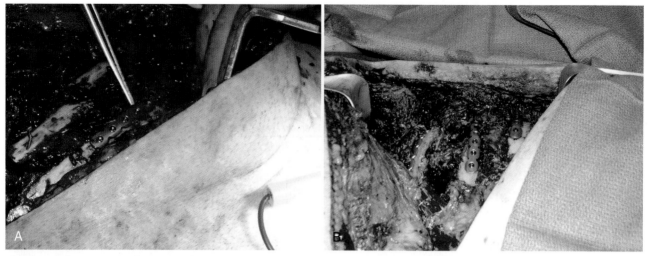

FIGURE 3   **A,** Intraoperative photograph of patient with flail chest. Severe overlap of a rib fractures is demonstrated. Operative fixation of rib fractures was accomplished by use of commercially available plates and locking screws specifically engineered to match the shape of the ribs. **B,** Operative stabilization of flail segment. Note the severe damage to the intercostal muscles.

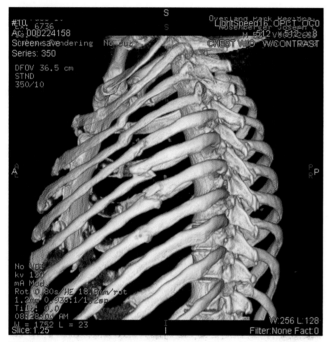

FIGURE 4   Computed tomography scan of the chest wall with three-dimensional reconstructions demonstrating chronic nonunion (pseudoarthrosis) of two ribs. Operative resection of pseudoarthroses and rib fixation resulted in marked improvement of chronic pain and disability.

a standardized protocol of mechanical ventilation, analgesia, and pulmonary toilet for 5 days. If patients were not stable for extubation after 5 days of mechanical ventilation, patients were randomized to either a surgical arm or continued nonoperative management. The surgical group had statistically significant fewer days of mechanical ventilation and decreased ICU length of stay. Additionally the group treated with operation had increased vital capacity after 1 month compared to the nonsurgical group. This difference was also statistically significant. More recently, Solberg et al described their experience with "chest wall implosion injury" due to side impact blunt trauma. Over a 7-year period this group evaluated 22 patients with severe lateral chest wall injuries. Nine patients were treated

operatively and the remaining patients were treated nonoperatively. Patients treated surgically were observed to have earlier extubation and decreased ICU length of stay. Collins et al have recently reported a 60-month retrospective review of 15 patients treated operatively compared to a nonoperative group of 18 patients. Operative and nonoperative groups were similar in age, gender, Injury Severity Score, and Glascow Coma Scale score. Operatively treated patients had decreased ventilator days (6.3 vs. 11.8, $P = .036$) and showed trends toward decreased ICU and total hospital length of stay. Our group has performed operative treatment in 36 patients over the last 5½ years. Twenty-four of these procedures were performed for acute flail chest and 12 were performed for chronic pain secondary to fracture nonunion causing severe disability. Results have been favorable, but in two cases, failure of implants required follow-up operations.

STERNAL FRACTURES

Sternal fractures usually occur in unrestrained drivers involved in deceleration motor vehicle crashes. Sternal fracture occurs in approximately 5% of patients with blunt chest wall injury. Rib fractures are associated with sternal fractures in up to 40% of patients. These injuries were once thought to be highly morbid with mortality rates in the range of 25% to 45% from associated injuries. More recent literature, however, has demonstrated lower morbidity and mortality rates. Sternal fractures do not usually require operative treatment. Nonunion of sternal fractures is rare. However, painful pseudoarthrosis or overlap deformities may require surgical repair. It is important to assess these patients for underlying cardiac, pulmonary, and thoracic spine injuries.

Patients with sternal fractures usually present with point tenderness over the sternum. Most sternal fractures are transverse and are located at the sternomanubrial junction. These fractures may be diagnosed by lateral chest radiograph or by CT scan of the thorax. The majority of these patients respond to supportive care consisting of analgesics and pulmonary toilet. Patients with significant overlap of fracture fragments may benefit from early operative repair. Operative repair results in markedly reduced pain, improves cosmesis, and improved pulmonary function in patients with overlapping sternal fractures.

CONCLUSIONS

Multiple rib fractures and flail chest cause significant morbidity and fatality following blunt trauma. The majority of patients with rib fractures and with flail chest do not require operative management. A carefully selected group of patients appears to benefit from early operative fixation. Some patients with chronic pain secondary to pseudoarthrosis also benefit from operative treatment. Technological advances that have resulted in the development of new implant systems have enhanced the surgeon's ability to repair flail segments.

Operative repair of sternal fractures is useful in a small group of patients. Operative treatment of chest wall injury should not be performed without the recognition that operative complications and device failure will be encountered.

For the chapter's Suggested Readings list, please visit the book at www.ExpertConsult.inkling.com.

TRACHEAL AND TRACHEOBRONCHIAL TREE INJURIES

Preston R. Miller and J. Wayne Meredith

Tracheobronchial injuries can lead to a multitude of sequelae, many of which are fatal. If they are diagnosed and treated appropriately, however, generally good outcomes can be obtained in patients surviving to present to a trauma center or other hospital. Such outcomes require a familiarity with signs and symptoms of injury, diagnostic techniques, appropriate airway management, and types of repair.

INCIDENCE AND MECHANISMS OF INJURY

Injury to the tracheobronchial tree is an uncommon but well-recognized complication of both penetrating and blunt chest trauma. Many victims die prior to emergency care from associated injuries to vital structures, hemorrhage, tension pneumothorax, or respiratory insufficiency. Thus, a substantial number of diagnoses are established only after death. At other times, the diagnosis is not readily apparent and is not made until late symptoms indicating tracheobronchial injury have developed. Thus, the true incidence of injury to the tracheobronchial tree is difficult to discern. In a review of autopsies of 1178 persons dying from blunt trauma to the chest, Bertelsen and Howitz found that tracheobronchial disruptions occurred in only 33 patients, for an incidence of 2.8%; 27 of these died immediately. In a review of survivors and nonsurvivors, Campbell reported on 15,136 patients diagnosed with blunt chest trauma. Forty-nine (0.3%) had a tracheobronchial injury. This series showed an extremely high mortality rate (67%), but did not describe the severity of associated injuries. Asensio in a review of the literature described the incidence in penetrating neck trauma with 331 of 4193 patients (8%) presenting with laryngotracheal injuries. Greater than 80% of blunt tracheobronchial ruptures occur within 2.5 cm of the carina. Main bronchi are injured in 86% of patients, distal bronchi in only 9.3%, and complex injuries are seen in 8%.

Penetrating injury is a straightforward mechanism and consists basically of the hole created by the path of a knife or bullet. Knife wounds occur almost exclusively in the cervical trachea, whereas gunshot wounds occur at any point along the tracheobronchial tree. Intrathoracic injury to the tracheobronchial tree occurs more commonly from blunt trauma but may also result from bullet wounds. These injuries occur at a higher incidence when the projectile crosses the mediastinum. Associated injuries to other mediastinal structures, including the heart, great vessels, and esophagus, are common and contribute significantly to the morbidity and mortality rates.

There are several mechanisms by which blunt trauma may injure the trachea and bronchus, including direct blows, sheer stress, and burst injury. A direct blow to the neck may produce a clothesline injury, crushing the cervical trachea against the vertebral bodies and transecting the tracheal rings or cricoid cartilage. Shear forces on the trachea create damage at its relatively fixed points, the cricoid and the carina. A common factor in burst injury along the tracheobronchial tree is rapid anteroposterior compression of the thorax. This compression causes a simultaneous expansion in the lateral thoracic diameter, and the negative intrapleural pressure stretches the lungs laterally along with the chest wall, thereby placing traction on the carina. When the plasticity of the tracheobronchial tree is exceeded, the lungs are pulled apart and the bronchi avulsed. Closure of the glottis before impact may convert the trachea into a rigid tube with increased intratracheal pressure, which may cause a linear tear or blowout of the membranous portion of the trachea or cause a complex disruption of the trachea and bronchi. As predicted by the law of LaPlace, this type of burst injury occurs where the airway diameter is greatest, usually within 2.5 cm of the carina, but may occur anywhere along the airway. A combination of these mechanisms is probably responsible for producing most injuries. Given the protected nature of these structures, a significant amount of high-energy transfer is usually required to create these injuries.

DIAGNOSIS

Presentation

A variety of clinical presentations result after injury to the tracheobronchial tree, with most depending on the severity and the location of the injury. Patients with cervical tracheal injuries may present with stridor and severe respiratory distress or with hoarseness, hemoptysis, or cervical subcutaneous emphysema. The presentation of thoracic tracheobronchial injury depends on whether the injury is confined to the mediastinum or communicates with the pleural space. Thoracic tracheobronchial injuries confined to the mediastinum usually present with massive pneumomediastinum. Pneumopericardium is occasionally described. Injuries that perforate into the pleural space usually create an ipsilateral pneumothorax that may or may not be under tension. A pneumothorax that persists despite adequate placement of a thoracostomy tube and has a continuous air leak is suggestive of tracheobronchial injury and bronchopleural fistula. Dyspnea may actually worsen after insertion of the chest tube due to the loss of total volume via the tube. Other radiographic clues to possible airway injury are seen with endotracheal intubation and show abnormal migration of the tube tip or overdistention of the endotracheal tube balloon outside the confines of the normal tracheal diameter.

Some retrospective reports show that up to two thirds of these intrathoracic tracheobronchial tears will go unrecognized longer than 24 hours and up to 10% of tracheobronchial tears will not produce any initial clinical or radiologic signs and are recognized months later after stricture occurs. Immediate intubation of patients with multisystem trauma can mask laryngeal or high cervical tracheal injuries and contribute to a delay in the diagnosis. Following tracheobronchial transection, the peribronchial connective tissues may remain intact and allow continued ventilation of the distal lung analogous to the way perfusion is maintained after traumatic aortic transection. If unrecognized, this injury heals with scarring and granulation tissue and may possibly create bronchial stenosis or obstruction. After a latent period, granulation tissue and stricture of the bronchus will develop. Distal to the stricture, pneumonia, bronchiectasis, abscesses, and even empyema can result. Complete obstruction without infection leads to prolonged atelectasis and diminished pulmonary function.

Although concomitant injury is the rule rather than the exception, patterns of associated injuries vary widely. Major vascular, cardiac, pulmonary, esophageal, bony thoracic, and neurologic injuries are common and reflect the site, magnitude, and mechanism of the trauma. The mechanisms of trauma may alert one to search for the presence of injury. For example, transcervical and transmediastinal penetrating injuries pose particular danger to the respective traversing structures. Associated injuries may be severe, and in at least one series, were responsible for all of the deaths. It has been suggested that corresponding rib fractures would be seen in all patients over 30 years old who had a rupture of the tracheobronchial tree, but this is not always true. The absence of a chest wall injury does not exclude serious chest trauma, but the presence of such an injury should alert one to investigate further for a major underlying injury. A high index of suspicion must be maintained in order to diagnose and treat an injury promptly and appropriately.

Evaluation

Diagnosis should be suspected based on the clinical history and the constellation of signs and symptoms previously listed. Evaluation of the patient with a suspected injury to the tracheobronchial tree is shown in the algorithm in Figure 1. Advances in computed tomography (CT) have resulted in reports of diagnosis and evaluation of injury with this technique. Three-dimensional reconstruction has been used to demonstrate the site and extent of injuries in case reports. Although tracheobronchial injury may be well demonstrated on CT in some cases, this diagnostic technique does not obviate the need for diagnostic bronchoscopy for diagnosis and planning of treatment. CT scan suggesting injury should prompt bronchoscopy for definitive diagnosis. In addition to visualization of possible tracheal injury on CT, indications for bronchoscopy include extensive

pneumomediastinum, refractory pneumothorax, or persistent air leak. Bronchoscopy, whether rigid or flexible, is the best studied means of establishing the diagnosis and determining the site, nature, and extent of the tracheobronchial disruption. Flexible bronchoscopy, the most commonly used method, may be performed without general anesthesia and can be done at the bedside. If the patient is not already intubated, it offers the potential for controlled insertion of a nasal or orotracheal tube while maintaining cervical stabilization. Rigid bronchoscopy does provide the advantage of the ability to provide ventilation. Lesions may be missed initially or their severity may be underestimated. These lesions may evolve into more obvious or severe injuries, and for this reason bronchoscopy should be liberally repeated as needed.

MANAGEMENT

Initial Management

Airway management, as with all injuries, is the first priority in the management of a patient with injury to the tracheobronchial tree. If the patient is maintaining his or her own airway and is ventilating adequately, a cautious approach of nonintervention is probably the best initial choice until further diagnostic workup can be completed or other life-threatening injuries can be stabilized. Careless handling or mishandling of the airway, such as inadvertently placing an endotracheal tube through a transected or ruptured airway into the soft tissue may compound the injury. If the injury is suspected, the airway should be evaluated carefully with the patient awake in order to plan for appropriate intervention. A bronchoscope may be passed into the trachea to evaluate for injury. In the case of less severe injuries, an endotracheal tube may be carefully passed distal to the injury over the bronchoscope. Blind nasal intubation or use of standard rapid sequence intubation (RSI)/endotracheal intubation should not be attempted in the case of known or suspected laryngotracheal injury because of the danger of creating a complete tracheal transection by pushing the tube against or through the injury.

Tracheostomy performed in the operating room is advocated by many as the safest and securest way to obtain airway control. This procedure may be done in the awake patient to avoid airway loss in those with adequate airway protection. If the trachea is completely transected, the distal trachea can usually be found in the superior mediastinum and grasped for insertion of a cuffed tube. The approach taken must vary with the resources and expertise available at each institution. One must also be aware that even though the airway is secured, the injury may still be worsened with mechanical ventilation if the injury is distal to the tube. Tube thoracostomies should be appropriately placed at this time and connected to suction. After the airway is controlled, there is time for an orderly identification of concurrent injuries, performance of interventions such as esophagoscopy, laryngoscopy, arteriography, and celiotomy as necessary and transport to definitive care areas. Guidelines for the management of tracheobronchial injuries are given in Figure 1.

Operative Management

As with emergency management of the airway, intraoperative management requires substantial coordination with the anesthesiologist. All of the same principles apply. After the airway is initially secured, manipulation during the repair creates additional challenges. A sterile anesthesia circuit and tube may be needed to pass off the table after regaining control of the airway at the level of transection, once the peritracheal connective tissue has been disrupted or entered for repair. If orotracheal intubation is performed, a single- or double-lumen endotracheal tube may be used. A double-lumen tube offers the benefit of independent lung ventilation but, because of the large

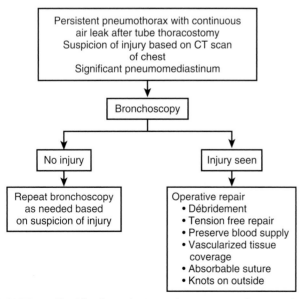

FIGURE 1 Algorithm for evaluation and management of suspected tracheobronchial injury. CT, Computed tomography.

size, it may create further disruption and is less desirable. A long, single-lumen tube may be passed beyond the area of injury for proximal levels of rupture, or for distal injuries, may be advanced into the contralateral main bronchus for single-lung ventilation. Intubation over a flexible bronchoscope adds safety and diagnostic capability to the procedure. If a tracheostomy is performed, it should be placed two to three rings caudally to high tracheal or laryngeal injuries and brought out through an incision separate from the surgical repair wound. Tracheostomy proximal to an injury is probably not necessary to protect the suture lines after repair of the thoracic trachea or major bronchus, and its prophylactic use is discouraged for distal tracheobronchial injuries. In the most difficult of cases, in which airway management is unsatisfactory, or during complex repairs, cardiopulmonary bypass may be instituted. The potential risks and benefits of this procedure must be weighed, including the need for systemic anticoagulation, especially in the multitrauma patient.

After repair, airway management ideally should be accomplished by removal of the endotracheal tube immediately following the operation. Otherwise, it should be removed and spontaneous respirations resumed as soon as the patient can breathe effectively. Occasionally, the patient will require ongoing positive-pressure ventilation, which may require creative techniques of critical care and ventilation, such as positioning of the endotracheal tube distal to the repair, single-lung ventilation, high-frequency ventilation, or extracorporeal membrane oxygenation. Every effort must be made to improve lung compliance by providing good pulmonary toilet, appropriate fluid management, and aggressive treatment of pneumonia.

Most extrathoracic airway injuries can be approached through a transverse collar incision. Occasionally, for added exposure, this incision may be extended up the neck for carotid repair or teed off (extend vertically downward from the collar incision) down the sternum, with partial or complete sternotomy being performed for more central exposure. Intrathoracic tracheal, right bronchial, and proximal left main bronchus injuries are best repaired through a right posterolateral thoracotomy at the fourth or fifth intercostal space. This approach avoids the heart and aortic arch. Complex or bilateral injuries should be approached through the right side of the chest for this same reason. Distal left bronchial injuries greater than 3 cm from the carina are approached through a left posterolateral thoracotomy in the fifth intercostal space.

Optimal repair includes adequate débridement of devitalized tissue, including cartilage, and primary end-to-end anastomosis of the clean tracheal or bronchial ends. This anastomosis can be accomplished free of tension by mobilizing anteriorly and posteriorly, thereby preserving the lateral blood supply. Tension may also be released with cervical flexion. This may be maintained postoperatively by securing the chin to the chest with a suture. Many investigators have recommended completion of the anastomosis with interrupted absorbable suture. We have found, however, that the use of a running, continuous, absorbable monofilament suture offers a secure repair and better visibility during construction of the anastomosis. The membranous portion may be repaired without tension and then brought together as the cartilaginous portion is begun. Sutures may be placed around or through the cartilage but must assure approximation of mucosa to mucosa. Tying the suture knots on the outside of the lumen helps prevent suture granulomas and subsequent stricture. To prevent subsequent leak and fistula formation, the suture line may be reinforced with a patch of pericardium, a vascularized pedicle from the pleura, intercostal muscle, strap muscles, omentum or vascularized pleura in late repairs to protect the repair and to aid in bronchial healing. During early repairs, the pleura is flimsy and usually not suitable as reinforcement. The vascularized pedicle of intercostal muscle offers both better protection and added healing potential for the repair. For this reason, the intercostal muscle should routinely be preserved during thoracotomy with the corresponding vein, artery, and nerve. This is accomplished by entering the chest through the bed of the rib. The rib may be preserved or sacrificed. An incision is made directly over the rib and the periosteum stripped off. At the superior border of the rib, the incision is carried

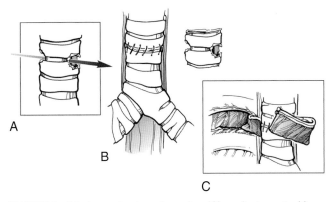

FIGURE 2 Injuries to the thoracic trachea (**A**) are best repaired by débridement of devitalized tissue and repair with absorbable suture (**B**). Débridement may include removal of several rings if necessary. The repair is protected with a vascularized pedicle of intercostal muscle (**C**).

through the posterior layer of the periosteum to enter the pleural space. The intercostal muscle is then divided from the ribs above and below and used as a flap to be wrapped around and tacked to the trachea. In this manner, viable tissue is placed between the repair and surrounding vital structures and blood supply in the area of the repair is increased, facilitating healing (Fig. 2).

Injuries to the cervical trachea may be managed by repair with or without tracheostomy. Simple anterior lacerations may undergo primary repair without tracheostomy if possible. Placement of a tracheostomy through these injuries should be avoided except in the case of short-term need for airway control via such a maneuver. In patients with severe injury to the proximal trachea, immediate repair with protective distal tracheostomy should be performed. Consideration should be given to stenting laryngeal injuries. Occasionally, the injury may cause extensive devitalization of the trachea and contamination of the field. In these rare instances, end tracheostomy, oversewing of the proximal trachea, and drainage may be the most prudent course of action. This allows for possible definitive repair later, after resolution of scarring and inflammation. However, attempts at primary repair should be exhausted first.

Nonoperative management has been described for some tracheal injuries. Criteria and techniques for this type of management are not well delineated, partially due to lack of data. For these reasons, nonoperative management of these patients should be undertaken only in highly selected patients by those with experience in this type of management.

OUTCOMES

The best results are obtained with early identification, débridement, and early primary repair of tracheobronchial injuries. Excellent anatomic and functional results should be expected with normal pulmonary function and voice characteristics after early repair. Early repair also results in fewer tracheal revisions to correct stenosis.

Reported mortality rate varies from 3.5% to 67% with most modern series reporting less than 30%. Most early fatalities are due to lack of airway control and to multiple associated injuries (e.g., vascular and esophageal injuries).

If there is a delay in diagnosis, repair should proceed as soon as the diagnosis is made or when practical after treatment of other life-threatening injuries. Regardless of the length of delay, reconstruction of the tracheobronchial tree should be attempted if there is no distal suppuration. Total bronchial disruption, if unrecognized, leads to complete occlusion and sterile atelectasis that may be amenable to repair later. The occluded segment is resected and repaired in a manner similar to that of the acute injury or as one would treat a benign stenosis. Although pulmonary function suffers with such delayed treatment, it can be expected to improve with repair. Incomplete bronchial obstruction ultimately leads to suppuration and irreversible pulmonary parenchymal destruction. Therapy in this case may require lobectomy or pneumonectomy, depending on the patient and degree of parenchymal damage. Thus, although bronchial rupture can be treated successfully in the acute or the delayed phase, early diagnosis and treatment minimize the risk of infection and other complications.

Although uncommon, tracheobronchial injuries will be encountered at most busy centers. These are challenging cases in which outcome depends on successful initial airway management as well as the level of suspicion by the astute clinician in investigating patients with signs and symptoms of the injury. These may range from severe presentations such as airway disruption or pneumothorax unresponsive to adequate tube thoracostomy to mediastinal emphysema or subtle findings on chest CT. Airway management efforts must be appropriate with overly aggressive techniques such as blind nasal intubation or RSI in those suspected of tracheal injury having potentially disastrous outcomes. With well-thought-out airway management and early operative intervention, good results can be expected in most cases.

For the chapter's Suggested Readings list, please visit the book at www.ExpertConsult.inkling.com.

OPERATIVE MANAGEMENT OF PULMONARY INJURIES: LUNG-SPARING AND FORMAL RESECTIONS

Juan A. Asensio, Patrizio Petrone, Alejandro Perez-Alonso, Thomas Templin, Shreya Shetty, Gerd Daniel Pust, Kirby R. Gross, and Marcus Balters

Chest injuries were reported in the Edwin Smith Surgical Papyrus as early as 3000 BC. Ancient Greek chronicles reveal examples of penetrating chest wounds and pulmonary injuries; the Greeks had anatomic knowledge and were cognizant of the thoracic structures and the position of the lungs inside the hemithoracic cavities. In Homer's *Iliad*, there is a vivid description of the death of Sarpedon by Patroclus: "[H]e penetrated him with his spear and while taking it out, his diaphragm came along with it. . . ." Homer emphasized the importance of the diaphragm, anatomically related to the lungs and the "beating heart." Although pneumothorax was a well-known entity, the Greeks realized the special problems related to thoracic penetration and considered open chest wounds fatal. Although the success of these early treatment modalities remains unknown, it seems that during Olympic competitions, physicians in ancient Greece were at least able to identify potentially lethal chest injuries, and most likely attempt their treatment.

Pausanias, a Greek traveler during the height of Roman rule, described a penetrating injury to the chest, inflicted to Creugas of Epidamnus by Damoxenos of Syracuse, with the presence of what seems to be an obvious pulmonary injury. Eusebius described in Evangelical Preparation, the match of Cleomedes of Astypalaia against Ikkos of Epidauros: "Why did they deify Cleomedes? For opening his opponent's rib, inserting his hand inside and eviscerating his lung."

Galen (130–200 AD), one of the most prominent physicians of antiquity, described packing of chest wounds in gladiators with thoracic and possibly lung injuries. A description of a lung injury was found in a treatise of Theodoric in 1226: "[W]hile I was living in Bolonia, a certain Domicellus, a Bolognan of normal birth, was cured by the hand of Master Hugo, part of his lung being torn away and Master Roand was there to witness it. . . ."

Even in the ancient world, most of the therapeutic modalities for chest wounds and traumatic pulmonary injuries were developed during wartime. In 1635, Alvar Nuñez Cabeza de Vaca, a Spaniard, while traveling from the Mexican northern territory to the capital of Nueva España (Mexico City), was captured by Indians. A wounded member of the tribe was brought to Cabeza de Vaca. With his assistant Esteban, Cabeza de Vaca made an incision to remove an arrowhead embedded in the man's chest, and sutured the wound. His innovation in surgical management won freedom from his captors for him and his friend.

During the 16th century, a few contributions were made to the management of traumatic pulmonary injuries. Ambroise Paré treated penetrating thoracic injuries by placing a scalding mixture of oil and treacle in the wound as the first dressing. John Hunter's initial experience dealing with penetrating thoracic injuries, caused by smooth-bore muskets firing round lead balls, led him to recognize that projectile velocity is a determinant factor dictating severity of the injury. Jean-Dominique Larrey and Pierre-Joseph Desault made important contributions to the surgical procedure known as débridement for the management of chest wall lacerations; however, the surgical treatment of intracavitary injuries did not evolve significantly during this time. Although Larrey described operative techniques for dealing with penetrating cardiac injuries, his contributions to the management of pulmonary injuries are not remarkable.

In 1822, William Beaumont, better known for Beaumont's gastric fistula observations than for his management of life-threatening chest injuries, treated a patient who sustained a gunshot wound to the chest and described the nature of the injury: "fracturing and carrying away the anterior half of the 6th rib, lacerating the lower portion of the left lobe of the lung, diaphragm and penetrating the stomach." During the 18th century, controversies emerged surrounding the benefit of surgical manipulation in the treatment of traumatic thoracic and pulmonary injuries. In Germany, Auenbrugger said: "opening the chest caused asphyxia because the lung collapsed." Dupuytren, a famous French surgeon, personally developed empyema in 1835. Although prepared to undergo a surgical intervention for its treatment, he decided, based on knowledge about Auenbrugger's description of "open-chest asphyxia," that "he would rather die at the hands of God than of the surgeons"; he survived for 12 days.

In the 1840s, the French Academy of Medicine studied the treatment of empyema to produce guidelines for its treatment based on war experiences. In the 18th century, Hewson called attention to the mechanism of pulmonary rupture after blunt trauma to the chest, and in 1886, Ashurt described rupture of thoracic viscera without rib fractures. In 1889, Holmes, consulting surgeon to St. George's Hospital in London, said: "All penetrating wounds to the chest, if small, should be closed at once and dressed antiseptically. If the wound is large and the lung evidently extensively injured, it is a better plan not to close the external wound completely, but to insert a large drainage tube to carry off the blood into an antiseptic dressing and so prevent its accumulation in the pleural cavity." In 1897, Duval described median sternotomy incision, which he described as a thoracolaparotomy, and in 1906, Spangaro, an Italian surgeon, described the left anterolateral thoracotomy incision. These incisions remain important contributions to the trauma surgical armamentarium to manage traumatic pulmonary injuries.

In 1916, Mentz reported removal of foreign matter from the lung and pointed out the relative safety of thoracotomy. The treatment of thoracic wounds in World War I started with many of the basic principles described in the 19th century. Specifically, hemothoraces were treated expectantly. Hemothoraces were not aspirated in the belief that tamponade of the injured lung had occurred. However, when surgery was required for thoracic injury, it was aggressive and largely successful following principles of airtight closure for wounds and removal of foreign bodies. In contrast to their surgical counterparts in the German Army, American surgeons with the Allied Expeditionary Force used positive-pressure anesthesia and a nitrous oxide/oxygen mixture, while practicing early thoracotomies following the principles for good exposure injuries, resection of affected anatomic structures, suture ligature, and irrigation of the thoracic cavity. Thoracotomies were closed airtight, traumatic wounds excised, and no drains were placed. This technique was associated with a 9% decrease in mortality rate. During this time Grey-Turner, Miles, Gask, Duval, and Bastianelli defined the technique of pulmonary decortication for the treatment of retained hemothorax after traumatic lung injuries (White).

In World War II, because of increased awareness of the high incidence of complications associated with hemothorax after wounding, an approach of aggressive conservatism for the management of hemothorax was adopted. Thoracentesis was used repeatedly until the thoracic cavity was totally evacuated. No air was permitted to enter the thoracic cavity. The injured lung was allowed to reexpand and tamponade bleeding, in hopes of returning pulmonary function to normal levels. Water-sealed intercostal catheters were placed in patients with tension pneumothoraces. Thoracotomy was reserved for continued hemorrhage or significant air leaks; additional indications included thoracoabdominal wounds, mediastinal injuries, traumatic thoracotomy, "the sucking chest wound," and removal of foreign bodies. Overall mortality rate with this treatment of war chest wounds was reported as 8%.

The Korean conflict created newer challenges for surgeons. Terrain characteristics and unfavorable tactical conditions, coupled with numerous incoming casualties, overloaded mobile army surgical hospitals (MASH units). Conservative management of traumatic hemothorax was thus a therapeutic strategy extremely suited to these conditions. Eighty percent of casualties from the Korean War were managed by repeated thoracentesis alone; however, there was limited experience with the use of chest tubes for drainage of hemothorax. The introduction of more advanced resuscitative techniques helped to compensate somewhat for the problems encountered with forward treatment.

In the Vietnam conflict, chest tube drainage for pulmonary injuries and hemothorax was widely practiced. Casualties were evacuated early at the hospital directly from combat. Well-organized "trauma centers" with cardiothoracic surgical capabilities operated under strict resuscitative protocols. Given the success of tube thoracostomy in this setting, early thoracotomy was indicated for fewer patients with hemothorax, although the former indications for its use remained. Tube thoracostomy remains the cornerstone for the treatment of traumatic hemothorax or pneumothorax, as well as for most traumatic injuries to the lung.

Recent awareness based on civilian and military experience has led to the recognition that complex procedures, such as anatomic resections and pneumonectomy in unstable patients, are poorly tolerated and potentially daunting. Critically injured patients often develop hypothermia, acidosis, coagulopathy, and dysrhythmias, resulting in irreversible physiologic injury. Control of such damage is also part of the trauma surgeon's armamentarium to deal with thoracic injuries. Progress in treating severe pulmonary injuries in critical patients has thus far relied on finding shorter, simpler, lung-sparing techniques, such as wedge and nonanatomic resections, and pneumonorrhaphy stapled and clamp tractotomy. In 1994, Wall et al described clamp pulmonary tractotomy to maximize pulmonary parenchymal salvage. Asensio and colleagues in 1997 described the technique of stapled pulmonary tractotomy. The applicability of stapled pulmonary tractotomy was subsequently confirmed as a safe, valuable, lung-sparing procedure in a series of 40 patients. Subsequently, Cothren and associates reported that lung-sparing techniques are associated with improved morbidity and mortality rates when compared with resectional techniques.

Rapid progress and advancement in technology, including endoscopic instrumentation anesthetic techniques, have revolutionized thoracic surgery and ushered in the era of video-assisted thoracoscopic surgery (VATS). VATS has provided the trauma surgeon with an alternative method for accurate and direct evaluation of the lung parenchyma, mediastinum, and diaphragmatic injuries, with the advantage of simultaneously allowing definitive treatment of such injuries. VATS also has been demonstrated to be an accurate, safe, and reliable operative therapy for complications of lung trauma, including posttraumatic pleural collections.

INCIDENCE

The true incidence of pulmonary injuries is unknown and difficult to estimate from the literature. The chest, in forming such a large and exposed part of the body, is particularly vulnerable to injury. The anatomic complex formed by the lungs, pulmonary vessels, and bronchial tree so completely fills the thorax that penetration or contusion of the chest rarely occurs without injury. The reported incidence of pulmonary injuries in the civilian arena varies according to authors and institutions. In 1979, Graham et al reported a 1-year experience, consisting of 373 patients sustaining penetrating pulmonary injuries; of these, 91 patients (24%) underwent thoracotomy, although operative interventions on the lung itself were only required in 45 (12%) patients. In this series, the mere presence of posttraumatic hemothorax or pneumothorax was considered by the authors as clear evidence of traumatic pulmonary injury, which justified the inclusion of these cases in the study.

In 1988, Robison et al described a 13-year civilian experience in the management of penetrating pulmonary injuries in 1168 patients sustaining penetrating chest injuries; however, only 68 patients required thoracotomy to manage traumatic lung injury. In 1988, Thompson et al reported a 5-year experience of 2608 patients with thoracic trauma. Of the total, 1663 patients sustained injuries from blunt trauma and only 11 (0.7%) required thoracotomy; 945 sustained penetrating injuries and 15 (1.6%) required thoracotomy. Wiencek and Wilson reported a series consisting of 161 patients requiring thoracotomy for civilian penetrating pulmonary injuries during a 7-year period, which translates to 23 cases per year. Wagner et al described a 4-year experience of 104 patients with significant blunt chest trauma; 115 pulmonary lacerations were detected in 75 patients, for an incidence of 72%; 86% of these injuries were diagnosed by computed tomography (CT) scan, and 14% were detected by surgery. Based on both radiologic and surgical findings, the authors reported a higher incidence of traumatic pulmonary injuries compared with other clinical series that report their results based only on surgical findings.

In 1993, Tominaga and colleagues described a 7-year single institutional experience of 2934 patients sustaining both blunt and penetrating chest trauma; 347 patients (12%) required thoracotomy, and 12 (3.5%) in this subgroup required pulmonary resections. The mechanism of injury was blunt in 25%, and penetrating in 75% of cases, for an incidence of 0.04%, translating into 1.7 cases per year. Wagner and associates in 1996 described an 8-year experience of 1804 patients admitted with chest trauma; 269 (15%) underwent thoracotomy, with 55 requiring operative interventions specifically for their pulmonary injuries, for an incidence of 3%, and an average of 6.9 patients per year.

In 1997, Stewart et al reported a 10-year experience consisting of 2455 patients with both penetrating and blunt chest trauma; 183

(7.4%) patients required thoracotomy, and 32 (17.4%) required pulmonary resection, which translates to 3.2 cases per year. Inci and colleagues in 1998 reported a 5-year experience consisting of 755 patients sustaining penetrating chest trauma, of whom 61 (8.1%) required thoracotomy; however, specific operative interventions for penetrating pulmonary injuries were required in only 3 patients (4.9%), for an incidence of 0.6 case per year.

In 1998, Wall et al described a 3-year experience of 236 patients requiring thoracotomy for penetrating chest trauma; 90 (38%) required repair or resection to manage their pulmonary lacerations, for an average of 30 patients per year. In 2001, Karmy-Jones and colleagues reported the findings of a multicenter 4-year review of five Level I trauma centers. A total of 43,119 patients were admitted for penetrating thoracic trauma, and 290 (2.8%) required thoracotomy; surprisingly, 115 patients (40%) in this subgroup underwent some type of lung resection. In a series of 4087 patients admitted for chest trauma, Cothren and associates reported that 416 patients (10%) patients required thoracotomy and 36 (9%) required surgical interventions on the lung, for an incidence of 1% and an average of 3.3 patients per year.

In the most recent report dealing with complex civilian lung injuries, in 2006, Asensio et al described 101 patients requiring thoracotomy for complex penetrating pulmonary injuries. In the military arena, Zakharia et al in 1985 reported 1992 casualties during the fighting in Lebanon; 1422 patients underwent thoracotomy for hemodynamic instability secondary to penetrating chest trauma, and pulmonary injuries were present in 210 (15%) patients, for an incidence of 11%. In 1997, Petricevic and associates reported on 2547 casualties from the most recent Balkan war experience. During a period of 4 years, 424 patients (16%) sustained both blunt and penetrating chest wounds; among these patients, 81 (19%) underwent thoracotomy for pulmonary injury, for an incidence of 20 cases per year.

ETIOLOGY

Most patients requiring thoracotomy for pulmonary injuries will have suffered penetrating mechanisms of injury—gunshot wounds, stab wounds, and shotgun wounds. Much less common are blunt thoracic injuries requiring operative intervention. In 2003, Huh et al reported a gradual rise in the incidence of blunt thoracic injuries, mostly from motor vehicle collisions requiring operative intervention, from 3% before 1994, to 12% in the latter period. In the series by Tominaga and colleagues, blunt mechanism of injury accounted for 25% of all pulmonary injuries requiring surgical treatment. In the civilian arena, gunshot wounds represent the major penetrating mechanism for patients requiring surgical treatment; several authors have reported that gunshot wounds account for 33% to 80% of cases with penetrating pulmonary injuries, and stab wounds account for 17% to 67% of these injuries. Karmy-Jones et al, in a multicenter study on managing traumatic lung injuries, reported an increasing rate of thoracotomy among these patients. Other mechanisms such as impalement and shotgun wounds are reported with a lower frequency of 1% to 5% of cases.

In a series from 2006, Asensio et al reported on 101 patients who required thoracotomy for treatment of civilian penetrating pulmonary injuries. In this series, gunshot wounds accounted for most cases (72% of cases); stab wounds and other mechanisms (e.g., impalement, shotgun wounds) accounted for 33% and 5% of cases, respectively. In the military arena, Zakharia et al reported from the experience in Lebanon that high-velocity gunshot wounds and shelling in urban battles were the major mechanisms of pulmonary injuries. Petricevic and colleagues reported the cause of pulmonary injuries during the war in Croatia, where explosive wounds prevailed (59%), followed by gunshot wounds (both high and low velocity, 37%), whereas other types of wounds—stabbing and falling—accounted for only 4% of cases.

CLASSIFICATION

The American Association for the Surgery of Trauma Organ Injury Scaling Committee (AAST-OIS) described the lung injury scale in 1994. This scale facilitates clinical research and provides a common nomenclature by which trauma surgeons may describe lung injuries and their severity. The grading scheme is fundamentally an anatomic description, scaled from 1 to 5, describing the least to the most severe injury. Thus far, studies have correlated injury grade with mortality rate for this study (Table 1).

DIAGNOSIS

The diagnosis of traumatic pulmonary injuries is established by physical examination and adjunctive diagnostic modalities.

Physical Examination

The clinical presentation of patients who sustain pulmonary injuries ranges from hemodynamic stability to cardiopulmonary arrest. Physical examination yields a wealth of diagnostic information, which is used to indicate emergent interventions on these patients.

Patients with pulmonary injuries may present with symptoms and signs of pneumohemothorax or an open pneumothorax with partial loss of the chest wall. They may also present with a tension hemothorax or pneumothorax, or rarely, with a pneumomediastinum upon auscultation. Hamman's crunch—a systolic crunch—may be detected upon auscultation in these patients. Similarly, they may also present with a pneumopericardium detected by auscultating Brichiteau's windmill bruit (bruit de moulin). Patients with penetrating pulmonary injuries may rarely present with true hemoptysis. Occasionally, these patients present with symptoms and signs of an associated cardiac injury.

During the evaluation of these patients, the trauma surgeon must be cognizant that the thoracic cavity is composed of both right and left hemithoracic cavity as well as the anterior, posterior, and superior

TABLE 1: Lung Injury: Organ Injury Scale, American Association for the Surgery of Trauma

Grade*	Injury Type	Description†
I	Contusion	Unilateral, <1 lobe
II	Contusion Laceration	Unilateral, single lobe Simple pneumothorax
III	Contusion Laceration Hematoma	Unilateral, >1 lobe Persistent (>72 hours), air leak from distal airway Nonexpanding intraparenchymal
IV	Laceration Hematoma Vascular	Major (segmental or lobar) air leak Expanding intraparenchymal Primary branch intrapulmonary vessel disruption
V	Vascular	Hilar vessel disruption
VI	Vascular	Total, uncontained transection of pulmonary hilum

*Advance one grade for multiple injuries up to grade III. Hemothorax is scored under thoracic vascular organ injury scale.
†Based on most accurate assessment at autopsy, operation, or radiologic study.

mediastinum, as often missiles or other wounding agents may traverse one or more of these cavities. Similarly, missile trajectories are often unpredictable and frequently create secondary missiles if they impact on hard bony structures (ribs, sternum, spine), thus creating the potential for associated injuries and greater damage.

Adjunctive Diagnostic Modalities

Adjunctive diagnostic modalities are divided into noninvasive diagnostic modalities and invasive diagnostic modalities.

Noninvasive Diagnostic Modalities

These diagnostic modalities include trauma ultrasound (focused assessment with sonography for trauma [FAST]), chest radiograph, CT, and electrocardiogram (ECG).

Trauma Ultrasound

Trauma ultrasound is performed as part of the secondary survey of the trauma patient, and remains a valuable diagnostic modality used to detect associated cardiac injuries as well as the presence of associated abdominal injuries in patients sustaining isolated chest trauma and multiply injured patients. In 2004, Kirkpatrick et al reported the use of sonography for detecting traumatic pneumothoraces and described this diagnostic strategy as extended FAST (E-FAST). Normal thoracic sonograms reveal comet-tail artifacts, originating from the sliding and reappositioning of the visceral pleura onto the parietal pleura during the ventilatory effort; posttraumatic pneumothoraces are diagnosed when comet-tail artifacts are absent. The authors enrolled 225 patients in this study, and concluded that E-FAST has comparable specificity (99.1% vs. 98.7%) to chest radiography, but was more sensitive (58.9% vs. 48.8%) for the detection of posttraumatic pneumothoraces. Knudson and colleagues in 2004 performed 328 thoracic evaluations in trauma patients and described thoracic sonography having a specificity of 99.7%, a negative predictive value of 99.7%, and an accuracy of 99.4% when used for diagnosing posttraumatic pneumothorax. However, thoracic sonography was noted to be more sensitive (100% vs. 88.9%) and with a higher positive-predictive value (100% vs. 88.9%) when used to diagnose posttraumatic pneumothoraces in patients sustaining penetrating versus blunt trauma, although the specificity (100% vs. 99.7%), negative-predictive value (100% vs. 99.7%), and accuracy (100% vs. 99.3%) are comparable. On the basis of these findings, Knudson et al concluded that ultrasound is a reliable modality for the diagnosis of pneumothorax in the injured patient, and thus, it may serve as an adjunct or precursor to routine chest radiography in the evaluation of injured patients.

Sonography has also been employed to detect the presence of traumatic hemothorax. The technique for this examination is similar to evaluate the upper quadrants of the abdomen. The transducer is advanced to identify the hyperechoic diaphragm and to evaluate both right and left supradiaphragmatic spaces for the presence or absence of fluid. Sisley and associates in 1998 evaluated 360 patients with suspected blunt or penetrating torso trauma, with 40 posttraumatic effusions, 39 (98%) of which were detected by sonography and 37 (93%) by chest radiography. The authors concluded that sonography is more sensitive (97.5% vs. 92.5%) than chest radiography for detecting posttraumatic effusions; however, a specificity of 97.5% in both studies is comparable. On the basis of these data, the authors concluded that surgeon-performed thoracic sonography is as accurate as, but significantly faster than, supine portable chest radiography for the detection of traumatic effusion.

Chest Radiograph

A standard supine posteroanterior chest radiograph is the most frequently used diagnostic modality in patients who sustain traumatic lung injury. Radiologic diagnosis of traumatic pulmonary injuries by chest radiography is based on the presence of pneumothorax, pleural fluid collections, intrapulmonary hematomas, traumatic pneumatoceles, and pulmonary parenchymal contusions. Although chest radiography has been demonstrated to be 99% specific, it is a relatively insensitive test (49%) for the detection of posttraumatic pneumothorax; chest radiography has been demonstrated to possess a sensitivity of 93% and a specificity of 99.7% to detect posttraumatic pleural effusions.

When compared with CT, the conventional chest radiograph underestimates or overlooks both parenchymal and pleural injuries, and has poor ability to determine the magnitude of pulmonary parenchymal compromise or pneumothorax size. Wagner et al demonstrated that pulmonary parenchymal lacerations are frequently missed by chest radiography.

Computed Tomography

CT is found to be more sensitive than chest radiography for diagnosing traumatic pulmonary injuries. The most common types of abnormalities seen on CT scans include parenchymal lacerations, posttraumatic hemothorax, posttraumatic pneumothorax, atelectasis, subcutaneous emphysema, pneumopericardium, and hemopericardium, and chest wall fractures. Additional diagnostic information related to the traumatic injury to the lung is usually supplied by CT scans, which can reliably detect the presence and extent of subtle or considerable parenchymal contusion.

As described by Karaaslan et al in 1995, CT scans are also able to detect the presence of associated thoracic and mediastinal vascular injuries, injuries to other thoracic great vessels, and extrathoracic injuries, associated cervical spine injuries, and intra-abdominal injuries in about 30% of cases.

Electrocardiogram

Nonspecific ECG abnormalities are often seen in trauma patients; some of these changes such as sinus tachycardia, and ventricular and atrial extrasystoles are related to systemic factors such as pain, decreased intravascular volume, hypoxia, abnormal concentration of serum electrolytes, and changes in sympathetic or parasympathetic tone; however, in some cases, ECG may exhibit changes caused by associated injuries—most commonly penetrating or blunt cardiac trauma consisting of findings related to myocardial injury like new Q waves, ST-T segmental elevation or depression, conduction disorders such as right bundle branch block, fascicular block, atrioventricular (AV) nodal conduction disorders, and other arrhythmias (atrial fibrillation, ventricular tachycardia, ventricular fibrillation, sinus bradycardia, and atrial tachycardia).

ECG findings may suggest the presence of pericardial tamponade in patients sustaining chest trauma and traumatic lung injuries. Low QRS voltage is closely associated with the presence of a large or moderate pericardial tamponade (sensitivity of 0%–42%, specificity of 86%–97%), although PR segment depression and electrical alternans commonly are also present in this setting.

Invasive Diagnostic Modalities

Chest Tubes

Chest tube placement may be diagnostic as well as therapeutic. After entering the pleural cavity, a finger is inserted, and depending on the position of the tract, the trauma surgeon may palpate the lung surface for the presence of contusion, the surface of the diaphragm for lacerations, and the pericardial sac to detect the presence of tamponade.

The nature and amount of the material draining from the tube are also important. The amount of blood evacuated upon initial placement of the chest tube may indicate the need for thoracotomy; persistent drainage of blood through the tube thoracostomy obligates the trauma surgeon to reassess the need for surgical intervention. Drainage of gastrointestinal contents implies an esophageal, gastric, or intestinal injury associated with a diaphragmatic laceration. An air leak implies an underlying lung laceration, and large air leaks may indicate bronchial disruption.

ASSOCIATED INJURIES

Associated injuries are commonly seen in conjunction with penetrating pulmonary injuries. From 5% to 65% of patients sustaining traumatic injuries to the lung present with associated thoracic or extrathoracic injuries; the average number of associated injuries reported in the literature ranges from 0.5 to 1.9 injuries per patient. The presence of an associated injury is an important determinant of outcome. Gasparri et al reported the presence of associated cardiac injury and the need for laparotomy for associated abdominal injuries as factors determining the mortality rate, and Asensio et al determined that the presence of an associated cardiac injury is an independent predictor of outcome.

Graham et al reported the presence of 73 associated thoracic injuries among 91 patients requiring thoracotomy for the management of penetrating pulmonary injuries, for an average of 0.8 associated thoracic injuries per patient; the most commonly injured organs included the heart, at 27%; intercostals, 16%; subclavian vessels, 9%; and superior vena cava, 7%. The authors also reported the presence of 175 associated abdominal injuries among 89 of the patients requiring laparotomy, for an average of 1.9 associated abdominal injuries per patient; the most frequently injured organs were the liver, 21%; spleen, 19%; stomach, 14%; and colon, 10%.

Robison and colleagues described the presence of 14 associated injuries in 11 of 28 patients sustaining traumatic lung injuries requiring thoracotomy and pulmonary resection or hilar repairs. In this series, the authors reported a morbidity rate of 39% and an average number of 1.3 injuries per patient. Cardiac injuries were present in 11% of cases; the remaining associated injuries follow: thoracic great vessel, 7%; spinal cord, 7%; hepatic, 7%; pancreatic, 4%; colonic, 4%; spleen, 4%; gastric, 4%; and peripheral nerve, 4%.

Wiencek and Wilson described the presence of 35 major associated injuries among 19 of 25 patients with central lung injuries, for an incidence of 76% and an average number of 1.4 injuries per patient, with the heart (26%) and thoracic great vessels (21%) as the most frequently injured organs. Associated abdominal injuries requiring laparotomy were found in 58% of cases. Tominaga and associates reported 10 associated injuries among 12 patients who required thoracotomy and lung resection for traumatic pulmonary injuries, for an average of 0.8 injuries per patient. Associated injuries included head injuries at 17%; intra-abdominal injuries requiring laparotomy, 33%; cardiac injuries, 25%; and great vessel injury, 8%. Petricevic et al reported a 4.5% incidence of associated injuries to visceral organs in patients sustaining chest trauma during the war in Croatia. Stewart and colleagues described the presence of 30 associated injuries in 21 of 32 patients (65%) requiring thoracotomy and pulmonary resection for traumatic injuries to the lung, for an average of 1.4 injuries per patient; these injuries were stratified into abdominal, 30%; musculoskeletal, 30%; neurologic, 17%; cardiac, 7%; and other injuries, 17%.

Gasparri et al reported associated injuries in 41 (58%) of 70 patients requiring thoracotomy for penetrating lung injuries, with heart (20%), diaphragm (17%), and liver (11%) as the most common organs involved. Karmy-Jones and colleagues reported 42 associated thoracic injuries among 115 patients requiring thoracotomy and lung resection for penetrating chest trauma, for an average of 0.36 injuries per patient.

Cothren et al reported 27 associated injuries in a series of 36 patients requiring thoracotomy for severe pulmonary injuries, for an average of 0.75 injuries per patient. Associated thoracic injuries were present in 33% of patients, and associated extrathoracic injuries represented 66% of the total. Huh and colleagues reported that 28% of patients requiring operative interventions on the lung required a concomitant laparotomy for intra-abdominal injuries.

Asensio and associates in 2006 reported a 169-month, single-center experience consisting of 101 patients requiring thoracotomy

for penetrating pulmonary injuries. In this series, there were 193 associated injuries for an average of 1.9 injuries per patient. There were 39 (22%) associated injuries to the thoracic organs, and 154 (79.7%) associated extrathoracic injuries. The most common thoracic organs involved were the heart (23.7%) and thoracic great vessels (14.8%), and the most common extrathoracic organs were the diaphragm (42.5%), liver (25.7%), and stomach (18.8%).

ANATOMIC LOCATION OF INJURY

The anatomic location of pulmonary injuries is not commonly reported in either clinical or radiologic series. Graham et al reported a predominance of left-sided lung injuries at 52% compared with right-side lung injuries at 36%, with bilateral injuries present in 12% of patients. Wiencek and Wilson, in a series focusing on central/hilar traumatic lung injuries, reported an incidence of 15% of hilar traumatic disruptions among 161 patients sustaining penetrating lung trauma. Robison and colleagues described the anatomic location of traumatic lung injuries requiring resective techniques for surgical management as follows: left lower lobe, 28%; right middle lobe, 22%; left upper lobe, including lingula, 22%; right upper lobe, 17%; and right lower lobe, 17%. The left pulmonary artery (25%) was the most commonly injured pulmonary vessel, followed by the right pulmonary artery (14%), right pulmonary vein (11%), and left pulmonary vein (7%). The results of this series showed that traumatic injuries presented a slight right versus left preference, although left-sided vascular injuries were more common compared with right-sided pulmonary vascular injuries, at 56% and 44%, respectively.

Huh and associates reported that the location of the traumatic pulmonary injuries requiring operative intervention showed a slight predilection for the left side (50%), followed by the right side (47%) and bilateral injuries (3%). Asensio et al, in a report consisting of 101 patients requiring thoracotomy for complex penetrating pulmonary injuries, found the left lung to be a predominant location of penetrating injuries compared with the right lung (65% vs. 35%, respectively). The authors also reported the specific location of these injuries: left lower lobe, 40%; left upper lobe, 21%; right middle lobe, 19%; right lower lobe, 11%; lingula, 5%; and right upper lobe, 5%.

MANAGEMENT

Although recent reports of thoracic injuries in military actions have advocated early thoracotomy and aggressive management of pulmonary injuries with resection as opposed to the more conservative and traditional treatment with tube thoracostomy, the vast majority of thoracic trauma patients—75% to 85%—are successfully managed with placement of chest tubes and supportive measures. The combination of lung expansion, low intravascular pressures, and high concentration of tissue thromboplastin provides adequate hemostasis in most instances; however, 9% to 15% of patients require thoracotomy to achieve surgical hemostasis or effect necessary repairs. Of patients undergoing thoracotomy for hemorrhage, 3% to 30% have been shown to require lung resection for control of injuries.

The indications for thoracotomy in patients sustaining penetrating pulmonary injuries include the following:

- Cardiopulmonary arrest
- Impeding cardiopulmonary arrest upon arrival at the emergency department (ED)
- Evacuation of 1000 to 1500 mL of blood upon initial placement of chest tube
- Evacuation of more than 1000 mL of blood upon placement of chest tube and ongoing blood loss
- Tension hemothorax
- Large retained hemothorax
- Massive air leak from the chest tube

Surgical Decisions

For patients who present in cardiopulmonary arrest, it is mandatory to proceed to ED thoracotomy (EDT). The placement of a chest tube in the right hemithoracic cavity is required. This may need to be extended into bilateral anterolateral thoracotomies. For patients who present with systolic blood pressure lower than 80 mm Hg, it is mandatory to insert bilateral chest tubes and resuscitate per the Advanced Trauma Life Support protocol. If the patient remains unstable, he or she should be immediately transported to the operating room (OR). If the patient stabilizes, a thorough workup should be instituted. For patients presenting with thoracoabdominal injuries, insertion of a chest tube or tubes is recommended. In patients who sustain abdominal and thoracic or thoracoabdominal injuries and require exploratory laparotomy, the trauma surgeon should reassess the need for thoracotomy in the operating room.

Operative Management

Emergency Department Thoracotomy

If the patient arrives at the ED in cardiopulmonary arrest, it is necessary to immediately proceed to EDT. The objectives of EDT follow:

- Resuscitation of agonal patients with penetrating cardiothoracic injuries
- Evacuation of pericardial tamponade if there is an associated cardiac injury
- Direct repair of cardiac lacerations if there is an associated cardiac injury
- Control of thoracic hemorrhage
- Prevention of air embolism
- Cardiopulmonary resuscitation, which may produce up to 60% of the normal ejection fraction
- Control of the pulmonary hemorrhage
- Cross-clamp of pulmonary hilum
- Cross-clamp of descending thoracic aorta

The technique for EDT is described here as it pertains to its use for patients sustaining penetrating pulmonary injuries arriving in cardiopulmonary arrest and should only be performed by surgeons who have had appropriate training in the performance of this procedure:

1. Immediate endotracheal intubation and venous access are performed; simultaneous use of rapid infusion techniques complements the resuscitative process. Chest tube insertion in the right hemithoracic cavity is also simultaneous.
2. The left arm is elevated and the thorax is prepped rapidly with an antiseptic solution.
3. A left anterolateral thoracotomy commencing at the lateral border of the left sternocostal junction and inferior to the nipple is carried out and extended laterally to the latissimus dorsi. In females, the breast is retracted cephalad.
4. The incision is carried rapidly through skin, subcutaneous tissue, and the pectoralis major and serratus anterior muscles until the intercostal muscles are reached.
5. The three layers of these interdigitated muscles are sharply transected with scissors. The pleura is then opened.
6. Occasionally, the left fourth and fifth costochondral cartilages are transected to provide greater exposure.
7. A Finochietto retractor is then placed to separate the ribs. At this time, the trauma surgeon should evaluate the extent of hemorrhage present within the left hemithoracic cavity. An exsanguinating hemorrhage with almost complete loss of the patient's intravascular volume is a reliable indicator of poor outcome.
8. The left lung is then elevated medially and the descending thoracic aorta is located immediately as it enters the abdomen via the aortic hiatus. The aorta should be palpated to assess the status of the remaining blood volume.

9. The descending thoracic aorta can be temporarily occluded against the bodies of the thoracic vertebrae.
10. Before cross-clamping the descending thoracic aorta, a combination of sharp and blunt dissection commencing at both the superior and inferior borders of the aorta is performed, so that the aorta may be carefully encircled between the thumb and index fingers.
11. Inexperienced surgeons usually commit the error of clamping the esophagus, which is located superior to the aorta. A nasogastric tube previously placed can serve as a guide in distinguishing the esophagus from the often somewhat empty thoracic aorta.
12. A Crafoord-DeBakey aortic cross-clamp should then be placed to occlude the aorta.
13. If a cardiac injury is present, the pericardium is then opened longitudinally above the phrenic nerve; pericardial clot and blood are evacuated and the cardiac injury repaired.
14. If a pulmonary hilar hematoma or active hemorrhage is present, cross-clamping of the pulmonary hilum with a Crafoord-DeBakey cross-clamp may be necessary.
15. If a parenchymal laceration is detected, it should be clamped with Duval clamps.
16. If the initial injury is located in the right hemithoracic cavity, or the previously inserted chest tube returns large quantities of blood, or injury is encountered in the contralateral hemithoracic cavity, the sternum is transected sharply and the left anterolateral thoracotomy is then converted to bilateral anterolateral thoracotomies.
17. Ligation of one or both internal mammary arteries may be necessary if the left anterolateral thoracotomy has been extended to the right hemithoracic cavity.
18. Aggressive ongoing resuscitation is needed with warm, pressure-driven fluids via rapid infusers while this procedure is ongoing.
19. Defibrillation with internal paddles may be needed, delivering 10 to 50 J.
20. Epinephrine may also be administrated into the right or left ventricle or systemically.
21. If air embolism is suspected, the ventricles will need to be aspirated with 16-G needles.
22. Occasionally the use of a temporary pacemaker might be needed but outcomes are very poor.
23. If the patient is successfully resuscitated, immediate and expedient transportation to the operating room is mandated for definitive repair of the pulmonary injury or injuries.

Effects of Pulmonary Hilar Cross-Clamping

Positive These effects include: (1) preservation and redistribution of remaining blood volume, (2) improvement in perfusion to contralateral uninjured lung, (3) control of hilar hemorrhage, and (4) prevention of air emboli.

Negative These effects include: (1) rendering the cross-clamped lung ischemic, (2) imposing a great afterload onto the right ventricle (RV), and (3) decrease in oxygenation and ventilation to cross-clamped lung.

Unknown These effects include the length of safe cross-clamp time and incidence of pulmonary reperfusion injury to both the injured and uninjured lung.

Effects of Thoracic Aortic Cross-Clamping

Positive These effects follow: (1) preservation and redistribution of remaining blood volume, (2) improvement of coronary/carotid arterial perfusion, (3) reduction of subdiaphragmatic blood flow, (4) increases in the left ventricular stroke work index (LVSWI), and (5) increased myocardial contractility.

Negative These effects include: (1) decreased blood flow to the abdominal viscera to approximately 10%, (2) decreased renal blood flow to approximately 10%, (3) decreased blood flow to the spinal cord to approximately 10%, (4) induction of anaerobic metabolism, (5) induction of hypoxia/lactic acidosis, (6) imposition of a great afterload onto the left ventricle (LV), and (7) in rare cases, paraplegia.

Unknown These effects include: (1) the length of safe cross-clamp time and (2) incidence of reperfusion injury.

Operating Room Thoracotomy

Instruments

Special instruments are needed to access the thoracic cavity as well as to retract, manipulate, and surgically intervene in the thoracic structures and lung (Fig. 1). These instruments include the following:

- Doyen costal elevators (Fig. 2)
- Alexander periosteotome (see Fig. 2)
- Cameron-Haight periosteal elevators (see Fig. 2)
- Bethune rib shears (Fig. 3)
- Stille-Horsley bone-cutting rongeurs (see Fig. 3)
- Lebsche knife and mallet (see Fig. 3)
- Rib raspatory
- Finochietto retractor

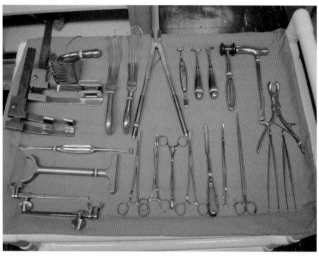

FIGURE 1   Thoracic instrument tray.

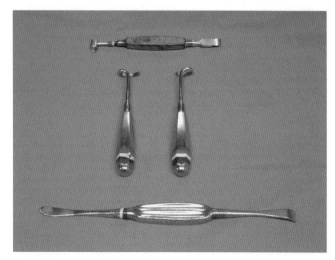

FIGURE 2   Alexander periosteotome, right and left Doyen costal elevators, and Cameron-Haight periosteal elevator.

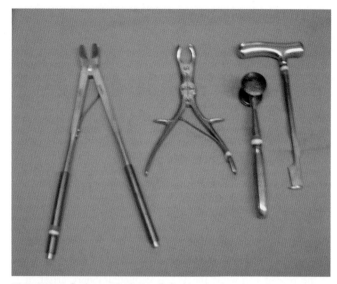

FIGURE 3   Bethune rib shears, Stille-Horsley bone-cutting rongeurs, and Lebsche knife and mallet.

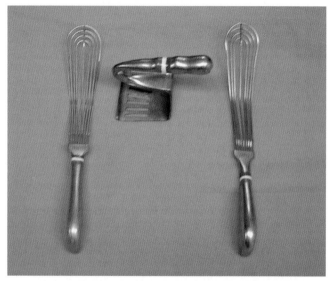

FIGURE 4   Allison lung retractors and Davidson scapular retractor.

- Davidson scapular retractor (Fig. 4)
- Allison lung retractors (see Fig. 4)
- Semb lung retractors
- Nelson lung dissecting lobectomy scissors (Fig. 5)
- Metzenbaum long dissecting scissors (see Fig. 5)
- Tuttle thoracic tissue forceps (see Fig. 5)
- Duval lung forceps (Fig. 6)
- Davidson pulmonary vessel clamps
- Sarot bronchus clamps
- Bailey's rib approximator (Fig. 7)
- Berry sternal needle holder
- Vascular clamps

Adjuncts

Double-lumen tubes are invaluable adjuncts in the management of penetrating pulmonary injuries (Fig. 8). Although more difficult to insert by the anesthesiologists, double-lumen tubes are designed to ventilate the right or left lung selectively. There are two types of double-lumen tubes; one is designed for the left main bronchus and the other for the right main bronchus. By inflating the balloon that occludes either the right or left main bronchus, the lung can

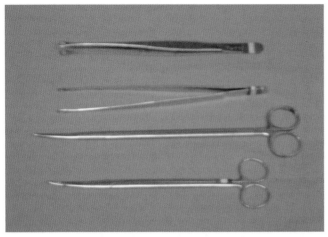

FIGURE 5   Tuttle thoracic tissue forceps, Nelson lung-dissecting lobectomy scissors, and Metzenbaum long dissecting scissors.

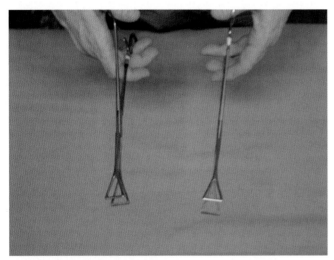

FIGURE 6   Duval lung forceps.

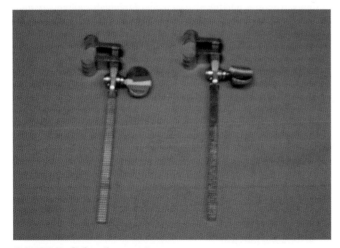

FIGURE 7   Bailey rib approximator.

be collapsed, thus allowing the trauma surgeon to operate on a collapsed and still lung. Bronchoscopy is also an invaluable adjunct when used intraoperatively. It can serve as a diagnostic tool by locating injured bronchi at the lobar and even segmental levels. It can also be therapeutic by removing blood within the tracheobronchial tree, which tends to cause bronchospasm.

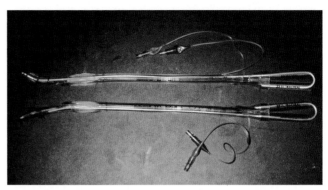

FIGURE 8   Double-lumen endotracheal tubes.

Ventilation

There are two types of ventilation that can be employed in the operating room. The conventional method intermittently allows for a periodic inflation/deflation of the lung, and High-Frequency Jet Ventilation allows the trauma surgeon to operate on a nonmoving still lung. The VDR-4 (Fig. 9) provides a modified form of jet ventilation know as Pulsatile Flow Ventilation.

Surgical Incisions and Exposures

No single incision will allow the surgeon to access all compartments of the thoracic cavity. The incisions used to access the thorax for the management of penetrating pulmonary injuries include anterolateral thoracotomy (Spangaro's incision), posterolateral thoracotomy, right posterolateral thoracotomy, left posterolateral thoracotomy, and median sternotomy (Duval-Barasty incision).

Anterolateral Thoracotomy (Spangaro's Incision)   This incision is the most frequently used to access the right or left hemithoracic cavity, as most of these patients will be transported to the operating room with some degree of hemodynamic instability. This incision

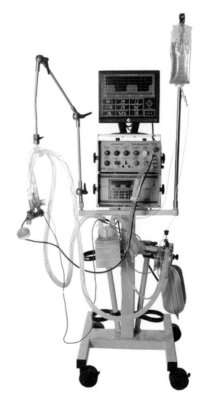

FIGURE 9   The VDR-4, which provides Pulsatile Flow Ventilation. *(Courtesy of Percussionaire® Corp.)*

allows the trauma surgeon to operate on either the right or left lung, although it provides for a very limited operating field. It does not allow access to the posterior structures of the right or left hemithoracic cavity. The left anterolateral thoracotomy will provide access to the heart and the descending thoracic aorta should cross-clamping be necessary if the patient's hemodynamic instability or cardiopulmonary arrest demands it.

The anterolateral thoracotomy is also the incision of choice when the thoracic cavity needs to be accessed in the presence of an associated abdominal injury. Anterolateral thoracotomy may be extended into bilateral anterolateral thoracotomies if associated injury is found in the contralateral hemithoracic cavity.

Posterolateral Thoracotomy This incision provides for the very best exposure for the management of penetrating pulmonary injuries. The disadvantage of this incision is that it is time consuming, as it requires a special positioning of the patient on the operating table. Most of these patients are usually transported to the operating room with hemodynamic instability and cannot afford the luxury of being placed in this position. This incision provides suboptimal access for the management of associated cardiac injuries.

Right Posterolateral Thoracotomy This incision provides access to the right lung and the thoracic esophagus up to its most distal portion when it crosses anterior to the thoracic aorta into the left hemithoracic cavity and superior to the descending thoracic aorta. It provides access to the azygous and hemiazygous veins, and is the incision of choice for the management of most, if not all, tracheal injuries.

Left Posterolateral Thoracotomy This incision provides access to the left lung, descending thoracic aorta, and the distalmost portion of the esophagus as it crosses from the right into the left hemithoracic cavity and superior to the descending thoracic aorta.

Median Sternotomy (Duval-Barasty Incision) This is the incision of choice for the management of patients with associated cardiac injuries who arrive with vital signs in the operating room. The right or left hemithoracic cavities can be accessed if the mediastinal pleura is sharply transected. This provides access to the anterior portions of either the right or left lung, although exposure of the posterior aspects of the pulmonary lobes is suboptimal. Care must be exercised when a significant portion of the lung is mobilized medially into this incision as the pulmonary hilar vessels can be rotated at a 90-degree angle, occluding both the inflow and outflow, causing significant hemodynamic compromise to the patient. Similarly, extreme caution must be exercised when mobilizing the inferior pulmonary ligaments, as an inadvertent iatrogenic injury to the inferior pulmonary vein may ensue.

Adjunct Maneuvers

Important adjunct maneuvers used in the management of pulmonary injuries include (1) aortic cross-clamping, (2) pulmonary hilar cross-clamping, (3) complete inflow occlusion (Shumacker maneuver), (4) pulmonary hilar vessel control, (5) control of the main right or left pulmonary artery, and (6) pulmonary vein control.

Aortic Cross-Clamping The aorta can be cross-clamped only through a left anterolateral thoracotomy. This requires a meticulous combination of sharp and blunt dissection of this vessel before its entrance into the abdominal cavity via the aortic hiatus. The aorta should be digitally encircled; however, lateral digital dissection must be gentle and limited to prevent iatrogenic injuries to the intercostal arteries. The esophagus, which lies immediately superior to the anterior border of the aorta, must be separated before placement of a Crafoord-DeBakey aortic cross-clamp. Esophageal identification is facilitated by the prior insertion of a nasogastric tube.

Pulmonary Hilar Cross-Clamping This maneuver is used when there is a central hilar hematoma or active bleeding from the pulmonary hilum. The hilum of the lung can be isolated using a meticulous combination of sharp and blunt dissection of the perihilar tissues to allow for the digital encirclement of all the structures. A Crafoord-DeBakey aortic cross-clamp is then placed as close to the pericardium as possible.

Complete Inflow Occlusion (Shumacker Maneuver) The Shumacker maneuver may occasionally be used if there is an associated cardiac injury either to the lateralmost aspects of the right atrium or to the atriocaval junction. This involves placement of Crafoord-DeBakey aortic cross-clamps in the intrapericardial portions of the superior vena cava as well as the inferior vena cava at the space of Gibbons. This will allow for immediate emptying of the heart. Although it is estimated that the safe period for this maneuver ranges from 1 to 3 minutes, the actual safety period is unknown.

Pulmonary Hilar Vessel Control This maneuver is necessary to control hemorrhage from the pulmonary artery or vein. The dissection and ligation or stapling of pulmonary arteries and veins requires a different technique than for systemic vessels. The pulmonary vessels are thin-walled and fragile. They tear easily and cannot be clamped with standard hemostats. The dissection must be gentle and meticulous. There is almost always a perivascular plane that permits rapid and safe dissection in a vascular area. Before encirclement of either the pulmonary artery or vein, three sides of the vessels should be dissected completely before an attempt is made to pass a Mixter right-angle forceps beneath the vessel. If this is not done, perforation is likely. Pulmonary vessels should not be held with vascular forceps as they may tear; only the adventitia should be grasped. Either of these vessels may be safely held or retracted with Kittner dissectors.

Control of Main Right or Left Pulmonary Artery This control can be extrapleural at the hilum or intrapericardial, which requires lateral cardiac displacement and occasionally transection of the pericardium.

Pulmonary Vein Control This control can be extrapleural at the hilum or intrapericardial, although the latter maneuver is quite difficult.

Uniform Approach to Management of Pulmonary Injuries

A uniform approach to the management of traumatic pulmonary injuries has been described. This approach includes the following steps:

1. Evacuate blood and clots from the thoracic cavity.
2. Expose the injured lung.
3. Pack, if necessary, to allow for restoration of depleted intravascular blood volume.
4. Evaluate for evidence of a hilar or central hematoma or hemorrhage.
5. Decide whether pulmonary hilar cross-clamping is necessary. If this is necessary, place a Crafoord-DeBakey aortic cross-clamp across the pulmonary hilum.
6. Proceed to identify bleeding structures within the pulmonary parenchyma and control hemorrhage proceeding to sequential declamping of the pulmonary hilum.
7. If the pulmonary parenchymal hemorrhage is away from the hilum, clamp the pulmonary injury with Duval lung forceps.
8. Evaluate pericardium and mediastinum.
9. Proceed to repair.

SURGICAL TECHNIQUES OF REPAIR AND RESECTION

The high mortality rates reported for lobectomy and pneumonectomy when performed for the management of traumatic lung injuries has served as the impetus to develop quicker and less extensive resection techniques. These techniques have been denominated "lung-sparing techniques" and include suture pneumonorrhaphy, stapled and clamp pulmonary tractotomy with selective deep vessel ligation, and nonanatomic resection. In 2006, Asensio et al reported that lung-sparing techniques were used in 80% of 101 patients requiring thoracotomy for the management of traumatic pulmonary injuries. The use of adjunct intraoperative tools including the argon beam coagulator and fibrin glue are valuable adjuncts in the trauma surgeon's armamentarium.

The surgical armamentarium to manage the penetrating pulmonary injuries discussed next is organized into two broad categories: tissue-sparing techniques and resectional procedures.

Tissue-Sparing Procedures

These procedures include (1) suture pneumonorrhaphy, (2) stapled pulmonary tractotomy with selective deep vessel ligation, (3) clamp pulmonary tractotomy with selective deep vessel ligation, and (4) nonanatomic resection. It is estimated that approximately 85% of all penetrating pulmonary injuries can be managed with these techniques.

These procedures are indicated for control of hemorrhage, control of small air leaks, and preservation of pulmonary tissue. They are also useful when the pulmonary injury is amenable to reconstruction.

Suture Pneumonorrhaphy

The lung is stabilized with Duval lung forceps. Stay sutures of 3-0 chromic or other absorbable sutures are placed in the superior and inferior aspect of the wound as well as in the lateral aspects, and they are used to gently retract the edges. Very fine malleable ribbon retractors are placed to separate the wound and to provide for visualization of the injured vessels, which are then selectively ligated with 3-0 chromic sutures or other similarly sized absorbable sutures. The same is done for small bronchi. The edges of the wound are then approximated with a running locked suture of 3-0 chromic.

Stapled Pulmonary Tractotomy

In 1997, Asensio et al described a technique for the management of penetrating pulmonary injuries, which included the use of a linear Endo GIA stapler (Ethicon, Somerville, N.J.) to perform pulmonary tractotomy with selective vascular ligation. Clamp tractotomy was previously described by Wall et al in 1994, using aortic clamps. The lung is stabilized with Duval lung forceps and orifices of entrance and exit are defined. If need be, the overlying visceral pleura is sharply incised with Nelson scissors. A GIA 55 or 75 stapler is used to place 3.8-mm staples through the orifices of entrance and exit (Figs. 10 and 11). This will open the tract traversed by the missile or other wounding agent, effectively exposing the injured vessels and bronchi, which are then selectively ligated utilizing 3-0 chromic or similarly sized absorbable sutures (Fig. 12). The lung parenchyma can then be approximated with a single running locked suture of 3-0 chromic or the same size of absorbable suture. The orifices of entry and exit are left open for the egress of air and blood. The integrity of the suture line is tested by having the anesthesiologist inflate the lung. Air leaks are then detected and repaired.

Clamp Pulmonary Tractotomy

The pulmonary tractotomy with selective vascular ligation described by Wall et al consists of the same technique as stapled pulmonary tractotomy; however, instead of a stapler, two Crafoord-DeBakey clamps are placed through the orifices of entrance and exit, and the pulmonary tissue between the clamps is sharply transected with either Nelson or Metzenbaum scissors.

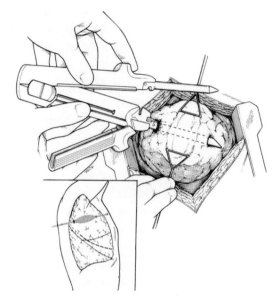

FIGURE 10 Depicts cavitary effect created by a missile traversing the lung. The GIA 55 is then inserted through the orifices of entry and exit. *(From Asensio JA, Demetriades D, Berne JD, et al: Stapled pulmonary tractotomy: a rapid way to control hemorrhage in penetrating pulmonary injuries. J Am Coll Surg 185:504–505, 1997.)*

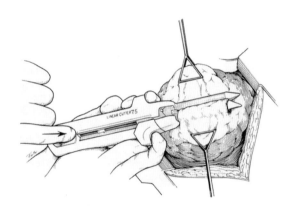

FIGURE 11 The GIA is then closed and fired to open up the missile tract. *(From Asensio JA, Demetriades D, Berne JD, et al: Stapled pulmonary tractotomy: a rapid way to control hemorrhage in penetrating pulmonary injuries. J Am Coll Surg 185:504–505, 1997.)*

Nonanatomic Resection

This procedure is indicated when a very small and peripheral portion of a lobe or a segment is devitalized. The area of resection is stabilized between Duval lung forceps and a GIA 55 or 75 stapler with 3.8-mm staples is fired across, thus resecting the injured portion of the lung. The staple line may be oversewn with a running locked suture of 3-0 chromic or the same size of absorbable suture, although this is not generally necessary. Nonanatomic resections can also be complex and require resections of major segments with complex reconstruction. This procedure will require meticulous attention in the reconstruction of an injured lobe.

Resectional Procedures

Resectional procedures include formal lobectomy and formal pneumonectomy. These procedures are indicated for (1) control of

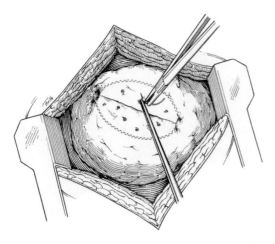

FIGURE 12 The tract is open, and the deep bleeding vessels are ligated. *(From Asensio JA, Demetriades D, Berne JD, et al: Stapled pulmonary tractotomy: a rapid way to control hemorrhage in penetrating pulmonary injuries. J Am Coll Surg 185:504–505, 1997.)*

hemorrhage, (2) resection of devitalized or destroyed pulmonary tissue, (3) control of major air leaks from lobar bronchi or main bronchi not amenable to repair, and (4) control of life-threatening hemorrhage.

Formal Lobectomy

Formal lobectomy is indicated when there is total lobar tissue destruction, or uncontrollable hemorrhage from the lobar vessels or a large lobar bronchial injury, which is destructive and not amenable to repair. To perform a lobectomy the fissures must be separated. Vascular dissection should be initiated extrapleurally at the hilum through a perivascular plane to find the major pulmonary vessels. Vascular dissection in the fissures identifies the lobar vessels. Transection of the inferior pulmonary ligament distally will allow greater mobility of the lower lobes of both lungs. All pulmonary vessels, whether they be the main lobar vessels or segmental vessels, can be ligated in continuity and transfixed with nonabsorbable sutures. Alternatively, they may be stapled with a TA-30, TA-45, or TA-90, with 3.5-mm staples, or an endovascular stapler. All pulmonary vessels may also be oversewn with 4-0, 5-0, or 6-0 monofilament polypropylene sutures.

The bronchi, whether they be the main, lobar, or segmental, should be stapled and transected with a TA-30, TA-45, or TA-90 stapler, with 4.8-mm staples. This is the preferred method for handling all bronchial structures. Bronchi may also be transected utilizing Sarot lung clamps and sutured with 4-0 Tevdek synthetic sutures. Should a suture technique be chosen, the trauma surgeon should avoid grasping the cut end of a bronchus with any instrument. The suture technique involves clamping the bronchus distal to the intended point of transection. The bronchus is cut transversely for 4 to 5 mm, and the cut end is sutured with 4-0 Tevdek. These sutures should be tied very carefully to avoid cutting or unnecessary devascularization. After placement of two sutures, the cut end is extended and additional sutures are placed. The sutures should be 2 to 3 mm apart. For a main bronchus, more than six sutures are seldom required. For a lobar bronchus, three or four sutures are usually enough. Too many sutures devascularize the transected bronchus. After closure is complete, the suture line is immersed in saline, and the lung is inflated by the anesthesiologist with up to 45 cm H_2O of inflation pressure. Additional sutures are placed if an air leak is detected.

After a lobectomy is performed, the remaining lobes are pexed to the thoracic wall with 2-0 chromic sutures to prevent lung torsion; this is very important. The bronchial stump may be covered with a pleural flap or pericardial fat, known as Brewer's patch. These

techniques are of unproven value. An intercostal pedicled muscle flap is probably superior, but it is time consuming.

Right Upper Lobectomy

To perform a right upper lobectomy, both the pulmonary artery and the vein are dissected peripherally toward the right upper lobe to carefully delineate the lobe's individual blood supply. First, the anterior and apicoposterior segmental branches of the main pulmonary artery to the upper lobe are ligated in continuity with 2-0 silk sutures, divided, and transfixed proximally with 3-0 silk suture ligatures. Within the major fissure, the posterior segmental branch of the upper lobe is identified, ligated, transfixed, and divided in a similar fashion. Within the minor fissure that exists between the upper and middle lobes, the pulmonary venous drainage from the upper lobe is identified and carefully dissected. The vein is ligated in continuity with 0 silk sutures, transfixed with 2-0 silk suture, and divided. At this point, the lung is retracted forward to gain access to the posteriorly placed bronchus. The right main bronchus and the carina are identified. The upper lobe bronchus is identified and transected with a TA-30 or TA-45 stapler with 4.8-mm staples.

Right Middle Lobectomy

For a right middle lobectomy, the pulmonary artery branch to the middle lobe is identified, ligated with 0 silk sutures, transfixed with 2-0 silk sutures, and divided. The middle lobe division of the superior pulmonary vein is similarly ligated with 0 silk sutures, transfixed with 2-0 silk sutures, and divided. With these two vessels addressed, the trauma surgeon carefully isolates the middle lobe bronchus, which is then transected with a TA-30 or TA-45 stapler with 4.8-mm staples.

Right Lower Lobectomy

To perform a right lower lobectomy, the main pulmonary artery is followed in the major fissure, and the segmental branches to the lower lobe are identified. The superior and basal segmental branches to the lower lobe are carefully identified, ligated in continuity with 0 silk sutures, transfixed with 2-0 silk sutures, and divided. Particular care is taken to avoid injury to the middle lobe arteries. Next, attention is directed to the inferior pulmonary vein, where, after the surgeon has ensured that any drainage from the middle lobe is protected, the inferior pulmonary vein is ligated in continuity with 0 silk sutures and transfixed with 2-0 silk sutures and transected. Again, within the same major fissure, the superior segmental and the basal segmental bronchi are individually identified and transected with a TA-30 or TA-45 stapler with 4.8-mm staples.

Left Upper Lobectomy

To perform a left upper lobectomy, the interlobar fissure is separated by a meticulous combination of sharp and blunt dissection. If the interlobar fissure is not complete, it can be divided with a TA-30 or TA-45 with 3.8-mm staples. Arterial dissection is begun at the junction of the upper third with the middle third of the fissure. The artery is exposed. The perivascular plane is entered, and the individual segmental branches to the upper lobe are identified, carefully dissected, ligated in continuity with 0 silk sutures, and then transfixed with 2-0 silk sutures. Similarly, the superior pulmonary vein and branches to the left upper lobe are identified, ligated in continuity with 0 silk sutures, and transfixed with 2-0 silk sutures. The left upper lobar bronchus is then identified and transected with a TA-45 with 4.8-mm staples.

Left Lower Lobectomy

To perform a left lower lobectomy, the same steps are taken as for a left upper lobectomy; however, the arterial and venous dissections are directed toward the appropriate left lower lobar vessels. The lingular artery or arteries, as there may be two identified, are ligated in continuity with 0 silk sutures and transfixed with 2-0 silk sutures. The left lower lobar bronchus is then identified and transected with a TA-30 or TA-45 with 4.8-mm staples.

Pneumonectomy

Right Pneumonectomy

Exploration of the right hemithoracic cavity is carried out, and the azygous vein is identified. The right pulmonary hilum is located. Using a meticulous combination of sharp and blunt dissection, the right main pulmonary artery is identified and encircled with a vessel loop; avoidance of undue traction is key. The right inferior pulmonary ligament is sharply transected. Both superior and inferior pulmonary veins are identified and encircled with vessel loops. All vessels may be either ligated in continuity or stapled individually utilizing a TA-30 or TA-45 stapler with 3.5-mm staples or an endovascular stapler. The right main bronchus is then identified and encircled. The trauma surgeon must be careful not to apply undue traction to avoid tearing subcarinal structures. The bronchus is then transected with a TA-30 or TA-45 stapler with 4.8-mm staples.

Left Pneumonectomy

A thorough exploration of the left hemithoracic cavity is carried out. The phrenic, vagus, and left recurrent laryngeal nerves are identified and preserved. The left pulmonary hilum is located. Using a meticulous combination of sharp and blunt dissection, the left main pulmonary artery is identified and encircled with a vessel loop; avoidance of undue traction is key. The left inferior pulmonary ligament is sharply transected. Both superior and inferior pulmonary veins are identified and encircled with vessel loops. All vessels may be either ligated in continuity or stapled utilizing a TA-30 or TA-45 stapler with 3.5-mm staples or an endovascular stapler. The left main bronchus is then identified and encircled. The trauma surgeon must be careful not to apply undue traction to avoid tearing subcarinal structures. The bronchus is then transected with a TA-30 or TA-45 stapler with 4.8-mm staples.

Alternate Technique for Pneumonectomy (Right or Left)

If the patient is exsanguinating from a central hilar vascular injury, the pulmonary hilum may be digitally encircled and compressed to allow the anesthesiologist to replace the lost intravascular volume. A Craafoord-DeBakey aortic cross-clamp is then placed a few centimeters from the mediastinal pleura. If this maneuver controls the life-threatening hemorrhage, extrapleural dissection of hilar vessels may be carried out and individual vessels ligated. If this maneuver cannot be performed, if it does not contain the hemorrhage, or if the cross-clamp is required in a very proximal location, the pericardium may have to be opened to control the pulmonary artery and the pulmonary veins. Intrapericardial control of the pulmonary veins is quite difficult and requires lateral displacement of the heart. This can be accomplished using a Satinsky clamp placed in the right auricle. It may even require total inflow occlusion with a Shumacker maneuver.

Alternatively, a TA-90 stapler with 4.8-mm staples may be placed across the pulmonary hilum and fired transecting the pulmonary artery, pulmonary veins, and main bronchus. In most cases, this controls the hemorrhage if the injuries to the pulmonary artery or veins are found in an extrapericardial location. If this does not control the bleeding, then intrapericardial control of the pulmonary vessels will be needed.

PROGNOSTIC FACTORS AND OUTCOMES

Factors associated with survival for pulmonary injuries requiring surgical intervention include the following: mechanism of injury and

type of wounding agents; prehospital transport time; presence of shock at the scene or upon arrival; loss of the airway; presence of associated injuries; complexity of the surgical procedure; and location of the injury.

Mechanism of Injury and Type of Wounding Agents

It is known that pulmonary injuries in civilian life are caused by both blunt and penetrating mechanisms. Most commonly, penetrating pulmonary injuries are produced by knives and low-velocity missiles; although the incidence of injuries caused by high-velocity missiles is increasing. Civilian penetrating injuries to the lung secondary to high-velocity missiles are associated with higher mortality rates than low-velocity missiles and stab wounds.

In a multicenter study dealing with traumatic pulmonary injuries in the civilian arena, Karmy-Jones and colleagues reported that blunt mechanism of injury tends to provide more extensive injury to pulmonary parenchyma requiring extensive resections in case of need for surgery. Blunt trauma is associated with a 3 to 10 times greater risk of death when compared with penetrating trauma.

In warfare, most pulmonary injuries are caused by penetrating mechanisms, such as shell fragments, shrapnel, and high-velocity missiles, although extensive damage is also observed with explosive wounds. Zakharia et al and Petricevic and colleagues reported a higher mortality rate among patients sustaining pulmonary lesions secondary to explosive devices and destructive injuries inflicted by high-velocity missiles than in those patients sustaining stab wounds or falls.

Prehospital Transport Time

The "scoop-and-run" doctrine of Gervin and Fischer might improve the survival prospects of some patients with time-related deterioration resulting from torso injuries. Wagner et al reported that rapidity of prehospital transport of patients with severe penetrating pulmonary injuries results in better outcomes, concluding that a well-organized trauma service caring for patients within the framework of well-defined protocols increases the survival rate. This fact was also reported by Petricevic and colleagues, who pointed out that the key for success in the treatment of patients sustaining traumatic pulmonary injuries during wartime is rapid transportation of the wounded to surgical centers.

Presence of Shock at Scene or Upon Arrival

Well-known physiologic factors predictive of high mortality rate in patients with traumatic pulmonary injuries include prehospital and ED absence of both vital signs and cardiac rhythm. Similarly, the absence of a palpable pulse in the presence of cardiopulmonary arrest is also predictive of high mortality rate. Robison et al reported a mortality rate of 85% among patients presenting with cardiopulmonary arrest upon arrival to the ED, and Wagner and colleagues reported that hypotensive patients sustaining penetrating pulmonary injuries with systolic blood pressures less than 90 mm Hg had a mortality rate of 90%.

Buckman et al, using the cardiovascular and respiratory components of the trauma score (CVRS) on admission of patients sustaining penetrating cardiac injuries, concluded that prospective physiologic scoring is helpful in predicting outcomes. Physiologic factors and CVRS have been further validated by Asensio et al as important predictive factors of outcome in two prospective studies dealing with this type of lethal injuries. It would be appropriate to extrapolate that these physiologic variables can play the same significant role among patients sustaining traumatic pulmonary injuries.

Loss of Airway

It is known that the highest priority in the resuscitation of the critically injured patient lies in achieving a rapid and secure airway regardless of setting wherever performed, and this dictum includes, of course, patients sustaining traumatic pulmonary injuries. Unsolved loss of the airway is uniformly fatal. As reported by Asensio et al, the vast majority of trauma patients treated at the ED in certified trauma centers in which endotracheal intubation is indicated will have a secured airway by means of this procedure. Occasionally endotracheal intubation is unsuccessful or contraindicated, and a surgical airway is required; in this case, emergency surgical cricothyroidotomy should be performed. Inoue and colleagues reported a strategy to secure the airway in patients with traumatic pulmonary injuries, consisting of selective exclusion of the injured lung by using endotracheal tubes with a movable bronchial occlusion cuff (Univent, Fuji Systems Corporation, Tokyo). By means of this strategy, occlusion by blood of the airways of the noninjured lung is prevented.

Presence of Associated Injuries

The presence of associated injuries, particularly cardiac or thoracic vascular injuries, uniformly increases mortality rate. Similarly, the presence of complex associated abdominal injuries is also known to increase mortality rate in these patients.

Complexity of Surgical Procedure

Several authors have pointed out that the complexity of the surgical procedure is closely related to the mortality rate. Wall et al, Velmahos and colleagues, and Cothren et al have established that the use of lung-sparing procedures correlates with lower rates of mortality than more extensive resective procedures. The mortality rate reported in the literature for pneumonorrhaphy, stapled tractotomy, clamp tractotomy, and wedge/nonanatomic resections varies. In contrast, the mortality rate reported for anatomic lobectomy is 40% to 50%, and for pneumonectomy, 60% to 100%.

Wagner and colleagues reported a 50% mortality rate among patients requiring pneumonectomy for trauma, and Thompson and associates reported 54.5% mortality rate for lobectomy and 100% for pneumonectomy; the overall mortality rate for this series was 28%, and the mortality rate for pneumonorrhaphy was 3% and for tractotomy, 17%. In 1993, Tominaga et al reported an overall mortality rate of 33%; the authors correlated the complexity of the surgical procedure on the lung with mortality rate, reporting a rate of 20% for nonanatomic resections, 33% for lobectomy, and 50% for pneumonectomy. In 1991, Velmahos et al reported an overall mortality rate of 5% among patients requiring thoracotomy for penetrating lung injuries. In this study, the authors focused on techniques employed to deal with these injuries. The mortality rate among patients requiring lung-sparing surgery was 3%, compared with 20% for those requiring resective techniques. Stewart et al reported an overall mortality rate of 12.5% among patients requiring pulmonary resection for pulmonary injuries and concluded that the use of stapled resections could be a factor related to the low mortality rate in the series. Karmy-Jones et al reported that mortality rate increased with each step of increasing complexity of the surgical technique, with pneumonorrhaphy at 9%; stapled tractotomy, 13%; wedge resection, 30%; lobectomy, 43%; and pneumonectomy, 50%. In 2002, Cothren et al reported an overall mortality rate of 30% among 36 patients requiring thoracotomy for severe lung injuries, and compared mortality rates for patients requiring anatomic resection at 77%, versus a 4% mortality rate for those patients that underwent nonanatomic resections. The authors reported that stapled tractotomy correlated with a significant

reduction in mortality rate. Huh and colleagues, also focusing on the level of complexity of the lung intervention, described a mortality rate of 24% for pneumonorrhaphy, 9.1% for tractotomy, 20% for wedge resection, 35% for lobectomy, and 69.7% for pneumonectomy.

Location of Injury

Wagner and associates pointed out that injury to the hilar pulmonary vasculature is associated with greater than 70% of mortality rate. Wiencek and Wilson reported a mortality rate of 63% among patients sustaining central/hilar lung injuries secondary to gunshot wounds, and the mortality rate among patients with hilar injuries resulting from stab wounds was 44%. The major causes of death in this series were exsanguination, and possibly air embolism. These authors also reported an overall mortality rate of 56% among patients with penetrating central pulmonary injuries. Petricevic and colleagues pointed out that the mortality rate is much higher if lung injury is combined with one or more extrathoracic lesions (from 6% to 14% to as much as 55%).

MORBIDITY

According to Asensio et al, complications related to the presence of a traumatic pulmonary injury or surgical management are classified into three main categories: intraoperative, short-term postoperative, and long-term postoperative complications.

Intraoperative Complications

These complications comprise univentricular failure (usually right ventricular failure) and biventricular failure.

Short-Term Postoperative Complications

Technical short-term complications are as follows:

- Lung hernia
- Lung torsion
- Bronchopleural fistulas
- Arteriovenous fistulas
- Bronchial stump leaks
- Bronchial stump blowouts

Physiologic short-term complications include the following:

- Right ventricular failure
- Pulmonary artery hypertension
- "Runaway" pulmonary artery hypertension
- Biventricular failure

Long-Term Postoperative Complications

These complications are classified as follows:

- Persistent bronchopleural fistula
- Bronchial stenosis
- Empyema
- Lung abscess
- Bronchiectasis
- Arteriovenous fistula

In 1979, Graham et al described the presence of 155 postoperative complications among 108 of 373 patients sustaining penetrating injuries to the lung for a morbidity rate of 29% and an average number of 1.43 complications per patient. The most common causes of morbidity included postoperative hemorrhage, at 32%; atelectasis, 13%; recurrent pneumothorax, 10%; persistent air leak, 9%; wound infection, 8%; and pneumonia, 6%. Postoperative hemorrhage and persistent air leak were major indications for surgical reintervention. Robison reported a morbidity rate of 70% among patients requiring thoracotomy for resective surgery of lung injuries. The most frequent postoperative complications included hemoptysis, bronchopleural fistula, air embolism, sepsis, and respiratory insufficiency.

MORTALITY

The overall mortality rate reported in the literature for patients with traumatic pulmonary injuries ranges from 1.7% to 37%. There are many factors significantly associated with mortality rate. The factors repeatedly mentioned in various series as outcome determinants are the physiologic status of the patient after injury, complexity of the pulmonary surgical intervention, number of associated injuries (especially cardiac injury), and need for additional surgical interventions.

In 1979, Graham et al reported an overall mortality rate of 8% among patients sustaining penetrating pulmonary injuries. The mortality rate among patients requiring only tube thoracostomy was 3% versus 6% for those requiring thoracotomy. Major causes of death were respiratory insufficiency, at 36%; shock/hemorrhage, 32%; sepsis, 11%; central nervous system injury, 11%; air embolism, 7%; and tracheoesophageal fistula, 4%. Robison in 1988 reported an overall mortality rate of 2.4%, with sepsis, the presence of associated injuries, air embolism, and exsanguination (notoriously common in central lung injuries) determined to be major causes of fatality.

In 1988, Wiencek and Wilson reported a mortality rate of 56% among patients sustaining central/hilar vascular injuries to the lung and concluded that exsanguination and air embolism play a cardinal role as cause of death in these patients. In 1993, Tominaga et al reported an overall mortality rate of 33% and noticed the role that complexity of the pulmonary surgical procedure played on mortality rate, describing a mortality rate of 20% for nonanatomic resections, 33% for lobectomy, and 50% for pneumonectomy. Velmahos and colleagues reported in 1999 an overall mortality rate of 5% among patients who underwent thoracotomy for penetrating lung injuries; the authors focused on the techniques employed to deal with these injuries and reported that mortality rates among patients requiring lung-sparing surgery was 3% versus 20% for those requiring resective techniques.

In 1997, Petricevic and colleagues reported an overall mortality rate of 1.7% among patients sustaining traumatic pulmonary injuries during the war in Croatia; causes of death were identified as hemorrhage and irreversible shock, 30%, and septic complications, 70%. Stewart et al reported an overall mortality rate of 12.5% among patients requiring pulmonary resection for lung trauma, concluding that the use of stapled resections could be a factor related to the low mortality rate in the series.

In 2001, Karmy-Jones et al, in a retrospective multicenter 4-year study, reported an overall mortality rate of 9% among 451 patients requiring thoracotomy for traumatic pulmonary injuries. Stratified by mechanism of injury, blunt trauma accounted for 68% and penetrating trauma 19%. Mortality rate increased with complexity of the surgical technique required to manage these injuries: for pneumonorrhaphy, the mortality rate was 9%; stapled tractotomy, 13%; wedge resection, 30%; lobectomy, 43%; and pneumonectomy, 50%. Blunt injuries were associated with a 10 times greater risk of death compared with penetrating trauma. Factors identified by univariate analysis as being significantly associated with fatality included mechanism—blunt versus penetrating trauma, high head/neck Abbreviated Injury Score, need for laparotomy, and presenting systolic blood pressure on arrival in operating room. When these factors were entered along with type of lung repair/resection—suture, stapled tractotomy, wedge resection, lobectomy, and pneumonectomy—into a stepwise model regression analysis, factors that retained significance were mechanism of injury, presenting systolic blood pressure on arrival in operating room, and increasing degree of pulmonary resection.

In 2001, Gasparri et al described an overall mortality rate of 16% among patients requiring pulmonary parenchymal interventions for lung trauma. Mortality rate was significantly higher in the presence of low systolic blood pressure, low temperature, high Injury Severity Score, large estimated blood losses, associated cardiac injuries, and the need for laparotomy. However, the authors did not find a correlation between the complexity of the operative intervention on the lung and the outcome. Cothren and colleagues reported an overall mortality rate of 30% among 36 patients requiring thoracotomy for severe lung injuries. The mortality rate for patients with anatomic resection was 77% compared with 4% among patients who underwent nonanatomic resection. The authors reported that stapled tractotomy was related with a significant reduction in mortality rate. Huh et al reported an overall mortality rate of 28% among patients requiring thoracotomy for traumatic pulmonary injuries and reported that if a concomitant laparotomy was required, mortality rate increased to 33%. The authors focused on the level of complexity of the lung intervention, and described a mortality rate of 23.9% for pneumonorrhaphy, 9.1% for stapled tractotomy, 20% for wedge resection, 35% for lobectomy, and 69.7% for pneumonectomy. In 2006, Asensio and colleagues reported an overall mortality rate of 37% among 101 patients requiring thoracotomy for penetrating pulmonary injuries; 7 of these patients (19%) required an EDT and did not reach the operating room.

CONCLUSIONS

Pulmonary injuries requiring thoracotomy are uncommon even in busy urban trauma centers. Their operative management requires excellent surgical technique to prevent postoperative complications. Simpler surgical techniques such as pneumonorrhaphy and wedge resections are frequently used for their management. Stapled pulmonary tractotomy has become the most frequently used lung-sparing procedure and can be used effectively to manage 85% of all pulmonary injuries requiring surgical intervention. Despite recent advances in trauma surgery and surgical critical care, pulmonary injuries, particularly those requiring resective procedures, are marked by high morbidity and mortality rates.

For the chapter's Suggested Readings list, please visit the book at www.ExpertConsult.inkling.com.

COMPLICATIONS OF PULMONARY AND PLEURAL INJURY

Thomas K. Varghese, Jr., Riyad Karmy-Jones, and Gregory J. Jurkovich

It has been stated that chest trauma is the primary cause of death in up to 25% of fatalities following traumatic injury, and a major contributing factor in another 25%, although as few as 5% to 15% require acute operative intervention. Based on these generalizations, it is accepted that overall chest injury is common, that acute operative intervention is uncommon, and that a significant, although ill-defined, number of thoracic operations are performed for delayed complications. The actual incidence of each of these varies from center to center based on ratio of blunt to penetrating admissions as well as overall volume. Pulmonary complications can result from direct injury to the lung, or secondarily as a result of response to trauma outside the thorax. Significant change in lung function that occurs as a result of these injuries can lead to interference in ventilation or pulmonary perfusion. Management strategies hence include acute resuscitation efforts, high degree of suspicion of pulmonary injuries, active treatment, and prevention of complications.

PULMONARY COMPLICATIONS

Pulmonary Contusion

It has been reported that up to 75% of patients who sustain blunt trauma to the chest will suffer a pulmonary contusion, with mortality rates of up to 40% documented in the literature. Bleeding into the lung parenchyma as a result of the injury sets up a cascade of pathophysiologic changes that typically are worst in the first 48 hours after injury, and most commonly subside by 7 days. As radiologic findings also follow this lag period from the time of injury, a high degree of suspicion is needed in the management of these injuries. Computed tomography (CT) is a more sensitive imaging modality as compared to plain chest radiographs. Factors that influence the degree of injury include mechanical forces such as the tearing of lung tissue by rib fractures or chest wall compression; bleeding into lung segments surrounding the direct impact area leading to bronchospasm; atelectasis adjacent to contused lungs; and pulmonary dysfunction as a result of increased mucus production and decreased production of surfactant by injured alveolar tissues. Alveolar ventilation is reduced in the contused lung. Ventilation-perfusion mismatch in the areas of lung contusion can lead to increase in intrapulmonary shunt (from local vasoconstriction) and subsequent loss of lung compliance. At the cellular level, impairment of the mucociliary function and impaired pulmonary macrophage and lymphocytic activity make the patient susceptible to pneumonia.

Management of patients with pulmonary contusions is primarily supportive. The objectives of pulmonary physiotherapy measures are to improve respiratory mechanics, help clear the bronchopulmonary tree from secretions, and decrease the areas of lung with atelectasis surrounding the contusion. Judicious fluid administration, control of pain associated with chest wall injuries, and careful hemodynamic monitoring are critical in the first few days after injury. The larger the area of pulmonary contusion, the higher the likelihood the patient will require mechanical ventilation. Severe unilateral pulmonary contusions may need the aid of independent mechanical ventilation via a double-lumen endotracheal tube to prevent barotrauma to the unaffected lung and undertreating the affected lung. While using mechanical ventilation, tidal volume and positive end-expiratory pressure (PEEP) should be adjusted by following serial measurements of intrapulmonary shunt (Qs/Qt). Although the use of noninvasive positive-pressure ventilation (NPPV) has been described for nontrauma patients with acute hypoxic respiratory failure, as repeated from a series from Australia consisting of 75 patients, caution is needed for the use of such therapies in the acutely injured trauma patient. Intermittent positive-pressure breathing pushes a set volume of air to a preset pressure. Complications with such a modality include increased incidence of pneumothoraces in those with underlying lung disease, worsening of air leaks from parenchymal injuries, and associated abdominal distention and bloating as air can go down into the gastrointestinal tract. Hence, trying to find the small category of trauma patients who may benefit from NPPV is very difficult in the acute trauma setting. Current Advanced Trauma Life Support (ATLS) protocols recommend that patients with significant hypoxia ($Pao_2 < 70$ mm Hg on room air, $Sao_2 < 90\%$), hypoventilation ($Paco_2 > 45$ mm Hg), or altered mental status should be intubated within the first hour of injury.

Persistent Air Leak

There are three scenarios in which persistent air leaks occur in the trauma patient: after parenchyma injury; after anatomic lung resection; and in mechanically ventilated patients.

Persistent Air Leak After Parenchymal Injury

Injuries to the lung parenchyma can occur as a result of penetrating injury, blunt trauma with maceration or rib penetration, or in patients with underlying predisposing parenchyma lesions such as bullous emphysema. Principles of management follow the algorithm for management of spontaneous pneumothorax. Simple tube thoracostomy with reexpansion of the collapsed lung is sufficient treatment in more than 80% of cases. Prospective studies have shown that placing the chest drain to water seal after 48 hours will hasten resolution of the air leaks as the transpleural gradient is diminished. After ruling out technical factors (tube dislodgment or disconnection), air leaks lasting more than 3 days or associated with recurrent pneumothorax appear to be most efficiently managed by thoracoscopic approaches than persistent chest drainage. Schermer and colleagues reviewed the course of 39 trauma patients who, except for air leak, were ready for discharge (air leak > 3 days' duration). Twenty-five agreed to video-assisted thoracoscopic surgery (VATS) with reduced chest tube duration (total 8 vs. 12 days) and length of stay (10 vs. 17 days).

CT scans can help define local lesions that may be amenable to thoracoscopic wedge resection or application of biologic sealants, which may also prompt earlier VATS. Carrillo and associates reported a series of 11 patients who had persistent air leak (mean 6 days) following trauma (10 blunt). In 10 patients the source of the air leak was identified, and a segmental stapled resection was performed, and the last patient had a chemical pleurodesis. All chest tubes were removed within 48 hours, and nine patients were discharged home in 72 hours. In many instances, simply breaking down soft loculations and placing a chest drain under direct vision is the primary therapeutic benefit of thoracoscopy. We prefer to not use chemical pleurodesis, but rather pleural abrasion because it reduces the risk of parenchyma trapping and the uncertain long-term impact of chemical agents in younger patients. Patients with underlying lung lesions should be managed as they would in nontrauma circumstances. A final option in patients with prohibitive operative risks or small leaks is to convert the patients to Heimlich valve and manage them as outpatients. As many as 80% will seal within 3 weeks using this approach.

Persistent Air Leak After Pulmonary Resection

As lobectomy and pneumonectomy are rarely performed for traumatic injury, it follows that the incidence of air leak (bronchopleural fistula, or BPF) is also small. However, the nature of acute lung resections are such that the risk is higher than after elective resection. Risk factors include long stumps, devascularization, and contaminated hemothorax. Ideally after lobectomy/pneumonectomy the stump should be reinforced at the time of original resection or during second-look exploration with pleural, intercostal, or other flap. Once an air leak occurs, management is determined by timing (less than or more than 7 days postoperatively), degree (ventilatory compromise and whether the defect can be visualized endoscopically), physiologic status, and whether or not the patient is ventilated. BPF may present in stable patients as a new productive cough, with a drop in pleural fluid levels (after pneumonectomy) of two or more rib spaces, or new air-fluid level. In ventilated patients, empyema and loss of tidal volume may predominate. The primary goal is to prevent aspiration. In nonintubated patients this is best accompanied by positioning upright or with affected side down. Then drainage should be instituted if a chest drain is not in place. If there is not a drain in place, the new drain should be placed above the thoracotomy scar because the diaphragm tends to rise to the level of the scar and adhere. If the leak is small, and endoscopically the hole cannot be visualized clearly, it is reasonable to attempt bronchoscopic glue application.

Reoperation and stump closure are possible within 7 days, but the associated empyema increases the risk of failure. The longer the interval between the initial and second operations, the greater the difficulty. After pneumonectomy the mediastinum becomes inflamed and the stump can be visualized only with difficulty, and mobilization is essentially impossible. Thus, after pneumonectomy the best option is probably to occlude the stump with omentum, pack the chest with packs, and plan serial washouts until the leak scarifies closed. An alternative approach, particularly after right-sided pneumonectomy, is to perform transcarinal right main bronchus resection. The residual stump cannot be removed as it tends to be fixed, but the mucosa should be cauterized and omentum or other viable tissue used to reinforce the new stump. The empyema cavity can then be treated by the drainage procedure of the surgeon's choice. After lobectomy, similar options are possible, but further resection may be required (e.g., right middle lobectomy after right lower lobe stump leak). The management of the residual space may involve open chest drainage or a variety of space-filling options, as will be discussed in the section dealing with empyema.

Persistent Air Leak in the Mechanically Ventilated Trauma Patient

Persistent air leak in a ventilated patient without a discrete lesion is better thought of as an alveolar-pleural fistula rather than a BPF. Clearly the underlying lung injury affects outcome, with alveolar-pleural leak in acute respiratory distress syndrome (ARDS) patients associated with up to 80% mortality rate. Whatever the underlying anatomy, air leak in ventilated patients can be a significant marker of increased mortality rate. Pierson and colleagues reviewed the course of 39 patients (out of a population of 1700 mechanically ventilated patients) who presented with air leaks lasting more than 24 hours, of whom 27 were trauma patients. The risk factors for fatality correlated with the following: air leak not present on admission or shortly thereafter (45% early vs. 94% if developed later); leak greater than 500 mL/breath (57% if less vs. 100% if greater); and chest trauma (56% for trauma admissions vs. 92% for nontrauma admissions).

These findings illustrate that although the course in trauma admissions is more benign, it still represents a major concern. On the other hand, the air leak itself is rarely the cause of death. These air leaks can lead to persistent or even tension pneumothorax that compromises ventilation. Pleural tubes (at times multiple) may be required. Less commonly, air leak is significant enough to affect oxygenation. The primary treatment is to minimize alveolar pressure, using end-inspiratory plateau pressure as an admittedly crude reflection of this. Ideally the end-inspiratory plateau pressure should be less than 30 cm H_2O. The most common method of attaining this is to combine low tidal volume and permissive hypercapnia. Marchenkov and colleagues described using periodic bilevel positive airway pressure (BiPAP) or synchronized intermittent mandatory ventilation (SIMV) in 74 patients with persistent air leak following blunt trauma who had developed ARDS. Using SIMV or BiPAP three to five times per day, with peak pressure 33.4 ± 0.2 cm H_2O and PEEP 16.1 ± 0.2 cm H_2O, they argued that they could demonstrate a more rapid resolution of air leak that allowed earlier more aggressive airway recruitment maneuvers. Alternative methods if this approach fails are high-frequency jet ventilation or independent lung ventilation. It should be stressed that high-frequency jet ventilation, although used successfully in patients with central airway disruption, and in the operating room, does not reduce mean airway pressure consistently, nor does it uniformly reduce air leak nor improve oxygenation. Thus, it should not be used routinely in patients with alveolar-pleural fistula.

A temporizing technique is to isolate the lobe that is the primary source of leak with bronchoscopic techniques. This is done by sequentially occluding bronchi with a Swan-Ganz or other balloon catheter. If this results in elimination or significant reduction in air leak, occlusive material (Gelfoam, fibrin glue, blood mixed with tetracycline, etc.) can be injected. Recently, the use of retrievable one-way valves, placed via flexible bronchoscopy, has been suggested as a minimally invasive and better controlled approach. In the majority of cases the air leak will diminish as airway pressure decreases. Surgery can be performed, as described earlier, but in the setting of diffuse parenchyma injury, lung inflammation, severe emphysema, or steroids, the risk is that staple lines will fail and the leak will be even worse. If surgery is felt to be needed, reinforced staple lines (i.e., with bovine strips), apical tents (mobilizing the apical pleura so that it falls onto the area of resection), and anatomic lobectomy (if predominantly one lobe) should be considered.

Pneumatocele and Pulmonary Hematoma

Pneumatoceles occur when disruption of lung parenchyma leads to internal rather than external leak of air or blood. They occur more commonly following blunt injury, but can be seen occasionally with deep stab or low-caliber missile injuries. These lesions are thus best described as pulmonary lacerations or as resulting from pulmonary lacerations. They are usually solitary, at times multilobulated, and occasionally multiple. They are typically not apparent on initial radiographs, either due to small size or because superimposed contusion or hemorrhage obscure them. Over time, they evolve into thin-walled cavities, with air or fluid. The location and size are affected by mechanism. Compression leading to rupture, the most common mechanism, tends to be associated with central lesions. Compression, leading to shear forces, tends to present as an elongated paramediastinal cavity extending from hilum to diaphragm and may be confused with loculated pneumothorax. Rib penetration forms pneumatoceles that tend to be small and peripheral. Adhesion tears are the least common. In the vast majority of cases pneumatoceles are benign. In rare cases they may result in persistent air leak or become infected, in which case they are treated as abscesses.

Hematomas are formed by the same mechanisms that result in pneumatoceles. They may remain solid, or with partial evacuation they can develop an air-fluid level, or even a fibrin wall resulting in a crescent of air on the superior surface that mimics a fungus ball. Usually these lesions resolve over 3 to 6 months, and recognizing the shrinking process is one method to avoid confusing these with malignant processes.

Pneumonia

Pneumonia may be the most common complication of chest trauma. Risk factors include aspiration, need for ventilation, direct injury, pulmonary contusion, and persistent atelectasis secondary to pain. The incidence is as low as 6% in nonintubated patients to as high as 44% in ventilated patients. Despite the high incidence, there are no data supporting prophylactic antibiotics. Of all patients admitted with a diagnosis of pulmonary contusion, nearly 50% will develop pneumonia, barotrauma, or major atelectasis. One fourth will progress to ARDS. Ventilator-associated pneumonia (VAP), defined as pneumonia arising more than 48 hours after initiation of mechanical ventilation, is difficult to define and to diagnose. At Harborview Medical Center we have found that the incidence in patients ventilated for more than 7 days is around 20%, and that prehospital intubation of patients with trauma was not associated with a higher risk of VAP. Clinical suspicion is often raised by new infiltrates, recurring fever, rising leukocytes, or a change in endotracheal secretions. However, distinguishing between colonization and infection may require specialized techniques. Quantitative cultures obtained from a variety of approaches increase the specificity (although perhaps with reduced sensitivity) of endobronchial cultures, and each institution must define cutoff values based on whether or not the patient is already receiving antibiotics (Table 1).

Necrotizing Lung Infection

Necrotizing lung infections comprise a triad of clinical scenarios that overlap or can be present concomitantly: lung abscess, necrotizing pneumonia, and lung gangrene. All three are similar in that lack of perfusion is combined with tissue devitalization. In simplistic terms, lung abscess can be described as a region of necrosis less than a lobe

TABLE 1: Yields of Diagnostic Tests for Ventilator-Associated Pneumonia

Sample	Threshold	Sensitivity (%)	Specificity (%)
Endotracheal aspirate	Any pathogen	70–95	<50
	≥10^6 CFU/mL	25–70	70–85
Endotracheal aspirate	≥10^3 CFU/mL	30–100	80–100
	≥10^4 CFU/mL	55–95	70–100
Bronchoscopy	2–7% CAB	30–85	65–100
PSB culture	10^3 CFU/mL	60–100	75–100
BAL culture	10^4 CFU/mL	70–100	65–95
BAL cytologic specimen			
Nonbronchoscopic PSB			
BAL			

From Skerrett SJ: The diagnosis of ventilator-associated pneumonia. In Karmy-Jones R, Nathens A, Stern E, editors. *Thoracic trauma and critical care.* Boston, Kluwer Medical Publishers, 2002, pp 397–402.
BAL, Bronchoalveolar lavage; CAB, cell-associated bacteria; CFU/mL, colony-forming units per milliliter; PSB, protected specimen brush.

with viable surrounding or bordering parenchyma. Lung gangrene represents complete lobar or entire lung destruction, often with only a rim of tissue remaining. Lung necrosis is best represented by patchy, often nonanatomic, loss of perfusion with variable parenchyma destruction, often seen on radiograph as multiple small abscess-like cavities. Although the three can be discussed separately, in the majority of cases two or three coexist and so the management can also overlap.

The cause(s) of lung abscess in the surgical intensive care unit (ICU) population include aspiration, complications of pneumonia, retained foreign body, septic emboli, and infected traumatic injury. More specific causes in the trauma population include aspiration (with or without bronchial obstruction), infected pneumatocele, infected site of resection (in particular emergent tractotomy), and late complications of VAP. As a whole these are less common in trauma patients than nontrauma patients. Of 45 thoracotomies performed at Harborview Medical Center over 7 years for abscess, necrotizing pneumonia, and lung gangrene, only 4 were in patients initially admitted following traumatic injury.

The diagnosis of lung abscess may be relatively simple. Fever, purulent sputum production, or hemoptysis may prompt chest radiograph, which will identify an air-fluid cavity. On the other extreme, a persistently febrile patient in the ICU with dense consolidation may require CT scan before the underlying cavity can be recognized.

Over the 3 decades during the 1950s to the 1970s, there were a number of advances that reduced the mortality rate from approximately 50% to 10%. These advances included recognizing the importance of antibiotics, the role of aspiration, the need for pulmonary toilet (including liberal use of bronchoscopy), image-guided catheter drainage, and operative intervention in selective situations. Percutaneous catheter drainage can be performed even in ventilated patients and has reduced the number of thoracotomies required. Although there is always concern about the risk of empyema and BPF, the former usually can be managed easily by chest drainage, and the latter is rarely so significant as to impair oxygenation. Some patients will require surgical intervention such as those with persistent sepsis from undrained fluid collections when there is inability to place a percutaneous catheter, incomplete drainage, hemoptysis, or persistent or major BPF. In these situations, the two primary operations are lobectomy, for large central cavities, or débridement (with/without muscle flap to help close the space) for smaller peripheral cavities. These are technically challenging surgical situations, and several technical points can help reduce complications: prevent aspiration by isolating the affected lung prior to posterolateral positioning; expose the main pulmonary artery early in the case so that should hemorrhage result control can be achieved; place a nasogastric tube or esophagoscope in the esophagus because the anatomy may be obliterated; and refrain from resecting small abscesses (<2 cm) that are in otherwise viable parenchyma. Air leak is not uncommon, and as will be discussed under empyema, a residual space can be managed with continuous postoperative irrigation.

The distinguishing characteristics of lung gangrene are central vascular thrombosis and bronchial obstruction, leading to significant cavitation and lobar or whole-lung liquefaction. As opposed to lung abscess, there is not a firm, well-defined capsule. Both these features are defined by CT with intravenous contrast agent and either one predicts the failure of medical therapy. This is because medical therapy relies on both blood supply for antibiotic therapy to be effective and bronchial patency to allow expectoration of purulent material. In a historical study, Schamaun and colleagues followed 14 patients with unilateral complete lung gangrene. Four were treated medically and all died, but 10 underwent surgical resection with 100% survival rate. Some patients have diffuse bilateral disease. In the face of persistent signs of infection, if there is a primary target site, surgery is still possible, and can be performed even if the patient cannot tolerate independent lung ventilation. Interestingly, the dissection in the fissures and of the vessels are relatively easy as the necrotic tissue tends to be easily swept aside. However, surgery resection should not be performed if the patient is pressor dependant. In this setting it is better to temporize with pleuroscopy to treat associated empyema and percutaneous drainage of the large cavitary lesions.

Necrotizing pneumonia is characterized by areas of dense consolidation, patchy perfusion, and often multiple small cavitary changes. Percutaneous drainage does not help in this setting. Generally parenchyma resection is not indicated. However, serial CT scans can identify areas that are developing demarcation lines and in the setting of persistent pulmonary sepsis resection can be a reasonable option.

Bronchial Stricture

Of patients with blunt traumatic injury to the distal trachea or bronchi, 10% to 20% are not diagnosed acutely, but in a delayed fashion as stricturing occurs. In approximately two thirds of these cases, suppuration, persistent atelectasis, and hemoptysis develop within 1 to 2 weeks of injury. In the remainder, presentation may be delayed years until "asthma," dyspnea on exertion, or delayed parenchyma necrosis develops. Any young patient with new-onset asthma should be considered for airway evaluation if this develops 1 to 2 years after blunt traumatic chest injury, even if initial radiographic and bronchoscopic workup was previously done and was normal. Bronchoscopy, CT scan, CT (or "virtual") bronchography, and flow-volume loops can help make the diagnosis, depending on the clinical circumstances. If postobstructive parenchymal destruction has occurred, then distal lung resection is required. If not, airway resection and reconstruction can salvage the distal lung. In chronic settings, there may be a suggestion of lack of perfusion to the affected lung. In the absence of clinical signs of sepsis and evidence of lung necrosis, attempts should be made to reconstruct the airway as in the majority of cases this lack of perfusion is a hypoxic vasoconstrictive response that reverses once ventilation had been restored. In patients who are too unstable, airway stenting can be tried to maintain airway patency as a temporizing measure. In those patients who present years later with a chronic fibrotic stricture, balloon dilation and repeat stenting may be an alternative to operative repair.

Pulmonary Torsion

Lobar torsion is exceedingly rare after trauma, and is reported more commonly after upper lobectomy when the middle lobe can swing freely in the residual space. Recognizing this potential, surgical fixation of the middle lobe to the lower lobe with the aid of a stapler or with sutures as pneumopexy can prevent this from occurring. Alternatively, torsion may occur during thoracotomy while retracting the lung to expose posterior mediastinal structures, particularly if the inferior pulmonary ligament has been divided. The key to prevent this complication is to observe that the lung expands properly before closing the chest. Primary pulmonary torsion is exceedingly rare, but not unheard of. Schamaun reviewed 26 cases of torsion in the literature and found that five were posttraumatic. Possible mechanisms include focal injury to one lobe, in the setting of a complete fissure, resulting in a focal immediate twisting or delayed torsion as hemorrhage and edema create a lead point. The diagnosis may be suggested by lobar consolidation, the development of fever, and hemoptysis, eventually developing into frank pulmonary sepsis. The diagnosis can be confirmed by bronchoscopy, which documents a "fish mouth" appearance of the affected bronchus, occasionally with blood or purulent material intermittently draining. When diagnosed, immediate operation is required. If not frankly gangrenous, the lobe should be "detorsed" to assess viability. If not viable, lobectomy is required. If viable, it should be stapled to an adjacent lobe to prevent retorsion or secured to the adjacent lobe with absorbable sutures as a pneumopexy.

Retained Parenchyma Missiles

The need for removal of parenchymal foreign objects is based on the risk of developing complications, which appear to be more common with irregularly shaped missiles compared to smooth objects. The University of Heidelberg reviewed the course of 55 patients who had retained bullets. Thirty-four experienced recurrent hemoptysis (single episode in eight). A Finnish review of 502 patients over several years noted that 20% developed complications requiring surgery. These complications included chronic bronchitis (39), lung abscess (31), bronchiectasis (5), empyema (24), and BPF (10). Much of contemporary recommendations are based on data from World War II and in the 2 decades following, including the aforementioned studies. In World War II early removal of retained missiles was associated with a 0.9% mortality rate and late removal of symptomatic objects was associated with 7.3% mortality rate. However, it was noted then and subsequently that waiting 2 to 6 weeks to allow parenchymal inflammation to resolve was also associated with easier removal with reduced complications, notably bleeding, air leak, and empyema. The technique of removal obviously depends on the location and nature of the missile. Peripheral objects can be removed by wedge resection. Deeper objects can be retrieved via tractotomy, or occasionally lobectomy if there is significant associated destruction, necrosis, or infection. Uncommonly, over time, central foreign objects can erode into the bronchi, leading to obstructive pneumonitis and abscess formation. These may be retrieved endoscopically, although severe tissue destruction, if present, mandates lobectomy. Alternatively, these objects may migrate peripherally, resulting in empyema. These can be retrieved and the empyema managed by VATS or thoracotomy.

PLEURAL COMPLICATIONS

Retained Hemothorax

Tube thoracostomy fails to completely evacuate hemothorax in approximately 5% of cases. Complications that may arise include empyema and fibrothorax. Conditions that predispose patients to both include prolonged ventilation, development of pneumonia, break in the pleura with residual blood (as is the case following tube thoracostomy), and other sites of infection. On the other hand, stable, nonventilated patients with small effusions (<25% hemothorax) following blunt trauma with no obvious pleural disruption usually will resolve without sequelae. In these patients the cornerstone of therapy should be observation.

The use of antibiotics at the time of chest tube placement, in particular with gram-positive coverage, has been shown to reduce the risk of empyema in many, but not all, reviews. However, even those papers that support prophylactic antibiotics do not show further advantages to giving more than one dose, 24 hours' worth of coverage, or administering antibiotics until all the drains are removed.

Early evacuation of hemothorax has been shown to reduce the incidence of complications preferably within 7 days when loculations begin to complicate pleural débridement. In particular, the risk of empyema is reduced. However, recognizing the extent of hemothorax can be difficult. Chest radiography can underestimate both the extent of parenchymal consolidation and the volume of retained blood, particularly in ventilated patients. Chest CT is much more accurate in this setting, but interpretation requires some individualization (Fig. 1). Moderate effusions in ventilated patients or those with other risk factors should be aggressively drained when detected by CT.

When recognized acutely following injury, the simplest and most expeditious treatment is to place a second chest tube. When recognized after 1 to 2 days, this may not be helpful in that it may simply increase pain, splinting, and the risk of pneumonia with subsequent seeding of the pleural space. Intrapleural streptokinase, urokinase, or more recently recombinant tissue plasminogen activator has an

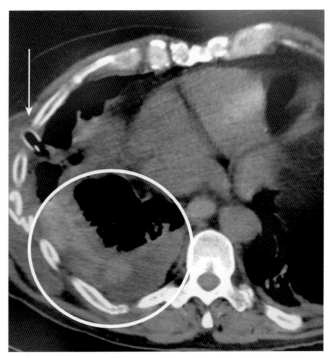

FIGURE 1 Computed tomography (CT) scan of retained hemothorax. This patient sustained blunt trauma with rib fracture and hemothorax. Plain chest radiograph suggested right lower lobe consolidation. The CT scan shows a chest tube in place *(arrow)* with consolidated lower lobe and retained complex effusion *(circle)*. Six days following admission, the patient was experiencing low-grade fever and had a mildly elevated white blood cell count.

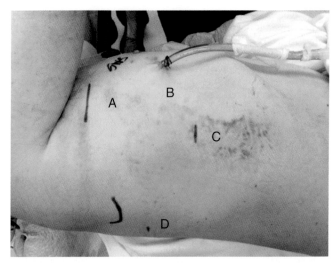

FIGURE 2 Video-assisted thoracoscopic surgery (VATS) approaches. There are a number of approaches possible. This figure illustrates the same patient as depicted in Figure 1. Ideally the first port should be placed "open," as the lung can be densely adherent to the chest wall. Although in many cases, especially if done early, VATS can be performed through one or two ports, the more chronic the setting, the wider the exposure must be. *A:* Accessory non–rib-spreading minimal incision allows wide débridement and manipulation, similar to that used for VATS lobectomy. The latissimus dorsi is spared. *B:* An anterior port is often the first placed. The intercostal spaces are wider and it is easier to dissect to the space with a small incision to avoid injuring the heart, diaphragm, and lung. In this case the chest tube site was used to gain initial entry, and the pleural space was cleared digitally to create the initial space to perform the procedure. *C:* Midaxillary port, placed under direct vision from port *B.* Often ideal for camera placement, this can be a 5-mm port, depending on the findings. *D:* Posterior port if needed. Often 5 mm, or if intrathoracic instruments are bigger than that, use without a port to minimize intercostal nerve irritation.

efficacy rate of 65% to 90%. Complications include fever and pain, but the risk of restarting bleeding is negligible. The downside of this approach is that it takes several days longer than more direct operative drainage and will not break down loculations. Furthermore, the cost of failed attempts of lysis are significant. Thus, it may be more useful following débridement when it is suspected that the clot is relatively "soft."

Thoracoscopy offers the advantage of complete removal of all clot without the excess morbidity of a formal thoracotomy. Meyer et al compared placement of a second chest tube versus thoracoscopy for treatment of retained traumatic hemothorax. Patients undergoing thoracoscopy had a shortened length of time requiring chest tube drainage, a shortened hospital stay (2.7 days less), and a decreased total hospital cost ($6000 less) compared to those patients treated with a second chest tube. There were no failures, no complications, and no patients required conversion to a formal thoracotomy in the group randomized to early thoracoscopy. In contrast, a second chest tube failed to completely evacuate the retained hemothorax requiring operative treatment in over 40% of the patients.

In highly selected cases, thoracotomies through "mini" approaches are often sufficient to allow removal of soft gelatinous visceral and pleural rind, permitting full lung expansion (Figs. 2 and 3). Irrigation with warm saline facilitates clot removal. The denser the adhesions the greater the exposure must be, and if a formal decortication of a formed visceral peel is anticipated, a standard approach is required. This can be facilitated by excising a rib subperiosteally to allow safe identification of the pleura.

In summary, patients with retained hemothorax, at risk of empyema, should be managed aggressively, preferably by early thoracoscopic drainage. There are occasional patients who present with delayed effusions, days after blunt injury, presumably partially due to missed small hemothorax and partially secondary to reactive

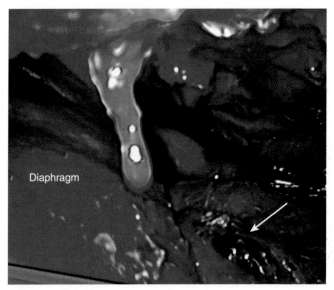

FIGURE 3 Camera view from VATS in the same patient as shown in the Figures 1 and 2. The right lower lobe is densely consolidated and has a small rent *(arrow)*. The pleural space after evacuation of free fluid remains full of debris, which was cleaned out by grasper and irrigation. The lung rent was no longer actively leaking air. Once the chest was evacuated positive pressure allowed the right lower lobe to fully expand. The patient responded rapidly, had the surgically placed thoracostomy tube removed on postoperative day 2, and quickly recovered with return of pulmonary function and toilet.

fluid accumulation. If these patients have adequate pain control, have small effusions (less than 25% of the hemithorax), and have no signs of infection, tube thoracostomy does not need to be performed as the risk of fibrothorax is negligible. Patients who present late (usually >3 months following injury) with an element of fibrothorax (but with no infection) should be managed nonoperatively as at 6 to 9 months in the majority of cases there is some remodeling and adaptation, and if surgery is required there is no increased difficulty if it is undertaken at a later date.

Empyema

Empyema occurs in 2% to 7% of patients who undergo tube thoracostomy following trauma. Patients at risk include those with residual hemothorax noted on chest radiograph, concurrent pneumonia, pain with diminished cough, and extrathoracic sites of infection, and possibly those who are ventilated and who have a chest tube in place. Trauma patients are at risk of developing gram-positive empyema, characterized by early loculations and formation of dense adhesions because of hemothorax, which offers both a rich supply of bacterial nutrients as well as fibrin. These factors also tend to make empyema in trauma patients less amenable to simple drainage than the more common parapneumonic empyema seen in medical patients.

The diagnosis of empyema is based on the documentation of an exudative effusion, characterized in particular by an elevated pleural/serum lactate dehydrogenase (LDH) ratio (>0.6). In approximately 25% to 30% of cases, cultures will be negative owing to suppression but not eradication by antibiotics. It is not uncommon for patients to present with indolent courses, often characterized by a failure to wean from ventilation, with persistent fluid noted by CT or chest radiograph, despite tube drainage. Contrast CT scans often reveal a "rim sign" of enhancing pleura, indicative of ongoing inflammation. In many cases once these "contaminated hemothoraces" are drained, the clinical picture rapidly improves.

Empyema has been described as having three stages. The first, usually within 1 to 7 days, is referred to as the "acute" or "serous" phase. This distinction is important because at this stage there is the best chance for draining the thin, exudative fluid by simple thoracostomy. There have been attempts to treat this early stage by simple aspiration. Evidence of vigorous inflammation (pH < 7.0) almost universally predicts failure of this technique. Tapping may be appropriate in patients who have complex effusions, with or without loculations, but who have other potential sites of infection. However managed, it is imperative that complete drainage be achieved, or failing that, early operative drainage is performed before progressive pleural obliteration occurs, characteristic of progression to the second or "subacute" phase and thence the final or "chronic" phase. Palpation at the time of thoracostomy or loculations noted on CT can alert the surgeon to the presence of loculations that would indicate that simple tube drainage will fail.

Probably the major reason for earlier intervention is that minimally invasive approaches are more successful early, whereas with the passage of time, the combined impact of pleural space obliteration and visceral peel lead to parenchyma trapping, increasing both the likelihood of requiring thoracotomy as well as the incidence of primary failure. As noted earlier, compared to nontrauma patients, empyema following trauma is much more likely to require operative intervention.

The primary treatment of empyema is to both completely drain the thorax and to permit full lung expansion. There are several "local" considerations that may impact operative approach and outcomes (Table 2). Predominant among these are whether or not loculations and a restrictive visceral peel have formed. In the acute setting, particularly when clinical signs suggest active infection, the primary goal is simply to drain the pleura. Evidence of loculations suggests that

TABLE 2: Considerations When Treating Empyema

Residual space
Quality of lung parenchyma
Trapped lung
Density of loculations
Patient ventilated
Air leak currently or anticipated
Lung abscess

simple tube drainage will fail. Alternative approaches could include image-directed catheter placement, thoracoscopic drainage, and "mini" or full thoracotomy. Thrombolytic therapy has been advocated as an alternative to operative intervention, but current data suggest that when compared to thoracoscopic approaches as primary intervention, thrombolytic therapy is associated with a higher failure rate, increased length of stay, and greater cost. Thrombolytic therapy is a reasonable alternative in patients who are deemed at high risk for operative intervention, and whose loculations may be diaphanous. In essence, these criteria would be in the uncommon scenario of a patient who is clinically infected and frail but not yet intubated, as once a patient is on the ventilator, the primary complication of operative approaches (respiratory failure) has already occurred. Thrombolytic therapy does have a role in the early postoperative period when after operative decortication residual loculated fluid collections are present. In this setting the fibrinous adhesions are "soft" and may be lysed.

Thoracoscopy, both VATS and pleuroscopy (using a mediastinoscope), have been compared to thoracotomy in a variety of series, which tend to be nonrandomized. VATS appears to be associated with decreased morbidity and shorter length of stay, but it is usually performed much earlier in the hospital course when loculations are less formed and the patients are clinically more stable. VATS may not be technically possible because of high ventilator requirements precluding lung isolation and dense pleural symphysis. An alternative approach is "rigid" thoracoscopy or pleuroscopy. Pleuroscopy can be performed on these patients, using CT imaging to direct the initial approach. The wider port allows easier débridement and suctioning, and visceral decortication is possible except in the most fibrotic cases.

Irrigation postoperatively is a useful adjunct in certain cases. The goal of irrigation may be to wash out blood from the operation, thus preventing new, vigorous adhesions. In addition, antibiotics can be added to improve local treatment of resistant organisms (such as *Candida* or methicillin-resistant organisms). Irrigation systems can be modified according to circumstances (e.g., a Jackson-Pratt drain connected to intravenous tubing via a three-way stopcock). The actual volume of irrigation is flexible, although we generally use 100 mL/hour. To avoid excessive drainage through the incision or drain sites, these tubes need to be closed tightly. When the pleural effluent is clear and culture negative, the irrigation can be discontinued. One potential disadvantage of postoperative irrigation is that pleural symphysis may be prevented, resulting in residual spaces. On the other hand, if a residual space is anticipated, irrigation is particularly effective. In fact, in some cases as the chest tubes are removed, it is possible, for example, to convert the Jackson-Pratt drain back into a simple bulb drain, which is better tolerated by the patient.

The residual pleural space remains a problem, requiring a flexible approach, depending primarily on whether or not the lung is capable of expanding (Table 3). In the trauma population the primary reason for failure of lung expansion is visceral peel, but in nontraumatic empyema, the cause is relatively equally divided between visceral peel, parenchymal consolidation, and pleural space following lung resection.

TABLE 3: Managing the Residual Space

Irrigation plus antibiotics
Positive-pressure ventilation to expand consolidated lung
Bronchoscopy to rule out and treat endobronchial obstruction
Visceral decortication
Open drainage for chronic treatment, particularly if patient
   debilitated
Tissue flaps
Combination: Clagett procedure

When performing thoracotomy for empyema, it may be advisable to avoid "counting ribs" beneath the scapula. This reduces contamination and the potential for a subscapular abscess. If a dense parietal pleural or significant pleural symphysis is anticipated, subperiosteal rib resection provides a safer avenue of entering the thorax. Visceral decortication may actually be simpler and safer with the affected lung being ventilated, as the "peel-parenchyma" interface is easier to define. Significant peripheral lung leaks are acceptable if it looks like the lung will expand and significantly fill the thorax. If the parenchyma is too consolidated to expand, or if visceral pleurectomy is proceeding poorly (technically difficult, large air leaks, bloody), it may be necessary to abandon pleurectomy in favor of a strategy aimed at treating a residual space, such as drainage, irrigation, tissue flaps, and open drainage.

However the empyema is drained, it is important to recognize that the underlying lung may have to be reevaluated. Once expansion has occurred, it may be apparent that there was a lung abscess or other necrotizing process that may require further intervention. In addition, in most cases the pleural space will appear radiographically much as it did prior to operation. This may make clinical assessment of whether or not there is ongoing pleural sepsis difficult. One possible method to help sort this out is to follow serial LDH levels from the chest tubes. A falling LDH level implies a reduction in pleural inflammation and success; a rising LDH implies the opposite.

In summary, the principles of treating empyema are as follows: drain the pleura; débride the pleura; maximize lung expansion; if lung expansion is not possible, consider either tissue flaps (if small) or chronic open drainage; and close significant BPFs. Earlier intervention allows less invasive procedures to be performed with higher likelihood of success. Thoracoscopy using "rigid" techniques is still possible in patients who are not VATS candidates, but thoracotomy should not be delayed.

Chylothorax

Primary traumatic chylothorax is exceedingly uncommon. It can occur following penetrating injuries to the thoracic inlet, after transmediastinal injuries, or after blunt trauma. Of interest, chylothorax is associated with spine fractures in only 20% of cases. Chylothorax can manifest in a delayed fashion with recurrent effusions, as persistent milky pleural output, or rarely as a tension chylothorax. Chylothorax is more commonly seen as a complication following repair of aortic injury or esophageal resection. The diagnosis can be established by documenting triglyceride levels greater than 110 mg/dL and predominant lymphocytes in the effusion. If noted acutely, it is important to consider the possibility of associated injury to adjacent structure, especially esophagus or aorta. The primary complication is nutritional and immunologic compromise. Initial management includes drainage, assuring complete lung expansion (with increased PEEP in ventilated patients), and parenteral nutritional support. Although low-fat diets do reduce the flow of chyle, even oral water has been noted to increase chyle flow. How long medical therapy should be tried is not clear, but generally 4 weeks is the maximum duration,

depending on the physiologic reserves of the patient. Chylothorax noted immediately after operation may be best treated by reoperation and maneuvers as described later.

Lymphangiography (either by CT, nuclear studies, or formal lymphangiogram) may be helpful in determining the site of the leak, the presence of collaterals, and the volume of the leak, all of which may predict success or failure of medical therapy. If no specific leak is documented, and collaterals are noted to drain into the venous system, medical management has a much higher success rate. With parenteral nutrition and strict NPO (nothing by mouth) an almost immediate cessation of chyle flow is a good prognostic sign that supports medical management. Octreotide has also been used as an adjunct. If the duct can be identified, then transabdominal coil embolization has been successful. A persistent space (especially after pneumonectomy), widespread disruption (after esophagectomy for example), or persistent high output with medical therapy is associated with an extremely high failure rate, and earlier intervention is warranted. Ultimately, operation should be considered if the leak persists after 2 weeks, and certainly by 4 weeks; if the patient is deteriorating immunologically or nutritionally; and clearly if there is another indication for operation. Patients who present in a delayed fashion are managed similarly. Our bias is that if after 1 week of maximal medical therapy the patient continues to drain more than 1500 mL/24 hours and is clearly losing ground nutritionally, then in the vast majority of cases we would try coil embolization and if this is not possible or unsuccessful, perform open ligation.

Operation can be performed by thoracoscopy or thoracotomy. The site may be directly visualized, in which case direct ligation (usually with pledget sutures) or glue application should be used. Localization can be assisted by feeding the patient cream just prior to operation. Mass ligation at the level of the diaphragm on the right side can resolve both right and left leaks. It is critical to recognize that the duct and surrounding tissue can be very friable, and thus ligation can lead to another site of leak. In addition, collaterals may exist that bypass the site of ligation. We have thus found that a critical component is to assure complete decortication (to allow lung expansion), pleural abrasion or decortication, and if in doubt, continue ventilation for 24 hours to assist full lung expansion. We maintain patients strictly on an NPO status for 7 days following surgery.

Fibrothorax

As mentioned in the discussion of retained hemothorax, symptomatic fibrothorax is more feared than real. Patients who have had an infected hemothorax are at the greatest risk, and usually present much sooner in their hospital course. The problem with deciding whether or not to operate for fibrothorax associated with chronic respiratory complaints includes the following: in many cases the decision is based on CT findings of pleural thickening, and invariably the postoperative films look identical to the preoperative films; patients who have sustained multiple chest wall injuries are actually symptomatic from that rather than fibrothorax, including chronic pain, which will be aggravated rather than relieved by thoracotomy.

▌ SURGICAL THERAPY POINTS

- Early thoracoscopy can shorten hospital stay for patients with persistent air leak or hemothorax
- The diagnosis of VAP is difficult and is based on clinical suspicion and an understanding that confirmatory tests have differing sensitivities and specificities, the thresholds of which may have to be decreased if the patient is receiving antibiotics.
- Pneumatocele and hematoma are in the majority of cases radiographic findings that do not require intervention.
- Necrotizing lung infections require an individualized approach. However, demonstration of a lack of perfusion is associated with

a failure of medical management and usually surgery is required. If the patient is, however, requiring vasopressors due to septic shock, parenchymal resection should be delayed, using percutaneous drainage or thoracoscopy.

- Risk factors for empyema in the trauma population include residual fluid seen by chest radiograph after tube placement. This should prompt consideration for thoracoscopic drainage early before vigorous adhesions develop.
- Patients who present with new-onset asthma following chest injury should be evaluated for bronchial stricture. In the absence of lung necrosis, either airway stents or direct reconstruction results in good outcomes.

- Retained parenchymal foreign bodies, particularly if irregular, tend to be associated with long-term complications. Large, central, and irregular fragments should be removed 2 to 3 weeks after injury to allow surrounding inflammation to resolve.
- Chylothorax can be managed medically or with other interventional techniques. Persistent leak or nutritional deterioration mandates an aggressive operative approach, of which the cornerstone is not simply duct ligation, but ensuring full lung expansion.

For the chapter's Suggested Readings list, please visit the book at www.ExpertConsult.inkling.com.

CARDIAC INJURIES

Juan A. Asensio, Patrizio Petrone, Alejandro Perez-Alonso, Zachary Torgersen, Brian Biggerstaff, Brittney J. Maloley-Lewis, Pulkesh Bhatia, Jeffery A. Bailey, Juan A. Sanchez, and Elias Degiannis

PENETRATING CARDIAC INJURY

Historical Perspective

The earliest descriptions of a cardiac injury are found in the *Iliad* and in the *Edwin Smith Papyrus*, written in approximately 3000 BC. Hippocrates stated that all wounds of the heart were deadly. Ambrose Paré, the famous French trauma surgeon, described two cases of penetrating cardiac injuries, both detailed from autopsy studies. Wolf, in 1642, was the first to describe a healed wound of the heart, and Senac, in 1749, concluded that although all wounds of the heart were serious, some wounds might heal and not be fatal. Larrey was the first to describe the surgical approach to the pericardium to relieve a pericardial effusion and is credited with pioneering the technique for pericardial window. Billroth, in 1875 and in 1883, proclaimed his strong resistance to any attempt at cardiac injury repair. Block, in 1882, created cardiac wounds in a rabbit model and was successful in achieving repair, thus demonstrating successful recovery and suggesting that the same techniques could be applicable to humans. Also, Del Vecchio demonstrated cardiac injury healing after suturing the heart in a canine model.

However, it took the courage of Cappelen from Norway to attempt cardiac injury repair in a human; in 1895 he repaired a 2-cm left ventricular laceration including ligation of a large branch of the distal left anterior descending coronary artery. This was followed by Farina in Italy in 1896, who also attempted to repair a left ventricular wound; however, both patients succumbed. Rehn in Germany in 1896 was successful in repairing a wound of the right ventricle, and Hill, in 1902, was the first surgeon in the United States to successfully repair a left ventricular injury.

Duval described the median sternotomy incision, and Spangaro, in 1906, described the left anterolateral thoracotomy incision. Peck in 1909 was the first to describe successful repair of a stab wound of the right atrium, and he reported a total of 11 patients. Smith was the first to develop a comprehensive plan for cardiac injury management, and for the first time pointed out the dangers of dysrhythmias occurring during cardiac manipulation. He also described the use of an Allis clamp near the apex to stabilize and hold the heart during suture placement.

Beck in 1942 described the technique of placing mattress sutures under the bed of the coronary arteries. During the same year, Griswold refined the techniques in the management of cardiac injuries and recommended that every large general hospital should have available a sterile set of instruments plus an available operating room 24 hours a day. Elkin in 1944 recommended the administration of intravenous infusions before operation and pointed to the beneficial effects of increasing blood volume and thus cardiac output. Beall and colleagues were the first to describe the technique of emergency department (ED) thoracotomy. Meanwhile, Mattox et al refined and protocolized ED thoracotomy and cardiorrhaphy, inclusive of the use of emergency cardiopulmonary bypass in the management of these injuries. These hallmark contributions have made it possible for patients sustaining penetrating cardiac injuries to survive today.

Incidence

Feliciano et al in 1983 described a 1-year experience consisting of 48 cardiac injuries at Ben Taub Hospital in Houston. Mattox and associates in 1989 described a 30-year experience from the same institution reporting 539 cardiac injuries (18 cardiac injuries per year). Asensio and colleagues reported two prospective consecutive series reporting a total of 165 cardiac injuries in a 3-year period (55 cardiac injuries per year) at Los Angeles County/USC Medical Center in Los Angeles. In 2006 a review by Asensio et al, which focused on the National Trauma Databank (NTDB) of the American College of Surgeons (ACS), identified a total of 2016 patients sustaining penetrating cardiac injuries, and calculated the national incidence of 0.16% for these injuries. Thus, penetrating cardiac injuries are uncommon and are usually seen only in busy urban trauma centers.

Etiology

In the civilian arena, penetrating cardiac injuries are usually caused by gunshot wounds (GSWs), stab wounds (SWs), and rarely by shotgun wounds and ice picks. According to a recent review, 63% of all reported cardiac injuries in America are caused by gunshot wounds and 36% are caused by stab wounds; shotgun and impalement injuries accounted for approximately 1% of these injuries. In the military arena, Rich and Spencer reported 96 cardiac injuries from the Vietnam conflict. Most of these patients sustained injuries from grenade fragments or shrapnel, and a few of these patients were impaled by flechettes.

Clinical Presentation

Beck's triad—muffled heart tones, jugular venous distention, and hypotension—describes the classical presentation of a patient with pericardial tamponade. Kussmaul's sign, described as jugular venous distention upon inspiration, is another classic sign attributed to pericardial tamponade. In reality, the presence of Beck's triad and Kussmaul's sign represents the exception rather than the rule. It is estimated that Beck's triad is present in only approximately 10% of patients.

The clinical presentation of penetrating cardiac injuries may range from complete hemodynamic instability to cardiopulmonary arrest; in fact, some penetrating cardiac injuries can be very deceptive in their presentation. The clinical presentation of penetrating cardiac injuries may also be related to other factors, including the wounding mechanism; the length of time elapsed before arrival at a trauma center; and the extent of the injury, which if sufficiently large in terms of myocardial destruction will invariably lead to exsanguinating hemorrhage into the left hemithoracic cavity. The presentation of these injuries is also related to blood loss, as patients who lose between 40% and 50% of intravascular blood volume develop cardiopulmonary arrest. The muscular nature of the left ventricle, and to a lesser extent that of the right ventricle, may seal penetrating injuries and prevent exsanguinating hemorrhage, allowing these patients to arrive with some signs of life at a trauma center.

The most unique presentation of a penetrating cardiac injury is pericardial tamponade. The tough fibrous nature, lack of elasticity, and noncompliance of this structure translate to acute rises in intrapericardial pressure leading to compression of the thin wall of the right ventricle, impairing its ability to accept the returning blood volume, resulting in a concomitant decrease in left ventricular filling and ejection fraction. This results in a drastic decrease in cardiac output (CO) and stroke volume (SV). The impaired ability to generate both right and left ventricular ejection fractions increases cardiac work and myocardial wall tension. This results in an increase in myocardial volume of oxygen consumption (MVO_2) which cannot be met, leading to myocardial hypoxemia and lactic acidosis.

It is well known that the pericardium is able to accommodate gradual quantities of blood, provided that the rate of hemorrhage is slow and does not cause acute rises in intrapericardial pressures exceeding the right ventricle and subsequently the left ventricle's ability to fill. Pericardial tamponade can have both deleterious and protective effects. Its deleterious effects can lead to a rapid rise in pericardial pressure and cardiopulmonary arrest, whereas its protective effect will limit extrapericardial hemorrhage into the left hemithoracic cavity, preventing exsanguinating hemorrhage. Moreno et al, in a retrospective study consisting of 100 patients presenting with penetrating cardiac injuries, reported 77 patients who presented with pericardial tamponade. The authors reported that for patients presenting with pericardial tamponade, the survival rate was much higher—73% versus 11%—thereby ascribing tamponade a protective effect. These findings were statistically significant, leading the authors to conclude that pericardial tamponade is a critical independent factor in patient survival.

Asensio et al, in a prospective 2-year study reporting 105 patients, failed to find any statistical significance to the presence of pericardial tamponade in terms of survival, and were not able to identify it as a critical independent factor for survival. What remains undefined is the actual period of time after which the protective effect of pericardial tamponade is lost and when exactly this transition occurs, causing its adverse effect on cardiac function.

Diagnosis

Physical Examination

The clinical presentation of patients with penetrating cardiac injury may range from hemodynamically stable to cardiopulmonary arrest. Frequently, these patients present with associated pneumohemothoraces and decreased breath sounds in the ipsilateral hemithoracic cavity. Occasionally, patients presenting with precordial injuries are restless and refuse to lie down; this may be a subtle indicator denoting the presence of hemopericardium or incipient pericardial tamponade. The most dramatic presentation for a patient sustaining

a penetrating cardiac injury is, of course, cardiopulmonary arrest, which will require ED thoracotomy as a lifesaving intervention. Pericardiocentesis is mentioned only to note that it currently has no role in establishing the diagnosis of cardiac injuries.

Subxiphoid Pericardial Window

The original technique of pericardial window was described by Larrey in the 1800s, and only small variations in the original technique have been added to this procedure. This technique has seen a marked diminution in its role during recent times because of the advent of two-dimensional echocardiography as part of the focused assessment with sonography in trauma (FAST) examination. Nevertheless, the technique is still widely employed in many countries where medical personnel do not have access to ultrasound equipment.

Pericardial window must be performed in an operating room under general anesthesia. A 10-cm incision is made in the midline over the xiphoid process. Blunt and sharp dissection after digitally palpating the transmitted cardiac impulses is used to locate the pericardium, which is then isolated and grasped between two Allis clamps and placed under gentle downward traction. A longitudinal incision measuring approximately 1 to 2 cm is made in the pericardium sharply, with meticulous care taken to avoid an iatrogenic injury to the underlying myocardium. After this longitudinal aperture is made, fluid in the pericardium will escape; the field is flooded either with clear straw-colored pericardial fluid, which signifies a negative window, or with blood, indicative of a positive window and, thus, an underlying cardiac injury. A positive pericardial window mandates proceeding with median sternotomy. Finally, the field may remain dry if blood has clotted within the pericardium.

The advantages of this technique are safety and reliability for the detection of penetrating cardiac injuries. This relatively simple surgical technique belongs in the surgical armamentarium of every trauma surgeon. Disadvantages consist of having to subject the patient to a general anesthetic and a surgical procedure.

Two-Dimensional Echocardiography

Echocardiography as part of FAST has become the gold standard in the evaluation of patients with penetrating thoracic injury. Major benefits of echocardiography include being noninvasive, rapid, and accurate; its ability to be repeated at any time; and most importantly, its painlessness. Data from two multicenter studies conclusively support the role of FAST as the initial investigative tool for the evaluation of patients with penetrating cardiac injuries, given its accuracy and ease of performance. Other techniques such as transesophageal echocardiography (TEE) have no role in the immediate evaluation of patients sustaining penetrating precordial injuries.

Minimally Invasive Methods

Thoracoscopy

Morales et al reported a 31% incidence of positive windows describing a technique that was both accurate and well tolerated without any complications, and the authors recommend this technique to be used in patients also requiring evacuation of a retained hemothorax. In our opinion, thoracoscopic pericardial window has no role in the acute evaluation of penetrating cardiac injuries.

Laparoscopy

Similarly, laparoscopy has been used to detect peritoneal violation in patients sustaining penetrating abdominal trauma. It has been used to evaluate patients with thoracoabdominal injuries to evaluate presence of diaphragmatic or solid organ injuries. During laparoscopy, the pericardium can also be evaluated. Although this technique can be used, it is the opinion of the authors that it has no role in the acute evaluation of penetrating cardiac injuries.

Management

Prehospital

Emergency medical systems in large urban areas providing rapid transport to trauma centers have allowed patients with penetrating cardiac injuries an opportunity to undergo lifesaving surgical procedures. Field stabilization of patients with penetrating cardiac injuries should consist of intubation and closed cardiopulmonary resuscitation for patients found in cardiopulmonary arrest. Several studies strongly support and advocate for the need of immediate transport of patients with penetrating thoracic injuries to a trauma center, with the only predictors of outcome being the achievement of an airway via endotracheal intubation. Endotracheal intubation has been proved to increase both duration and tolerance of cardiopulmonary resuscitation administered for a period of less than 5 minutes. The return of organized cardiac electrical activity will provide the best opportunity for survival for these patients.

Emergency Department

All patients with penetrating cardiac injuries should undergo rapid initial assessment and resuscitation following Advanced Trauma Life Support (ATLS) protocols. Patients will usually self-stratify into those who are hemodynamically stable and may undergo diagnostic studies, those who are hemodynamically unstable but will respond to fluid resuscitation and allow for rapid transport to the operating room (OR), and those who present in cardiopulmonary arrest and will necessitate lifesaving surgical interventions such as ED thoracotomy. Patients can be initially and rapidly evaluated with FAST, chest radiograph, and optionally an electrocardiogram (ECG). Volume resuscitation with lactated Ringer solution and O-negative or type-specific blood should be initiated. An arterial blood gas analysis to determine initial pH and base deficit and lactic acid level should also be obtained. However, a significant majority of these patients will arrive in extremis, requiring lifesaving interventions.

Emergency Department Thoracotomy

ED thoracotomy is a surgical procedure of great value if undertaken after strict indications for its performance. This procedure is routinely performed in urban trauma centers that receive patients in extremis. When performed in an expedient fashion, ED thoracotomy, aortic cross-clamping, and cardiorrhaphy are successful in salvaging approximately 10% of all penetrating cardiac injuries. Open cardiopulmonary massage after definitive repair of penetrating cardiac injuries is more effective in producing a greater ejection fraction. Similarly, lacerations of major thoracic blood vessels can also be controlled by means of vascular clamps.

Prehospital factors predictive of poor outcome include absence of vital signs, fixed and dilated pupils, absence of cardiac rhythm, absence of motion in the extremities, absence of a palpable pulse, and the presence of cardiopulmonary arrest.

Generally accepted indications for this procedure include cardiopulmonary arrest secondary to penetrating thoracic injuries and profound shock with systolic blood pressures of less than 60 mm Hg because of exsanguinating hemorrhage or pericardial tamponade. Cardiopulmonary arrest secondary to blunt injury is generally a contraindication to the performance of this procedure.

Objectives to be achieved with this procedure include resuscitation of agonal patients arriving with penetrating cardiothoracic injuries, evacuation of pericardial tamponade, control of massive intrathoracic hemorrhage secondary to cardiovascular injuries, prevention of air emboli, and restoration of cardiac function using open cardiopulmonary massage. Other objectives to be accomplished include definitive repairs of penetrating cardiac injuries and control of exsanguinating thoracic vascular injuries. Similarly, cross-clamping of the descending thoracic aorta, redistributing the remaining blood volume to perfuse the carotid and coronary arteries, is achieved with this technique.

ED thoracotomy should be performed simultaneously with the initial assessment evaluation and resuscitation, using the ATLS protocols by trained trauma surgeons. Similarly, immediate venous access with simultaneous use of rapid infusion techniques complements the resuscitative process. A left anterolateral thoracotomy commencing at the lateral border of the left sternocostal junction and inferior to the nipple is carried out and extended laterally to the latissimus dorsi. In females, the breast is retracted cephalad. This incision is rapidly carried through skin until the intercostal muscles have been reached and sharply transected. A Finochietto retractor is then placed to separate the ribs. The lung is then elevated medially, and the thoracic aorta is located immediately as it enters the abdomen via the aortic hiatus. The aorta should then be palpated to assess the status of the remaining blood volume. It can also be temporarily occluded digitally against the bodies of the lower thoracic vertebrae. To fully cross-clamp the aorta, a combination of sharp and blunt dissection commencing at both the superior and inferior borders of the aorta is performed so that the aorta may be encircled between the thumb and index fingers; this facilitates the aortic cross-clamp to be placed safely. Trauma surgeons should then observe the pericardium and search for the presence of an injury. The pericardium is usually tense and discolored in the presence of tamponade. A longitudinal opening in the pericardial sac is then made anterior to the phrenic nerve and extended both inferiorly and superiorly. Usually it is necessary to grasp the pericardium and then make a small incision sharply, followed by opening the pericardium with Metzenbaum scissors.

After opening the pericardium, clotted blood is evacuated. The trauma surgeon should immediately note the presence or absence and type of underlying cardiac rhythm as well as location of the penetrating injury or injuries. The finding of a flaccid heart, devoid of any effective forward pumping motion is a strong predictor of poor outcome. Other predictors of poor outcome are empty coronary arteries and presence of air, indicating air emboli in the coronary veins.

Digital control of penetrating ventricular injuries as they are simultaneously sutured prevents further hemorrhage. We generally recommend the use of monofilament suture, such as 2-0 polypropylene. If the injury or injuries are quite large, balloon tamponade using a Foley catheter can temporarily arrest the hemorrhage either to allow the performance of cardiorrhaphy or to gain time so that the patient may be transferred expeditiously to an OR for a more definitive surgical procedure. We do not recommend the use of bioprosthetic materials such as Teflon patches in the ED. This is a time-consuming technique that, if needed, should be performed in the OR.

In our experience, staples do not effectively control hemorrhage, tend to enlarge the cardiac injury, and prove to be rather difficult to remove, although they have worked in the hands of others.

Strict pharmacologic manipulation coupled with directly delivered countershocks of 20 to 50 J is frequently needed to restore a normal sinus rhythm. At times a rhythm can be restored, but no effective pumping mechanism is observed. Progressive myocardial death can be witnessed, first by dilatation of the right ventricle with accompanying cessation of contractility and motion, followed by the same process in the left ventricle.

Outcomes of Emergency Department Thoracotomy for Penetrating Cardiac Injuries

Wide disparity in the reporting of outcomes exists in the literature, ranging from 0% to 72%. Most of these series are retrospective, and the patients reported have been injured because of stab wounds. Asensio, Wall, and others in the Working Group of the Committee on Trauma of the American College of Surgeons, after an extensive analysis of the literature, generated practice management guidelines for ED thoracotomy (Table 1).

TABLE I: Emergency Department Thoracotomy for Cardiac Injuries

Lead Author and Year	Type of Study	Survivors/ Penetrating Trauma	Survivors/Total Number of EDTs
Boyd, 1965	R	0/0	17/25
Beall, 1966	R	3/16	42/197
Sauer, 1967	R	12/0	12/13
Sugg, 1968	R	0/0	63/459
Yao, 1968	R	0/0	61/80
Steichen, 1971	R	7/21	35/58
Beall, 1971	R	29/52	42/66
Borja, 1971	R	0/0	24/145
Carrasquilla, 1972	R	8/30	20/245
Beall, 1972	R	0/0	67/269
Bolanowski, 1973	R	0/0	33/44
Trinkle, 1974	R	0/0	38/45
Mattox, 1974	R	25/37	31/62
Harvey, 1975	R	0/0	22/28
Symbas, 1976	R	0/0	50/98
Beach, 1976	R	0/4	26/34
Asfaw, 1977	R	0/0	277/323
Sherman, 1978	R	32/41	31/92
Trinkle, 1979	R	0/0	89/100
Evans, 1979	R	0/4	29/46
Breaux, 1979	R	39/44	78/197
Mandal, 1979	R	0/38	26/55
Gervin, 1982	R	4/21	4/21
Demetriades, 1983	R	2/16	40/125
Demetriades, 1984	R	1/11	0/45
Tavares, 1984	R	21/37	64
Feliciano, 1984	R	5/15	2/3
Mattox, 1985	R	50/119	204
Demetriades, 1986	R	1/18	70
Moreno, 1984	R	4/69	100
Ivatury, 1987	R	28/91	—
Jebara, 1989	R	4/17	—
Attar, 1991	R	21/55	—
Knott-Craig, 1992	R	5/13	—

TABLE I: Emergency Department Thoracotomy for Cardiac Injuries—cont'd

Lead Author and Year	Type of Study	Survivors/ Penetrating Trauma	Survivors/Total Number of EDTs
Buchman, 1992	R	1/2	23
Benyan, 1992	R	1/13	—
Macho, 1993	R	12/24	—
Mitchell, 1993	R	7/47	—
Kaplan, 1993	R	2/23	
Henderson, 1994	R	6/122	215
Coimbra, 1995	R	0/20	
Arreola-Risa, 1995	R	11/40	
Karmy-Jones, 1997	R	3/6	16
Rhee, 1998	R	15/58	41/96
Asensio, 1998c	P	6/37	6/37
Asensio, 1998a	P	10/71	10/71
Tyburski, 2000	R	12/152	12/152
Asensio, 2006	R	47/830	47/830

EDTs, Emergency department thoracotomies; P, prospective; R, retrospective.
Note: There were no survivors of blunt trauma.

Techniques for Cardiac Injury Repair

Incisions

Two main incisions are used in the management of penetrating cardiac injuries. Median sternotomy described by Duval is the incision of choice for patients admitted with penetrating precordial injuries who arrive with some degree of hemodynamic instability and may undergo preoperative investigation with either FAST or chest radiography. The left anterolateral thoracotomy described by Spangaro is the incision of choice in the management of patients who arrive in extremis. This incision is used in the ED for resuscitative purposes, and it can also be extended across the sternum as bilateral anterolateral thoracotomies. Extension into bilateral anterolateral thoracotomies is also the incision of choice for patients who are hemodynamically unstable after incurring mediastinum-traversing injuries (Fig. 1). It is important to note that upon transection of the sternum, both internal mammary arteries are also transected and must be ligated after restoration of perfusion pressure. For patients who sustain thoracoabdominal injuries, the left anterolateral thoracotomy is also the incision of choice if patients deteriorate in the OR while undergoing a laparotomy.

Adjunct Maneuvers

Trauma surgeons must possess several maneuvers in their armamentarium to deal with penetrating cardiothoracic injuries. Total inflow occlusion to the heart is a complex maneuver that entails cross-clamping both the superior vena cava (SVC) and inferior vena cava (IVC) in their intrapericardial location to arrest total blood flow to the heart (Fig. 2). It is indicated for the management of injuries in the lateralmost aspect of the right atrium or the superior or inferior

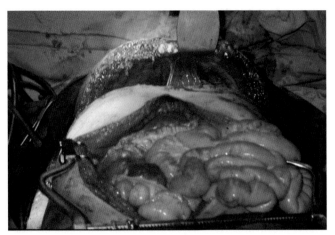

FIGURE 1 Bilateral thoracotomy and laparotomy in management of patients with thoracoabdominal injuries arriving in extremis.

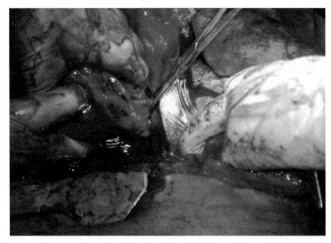

FIGURE 3 Vascular clamps in the pulmonary hilum. This maneuver is helpful to control penetrating pulmonary injuries with profuse bleeding or with a big hematoma in the pulmonary hilum.

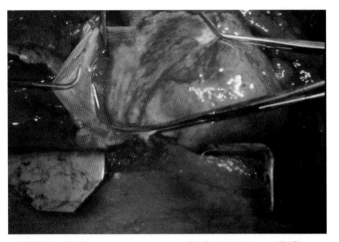

FIGURE 2 Both superior vena cava and inferior vena cava (IVC) clamped. The IVC is clamped at the Gibbon space. Note the clamp on the right auricle providing better exposure.

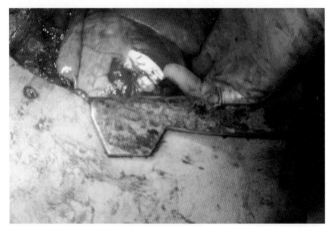

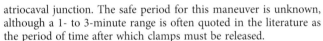

FIGURE 4 Gunshot wound to the left ventricle repaired with Teflon strips.

atriocaval junction. The safe period for this maneuver is unknown, although a 1- to 3-minute range is often quoted in the literature as the period of time after which clamps must be released.

Cross-clamping of the pulmonary hilum is another valuable maneuver indicated for the management of associated pulmonary injuries, particularly those that present with hilar central hematomas or active bleeding (Fig. 3). This maneuver arrests bleeding from the lung and prevents air emboli from reaching the systemic circulation. However, in the presence of acidosis, hypothermia, and ischemia, the right ventricle may not be able to tolerate this maneuver, leading to fibrillation and arrest.

At times, a trauma surgeon will need to elevate the heart out of the pericardium in order to repair certain injuries. If hemorrhage can be digitally controlled, gradual elevation of the heart by placing multiple laparotomy packs will allow better tolerance of this maneuver while decreasing the chances for development of dysrhythmias.

Repair of Atrial Injuries

Atrial injuries can usually be controlled by placement of a Satinsky partial occlusion vascular clamp. Control of the wound will allow the trauma surgeon to perform cardiorrhaphy. We recommend utilizing monofilament sutures of 2-0 polypropylene on an MH (medium half) needle either in a running or in an interrupted fashion. It is

important to visualize both sides of the atrial injury, particularly those caused by missiles, as they can cause a significant amount of tissue destruction, which might require meticulous débridement before closure. The use of bioprosthetic materials in the form of Teflon pledgets is not recommended for the management of these injuries.

Repair of Ventricular Injuries

Ventricular injuries usually cause significant hemorrhage. They should be occluded digitally while simultaneously repaired by either simple interrupted or horizontal mattress sutures of Halsted. Performing cardiorrhaphy for ventricular stab wounds is usually less challenging than for gunshot wounds. Missile injuries often produce some degree of blast effect that causes myocardial fibers to retract and frequently require multiple sutures to control significant hemorrhage. In this scenario, bioprosthetic materials such as Teflon strips and pledgets are often needed to buttress the suture line (Fig. 4). We recommend 2-0 monofilament sutures of polypropylene on an MH needle.

Coronary Artery Injuries

The repair of ventricular injuries adjacent to coronary arteries can be very challenging. In order to avoid potential narrowing and occlusion of a coronary artery or one of its branches, it is recommended that sutures be placed underneath the bed of the coronary artery. Coronary arteries are usually divided into three segments: proximal, middle, and distal. Injuries to the proximal and middle segments will usually require cardiopulmonary bypass for repair, and the institution of intra-aortic balloon counterpulsation followed by aortocoronary bypass, respectively. Lacerations of the distal segment of the coronary artery, particularly in the distalmost third of the vessel, are managed by ligation.

Complex and Combined Injuries

A significant number of patients arrive harboring multiple associated injuries in addition to their penetrating cardiac injuries. Complex and combined cardiac injuries can be defined as a penetrating cardiac injury plus associated neck, thoracic, thoracic vascular, abdominal, abdominal vascular, or peripheral vascular injuries (Figs. 5 and 6). These injuries are quite challenging to manage. Priority should be given early to the injury causing the greatest blood loss or threatening the patient's life.

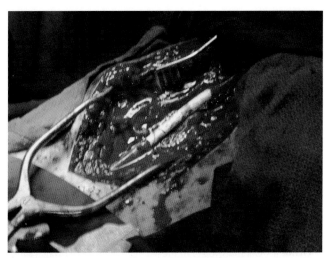

FIGURE 5 Patient with a femoro-femoral bypass with polytetrafluoroethylene, and after ligation of femoral vein. This patient sustained a gunshot wound to the left ventricle, and concomitantly left lung, left femur, and right hand injuries.

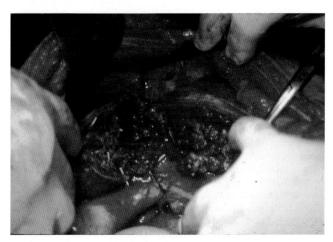

FIGURE 6 Liver injury American Association for the Surgery of Trauma Organ Injury Scale grade IV concomitantly with a cardiac injury. Complex hepatotomy and hepatorrhaphy were performed. Note the clips used to control bleeding.

Anatomic Location of Injury

A great deal of variability exists in the literature when it comes to reporting the breakdown of cardiac injuries by chambers (Table 2). Ventricular injuries occur with an incidence ranging from 37% to 67% of all cardiac injuries, whereas left ventricular injuries occur with an incidence ranging from 19% to 40%. Right atrial injuries appear to occur with greater frequency ranging from 5% to 20%, whereas the left atrium, the most recessed chamber of the heart, is injured between 2% and 12% of the time.

Associated Injuries

Penetrating cardiac injuries resulting from stab wounds are generally isolated and usually only involve one chamber because of their precordial penetration. However, missile injuries may injure the heart either from precordial or from extraprecordial locations, and thus have a greater propensity for causing multiple-chamber and associated injuries.

Prognostic Factors

The American Association for the Surgery of Trauma Organ Injury Scale (AAST-OIS) committee has developed a scale to uniformly describe cardiac injuries (Table 3). This scale comprehensively describes these injuries, but although the scale has been available since 1994, few studies have correlated cardiac injury grade with mortality rate.

Asensio and colleagues, in a 2-year prospective study of 105 patients, correlated AAST-OIS for cardiac injuries with mortality rate, in which 99 (94%) of the 105 patients incurred grade IV to VI injuries. Mortality rate progressively increased with injury grade. Grade IV injuries incurred a mortality rate of 56%, grade V 76%, and grade VI 91%. Although findings of both these studies would appear to validate the correlation between mortality rate and organ injury grade, the authors feel that further work is necessary to confirm their findings. Furthermore, the authors strongly believe that all cardiac injuries should be graded according to this scale.

Prognostic factors such as mechanism of injury; physiologic parameters at the scene of the traumatic incident, during transport, and upon arrival such as pupillary response, spontaneous ventilation, presence of a carotid pulse, presence of a measurable blood pressure, sinus rhythm, any extremity movement, and need for intubation and cardiopulmonary resuscitation; as well as scene times greater than 10 minutes have been prospectively validated in many studies. The presence of cardiopulmonary arrest upon arrival as a poor predictor of outcome has been confirmed. Similarly, physiologic parameters upon arrival such as these measured by the cardiovascular respiratory score (CVRS) component of the trauma score (TS) have been validated by Buckman et al.

BLUNT CARDIAC INJURY

Historical Perspective

The first unquestionable case of myocardial contusion was reported in 1764 by Akenside, and the first recorded case of blunt cardiac chamber rupture was reported in 1679 by Borch. According to Warburg, for almost 200 years, from 1676 to 1868, only 27 cases of blunt traumatic cardiac injuries were reported in the literature.

In 1958, Parmley et al reviewed 207,548 autopsy cases from the Armed Forces Institute of Pathology (AFIP) and described 546 patients with nonpenetrating traumatic injury to the heart, reporting an incidence of 0.1%. In this hallmark study, the authors reported 353

TABLE 2: Anatomic Location of Injuries

Lead Author	Year	Span (Years)	No. of Patients	CARDIAC CHAMBERS (#/%)				Multiple Chambers	Associated Coronary Arteries
				RV	LV	RA	LA		
Ivatury	1987	20	228	90 (39.4%)	44 (19.2%)	15 (6.5%)	6 (2.6%)	38 (16.6%), Location NR 20 (8.8%)	11 (4.8%)
Buckman	1993	2.25	66	Single chamber 42 (63.6%)				24 (36.3%)	NR
Henderson	1994	6	251	96 (38.2%)	98 (39.8%)	57 (22.7%)	31 (12.3%)	101 (40.2%)	NR
Arreola-Risa	1995	7	55	29 (52%)	17 (30%)	7 (12%)	2 (3%)	11 (20%)	1 (1.5%)
Wall	1997	20	711	284 (40%)	284 (40%)	171 (24%)	21 (3%)	14 (1.9%)	39 (5.4%)
Asensio	1998c	1	60	40 (66.6%)	15 (25%)	11 (18.3%)	3 (5%)	NR	5 (8.3%)
Asensio	1998a	2	105	39 (37.1%)	26 (24.7%)	8 (7.6%)	5 (4.7%)	23 (21.9%)	9 (8.5%)
Tyburski	2000	17	302	121 (40%)	75 (24.8%)	17 (5.6%)	6 (1.9%)	83 (27.4%)	NR
Totals			1778	699	559	328	74	314	65

LA, Left atrium; LV, left ventricle; NR, not reported; RA, right atrium; RV, right ventricle.

TABLE 3: American Association for the Surgery of Trauma Organ Injury Scale: Cardiac Injury

Grade*	Injury Description
I	Blunt cardiac injury with minor electrocardiographic abnormality (nonspecific ST-segment or T-wave changes, premature atrial or ventricular contraction, or persistent sinus tachycardia) Blunt or penetrating pericardial wound without cardiac injury, cardiac tamponade, or cardiac herniation
II	Blunt cardiac injury with heart block (right or left bundle branch, left anterior fascicular, or atrioventricular) or ischemic changes (ST-segment depression or T-wave inversion) without cardiac failure Penetrating tangential myocardial wound up to, but not extending through, endocardium, without tamponade
III	Blunt cardiac injury with sustained (≥6 beats per minute) or multifocal ventricular contractions Blunt or penetrating cardiac injury with septal rupture, pulmonary or tricuspid valvular incompetence, papillary muscle dysfunction, or distal coronary arterial occlusion without cardiac failure Blunt pericardial laceration with cardiac herniation Blunt cardiac injury with cardiac failure
IV	Penetrating tangential myocardial wound up to, but not extending through, endocardium, with tamponade Blunt or penetrating cardiac injury with septal rupture, pulmonary or tricuspid valvular incompetence, papillary muscle dysfunction, or distal coronary arterial occlusion producing cardiac failure Blunt or penetrating cardiac injury with aortic or mitral valve incompetence Blunt or penetrating cardiac injury of the right ventricle, right atrium, or left atrium
V	Blunt or penetrating cardiac injury with proximal coronary arterial occlusion Blunt or penetrating left ventricular perforation Stellate wound with <50% tissue loss of the right ventricle, right atrium, or left atrium
VI	Blunt avulsion of the heart; penetrating wound producing >50% tissue loss of a chamber

Modified from Moore EE, Malangoni MA, Cogbill TH, et al: Organ injury scaling IV: thoracic, vascular, lung, cardiac, and diaphragm. *J Trauma* 36:229–300, 1994.
*Advance one grade for multiple penetrating wounds to a single chamber or multiple chamber involvement.

cases of cardiac chamber rupture, of which 273 were isolated and 80 associated with combined aortic ruptures. The breakdown per chamber included 66 ruptured right ventricles, 59 ruptured left ventricles, 41 ruptured right atria, and 26 ruptured left atria. A total of 106 patients sustained multiple-chamber injuries.

Mechanism, Pathophysiology, and Incidence

Establishing a firm definition for what blunt cardiac injury (BCI) is has remained somewhat elusive. In fact, this entity was for quite some time known as myocardial contusion and has even been described as myocardial concussion. The exact definition of BCI has remained difficult to pinpoint because it is not really a single entity but rather a spectrum of entities.

BCI can range from a mild myocardial contusion to frank cardiac chamber rupture including the rare entity of *comotio cordis* described as sudden cardiac arrest from a sternal blow, leading to cardiogenic shock. Blunt cardiac injuries may occur secondary to compression, deceleration, blast, and direct forces applied to the chest, or transmitted increases in intravascular abdominal pressures associated with compression of the abdominal contents. High-speed motor vehicular collisions, causing crushing injuries to the thoracic cage, or objects of great weight falling directly onto the sternum or thoracic cage will directly compress the heart against the vertebral column causing BCI. Similarly, accidental falls from great heights as well as blast injuries can also cause BCIs. The true incidence of BCIs remains difficult to estimate from the literature.

Clinical Presentation

BCI encompasses an entire spectrum of different processes; therefore, clinical presentation for patients sustaining BCI may range from complete hemodynamic instability to cardiopulmonary arrest. These patients may also present with the classical syndrome of pericardial tamponade. Chest pain experienced by some of these patients and its distribution may be indistinguishable from the classical pain of myocardial infarction. Physical findings may include pain and tenderness over the anterior chest wall, contusion, ecchymosis, anterior rib fractures, and even a central flail chest.

Diagnosis

A number of different modalities have been employed to establish a diagnosis of BCI including chest radiography, ECG, Holter monitoring, measurement of cardiac enzymes, transthoracic (TTE) and TEE echocardiography, and nuclear medicine scans including radionuclide angiography (RNA), thallium 201, single-photon emission computed tomography (SPECT), and multiple-gated image acquisition scans (MUGAs). Chest radiographs are routinely obtained in all trauma patients; they may detect the presence of fractured ribs and flail chest and rarely may reveal a globular cardiac silhouette. ECG is used to screen patients and detect conduction disturbances. However, there is no pathonogmonic finding that can reliably establish the diagnosis of BCI.

The measurement of creatine phosphokinase (CPK) or creatine kinase (CK) with measurement of the myocardial band (MB) was for a time used to establish the diagnosis of BCI. However, more specific measurements of contractile proteins of different muscle types including cardiac troponin (cTn) have emerged as tools to diagnose BCI as both troponin T and I belong to a group of proteins of the contractile apparatus that are unique to cardiac muscle. Fulda et al prospectively evaluated 71 patients with thoracic wall injuries utilizing signal-averaged ECG, serum troponin T levels, standard ECG, and CPK-MB measurements. Patients were monitored electrocardiographically and by serial measurements of troponin T and CPK-MB fractions. The authors reported that the sensitivity and specificity of troponin T in predicting clinically significant abnormalities were 27% and 91%, respectively. From the findings of this study, the authors concluded that the best predictors for the development of significant electrocardiographic changes are an abnormality detected in the initial ECG as well as an elevated serum troponin T level, recommending that both of these tests be obtained to diagnose BCI.

Salim and colleagues investigated the role of serum cardiac troponin I (cTnI) and ECG to identify patients at risk for the development of cardiac complications after blunt cardiac trauma. In this prospective 115-patient study, the authors identified patients at risk for significant BCI defined as cardiogenic shock, arrhythmias requiring treatment, or structural cardiac abnormalities directly related to blunt cardiac trauma. All patients were evaluated with ECG upon admission, which was repeated at an 8-hour interval. Cardiac troponin I was obtained at admission and also at 4 and 8 hours. Two-dimensional ECGs were obtained when clinically indicated. Nineteen patients (16.5%) had significant BCIs. In 18 of the 19, symptoms were present within 24 hours. Of the 115 patients, 58 (50%) had abnormal ECGs and 27 (23.5%) had increased cTnI. From these data, the authors concluded that the combination of ECG and troponin I reliably identified the presence or absence of significant BCIs.

The use of two-dimensional echocardiography (TTE) has been extensively used as diagnostic modality for the evaluation of patients with suspected BCI. Patients are selected for evaluation by this modality after abnormal ECG and abnormal cardiac enzymes and troponin level measurements are detected. TTE evaluates segmental wall abnormalities and valvular dysfunction. However, although useful, it has not been shown to correlate with complications or eventual outcome in BCI, and whereas it may detect and identify structural defects and abnormalities with wall motion, it is limited by chest wall edema and traumatic structural abnormalities, such as fractured ribs and flail chest; most importantly it cannot detect the electrical instability that is a hallmark for BCI.

TEE has been shown to be a useful adjunct to evaluate patients with BCI, as it is more versatile in its ability to detect BCI. However, it is an invasive procedure that is operator dependent and not always available around the clock.

A number of different radionuclide scans have been used in the past for the diagnosis of BCI, but none were sufficiently sensitive or specific to reliably establish the diagnosis of BCI and have been abandoned.

Spectrum of Blunt Cardiac Injury

Clinically, BCI can be divided into two types: acute and subacute. The acute type is usually the catastrophic injury that causes death immediately or rapidly if surgical intervention is not instituted, including cardiac chamber rupture with acute pericardial tamponade, combined chamber and pericardial rupture with hemorrhage into the pleural cavity, and acute myocardial injury with cardiogenic shock. Subacute cardiac injury may not lead to immediate death, but does impact cardiac hemodynamics, while placing the patient at risk for the development of significant arrhythmias and hemodynamic complications, and includes myocardial contusion, subacute pericardial tamponade, myocardial infarction, valvular injury, intracardiac shunts, mural thrombi, and of course, arrhythmias.

Pericardial Injury

Blunt rupture of the pericardium occurs from direct high-energy impact or from transmitted sudden and acute increases of intraabdominal pressure. The pericardium may rupture on the diaphragmatic or pleural surfaces usually parallel to the left phrenic nerve. In addition, the heart may eviscerate into the abdominal cavity; in rare cases it can cause torsion of the great vessels acutely. The clinical presentation of patients sustaining blunt pericardial rupture can range from hemodynamic instability to cardiopulmonary arrest, secondary torsion of the great vessels, or associated blunt cardiac chamber rupture. Patients should be investigated with a chest radiograph, which may reveal displacement of the cardiac silhouette, pneumopericardium, or an abnormal gas pattern secondary to herniated hollow viscera. If hemodynamically stable, the patients may be investigated with FAST and ECG. Diagnosis can also be confirmed via a subxiphoid pericardial window, which will reveal a hemopericardium. This should then be followed by median sternotomy.

Valvular, Papillary Muscle/Chordae Tendineae, and Septal Injury

BCI may rarely cause valvular injuries. The most frequently injured valve is the aortic, followed by the mitral. The classic signs associated with valvular dysfunction may not be immediately recognized because of the presence of more obvious life-threatening injuries. Important clinical findings include the presence of new cardiac murmurs, thrills, or loud musical murmurs. Similarly, acute left ventricular dysfunction with cardiogenic shock and associated pulmonary edema are important clinical findings.

Rapid displacement of blood secondary to crushing or compressive forces applied to the thoracic cage during ventricular diastole may lacerate cardiac valve leaflets, papillary muscles, or chordae tendineae, leading to valvular insufficiency. From this mechanism, the aortic valve is most frequently injured. Similarly, any sudden increases in intra-aortic pressure may lead to laceration or leaflet rupture and can also result in stretching and hematoma formation within the papillary muscle. Sudden alterations in papillary muscle anatomy will render it dysfunctional, and may cause valvular insufficiency.

Septal ruptures are also uncommon. Hewett in 1847 first described the rupture of the intraventricular septum caused by blunt trauma. Bright and Beck in 1935 described 11 patients with septal rupture in a series of 152 patients who sustained fatal cardiac injury.

Blunt Coronary Artery Injury

Blunt coronary artery injuries are extremely rare. Direct impacts may cause acute coronary thrombosis and may result in intimal disruption caused by significant application of blunt energy to the chest. Blunt coronary artery injuries are usually associated with severe myocardial contusions, generally along the distribution of the left anterior descending coronary artery (LAD). The clinical presentation of these patients cannot be distinguished from acute myocardial infarction. Long-term sequelae of these injuries may lead to the development of a ventricular aneurysm with its potential complications such as rupture, ventricular failure, and production of emboli or malignant arrhythmias.

Cardiac Chamber Rupture

Blunt cardiac rupture is relatively uncommon. Only a small number of patients sustaining these injuries survive to reach the hospital. Blunt chamber rupture is often the immediate cause of death at the scene of motor vehicular collisions and is frequently encountered during autopsy. Several mechanisms for blunt cardiac rupture have been postulated, including direct precordial impacts; hydraulic effect from retrograde transmission of force through the abdomen into the venous system, causing rapid rises of venous pressure transmitted to the heart, particularly the atria; compression; acceleration or deceleration injuries leading to tears of the heart at its attachment to the great thoracic vessels; blast effects; and concussive blows thought to be fatal secondary to the production of malignant arrhythmias.

Blunt cardiac chamber rupture usually presents with persistent hypotension and pericardial tamponade. Similarly, patients may present in cardiopulmonary arrest secondary to exsanguinating hemorrhage. These patients should be rapidly evaluated by FAST to detect pericardial fluid. For those who are hemodynamically stable, subxiphoid pericardial window remains an option to confirm the results of FAST; however, for those who present in cardiopulmonary arrest, ED thoracotomy may be the only chance at survival, albeit these patients have a dismal prognosis.

Türk and Tsokos reported that blunt atrial injuries are more common than ventricular injuries. The most frequently injured cardiac chamber is the right atrium, followed by the right ventricle. Left-sided chamber injuries occur with less frequency. Several patients have been reported with multiple chamber injuries; however, none survived.

Myocardial Contusion

Of all the BCIs, the least important and more difficult to define is myocardial contusion/concussion. The definition of myocardial contusion has evolved over several decades of discussion among trauma surgeons. This diagnosis is more often established out of proportion to its incidence, severity, and clinical relevance. Mattox et al suggested that the terms of myocardial contusion and concussion be eliminated in favor of a more reasonable definition for this entity, and proposed that they be defined as BCI either with cardiac failure, with the presence of complex arrhythmia, and with minor ECG or enzyme abnormality. On this basis, it is recommended that asymptomatic patients with anterior chest wall injuries should not be admitted to a surgical intensive care unit for continuous ECG monitoring, serial determination of CPK-MB enzyme levels, or further cardiac imaging.

Civetta and colleagues concluded that significant cardiac events are uncommon in young patients with chest trauma, and pointed out that initial ECG abnormalities are better indicators of cardiac complications in critically injured patients.

After a thorough review of the literature, Pasquale et al identified well-conducted primary studies or reviews involving the identification of BCI. On the basis of this literature review, the Eastern Association for the Surgery of Trauma (EAST) generated the following three recommendations:

Level I

An admission ECG should be performed for all patients in whom there is suspected BCI.

Level II

1. If the admission ECG results are abnormal, the patient should be admitted for continuous ECG monitoring for 24 to 48 hours. If the admission ECG results are normal, the pursuit of diagnosis should be terminated.
2. If the patient is hemodynamically unstable, an imaging study should be obtained. If an optimal TTE cannot be performed, then the patient should have a TEE.
3. Nuclear medicine studies add little compared with echocardiography and are not useful if an echocardiogram has been performed.

Level III

1. Elderly patients with known cardiac disease, unstable patients, and those with an abnormal admission ECG can be safely operated on provided that they are closely monitored. Consideration should be given to placement of a pulmonary artery catheter in such cases.
2. The presence of a sternal fracture does not predict the presence of BCI and does not necessarily indicate that monitoring should be performed.
3. Neither CPK analysis nor measurements of circulating cardiac troponin T are useful in predicting which patients have or will have complications related to BCI.

CONCLUSION

Cardiac injuries continue to be both challenging and fascinating entities. Only with serious scientific inquiry based on prospective collection and analysis of data can we extend the frontiers in the management of these critical injuries (Fig. 7).

For the chapter's Suggested Readings list, please visit the book at www.ExpertConsult.inkling.com.

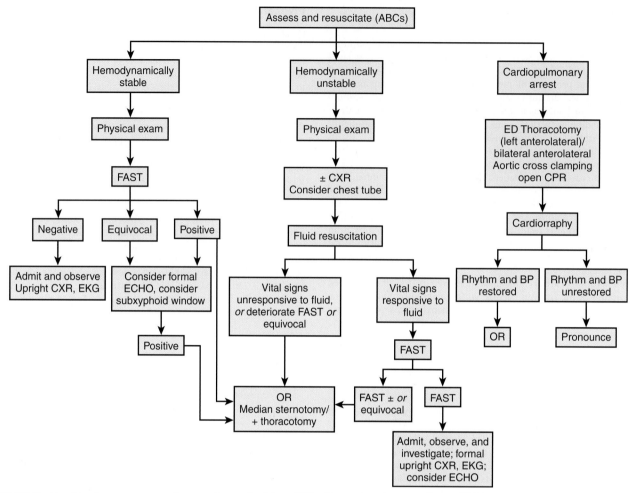

FIGURE 7 Algorithm for management of penetrating cardiac injury. ABCs, Airway, breathing, circulation; BP, blood pressure; CPR, cardiopulmonary resuscitation; CXR, chest x-ray; ED, emergency department; ECHO, echocardiography; EKG, electrocardiogram; FAST, focused assessment with sonography in trauma; OR, operating room.

THORACIC VASCULAR INJURY

Peter I. Tsai, Ramyar Gilani, Kenneth L. Mattox, and Matthew J. Wall, Jr.

The heart, aorta, and its great vessels are for the most part encased in the chest cavity, protected by the vertebral bodies, rib cage, clavicle, manubrium, and sternum. Penetrating trauma to the great vessels can lead to a pattern similar to blunt trauma resulting in complete disruption followed by immediate hemorrhage, transection with pseudoaneurysm, intramural hematoma, and intimal flap with subsequent thrombosis. One of the earliest reports of thoracic vascular injury was described by Vesalius in 1557 of a fatal, blunt traumatic rupture of the aorta in a man who was thrown from a horse. It was not until 1959 that Passaro and Pace reported the first successful primary repair of traumatic aortic rupture performed by Klassen in 1958.

Before the development of modern trauma centers, most individuals with thoracic vascular trauma died before reaching the hospital. With the advent of rapid-response trauma systems, the number of those with thoracic vascular injury surviving to the hospital is increasing and the complexity of their injuries is becoming more challenging. This is reflected by Mattox et al reporting 5760 cardiovascular injuries in 4459 patients over a 30-year period from 1958 to 1987 in Houston, Texas.

Thoracic vascular injury presents a particular challenge to trauma surgeons as exposure for proximal and distal control of these vascular injuries is not straightforward. Poorly planned incisions can potentially lead to devastating consequences. Because of the increasing complexity of thoracic vascular injuries reaching trauma centers, it is important for the surgeons caring for them to have a systematic approach and a plan of action formulated in order to avoid the associated morbidity and fatality of such injuries. Additionally, advances in technology continue to provide increasing capability in diagnosis and management but must be continually evaluated objectively prior to proclaiming changes in patient care algorithms.

INCIDENCE

Thoracic trauma is responsible for 50% of all trauma deaths nationally. In a large series of thoracic trauma patients, the aorta and great vessels were injured in 4% of cases. More than 90% of the thoracic great vessel injuries are due to penetrating trauma. With penetrating trauma, all thoracic vessels are potentially susceptible to injury. The anatomic location of the ascending aorta makes it the most commonly injured large thoracic vessel from stab wounds, whereas gunshot wounds usually cause descending thoracic aortic injury. Blunt trauma can potentially cause injury to all thoracic arteries and veins, but specifically to the innominate artery origin, pulmonary veins, vena cava, and most commonly descending thoracic aorta.

MECHANISM OF INJURY

A large number of thoracic great vessel injuries are caused by penetrating or iatrogenic trauma. The mechanism of injury for penetrating thoracic vascular trauma is usually direct laceration or penetration of blood vessels. This type of injury can often present with external or internal hemorrhage, vascular thrombosis from intimal flap, or pseudoaneurysm. Because of the various types of missiles involved in penetrating vascular trauma, all thoracic vascular structures are at risk. The bony structures, interestingly, can also provide unique patterns of injuries as they cause a ricocheting of bullets/fragments or alter vectors of the original direction of penetration. External bleeding from skin tracts usually occurs with injuries to vessels at the thoracic outlet, whereas internal hemorrhage commonly occurs with aortic and caval injuries. Intrathoracic great vessel injuries can present with internal bleeding into the mediastinum, pleural space, or pericardial sac. It is important to note that the presence of a normal palpable distal pulse does not rule out a proximal vascular injury. Penetrating vascular injuries can be completely contained by perivascular adventitia with blood flow preserved distally.

The absence of a significant amount of bleeding does not rule out vascular injury from penetrating trauma. Vascular injuries from stab wounds can often cause an intimal flap or dissection, which may eventually lead to partial or complete thrombosis of injured vessels. Small vascular disruptions may not present initially with bleeding but can present with delayed formation of a pseudoaneurysm. Gunshot blast vascular injuries are often underestimated because intimal disruption sometimes extends beyond external signs of injury. For this reason, meticulous intimal inspection from inside of the blood vessel is helpful during thoracic vascular reconstruction.

Because of the large diameter of thoracic vessels, bullets can directly enter vessels and migrate distally (Fig. 1). The diagnosis of bullet embolism is often delayed because the course of the bullet may not be obvious. Bullet embolism for thoracic missiles usually lodges in the iliac and femoral vessels. The site of entry should be controlled for hemorrhage first, followed with attempts at removing the bullet emboli with endovascular intervention or separate arteriotomy.

There are two proposed mechanisms for blunt trauma injuries to thoracic aorta and great vessels. During anteroposterior impact in the thorax, the aorta and its branched vessels may be "pinched" between the sternum and the vertebral column, resulting in vascular disruption. In rapid-deceleration thoracic injuries from either frontal or side impact motor vehicle accidents, the point of attachment of pulmonary veins and vena cava and the relative immobility of the descending aorta at the level of the ligamentum arteriosum and diaphragm increase their susceptibility to rupture. In contrast to patients with aortic intimal disease in which adventitia is the restraining barrier, it is the intact parietal pleura that contains the hematoma and prevents massive hemothorax.

DIAGNOSIS

Patients with penetrating thoracic vascular trauma often exsanguinate and die at scene. With advancement in emergency medical system (EMS) transport, more patients remain alive on transport and arrival to emergency room. These patients can present with hemodynamic instability from uncontrolled hemorrhage into the

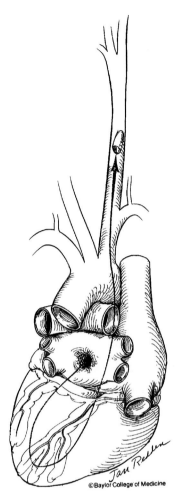

FIGURE 1 Bullet embolism from the left atrium to the left carotid artery. *(Courtesy of Jan Redden, Baylor College of Medicine, 1980.)*

mediastinum, pleural space, or pericardial sac, and are taken emergently to the operating room for surgical management. These injuries are typically diagnosed intraoperatively during resuscitative thoracotomy. In contrast, patients with blunt thoracic trauma are often initially hemodynamically stable with multiple other injuries that may mask a significant concomitant vascular injury.

Focused history and physical examination in the trauma room are helpful in arriving at a specific vascular injury diagnosis. In penetrating trauma, it can be helpful to note the type of instrument used, length of the knife, caliber of the gun, and patient's distance from the firearm. Although often unreliable, this information may help the surgeon to develop a mental picture of the trajectory of penetrating missile injury and to formulate a surgical treatment plan. In blunt thoracic trauma, the mechanism of injury is of particular importance to allow the surgeon to estimate the amount of kinetic energy transferred as it relates the geometry of the patient's body upon impact. Emergency medical personnel can also provide information regarding amount of blood loss in the field and hemodynamic stability during transport.

Indicators of possible thoracic vascular injury are outlined in Table 1. The single most important screening tool for thoracic vascular trauma is the anteroposterior chest radiograph. There are numerous chest radiograph findings suggesting thoracic vascular injury as outlined in Table 2. One of the most reliable radiographic findings suggestive of blunt thoracic vascular injury is alteration of the aortic knob contour on chest radiograph.

Arteriography remains the "gold standard" imaging study for evaluation of suspected thoracic vascular injury. It is important to note

TABLE 1: Indicators of Possible Thoracic Vascular Injury

Mechanism of Injury

Severe deceleration caused by falls, motor vehicle accidents, and pedestrian versus motor vehicle

Crush injuries

Penetrating injuries to chest with suggestive trajectories, including mediastinal traverse gunshot wounds

Suggestive Physical Signs

Thoracic outlet hematoma

Unequal peripheral pulses or blood pressures

Steering wheel contusion on anterior chest

Palpable sternal fracture

Focal neurologic deficits

Findings on Chest Radiographs

Abnormal or widened mediastinum

Obliteration of aortic knob contour

Lateral deviation of trachea or nasogastric tube

TABLE 2: Radiologic Findings Suggesting Great Vessel Injury

Widening of the superior mediastinum > 8 cm

Depression of the left main bronchus > 140 degrees

Loss of the aortic knob

Deviation of nasogastric or endotracheal tubes, or trachea to the right

Fracture of the first or second rib, scapula, or sternum

Left apical pleural cap

Obliteration of the aortopulmonary window on lateral chest radiograph

Anterior displacement of trachea on lateral chest radiograph

Fracture dislocation of thoracic spine

Calcium layering in aortic knob area

Obvious double contour of aorta

Multiple left rib fractures

Massive hemothorax

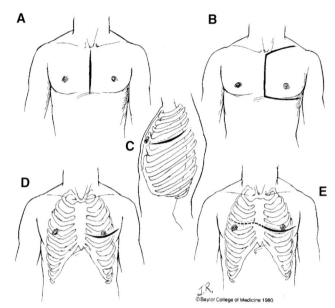

FIGURE 2 Various thoracic incisions that may be employed to manage thoracic vascular injuries. **A,** Median sternotomy. **B,** Combined anterolateral thoracotomy and supraclavicular incision (less commonly with sternotomy to form "trapdoor" thoracotomy). **C,** Posterolateral thoracotomy. **D,** Anterolateral thoracotomy (the universal incision for patients in extremis). **E,** Extension of left anterolateral thoracotomy to right from clamshell incision. *(Courtesy of Jan Redden, Baylor College of Medicine, 1980.)*

make for proximal control of these branched aortic vessels (Fig. 2). Furthermore, the proximity of missile trajectory to brachiocephalic vessels is an indication for arteriography in order to definitively rule out an injury. In blunt thoracic trauma, the need for arteriography is determined by physical examination, screening chest radiograph, and a high index of suspicion for mechanism of injury. Fifty percent of patients with blunt thoracic vascular injury present without any external signs of injury. Seven percent of patients with blunt injury to the aorta and its branched vessels have a normal-appearing mediastinum on screening chest radiograph. Therefore, additional imaging studies are indicated in this subgroup based on high index of suspicion from mechanism of injury.

Contrast-enhanced spiral computed tomography angiography (CTA) of the chest is being used more frequently for evaluating thoracic trauma. The sensitivity of chest CTA for thoracic vascular injury ranges from 54% to 80%. The negative predictive value of a chest CTA is close to 100% in evaluating thoracic vascular injury. Therefore, it is also reasonable to use chest CTA as a screening tool in stable patients with significant mechanism of injury, normal-appearing admission chest radiograph, and benign physical examination to rule out an underlying thoracic vascular injury. However, positive or equivocal CTA results should be followed by additional imaging, most commonly angiography for definitive diagnosis of thoracic vascular injury before operative intervention. CTA is also used for preoperative endovascular repair planning. Detailed information regarding access vessels and seal zones can be readily obtained. With this information, the feasibility of an endovascular repair can be determined as well as proper device selection. In addition, individual patient anatomy can be assessed for extent of coverage and need for adjuvant procedures such as a carotid-subclavian bypass.

However, CTA is not without limitations as it relates to thoracic vascular trauma. Injuries of the aortic root and ascending aorta are often not well visualized with standard CTA secondary to cardiac motion. Cardiac-gated CTA is an emerging technology that serves to mitigate motion artifact and is becoming increasingly used for imaging of the most proximal aorta with a potential application for

that preoperative angiography is never indicated in hemodynamically unstable patients with suspected thoracic vascular injury. In hemodynamically stable patients with suspected penetrating injury to the innominate, carotid, or subclavian arteries, preoperative arteriography is indicated to provide information on the type of incisions to trauma. In addition to abnormal findings on CTA, there are many normal variants such as ductus bumps, infundibulum of the superior intercostal artery, or diverticula of Kommerell, which can mimic aortic injury and do not require treatment. Lastly, hemodynamically unstable trauma patients have transiently reduced vessel diameters, which can theoretically lead to endograft undersizing and device failure. Intravascular ultrasound (IVUS) provides 360-degree real-time images that can provide information on vessel wall and lumen abnormalities. The images are not sensitive to motion, which creates an application for imaging the proximal aorta. Intimal injuries masked by intraluminal contrast agent as well as intramural hematomas that are not seen with contrast angiography can be seen with real-time IVUS. Furthermore, when evaluating patients with equivocal CTA, IVUS has been shown to be better than traditional angiography in the diagnosis of blunt aortic injury (BAI).

Magnetic resonance angiography (MRA) is neither ideal nor practical in evaluating for acute injury because of the difficulty in monitoring and managing patients in the magnetic resonance coil suites, and therefore, MRA is not recommended in evaluating trauma patients.

Transesophageal echocardiography (TEE) offers several potential advantages to arteriography in evaluating thoracic vascular injury. Avoidance of intravenous contrast material, the concomitant information gained on cardiac function, and its portability are potential advantages compared with arteriography. However, published literature reports sensitivity and specificity of 85.7% and 92.0% for TEE compared with 89.0% and 100% for arteriography, respectively, in diagnosing aortic injury. TEE is also heavily technician and operator dependent. Furthermore, the ascending aorta, proximal aortic arch, and branch aortic vessels are extremely difficult to visualize with TEE, made worse by the concomitant chest wall injury/hematoma. Therefore, its use in evaluating thoracic vascular injury is not routinely recommended.

AMERICAN ASSOCIATION FOR THE SURGERY OF TRAUMA, ORGAN INJURY SCALE

The American Association for the Surgery of Trauma (AAST) designates an organ injury scale for thoracic vascular injury from grade I to VI, as outlined in Table 3, based on the size and severity of the injury.

Grade I injuries generally involve small thoracic vessels. Grade II injuries involve named venous tributaries of the superior vena cava such as the innominate vein, internal jugular veins, subclavian veins, and azygous vein. Branched aortic vessels such as innominate artery, carotid arteries, and subclavian arteries make up grade III injuries. Grade IV injuries include large extrapericardial vascular structures, whereas grade V injuries include major intrapericardial vascular structures. Grade VI injuries are uncontained, complete transection of the thoracic aorta or pulmonary hilum.

SURGICAL MANAGEMENT

Indications for urgent surgical intervention for thoracic vascular injuries are outlined in Table 4. The choice of incisions varies depending on the location of injury (see Fig. 2). For unstable patients with presumed but undiagnosed thoracic vascular injury, the most appropriate incision is a left anterolateral thoracotomy in the supine position. This incision allows excellent exposure to the heart and aorta for resuscitative efforts. Furthermore, it can be converted easily to a clamshell incision by extending transsternally to the contralateral side to provide exposure to the right lung hilum, ascending aorta, and right subclavian vessels. Median sternotomy is the incision of choice for innominate, right subclavian, right carotid, and proximal left carotid arterial injuries. Oblique cervical or transverse supraclavicular extensions can be added to provide further exposure. Left posterolateral

TABLE 3: Thoracic Vascular Injury Scale

Grade*	Description of Injury
I	Intercostal vessels Internal mammary vessels Bronchial vessels Esophageal vessels Hemiazygos vein Unnamed vessels
II	Azygous vein Internal jugular vein Subclavian vein Innominate vein
III	Carotid artery Innominate artery Subclavian artery
IV	Descending thoracic aorta Intrathoracic inferior vena cava Pulmonary artery/vein, primary intraparenchymal branch
V	Ascending aorta Aortic arch Superior vena cava Main pulmonary artery trunk Pulmonary vein, main trunk
VI	Uncontained complete transection of thoracic aorta or pulmonary hilar vessels

Modified from American Association for the Surgery of Trauma (AAST).
*Increase one grade for multiple grade III injuries or >50% circumference involvement in grade IV injuries. Decrease one grade for grade IV injuries if <25% circumference involvement.

TABLE 4: Indications for Operative Repair of Thoracic Great Vessel Injury

Initial loss of 1500 mL of blood from chest tube

Continuing hemorrhage >200 mL/hour from tube thoracostomy

Posttraumatic hemopericardium

Pericardial tamponade

Expanding hematoma at thoracic outlet

Exsanguinating hemorrhage presenting from supraclavicular penetrating wound

Imaging evidence of acute thoracic great vessel injury

Radiographic or other imaging evidence of chronic thoracic great vessel injury complications

thoracotomy in the lateral decubitus position provides the best exposure for known injuries to the descending thoracic aorta and left lung hilum.

Patients with ascending/transverse aortic injury rarely survive long enough to be transported to the trauma center. Most of these blunt injuries require the use of interposition grafts with cardiopulmonary bypass or circulatory arrest for repair. In selected patients with penetrating trauma small anterior or lateral lacerations of the ascending aorta can be primarily repaired without the use of cardiopulmonary bypass. Complex injuries involving posterior aspects of the ascending aorta and pulmonary artery are also repaired with cardiopulmonary bypass. Exposure of the transverse arch can be improved by extending the median sternotomy incision to the neck and dividing the innominate vein.

Much focus has been recently placed on BAI in terms of proper management. Evidence is now accumulating that, in hemodynamically stable patients, purposeful delay of surgery combined with pharmacologic anti-impulse (dP/dT) therapy using intravenous beta blockers and close monitoring may be a safe alternative to emergent repair. In addition, "minimal" BAIs, such as a small intimal flap or intramural hematoma, may be amenable to nonoperative management.

The operative principles for managing descending thoracic aortic injuries are proximal/distal control, addressing the injured segment, and reestablishing continuity of blood flow. Most blunt traumatic injuries in the descending thoracic aorta originate medially at the level of the ligamentum arteriosum. The most expeditious way of obtaining proximal control is to follow the left subclavian artery proximally to the aortic arch and place an umbilical tape around the aortic arch between the takeoff of the left common carotid artery and the left subclavian artery. An umbilical tape is also passed around the left subclavian artery. Care should be taken to try to avoid injury to the left recurrent laryngeal nerve as it courses posteriorly around the aortic arch near the ligamentum arteriosum. The next maneuver is to achieve vascular control distal to the anticipated injury. It is important to examine the entire length of the descending thoracic aorta in order to identify any additional tears, especially at the level of the diaphragm. There are several approaches to the basic vascular repair of the descending thoracic aorta. First is the simple clamp-and-sew technique without the use of left-sided heart bypass. Some surgeons advocate the use of active partial left-sided heart bypass for repairing descending thoracic aortic injuries (Fig. 3). This procedure is mostly done in elderly patients with known coronary artery disease and compromised ejection fraction. All of these adjunct techniques should be familiar to surgeons managing this type of injury. The hematoma is entered after proximal and distal control is established. Intercostal vessels are not routinely oversewn. The extent of the injury is inspected from both external and internal aspects of the aorta. Simple partial lacerations of the aorta can be primarily closed with running sutures using 4-0 polypropylene. Complex injuries often require an interposition graft.

Heated debate continues in the literature on whether active distal perfusion decreases the dreaded morbidity of paraplegia. The length of aortic cross-clamp time has been argued as an independent factor contributing to increased incidence of postoperative paraplegia. Numerous studies, however, have shown that the incidence of postoperative paraplegia is multifactorial and cannot be attributed to any single cause. All distal perfusion techniques have potential complications including those from cannulation sites or from systemic heparinization. Regardless of the technique used, the overall incidence of postoperative paraplegia averages 8% according to various studies.

Within the last decade, there have been major shifts in the management of descending thoracic BAI. Demetriades et al, in 2008 and subsequently two follow-up reports of the AAST multicenter study, documented a shift in initial diagnostic modality of choice to CTA. Also, thoracic endovascular aortic repair (TEVAR) has gained popularity in recent years and has become the repair method of choice at most centers. There are no randomized control trials comparing TEVAR to open repair; however, TEVAR has been shown to have lower mortality rate, less blood loss, less paraplegia, and decreased stroke rates in comparison to open repair. There remains some concern for TEVAR as device complication rates of 20% have been reported and long-term follow-up remains limited. As a result devices

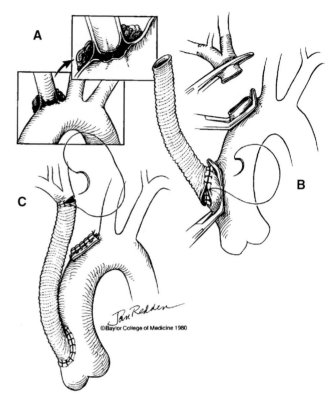

FIGURE 3   Bypass-exclusion technique for management of innominate artery injuries. **A,** Severe intimal disruption may be associated with minimal external hematoma. **B,** A site is selected for aortotomy along the ascending aorta, and a prosthetic graft is sewn end to side. A partial occluding vascular clamp is placed at the origin of the innominate artery and a vascular clamp is placed across the distal innominate artery. The artery is divided between the clamps. **C,** The repair is completed by an end-to-end anastomosis of the graft to the distal innominate artery and by oversewing the native origin of the innominate artery on the aorta. *(Courtesy of Jan Redden, Baylor College of Medicine, 1980.)*

have undergone several generations of modification although commercially available devices still remain less than ideal for use in young trauma patients. These trends are mirrored by our own institution's experience over the last 3 years.

TEVAR for BAI is performed similarly as for aneurysm disease. Given the most common location of BAI, coverage of the left subclavian artery is often required to achieve adequate proximal seal. If coverage is required, the need for revascularization should be evaluated on an individual basis referencing published guidelines. Systemic heparinization may be contraindicated in the polytrauma patient and is not mandatory. Postprocedural follow-up guidelines are not well established, but it appears acceptable to use similar protocols as for aneurysm repair.

Innominate artery and proximal left common carotid artery injuries are best approached via median sternotomy incision with cervical extension, if necessary. Division of the innominate vein provides excellent exposure to the transverse aortic arch for proximal control. In patients with small, partial tears of the distal innominate artery, primary repair with 4-0 polypropylene suture is often possible. In most cases, innominate artery injuries are best managed using the bypass exclusion technique (Fig. 4). This approach allows management without the use of systemic heparinization, cardiopulmonary bypass, or hypothermic circulatory arrest. A 10-mm knitted tube graft is used to create a proximal ascending aorta to distal innominate artery bypass. After the bypass is completed, the injury at the origin of the aortic duct is oversewn. Injuries to the proximal left common carotid artery can also be managed in a similar fashion.

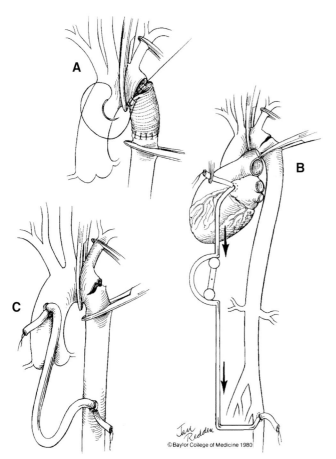

FIGURE 4 Adjuncts in the management of descending thoracic aortic injuries. **A,** Simple clamp and sew technique with proximal and distal control using vascular clamps. **B,** Active left atriofemoral bypass with partial left-sided heart bypass. **C,** Passive ascending to descending thoracic aorta with shunt. *(Courtesy of Jan Redden, Baylor College of Medicine, 1980.)*

Median sternotomy with right-sided cervical extension is the incision of choice for right subclavian artery injury. Proximal left subclavian artery injury is best repaired through a left posterolateral thoracotomy in the fourth intercostal space. Exposure of the distal left subclavian artery can be obtained through a left supraclavicular incision with proximal control via a third interspace anterolateral incision. Although seldom seen, injury to multiple segments of the left subclavian artery can be managed by combining the two incisions to create a "trapdoor" incision. Injury to the phrenic nerve, lying anterior to the scalenus anticus muscle, should be avoided during exposure of the subclavian artery. The left clavicle can be divided or resected to provide better exposure if necessary. After obtaining proximal and distal control, either primary repair or interposition knitted or polytetrafluoroethylene grafts may be used, depending on the extent of injury. Because of the soft nature of the subclavian artery, mobilization for end-to-end anastomosis is generally difficult. Subclavian artery injuries are often associated with concomitant brachial plexus injuries; therefore, it is helpful to note the preoperative neurologic examination. Subclavian venous injuries are exposed similarly as subclavian artery injuries. Venous injuries are repaired by either primary venorrhaphy or ligation.

Endovascular techniques are certainly applicable in managing great vessel injuries and serve to mitigate difficulties with accessibility and morbidity associated with exposure. Regardless of specific method, endovascular surgery for such injuries must adhere to similar vascular trauma dogma as open surgery. The feasibility of endovascular repair is established in early series within properly selected patients. Despite early success, open surgery remained advocated

for hypotensive patients, complete transection, or thrombosis. However, more recent reports describe overcoming such barriers and achieving acceptable clinical results rivaling open repair. In certain situations, it may be advantageous to take an endovascular vascular approach to achieve proximal and distal balloon control before proceeding with open surgical repair. These hybrid procedures attest to the importance of being facile with both open and endovascular techniques to best manage these complex injuries.

Intrapericardial pulmonary artery injuries are best approached with a median sternotomy incision. Main pulmonary artery and proximal left pulmonary artery are readily accessible upon opening the pericardium. The proximal right pulmonary artery is exposed by dissecting between the superior vena cava and the ascending aorta. Small anterior injuries are primarily repaired with running 4-0 polypropylene sutures with the use of a partial occluding vascular clamp. More complex and posterior injuries may require the use of cardiopulmonary bypass. Distal extrapericardial pulmonary artery injuries are approached with thoracotomy incisions. In selected patients, pneumonectomy may be the lifesaving procedure of choice for major hilar injuries.

Injuries to the thoracic vena cava are extremely difficult to manage surgically because of its anatomic location. A median sternotomy incision provides optimal exposure. Simple anterior lacerations can be primarily repaired with a partial occluding vascular clamp. Posterior injuries may require the use of total cardiopulmonary bypass or circulatory arrest. Subsequent repair is accomplished from inside the right atrium. Occasionally, an intracaval shunt may be a useful adjunct.

Intrapericardial pulmonary venous injuries are rare and diagnosed intraoperatively during an empiric emergent thoracotomy. The optimal incision is a left anterolateral thoracotomy that allows access to the posterior aspect of the heart. Extrapericardial pulmonary venous injuries in stable patients are approached from posterolateral thoracotomy incisions. Simple lacerations can be closed primarily. Massive hemorrhage can be controlled with temporary hilar occlusion. If a pulmonary vein must be ligated for lifesaving measures, appropriate pulmonary lobectomy should follow.

Because the azygous vein drains directly into the superior vena cava, injuries to the azygous veins can be potentially fatal. This type of injury is rarely diagnosed or suspected preoperatively. When seen in the operating room, azygous venous injuries are best managed by primary repair or division and suture ligation of both ends. Similarly, internal mammary arterial and venous injuries can cause massive hemorrhage and are often diagnosed intraoperatively. The best treatment option is simple ligation and proper documentation in the operative notes in order to eliminate the possibility of using internal mammary arteries as conduits for potential future coronary artery bypass operations.

In a dying patient with thoracic vascular injury, damage control thoracotomy is a treatment option. A left anterolateral thoracotomy incision provides the best initial exposure. The principle of damage control thoracotomy consists of the use of simpler techniques to achieve expeditious control of hemorrhage in a single setting, or temporary measures for hemorrhage control with planned second operation for definitive repair as the patient's physiologic status is restored to a more survivable level. Hilar vascular injuries can be controlled quickly by performing pneumonectomy or lobectomy with a stapling device. For vessels greater than 5 mm, synthetic grafts may be used to avoid delays in harvesting vein grafts. Temporary ligation and placement of intravascular shunts can control hemorrhage until the patient's physiologic status is restored to a more appropriate level for definitive repair. Ligation of the subclavian artery is often well tolerated and can be used in a damage control setting. Thoracotomy incisions can be closed quickly with towel clips; however, en mass closure using large needles encompassing all muscle layers are more hemostatic. A Bogota bag or patch closure can also be used as temporary closures in patients with cardiac dysfunction in order to prevent compression of the heart.

Young patients usually have very soft medium-sized and large named arteries in the chest without atherosclerotic disease. During surgical repair of thoracic vessels, any slight lateral deviation from the natural curve of the suture needle translates to increasing hemorrhage from needle holes, which on some occasions may lead to further tears in the artery and result in a fatal outcome. Also, vasospasm in the hypotensive patient can be significant and should be considered when sizing graft prosthesis. Gentle, precise technique provides the best repairs.

MORBIDITY AND MANAGEMENT COMPLICATIONS

Neurologic deficits often accompany injuries to thoracic vascular structures either as additional associated injuries or as postoperative morbidities. Therefore, proper preoperative documentation of the patient's neurologic status is important. As mentioned previously, the overall average incidence of postoperative paraplegia is 8% for descending thoracic aortic repair. Endograft repair has significantly decreased the paraplegic rate to 1%. The anatomic proximity of the brachial plexus to the subclavian vessels is the reason for the high incidence of brachial plexopathy associated with subclavian vessel injuries. Detailed discussion with the patient and family members of these associated neurologic morbidities is warranted. Some patients experience persistent postthoracotomy pain, which can be socially and emotionally devastating. Thus, early mobility and rehabilitation are important adjuncts to the care of these patients. In selected patients, intercostal nerve blocks may be beneficial.

A majority of patients with thoracic vascular trauma have associated multiorgan injury. As a result, a significant portion of these patients remain critically ill in the intensive care unit setting. Various pulmonary complications such as atelectasis, pneumonia, and acute respiratory distress syndrome are becoming some of the most common complications in the early postoperative period. Patients with concomitant pulmonary contusions are at an increased risk of developing acute respiratory distress syndrome. Aggressive pulmonary toilet, adequate pain control, and detailed critical care are all essential elements in preventing these complications.

MORTALITY

Thoracic vascular injuries have one of the highest mortality rates of any organ system trauma because of the high incidence of other concomitant injuries in other body compartments. Patients with ascending aortic injuries rarely reach the hospital alive. The mortality rate remains as high as 50% for patients with ascending aortic injuries with stable vital signs on arrival to trauma centers. Injuries to the central pulmonary artery and vein are highly lethal with mortality rates in excess of 70%. Similarly, thoracic vena cava injuries are infrequent but extremely difficult to control and carry a mortality rate greater than 60%. Regardless of the surgical technique used, the mortality rate of descending thoracic aortic injuries ranges from 5% to 25%. The overall mortality rate for innominate artery injuries is reported to be 25% from 1960 to 1992. Subclavian artery injuries have the best prognosis with an overall mortality rate of less than 5% as reported by Graham et al.

CONCLUSIONS

Managing patients with thoracic vascular injuries requires technical expertise and excellent surgical judgment. For this reason, taking care of patients with this type of injury can be both extremely challenging and rewarding.

Unlike abdominal injuries, in which midline vertical incision is the standard exploratory incision, patients with stable thoracic vascular injuries require careful preoperative planning. Because of the rigid chest wall, ill-placed incisions and incorrect intercostal space entry significantly compromise exposure for proximal/distal control of hemorrhage from thoracic vascular injuries. Endovascular repair requiring femoral or brachial access can avoid the different thoracic exposures, but demand skilled techniques. Although thoracic vascular injuries have one of the highest mortality rates of any trauma, superb surgical judgment along with operative precision will translate to improved patient care and outcome.

For the chapter's Suggested Readings list, please visit the book at www.ExpertConsult.inkling.com.

OPEN AND ENDOVASCULAR MANAGEMENT OF THORACIC AORTIC INJURIES

K. Shad Pharaon and Donald D. Trunkey

and knowing which incision is best is not always obvious. Knowledge of normal anatomy, variant anatomy, and orientation are important for any surgeon, whether an open or catheter-based therapy is chosen. Open repair for thoracic aortic injury (TAI) is associated with significant morbidity and mortality risks. Although the quality of evidence is very low, thoracic endovascular aortic repair (TEVAR) is now chosen as the preferred technique because of its improved outcomes compared with open repair, especially its lower mortality rate and incidence of spinal cord ischemia (Figs. 1 to 4).

I n 1557, Vesalius first described blunt traumatic aortic rupture, reporting his findings of a man who was killed after being thrown from his horse. In 1946, DeBakey and Simeone reported on thoracic vascular injuries that occurred during World War II. In 1959, Passaro and Pace reported the first successful primary repair of a traumatic aortic rupture, and in 1994, Dake et al first reported endovascular repair of a descending thoracic aortic aneurysm.

An injury to the aorta presents a particular challenge to trauma surgeons because portions of the aorta can be accessed through a median sternotomy, a left thoracotomy, and a midline laparotomy,

INCIDENCE

The incidence of TAI is not well known. Some estimates are based on autopsy studies. Motor vehicle crash (MVC) is the most common mechanism of injury leading to TAI, followed by pedestrian struck by automobile and motorcycle collision. The majority of patients killed are men (71%), and alcohol or illicit drug use is associated with 39% of cases. A thoracic aortic rupture is found in 34% of those killed, and the most frequent site of injury is the isthmus/descending thoracic aorta (66%). Patients with TAI are also found to have associated

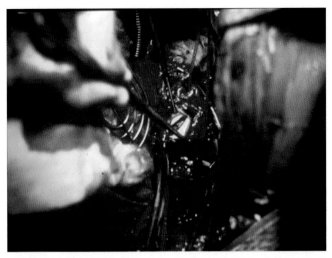

FIGURE 1 Thoracic aortic repair with Dacron graft flap. *(Courtesy of J.A. Asensio, MD.)*

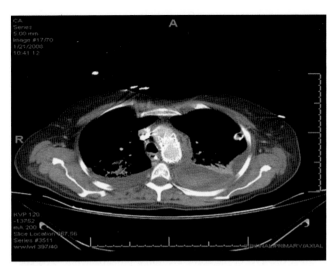

FIGURE 4 Computed tomography scan of thoracic endograft after thoracic endovascular aortic repair completed. *(Courtesy of J.A. Asensio, MD.)*

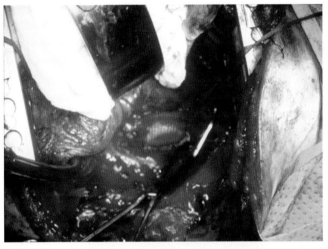

FIGURE 2 Left posterolateral thoracotomy depicting the rupture. *(Courtesy of J.A. Asensio, MD.)*

cardiac injury, hemothorax, rib fractures, intra-abdominal injury, and pelvic fractures. Despite improvements in both automobile safety and in our prehospital care system, it is estimated that approximately 80% of patients with these injuries die immediately at the scene from exsanguination.

MECHANISM OF INJURY

Because of their anterior location, the arch of the aorta, the innominate artery, and the carotid arteries are at risk for injury after a penetrating injury such as a stab wound. The descending thoracic aorta has a posterior location but is particularly susceptible to injury from blunt trauma such as that sustained in motor vehicle accidents, plane crashes, and falls. The descending thoracic aorta is fixed at the ligamentum arteriosum and diaphragm and is likely the site of most injuries occurring in the proximal descending aorta.

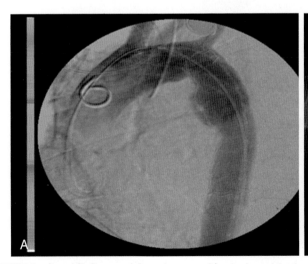
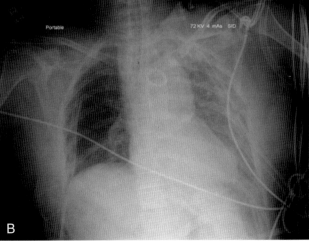

FIGURE 3 **A** and **B,** Ruptured thoracic aorta with wire in anticipation of thoracic endovascular aortic repair. *(Courtesy of J.A. Asensio, MD.)*

DIAGNOSIS

A supine chest radiograph should be obtained in the emergency department as part of the workup of a patient with suspected blunt or penetrating trauma to the torso, and traumatic aortic injury should be considered in any patient who has suffered a deceleration accident. For penetrating injuries of the chest, placement of radiopaque markers to identify entrance and exit wounds can often aid in radiographic interpretation. Furthermore, the chest radiograph may provide evidence of pneumothorax, hemothorax, and foreign bodies such as bullets and shrapnel. Radiographic findings suggesting possible traumatic aortic injury include widened mediastinum, abnormal aortic arch, a left apical cap, depression of the left main bronchus, deviation of a nasogastric tube in the esophagus, and lateral displacement of the trachea.

The mediastinum includes the heart, great vessels, esophagus, trachea, phrenic nerve, thoracic duct, thymus, and lymph nodes. The most sensitive indicator of blunt aortic injury remains an abnormal or widened mediastinum, which is defined as a mediastinal width greater than 8 cm at the level of the aortic arch on a posteroanterior (PA) chest radiograph. Normally, a clear aortic outline from the arch down to the diaphragm should be seen. Loss of this clear line is another potential radiographic finding suggesting TAI. A left apical cap (accumulation of blood in the extrapleural space overlying the lung), depression of the left main bronchus, or lateral displacements of the trachea are other clues that make one suspicious of a thoracic great vessel injury.

CLASSIFICATION

TAIs are best diagnosed with computed tomography angiography (CTA) and, for the purposes of treatment, are classified into one of four grades (grades I–IV). Grade I injuries present with an intimal tear only and are managed with blood pressure control. A repeat CTA should occur in approximately 6 weeks in order to follow the injury. Grade II injuries present with injury to the media, presenting with intramural hematomas. Once a hematoma develops within the media, it often changes the contour of the vessel. Grade II injuries should be considered for an endograft repair. Grade III injuries extend to the adventitia and lead to pseudoaneurysm formation. Grade II and III injuries should be considered for urgent, rather than emergent, repair. Grade IV injuries, however, are emergent. Because of free rupture of the aorta they are associated with high mortality risk (Fig. 5).

TAIs can be complicated by concurrent injuries to the spleen, liver, bowel, mesentery, pancreas, or gallbladder, and these injuries, if present, are often addressed first with laparotomy. Once the patient survives repair of the intra-abdominal injuries, treatment of the aortic injury can be performed with an endograft. Traditionally, repair of the aorta was accomplished through a median sternotomy or thoracotomy (depending on location) with a "clamp and sew" technique.

Classification of
TRAUMATIC AORTIC INJURY

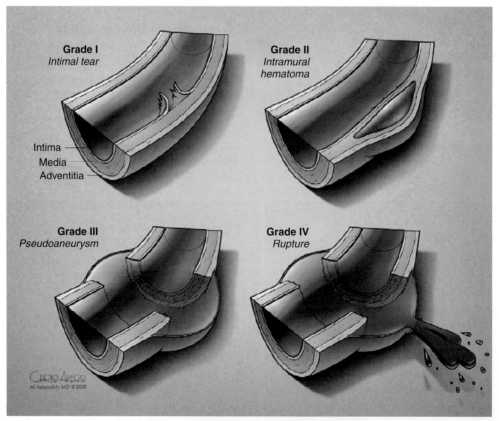

FIGURE 5   Classification of traumatic aortic injury, grades I to IV. *(From Dua A, Desai SS, Holcomb JB, et al, editors: Clinical review of vascular trauma. New York, Springer, 2014, p 160.)*

INITIAL EVALUATION AND MANAGEMENT

Most patients with TAI die at the scene from exsanguination. The patients who do survive the initial aortic injury may have other injuries that pose a more immediate threat to their lives. Once a TAI is found, the tendency is to focus on the aorta and overlook other life-threatening injuries. Therefore, if a patient survives to emergency room presentation, the initial management should begin with the Advanced Trauma Life Support (ATLS) guidelines, as stabilization is the first priority. Assessment of the patient's airway, breathing, circulation, disability, and exposure should be done. There should be an appropriate balance between permissive hypotension and maintaining a satisfactory cerebral perfusion pressure. A mean arterial pressure of 80 mm Hg should be the target. Patients who are hemodynamically stable generally undergo a primary and secondary survey, plain films of the chest and pelvis, and then CT of their chest, abdomen, and pelvis. Recent evidence suggests that some TAIs do not need repair at all.

NONOPERATIVE MANAGEMENT

Patients with grade I TAI can be treated medically. The blood pressure can be lowered with nicardipine or an esmolol drip. The ideal heart rate is below 100 beats per minute and the diastolic blood pressure below 100 mm Hg. Transition from an intravenous (IV) drip to an oral regimen can subsequently occur. Follow-up imaging in 6 weeks is suitable for patients with grade I injures.

ENDOVASCULAR REPAIR

TEVAR is more commonly being performed in operating rooms with more permanent imaging technology, sometimes referred to as "hybrid" operating rooms. TEVAR has a markedly improved outcome compared to nonoperative management of TAI for certain grades of injury, and most consider it the preferred approach over an open surgical repair. CTA is the method of choice for diagnosis and treatment planning. Magnetic resonance imaging (MRI) is not widely used in the acute setting. Conventional angiography is no longer recommended as a routine diagnostic procedure. Once the CTA has been obtained, sizing has occurred, and the graft chosen, the patient can be taken to the hybrid operating room for insertion of the endograft. The chest, abdomen, bilateral groins, and both legs down to the knees are prepped. A diagnostic aortogram (Fig. 6) is obtained through percutaneous femoral artery access. The patient is anticoagulated with IV heparin. A thoracic stent graft is selected based on cross-sectional measurements of the aorta. Four types of stent grafts are available: Valiant (Medtronic), TX2 (Cook), TAG (W.L. Gore), and Relay (Bolton). Currently the smallest graft available is 21 mm and can be used in a 16-mm aorta. When the graft is placed, the left subclavian artery can be covered if necessary to achieve a proximal seal. Immediate endovascular treatment is indicated in patients with complete transection of the aortic wall and free bleeding into the mediastinum, although some still claim this to be the last remaining indication for an open repair (Fig. 7).

OPEN REPAIR

Traditionally, for a patient with a descending TAI, the most appropriate incision was a left anterolateral thoracotomy in the supine position. Although many surgeons have used the "clamp and sew" technique, obviating the need for shunts or bypass, aortic perfusion

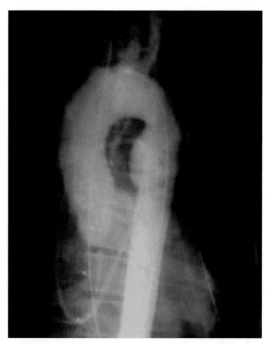

FIGURE 6 Thoracic aortogram depicting a thoracic aortic rupture intimal. *(Courtesy of J.A. Asensio, MD.)*

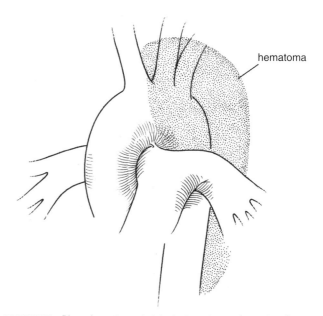

FIGURE 7 Blunt thoracic aortic injuries in patients who arrive alive at a trauma center are usually contained by the adventitia and have a large surrounding hematoma. Today the vast majority are treated with thoracic endovascular aortic repair. However, rarely, they require open techniques requiring cardiopulmonary bypass or partial bypass.
Because this is rarely performed, the authors sought to illustrate the open technique.

distal to the arch can be achieved with cardiopulmonary bypass (Fig. 8). Outflow cannulation is from the heart or ascending aorta to either the distal descending aorta or left common femoral artery. Principles of managing descending thoracic aortic injuries are proximal/distal control, addressing the injured segment, and

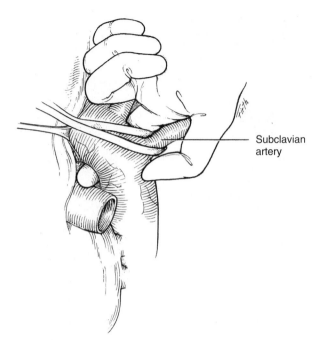

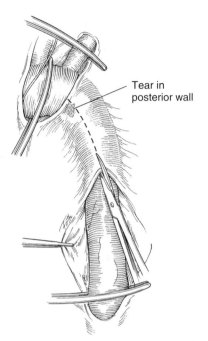

FIGURE 8 After placing the patient on partial or full cardiopulmonary bypass, the aorta is approached via a left posterolateral thoracotomy. The aortic arch is meticulously dissected. This figure depicts encirclement of the left subclavian artery at its origin. The hematoma is often very large and extends superiorly and laterally. The clamp and sew technique has been abandoned because of its large number of complications, particularly paraplegia.

FIGURE 10 The descending thoracic aorta is dissected, and the hematoma is entered by incising the pleura over the aorta prior to obtaining proximal and distal control.

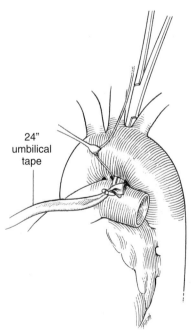

FIGURE 9 The thoracic aorta is encircled between the origin of the distal carotid and left subclavian artery. This maneuver is performed to secure proximal control prior to the application of vascular clamps. The left recurrent laryngeal nerve is located and preserved as it encircles the aortic arch and curves superiorly.

reestablishing continuity of blood flow. The patient is therapeutically heparinized. Proximal control is obtained by passing umbilical tape around the aortic arch between the takeoff of the left common carotid artery and the left subclavian artery (Fig. 9). Umbilical tape is also passed around the left subclavian artery. Injury to the left recurrent laryngeal nerve should be avoided as it courses posteriorly around the aortic arch near the ligamentum arteriosum. Next, vascular control is achieved distal to the descending thoracic aorta (Figs. 10 and 11). Simple partial laceration of the aorta can be primarily closed with 4-0 Prolene (Ethicon). Complex injuries often require an interposition Dacron tube graft (Fig. 12). Regardless of the technique chosen, the overall incidence of postoperative paraplegia averages 8%.

Median sternotomy provides access to the superior mediastinum. Dividing the left innominate vein improves exposure and gives the surgeon access to the aortic arch and its branches. Repair of the aortic arch often requires cardiopulmonary bypass. Occasionally, minor injuries to the innominate artery can be repaired primarily. More often, injuries to the innominate artery require repair via the bypass exclusion technique. A piece of synthetic interposition graft is sewn from the ascending aorta to the distal innominate artery. The proximal innominate artery is oversewn. With transection of the left common carotid artery, a bypass to the aorta using polytetrafluoroethylene (PTFE) is preferred over end-to-end anastomosis. The superficial femoral-popliteal vein has been used in the reconstruction of the innominate artery and common carotid artery.

The right and left subclavian arteries are exposed differently depending on the location of injury with respect to the vertebral artery. The right subclavian artery can be exposed with a right supraclavicular incision, and the incision can be extended to a median sternotomy if more proximal exposure is needed. The left subclavian artery can be exposed with a supraclavicular incision with clavicle resection, a left anterolateral thoracotomy, and a sternoclavicular flap (trap door) as a last resort.

FIGURE 11 **A,** Obtaining meticulous proximal control is of the utmost importance. Often the space between the origin of the left common carotid artery and left subclavian artery is small. Double clamping the aorta and origin of the left subclavian artery is required until the injury is better defined. **B,** Clamps can then be repositioned prior to resection of the injured descending aortic segment.

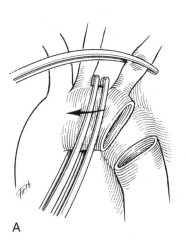
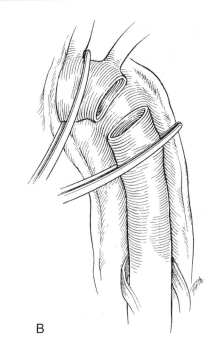

A

B

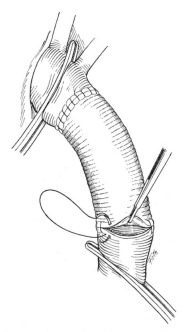

FIGURE 12 The injured descending thoracic aorta is reconstructed with a knitted Dacron graft. The size of the graft is selected after measuring the aorta. Most adult aortas measure between 18 and 29 mm. Monofilament sutures of 2-0 or 3-0 polypropylene are used to perform the end-to-end anastomosis. Bleeding from the intercostal arteries must be controlled.

MORBIDITY AND MANAGEMENT COMPLICATIONS

The most feared complication of the open technique is paraplegia. Ischemic bowel and renal failure may also result from prolonged clamping. Almost nonexistent paraplegia risk makes the use of TEVAR very attractive. Patients who undergo TEVAR require long-term follow-up. They should be monitored with CT imaging at 1 month, 6 months, 1 year, and every other year thereafter. Complications specific to TEVAR are endoleaks, stent migration, stent graft patency, and device integrity. TEVAR is associated with a lower spinal cord ischemia, end-stage renal disease, and systemic and graft infections as compared to open repair. TEVAR patients have associated secondary interventions for device-related complications, yet the costs of TEVAR compared to open repair are not significantly different.

MORTALITY

TAIs have very high mortality rates, partially due to the high incidence of other concomitant injuries in other body compartments. Patients with ascending aortic injuries rarely survive the causative event. There is a significantly higher mortality rate for nonoperative management of high-grade injuries and open repair compared to TEVAR. The mortality rate remains as high as 50% for patients with ascending aortic injuries with stable vital signs on arrival to trauma centers.

CONCLUSIONS

TAIs occur in almost one third of blunt traumatic fatalities, with the majority of deaths occurring at the scene. For survivors of TAIs, ATLS assessment should occur, and the patient should be fully evaluated for other concomitant life-threatening injuries, as many patients with TAI will have other intra-abdominal injuries that require laparotomy before treatment of the aortic injury is performed. Grade I TAI can be treated with blood pressure control alone. For most patients who do require treatment of aortic injuries, TEVAR is considered the treatment of choice, although in a dying patient with thoracic vascular injury, damage control thoracotomy remains a treatment option. Open repair carries with it higher mortality rate including higher paraplegic rates, higher incidence of bowel ischemia, and more acute kidney injury.

For the chapter's Suggested Readings list, please visit the book at www.ExpertConsult.inkling.com.

TREATMENT OF ESOPHAGEAL INJURY

A. Britton Christmas and J. David Richardson

INCIDENCE

The incidence of esophageal injuries is low with most resulting from penetrating trauma. Esophageal trauma received little notice until the completion of World War II, with only 18 esophageal injuries recorded in the military records reviewed from that war and the Korean and Vietnam Wars combined. Numerous reports in the literature document the incidence of esophageal trauma to be less than 1%. Penetrating injuries of the esophagus far outnumber blunt esophageal injuries. The predominant mechanism responsible for esophageal trauma injury is gunshot wounds (70% to 80%) followed by stab wounds (15% to 20%) and shotgun wounds (3% to 5%). Esophageal injuries resulting from blunt trauma account for less than 1% of all esophageal injuries and are quite rare. These injuries are most often located in the cervical esophagus as the result of an anterior blow with the neck in a hyperextended position. An acute blow to a distended stomach may produce tears of the distal esophagus, with the most common cause being penetrating injuries sustained from stab and gunshot wounds.

The cervical esophagus represents the most common site of injury followed by thoracic and abdominal esophageal injuries. Virtually all patients who sustain an esophageal injury also incur associated injuries to other respiratory, gastrointestinal, and vascular structures. As a result, trauma surgeons must maintain a high index of suspicion so that untoward diagnostic delays may be avoided. Although these wounds occur relatively infrequently, they continue to be associated with high mortality rate ranging from 20% to 30%.

DIAGNOSIS

Diagnostic delays are often cited as significant factors in the high morbidity and mortality rates associated with injuries to the esophagus. Several factors contribute to this diagnostic delay including the uncommon occurrence of these injuries. Because associated injuries are common, delays may occur before the initiation of specific diagnostic tests to evaluate the esophagus. All the while, even a "simple" perforation elicits a massive inflammatory response with mediastinal tissue destruction that may further complicate the integrity of repair.

Esophageal injuries must be suspected in penetrating neck injuries that violate the platysma, in transmediastinal gunshot wounds, and following significant chest trauma with associated tracheobronchial injuries. The clinical findings most commonly associated with cervical esophageal injuries include neck pain and dysphagia. Tenderness to palpation and with passive motion, dyspnea, and hoarseness may be present. Hematemesis, hemoptysis, or bloody nasogastric tube aspirate in the absence of obvious oral or pharyngeal trauma should suggest the possibility of esophageal injury. Expanding cervical hematoma is certainly a cause for concern as are the subsequent development of fever, cough, and stridor. Palpable crepitus or air within the soft tissues or a wide prevertebral shadow on neck or cervical spine radiographs may provide the initial suggestion of an esophageal injury. Computed tomography examination may demonstrate subcutaneous emphysema within the soft tissues or in the upper mediastinum.

The clinical findings associated with thoracic esophageal injuries may be nonspecific and initially absent. They may include abdominal tenderness or rigidity, cervical crepitus from tracking of mediastinal emphysema, and Hamman sign (mediastinal crunch on auscultation). The presence of mediastinal emphysema and pleural effusion in the face of penetrating thoracic trauma should elevate awareness for the possibility of a thoracic esophageal injury.

Subdiaphragmatic esophageal injuries often present with abdominal tenderness or rigidity. Patients frequently complain of abdominal pain and may progress to signs of frank peritonitis. Upright chest radiographs or computed tomography scans may demonstrate pneumoperitoneum.

Although penetrating neck or thoracic wounds with hemodynamic instability often necessitate immediate exploration for associated injuries, the hemodynamically stable patient often presents a diagnostic challenge. In the past, all penetrating neck wounds that violated the platysma were routinely explored. However, many trauma centers now practice selective management of neck wounds. Selective management necessitates some type of study to exclude esophageal injury. We recommend a water-soluble contrast esophagogram in stable patients. If no injury is seen, addition of dilute barium adds a measure of safety in excluding an injury. Because contrast studies yield a false-negative rate of up to 25%, esophagoscopy may be added in patients regarded as high risk for injury. The specificity of a negative esophagogram accompanied by negative esophagoscopy approaches 100%. Even in hemodynamically stable patients with cervical hematomas who undergo exploration, we advocate esophagoscopy, as the injury may be further localized by the appreciation of blood or hematoma within the esophagus. It is often difficult to identify an esophageal injury during exploration due to extensive blood staining of the tissues. All studies should be obtained in an expeditious manner as prolonged time to diagnosis has been widely correlated with increased morbidity and mortality rates. Once an esophageal injury has been diagnosed, all oral intake is held, careful nasogastric tube decompression is performed, and intravenous fluid resuscitation and broad-spectrum antibiotics are initiated before prompt surgical intervention.

SURGICAL TREATMENT

Although some penetrating cervical wounds may be managed nonoperatively, all confirmed esophageal injuries should be managed operatively in expedient fashion. The preferred surgical management of esophageal injuries is dictated by the location of the injury, stability of the patient, time to diagnosis, and associated injuries.

In our opinion, all esophageal injuries should be treated by general unifying principles regardless of location. These principles include (1) attempted closure of all defects by some method; (2) the use of onlay flaps, preferably muscular, as a buttress or for primary closure; and (3) tube drainage near the repair. Given the lack of a serosa, primary healing of the esophagus is not uniform. Therefore, the use of a buttress often enhances healing without fistula development. Local muscle flaps, in particular, are useful for either buttress or as a primary onlay repair.

Injuries to the cervical esophagus may be approached either by a collar incision or by an incision anterior to the sternocleidomastoid. An anterior unilateral incision should be made for unilateral cervical and single injuries, whereas a collar incision is indicated for midline, multiple, or bilateral cervical injuries. The esophagus is located deep to the trachea and placement of a nasogastric tube often facilitates localization by palpation. Throughout the dissection, great care must be taken to identify and avoid injury to the recurrent laryngeal nerves, which are located in the tracheoesophageal groove. If further exposure is needed, the omohyoid muscle may be divided. After blunt dissection, the esophagus should be encircled by a Penrose drain in order to further facilitate the dissection.

Thoracic esophageal injuries are best approached through thoracotomy incisions based on the suspected level of the injury. Following initial studies, the decision for the incision should be determined by the presence of pleural effusion or defined leak identified on esophagogram. Injuries to the upper two thirds of the thoracic esophagus are best approached through a right posterolateral thoracotomy though the fifth intercostal space. Injuries to the lower third of the thoracic esophagus are best approached through an incision in the left sixth intercostal space.

Injuries to the most distal portion of the esophagus should be approached through a laparotomy incision, with the left side of the chest prepped into the operative field should a thoracic approach be necessitated. Additional exposure can be achieved by placing the patient in the Trendelenburg position and by mobilizing the left lobe of the liver. The midline incision can be extended superiorly and to the left of the xiphoid process for an additional 1 to 2 cm of exposure. The esophagus should be exposed with blunt manual dissection at the gastroesophageal junction and encircled with a Penrose drain. The hiatus can be widened, if necessary, to expose wounds near the gastroesophageal junction.

Most injuries of the esophagus can be primarily repaired if promptly diagnosed. Small injuries may be closed transversely, whereas injuries larger than 2 to 3 cm can be closed longitudinally in order to avoid undue tension. Unfortunately, diagnostic delay often yields significant mediastinal inflammation and sepsis. Furthermore, the lack of a serosal layer complicates primary reapproximation as the esophageal tissues are extremely friable especially under these circumstances. Numerous strategies have been proposed including nonoperative management with drainage, esophageal resection, and diversion with exclusion. The use of pleural and pericardial flaps has been widely described for buttressing primary repairs. More recently, various muscle flaps have been advocated for primary repair of esophageal defects. However, adequate esophageal tissue débridement, tension-free repairs, and effective drainage remain the mainstays of successful operative management.

CERVICAL ESOPHAGUS

The presence of a cervical esophageal injury mandates exploration of the neck. Careful examination of the esophagus should be performed to locate the site of esophageal injury as well as possible concomitant injuries to the trachea or vascular structures. Once identified, any nonviable or necrotic tissue should be débrided until viable edges are obtained. The defect should be closed in two layers if possible. An absorbable mucosal repair is preferable with a nonabsorbable suture closure of the muscular layer. In cases of significant inflammation, single-layer closure may be the only feasible option. All wounds of the cervical esophagus may be buttressed or closed primarily by a sternocleidomastoid muscle flap. The muscle flap is created by mobilizing the sternal attachment of the sternocleidomastoid and positioning it over the suture line. Absorbable sutures are used to secure the muscle flap over the defect or repair. All repairs should be drained with either Penrose or Silastic tube drains. In the presence of associated carotid artery injuries, drainage should be performed from the opposite side of the neck so as to divert leakage and avoid late vascular complications.

Occasionally, diagnostic delays of an injured esophagus cause intense inflammation in the neck. If the site of injury is not obvious, the esophagus may be insufflated with air under a layer of sterile water. Methylene blue may also be instilled into the esophagus in an attempt to localize the injury. If the injury cannot be localized, then drainage and broad-spectrum antibiotics will often provide satisfactory results.

The delayed diagnosis of cervical esophageal injuries necessitates adequate débridement, irrigation, and drainage. In these instances, primary repair will often not suffice. Therefore, the defect may be primarily closed with a sternocleidomastoid muscle flap. The paraesophageal and precervical planes must also be inspected, irrigated, and drained to decrease contamination. We have treated several patients with large defects that could not be closed primarily with muscle flaps. Likewise, we have treated several patients with delayed recognition of an injury with onlay sternocleidomastoid flaps.

THORACIC ESOPHAGUS

Once the diagnosis of a thoracic esophageal injury has been identified, surgical exploration should ensue through an appropriate thoracotomy as previously described. These injuries are frequently associated with acute coagulation necrosis, diffuse tissue hemorrhage, and significant inflammation. The mediastinum should be opened and thoroughly irrigated. Occasionally, the inflammation is so severe that the defect is difficult to identify. In such cases, the esophagus can be encircled in an area remote from the injury. The esophagus can then be mobilized toward the area of injury. Diligent exploration should be performed until the injury is visualized. Both mucosal and muscular layers should be identified, and one should recognize that the mucosal tear is usually larger than the muscular defect. Subsequently, it is often necessary to open the muscular layer more proximally and distally to fully appreciate the mucosal defect. Failure to completely expose the mucosal defect may result in incomplete closure and subsequent leakage from the site of repair. If possible, a double-layered closure should be performed with reapproximation of both mucosa and muscularis. The repair should always be buttressed with adjacent tissue for additional reinforcement.

Primary repairs of the thoracic esophagus tend to fail in a significant percentage of cases. The lower esophageal blood supply and the lack of a serosal layer make primary closure much more tenuous. As a result, several adjacent tissues have been used to buttress or primarily repair these injuries with variable success. Pleural flaps have been widely used but are often too friable and sometimes provide inadequate tissue coverage. Pleural flaps are more reliable if there have been inflammatory changes to thicken the pleura. The use of pericardial flaps seems unwise, as this would expose the pericardial sac to contamination. In our experience, we have found muscle flaps to be more reliable both in terms of buttressing and primary repair of esophageal defects.

Adequate tissue coverage is especially important in close proximity to the trachea in order to reduce the incidence of later fistula development. If both trachea and esophagus are injured, we attempt to interpose a muscle flap between the suture lines of the two injuries. Muscle flaps tend to be less friable and provide greater bulk of tissue coverage of the defect. Intercostal bundles are frequently mentioned as muscle flaps, but we often find they provide inadequate tissue for buttress and especially for primary repair.

We have demonstrated that injuries to the esophagus involving up to two thirds of the circumference can be adequately closed with muscle flaps without increased incidence of stricture. The rhomboid muscle may be mobilized for repair of upper esophageal and midesophageal injuries (Fig. 1). The muscle is dissected from its attachment of the scapula through a parascapular incision and transferred as a pedicle flap into the thoracotomy. For distal esophageal lesions that are too proximal to be buttressed with the gastric fundus, we advocate the use of a diaphragm muscle flap (Fig. 2). The central portion of the diaphragm is excised as a pedicle flap and sutured over the defect or buttressed to the repair. The flap should be posteriorly based and great care should be taken to avoid the phrenic nerve. Diaphragm pedicle flaps may reach to the level of the azygous vein. The edges of the diaphragm are then reapproximated with heavy nonabsorbable sutures. A two-layer closure is performed if feasible. This has the additional benefit of plicating the diaphragm.

Delayed diagnosis of thoracic esophageal injuries presents a significant surgical challenge. Prolonged perforations are often difficult to visualize secondary to mediastinitis and subsequent empyema. Successful management of uncontained esophageal leaks requires

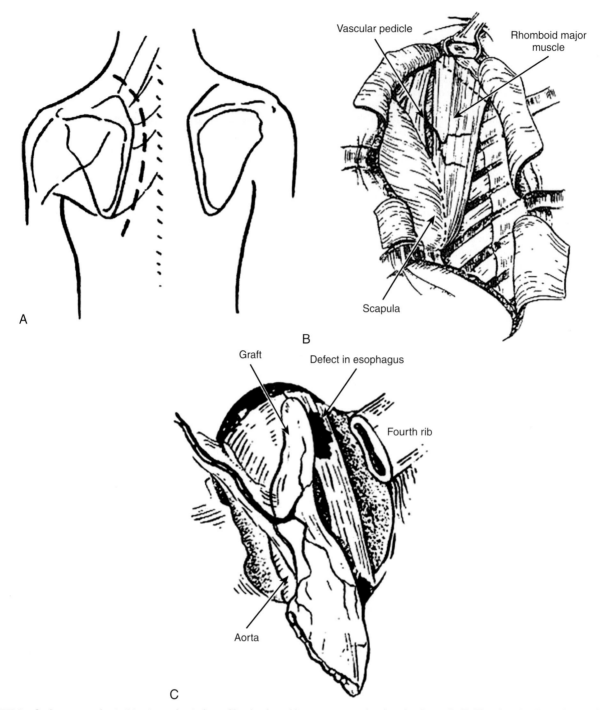

FIGURE I   A, A parascapular incision is used as indicated by the dotted lines to expose the rhomboid muscle. **B,** The rhomboid muscle is isolated and carefully dissected to preserve its vascular pedicle. **C,** A rib resection allows the muscle to be transposed into the thoracic cavity where it is sutured over the esophageal defect as an onlay flap. *(From Richardson JD, Tobin GR: Closure of esophageal defects with muscle flaps. Arch Surg 129:541–548, 1994.)*

débridement of necrotic tissue, copious irrigation, and complete mediastinal and pleural drainage. Often, a decortication must also be performed at the time of operation if the diagnosis has been delayed for several days. Although primary repair remains the preferred method of management, we have found that this is essentially futile after delayed diagnosis and treatment.

All thoracic esophageal injuries should be widely drained. The mediastinal pleura should be widely incised, and a large-bore chest tube should be placed in the mediastinum adjacent to the repair. In those with large esophageal injuries, those with delayed diagnosis

of the injury, or those believed at high risk for failure, we support the routine placement of a gastrostomy tube for gastric decompression. The placement of a jejunostomy tube for distal feeding should also be considered in order to maintain adequate nutrition.

ABDOMINAL ESOPHAGUS

Injuries to the abdominal esophagus are often accompanied by extensive intra-abdominal or intrathoracic injuries. These injuries are best

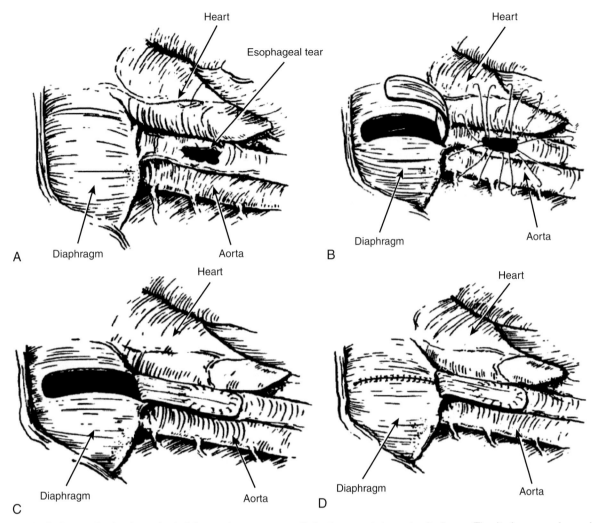

FIGURE 2 **A,** Defects in the distal one third of the esophagus are generally in close proximity to the diaphragm. The diaphragm can be used to close midthoracic defects. **B,** The edges of the esophageal defect are débrided and a diaphragm flap is elevated. Double-armed sutures can be passed through the defect and then sutured to muscle to ensure a complete onlay graft. **C,** The flap is then sutured in position. **D,** The diaphragmatic defect is closed in two layers with heavy sutures. *(From Richardson JD, Tobin GR: Closure of esophageal defects with muscle flaps. Arch Surg 129:541–548, 1994.)*

approached through a laparotomy incision with the left side of the chest prepped into the operative field should a thoracotomy be necessary. Perforations or injuries to the distal esophagus should be closed primarily in two layers with nonabsorbable sutures. The layered closure should then be buttressed with either a Nissen fundoplication over a 50 to 60 F bougie, a Thal patch, or with a diaphragm flap. Injuries that are not amenable to primary closure should be primarily closed with the diaphragm flap. The area of repair should be adequately drained with a Silastic tube drain. A gastrostomy tube should be placed for gastric decompression, and a jejunostomy tube should be placed for distal enteric feeding.

DEVASTATING INJURIES

Occasionally, devastating injuries of the esophagus occur. If repair is not feasible, there are several less than desirable options, including resection, T-tube placement, and cervical esophagostomy with or without esophageal exclusion.

Esophageal resection may be indicated in some unusual circumstances, but the senior author has never been forced to resect the esophagus for trauma in 35 years of experience. Clearly, injuries to a damaged esophagus or caustic injuries may require emergency esophagectomy.

If this unusual circumstance arises, delayed reconstruction using stomach or colonic bypass would likely be the treatment of choice.

Occasionally, large defects in the esophagus are encountered that cannot be closed. Although we attempt to cover such injuries with an onlay muscle flap, creation of a controlled fistula with a T-tube has been reported. In this technique, the short limb of the T-tube is placed in the defect and the long limb is brought out through the chest. In our experience, if a perforation is amenable to closure around a tube, it can be closed with a tissue flap even if the treatment is delayed.

Cervical esophagostomy should not be used routinely because it presents extremely difficult problems to reconstruct. In our experience, a diversion should be performed for an uncontrolled leak that results in sepsis or a life-threatening problem. If possible, a loop esophagostomy should be performed. This permits the possibility of a one-stage closure of the esophagostomy if and when the esophageal injury has healed. End esophagostomy invariably requires complex reconstruction.

If diversion is performed, we rarely use esophageal exclusion in which the distal esophagus is ligated. This creates a distal obstruction and permits bacterial overgrowth in an organ whose only egress is through the original injury. For this reason, we do not attempt to exclude the esophagus even if a proximal diversion is performed.

An esophagus damaged badly enough to require exclusion is best treated by resection. Using muscle flaps, we have been able to preserve esophageal function in many patients with complex injuries.

USE OF ESOPHAGEAL STENTS

In the past decade, over 300 reports on the use of esophageal stents have been published; stents have been used to treat a variety of problems resulting in esophageal perforations including iatrogenic injuries, anastomotic leaks, complications of bariatric procedures, and spontaneous perforations among others. Stents have proved effective in the treatment of complex delayed leaks as well. Although most of these reports are isolated cases, series of collected cases are emerging, though none of these larger reports have included any trauma patients. To date, less than five cases of traumatic injuries (noniatrogenic) managed by stents have been reported. Given the infrequency of esophageal trauma and the need to address associated injuries, it is highly unlikely that large series of such cases will be reported. A more likely use of stents will be in the treatment of ongoing leaks after ineffective repair of injuries to the esophagus.

There are certainly no evidenced-based recommendations for the appropriate use of covered stents for traumatic injuries at this time. Intuitively one would suspect isolated injuries in a stable patient would be appropriate to consider for such approaches. However, as previously described, traumatic lesions are inherently complex, particularly in terms of the potential for other associated injuries.

MANAGEMENT OF COMPLICATIONS

The morbidity associated with cervical esophageal injuries has been estimated as high as 16%, with most complications related to the duration of diagnostic delay and subsequent contamination from esophageal contents. Gunshot wounds exhibit a greater preponderance for complications, whereas stab wounds often fare better secondary to less tissue destruction.

Increased morbidity from diagnostic delays and subsequent delays in operative treatment has been well established. However, little literature exists addressing long-term complications and esophageal function after traumatic esophageal injuries. Certainly, the most concerning complications associated with esophageal injuries are major vascular or airway injuries producing massive hemorrhage or acute respiratory decompensation. The development of anastomotic leaks with subsequent mediastinitis, sepsis, and pulmonary failure presents significant management challenges. Shock, extensive mobilization, inadequate débridement, and tension are well-known risk factors for suture line breakdown and subsequent esophageal leakage. Approximately 50% of esophageal leaks are asymptomatic, being noticed only on postoperative esophagograms. Once a leak is identified, the initiation of adequate drainage, wide-spectrum antibiotics, parenteral or distal enteral nutrition, and limited oral intake are the mainstays of therapy. The development of interventional radiologic techniques with the advent of percutaneous drainage has certainly assisted in the management of these complicated injuries. Most leaks will subsequently resolve without the need for further operative intervention. Increasingly, endoluminal stents have been used to manage esophageal leaks. We have no experience using stents as primary treatment, but we have used them on two occasions for the treatment of delayed leaks resulting from trauma.

CONCLUSIONS

Esophageal injuries, although uncommon, mandate a high degree of suspicion especially for penetrating injuries to the neck or thorax. Many of these patients have concomitant vascular, airway, or intra-abdominal injuries that often require emergent operative intervention. For those who remain hemodynamically stable, prompt diagnostic evaluation should ensue to avoid delays in treatment. A water-soluble esophagogram should be performed followed by dilute barium if no leak is visualized. A false-negative rate as high as 25% has been reported with esophagogram alone. Therefore, radiographic studies should be complemented with esophagoscopy for verification. The combination of esophagography in combination with esophagoscopy approaches a specificity of nearly 100%. In the presence of cervical hematoma, we advocate the use of intraoperative esophagoscopy to localize the injury before operative exploration. This should be performed in the operative suite in the event of hemorrhage, loss of airway, or hemodynamic collapse. After diagnosis, wide-spectrum antibiotics, meticulous surgical technique with adequate débridement, and wide drainage are the mainstays of successful management.

For the chapter's Suggested Readings list, please visit the book at www.ExpertConsult.inkling.com.

DIAPHRAGMATIC INJURY

Charles E. Lucas and Anna M. Ledgerwood

ANATOMY AND PHYSIOLOGY

This diaphragm arises from the confluence of the abdominal peritoneum and the parietal pleura as a circumferential extension from the posterior sternal border, the lower six costal cartilages, and the posterior lumbocostal arches. These muscular groups join as a central tendon with left, right, and central leaflets (Figs. 1 and 2). The most medial posterior margins are formed by the crura. The central leaflet contributes to the pericardial fibers. Incomplete closure of the right or left posterior lateral leaflet results in herniation in the foramen of Bochdalek. Partial closure may result in pleural and peritoneal apposition without union as a central tendon, namely, eventration (Figs. 3 and 4).

The diaphragm changes contour during ventilation. The dome extends high in the thorax during full expiration but is pulled inferiorly and becomes platelike with deep inspiration. The range of movement exceeds three intercostal spaces. The most inferior extension occurs posteriorly to the level of the second and third lumbar vertebrae. The posterior sulcus extends inferiorly to the midportion of the kidneys. Patients with upper abdominal gunshot wounds or stab wounds often have a missed diaphragm perforation at the posterior sulcus. The resultant hemothorax is diagnosed and treated after laparotomy.

The diaphragm has three major foramina, permitting passage of the aorta, the esophagus, and the inferior vena cava (see Fig. 1). The minor anterior foramen of Morgagni, through which the internal mammary vessels course, is retroxiphoid. The median plane of the diaphragm extending from the foramen of Morgagni to the esophageal foramen, the so-called median raphe, is less vascular and can be divided to provide better exposure to the inferior mediastinum (see Fig. 2). The phrenic vein may cross this median plane about 1 cm above the esophageal hiatus; inadvertent injury can cause major hemorrhage. The phrenic nerves arising from the cervical vertebrae C3, C4, and C5 descend medially through the mediastinum to the diaphragm, where they fan out to their anterior, lateral, and posterior attachments (see Fig. 1).

INCIDENCE

Asensio and coworkers, in a multicenter review, noted a 3% incidence for all patients sustaining torso trauma with a range of 0.8% to 5.8%; this wide range reflected the different types of injuries treated at each institution and the diligence one places on confirming a diaphragmatic perforation. Rural centers see more blunt injuries, whereas penetrating injury predominates in the inner city centers. The reported incidence of diaphragmatic rupture also reflects the different therapeutic approaches to patients with penetrating abdominal wounds. Most patients with penetrating stab wounds to the abdomen are now being treated by nonoperative management (NOM) when the patient exhibits no signs of peritonitis or hemoperitoneum. This category includes lower thoracic stab wounds with hemopneumothorax; presumably, an associated diaphragmatic perforation would, in the past, be diagnosed during exploratory laparotomy. Treatment by tube thoracostomy alone results in the diaphragmatic perforation going unrecognized (Fig. 5). Finally, patients with right upper quadrant gunshot wounds with right-sided hemopneumothorax are treated by tube thoracostomy alone, even though there may be at least two diaphragmatic perforations along with a through-and-through liver injury. These unrecognized diaphragmatic perforations are not coded in the trauma registry. When diagnostic peritoneal lavage (DPL) was performed routinely for patients with lower thoracic penetrating wounds, a pink effluent with a red blood cell count less than 100,000 cells/cm^3 would predict diaphragmatic perforation; this would be confirmed and treated at subsequent laparotomy. Ultrasonography (US) replaced DPL and is less sensitive for identifying small amounts of blood. Penetrating diaphragmatic perforation after upper abdominal wounds may also go unrecognized during laparotomy, for which the missile is thought to have penetrated only the transversalis abdominis muscle. A postoperative hemothorax confirms a missed diaphragmatic injury, which is then treated by tube thoracostomy. During the 1970s when routine laparotomy was performed for most penetrating abdominal wounds, the incidence of diaphragmatic perforation was 19% for gunshot wounds and 11% for abdominal stab wounds; since the era of NOM, the incidence of diaphragmatic perforation is about 8% for gunshot wounds and 2% for stab wounds. Patients with blunt injury are less likely to have a diaphragmatic injury that is not recognized during the same hospitalization (Fig. 6). However, a number of patients present with a diaphragmatic hernia years after major blunt torso trauma when diaphragmatic injury was not recognized initially. Likewise, the incidence of diaphragmatic injury in patients with blunt torso injury is now less than 1%; those undergoing laparotomy for blunt injury have about a 3% incidence of diaphragmatic rupture.

MECHANISM AND LOCATION OF INJURY

The site of diaphragmatic perforation varies with mechanism of injury. Lopez and coworkers noted more than a fourfold (13% to 66%) increase in the incidence of blunt rupture after initiating a policy of NOM for asymptomatic penetrating abdominal wounds. The classic scenario for blunt injury is a head-on motor vehicle collision

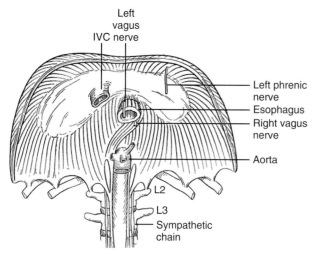

FIGURE 1   Inferior view of the diaphragm highlighting the posteriorly located foramina and central tendon. IVC, Inferior vena cava. *(From Asensio AA, Petrone P, Demetriades D:* Diaphragmatic injuries: operative techniques in general surgery, *Philadelphia, 2000, Saunders.)*

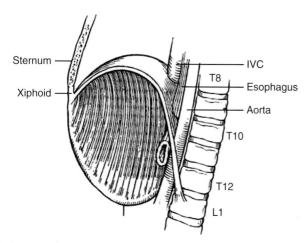

FIGURE 2   Lateral view of the diaphragm. Note xiphoid and sternal attachments anteriorly and the extension of the crus posteriorly. IVC, Inferior vena cava. *(From Asensio AA, Petrone P, Demetriades D:* Diaphragmatic injuries: operative techniques in general surgery, *Philadelphia, 2000, Saunders.)*

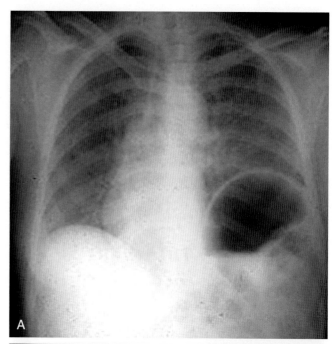

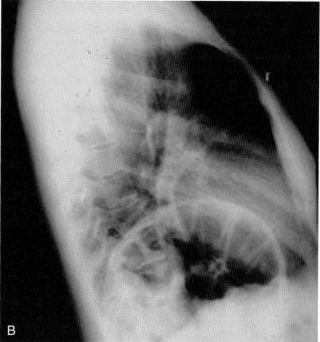

FIGURE 3   **A** and **B,** Preoperative anteroposterior and lateral views of eventration misdiagnosed as ruptured diaphragm after motor vehicle collision.

(MVC) or a broadside (t-bone) impact causing a marked increase in the intra-abdominal pressure, thereby stretching the diaphragm to the point of rupture. The rupture typically occurs in the posterolateral segment in the central tendon of the left hemidiaphragm, often with extension into the muscular portion. Blunt rupture can also be caused by assaults, stampings, falls from a height, and explosions. Although the posterolateral location is most common, rupture may occur adjacent to the esophageal hiatus, near the bare area of the liver on the right side, and in a subxiphoid location on either side with intrapericardial herniation. Asensio and coworkers, in a review of 32 published series with 1589 patients, showed a distribution of left-sided rupture in 1187 patients (75%), right-sided ruptured in 363 patients (23%), and bilateral rupture in 39 patients (2%). The relative protection of the right hemidiaphragm has been historically attributed to the liver, which blunts the rapid transmission of force against the right hemidiaphragm. A relative weakness of the left hemidiaphragm has been proposed but has never been documented. The site of penetrating perforations may be anywhere. Bilateral perforations are more

likely with missiles. Stab wounds are more commonly located along the periphery of the diaphragm.

SEVERITY OF INJURY

The severity of diaphragmatic rupture is best judged by the five-grade organ injury scale developed by the American Association for the Surgery of Trauma. Grade I injury is a contusion or hematoma without rupture. Grade II injury is a laceration less than 2 cm in diameter. Grade III rupture is a laceration 2 to 9 cm in magnitude. Grade IV is a 10 to 25 cm rupture. Grade V injury is greater than 25 cm. Patients

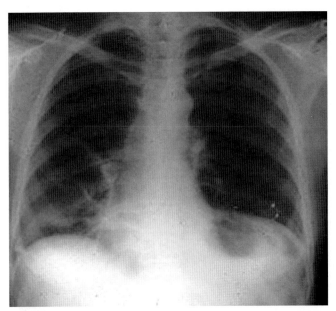

FIGURE 4 Postoperative view after plication of eventration misdiagnosed as ruptured diaphragm.

with penetrating stab wounds and low-velocity gunshot wounds likely have minor injuries (grades I and II). Patients with blunt injury are more likely to have grade III or grade IV lacerations. The massive injuries with extensive tissue loss (grade V) are seen after close-range shotgun blasts, high-velocity rifle perforations, or explosions.

DIAGNOSIS

The diagnosis of diaphragmatic rupture after blunt injury is typically made on a chest radiograph that demonstrates the gastric bubble in the left hemithorax (see Fig. 6). Contrast agent injected through the nasogastric tube will flow into the thorax and fill the herniated stomach. Associated findings include obfuscation of the costal phrenic angle, apparent elevation of the hemidiaphragm, and the presence of the colon in the left thorax (see Fig. 6). Hypotensive patients with multisystem injuries involving the chest and pelvis are more likely to have an associated diaphragmatic injury. When the diagnosis is not appreciated on the initial chest radiographs, a subsequent computed tomography (CT) scan of the trunk may show the injury; the diagnosis of diaphragmatic rupture by CT, however, is not that sensitive.

When the blunt injury occurs on the right side, the liver may prevent abdominal visceral from entering the right hemithorax. Patients presenting with blunt trauma and significant bleeding from a right-sided pneumothorax, however, should be suspected of having a right-sided diaphragmatic tear near the bare area of the liver that is also injured and is the source of bleeding (Fig. 7). Bilateral diaphragmatic rupture is much less frequent but, when present, may lead to a delay in diagnosis due to the apparent lack of diaphragmatic elevation on either side. Both costophrenic angles, however, show lack of clarity (Fig. 8). Repeat chest radiographs in such patients will typically show further elevation of one or both hemidiaphragms (see Fig. 8). When the chest radiograph shows what appears to be a large rupture of the left hemidiaphragm in a patient who has minimal symptoms, one should obtain a good history to rule out previous anatomic changes of the left hemidiaphragm and, if possible, obtain old chest radiographs that might identify the presence of an eventration (see Fig. 3).

When the chest radiograph does not confirm a diaphragmatic rupture, a number of other studies may be obtained. A CT scan of the torso may help but does not have a high sensitivity; laparoscopy has become more popular for identifying diaphragmatic injury, especially after penetrating wounds. Likewise, technetium scanning has been employed but has been of limited value. DPL may lead to suspicion of diaphragmatic injury in patients with associated penetrating wounds to the lower thorax but has not been too reliable in patients with blunt torso injuries. Thoracoscopy has been used in patients with late manifestations of a previously missed diaphragmatic injury. Finally, magnetic resonance imaging has been attempted but is of limited value.

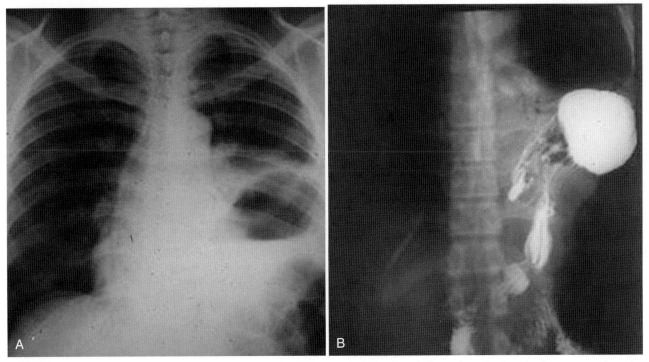

FIGURE 5 **A,** Anteroposterior view of chest showing diaphragmatic hernia in patient treated 18 months earlier by tube thoracostomy for stab wound of left chest. **B,** Gastrografin confirms the presence of stomach in the left hemithorax.

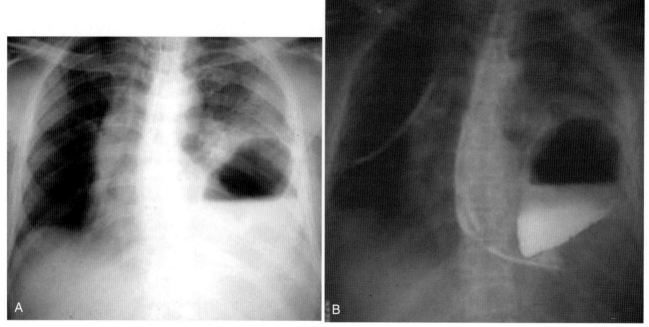

FIGURE 6 **A,** Anteroposterior chest radiograph demonstrates an apparent gastric bubble in the left hemothorax after blunt trauma. **B,** Injection of contrast agent through the nasogastric tube confirms the gastric filling.

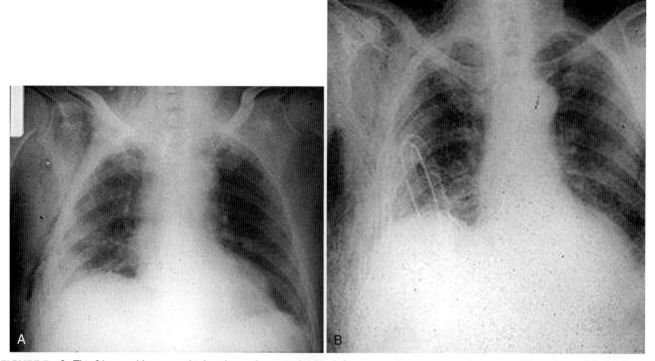

FIGURE 7 **A,** This 86-year-old man was hit by a bus and sustained right rib fractures, subcutaneous emphysema, and hemothorax. Note lack of clarity of the right costal phrenic angle. **B,** Right chest tube yielded 500 mL blood with continued bleeding of 300 mL during the next hour. Laparotomy revealed a large rent in the dome of the diaphragm and a type IV liver injury, which was repaired.

The diagnosis of a penetrating injury is usually made at the time of laparotomy performed for the treatment of other organ injuries. Thus, many diaphragmatic perforations are not being diagnosed due to the rise in NOM after most torso stab wounds and some gunshot wounds. When an inferior stab wound to the chest causes a hemothorax in an asymptomatic patient, a DPL yielding a small amount of hemoperitoneum strongly suggests diaphragmatic perforation. Laparoscopy permits confirmation and primary repair of a minor perforation. A missed injury in such patients may lead to a later diaphragmatic hernia (see Fig. 5). Repair of these injuries may be

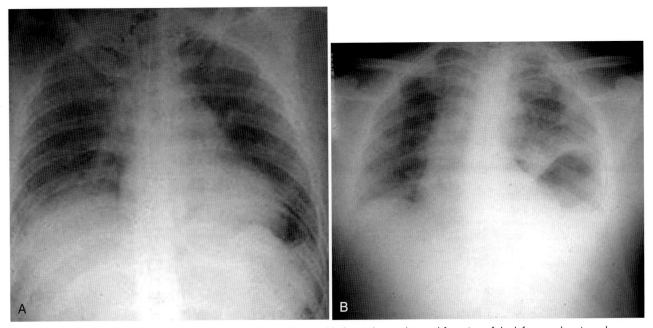

FIGURE 8 **A,** Chest radiograph following steering wheel impact in an elderly gentleman shows obfuscation of the left costophrenic angle without diaphragmatic elevation when compared to the right side. **B,** Two hours later, both hemidiaphragms are elevated, and both costophrenic angles are obfuscated. Laparotomy revealed bilateral hemidiaphragmatic rupture.

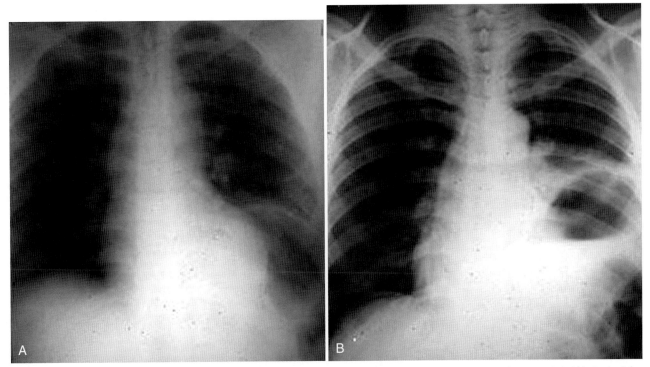

FIGURE 9 **A,** Postoperative chest radiograph, 1 day after laparotomy and repair of a grade III blunt liver injury, shows an air bubble in the left side of the chest thought to be an eventration. **B,** This air bubble increased 1 day later, resulting in reoperation, which demonstrated a missed 4-cm vertical tear of the diaphragm posterior to the left triangular ligament and adjacent to the esophageal foramen.

complicated because of associated adhesions but can usually be accomplished through a transabdominal approach. When the perforation occurs along the medial portion of the diaphragm near the esophageal foramen, the herniated viscus may also extend into the pericardium, which makes the diagnosis somewhat more difficult.

The location of diaphragmatic rupture along the more medial portion of the diaphragm increases the likelihood that the rupture will be missed at the time of laparotomy performed for repair of other injuries (Fig. 9). After completing therapy for associated intra-abdominal injuries, the surgeon should carefully examine all surfaces of the diaphragm, including the posterior portions behind the triangular ligaments.

MANAGEMENT

The severity of diaphragmatic injury plus the magnitude of the associated injuries determine the optimal approach to surgical treatment. The decisions regarding resuscitation and prioritization of specific organ injury treatment are discussed elsewhere in this text. Antibiotics should be administered. Most patients with grade I injury (contusion or hematoma) are diagnosed at the time of laparotomy or thoracotomy performed for some other reason. These injuries require no surgical treatment. The surgeon should make sure that the hematoma or contusion is not hiding a full-thickness perforation. When a small full-thickness perforation is seen, simple closure is recommended (Fig. 10). When diagnosed by laparoscopy, minor perforations may be repaired through the scope. The type of suture used for closure of diaphragmatic perforations varies according to surgical preference; the authors prefer 2-0 or 1-0 absorbable polyglycolic sutures. When the perforation is posterior, suture placement may be facilitated by hooking the diaphragm through the perforation with a long right-angle clamp, thus, exposing the perforation for suture placement. The first suture becomes the handle to expose the diaphragm for placement of subsequent sutures (Fig. 11).

Larger grade III rents of 2 to 10 cm can be closed primarily using the same techniques described previously when the tear is linear, as might be caused by a large knife or, in some patients, after blunt injury (see Fig. 11). The grade III tears seen after large high-velocity missiles or with blunt injury, however, are often irregular. Once the perforation is exposed, the initial placement of strategic sutures designed to reapproximate the irregular borders helps with the subsequent closure. Minimal débridement of irregular fragments helps preserve enough tissue for approximation. The authors prefer to use interrupted 1-0 absorbable suture for approximation along the irregular borders followed by the placement of running 1-0 absorbable sutures for the definitive closure.

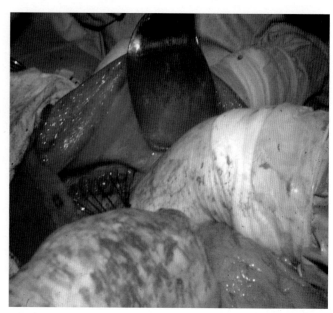

FIGURE 11   Running 0 nonabsorbable suture repair shown for grade III perforation following blunt injury.

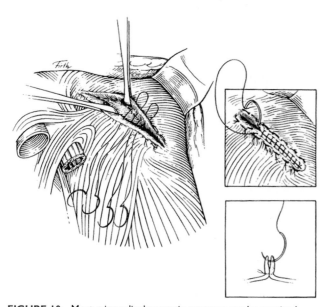

FIGURE 10   Most minor diaphragmatic ruptures can be repaired with either a running or an interrupted suture technique. The authors prefer a running 0 absorbable polyglycolic suture for most minor injuries. This is reinforced with strategically placed interrupted sutures for major injuries. *(From Asensio AA, Petrone P, Demetriades D: Diaphragmatic injuries: operative techniques in general surgery, Philadelphia, Saunders, 2000.)*

The reconstruction of grade IV lacerations greater than 10 cm and associated with modest tissue loss is more challenging. These larger injuries usually are associated with herniation of abdominal viscera into the left hemithorax. Classically, the stomach, spleen, and colon are herniated; omentum and small bowel may also be in the thorax. Once exposed, these organs need to be relocated within the abdomen. Gentle traction should be tried initially. If the viscera resist gentle traction, the surgeon should place a hand within the thorax, cup the spleen, and gently push the viscera into the peritoneal cavity. When the diaphragmatic rent is too tight around the herniated viscera, opening the rent further in a radial direction will allow the surgeon's hand to get superior to the viscera and successfully restore them into the abdomen. This precaution protects the herniated spleen which, surprisingly, is seldom injured in these patients. Most grade IV injures, however, can be closed primarily without using mesh or fascia lata and without altering diaphragmatic attachments. The diaphragm has significant redundancy in the relaxed state, so this approximation can be achieved without tension. Although there will be decreased excursion of the repaired hemidiaphragm after primary closure in this setting, there is seldom long-term impairment. When approximation of ragged borders is difficult, a modified Z-plasty is helpful. In theory, the incisions made in creating the Z-plasty should be radial, extending from the medial plane to the periphery, thus preserving the branches of the phrenic nerve; however, the long-term result of successful approximation of a viable diaphragm is almost always excellent, even when branches of the phrenic nerve are severed. When repairing large defects, one should reapproximate the midportions of the defect, so that the lateral portions can be accurately reapposed without creating a dog-ear type of closure.

The grade V diaphragmatic injury with tissue loss exceeding 25 cm presents a major surgical challenge. Many of these large defects with major tissue loss, however, can be closed primarily if the adjacent chest cage and abdominal wall are intact. When the central defect precludes a tension-free approximation, even in the relaxed state, the peripheral diaphragmatic attachments can be severed anteriorly, laterally, and posteriorly from their costal origins so that the defect can be closed and the diaphragmatic edges reattached two or three interspaces more cephalad. This permits a generous advancement of healthy tissue and allows a tension-free primary closure. The long-term results are good.

MORTALITY

The reported morbidity and mortality rates following diaphragmatic injury vary with the cause, severity of injury, and the extent of injury to other organs. Most serious complications and deaths are caused by the associated injuries. Lopez and coworkers noted a marked increase in mortality rate after diaphragmatic rupture due to higher percentage of blunt rupture now that most penetrating torso wounds are treated by NOM, thus missing minor penetrating diaphragmatic wounds. Patients sustaining blunt diaphragmatic rupture often have associated injury to the liver, spleen, or more importantly, the underlying lung. The association of multiple rib fractures and pulmonary contusion often causes respiratory compromise and prolonged ventilatory support; a fatal outcome is not unusual.

The collective review by Asensio and coworkers described an overall mortality rate of 4.3% to 41% with the average morality rate being 13.7%. The lower mortality rate is noted in patients treated for penetrating wounds; the higher mortality rate, reported by Boulanger and coworkers, reflected treated patients with associated injury to rib cage, lung, and brain. During this same interval, the authors observed a mortality rate of well under 4% in patients treated with penetrating diaphragmatic wounds. Because operation for penetrating torso wounds is reserved for patients with hypotension or peritonitis, the incidence of life-threatening injuries to other organs is much higher, and the diaphragmatic perforation represents the minor injury. Consequently, the mortality rate may exceed 30% for penetrating diaphragmatic injuries; the deaths are related to hemorrhage from associated injures.

The mechanism of injury also affects the manner of treatment and the likelihood for life-threatening associated injuries following blunt trauma. Patients presenting after high-speed MVCs, are the most likely candidates for life-threatening injuries to the lung, brain, and pelvis. The increased protection by airbags reduced diaphragmatic injury in the inner city. In contrast, patients presenting after a fall or a stamping brought about by not repaying drug-related loans are more likely to have isolated injures. This is reflected in the reduced mortality rate for patients treated for blunt rupture in the inner city. The authors found no deaths in 11 patients treated for blunt rupture in 2004 but had six patients presenting with no vital signs whose autopsies showed multiple injuries including blunt diaphragmatic rupture in 2010.

MORBIDITY

Like fatality, the observed morbidity following diaphragmatic injury results primarily from injuries to other organs. Pulmonary insufficiency due to atelectasis, pneumonia, and contusion follows multiple rib fractures. An intrapulmonary hematoma that becomes infected and develops into a lung abscess is more common after a gunshot wound. Occasionally, there will be a surgical disruption of a diaphragmatic repair after one has performed extensive mobilization in order to achieve primary closure for a grade IV or grade V injury. Breakdown of the diaphragmatic repair, however, is an unusual occurrence. Other complications that occur with diaphragmatic injury include phrenic nerve paralysis, supradiaphragmatic empyema, and subdiaphragmatic abscess. Rodriguez-Morales and coauthors reported a 65% incidence of atelectasis and a 5% incidence of empyema.

COMPLICATED DIAPHRAGMATIC REPAIR WITH THORACIC INJURY

The greatest technical challenge with the treatment of grade V diaphragmatic injuries occurs when there are associated injuries to the chest wall or abdominal wall. These massive injuries are usually caused by close-range shotgun blasts or high-velocity rifle wounds.

There are a few descriptions of the technical challenges associated with these rare injures, probably because the mortality rate is extraordinarily high. Successful care of these huge defects requires the combined reconstruction of the diaphragm and the torso wall; this reconstruction may take place in multiple phases.

These patients typically present in shock because of associated injuries to major vessels, lung, or intraperitoneal viscera, especially the liver. During the rapid resuscitation, the surgeon must remember that a complicated repair of the torso wall in conjunction with a large diaphragmatic rupture is facilitated by having separate airway control of both main bronchi. Intubation with a double-lumen tube allows for the injured lung to be deflated while the abdominal or thoracic wall reconstruction is performed in conjunction with the diaphragmatic repair. Likewise, the double-lumen airway tube prevents blood from flowing, by gravity, from the injured side, across the carina into the dependent uninjured side, thus causing a lethal postoperative respiratory insufficiency. The primary intraoperative objective is to get rapid control of hemorrhage, which may require pulmonary lobectomy for a massively injured lung (Fig. 12). This is followed by débridement of devitalized tissues of the chest wall and diaphragm (Fig. 13). Often the resultant defect after massive injury precludes successful primary closure. When the wound occurs solely in the abdomen, the abdominal wall pack technique can be used. However, when the wound involves the thorax, it is impossible to pack the thorax open, so some type of imaginative reconstruction must take place. Sometimes it is possible to relocate the diaphragm to a more superior position in the thorax (Fig. 14). This is accomplished by detaching the anterior, lateral, and posterior attachments from their peripheral origins and reattaching them superiorly to an inner space above the destroyed chest wall (Fig. 15). This allows for the thoracic cavity to be closed, and the defect, which is in the rib cage, exposes the abdominal cavity; this defect can be treated by the abdominal wall pack technique. Continued dressing changes will allow for granulation tissues to develop over the abdominal viscera, after which a split-thickness skin graft can be placed over the granulation tissues (Fig. 16). Later construction of the defect can be accomplished by rotating fascia grafts after the patient has recovered from the underlying insult.

The diaphragm is a large muscular organ with an excellent medially based blood supply, thereby facilitating easy detachment and resuturing. Being native tissue, there is less risk of infection. Even

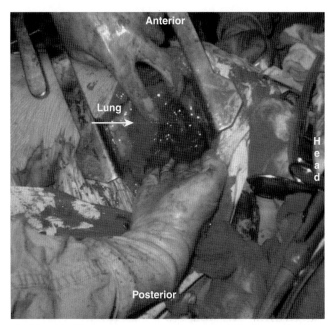

FIGURE 12 This man presented with a massive left chest wall and left lower lung injury from a close-range shotgun blast.

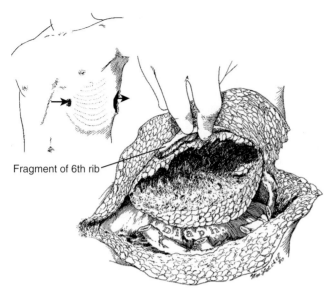

Fragment of 6th rib

FIGURE 13   After left lobectomy for hemostasis and débridement of extensive chest wall tissue, this patient was left with a full-thickness chest wall defect.

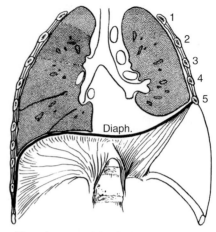

Diaph.

FIGURE 15   The relocation of the diaphragm to an inner space superior to the full-thickness chest wall defect converts the chest wall defect into an abdominal wall defect, which is then packed.

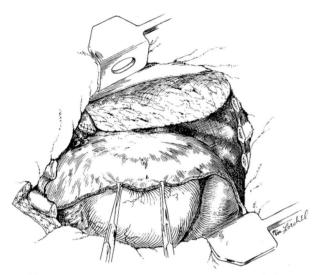

FIGURE 14   Following the extensive débridement shown in Figure 13, the diaphragm was detached anteriorly, laterally, and posteriorly in order that it could be reattached three inner spaces higher, thus, converting a chest wall defect into an abdominal defect.

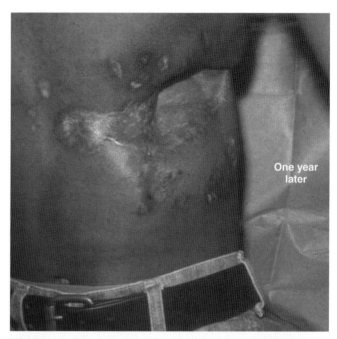

One year later

FIGURE 16   The chest wall defect, which now covers abdominal visceral, has been successfully skin grafted; later reconstruction is performed after the patient has recovered from his underlying insult, which is best judged by restoration of normal activity and weight gain.

if the diaphragm has been partially destroyed by the blast, the redundancy should allow for relocation. This technique is ideally suited for lower thoracic full-thickness chest wall defects. This technique is not suited for superiorly located chest wall defects. More superiorly located full-thickness defects from shotgun blasts can be managed by upper lobectomy combined with wound coverage by a thoracoplasty or rotation of a latissimus dorsi muscle flap. An anteriorly located wound that dismembers the ipsilateral breast and underlying chest wall can be managed by relocation of the uninjured contralateral breast or ipsilateral pectoralis major.

COMBINED CHEST WALL AND ABDOMINAL DEFECT WITH DIAPHRAGMATIC RUPTURE

The challenge is greater when the massive injury to both the chest wall and abdominal wall is associated with diaphragmatic rupture. The

technical challenges of successful treatment of such an injury are best illustrated by the care provided to a young man who presented minutes after sustaining a close-range shotgun blast of the right inferior and lateral chest wall plus the superior and lateral abdominal wall (Fig. 17). During rapid resuscitation, a double-lumen endotracheal tube was inserted to prevent blood aspiration into the left lung. The presence of a large combined injury of the abdominal wall, chest wall, and hemidiaphragm should not influence the surgeon to minimize débridement of devitalized tissue in order to achieve primary closure. The likely result will be tissue ischemia, infection, and an exposed lung; this result is fatal. When mature and proper débridement results in a huge defect of the chest and abdomen walls, unusual techniques must be used to achieve a tension-free closure. Different types of mesh may be tried but are doomed to failure if there is associated colon spill. Successful closure of this combined defect may be

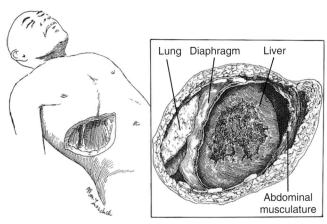

FIGURE 17 This young man sustained a close-range shotgun blast to the right upper quadrant and right lower chest wall. After débridement of nonviable liver, diaphragm, right lower lobe of lung, and chest wall, the combined defect measured 25 × 18 cm.

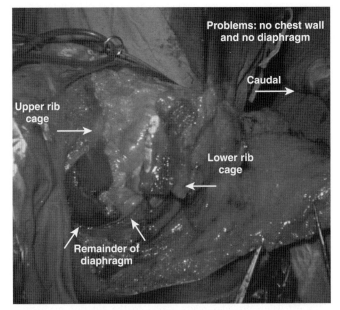

FIGURE 18 Part of the chest defect was closed by detaching the anterior confluence of ribs 7 through 10 from the sternum and rotating it superiorly and laterally to approximate a portion of the diaphragm. The posterior segment of diaphragm that remained was relocated to a higher inner space, thus, allowing for diaphragmatic closure. The remaining chest wall and abdominal defect were closed by rotating a full-thickness abdominal wall musculature flap off the linea alba medially to a superior and lateral location. The right-sided abdominal defect was covered with the skin and subcutaneous tissue.

achieved with native tissues by a number of rotation flaps of chest wall with rib fragments and abdominal wall musculature (Figs. 18 to 20). The primary concern is coverage; resultant hernias can be repaired later when the patient has recovered. The exposed tissues without skin coverage are treated with frequent dressing changes until later skin graft coverage (Fig. 21). After removal of the skin graft and primary closure, the patient described herein elected not to have his full-thickness abdominal wall defect repaired (Fig. 22).

For the chapter's Suggested Readings list, please visit the book at www.ExpertConsult.inkling.com.

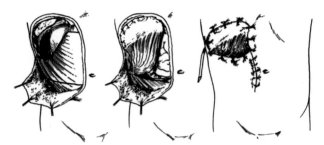

FIGURE 19 The full-thickness right-sided abdominal wall muscular flap with preserved blood supply laterally is rotated superiorly to cover the abdominal visceral and create a new costal arch.

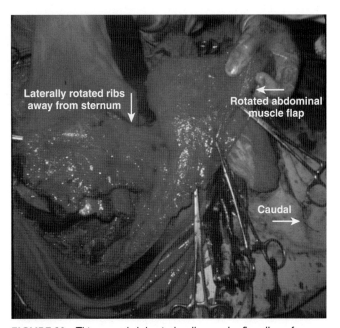

FIGURE 20 This rotated abdominal wall muscular flap allows for a tension-free closure of the exposed lower thorax and upper abdomen.

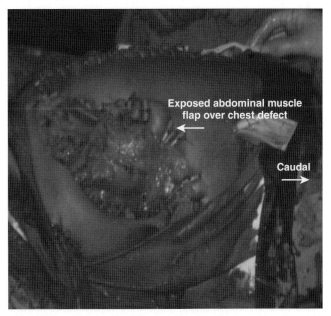

FIGURE 21 The exposed rotated muscle flap of the patient in Figure 16 was treated with frequent dressing changes and later skin grafted.

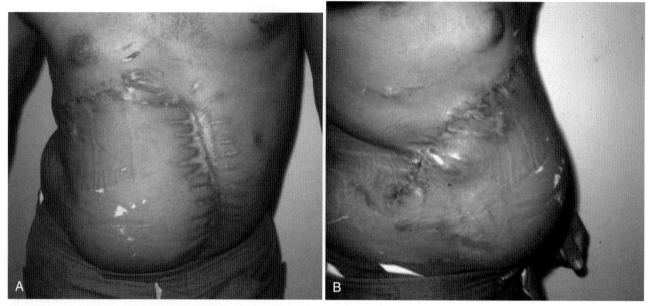

FIGURE 22 **A** and **B**, One year later, split graft was removed, and skin was closed primarily; the patient declined to have repair of his full-thickness abdominal wall defect, preferring a corset.

SURGICAL ANATOMY OF THE ABDOMEN AND RETROPERITONEUM

Joe DuBose and Thomas M. Scalea

The abdominal cavity and the retroperitoneum lie immediately adjacent to one another, separated by a peritoneal lining. Some organs, such as the small bowel and the colon, have portions that lay within both the abdominal cavity and the retroperitoneum. Vascular structures such as the superior mesenteric artery and vein course through both body compartments as well. A thorough knowledge of the anatomy of both the abdomen and retroperitoneum is critical for a rational operative approach to torso injuries.

The majority of injuries to both the abdomen and retroperitoneum are approached via the same incision, a midline laparotomy. Injuries in some areas, such as the supraceliac aorta or the pelvic vasculature, may best be approached when the midline incision is combined with a counterincision or a separate incision such as a thoracotomy, a groin exploration, or a direct retroperitoneal incision to identify and repair specific injuries. In this chapter, we will review the pertinent anatomic considerations of both the abdomen and retroperitoneum. In particular, we will stress functional anatomic considerations that are important during operative trauma surgery.

MAKING THE INCISION

The abdomen and retroperitoneum are generally explored via a generous midline incision, usually made from the xiphoid to pubis in order to facilitate effective exposure. A less extensive incision may be useful only if a specific diagnosis has been established prior to

operation. An adequate midline laparotomy incision will provide the greatest access to all of the structures in the abdomen and retroperitoneum. Additional incisional options exist that may augment exposure to specific areas.

A thoracoabdominal approach gives access to certain structures high in the abdomen. This generally involves a seventh or eighth interspace anterolateral thoracotomy that is brought down to the sternum. The ribs are divided flush with the sternum. The diaphragm is then taken down off the chest wall radially. Approximately 1 to 2 inches should be left on the chest wall for later diaphragmatic reconstruction. The diaphragm should be taken down all the way to the aorta on the left and the vena cava on the right. A left-sided thoracoabdominal approach is probably the best exposure for the supraceliac aorta. A right-sided thoracoabdominal incision increases the exposure of the posterior portion of the right lobe of the liver, as well as the retrohepatic vena cava.

A midline incision can be extended into a median sternotomy. This extension provides ready access to the anterior mediastinal structures. If an atriocaval shunt is to be used to treat a retrohepatic caval injury, a sternotomy will most expeditiously facilitate this maneuver, providing access to the right atrial appendage. In addition, if one wishes to control the inferior vena cava (IVC) within the pericardium to achieve complete vascular isolation of the liver, a sternotomy or a right-sided thoracoabdominal incision will give the surgeon good access to perform this maneuver.

Exposure of the deep pelvic vasculature can also be difficult through a standard laparotomy, and may require additional exposure maneuvers. Several options exist to improve access. A groin incision allows for vascular control of the common femoral artery and vein at the level of the inguinal ligament. A combination of a full laparotomy and groin incision can aid in repair of a vascular injury immediately adjacent to the inguinal ligaments.

The inguinal ligament can be retracted or divided to give access to the distal external iliac vessels. Another option is to perform a retroperitoneal incision similar to those used for renal transplant. This "hockey stick" incision, which comes down through the retroperitoneum, exposes the distal iliac artery and vein well but is only useful in a stable patient. Distal pelvic vascular repair can then be accomplished. Although rarely required, if a transplant incision is combined with a midline incision, the bridge of skin, subcutaneous tissue, and fascia between the two incisions can become ischemic or an infarct.

EXPLORING THE ABDOMEN

As the fascia is divided at the time of laparotomy, it is helpful to pay careful attention to the superficial peritoneum. If it is bulging, and has a bluish discoloration, that generally indicates that a tense hemoperitoneum will be released as the peritoneum is opened. Preparations should be made to collect the blood for potential autotransfusion using a cell saver circuit. The most commonly injured organs after blunt trauma are the liver and spleen. These organs can be quickly assessed for injury by palpating the right upper quadrant and left upper quadrant. The surgeon can then sweep the small bowel and colon medially, which provides for identification of any large retroperitoneal hemorrhage. Examination of the small bowel mesentery facilitates the identification of mesenteric injury.

It is imperative to fully mobilize the spleen in order to be able to fully inspect all surfaces. This allows for intelligent decision making regarding the need for splenectomy or splenorrhaphy (Fig. 1). All of the ligamentous attachments must be divided in order to deliver the spleen toward the midline of the anterior abdominal wall in order to facilitate decision making.

Similar care must be taken when mobilizing the injured liver. The falciform ligament should be taken down all the way to the level of the vena cava. Both triangular ligaments must be completely incised. These combined maneuvers should leave the liver suspended only on the hepatic veins and the portal structures, and allows the surgeon to rotate the liver up and out of the deep recesses of the right upper quadrant. This mobilization is particularly important when evaluating injuries to the posterior right lobe. At this point, one should consider the need for sternotomy or right thoracotomy with takedown of the diaphragm to facilitate exposure.

Although many blunt liver injuries in the modern era may be managed nonoperatively, bleeding from higher-grade liver injury is often persistent and of significant volume. In these instances, manual compression by direct pressure or packing will often temporize the bleeding. The Pringle maneuver is often both diagnostic and therapeutic because it can help achieve temporary hemostasis. The Pringle maneuver involves placing a vascular clamp across the hepaticoduodenal ligament, thereby occluding both portal venous and hepatic arterial inflow. Application of this vascular control maneuver allows the surgeon to reinspect and repair the liver in a field less compromised by ongoing hemorrhage. If bleeding persists despite portal

compression, the surgeon must suspect a retrohepatic IVC injury, hepatic vein injury, or anomalous hepatic arterial anatomy, which occurs in 10% to 25% of patients. The main or right hepatic artery comes off the superior mesenteric artery (SMA) in 10% to 20% of cases and the accessory right hepatic artery comes off the SMA in approximately 5% of cases. In addition, an anomalous left hepatic artery comes off the left gastric artery in nearly 5% of cases.

Although often quite effective, the Pringle maneuver can produce global ischemia of the liver, potentially worsening hepatic function in the postoperative period. Although some evidence suggests that the liver can withstand several hours of warm ischemia during elective hepatic resection when there has been time for the development of collateral circulation, the same may not be true for the patient in shock as the acutely injured liver has no collateral circulation between the lobes. The Pringle maneuver can also be cumbersome. The clamp combined with the surgeon's hand and the assistant's hand may result in limited exposure. In addition, in severe liver injuries there almost always is a component of hepatic venous injury limiting the utility of the Pringle maneuver.

In more severe cases of liver injury, one may also consider the Heaney maneuver, which involves complete vascular isolation of the liver. In this technique, vascular clamps are placed on the cava, above and below the liver. When combined with the Pringle maneuver or supraceliac aorta clamping, this should provide for hepatic vascular exclusion and produce a relatively dry field, allowing the surgeon to repair the liver and deal with hepatic venous injury; collaterals into the retrohepatic vena cava will continue to bleed, but this is usually manageable. Although this exclusion technique may prove effective, the required dissection of the suprahepatic vena cava in order to place a clamp may prove difficult, unless the diaphragm has been divided or the pericardium opened via a thoracotomy or sternotomy. The infrahepatic cava must also be occluded distal to the junction of the renal vein. If the clamp is placed too low, flow from the renal vein into the cava will perpetuate bleeding and continue to make exposure difficult.

Occlusion of the vena cava with total vascular exclusion of the liver causes a significant decrease in cardiac preload. This may not be well tolerated by a hypovolemic patient, resulting in pronounced cardiac dysfunction and even fatal arrhythmia and cardiopulmonary arrest. All venous infusion resuscitation lines should be placed in subclavian or internal jugular positions. Compensatory increase in afterload, via compression or clamping the aorta above the celiac, may improve tolerance and mitigate the risk of total cardiovascular collapse. For the same reason, complete vascular isolation can also be combined with a venous bypass circuit to allow for venous return to the heart (Fig. 2). This is not immediately available in most centers, limiting its use.

An intermediate solution to injuries with a hepatic vein component is manual compression medial to the injury. This should control all inflow to the injured segment. The injured liver can then be débrided. The hepatic vein can be identified and ligated when pressure is relaxed. The more central hepatic arterial and portal venous branches can be ligated as well using the same temporary relaxation of handheld pressure (Fig. 3).

The anterior portions of the duodenum and the head of the pancreas are located within the abdomen. The posterior portion of the duodenum and the head of the pancreas are positioned in the retroperitoneum. A full Kocher maneuver (incising the lateral peritoneal reflection and completely mobilizing the duodenum and pancreas) is necessary to evaluate both structures for injuries. The body of the pancreas lies within the lesser sac. It is necessary to widely open the lesser sac to examine the posterior stomach, as well as the anterior aspect of the body of the pancreas. This is best accomplished by dividing the gastrocolic omentum.

The gastrocolic omentum can be divided all the way up the greater curvature of the stomach to the level of the gastroesophageal (GE) junction. This requires taking the short gastric vessels adjacent to the spleen. When the gastrocolic omentum has been completely

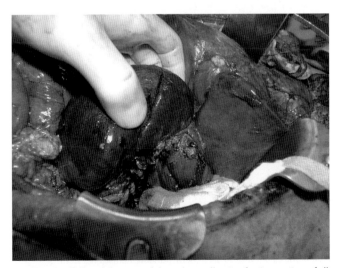

FIGURE I Full mobilization of the spleen, allowing for inspection of all surfaces.

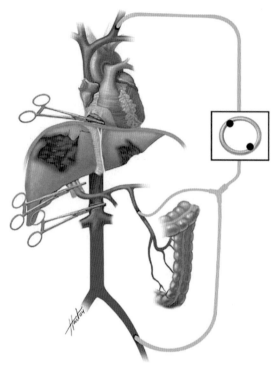

FIGURE 2   Hepatic venous exclusion and venovenous bypass. *(Courtesy of ATOM, Dr. L. Jacobs, Cine-Med, 2004.)*

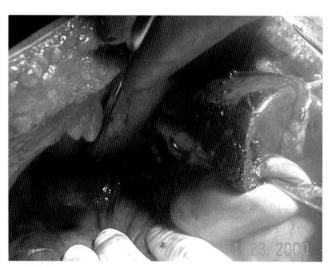

FIGURE 3   Liver after right débridement hepatectomy. Note the hemoclips on the cut surface.

divided, the surgeon is provided good access to the lesser sac, allowing inspection of the posterior wall of the stomach. It is necessary to carefully inspect the stomach, particularly around the area of the GE junction in order to avoid missing small injuries. If necessary, the intra-abdominal portion of the esophagus can be mobilized on a Penrose drain, and inferior retraction used to aid in exposure. An attempt to triangulate the stomach using sponge sticks to flatten out both the anterior and posterior aspect of the stomach adjacent to the GE junction may also prove useful. This approach allows for comprehensive inspection and minimizes the risk of missing a subtle injury high up on the stomach.

The area of the porta hepatis contains the hepatic artery, portal vein, and common bile duct. The portal structures are covered with

peritoneum. When the peritoneum is opened, the common bile duct is generally the first structure encountered. The hepatic artery can be identified by its palpable pulse and the thrill usually present within it. The hepatic artery is most commonly located medial to the common bile duct, although anatomic anomalies may be present. The portal vein lies posterior to the common bile duct. Each of these structures can be individually isolated, examined for injury, and repaired as required.

Once major vascular injuries and solid visceral injuries are controlled, the small bowel should be examined next. It is necessary to completely evaluate the small intestine to avoid missing an injury. Complete evaluation of the bowel involves running the small bowel using a hand-over-hand technique. The bowel should be flipped with each inspection to be sure both sides have been completely evaluated. Spreading the bowel out allows for inspection of the corresponding mesentery. All mesenteric hematomas adjacent to the bowel must be explored. It is a prudent practice to reexamine the small bowel prior to closing to avoid missing an injury.

EXPLORING THE RETROPERITONEUM

The retroperitoneum is generally divided into three zones (Fig. 4). Zone 1 is the central portion of the retroperitoneum containing the aorta, vena cava, and the major branch vessels, as well as the superior mesenteric vein (SMV) and splenic vein. Any retroperitoneal hematoma in zone 1 is generally explored. Zone 2 is the lateral perinephric area above the pelvis. Zone 2 houses the kidney, ureters, and renal

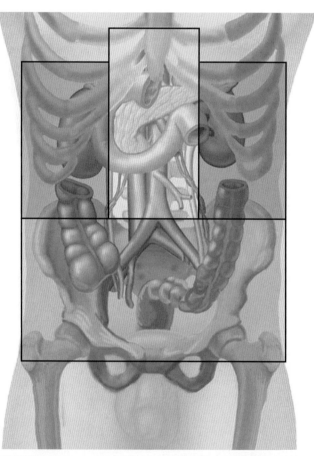

FIGURE 4   Retroperitoneal hematoma. Zone 1 *(center box)*: mandatory exploration. Zone 2 *(side portions)*: explore in all penetrating injury and blunt injury with expanding or pulsatile hematoma. Zone 3 *(bottom box)*: explore in penetrating injury only. *(Courtesy of ATOM, Dr. L. Jacobs, Cine-Med, 2004.)*

artery and vein. In general, zone 2 hematomas are explored after all penetrating injuries. In selected cases in which preoperative imaging had been performed, peripheral kidney injuries can be observed and the hematoma left intact. Zone 2 hematomas in blunt trauma can be managed expectantly unless there is a known injury requiring operation such as a ruptured ureter or if the hematomas are expanding or pulsatile. Zone 3 houses all pelvic organs, including the common and external iliac arteries and the hypogastric artery. The lower portion of the sigmoid colon is in zone 3 as well as the distal ureters.

Zone 3 hematomas are generally explored in penetrating injury only. In general, surgical exploration of a pelvic retroperitoneal hematoma after blunt trauma is discouraged. The internal iliac artery is short and branches into a large number of small vessels. Unroofing the pelvic hematoma risks loss of tamponade. Other techniques such as external compression or angiographic embolization generally are a wiser course to treat bleeding in zone 3 following blunt trauma. Extraperitoneal pelvic packing is an option currently being used for hemostasis after blunt trauma. This approach involves a counterincision into the retroperitoneal space, not exploration from the abdominal cavity.

There are several surgical maneuvers to allow access to the retroperitoneum. They involve medial visceral rotation on either the left or right side. The viscera can be rotated medially by incising the white line of Toldt. A small incision can be made in the white line and then the white line may be divided using cautery or a pair of scissors over a finger inserted into the retroperitoneum to protect the deeper structures. The incision should be brought around the hepatic or splenic flexure of the colon. We generally hold the colon up with a hand and then sweep the retroperitoneal contents downward either with a laparotomy sponge, sponge stick, or hand. This protects the mesentery of the colon and allows for rapid access to the retroperitoneum.

The original left medial visceral rotation maneuver was described by Creech and DeBakey in 1956 for the management of thoracoabdominal and suprarenal aortic aneurysms. It involves taking down the white line of Toldt of the left colon all the way to the splenic flexure and sweeping the spleen, tail of the pancreas, and stomach medially to the aorta, celiac axis, and SMA.

The so-called "Mattox maneuver" involves medial visceral rotation on the left side (Fig. 5). The left colon is mobilized as described previously. This brings the surgeon down into the retroperitoneum. At the base of the mesentery, the surgeon will then encounter the aorta. The aorta can be followed up on its lateral margin at the 3 o'clock position quickly as there are no branches until one encounters the left renal artery and vein.

The Mattox maneuver is the same as the Creech and Debakey maneuver with the exception that it involves mobilizing the kidney with the remainder of the viscera (see Fig. 5). We generally prefer to leave the kidney in situ and mobilize it later if necessary. The splenic flexure must be completely mobilized into the lesser sac. The spleen and tail of pancreas can be mobilized, which exposes the aorta up to the level of the hiatus. This is our preferred method of achieving aortic control at the level of the diaphragm. Often, the diaphragmatic crura come down lower than the surgeon expects. It is usually necessary to divide some of the diaphragmatic fibers to control the supraceliac aorta. The left-sided medial rotation also provides good access to the left renal artery and vein. If exploring a patient for a penetrating injury to the pelvis, left-sided medial visceral rotation allows aortic control above the bifurcation. This is also a reasonable exposure to control the SMA at its origin. If one must expose a longer length of the SMA, we generally combine a lesser sac exposure with the left-sided medial rotation.

We strongly believe that supraceliac aorta control must be accomplished by completely encircling the aorta. Blindly placing a clamp either from the anterior or lateral aspect of the aorta almost certainly results in the clamp slipping off. We mobilize the esophagus off the aorta anteriorly and insert a finger from the left side around to the right. It is then possible to bluntly dissect the fibers holding the aorta down to the spine. With a finger completely encircling the aorta, the

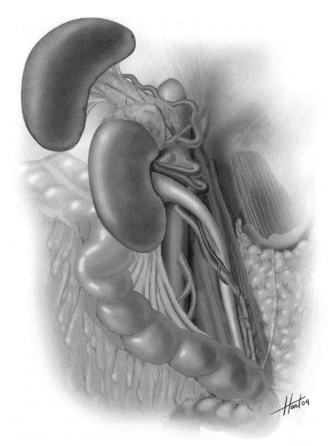

FIGURE 5   Aortic exposure: Mattox maneuver. *(Courtesy of ATOM, Dr. L. Jacobs, Cine-Med, 2004.)*

surgeon may then gently place the cross-clamp around the aorta and occlude the aorta.

Supraceliac aortic control can also be obtained via a lesser sac approach (Fig. 6). The lesser sac is opened widely by dividing the gastrohepatic ligament or lesser omentum, and the surgeon then dissects down onto the superior aspect of the pancreas. The pancreas is mobilized and the esophagus and stomach bluntly dissected. This will bring the surgeon down onto the aorta. Again the diaphragmatic crura may have to be divided in order to gain good access to the aorta. With the aorta exposed, a cross-clamp can be applied. Alternatively temporary supraceliac aortic control can be achieved with a Conn aortic compressor.

We prefer the left-sided visceral rotation for several reasons. There are a number of esophageal branches coming off the anterior aorta. The lesser sac approach risks injuring these branches as the dissection is somewhat blind. In addition, we have found it more difficult to completely encircle the aorta through the lesser sac. Using this approach, the clamp is generally applied somewhat blindly down onto the aorta and often slips off.

A right-sided medial visceral rotation, the so-called Cattell-Braasch maneuver, exposes the right-sided retroperitoneal structures (Fig. 7). The right colon is mobilized in a technique exactly similar to what was described on the left side. Similarly, the dissection should be brought around the hepatic flexure and into the lesser sac. The duodenum and head of the pancreas should be completely mobilized via a Kocher maneuver. This maneuver also involves a diagonal transection of the small bowel mesentery along with cephalad displacement of the transverse colon. This brings the surgeon down onto the IVC. The IVC can be controlled and traced up to the confluence of the left and right renal veins. There is a short suprarenal segment of the cava and then the vena cava becomes retrohepatic in location.

PROXIMAL AORTIC CONTROL

FIGURE 6   Proximal aortic control.

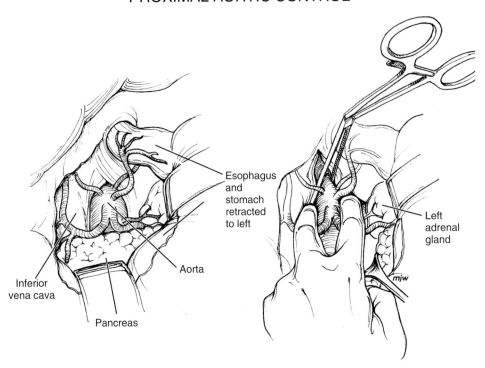

Esophagus and stomach retracted to left

Aorta

Inferior vena cava

Pancreas

Left adrenal gland

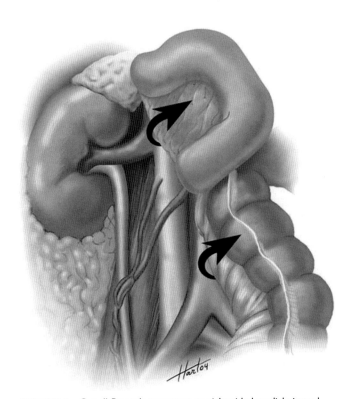

FIGURE 7   Cattell-Braasch maneuver or right-sided medial visceral rotation. Kocher maneuver. Mobilize the right colon along the equivalent of the white line of Toldt. *(Courtesy of ATOM, Dr. L. Jacobs, Cine-Med, 2004.)*

The Cattell-Braasch maneuver is ideal exposure for the vena cava and the right kidney with its vasculature. When combined with the Kocher maneuver, the duodenum and head of the pancreas can be completely explored. In addition, the right-sided pelvic vasculature can be exposed via this maneuver. The Cattell-Braasch maneuver gives better access to the pelvic vasculature than does a left-sided approach. The mesentery of the left colon can limit exposure with the Mattox maneuver. As there is no mesentery to obscure the view, the Cattell-Braasch maneuver gives wider exposure.

The mesentery of the small bowel can also be incised and lifted off the aorta and vena cava in a maneuver similar to that used by vascular surgeons during aortic surgery. When combined with the Cattell-Braasch maneuver, it gives the widest exposure of the retroperitoneal vasculature from the aorta and cava down into the pelvis.

Retroperitoneal arterial injuries are handled using the standard technique. Proximal and distal control must be obtained, and a decision made about direct repair, bypass grafting, or shunting. Injuries to the external iliac artery at the junction with the common iliac and hypogastric arteries can sometimes be managed by using the proximal hypogastric artery as a conduit. The hypogastric artery is mobilized out of the pelvis and ligated. An end-to-end anastomosis then can be performed between the hypogastric artery and the external iliac artery.

Retroperitoneal venous injuries can be among the most difficult to treat, particularly if located at the confluence of the vena cava and external iliac vein or in the juxtarenal IVC. Many techniques have been described for temporary vascular control, including the use of sponge sticks, vascular clamps, and direct finger pressure to control bleeding. We have preferred the use of intestinal Allis clamps (Figs. 8 to 10). The vascular injury is first controlled with digital pressure and an Allis clamp is applied at the apex of the injured vessel. The clamps are then sequentially stacked for the length of the injury. The clamps can then be lifted. This allows for restoration of venous return to the heart. A decision can be made about ligation or repair. Vascular repair can be accomplished by running a suture below the clamp.

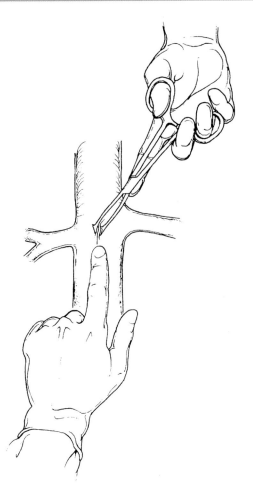

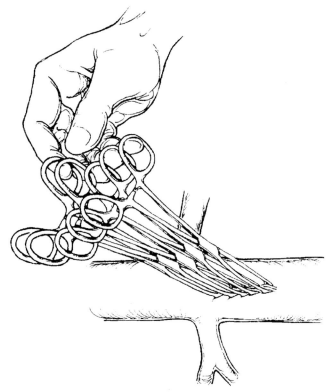

FIGURE 9 Temporary venous control is obtained with digital pressure. Intestinal Allis clamps are stacked and the vein is repaired by running a suture under them. *(From Henry SM, Duncan AO, Scalea TM: Intestinal Allis clamps as temporary vascular control for major retroperitoneal venous injury. J Trauma 51:170–172, 2001.)*

FIGURE 8 Temporary venous control is obtained with digital pressure. Intestinal Allis clamps are stacked and the vein is repaired by running a suture under them. *(From Henry SM, Duncan AO, Scalea TM: Intestinal Allis clamps as temporary vascular control for major retroperitoneal venous injury. J Trauma 51:170–172, 2001.)*

Exposure of the SMV within the lesser sac can be extraordinarily problematic. The SMV courses behind the pancreas and joins the splenic vein to become the short portal vein. SMV injuries often present with torrential blood loss. Occasionally, the pancreas can be mobilized up off the SMV and the injury isolated. There are many small branches off the SMV that must be individually ligated. If these vessels are torn, the bleeding only becomes more difficult to control.

Occasionally, identification of the location of an SMV injury is impossible, particularly if it is directly behind the pancreas or adjacent to the confluence of the splenic vein. In those cases, we generally divide the pancreas at the level of the SMV. This is done by gently inserting a finger behind the pancreas and above the SMA and SMV (in this space there are two anterior branches of these vessels) and mobilizing the pancreas off the SMV. A GIA (gastrointestinal anastomosis) stapler can be guided using a Penrose drain and the pancreas divided. This gives excellent exposure to the SMV proper and its junction with the splenic and portal veins. Virtually any injury can be identified and repaired. The distal pancreatic remnant can be resected later or inserted into a loop of jejunum, depending on the surgeon's preference.

Exposing the pelvic vasculature is a particular challenge (Fig. 11). It is essential to identify the aorta proximally and be sure of its identification. Young patients in profound hemorrhagic shock can become intensely vasospastic. The common iliac artery may be mistaken for the external iliac artery or even the aorta. With the aorta and cava clearly identified and controlled, the surgeon must sequentially expose the common, external, and hypogastric arteries. All of these should be individually controlled. The ureter runs through the retroperitoneum and into the pelvis at the confluence of the iliac arteries. This is a constant anatomic relationship. The ureter should be identified and protected during any pelvic exposure.

The pelvic veins are very large and fragile. They generally course behind the arteries. Iatrogenic injury to these can be devastating. Even if patients are in deep shock, the surgeon must be deliberate enough to avoid adding to the problem. Temporary venous control can be obtained by packing and the veins individually identified and looped. Access to the proximal hypogastric vein is limited by the hypogastric artery. Exposure can be improved by dividing the hypogastric artery. Once the vein is repaired or ligated, the artery can generally be ligated with impunity.

FUTURE CHALLENGES

Operative trauma cases are declining. NOM has become the norm for the vast majority of blunt solid visceral injuries. Even operative cases following penetrating injury are fewer in number and are concentrated in a few centers. How then will we train the surgeons of the future to understand these complex anatomic relationships and operative techniques?

The average general surgeon spends little time in the retroperitoneum, the lesser sac, or near the GE junction. Conditions that were once treated with open operations by general surgeons are now treated nonoperatively because of better pharmacologic agents or using minimally invasive and endoscopic techniques. General surgical procedures are increasingly being performed via a laparoscope. Finally, the average general surgery resident finishes his or her residency with fewer than 700 operative cases, a number far fewer than residents

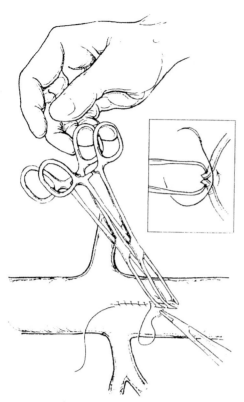

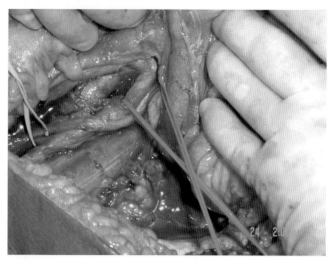

FIGURE 11 Pelvic vascular anatomy. Note the ureter coursing over the iliac bifurcation.

FIGURE 10 Temporary venous control is obtained with digital pressure. Intestinal Allis clamps are stacked and the vein is repaired by running a suture under them. *(From Henry SM, Duncan AO, Scalea TM: Intestinal Allis clamps as temporary vascular control for major retroperitoneal venous injury.* J Trauma 51:170–172, 2001.)

performed in the past. Although community surgeons may opt to transfer moderately injured patients to a higher level of care, it simply is not feasible if the patient is hemodynamically unstable.

Clearly we must devise a different training scheme so that surgeons of the future are prepared to deal with operative trauma. A number of solutions have been proposed. Simulators offer some advantages, although the technology is not yet robust enough to replace hands-on operating. Cadaver courses can be helpful, allowing the surgeon to understand anatomic relationships. Unfortunately, cadaveric tissues handle much differently than in a hemorrhaging trauma patient. The cadaver course is a static experience; it has none of the urgency of operating on a real-life trauma surgery.

We have embraced the Advanced Trauma Operative Management (ATOM) course, which was developed in Hartford, Connecticut, by Dr. Lentworth Jacob and a cadre of other well-known and respected trauma surgeons. The students must repair injuries in a 50-kg swine. These injuries encompass all organ systems in the abdomen and some in the chest. For instance, the student must successfully repair the bladder, ureter, and the pancreas as well as more common liver, spleen, and bowel injuries. The final two scenarios involve a large injury to the IVC and a right ventricular stab wound. The course is conducted in a full operating room atmosphere with real instruments, drapes, and a scrub tech. It does not take long to forget that this is an animal exercise and fall into the rhythm of repairing injury.

Another recently developed cadaver-based course, Advanced Surgical Skills for Exposure in Trauma (ASSET), provides an anatomic based review of vascular exposures within the retroperitoneum and also has the potential to improve experience with the maneuvers required to facilitate adequate exposure of vascular structures in this anatomic space. We highly recommend both of these courses for senior residents and community surgeons who take calls for the emergency department.

SUMMARY

A complete knowledge of anatomic relationships in the abdomen and retroperitoneum is absolutely essential to being able to rapidly and effectively control hemorrhage and repair injuries. It is critical that the general surgeon understand these relationships and be comfortable with them before being called to see a patient with a serious torso injury. Operative trauma case volume is diminishing. Thus, surgical residents are exposed to fewer and fewer trauma operations. Other training paradigms exist, and we strongly urge that they be incorporated into residency training and special postresidency courses to be sure that surgeons of tomorrow are adequately prepared to meet the challenge of operative trauma surgery.

For the chapter's Suggested Readings list, please visit the book at www.ExpertConsult.inkling.com.

Diagnostic Peritoneal Lavage and Laparoscopy in the Evaluation of Abdominal Trauma

Amy Rushing and David T. Efron

Current technology provides several diagnostic modalities for the trauma surgeon. The challenge lies in selecting the appropriate test that will identify injuries quickly and accurately. Almost 50 years ago, Root and colleagues introduced diagnostic peritoneal lavage (DPL) to evaluate for occult hemorrhage. This soon became one of the standard diagnostic tests for the identification of abdominal visceral injuries and remains a learning objective in the American College of Surgeons' Advanced Trauma Life Support (ATLS) course. With the development of advanced computed tomography (CT) and ultrasonography, many surgeons believe that DPL no longer has a role in the evaluation of the injured patient. In spite of the decline in its use, DPL may still have a role in certain clinical scenarios, and a review of the technique is thus worthwhile.

Diagnostic laparoscopy has also allowed trauma surgeons to evaluate patients for potential intraperitoneal and diaphragmatic injuries while avoiding complications associated with nontherapeutic laparotomies. In this chapter, we will review the evolution of laparoscopy in penetrating abdominal trauma and its impact on current practices.

DIAGNOSTIC PERITONEAL LAVAGE

First described in 1965 by Root and colleagues, DPL was developed to diagnose intra-abdominal vascular and visceral injuries in patients who were otherwise deemed difficult to assess because of altered mental status or concomitant spinal cord injury. The advantages of DPL are that it can be performed quickly, it does not require the patient to be transported to a specific procedural suite, and it is highly sensitive. The disadvantages are that it has a low specificity, the test cannot be repeated, and the lavaged fluid may obscure future CT imaging. The American College of Surgeons recommends DPL as an alternative to FAST (focused assessment with sonography in trauma) in the workup of abdominal trauma for the following clinical scenarios involving the hemodynamically labile patient with blunt injuries:

- Altered mental status secondary to brain injury, alcohol intoxication, or illicit drug use
- Diminished sensation due to spinal cord injury
- Associated injuries to the lower ribs, pelvis, and lumbar spine
- Equivocal physical examination findings
- Anticipation of suspended serial physical examinations due to general anesthesia for extra-abdominal injuries or angiography
- Lap-belt sign with suggestion of bowel injury

Table 1 delineates the relative advantages and disadvantages of DPL, FAST, and CT scan in the workup of abdominal trauma.

There are several approaches to performing a DPL—open, semi-open, and percutaneous. Root describes the open approach as the safest practice. Prior to starting the procedure, the stomach and bladder are decompressed with a nasogastric tube and Foley catheter, respectively. A 2-cm incision is then made either above or below the umbilicus to expose the linea alba. In patients sustaining pelvic fractures, the incision is always made supraumbilically. Once the fascia is

TABLE 1: Advantages and Disadvantages for DPL, FAST, and CT Scan in the Workup of Abdominal Trauma

Test	Advantages	Disadvantages
DPL	Rapidly available No need for transport Specific for hollow viscus injury	Invasive Not repeatable Misses retroperitoneal and diaphragm injuries
FAST	Rapidly available No need for transport Repeatable	Misses retroperitoneal and diaphragm injuries Very operator dependent
CT scan	Most sensitive Best anatomic information (including retroperitoneum)	Needs transport from resuscitation area Expensive Requires hardware

CT, Computed tomography; DPL, diagnostic peritoneal lavage; FAST, focused assessment with sonography in trauma.

identified, it is divided and the peritoneum is isolated and divided as well. A peritoneal dialysis catheter is inserted into the peritoneal cavity and directed inferiorly into the pelvis. Catheters of similar size are essential and there are several commercially available kits to perform this. The fascia is then closed with a purse-string suture. Next, the surgeon proceeds with aspiration of peritoneal fluid; recovery of greater than 10 mL of blood, bile, succus entericus, or vegetable matter is considered a positive test. If less than 10 mL of blood is aspirated, lavage is performed using 1 L of saline and the fluid is then siphoned by placing the empty saline bag on the floor. A minimum of 300 mL of fluid must be recovered and the fluid is subsequently sent for testing. A positive test may yield one of the following: more than 100,000 red blood cells (RBCs) per milliliter, more than 500 white blood cells (WBCs) per milliliter, or a Gram stain with bacteria present. When performed correctly, DPL has a sensitivity of 83% to 96% and specificity of 87% to 99% (Table 2).

Although DPL revolutionized the diagnosis of intra-abdominal injuries in the 1960s, the development of multidetector CT and ultrasound has made DPL a seldom used diagnostic modality. Critics of DPL claim that its lack of specificity can yield a nontherapeutic laparotomy rate of up to 36%. False-positive findings may result from pelvic fractures as well as splenic or hepatic lacerations, which are typically managed nonoperatively. Expanding retroperitoneal hematomas and diaphragmatic lacerations often fail to yield positive DPL results, yet both mandate operative intervention. Additionally, DPL carries a complication rate ranging from 0.8% to 1.7%—these numbers are derived from a report of 2500 DPLs and include the following adverse events: bowel and bladder injuries, minimal fluid recovery, abdominal wall infusion, and wound healing problems. Finally,

TABLE 2: Definition of a Positive Diagnostic Peritoneal Lavage

Immediate aspiration of 10 mL of at least one of the following:	Laboratory test confirming the presence of at least one of the following:
Blood	>100,000 RBCs/mL
Bile	>500 WBCs/mL
Succus entericus	
Undigested particulate matter	Gram stain with bacteria present

RBCs, Red blood cells; WBCs, white blood cells.

DPL has a longer list of contraindications when compared to modern diagnostic imaging including prior abdominal surgery, known coagulopathy, cirrhosis, and morbid obesity. Pelvic fractures and pregnancy may also preclude a safe DPL.

The question remains: Does DPL have a role in modern trauma care? Wang and colleagues recently studied 64 patients who had sustained blunt abdominal trauma and underwent DPL. These patients were originally allocated to undergo conservative management based on CT scan findings yet received DPL to evaluate for possible hollow viscus injuries. Of the 19 patients who had positive DPL findings, 4 patients had small bowel injuries. Overall sensitivity and specificity was 100% and 75%, respectively. No hollow viscus injuries were missed. In contrast, the sensitivity of CT imaging for the diagnosis of hollow viscus injury following blunt trauma ranges from 64% to 95% and all 4 cases of small bowel injury went undiagnosed via CT scan though it must be recognized that patient selection was altered as a result of prior CT imaging. The stipulation to Wang's study lies in the use of a cell count ratio to qualify a DPL as positive. The cell count ratio was developed by Fang and colleagues to improve the specificity of DPL and reduce the incidence of nontherapeutic laparotomy. It is defined by the following formula:

$$(\text{Lavage WBCs}/\text{Lavage RBCs}) : (\text{Peripheral WBCs}/\text{Peripheral RBCs})$$

If the cell count ratio is greater than or equal to 1, the DPL is considered positive. Although the cell count ratio allowed Fang et al to report a positive-predictive value of 89%, the original studies had certain limitations regarding specimen collection. Specifically, the timing of DPL to yield a cell count ratio greater than 1 was 3 hours. This delay in testing is not practical when triaging patients in a timely fashion to the operating room. In spite of this, the authors' novel approach to DPL illustrates that this modality may still serve as an adjunct to CT imaging when the radiographic interpretation is equivocal.

Cha and colleagues recently reported on a 10-year history of DPL practices in a Level I trauma center. They showed that although the overall accuracy of DPL for predicting therapeutic laparotomy for patients was 77%, in the group of hemodynamically unstable patients, it was 100%. Among the unstable patients who required laparotomy, only 46% had a positive FAST examination. Alternatively, Cha reported that 7% of patients with a negative DPL came to a therapeutic laparotomy, illustrating that this technique maintains a place in the assessment of trauma patients when ultrasonography may fall short. Based on the data, the authors recommend that hemodynamically unstable patients with a negative FAST examination, as well as patients who sustain anterior abdominal stab wounds with questionable peritoneal violation, should undergo immediate DPL.

There are many surgeons who have put DPL "to rest." The best example is an article written by Jansen and Logie entitled, "Diagnostic peritoneal lavage—an obituary," in which the authors depicted DPL as an antiquated test that has largely been replaced by CT imaging and ultrasonography. It is true that these studies are noninvasive and demonstrate higher specificities—up to 98% for both in some literature. Nevertheless, one test requires that the patient travel to the radiology suite but the other is directly operator-dependent. For the unstable, comatose patient who may be in a facility without 24-hour ultrasonography available, DPL may answer the diagnostic question at hand.

DIAGNOSTIC LAPAROSCOPY

There are few technological advancements that have revolutionized surgical practice like laparoscopy. In 1976, Gazzaniga and colleagues described their experience with laparoscopy in the evaluation of abdominal trauma and found that it carried a high sensitivity and specificity in the diagnosis of splenic and small bowel injuries. Since then, surgeons have further defined the role of laparoscopy in trauma to the diagnosis of diaphragmatic laceration via blunt or penetrating mechanisms. As a result, this technique has greatly reduced the number of nontherapeutic laparotomies and their associated morbidities.

Indications for diagnostic laparoscopy include hemodynamically stable patients who sustain penetrating abdominal or thoracoabdominal trauma and do not have the classic signs that mandate laparotomy such as evisceration or peritonitis. For patients who have evidence of thoracoabdominal trauma, particularly a penetrating mechanism, diagnostic laparoscopy is indicated to assess for diaphragmatic injuries. This is key as it has been shown that delayed recognition of diaphragmatic hernias with subsequent incarceration of abdominal viscera carries a mortality rate of up to 36%. Given that over 20% of penetrating injuries to the thoracoabdominal region result in diaphragmatic lacerations, there is little question that further evaluation is necessary.

The technical aspects of laparoscopy for trauma are essentially no different than those considered in general minimally invasive procedures. Access to the peritoneal cavity is obtained via insertion of a Veress needle or Hasson trocar through the periumbilical region of the anterior abdominal wall. Selection of either method depends on the surgeon's preference as well as the patient's past surgical history. Following entry into the peritoneal cavity, a pneumoperitoneum is established with instillation of carbon dioxide gas. This can only occur if the patient remains hemodynamically stable as extrinsic pressure on the inferior vena cava would only exacerbate preexisting hypotension. Next, a 30-degree laparoscope is inserted through the cannula to evaluate the peritoneal cavity. Care must be exercised during the initial inspection so as to examine the site of peritoneal entry following gunshot or stab wounds. Additional trocars may be placed as needed to retract and run the small and large bowel. In order to fully assess the diaphragm, the patient must be placed in steep reverse Trendelenburg position to allow the viscera to fall inferiorly. If an injury is identified that requires further operative intervention, the surgeon may convert to laparotomy and proceed with definitive repair.

In studies looking at patients with penetrating abdominal injuries and normal hemodynamics, up to 60% have no evidence of peritoneal violation on laparoscopy and avoid nontherapeutic laparotomy in those patients that cannot be selected for observation. This situation is typically true for patients who sustain stab wounds to the anterior abdominal wall. Although laparoscopy has been shown to have a 100% sensitivity in the diagnosis of peritoneal penetration, it has been less successful in diagnosing hollow viscus injuries. Historically, laparoscopy has as low as 18% sensitivity in recognizing bowel injury; however, this finding may be due to the surgeon's comfort with laparoscopic technique. Now that minimally invasive surgery has become a mainstay in modern surgical training, we may see that future surgeons can easily recognize hollow viscus injury and proceed with laparoscopic repair in the hemodynamically stable patient (Fig. 1).

Combining DPL and laparoscopy to develop a novel diagnostic approach, Vinces and Madlinger recently reported on a series of patients who underwent laparoscopic exploration and lavage (LELA) to exclude hollow viscus injuries. Twenty-eight patients with anterior abdominal stab wounds underwent laparoscopy to evaluate for peritoneal violation. Of the 17 patients who had evidence of peritoneal penetration, 8 patients had injuries that mandated immediate conversion to laparotomy. The remaining 9 patients underwent LELA with a positive lavage defined as RBC count higher than 5000/mL or WBC count higher than 150/mL in the absence of gross bile, blood, succus entericus, or vegetable matter. Four patients had positive lavage results and underwent laparotomy to reveal injuries to the colon or small bowel. The remaining 5 patients had negative lavage results and avoided laparotomy without missed injuries. This particular study illustrates how two diagnostic modalities with inherent weaknesses can be combined to offer a novel and perhaps more thorough test in the evaluation of penetrating abdominal trauma.

As for the evaluation of diaphragmatic injuries, it is clear that laparoscopy offers adequate visualization for the diagnosis of occult lacerations. At maximum expiration, the apex of the diaphragm comes to the level of about the fifth intercostal space, exposing it to the risk of injury from wounds in the thoracoabdominal region. This area is defined on the surface anatomically by the sternal border anteromedially, superiorly by the line that connects the inferior border of the nipple wrapping laterally and posteriorly at the level of the scapular tip to the lateral edge of the paraspinous muscles posteromedially. Inferiorly

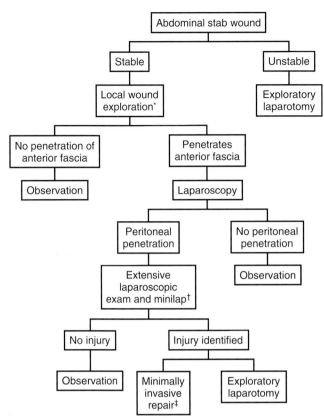

FIGURE 1 Proposed algorithm for the management of hollow viscus injuries. *Local wound exploration performed in the emergency room. †Majority of examination is performed by laparoscopy; examination of the small bowel is performed via a 4-cm minilaparotomy incision. ‡Limited injuries may be repaired laparoscopically depending on the capability of the surgeon.

the border is defined by the costal margin front, side, and back. This trapezoid defines the area through which penetrating injury carries a high risk for diaphragmatic injury.

Most trauma surgeons agree that laparoscopy for potential diaphragmatic injury should be reserved for left thoracoabdominal wounds. This procedure is performed to identify and repair a diaphragmatic rent, thereby preventing subsequent development of symptomatic herniation of abdominal contents. On the right this is prevented by the natural buttress of the liver. Ideally some time of observation should occur prior to exploration to allow for the potential evolution of signs of hollow viscus injury. If this does not develop, then the surgeon is more reassured that the diaphragmatic injury can be repaired laparoscopically, avoiding conversion to laparotomy (Fig. 2). In reality, a period of observation may not be practical given patients who are unable to be safely observed (altered mental status), busy clinical work flows with limited resources, or immediate high clinical suspicion of injury (gunshot wound or CT findings that are worrisome).

Friese and colleagues performed a prospective case series of 34 patients with thoracoabdominal penetrating injuries who were asymptomatic upon initial presentation. All patients underwent diagnostic laparoscopy followed by either laparotomy or video-assisted thoracoscopy to confirm the presence or absence of injuries. They demonstrated laparoscopy to yield a sensitivity and specificity of 87.5% and 100%, respectively. Reporting on a larger series of patients, Powell and colleagues evaluated 108 patients who sustained penetrating thoracoabdominal injuries over a 3-year period. These patients subsequently underwent diagnostic laparoscopy and 22 (20%) patients were found to have diaphragmatic lacerations. Interestingly, chest radiographs were unremarkable among 15 (68%) of the 22 with injuries. No patients demonstrated evidence of a herniated viscus on chest radiograph. These studies show that laparoscopy has a valuable role in the realm of trauma surgery, a specialty that is not often associated with minimally invasive technique.

In conclusion, DPL and diagnostic laparoscopy have their own advantages in the evaluation of abdominal trauma. DPL remains one of the most sensitive tests for intraperitoneal injury and can be performed quickly at the bedside. As for diagnostic laparoscopy, the presence of peritoneal violation with subsequent injury can be readily visualized. This allows the surgeon to exclude serious intraabdominal injuries that require operative intervention and save the patient from an unnecessary laparotomy and prolonged hospital stay. Additionally, laparoscopy is now a preferred approach for diagnosing occult diaphragmatic injuries that often go unrecognized by conventional chest imaging. These diagnostic modalities illustrate how trauma evaluation has evolved over the last 50 years and they continue to provide the trauma surgeon with options for managing the acutely injured patient.

For the chapter's Suggested Readings list, please visit the book at www.ExpertConsult.inkling.com.

FIGURE 2 Proposed algorithm for the management of left thoracoabdominal penetrating wounds.

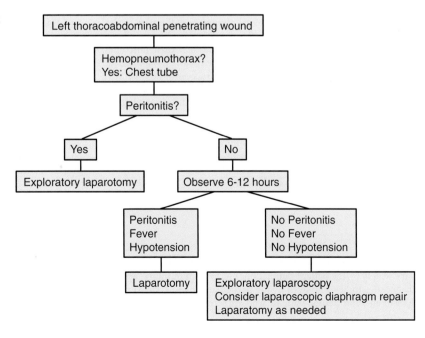

NONOPERATIVE MANAGEMENT OF BLUNT AND PENETRATING ABDOMINAL INJURIES

Matthew J. Martin and Peter Rhee

BLUNT ABDOMINAL INJURY

Key Surgical Therapy Points

1. Abdominal computed tomography (CT) with intravenous (IV) contrast agent is the most reliable and accurate means of evaluating the entire abdominal cavity.
2. However, the initial CT scan is not perfect and can miss some major injuries, particularly those of the pancreas.
3. Most abdominal solid-organ injuries can be managed successfully without celiotomy.
4. The decision for nonoperative management should be based mainly on patient physiology and available resources, not on the injury grade or radiologic appearance.
5. An initial decision for nonoperative management should be made and constantly reevaluated by an experienced trauma surgeon.
6. Interventional and minimally invasive techniques should be used as adjuncts in managing select injuries and complications.
7. Appropriate and timely conversion to operative management should be considered a lifesaving success and not a failure of nonoperative management.

Introduction

The evaluation and management of the abdominal cavity in the blunt trauma patient has undergone radical change over the past several decades, due both to significant technological advances as well as a critical reappraisal of management techniques and their outcomes. Early and rapid diagnosis of injuries coupled with the application of modern trauma care principles has made successful nonoperative management of most blunt abdominal injuries the rule rather than the exception. Although select patients may require immediate or delayed surgical intervention, nonoperative management can now safely be extended to the majority of patients with blunt abdominal injury regardless of age or associated injuries. However, the inappropriate use of nonoperative management and the failure to adhere to strict principles and protocols are associated with major adverse outcomes, including delayed therapy, increased morbidity, and preventable death.

Incidence

The incidence of intra-abdominal injury following blunt trauma will vary widely by the patient population, mechanism of injury, and the diagnostic studies employed by the particular center. Approximately 12% of all blunt trauma patients who are screened with CT have one

or more intra-abdominal injuries, with 46% being major injuries and 30% requiring surgical or angiographic intervention. The vast majority will be solid organ injuries to the spleen and liver, followed by injury to the kidney, mesentery, small bowel, colon, and pancreas. These injuries may be categorized as solid organ (liver, spleen, kidney), hollow viscus (stomach, duodenum, small bowel, colon, ureter, bladder), endocrine (pancreas, adrenal), or vascular. Overall, greater than 80% of blunt solid organ injuries may be managed without surgical intervention and with similar or lower complication rates compared with operative management.

Mechanism of Injury

Blunt trauma may produce abdominal injuries through a variety of mechanisms, including direct transmission of energy to abdominal structures causing tissue disruption or hollow viscus blowout, shearing from rapid deceleration, direct compression of abdominal organs against the vertebral column, and puncture or laceration from associated rib fracture, spine fracture, or foreign bodies. Although there is not a linear relationship between the degree of force and the amount of abdominal injury, mechanisms involving higher velocity and forces will result in more significant and extensive injuries to the abdominal organs. Direct transmission of force to the abdomen will predominantly be absorbed by the large solid organs, such as liver, spleen, and kidney, resulting in parenchymal disruption. Rapid deceleration forces tend to affect fixed or tethered structures such as the kidneys, duodenum, and bowel mesentery, resulting in lacerations or pedicle avulsion. Although seatbelt use has resulted in a decrease in traumatic brain injury and death, there is a twofold increase in the incidence of hollow viscus injuries among belted passengers. Organs and structures that are fixed to or in close proximity to the vertebral column may also be injured by direct compression and include the distal duodenum, pancreas, and great vessels. Fractures of the lower rib cage may directly lacerate upper abdominal structures including the diaphragm, liver, spleen, and kidneys.

Diagnosis

The diagnosis of intra-abdominal injury in the blunt trauma patient begins with the primary survey and focused examination of the abdomen. Hypotension should be assumed to be due to hemorrhage from an abdominal injury until proved otherwise. Physical examination of the abdomen may be limited by distracting injuries or depressed mental status, but should focus on the elicitation of peritoneal signs, localized tenderness, external bruising or evidence of a "seatbelt sign," and distention. Peritonitis should never be attributed to a solid organ injury, as isolated hemoperitoneum should not cause diffuse peritoneal irritation. Focused assessment with sonography in trauma (FAST) is now commonly performed as part of the initial evaluation. Although a "positive" FAST examination reliably identifies the presence of free fluid in the abdominal cavity suggestive of injury, a negative study does not exclude significant abdominal injury and should not be considered a definitive evaluation. Although ultrasound has been used to identify and grade specific organ injuries (i.e., liver and spleen), its reliability and reproducibility in this capacity has not been well demonstrated.

The utility of trauma ultrasound beyond the standard four-view FAST examination is becoming increasingly appreciated, particularly for blunt truncal trauma. An extended FAST examination (E-FAST) that includes thoracic imaging for pneumothorax and hemothorax can be performed with little additional time compared to standard FAST. The technical details of performing an E-FAST examination can be easily taught to staff and resident level providers, and has been shown to be more accurate than the chest radiograph. Additional helpful uses of ultrasound in the acute trauma setting include assessment of volume status and fluid responsiveness (using vena cava diameter and respiratory variation), as well as guidance of procedures such as percutaneous vascular access. Diagnostic peritoneal lavage (DPL) has largely been replaced by the FAST examination and CT scan and is infrequently indicated, although it may be useful in select cases in which there is suspicion for hollow viscus perforation with a compromised physical examination and equivocal CT scan findings. However, a diagnostic peritoneal aspirate (DPA), looking for the presence of gross blood only, can be very useful in the patient who is hypotensive with a negative FAST examination. A urinalysis should be obtained on all patients, and evaluation of the complete urinary tract (kidneys, ureters, bladder) should be performed in the presence of significant hematuria.

CT has become the standard of care for the definitive diagnosis of most blunt abdominal injuries and should be used liberally. Missed intra-abdominal injuries, typically resulting from an incomplete diagnostic evaluation, represent the most common cause of preventable deaths from trauma. Modern generation helical CT scanners provide excellent detailed imaging of the abdominal organs, including retroperitoneal structures and major vasculature. It has a sensitivity and specificity approaching 100% for solid organ injuries, and provides anatomic detail that is invaluable for injury grading. One often underappreciated exception to this is the limited ability of CT scan to identify and classify pancreatic injuries, particularly when performed immediately following the traumatic event. A recent American Association for the Surgery of Trauma (AAST) multicenter study found a sensitivity of only 60% for modern multidetector CT scan to detect pancreatic injury, highlighting the need for a high index of suspicion and adjunctive diagnostic methods. Serial measurement of amylase and lipase levels over the first 48 to 72 hours is effective for diagnosing major injuries, but these values may be normal in up to 30% of minor pancreatic injuries.

The abdominal CT scan should always be performed using IV contrast if possible, as a "contrast blush" can provide evidence of active bleeding or arteriovenous fistula. Although some older series have characterized CT as unreliable for hollow viscus perforation or major duodenal/pancreatic injury, more recent experience demonstrates that a high-quality CT scan will correctly identify most of these injuries. However, repeat CT imaging (if no other indication for laparotomy is present) or DPL should be considered in those infrequent situations with a high index of suspicion for missed injury or equivocal findings on the initial CT scan. We perform the abdominal CT scan with IV contrast only, as oral contrast has been shown to add little value in the trauma setting and may create undue delay as well as risk aspiration. Oral contrast may be useful when obtaining a delayed CT scan to evaluate for hollow viscus perforation, or to better delineate known or suspected pancreatic or duodenal injuries.

Anatomic Location of Injury and AAST-OIS Grading

The abdominal cavity can be divided into two main compartments, the peritoneal cavity and the retroperitoneum. The majority of injuries following blunt trauma are to the intraperitoneal structures such as the liver, spleen, small bowel, and mesentery, and frequently result in clinical signs and symptoms such as pain, tenderness, and distention. The main retroperitoneal structures of concern to the trauma surgeon are the kidneys, duodenum, pancreas, great vessels, and portions of the colon. Clinical signs and symptoms with retroperitoneal injuries may frequently be absent or significantly delayed, even in the presence of a severe injury. Fortunately retroperitoneal hollow viscous injuries are relatively rare.

Abdominal injuries identified by CT should be graded according to the American Association for the Surgery of Trauma Organ Injury Scale (AAST-OIS system, Table 1). This provides a commonly

TABLE 1: AAST-OIS Grading Scales for Selected Abdominal Organs

Grade Spleen*	Description
I	Laceration <1 cm Subcapsular hematoma <10% surface area
II	Laceration 1–3 cm Subcapsular hematoma 10–50% surface area Intraparenchymal hematoma <5 cm diameter
III	Laceration >3 cm or involving trabecular vessels Subcapsular hematoma >50% surface area or expanding/ruptured Intraparenchymal hematoma >5 cm or expanding/ruptured
IV	Laceration of segmental or hilar vessels with major devascularization (>25% of spleen)
V	Shattered spleen Hilar vascular injury with complete devascularization
Liver*	
I	Laceration <1 cm deep Subcapsular hematoma <10% surface area
II	Laceration 1-3 cm deep, <10 cm in length Subcapsular hematoma 10–50% surface area Intraparenchymal hematoma <10 cm diameter
III	Laceration >3 cm deep Subcapsular hematoma >50% surface area or expanding/ruptured Intraparenchymal hematoma >10 cm diameter or expanding/ruptured
IV	Parenchymal disruption involving 25–75% of hepatic lobe or 1–3 Couinaud segments within a single lobe
V	Parenchymal disruption >75% of lobe or >3 Couinaud segments Juxtahepatic venous injuries to vena cava or major hepatic veins
VI	Hepatic avulsion
Kidney*	
I	Hematuria with normal urologic studies Subcapsular hematoma
II	Laceration <1 cm deep without urinary extravasation Nonexpanding perirenal hematoma
III	Laceration >1 cm deep without collecting system rupture or urinary extravasation
IV	Laceration through renal cortex, medulla, and collecting system Main renal artery or vein injury with contained hemorrhage
V	Completely shattered kidney Renal hilar avulsion with devascularized kidney

Continued

TABLE I: AAST-OIS Grading Scales for Selected Abdominal Organs—cont'd

Grade Spleen	Description
Pancreas*	
I	Superficial laceration, no duct injury
	Minor contusion, no duct injury
II	Major laceration, no duct injury
	Major contusion, no duct injury
III	Distal transection or parenchymal injury with duct injury
IV	Proximal transection or parenchymal injury involving ampulla
V	Massive disruption of pancreatic head
Abdominal Vascular	
I	Non-named branches; phrenic, lumbar, gonadal, or ovarian artery/vein
II	Hepatic, splenic, gastric, gastroduodenal, inferior mesenteric or primary named mesenteric arteries/veins requiring ligation or repair
III	Superior mesenteric vein, infrarenal vena cava
	Renal, iliac, or hypogastric artery/vein
IV	Superior mesenteric artery, celiac axis, suprarenal vena cava, infrarenal aorta
V	Portal vein, extraparenchymal hepatic vein
	Retrohepatic or suprahepatic vena cava
	Suprarenal subdiaphragmatic aorta
Duodenum*	
I	Hematoma involving single portion
	Laceration, partial thickness
II	Hematoma involving more than one portion
	Laceration <50% of circumference
III	Laceration 50–75% circumference of D2 or 50–100% of D1, D3, or D4
IV	Laceration >75% circumference of D2
	Involvement of ampulla or distal common bile duct
V	Massive disruption of duodenopancreatic complex
	Devascularization of duodenum

Modified from Moore EE, Cogbill TH, Jurkovich GJ, et al: Organ injury scaling: spleen and liver (1994 revision). *J Trauma* 38:323–324, 1994; Moore EE, Cogbill TH, Jurkovich GJ, et al: Organ injury scaling III: chest wall, abdominal vascular, ureters, bladder, and urethra. *J Trauma* 33:337–339, 1992; Moore EE, Cogbill TH, Malangoni MA, et al: Organ injury scaling, II: pancreas, duodenum, small bowel, colon, and rectum. *J Trauma* 30:1427–1429, 1990; and Moore EE, Shackford SR, Pachter HL, et al: Organ injury scaling: spleen, liver, and kidney. *J Trauma* 29:1664–1666, 1989.

AAST-OIS, American Association for the Surgery of Trauma Organ Injury Scale.

*Advance one grade for multiple injuries, up to grade III.

understood language for discussion and study of these injuries, and may be used to guide the level and duration of monitoring for nonoperative management. The AAST-OIS for spleen, liver, and kidney has recently been validated through analysis of these injuries and associated outcomes in the National Trauma Data Bank. Although higher grade injuries are associated with higher rates of morbidity and failure of nonoperative management, the grade of injury should not be the primary factor in this decision. All grades of injury may be successfully managed nonoperatively in the appropriate clinical setting. Additional factors such as the amount of hemoperitoneum, patient age and comorbid conditions, presence of associated injuries (particularly traumatic brain injuries), and presence of a contrast "blush" should be noted and factored into subsequent management decisions.

Management

Initial management decisions in patients with a known or suspected intra-abdominal injury should be based on the clinical examination and hemodynamic status. Patients with peritonitis or hemodynamic instability that persists despite adequate fluid resuscitation should undergo prompt exploratory celiotomy. Fluid resuscitation in the early evaluation period should be administered judiciously and only if necessary. Overzealous volume resuscitation with elevation of the mean arterial pressure may exacerbate hemorrhage from the injured organ or may cause an iatrogenic drop in the hemoglobin by hemodilution, which may be difficult to differentiate from active bleeding. We prefer small volume boluses with immediate assessment of the patient's response by an experienced trauma surgeon. There is some controversial evidence that supports the positive resuscitation and immunomodulatory benefits of hypertonic crystalloid solutions over standard crystalloid or colloid formulas. Administration of small boluses of hypertonic fluid (100–250 mL of 3% to 7.5% saline) will result in decreased tissue edema with improved gas exchange and a decreased systemic and organ-specific inflammatory response, with an excellent safety profile. In patients with associated traumatic head injury, hypertonic saline has the added benefit of lowering intracranial pressure while volume resuscitating the patient. For patients with major injury requiring initiation of large volume blood products, a balanced resuscitation approximating a 1:1 ratio of packed red blood cells to plasma appears to be associated with improved survival. However, the need for initiation of large volume resuscitation or blood transfusion should almost always prompt abandoning attempts at nonoperative management and proceeding to the operating room.

The primary components of safely managing these injuries are appropriate monitoring and frequent reassessments of the patient's clinical examination and laboratory values. The level of inpatient care (intensive care unit [ICU] versus ward) and the frequency of monitoring should be dictated by the patient's clinical status, associated injuries, and the severity of the organ injury. All personnel caring for the patient should be made aware of the presence and type of abdominal injury, and a clear plan for monitoring and alerting the trauma team to any changes should be in place. The majority of injuries that fail nonoperative management will declare themselves within 48 hours of injury, and this should be the period of most intensive monitoring.

Additional important factors to be considered in guiding management are the age of the patient and the presence of comorbid conditions and associated injuries. Traditionally, nonoperative management of abdominal solid organ injuries was contraindicated in elderly patients and those with multiple associated injuries, particularly severe traumatic brain injuries. However, with improvements in imaging technology and monitoring capabilities, many centers are reporting favorable results of nonoperative management in these more difficult patient populations. Success rates for nonoperative management of over 90% have been reported among patients with multiple associated injuries, with similar complication rates to those with isolated injuries. This should only be attempted at centers with experience and expertise in managing complex, multisystem trauma and requires coordination and cooperation between the involved surgical services, such as neurosurgery and orthopedics. Although most comorbid conditions do not significantly impact the success of nonoperative management, the presence of cirrhosis should raise a red flag of caution following blunt abdominal trauma. Hemostasis of blunt liver or spleen lacerations in the presence of advanced cirrhosis may be significantly compromised by portosplenic hypertension, increased organ rigidity, hepatosplenomegaly, and systemic coagulopathy. In addition, these patients often have extremely poor physiologic reserve and have a high rate of mortality and morbidity with both nonoperative and operative management strategies. The failure of nonoperative management of splenic injury among advanced cirrhotics has been reported as high as 92%, with an associated increase in mortality rate versus immediate laparotomy.

Spleen and Liver

Patients with any identified injury of the spleen or liver should be admitted to the hospital for a minimum of 24 to 48 hours of observation. We recommend ICU or intermediate-level (step-down) admission for all high-grade injuries (grades III through V, Figs. 1 and 2). The primary purpose of observation is to identify the presence of any associated abdominal injuries and to monitor for ongoing or recurrent bleeding from the liver or spleen. The overall incidence of missed injuries in these patients appears to be low (around 2%), and should not influence the decision for nonoperative management. Serial physical examinations should focus on the patient's hemodynamic status and any evidence of worsening abdominal tenderness, distention, or the development of peritonitis. Serial laboratory evaluations should include a complete blood count at the minimum. Some measure of global tissue perfusion and acidosis, such as the lactate or base deficit, may be useful in making management and treatment decisions in these patients. The timing and appropriateness of blood transfusion in these patients remain an area of controversy. Although the need for transfusion was previously used as a guideline for operative intervention, this is no longer the case. For spleen injuries, we favor a low threshold for operative or angiographic intervention if the patient requires more than 1 to 2 units of transfused blood. We accept a higher threshold for surgical intervention on liver injuries that require transfusion, typically after 4 to 6 units of transfused blood. Ideally it would be preferred if one could avoid transfusion

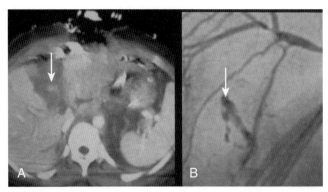

FIGURE 2 **A,** Abdominal computed tomography scan demonstrating intraparenchymal liver laceration (grade III) with an area of contrast extravasation or "blush" *(white arrow).* **B,** Hepatic angiogram of the same injury demonstrating contrast extravasation from the right hepatic arterial system *(white arrow).*

and surgery, but the exact timing of transfusion, surgery, or both for patients with solid organ injuries remains more an art than science. It requires the expert judgment of an experienced trauma surgeon to avoid the error of delaying a needed laparotomy until the patient is on the verge of hemodynamic collapse.

Bed rest and activity restriction have traditionally been recommended for these injuries, but there is no clinical data or science to support this practice. Prolonged immobility should be avoided and patients should be allowed to mobilize as early as possible. Although routine repeat imaging of all injuries with ultrasound or CT does not appear to be beneficial or cost-effective, we recommend reimaging in select patients such as those with high-grade injuries or those with above average activity levels, such as athletes, firefighters, and police officers. Age-appropriate immunizations against encapsulated organisms should be considered for all patients with grade IV or V splenic injuries as they may be functionally asplenic. Immunizations should be administered prior to patient discharge to ensure compliance.

Kidney

The kidneys are highly amenable to nonoperative management of most blunt injuries, with successful nonoperative management reported in over 90% of injuries and even in up to 50% of grade V injuries. This is particularly important for preserving renal function, as a significant number of surgical explorations for blunt renal injury will result in nephrectomy. Tamponade of hemorrhage from the renal parenchyma is enhanced by the tough, fibrous capsule of the kidneys (Gerota's fascia) and their retroperitoneal location. The principles of hospital admission, monitoring, and serial evaluations are the same as for liver and spleen injuries. In addition to serial hemoglobin assessments for bleeding, measures of renal function (blood urea nitrogen [BUN], creatinine, creatinine clearance) should be obtained at admission and intermittently throughout the hospital stay. A urinary catheter should be placed to quantify urine output and the degree of hematuria (if present) in the initial observation period. We recommend liberal use of repeat imaging, including renal function studies, in patients with grades III through V injuries to assess the extent of injury and amount of functional renal parenchyma remaining.

An additional distinction must be made between blunt renal parenchymal injuries and blunt renovascular injuries. Blunt renovascular injuries involve the renal artery, vein, or both and are typically a result of a stretch or tearing type mechanism with associated vessel thrombosis or disruption. In the absence of free bleeding that typically results in immediate laparotomy, these injuries often present in a more delayed fashion or as an incidental finding of renal infarction

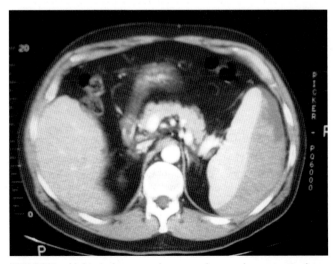

FIGURE 1 Abdominal computed tomography scan demonstrating large subcapsular splenic hematoma (grade III) with no evidence of active contrast extravasation.

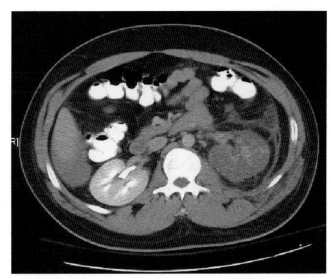

FIGURE 3 Abdominal computed tomography scan demonstrating a blunt left renal artery injury with an ischemic left kidney and normal, contrast-enhancing right kidney.

on CT scan (Fig. 3). Interventions to restore renal perfusion, via either open operative or endovascular approaches, have been associated with poor outcomes including repair failure, need for nephrectomy, infection, renovascular hypertension, and death. A multicenter study from the Western Trauma Association confirmed the poor outcomes with attempts at vascular repair and demonstrated superior results with either immediate or delayed nephrectomy. Most patients should either be observed nonoperatively or be considered for delayed nephrectomy after initial evaluation and management of more pressing injuries. Attempts at revascularization should usually be reserved only for those patients with an early diagnosis (within 2–4 hours) and with already borderline renal function, bilateral injuries, or solitary functioning kidneys.

Duodenum and Pancreas

Injury to the duodenum or pancreas is rare following blunt trauma, and appears to occur more frequently in children compared to adults. Diagnosis of these injuries is difficult due to their retroperitoneal location, often subtle clinical signs, and frequent poor visualization by CT scan. Unlike other abdominal organ injuries, the majority of identified duodenal and pancreatic injuries will require operative exploration for repair and drainage. However, select lower grade injuries may be amenable to successful nonoperative management. The majority of grade I injuries of the duodenum (hematoma or partial-thickness laceration) do not require laparotomy and will resolve spontaneously. Patients with a large intramural hematoma, particularly children, may experience obstructive symptoms and require hospitalization for nutritional management until the hematoma shrinks and obstruction resolves. Repeat imaging with oral contrast agent may be helpful in these patients to assess the degree of luminal obstruction and resolution or progression of the lesion.

The primary determinant of the need for operative intervention in pancreatic injuries will be the extent of parenchymal disruption and the presence or absence of ductal injury. Grades I and II injuries (contusions and lacerations without ductal injury) identified by CT scan may be occasionally managed by observation alone in the hemodynamically stable patient with minimal clinical symptoms. Serial physical examinations and measurement of pancreatic enzymes (amylase and lipase) should be performed to monitor the progression or resolution of pancreatic injury and inflammation. Repeat imaging with a contrast-enhanced dedicated pancreatic CT should be performed in

the face of clinical deterioration or laboratory evidence of worsening pancreatic injury. If a localized fluid collection or pancreatic abscess is identified, percutaneous drainage may be attempted in lieu of operative drainage. If ductal injury is suspected, endoscopic retrograde cholangiopancreatography (ERCP) may be performed to both diagnose the injury and perform a therapeutic intervention (stenting, sphincterotomy). However, laparotomy should be strongly considered if there is evidence of a significant ductal disruption. Similarly, there is limited experience with nonoperative management of blunt pancreatic injury.

Role of Angiographic Interventions

The increased abilities and availability of interventional radiology are now being widely applied to the management of traumatic abdominal injuries and may offer significant benefit in the nonoperative management of select injury types. The most common application of these techniques in the abdomen is to control active hemorrhage from the spleen or liver by angioembolization of either the bleeding vessel (selective) or the proximal main vessel supplying the bleeding area (nonselective). Although there was initial widespread enthusiasm for angioembolization of higher grade solid organ injuries, particularly splenic injury, this has been tempered after the accumulation of more experience. Multiple series have outlined the limitations of angioembolization for these injuries, including end organ necrosis leading to splenic abscesses and cysts and a significant rate of rebleeding. A multicenter report from the Western Trauma Association found a 20% incidence of major complications with splenic angioembolization, highlighting the need for careful consideration and patient selection for this therapy.

Patients with a contrast blush seen on the initial CT scan or evidence of ongoing hemorrhage should be considered for angiographic embolization if they are not volume dependent and remain hemodynamically stable enough to undergo the procedure. Although there are no well-defined criteria for prophylactic embolization, we recommend it in the nonoperative management of complex hepatic injuries (grades IV and V), which have a high rate of recurrent bleeding and failure of nonoperative management. Angiographic embolization is currently performed either with coil placement, which causes permanent clotting of the vessel, or with absorbable Gelfoam. Gelfoam usually provides only temporary occlusion of the vessel and as recanalization can occur in 8 to 96 hours, the patient should be monitored for recurrent hemorrhage.

Angiographic interventions such as catheter-directed clot lysis and vessel stenting may also have a very selective role in the management of selected blunt vascular injuries, particularly injury to the renal vasculature, if performed within several hours of injury. Although angiography is increasingly being integrated as a component of nonoperative management, it is an invasive procedure with a well-defined complication profile that should be factored in to any management decisions or algorithms. Further study and experience with these techniques are needed to clarify the indications and treatment-associated outcomes, as this is an evolving field.

Morbidity and Complications Management

The amount and degree of morbidity associated with nonoperative management of blunt abdominal injuries will be a function of the specific organ injured, the presence and degree of associated injuries, and patient factors such as age and comorbid disease. Avoiding a laparotomy does not equate to avoiding any morbidity, and in some cases may be associated with equal or greater morbidity than operative management. Although hemorrhage from a missed solid organ injury has classically been described as the most common cause of preventable morbidity and fatality in trauma patients, this should be an extremely rare occurrence in a modern, dedicated trauma center. Approximately 25% of patients with abdominal organ injuries managed nonoperatively will develop a significant complication requiring some form of intervention, and over 80% of these can be successfully managed without surgical intervention.

The most common sources of morbidity in this patient population will be those seen in any injured and hospitalized patient population. These include local and systemic infections, single and multiple organ failures, venous thromboembolism, prolonged hospital stay, and functional disability. Other complications specific to the injured organ may also be seen, such as delayed hemorrhage, organ necrosis or abscess formation, pseudoaneurysm or arteriovenous fistula, bile or pancreatic leak, hemobilia, urinary extravasation, and end-organ ischemia from arterial or venous thrombosis.

The key to optimizing patient outcomes following blunt abdominal injury is anticipation of the commonly associated complications, and institution of a multidisciplinary approach to diagnosis and management. Any change in the patient's clinical status or complaints suggestive of an abdominal complication (pain, fever, emesis, ileus, bleeding, jaundice) should prompt immediate investigation. CT is the study of choice for diagnosing the majority of these organ-specific complications, and can readily visualize organ necrosis or ischemia, fluid collections (abscess, biloma, urinoma, pseudocyst), biliary ductal dilation, and progression or resolution of the primary organ injury. The addition of IV contrast can delineate most vascular complications, such as pseudoaneurysm, arteriovenous (or portovenous) fistula, intimal dissection, and thrombosis. Arteriography should be performed if the diagnosis is unclear by CT, or to perform interventional therapy. Fluoroscopic contrast studies such as IV pyelography and retrograde urethrography may be indicated to evaluate the urinary tract for injury or urine leak. Suspected biliary or pancreatic trauma (leaks, fistulas) should be further studied using MRCP, ERCP or percutaneous transhepatic cholangiography (PTC).

The management of these complications will depend on the nature of the complication, the patient's clinical status, and the availability of resources and expertise. However, the majority of these complications may also be managed nonoperatively or with minimally invasive techniques. Although there is no role for prophylactic antibiotics in the nonoperative management of abdominal injuries, appropriate antibiotics should be started immediately when infection is diagnosed or strongly suspected. Percutaneous drainage of abdominal fluid collections can be performed using CT or ultrasound guidance and the fluid should be sent for Gram staining and appropriate microbiologic cultures. Additional studies such as total bilirubin, BUN, creatinine, and amylase and lipase levels may assist the diagnosis in cases of suspected biloma, urinoma, or pancreatic leak, and can be followed serially to assess for resolution. Major hepatic injuries with persistent biliary leak should undergo ERCP or PTC with biliary stent placement. Stenting across the ampulla may also decrease or resolve pancreatic ductal leaks. Similarly, persistent urinary extravasation can usually be treated successfully with percutaneous drainage and ureteral stent placement. Repeat imaging studies should be obtained to assess the efficacy of these interventions and the timing of drain or stent removal.

Parenchymal injury to any abdominal organ will result in some degree of tissue necrosis, which is usually followed by tissue regeneration, remodeling, or scar formation. A large volume of necrotic tissue or necrotic tissue that becomes secondarily infected may result in local and systemic complications. This may be particularly pronounced in patients who have decreased organ perfusion following angioembolization. Most patients can be managed successfully with IV fluids and antibiotics, and percutaneous drainage should be considered if there is a significant component of liquefied necrosis. However, select patients will require laparotomy with surgical débridement of all necrotic and infected tissue (Fig. 4). Finally, vascular complications following blunt abdominal trauma may manifest at any time following the injury, with many being identified years later. Small, asymptomatic pseudoaneurysms and arteriovenous fistulas may be managed by observation and repeat imaging

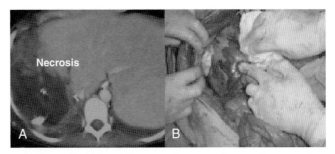

FIGURE 4   A, Abdominal computed tomography scan demonstrating necrosis of the lateral portion of the right hepatic lobe, which required operative débridement. **B,** Intraoperative findings demonstrate segmental area of necrosis in right hepatic lobe.

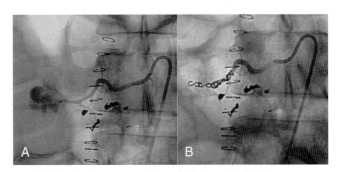

FIGURE 5   A, Arteriogram obtained 10 days after liver injury demonstrating a hepatic artery pseudoaneurysm. **B,** Repeat arteriogram after embolization demonstrating coils in position and obliteration of the pseudoaneurysm

(Fig. 5). Any significant or symptomatic lesion is best managed by angiographic embolization. Hemobilia should be suspected in any patient with evidence of upper gastrointestinal bleeding, right upper quadrant pain, and jaundice (Sandblom's triad) following a blunt hepatic injury and is also best managed by angiographic embolization.

Mortality

The mortality rates for nonoperative management of abdominal injuries will vary widely by the patient population being studied, the specific organ or organs involved, and the grade of organ injury. Death in these patients will most commonly be a result of associated injuries and comorbid conditions and not directly attributable to the abdominal organ injury. Over half of all deaths in this patient population are attributable to other associated injuries, most commonly closed head and thoracic injuries, with only about 10% of deaths related to hemorrhage from the injured organ. The overall mortality rate for nonoperative splenic injuries in modern series is approximately 6%, with the mortality rate doubling for patients older than 55 years. Failure of nonoperative management is also associated with increased mortality rates of 12% to 30%. Nonoperatively managed liver injuries are associated with higher rates of nonoperative failure, continued hemorrhage, associated injuries, and thus a higher overall mortality rate compared to splenic injuries. There is an approximate 12% mortality rate for all liver injuries managed nonoperatively, with increased death rates of up to 80% reported for high-grade liver injuries (grades IV and V). Failure of nonoperative management, continued organ-related hemorrhage, and overall mortality rate among these patients doubles when additional abdominal organ injury (spleen, kidney) is present. Similar mortality rates have been reported for renal and other blunt abdominal injuries managed nonoperatively but, again, are mainly a function of patient factors and associated injury patterns.

Conclusions

The overwhelming majority of trauma in most modern civilian settings is from blunt, high-velocity mechanisms that commonly result in abdominal organ injury. All trauma surgeons must be well versed in the epidemiology, diagnostic modalities, and modern management strategies to achieve optimal outcomes in the care of these often-complex patients. The multiplicity of factors and decision points that must be taken into account when performing nonoperative management of these injuries precludes a simple algorithmic approach, and requires the skill and constant vigilance of an experienced physician. Once hemodynamic stability has been determined, nonoperative management may be extended to the majority of patients with blunt abdominal organ injuries with a low rate of failure and adverse outcomes. The most important factor for maximizing the success and outcome among this patient population is management by an expert and dedicated trauma team.

PENETRATING ABDOMINAL INJURY

Key Surgical Therapy Points

1. All penetrating abdominal wounds require immediate and thorough evaluation to identify or rule out an intraabdominal injury.
2. Immediate laparotomy should be performed on all patients with hemodynamic instability or evidence of peritonitis.
3. Physical examination in the awake and alert patient can reliably identify those patients with a low likelihood of significant injury who should be considered candidates for selective nonoperative management.
4. CT with reconstruction of the missile tract should be performed in all patients selected for nonoperative management of an abdominal gunshot wound.
5. Diaphragm injury may be clinically silent but should be suspected in all lower chest and upper abdominal wounds.
6. Patients selected for nonoperative management of penetrating injuries should be closely monitored and serially examined for at least 24 to 48 hours.
7. Routine repeat imaging with abdominal CT should be considered for all penetrating solid organ injuries.
8. The majority of infectious and organ-specific complications can be managed nonoperatively using a multidisciplinary approach including interventional radiology and endoscopy.
9. Strict criteria should be established and a low threshold maintained for converting to surgical intervention.

Introduction

There are few situations in the field of surgery that generate as much excitement and adrenaline as a "crash laparotomy" in the trauma patient with a penetrating abdominal injury. Despite the omnipresence of these scenarios in movies and television programs, the overall incidence of penetrating trauma in both the civilian and military setting has sharply declined over recent decades. This has resulted in a paucity of experience with penetrating abdominal injuries among surgeons and residents in all but a few select, high-volume urban centers. In contrast to the revolutions seen in blunt trauma management, there has been relatively little change in the general approach to most

penetrating injuries over the past 50 years. Although penetrating abdominal trauma with suspicion or evidence of peritoneal violation has traditionally mandated an exploratory laparotomy, there is some experience with selective nonoperative management of civilian penetrating abdominal injuries. Although this approach has been well described and is becoming more widely accepted for stab wounds, the selective nonoperative approach to abdominal gunshot wounds remains an area of active study and controversy and has not been accepted by the vast majority of trauma surgeons or trauma centers.

Incidence

The overall incidence of penetrating trauma has declined sharply in modern times as a result of multiple factors. Penetrating mechanisms now account for less than 10% of all trauma presentations, even at most dedicated and high-volume trauma centers in the United States. Only a select few urban trauma centers continue to see penetrating trauma as a high (40% to 50%) proportion. The overall incidence of penetrating mechanisms among over 850,000 civilian trauma patients in the 2013 report from the National Trauma Data Bank was 4.34% for gunshot wounds and 4.51% for stab wounds, with the highest percentages documented in the 15- to 35-year-old age groups. Recent military experience in Iraq and Afghanistan has shown a shift away from single projectile gunshot wounds to the currently predominant blast mechanisms such as improvised explosive devices (IEDs), now accounting for up to 81% of injuries. Although the widespread use of body armor has resulted in a shift away from chest and abdominal injuries compared to prior conflicts, U.S. military surgeons can still expect to treat a large number of penetrating abdominal injuries.

The most important issue when discussing the validity of selective nonoperative management of penetrating abdominal wounds is the incidence and type of intra-abdominal organ injury. Abdominal stab wounds are much more amenable to selective nonoperative management compared to gunshot wounds and have a large body of supporting literature. Approximately half of all patients with anterior abdominal stab wounds and up to 30% of patients with proven peritoneal violation will not have any significant intra-abdominal injury. The incidence of intra-abdominal and retroperitoneal injury is significantly lower for flank or back stab wounds. Therefore, a policy of routine exploration for all stab wounds, or even just those with proven peritoneal violation, results in a nontherapeutic laparotomy rate of 30% to 50%.

Although there is an alleged greater than 90% to 95% incidence of organ injury requiring laparotomy following abdominal gunshot wounds, this statistic mainly applies to high-velocity injuries often seen in military combat or civilian trauma with moderate- to high-caliber handguns, which will not be specifically addressed in this chapter. According to a single study, approximately 30% to 40% of patients with anterior abdominal gunshot wounds and up to 70% with posterior wounds do not have clinically significant intra-abdominal injuries that require surgical therapy. Successful selective nonoperative management offers the benefit of avoiding the morbidity of an unnecessary laparotomy but must always be weighed against the risk of missed or delayed treatment of a significant intra-abdominal injury. According to a single study, approximately 20% to 40% of abdominal gunshot wounds and more than 50% of stab wounds can be successfully and safely managed without laparotomy. However, these findings are not universally accepted by most trauma surgeons.

Mechanism of Injury

Tissue and organ injury from penetrating wounds may occur by a variety of mechanisms, and will vary significantly by the type

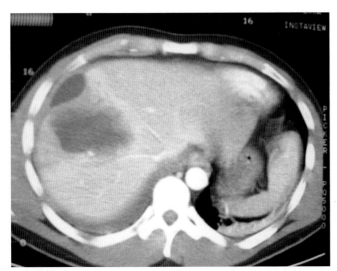

FIGURE 6 Abdominal computed tomography scan following an anterior abdominal stab wound demonstrates a grade III parenchymal injury to right lobe of liver.

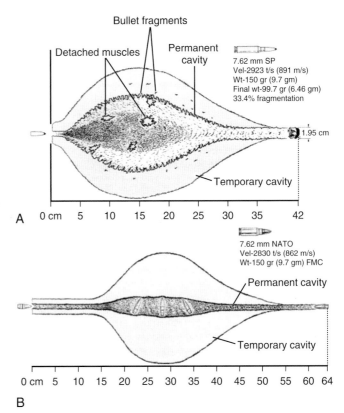

FIGURE 7 Wound profiles created by the 7.62 mm NATO cartridge loaded with a soft-point (SP) hunting bullet which expands and fragments upon impact (**A**), and 7.62 mm NATO standard rifle bullet (**B**). Note that despite having similar masses and velocities, the SP bullet in panel A produces a significantly larger primary wound cavity than the standard military round in panel B. FMC, Full metal case. (*Modified from Fackler ML: Civilian gunshot wounds and ballistics: dispelling the myths.* Emerg Med Clin North Am *16:17–28, 1998.*)

of weapon involved. Stab wounds are very low velocity and produce injury through primary tissue disruption or devascularization at the point of contact. The degree of tissue injury and clinical significance will largely depend on the exact location and depth of the wound. They produce relatively uniform injuries (punctures, lacerations) with little or no damage to surrounding tissue. Although the vast majority of stabbing injuries are direct and linear with forceful insertion and extraction of the blade, one must be aware that on occasion, there can be a pivoting and twisting motion during the injury. The point of pivot is at the skin, and this "jug" maneuver can cause seemingly minor injury at the skin but can have a larger lacerating injury within the abdomen (Fig. 6).

In contrast, missile wounds may vary widely in the mechanisms of injury and the amount of tissue involved. Projectiles typically create a tract or cavity as they travel through tissue, producing primary injury by mechanical disruption and laceration. Fragmentation of the missile after impact (or secondary to striking bone) may produce multiple smaller projectiles that increase the cavity size and area of tissue injured and explains the larger wounds produced by unjacketed bullets. Bullet deformation or spin upon impact will also significantly increase the extent of the primary wound cavity produced. In addition to the primary tissue injury, the energy imparted by the bullet to surrounding tissues creates a "shock wave" or temporary cavitation, which may result in tissue injury and devitalization over a much greater area.

Despite the long published experience with civilian and military gunshot injuries, there are many misconceptions regarding wound ballistics that have become widely propagated. Although high-velocity weapons do impart greater force to the involved tissue, the amount of tissue injury and cavitation will depend more on the properties of the projectile (jacketing, deformities, amount of spin and yaw, and the trajectory capabilities of the missile) than the velocity. As an example, a high-velocity jacketed round may pass cleanly through a tissue bed producing little injury, but a low-velocity unjacketed round, which easily deforms and fragments, may produce a significantly larger wound and greater tissue destruction. In addition, the size and clinical significance of the "temporary cavity" have been largely overstated, and appear to be much less than the oft-quoted 20 or 30 times the bullet diameter (Fig. 7). The dictum that all high-velocity wounds require extensive débridement of the temporary cavity area is not supported by animal or

clinical data, and the corollary that all low-velocity wounds require little débridement is equally unsupported.

Diagnosis

The diagnostic approach to the hemodynamically normal patient with a penetrating abdominal wound is controversial, and will vary by the injury mechanism, wound location, and the patient's clinical status. The diagnostic paradigm has rightly shifted away from determining whether the peritoneum has been violated and moved closer to determining whether there has been an injury that needs surgical therapy. The evaluation should focus on rapidly identifying those patients with injuries requiring immediate or urgent laparotomy, such as hollow viscus perforation or ongoing hemorrhage, and evaluation for significant extra-abdominal injuries.

The diagnostic evaluation of abdominal gunshot wounds has traditionally been minimal, with the diagnosis of most injuries occurring in the operating room during exploratory celiotomy. In the emergency department a thorough external survey should be performed to identify and mark the location of all wounds, and a radiologic survey (chest, abdomen, and pelvis radiograph) can rapidly identify the number and location of retained missiles or fragments. Patients who are hemodynamically stable, awake, and alert; have a reliable physical examination (no intoxication with alcohol or drugs or significant distracting injuries); and have no other indication for operation or general anesthesia are candidates for nonoperative management.

However, the vast majority of trauma patients do not fit this pattern of clinical presentation. These patients should then undergo an urgent CT scan of the abdomen, which is performed with fine cuts through the area of injury or wound tract. In addition to delineating solid organ and other injuries, the CT scan can be used to reconstruct the missile tract and determine the likelihood of injury to surrounding structures. Close monitoring by an experienced surgeon during the entire radiologic evaluation is important to identify any change in clinical status that will mandate urgent operative intervention. However, it is worthwhile to note that the reliabiltiy of CT scans for identifying injuries has not been definitively validated.

Upper abdominal stab wounds should have a chest radiograph performed, and any evidence of thoracic involvement (pneumothorax, hemothorax) should be considered diagnostic of a diaphragm injury. Flank or back stab wounds should undergo contrast-enhanced CT scan of the abdomen and pelvis unless they are clearly superficial in nature. Although some of the literature does recommend triple contrast CT (IV, oral, rectal), other studies refute the necessity of oral and rectal contrast. We have not found that triple contrast CT is required and prefer to use only IV-enhanced CT of the abdomen and pelvis. The role of CT scan for anterior abdominal stab wounds is not well defined but should be considered if there is a high suspicion for solid organ injury based on wound location, a positive FAST examination, or hematuria. However, most patients who are hemodynamically stable have an intact mental status and clear sensorium, and have no evidence of peritonitis do not require any further imaging studies. These patients may be safely observed with serial clinical assessments and surgical exploration for clinical deterioration or development of peritonitis. Local wound exploration (LWE) for anterior abdominal stab wounds has traditionally been advocated as a decisive factor in management, with observation or discharge if there is no evidence of fascial penetration and laparotomy if the exploration is positive for fascial penetration. Two multicenter Western Trauma Association trials have demonstrated that a negative LWE is reliable to exclude injury, but a positive LWE is not a reliable indicator of the need for laparotomy. Therefore, LWE may be performed to exclude injury, but patients with a positive LWE do not require mandatory laparotomy and may be triaged to surgical exploration or close observation based on their abdominal examination and clinical assessment.

Anatomic Location of Injury and AAST-OIS Grading

The anatomic location of injury will depend primarily on the wounding mechanism and the tract of injury. Stab wounds will most often be anatomically limited to one area or zone of the abdomen and usually involve only one organ or structure. Gunshot wounds may involve multiple areas of the abdomen, frequently cross into separate body cavities (thoracic, pelvis), and may also be transaxial (across the midline). Injuries or tracts that involve the upper abdomen or lower chest, defined as the area from the inferior border of the costal margin to the nipple line circumferentially, should be assumed to have penetrated the diaphragm until proved otherwise. Organ injuries should be assessed and scored according to the AAST-OIS scheme in the same manner as previously described for blunt abdominal trauma (see Table 1). Although anatomic delineation of the projectile tract by CT scan should not be the primary determinant of therapy, it may increase or lower the threshold for performing an exploratory celiotomy.

Management

The most important factors in safe and successful selective nonoperative management for penetrating abdominal injuries are proper patient selection and supervision by an experienced surgeon. Once the diagnostic evaluation has been completed as outlined earlier, the patient should be admitted to an area where close observation and monitoring can be easily accomplished for at least 24 hours. Serial laboratory evaluations and examinations should be performed as outlined in the section on blunt abdominal injuries. It is preferable that the serial physical examinations are performed by the same physician (attending or supervised resident) so that subtle changes can be more easily appreciated. Immediate laparotomy is performed at the first indicator of clinical deterioration or development of peritoneal signs. Other factors that should prompt consideration for celiotomy are persistent tachycardia, fever, rising white blood cell count, and worsening metabolic acidosis (base deficit or lactate). Although surgeons are classically taught that the physical examination is unreliable and can miss injuries, we have found that the physical examination is accurate and reliable in determining who requires surgical therapy.

Pain medication may be administered but should be administered judiciously and the patient immediately reevaluated in the presence of increasing abdominal pain. Clear liquids may be administered shortly after admission and prolonged periods of fasting in anticipation of a possible celiotomy should be avoided. There appears to be no benefit (and significant detriment) to prolonged immobility, so early ambulation is encouraged. The duration of intensive monitoring will vary by the type of abdominal injury and associated conditions, but any significant problems such as bleeding or the development of peritonitis will almost always occur within 24 to 48 hours from injury. Criteria for hospital discharge and instructions should be the same as previously described for blunt organ injuries. Outpatient follow-up and arrangements for emergency care if needed must be ensured prior to hospital discharge.

The role of angiography and other minimally invasive techniques in penetrating abdominal injuries has not been well studied. The indications and utility of interventional techniques such as angioembolization in the management of hemorrhage from solid organ injuries should be essentially the same as those previously described for blunt injuries (Figs. 8 and 9). In addition, angiography and prophylactic embolization should be considered for all high-grade liver injuries (grades IV and V) or if angiography is already being performed for other reasons. Even after the successful nonoperative management of a penetrating injury, laparoscopic

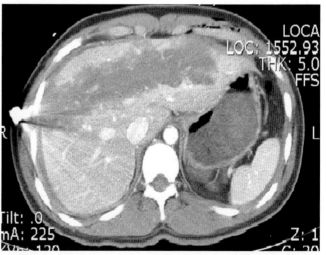

FIGURE 8 Abdominal computed tomography scan showing a transhepatic gunshot wound (grade IV) that was successfully managed nonoperatively.

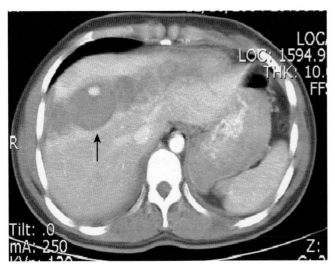

FIGURE 9 Routine repeat computed tomography scan of the injury depicted in Figure 8 at 1 week after injury demonstrates a large pseudoaneurysm with central contrast enhancement *(black arrow)* that was managed by angiographic embolization.

or thoracoscopic evaluation of the diaphragm may be required for select high-risk injury locations (as outlined previously) or in any patient with penetrating injury to the liver, spleen, or upper kidney. However, this should be considered an elective procedure and should not be done until the patient has been observed for long enough to ensure clinical stability and no other indication for celiotomy develops.

Morbidity and Complications Management

The most significant concern among this patient cohort is the incidence and outcome of failures of nonoperative management. Although there is an overall high incidence of injuries requiring laparotomy with penetrating abdominal wounds, there is an extremely low incidence of these injuries among the cohort of patients that qualify for selective nonoperative management as described previously. For both abdominal stab and gunshot wounds, approximately 4% of patients initially managed nonoperatively go on to require celiotomy, most commonly for the development of peritoneal signs. The morbidity and mortality rates associated with delayed celiotomy are low and are comparable to rates for those undergoing immediate laparotomy. However, there is a significant benefit of selective nonoperative management in reducing the incidence of nontherapeutic laparotomies from 30% to 50% down to 5% to 10%. This reduction will translate into a significant reduction in resource utilization, patient morbidity, and costs to the hospital and health care system.

The development of infectious and organ-specific complications and their management among patients managed nonoperatively are essentially the same as previously described for blunt injuries and will not be repeated here. The role of routine repeat imaging to identify important but clinically silent complications following penetrating solid-organ injuries has not been well defined and is at the discretion of the managing physician. Delayed imaging (7 to 10 days after injury) following severe solid organ injury will identify organ-related complications in up to 50% of patients, with half of these being among asymptomatic patients. Until further data are available on the natural history of these injuries, we recommend liberal use of routine repeat imaging with abdominal CT, which we perform prior to hospital discharge and at several months after injury.

The majority of identified complications such as fluid collections or vascular injuries (pseudoaneurysms, arteriovenous fistulas) can be managed nonoperatively, using interventional or minimally invasive adjuncts (Fig. 9). Although the movement toward nonoperative management may be disappointing to surgeons, in most cases it will be beneficial in improving patient outcomes.

Mortality

In the 2013 National Trauma Data Bank report, the overall case-fatality rate for gunshot wounds was 16% and for stab wounds it was significantly lower at 1.80%. Mortality rate will mainly be a reflection of the severity of injuries, patient factors (age, comorbid conditions), and the appropriate postinjury management. Several large series of abdominal stab wounds have reported no fatalities among patients initially selected for nonoperative management, even including those who failed and required celiotomy. Similarly, the reported mortality rates for nonoperative management of abdominal gunshot wounds is less than 1%, and is significantly lower than the 10% to 20% mortality rate among patients managed surgically. The most important factors for avoiding any preventable fatality from selective nonoperative management are proper patient selection and adherence to strict criteria for monitoring and conversion to operative management.

Although death resulting from a missed intra-abdominal injury has been a primary concern among skeptics of nonoperative management, the collective experience to date confirms that properly performed selective nonoperative management is safe and effective. In fact, it appears that the overall morbidity and resultant mortality rates will be significantly lowered by avoiding the high rates of nontherapeutic laparotomies associated with a policy of liberal celiotomy for penetrating injury. However, selective nonoperative management for gunshot wounds that have truly penetrated the peritoneal cavity should only be undertaken by an experienced trauma surgeon with close adherence to a strict policy of close observation with serial clinical assessments and immediate laparotomy for any deterioration or other concerning change in examination or clinical status. It should be noted that nonoperative management of gunshot wounds of the abdomen has not been accepted by the vast majority of trauma surgeons or trauma centers, and there are only several studies in the literature supporting this practice. The findings and results from these studies await further validation from other centers and with larger patient samples

Conclusions and Algorithm

Although the nonoperative management of most blunt abdominal organ injuries has become routine at all modern trauma centers, there is a very limited experience and willingness to extend this option to penetrating abdominal injuries. Selective nonoperative management can be performed safely in appropriate candidates, but should only be considered if adequate resources and experienced supervision are present. Strict adherence to the principles outlined previously is particularly critical to the safe nonoperative management of patients with abdominal gunshot wounds. We believe that as further experience is gained and published, there will be increased acceptance and utilization of selective nonoperative management. The avoidance of the costs and morbidities associated with nontherapeutic laparotomies will benefit the individual patient as well as the entire health care system.

Figure 10 outlines our current algorithm used for the triage of patients with penetrating abdominal trauma without peritonitis.

For the chapter's Suggested Readings list, please visit the book at www.ExpertConsult.inkling.com.

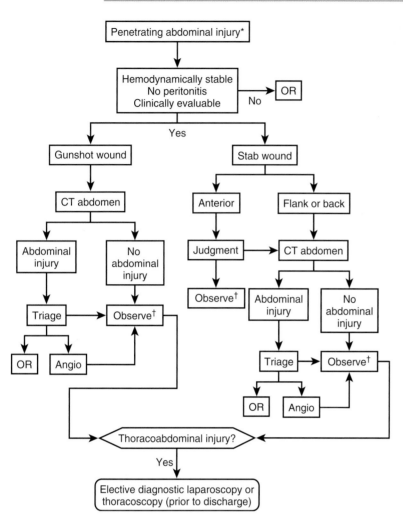

FIGURE 10 Algorithm for the initial evaluation and selective nonoperative management of patients with penetrating abdominal trauma. CT, Computed tomography; OR, operating room. *Evaluation and decision for nonoperative management made by attending trauma surgeon. †Observation in monitored setting with serial laboratory and clinical evaluations for at least 24 hours.

GASTRIC INJURIES

Lawrence N. Diebel

The stomach is a relatively thick-walled, well-vascularized organ that is variably positioned in the peritoneal cavity. Although partially protected by the lower rib cage, its size and location put the stomach at risk for injury, particularly injury from penetrating trauma to the abdomen or lower chest.

The generous blood supply to the stomach includes the left gastric artery, a branch of the celiac axis; the right gastric artery, a branch of the common hepatic artery; the right gastroepiploic artery, a branch of the gastroduodenal artery; the left gastroepiploic artery, a branch of the splenic artery; and the short gastric arteries, which also arise from the splenic artery. Because of the plentiful blood supply, gastric injuries can cause significant bleeding and require precise hemostasis in their repair. However, the excellent blood supply to the stomach contributes to the good results of the surgical repair of most gastric injuries in even the worst clinical circumstances.

The stomach has a number of important anatomic relationships, including the diaphragm, liver, spleen, pancreas, and transverse colon and mesocolon. Concomitant injuries to these adjacent structures often dictate the priority of management of the ultimate outcome for both blunt and penetrating gastric trauma.

INCIDENCE

Gastric injuries usually result from penetrating trauma and occur in approximately 20% of gunshot wounds and 10% of stab wounds. Blunt gastric trauma is much less common. The Eastern Association for the Surgery of Trauma (EAST) multi-institutional study on hollow viscus injury reported that the prevalence of blunt gastric rupture was 0.06% in patients undergoing evaluation for blunt abdominal trauma and 2.1% of all patients found to have hollow viscus injury.

MECHANISM OF INJURY

The stomach is at risk for injury after stab wounds to the left thoracoabdominal region of the body. A single perforation occurs in over 50% of these cases. However, injury to adjacent organs is common. Gunshot wounds result in two or more gastric wounds in 90% of cases. Although gunshot wounds are often associated with some surrounding tissue damage to the stomach, such damage is usually only significant with high-velocity missiles. Shotgun wounds at close range (<15 feet) often cause massive destruction of the abdominal wall, stomach, and other intra-abdominal organs.

Blunt injury to the stomach is most often the result of motor vehicle crashes, or motor vehicle–pedestrian trauma. Less common causes include falls, assaults, and improperly performed cardiopulmonary resuscitation. Blunt gastric injuries include linear lacerations and complete gastric rupture. The postulated mechanisms for blunt gastric injury include sudden increases in intraluminal pressure resulting in a balloon-bursting type of phenomenon of a full stomach, compression against the spine (seat-belt injury), or a deceleration injury with shearing forces resulting in a laceration of the anterior stomach wall.

DIAGNOSIS

Gastric perforations caused by blunt forces are often large, and intraperitoneal contamination is usually significant. Peritoneal signs are usually obvious, leading to early surgical intervention. Patients with blunt gastric rupture are frequently in shock related to other significant injuries including spleen and liver wounds.

Patients with stab wounds and hypotension, peritonitis, or both should undergo laparotomy immediately. Asymptomatic patients without central nervous system injury (brain or spinal cord injury) or drug or alcohol involvement may be observed with repeated physical examinations. In other patients, local wound exploration, diagnostic peritoneal lavage (DPL), and laparoscopy are alternatives. Laparoscopy is most helpful with thoracoabdominal stab wounds in identifying associated injuries to the diaphragm. Focused assessment with sonography in trauma (FAST) may not identify the small amount of fluid initially associated with hollow viscus injury, and thus may be misleading with isolated gastric injuries.

Early operation is indicated for symptomatic gunshot wounds to the abdomen. Occasionally, a tangential gunshot wound in a stable patient may be observed, or such a wound may be found after the patient undergoes either DPL or laparoscopy. Abdominal computed tomography (CT) is also helpful in this situation. In patients suspected to have either blunt or penetrating gastric injury, the placement of a nasogastric tube is helpful. Not only does proper placement of a nasogastric tube minimize the risk of aspiration, but a bloody aspirate when present is highly suspicious for a gastric injury. In patients with blunt gastric injury and no obvious peritoneal signs, a supine film of the abdomen discloses free air in less than 50% of cases. In this situation, abdominal CT is more sensitive in identifying free air.

SURGICAL MANAGEMENT

The abdomen is explored through a midline incision. Visualization of the stomach is facilitated by nasogastric tube decompression. Control of hemorrhage is the first priority, followed by control of enteric spill. Gastric wounds may be rapidly initially controlled by a running locking full-thickness closure with absorbable sutures. A seromuscular layer of nonabsorbable sutures is placed later in the operation. This not only affords hemostasis, but also controls further peritoneal contamination by gastric contents. Alternatively a TA (thoracoabdominal) stapler or Allis or Babcock clamp may be used for temporary control.

After attention to the more life-threatening injuries, the stomach wound may be addressed. The stomach should first be carefully inspected for ecchymosis or hematomas along either the lesser or greater curvature. Certain areas of the stomach are particularly difficult to assess: the gastroesophageal junction, high in the gastric fundus, the lesser curvature, and the posterior wall. Perixiphoid extension of the midline incision, the use of a self-retaining retractor, and positioning of the hemodynamically stable patient in the reverse Trendelenburg position may aid in exposure of these problematic areas. The gastroesophageal junction area may also be better exposed by division of the left triangular ligament and mobilization of the

TABLE 1: AAST Organ Injury Scale for Stomach

AAST Grade	Characteristics of Injury
I	Intramural hematoma <3 cm, partial thickness laceration
II	Intramural hematoma >3 cm; small (<3 cm) laceration
III	Large (>3 cm) laceration
IV	Large laceration involving vessels of greater or lesser curvature
V	Extensive (>50%) rupture; stomach devascularization

Modified from American Association for the Surgery of Trauma (AAST).

lateral segment of the left lobe. The posterior wall of the stomach is exposed by opening the gastrocolic ligament just outside the gastroepiploic arcade along the greater curvature of the stomach. Division of the short gastric vessels may be necessary to adequately expose the proximal gastric fundus. Occasionally, air insufflated into the stomach via the nasogastric tube with the stomach submerged in saline may help identify an occult injury to the stomach. Tangential wounds and single perforations of the stomach do occur, but this is a diagnosis of exclusion.

Gastric injuries thus identified are treated according to their severity (Table 1, Fig. 1). Most intramural hematomas (grades I and II) are treated by careful evacuation, hemostasis, and closure with seromuscular sutures made of nonabsorbable material. Small grade I and II perforations can be closed in one or two layers. Because of the vascularity of the stomach, I prefer a two-layer closure after hemostasis is achieved.

Large (grade III) injuries near the greater curvature can be closed by the same technique or by the use of a gastrointestinal anastomosis (GIA) stapler. Certain defects may also be closed using a TA stapler. The staple line may be protected with a seromuscular closure using nonabsorbable sutures. Care must be taken to avoid stenosis in the gastroesophageal and pyloric area. A pyloric wound may be converted to a pyloroplasty to avoid possible stenosis in this area. Extensive wounds (grade IV) may be so destructive that a proximal or distal gastrectomy is required. Reconstruction with either a Billroth I or II anastomosis is dictated by the presence or absence of an associated duodenal injury. In rare cases, a total gastrectomy and a Roux-en-Y esophagojejunostomy are necessary for severe injuries (grade V).

If a diaphragm injury occurs in association with a gastric perforation, contamination of pleural cavity with gastric contents can be problematic. Under most circumstances, it is sufficient to clear the pleural space through the diaphragmatic rent after closure of the gastric perforation. It may be necessary to enlarge the diaphragmatic injury to achieve complete evacuation of the pleural contamination. After surgical repair of the stomach, the diaphragm injury is closed, and a chest tube is placed. Occasionally, the contamination may be so severe, particularly if operation is delayed, that a separate thoracotomy to provide adequate drainage of the pleural space is necessary. Thoracoscopic evacuation of the gastric contamination of the pleural space followed by chest tube placement is another option.

MORTALITY

Mortality risk after gastric injury is related to the mechanism of injury and the presence of shock and transfusion requirements, as well as the number of associated injuries. The mortality rate associated with blunt gastric rupture has been reported to range from 0% to 66% and averages around 30%. Associated intraabdominal and extraabdominal injuries are usually present. The intraabdominal organs most

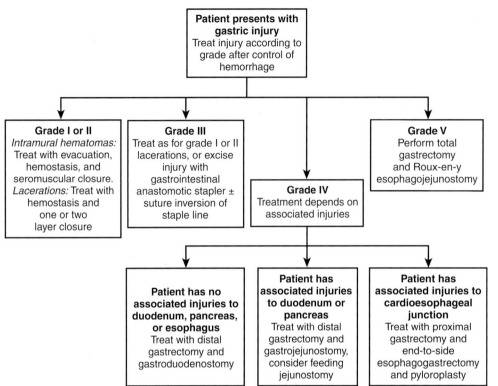

FIGURE 1 Algorithm for treatment of gastric injury.

frequently injured include the spleen, liver, small bowel, and pancreas. The most frequent extra-abdominal injuries are those involving the chest, extremity, and head. Hemorrhagic shock and complications related to the associated injuries account for the vast majority of deaths.

The overall mortality rate for penetrating gastric injuries is 14% to 20%. Early deaths are related to irreversible hemorrhagic shock from associated injuries. Mortality risk increases dramatically with the number of organs injured. The most common associated injuries include the liver, diaphragm, colon, lung, and small bowel. Injuries to the spleen, pancreas, and major blood vessels in the abdomen are also common. Fatality after either penetrating or blunt gastric injury rarely is the result of injury to the stomach. When it occurs, it is related to anastomotic dehiscence, abscess or fistula formation, and subsequent organ failure.

MORBIDITY

Major morbidity after gastric injury includes intraabdominal abscess formation, bleeding, anastomotic breakdown, and empyema formation. The severity of gastric injury and degree of contamination contribute to the development of intraabdominal abscess formation. Intraabdominal contamination is often significantly greater after blunt gastric injury.

After penetrating trauma, the incidence of intraabdominal abscess formation and surgical site infection is similarly low for both isolated gastric and colonic injury. The low incidence of intraabdominal abscess formation with either isolated stomach or colon injury increases dramatically when concomitant injuries to the liver, kidney, pancreas, or duodenum are present. There is even a greater synergistic effect on intraabdominal abscess formation with combined stomach and colon injuries. The risk of empyema increases significantly when there is a diaphragm injury in association with penetrating injuries to the stomach. Bleeding can occur from the surgical site or gastric suture line and may require reoperation. Occasionally suture line bleeding may be controlled using endoscopic techniques. In the rare instances of gastric injuries that require resection and anastomosis, anastomotic stenosis may require revision.

CONCLUSION

Most gastric injuries require débridement and closure. On rare occurrences, more complex procedures, including gastric resection and anastomosis, are required. Shock and associated injuries dictate overall outcome.

For the chapter's Suggested Readings list, please visit the book at www.ExpertConsult.inkling.com.

SMALL BOWEL INJURY

Kimball Maull

Injuries to the intestines have been described since antiquity. The statement "a slight blow will cause rupture of the intestines without injury to the skin" is attributed to Aristotle, and Hippocrates was the first to describe intestinal injury from penetrating trauma. In 1275, De Salicet was the first to report lateral suture repair of an intestinal wound. In 1686, Bonet described blunt intestinal injury in a hunter who was thrown violently against a tree by a stag. Autopsy showed rupture of the terminal ileum and cecum. In 1761, Morgagni reported several instances of blunt trauma to the small intestine caused by direct blows to the abdomen. He emphasized the slow and insidious nature of abdominal signs, an observation clinically pertinent to this day. The first long-term survivor after repair of a traumatic totally divided small intestine was reported in 1889 by Croft. In the early 20th century, the experience of Gedroitz during the Russo-Japanese War confirmed the advantage of early operative intervention for abdominal injuries. She positioned her operating theater close to the front lines and, by selecting casualties wounded within 4 hours, showed improved outcomes. In the late 20th century, awareness of the benefits of early repair, coupled with the technological advances in diagnosis, led to significant improvements in outcome. However, they also led to controversy and loss of consensus regarding both diagnostic and therapeutic approaches to patients at risk. As a result, there continue to be missteps in both diagnosis and management that require surgical vigilance.

INCIDENCE

Injuries to the small intestine must be differentiated by their means of wounding. Because the small intestine occupies the largest portion of the peritoneal cavity, injuries to the small intestine are overrepresented after penetrating trauma. Most series cite an incidence of involvement of the small bowel or its mesentery in 90% or greater after gunshot wounds and 25% to 30% after stab wounds. In blunt trauma, although the small bowel is acknowledged as the third most common organ injured, after the liver and spleen, the incidence has recently been shown to be much less than previously thought (Table 1). The 1% incidence after blunt trauma increases to 3% in patients with blunt abdominal trauma, with the incidence of free

TABLE 1: Prevalence of Blunt Small Bowel Injury

	BLUNT TRAUMA ADMISSIONS (*n* = 227,972)		BLUNT ABDOMINAL TRAUMA (*n* = 85,643)	
	Any Injury	Perforating Injury	Any Injury	Perforating Injury
All small bowel	1.1%	0.3%	2.9%	0.8%
Jejunum/ ilium	0.9%	0.3%	2.5%	0.7%

Modified from Fakhry SM, Brownstein M, Watts DD, et al: Relatively short diagnostic delays (<8 hours) produce morbidity and mortality in blunt small bowel injury: an analysis of time of operative intervention in 198 patients from a multicenter experience. *J Trauma* 48:408–415, 2000.

perforation after blunt abdominal trauma still less than 1%. These figures may be misleading. Nance et al, using data from the Pennsylvania Trauma System database, showed a strong statistical correlation between the number of solid organs injured and the likelihood of associated hollow viscus injury. The overall incidence was 9.6%, but climbed appreciably as the number of solid organs increased, reaching 34% with three or more solid organ injuries. Isolated injury to the pancreas was associated with a 33% incidence of hollow viscus injury. Only hollow viscus injuries with an Abbreviated Injury Scale (AIS) score of 3 or greater were included, but the database also included injuries to the gallbladder and urinary bladder.

MECHANISM OF INJURY

There are few anatomic areas, other than the hollow viscera, where the mechanism of injury plays as important a role in determining the ease or difficulty of diagnosis or where the treatment is so well defined or confused. The small bowel may be injured by penetrating forces, including gunshot or shotgun wounds, stabbings, and impalements. Although there are recent reports attesting to the validity of nonoperative management of gunshot wounds, most surgeons hold to the belief that operation is mandated for gunshot wounds of the abdomen or when the abdomen is in jeopardy, that is, lower thoracic entry or buttock wounds. Because the likelihood of surgically significant injury exceeds 80% for gunshot wounds of the abdomen, laparotomy is indicated. Further, even when penetration of the peritoneal cavity can be excluded, blast effect leading to perforation has been described from proximity wounds, especially if the offending firearm is of high velocity (>2000 feet/second). The injurious nature of shotgun wounds is directly related to the shot size and distance between the victim and the muzzle of the shotgun, with large shot size and close-range wounds being the most damaging. Stab wounds are considerably less lethal, but because most are managed selectively, the risk of missed injury is increased compared with those in which protocol demands operation.

The small bowel may be injured by nonpenetrating forces. High-speed modes of transport and the omnipresent use of safety restraints have enhanced the risk of blunt small bowel injury. Whereas traffic casualties died at the scene or sustained rapidly fatal central nervous system injuries in the past, road safety efforts have reduced traffic fatalities and created different patterns of injury, one of which is the seat-belt syndrome, which includes small bowel injuries. In fact, in the 2003 multiinstitutional report of Fakhry et al, a seat-belt mark was associated with an increased risk of perforated small bowel injury. In many cases, the mark represented incorrect use of the safety belt, that is, too loose, too high, or poor geometry related to body size, as in children restrained by adult belts.

The pathogenesis of small bowel rupture from blunt forces is still speculative, but has variously been ascribed to crushing, shearing, or bursting forces. A violent force directly applied to the abdomen can crush the intestines between the external force and the spine. This mechanism is commonly accompanied by injuries to other organs. Shearing injuries occur from sudden deceleration with typical injuries occurring at points of relative fixation such as the ligament of Treitz and terminal ileum or at sites of adhesive bands. Some investigators have minimized this as an injury mechanism, citing the relatively even distribution of small bowel injuries in some series. The small bowel may burst if force is applied to a distended segment where ends may be temporarily closed. This explains how the small bowel may rupture after relatively minimal force, and has actually been demonstrated in the canine model. In summary, gaping small bowel disruptions with mesenteric mutilation and extensive small bowel contusion suggests a crush injury mechanism (Fig. 1). Small bowel injuries with isolated clearly defined points of rupture probably represent burst injuries and shredding injuries, especially if near the ligament of Treitz, cecum, or other points of fixation, and are probably caused by shearing forces (Figs. 2 and 3).

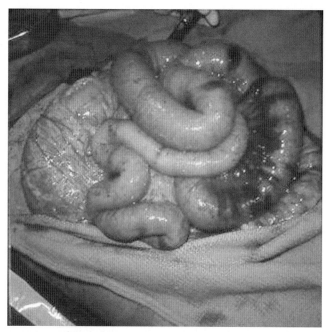

FIGURE 1   Small bowel injury from crushing force. Note extensive areas of nonviability.

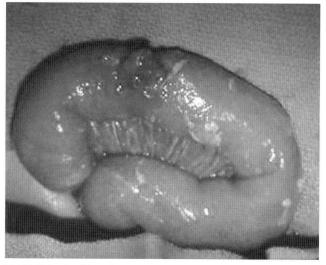

FIGURE 2   Small bowel segment showing burst injury.

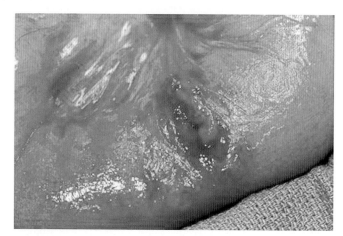

FIGURE 3   Small bowel demonstrating linear perforation, suggesting shear injury mechanism.

DIAGNOSIS

The diagnostic approach to penetrating wounds of the abdomen is slowly evolving based on newer technologies and minimally invasive surgical techniques. In 1960, Shaftan created controversy by suggesting that surgical judgment rather than mandatory laparotomy was the preferred approach to patients with penetrating trauma. His initial efforts slowly gained support in the management of stab wounds. Stab wounds follow the rule of thirds: one third do not penetrate the peritoneal cavity, one third penetrate the peritoneal cavity but do not create injury, and one third cause injury requiring operative repair. Recognizing that a mandatory policy of laparotomy resulted in negative or nontherapeutic celiotomy in two thirds of patients, selective management is now a common practice. In 2001, Chiu et al reported a prospective series of hemodynamically stable patients with penetrating trauma studied by triple-contrast computed tomography (CT). There were 75 consecutive patients and 60% sustained gunshot or shotgun wounds. Nonoperative management was successful in 96% of patients with a negative CT scan. Despite this impressive series, most surgeons employ laparotomy for the treatment of gunshot wounds and accept a 15% negative or nontherapeutic laparotomy rate. In some institutions, both operative and selective management coexist, with surgical judgment prevailing in instances when the suspicion of intraperitoneal penetration or injury is low, that is, flank wounds and wounds confined to the liver.

Indications for operation follow generally accepted algorithms (Figs. 4 and 5). When criteria are met, most surgeons proceed with operative treatment. The emergence of experienced minimally invasive surgeons is beginning to modify indications for celiotomy after

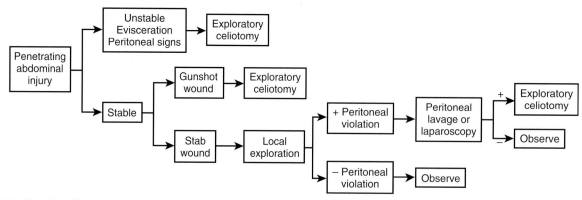

FIGURE 4   Algorithm for penetrating injuries to small bowel.

FIGURE 5 Algorithm for blunt injuries to small bowel. CT, Computed tomography.

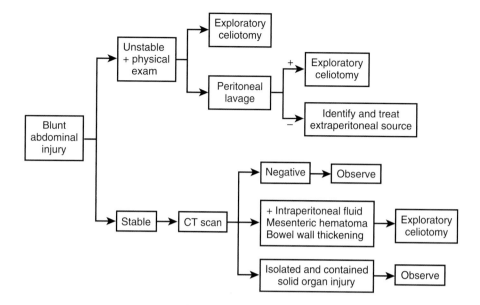

penetrating trauma, especially in wounds that potentially injure the hemidiaphragm or when abdominal penetration is in doubt. These enhanced skills have supported the evolution of laparoscopy from a primary diagnostic modality to both a diagnostic and therapeutic tool. Wounds to the diaphragm can be seen and repaired; wounds to other organ systems can be detected, characterized as to injury severity and, in many instances, repaired or controlled with hemostatics. Small bowel wounds remain problematic. Injuries obvious to the laparoscopic surgeon are probably detectable by other simple or less invasive techniques, that is, physical examination, CT, and diagnostic peritoneal lavage (DPL). Occult injuries may be initially missed regardless of the diagnostic approach, but exclusion of peritoneal penetration is useful whether by local wound exploration or direct visualization via a laparoscope.

Diagnosis of blunt small bowel injury is less obvious. Blunt small bowel injury ranges from contusion with or without serosal tear to intramural hematoma to loss of integrity of the bowel wall. The latter usually occurs immediately as a direct result of the injury, but there are many examples of delayed perforation, presumably as a result of posttraumatic ischemia leading to bowel wall necrosis. Trauma to the mesentery can have similar consequences or resolve only to cause posttraumatic stricture and delayed symptoms of intestinal obstruction. Injured patients with free perforation almost always present with abdominal pain and usually have signs of peritoneal irritation including percussion tenderness, tenderness to deep palpation, and direct and referred rebound tenderness. Operation is indicated in such situations without additional diagnostic studies. In many injured patients, the physical examination may be obscured by concurrent head injury, use of alcohol or other drugs, or associated injuries that distract the patient. In these instances, diagnostic studies, including CT, ultrasonography, DPL, or laparoscopy may play a role. The algorithm for the diagnosis of small bowel injury rests on certain caveats:

1. The alert patient is subject to reliable interpretation of physical findings.
2. There is no single diagnostic test, other than laparotomy, that can identify a small bowel injury with certainty.
3. There are injuries to the small bowel and mesentery that do not cause free perforation but still require operative management.

The reliability of CT scanning in the diagnosis of small bowel injury is subject to great debate. The technique of performing the CT, that is, whether or not oral contrast adds to the accuracy of the scan, is debated. What to do in the patient with free intraperitoneal fluid without solid organ injury is debated. The role of DPL as a complementary study to CT is debated. What is not debated, however, is the fact that patients can have a normal CT scan and still have significant small bowel injury, including perforation. CT findings suggesting small bowel injury occur in less than 50% of cases in some series (Fig. 6). Because abdominal CT has become the most widely used test to detect intra-abdominal injury, there is great potential, in the patient with a negative CT, to miss the diagnosis and delay appropriate operative therapy. In 2000, Malhotra et al cited the difference in the generations of CT scanners as impacting the ability to identify blunt small bowel injuries. Compared with early-generation scans, the newer helical scanners appeared to be more sensitive. Yet, there were 7 of 47 patients (15%) in his series who had negative scans and had small bowel or mesenteric injuries requiring operation. Malhotra's experience parallels that from the Eastern Association for the Surgery of Trauma (EAST) multi-institutional trial, which demonstrated a 13% false-negative rate for CT in the diagnosis of small bowel injury. In 2004, Allen et al reported sensitivity and specificity of 95% and 99%, respectively, for abdominal CT scans performed with intravenous (IV) contrast alone in the diagnosis of blunt small bowel and mesentery injuries. However, their sample of patients with actual injury was small. In 2001, Gonzalez et al reported the use of pre-CT DPL in a series of patients and compared

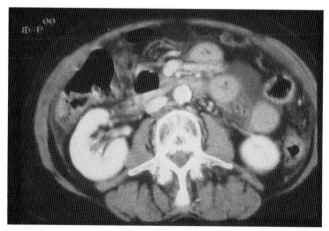

FIGURE 6 Positive computed tomography findings of wall thickening and adjacent free intraperitoneal fluid in patient with ruptured small bowel.

TABLE 2: Patient Management: No Solid Organ Injury, Free Fluid, Unreliable Examination

Management Option	Head Injury (%)	Intoxication (%)
Observe	28	51
Repeat computed tomography	12	11
Diagnostic peritoneal lavage	42	26
Operate	16	10

Modified from Brownstein MR, Bunting T, Meyer AA, Fakhry SM: Diagnosis and management of blunt small bowel injury: a survey of the membership of the American Association for the Surgery of Trauma. *J Trauma*48:402–407, 2000.

TABLE 3: Injury Grading for Small Bowel Injury

Grade*	Type of Injury	Description of Injury	AIS Score
I	Hematoma	Contusion or hematoma without devascularization	2
	Laceration	Partial thickness, no perforation	2
II	Laceration	Laceration <50% of circumference	3
III	Laceration	Laceration 50% of circumference without transaction	3
IV	Laceration	Transection of small bowel	4
V	Laceration	Transection of small bowel with segmental tissue loss	4
	Vascular	Devascularized segment	4

AIS, Abbreviated Injury Scale.
*Advance one grade for multiple injuries up to grade III.

the study group with a like group randomized to CT only. If the red blood cell count was higher than 20,000 cells/μL, a CT was performed. Those undergoing CT only and found to have free fluid without solid organ injuries were explored. Using this protocol of screening DPL, they found a low nontherapeutic laparotomy rate and improved cost-effectiveness. CT scanning has also been combined with laparoscopy in an attempt to improve diagnostic accuracy. In 2005, Mitsuhide et al reported the use of selective laparoscopy in patients suspected of small bowel injury, either by physical examination or CT scanning. The laparoscopic finding of bowel perforation or ischemia mandated conversion to open operation. They concluded that CT combined with laparoscopy could prevent nontherapeutic celiotomy and reduced delay in diagnosis. In 2000, a report of the American Association for the Surgery of Trauma (AAST) membership regarding diagnosis and management of small bowel injuries showed a lack of confidence in any of the available diagnostic approaches. There was considerable variation in how to manage the neurologically impaired patient with free fluid on CT in the absence of solid organ injury (Table 2). Options ranged from observation to operation with a plurality using DPL when in doubt. In children, the presence of abdominal tenderness and isolated free intraperitoneal fluid was highly predictive of small bowel perforation.

INJURY GRADING

The grading of small bowel injuries is uncomplicated, but the consequences of the injury are not. The reason for this is simple—bowel injuries occur and some are not initially diagnosed. Many proceed to heal without incident, some necrose and present as an intra-abdominal catastrophe, and others cause delayed symptoms, often requiring late operative treatment. The AAST Organ Injury Scale is depicted in Table 3. Note that grades II to IV correspond to free perforation and are likely to be encountered immediately or soon after presentation. Grade V injuries, transection with segmental tissue loss or devascularization, may be apparent or occult, but both cause loss of bowel integrity and require small bowel resection. Somewhere in the scheme of things, but still unclassified, rests the partial devascularization injury without full thickness necrosis that heals by stricture and causes delayed obstructive symptoms. Operation is almost always required to deal with this problem.

SURGICAL MANAGEMENT

In most instances, surgical management means operative management. Nonetheless, there is a definite role for surgical judgment to decide the need for resection, the extent of resection, and the method

of repair or resection. Small bowel injuries occur as isolated injuries but they more commonly coexist with other intra-abdominal injuries from both penetrating or blunt injury mechanisms. Surgical decision making is critical in the management of associated injuries and whether to employ damage control. In 2000, Hackam et al compared small bowel–injured patients both with and without other intra-abdominal injuries. Although the presence of other injuries led to earlier diagnosis and celiotomy, associated injuries adversely affected mortality rate, length of hospital stay (LOS), and intra-abdominal complications.

Injuries to the small bowel that require operative management include perforation, intramural hematoma, crush injury with loss of viability, laceration, and mesenteric trauma causing tears or avulsions of the mesentery, hemorrhage, expanding hematoma, and small bowel ischemia. The decision to repair, resect, or employ damage control techniques is based on the patient's clinical condition, the anatomy of the injury, whether the injuries are localized to a single wound site or intestinal segment, or if multiple wounds are dispersed over several segments of intestine. The surgeon should beware the finding of a single perforation or an odd number of intestinal wounds. Although this may be explained by a tangential wound or the finding of an intraluminal missile, perforation of the intramesenteric small bowel wall is more likely and easy to miss. All juxtaintestinal mesenteric hematomas should be opened to ensure integrity of the intestinal wall.

Repair is best performed by direct suture. If resection is indicated, stapler and hand-sewn techniques of anastomosis appear to be equally effective. However, both forms of resection have higher complication rates than repair. Therefore, injuries amenable to suture repair should be repaired rather than resected unless there are multiple proximity wounds that are technically easier to include in a limited resection than repair individually. In the damage control mode, wounds and lacerations are closed rapidly with a stapler to prevent continued soiling. No definitive anastomoses are performed.

Laparotomy for trauma must include an initial exploration to control active hemorrhage followed by a systematic inspection to identify all injuries. Injuries missed at celiotomy are the most lethal missed injuries. Therefore, every effort should be made to identify all intra-abdominal injuries, especially in a damage control situation in which continued contamination predicts poor outcome. Soiling from hollow viscus injuries should be isolated with noncrushing intestinal clamps or controlled with the assistant's thumb and forefinger. Alternately, Babcock clamps can be applied. After the intestinal tract is examined from gastroesophageal junction to rectum, injuries should be counted and mentally noted or identified with tag sutures. Areas of hematoma should be carefully inspected. Most are limited to serosal injuries and are best treated by imbricating the bordering serosal margins. True intramural hematomas require surgical judgment. If limited in extent and nonexpanding, the hematoma will likely resolve on its own and does not require specific therapy. Large or expanding intramural hematomas, or those in which the viability of the involved intestinal segment cannot be determined, require intervention. Both hematoma evacuation and resection of the involved segment have been recommended. This author favors the latter. Perforations should be carefully débrided back to viable tissue, splayed with corner stay sutures, and closed transversely in two layers (Figs. 7 to 9). Perforations that are closely opposed should be

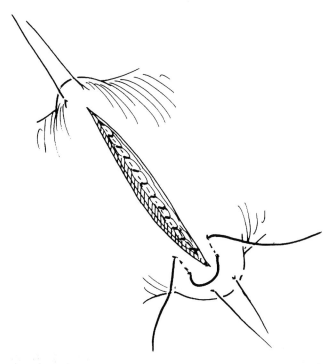

FIGURE 9 Perforations closed transversely in two layers. *(From Maull KI: Stomach, small bowel and mesentery injury. In Champion HR, Robbs JV, Trunkey DD, editors: Rob and Smith's operative surgery: trauma surgery, 4th ed, London, 1989, Butterworth-Heinemann, pp 401–413.)*

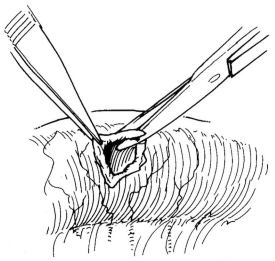

FIGURE 7 Perforations carefully débrided back to viable tissue. *(From Maull KI: Stomach, small bowel and mesentery injury. In Champion HR, Robbs JV, Trunkey DD, editors: Rob and Smith's operative surgery: trauma surgery, 4th ed, London, 1989, Butterworth-Heinemann, pp 401–413.)*

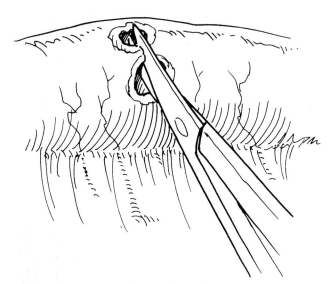

FIGURE 10 Perforations that are closely opposed should be converted to a single defect and closed in like manner. *(From Maull KI: Stomach, small bowel and mesentery injury. In Champion HR, Robbs JV, Trunkey DD, editors: Rob and Smith's operative surgery: trauma surgery, 4th ed, London, 1989, Butterworth-Heinemann, pp 401–413.)*

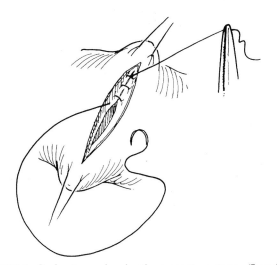

FIGURE 8 Perforations splayed with corner stay sutures. *(From Maull KI: Stomach, small bowel and mesentery injury. In Champion HR, Robbs JV, Trunkey DD, editors: Rob and Smith's operative surgery: trauma surgery, 4th ed, London, 1989, Butterworth-Heinemann, pp 401–413.)*

converted to a single defect and closed in like manner (Fig. 10). Multiple perforations within a short segment are best treated by resection and anastomosis (Fig. 11). The mesenteric defect should be closed in continuity (Fig. 12).

Injuries to the mesentery vary from small hematomas to extensive life-threatening avulsion injuries. Large or expanding mesenteric hematomas and those adjoining the intestinal wall should be explored

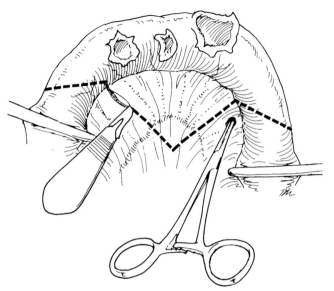

FIGURE 11 Multiple perforations within a short segment are best treated by resection and anastomosis. *(From Maull KI: Stomach, small bowel and mesentery injury. In Champion HR, Robbs JV, Trunkey DD, editors: Rob and Smith's operative surgery: trauma surgery, 4th ed, London, 1989, Butterworth-Heinemann, pp 401–413.)*

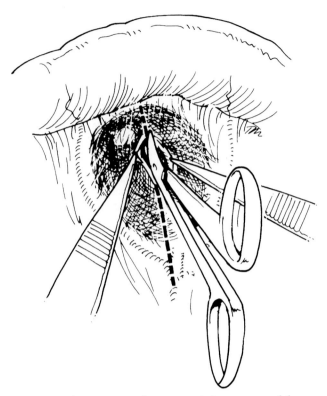

FIGURE 13 Large or expanding mesenteric hematomas and those adjoining the intestinal wall should be explored and direct vascular control established by suture ligature. *(From Maull KI: Stomach, small bowel and mesentery injury. In Champion HR, Robbs JV, Trunkey DD, editors: Rob and Smith's operative surgery: trauma surgery, 4th ed, London, 1989, Butterworth-Heinemann, pp 401–413.)*

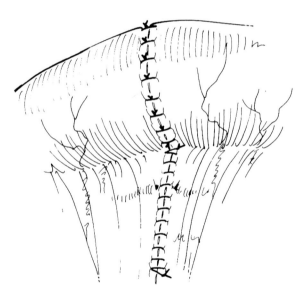

FIGURE 12 The mesenteric defect should be closed in continuity. *(From Maull KI: Stomach, small bowel and mesentery injury. In Champion HR, Robbs JV, Trunkey DD, editors: Rob and Smith's operative surgery: trauma surgery, 4th ed, London, 1989, Butterworth-Heinemann, pp 401–413.)*

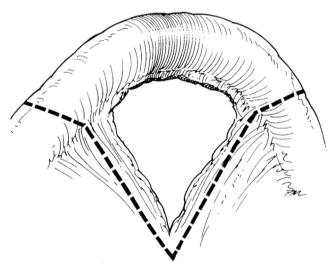

FIGURE 14 Mesenteric tears may cause ischemia of the involved intestinal segment, and resection may be necessary. *(From Maull KI: Stomach, small bowel and mesentery injury. In Champion HR, Robbs JV, Trunkey DD, editors: Rob and Smith's operative surgery: trauma surgery, 4th ed, London, 1989, Butterworth-Heinemann, pp 401–413.)*

and direct vascular control established by suture ligature (Fig. 13). The integrity of the intestinal wall should be confirmed or repaired, as needed. Mesenteric tears may cause ischemia of the involved intestinal segment and resection may be necessary (Fig. 14). All tears must be closed with sutures (Fig. 15).

It should come as no surprise that minimally invasive techniques have been reported with increasing frequency in the diagnosis and treatment of small bowel injuries, both blunt and penetrating. The successful use of minimally invasive methods rests heavily on the expertise of the surgeon and the stability of the patient. Because of the potential for missed injury, minimally invasive approaches to small bowel trauma must be used very selectively and only by those who possess special expertise with laparoscopy pending further evidence of their safety.

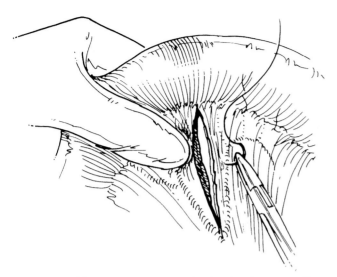

FIGURE 15 All mesenteric tears must be closed with sutures. *(From Maull KI: Stomach, small bowel and mesentery injury. In Champion HR, Robbs JV, Trunkey DD, editors: Rob and Smith's operative surgery: trauma surgery, 4th ed, London, 1989, Butterworth-Heinemann, pp 401–413.)*

COMPLICATIONS

Complications after small bowel injury differ by injury mechanism. In blunt trauma, the principal concern is delay in diagnosis. In 2000, Fakhry et al, in a study of eight trauma centers, reported a statistically significant increased risk of wound infection, wound dehiscence, intraabdominal abscess, acute respiratory distress syndrome (ARDS), and sepsis in patients with isolated small bowel perforations operated on more than 24 hours after injury compared with those undergoing operation less than 8 hours after injury. Fang et al reported a dramatic increase in complications if surgery was delayed more than 24 hours. In children sustaining blunt small bowel rupture, delay in diagnosis more than 24 hours did not result in increased morbidity or mortality risks as reported by Bensard et al.

Complications are also related to associated injuries and to whether management of the small bowel injury requires repair or resection. Associated multisystem injuries occur in as many as 70% of cases after blunt trauma, and often dictate not only the occurrence of complications, but also the eventual outcome (Fig. 16). Anastomosis-related complications include leaks, enterocutaneous fistula, and intraabdominal abscess. These complications are uncommon but exceed the incidence after simple repair. Damage control predicts an increased likelihood of anastomosis-related complications.

Late complications of bowel obstruction relate to adhesions and ischemic stenosis from unrecognized small bowel or mesenteric injury. In the latter circumstance, symptoms usually appear within 6 weeks after injury and vary from vague abdominal pain to frank obstruction. Resection is necessary to relieve the obstruction.

MORTALITY

Although reported mortality rates have reached 25% or higher in some series, the consensus mortality rate after blunt small bowel injury is approximately 10%. In the multicenter study reported by Fakhry et al in 2000, there was no difference in mortality risk between patients with isolated small bowel injury and those who incurred small bowel injury in the setting of multiple other injuries. Delays in diagnosis were directly related to almost half the deaths in this series. In fact, delays exceeding as little as 8 hours increased risks of morbidity and mortality. Fatality after penetrating injury is most commonly related to injury to other intraperitoneal and retroperitoneal injuries.

CONCLUSIONS

Small bowel injuries may follow blunt or penetrating trauma. The major concern in the patient who sustains blunt small bowel injury is recognizing the presence of the injury. In patients with associated injuries requiring operation or in those sustaining gunshot wounds, small bowel injuries are promptly discoverable. The trend toward

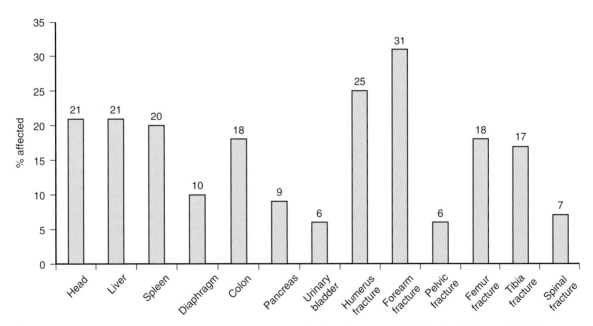

FIGURE 16 Typical injuries accompanying blunt small bowel trauma. *(Modified from Neugebauer H, Wallenboeck E, Hungerford M: Seventy cases of injury of the small intestine caused by blunt abdominal trauma: a retrospective study from 1970 to 1994. J Trauma 46:116–121, 1999.)*

CT-based nonoperative management and the inaccuracy of early postinjury CT places patients with isolated blunt small bowel injury at risk of delayed diagnosis and increased morbidity and mortality. The importance of injury mechanism and physical findings is often overlooked. Patients who are neurologically intact will demonstrate abdominal tenderness; many will have peritoneal findings at presentation. The presence of a seat-belt contusion should elevate concern.

Injuries that can be repaired by lateral enterorrhaphy rarely cause postoperative complications, which are more commonly related to associated injuries after both blunt and penetrating trauma. Surgical judgment is required to ensure early diagnosis and appropriate operative management.

For the chapter's Suggested Readings list, please visit the book at www.ExpertConsult.inkling.com.

Duodenal Injuries

Gregory J. Jurkovich

D uodenal injuries are uncommon, but not so rare as to preclude a comprehensive understanding of diagnostic and treatment strategies by surgeons and emergency physicians. A 6-year statewide review in Pennsylvania documented a 0.2% incidence of duodenal injury following blunt trauma (206 of 103,864 trauma registry entries), and only 30 of these patients had full-thickness duodenal injuries. Blunt duodenal injuries are the result of a direct blow to the epigastrium, which in adults is usually from a steering wheel injury in an unrestrained driver, and in children is the result of a direct blow from a bicycle handlebar, fist, or similar mechanism. Penetrating wounds are more common causes of duodenal injury, with about 75% of patients in published reports of duodenal trauma management sustaining penetrating trauma. This figure may primarily be a reflection of the experience of urban, academic trauma centers where penetrating mechanisms are more prevalent. Penetrating duodenal injury should be diagnosed as part of a laparotomy and careful and systematic following of the tract of the offending agent. Blunt duodenal injuries are more insidious in their presentation, making the initial diagnosis difficult. Despite this well-known observation, delays in the diagnosis of duodenal trauma continue to plague trauma surgeons and seriously compromise patient care.

DETERMINANTS OF OUTCOME

Directly attributable duodenal mortality rate ranges from 2% to 5% and is the result of the common complications of wound dehiscence, sepsis, and multiple-organ failure. Associated causes of mortality risk in patients with a duodenal injury can be garnered from large series of duodenal injuries reported during the late 20th century. These reports demonstrated an average mortality rate in patients with a duodenal injury of 18%, but with great individual report variability, ranging from 6% to 29%. Morbidity rates after duodenal injury range from 30% to 63%, although only about a third of these are directly related to the duodenal injury itself. Reasons for this variability in morbidity and mortality statistics include the mechanism of injury, associated injuries, and time to initial diagnosis. For example, Ivatury and colleagues reviewed 100 consecutive penetrating duodenal injuries and documented a 25% mortality rate, compared with mortality rates of 12% to 14% in patients with blunt injury mechanisms.

Early death from a duodenal injury, particularly with penetrating wounds, is caused by exsanguination from associated vascular, liver, or spleen injuries. The proximity of the duodenum to other vital structures makes isolated injuries uncommon, but not unheard of. Although exsanguinating hemorrhage and associated injuries are responsible for early deaths, infection and multiple-system organ failure are responsible for most late deaths. Up to one third of patients who survive the first 48 hours develop a complication related to the duodenal injury. Anastomotic breakdown, fistula, intra-abdominal abscess, pneumonia, septicemia, and organ failure are the common complications. Late deaths in patients with a duodenal injury typically occur 1 to 2 weeks or more after the injury, with about one third of the late deaths attributable to the injury itself.

The time from injury to definitive treatment is also an important factor in the development of late complications and subsequent fatality. Roman and colleagues identified 10 patients in whom the diagnosis of duodenal injury was delayed over 24 hours; 4 of the 10 died, and 3 of the 10 had duodenal fistulas. In a true trauma classic publication, Lucas and Ledgerwood demonstrated the remarkable importance (and frequency) of a delay in diagnosis of duodenal injury. In their report, a delay in diagnosis of more than 12 hours occurred in 53% of their patients, and a delay of more than 24 hours in 28%; mortality rate was 40% among the patients in whom the diagnosis was delayed greater than 24 hours, as opposed to 11% in those undergoing surgery within 24 hours. Snyder and coworkers confirmed these observations, noting that of the four patients with blunt duodenal trauma in their series, in whom the diagnosis was delayed, two died and the other two developed duodenal fistula. Cuddington and associates also noted that 100% of the deaths directly attributable to duodenal injury occurred in patients in whom there was a delay in diagnosing such injury.

The implication of these observations is that the first priority in managing duodenal trauma should be control of hemorrhage. The next priority is limiting bacterial contamination from colon or other bowel injury to prevent late infections. A clear identification of the extent of the duodenal injury should follow as the next priority, with an emphasis on determining the status of the pancreas as well, as this affects definitive treatment plans. Missing the diagnosis of a duodenal injury is lethal, hence awareness of mechanisms of injury and subtle early clinical presentations and imaging findings is a key responsibility of the trauma surgeon and emergency physician.

ANATOMY AND PHYSIOLOGY

The duodenum is the first portion of the small intestine, beginning just to the right of the spine at the level of the first lumbar vertebra and extending from the pyloric ring to the duodenojejunal flexure, commonly known as the ligament of Treitz. The duodenum is named from the Latin word *duodeni*, which means "twelve each," because it is in total 25 to 30 cm, or about 12 fingerbreadths, in length. For convenience of description, the duodenum is arbitrarily divided into four divisions, differentiated by the alteration in direction of the organ. The *superior* or first portion of the duodenum passes backward and upward toward the neck of the gallbladder, and most of this portion is intraperitoneal. The *descending* (vertical) or second portion forms an acute angle with the first portion and descends 7 to 8 cm. It contains the bile and pancreatic duct openings. This portion (and the remainder of the duodenum) is entirely retroperitoneal; this is the segment mobilized by a Kocher maneuver. The *transverse* or third portion of the duodenum runs 12 cm horizontally to the left in front of the ureter, inferior vena cava, lumbar column, and aorta, and ends at just at the left edge of the third lumbar vertebra. The superior mesenteric artery runs downward over the anterior surface of the third portion of the duodenum. The *ascending* or fourth portion of the duodenum runs upward and slightly to the left for only a short distance (2 to 3 cm) alongside the spine to the duodenal suspensory ligament of Treitz.

The arterial blood supply of the duodenum is derived from the pancreaticoduodenal artery. The superior branch comes off the hepatic artery, and the inferior branch from the superior mesenteric artery. These two arteries run in a groove between the descending (second) and transverse (third) portions of the duodenum and the head of the pancreas, with well-developed collateralization via a continuous marginal artery. The venous drainage parallels the arterial supply, with the posterosuperior arcade draining into the portal vein and the anteroinferior arcade draining into the gastrocolic trunk.

The duodenal mucosa resembles that of the remainder of the small bowel, with the characteristic histologic feature of the submucosal Brunner's glands in the most proximal (first) portion. The viscous, mucoid, alkaline secretion of these glands probably affords some protection to the duodenum from gastric acid and serves to begin neutralization of this acid. The mixing of pancreatic and bile juices with the gastric efflux also normally occurs in the duodenum. The duodenum sees an average of 2500 mL gastric juice, 1000 mL of bile, 800 to 1000 mL of pancreatic secretions, and 800 mL of saliva, for a total of about 5 L of combined flow through the duodenum per day. Such massive flow volumes make it clear that duodenal integrity is crucial, and helps to explain why duodenal fistulas can be such a difficult complication of injury to this organ.

DIAGNOSTIC ADJUVANTS

The radiologic signs of duodenal injury on the initial plain abdominal or upright chest radiograph are often quite subtle, with mild spine scoliosis or obliteration of the right psoas muscle being occasionally all that suggests a retroperitoneal duodenal injury. The presence of air in the retroperitoneum is a clear sign of duodenal injury, but this is often difficult to distinguish from the overlying transverse colon. Computed tomography (CT) remains the best method of early diagnosis of a duodenal injury, but it is not infallible. Ultrasound in the acute setting is largely useless. The key to accurate diagnosis involves the combined use of both oral and IV contrast. Because oral contrast is not a standard component of most trauma abdominal CT scan protocols, the onus is placed on the clinician to demand its use in selected settings in which a duodenal injury is possible (Fig. 1). In a 1997 report describing a 6-year statewide experience with duodenal injuries, Ballard et al reported that of 30 documented blunt duodenal injuries, the initial CT scan missed 27%. The examination must be interpreted with great suspicion for injury, and uncertainty in interpretation is adequate justification for operative exploration, not further delays and repeat imaging. False-negative examinations are known to occur. In one careful study of the accuracy of CT in diagnosing duodenal and other small bowel injuries, only 59% (10 of 17) of scans were prospectively (preoperatively) interpreted as suggestive for bowel injury, which increased to 88% (15 of 17 injuries) when evaluated retrospectively. These investigators emphasized that using CT for the diagnosis of blunt bowel rupture requires careful inspection and technique to detect the often subtle findings.

A more cumbersome alternative to CT is upper gastrointestinal (UGI) series with water-soluble contrast medium followed by barium if the initial examination is negative. Some have advocated this study if the initial CT scan is difficult to interpret, but I would argue that subtle findings on CT are adequate justification for operative exploration. In a series of 96 patients with CT findings suspicious for duodenal injury, the sensitivity of a subsequent duodenography was 54% with a specificity of 98%. For those injuries requiring operative repair, the sensitivity was only 25%, with a 25% false-negative rate. Allen et al demonstrated that 83% of the patients with a delay in the diagnosis of blunt duodenal injury had subtle CT findings, including pneumoperitoneum, unexplained fluid, and unusual bowel morphologic appearance, that were dismissed. These authors emphasized the point that subtle findings of duodenal injury on abdominal CT should mandate laparotomy.

Diagnostic peritoneal lavage (DPL) is unreliable in detecting *isolated* duodenal and other retroperitoneal injuries. Nevertheless, DPL is often helpful because approximately 40% of patients with a duodenal injury have associated intra-abdominal injuries that will result in a positive peritoneal lavage. The findings of amylase or bile in the lavage effluent are more specific indicators of possible duodenal injury. Serum amylase levels are nondiagnostic as well, but if these levels are elevated, additional investigation (CT or celiotomy) for the possibility of pancreatic or duodenal injury is warranted. At celiotomy, the presence of *any* central upper abdominal retroperitoneal hematoma, bile staining, or air mandates visualization and a thorough examination of the duodenum. In 1997, Asensio and colleagues published the unified maneuvers and approaches for the exposure of the duodenum and pancreas.

TREATMENT

Treatment principles are governed by the severity of duodenal injury and the likelihood of postrepair complications. Approximately 70% of

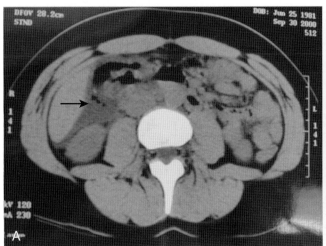
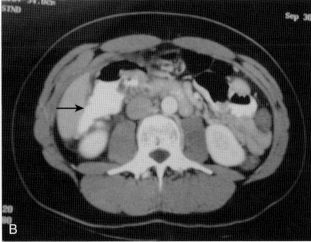

FIGURE 1   A and **B,** Duodenal perforation. A 19-year-old woman dropped a 185-lb barbell on her abdomen, and presented to the emergency department 4 hours later with mild abdominal pain and nausea, afebrile, hemodynamics stable, persistent epigastric tenderness without peritoneal signs, white blood cell count 16,000/mL, amylase 114 U/L. Arrows point to nonluminal air in the retroperitoneum and free extravasation of contrast agent.

duodenal wounds can be safely repaired primarily, and the remaining 30% are "severe" injuries that require more complex procedures, although there is a growing trend by some authors to advocate for primary repair of nearly all duodenal injuries (Asensio, Rickard et al, 2005; Talving et al, 2006; Velmahos et al, 2008). Snyder and colleagues are credited with cataloging the factors that determine whether a duodenal wound can be primarily repaired. In their review of 247 patients treated for duodenal trauma, they reported an overall duodenal fistula rate of 7% and a mortality rate of 10.5% in the 228 patients surviving for greater than 72 hours. These investigators felt that the first five factors listed in Table 1 most significantly correlate

with the severity of duodenal injury and subsequent morbidity and mortality risks. A more recent addition to this list of factors, as noted in the table, is the presence of a pancreatic injury, a significant predictor of late morbidity and mortality risks. Each of these factors, either individually or in combination, has been used to develop a variety of duodenal injury classification systems. Snyder and colleagues demonstrated that patients with "mild" duodenal trauma had 0% mortality rate and 2% duodenal fistula rate, as compared with 6% mortality rate and 10% fistula rate among those with severe duodenal injuries. In general, patients with a "mild" duodenal injury and no pancreatic injury can be primarily repaired.

Patients with more severe duodenal injuries may require more complex treatment strategies. A useful algorithm approach to the management of duodenal injuries is provided in Figure 2. A classification system for all organ injuries has been developed by the American Association for the Surgery of Trauma (AAST) and is known as the Organ Injury Scale (OIS). This classification for duodenal wounds is listed in Table 2, with duodenal injuries graded from I to V, minor to major injury. In a review of 164 duodenal trauma patients managed at eight trauma centers and to whom the AAST-OIS classification scheme was applied, there were 38 grade I, 70 grade II, 48 grade III, four grade IV, and four grade V injuries. Primary repair alone was performed in 117 cases (71% of all). Primary duodenal repair was performed in 90 of 108 patients with grade I or II injuries. More complex duodenal treatment strategies, including pyloric exclusion, duodenoduodenostomy, duodenojejunostomy, or pancreatoduodenectomy, were employed in 26 of 56 (46%) patients with grade III to V injuries, or 29% of the total population.

Primary repair is usually the simplest, fastest, and most appropriate way to manage duodenal injuries. Primary repair is appropriate for partial or complete transection of the duodenum if there is little tissue loss, if the ampulla is not involved, and if the mucosal edges can be débrided and closed without tension. The repair is done as with any small bowel repair. A two-layer closure, but a watertight, serosa-approximating single layer repair is equally acceptable. However, if adequate mobilization for a tension-free repair is impossible,

TABLE 1: Determinants of Duodenal Injury Severity

Parameter	Mild	Severe
Determinants of Injury Severity		
Agent	Stab	Blunt or missile
Size	<75% wall	≥75% wall
Duodenal site	3, 4	1, 2
Injury-repair interval (hour)	<24	≥24
Adjacent injury	No CBD	CBD
	No pancreatic injury	Pancreatic injury
Outcome		
Mortality rate (%)	6%	16%
Duodenal morbidity (%)	6%	14%

CBD, Common bile duct.

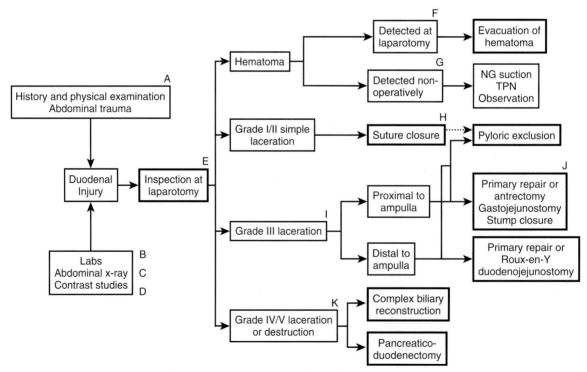

FIGURE 2   Algorithm for the management of duodenal injuries. NG, Nasogastric; TPN, total parenteral nutrition. *(From Jurkovich G: Duodenal injury. In McIntyre R, Van Stiegmann G, Eiseman B, editors: Surgical decision making, 5th ed, Philadelphia, 2004, Elsevier, pp 512–513.)*

TABLE 2: AAST-OIS Grading of Duodenal Injury Severity

Grade*	Type	Description
I	Hematoma Laceration	Single portion of duodenum Partial thickness
II	Hematoma Laceration	More than one portion <50% circumference
III	Laceration	50%–75% D2 50%–100% D1, D3, D4
IV	Laceration	≥75% D2 Involves ampulla or distal CBD
V	Laceration	Massive disruption of duodeno-pancreatic complex Devascularization

Modified from American Association for the Surgery of Trauma (AAST). AAST-OIS, American Association for the Surgery of Trauma Organ Injury Severity scoring system; D1, first position of duodenum; D2, second portion of duodenum; D3, third portion of duodenum; D4, fourth portion of duodenum.
*Advance one grade for multiple injuries to the same organ.

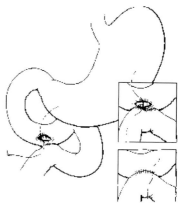

FIGURE 4 Serosal patch technique. Rarely indicated, this repair has been used in select circumstances in which loss of duodenal wall has occurred that cannot be primarily repaired or resected and repaired. The serosa of a loop of jejunum is sutured to the edges of the duodenal defect. *(From Asensio J, Feliciano D, Britt L, Kerstein M: Management of duodenal injuries.* Curr Probl Surg *11:1060, 1993, Fig. 6.)*

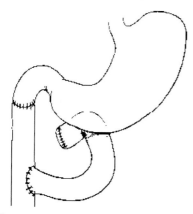

FIGURE 3 Extensive disruptions of the duodenum may be treated by resection with end-to-end Roux-en-Y duodenojejunostomy. *(From Asensio J, Feliciano D, Britt L, Kerstein M: Management of duodenal injuries.* Curr Probl Surg *11:1064, 1993, Fig. 9.)*

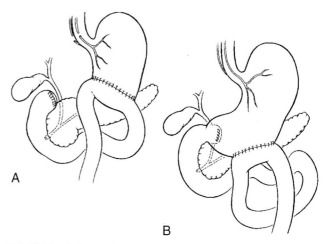

FIGURE 5 **A,** Berne diverticulization and **B,** pyloric exclusion. *(From Jurkovich GJ: Duodenum and pancreas. In Moore EE, Feliciano DV, Mattox K, editors:* Trauma, *5th ed, New York, 2004, McGraw-Hill, p 717.)*

or if the injury is very near the ampulla and mobilization risks common bile duct injury, a Roux-en-Y jejunal limb anastomosis to the proximal duodenal injury with oversewing of the distal duodenal injury is the most reasonable option (Fig. 3). A less desirable option may be the jejunal patch repair whereby the serosa of an adjacent loop of small bowel is sutured as a buttress over the duodenal defect (Fig. 4). Although some experimental evidence suggests that the duodenal mucosa may rapidly resurface over the serosal patch, this technique has been fraught with complications when applied clinically. It was not used in any patient in the most recent multicenter trial of severe duodenal injuries, in which only five patients (3%) had duodenoduodenostomy or duodenojejunostomy repairs. A 1985 report by Ivatury et al compared outcome of patients with a duodenal injury managed by primary repair versus repair with a decompressive enterostomy or serosal patch, and demonstrates why this type of reconstruction is not recommended. In this report of 60 patients with penetrating duodenal injuries, there was a 64% incidence of abdominal sepsis and a 27% death rate in 11 patients with duodenal gunshot wounds managed with a serosal patch or repair, compared with a 7%

abdominal sepsis and 0% mortality rate in 30 patients who had either primary repair or Roux-en-Y anastomotic repair of similar injuries. In 17 patients from that same series with duodenal stab wounds, the complication rate was also higher if the "sucker patch" repair of a duodenal wound was used. The "sucker patch" repair is a modification of the patch repair whereby the open end of a Roux-en-Y loop of small bowel is sutured to the duodenal defect. Given these findings, it is preferable to fully débride the wound, mobilize the edges, and perform a direct end-to-end duodeno-duodeno anastomosis. If adequate mobilization of the duodenal ends is not possible, an end-to-end Roux-en-Y anastomosis should be done. Several techniques may help protect a duodenal repair. Buttressing the repair with omentum (my preference) or a "serosal patch" from a loop of jejunum seems logical, but the benefit of such techniques is unproved. Diversion of gastric contents is another option, most commonly accomplished by the Vaughan/Jordan pyloric exclusion technique. Probably first described by Summers in 1904 as an adjunct to treatment of duodenal wounds, pyloric exclusion is a less disruptive procedure than true duodenal "diverticulization" advocated by Berne and associates and Donovan and colleagues (Fig. 5).

Duodenal diverticulization employs primary closure of the duodenal wound, antrectomy, vagotomy, end-to-side gastrojejunostomy,

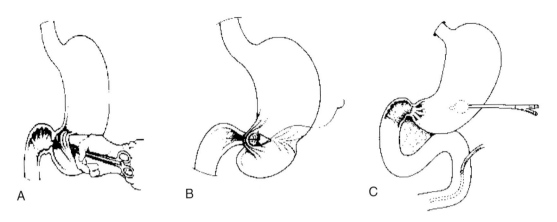

FIGURE 6 **A** to **C,** Pyloric exclusion technique.

T-tube common bile duct drainage, and lateral tube duodenostomy. The concept is to completely divert both gastric and biliary contents away from the duodenal injury, provide enteral nutrition via the gastrojejunostomy, and convert a potential uncontrolled lateral duodenal fistula to a controlled fistula. A less formidable and less destructive alternative is the "pyloric exclusion," which does not employ antrectomy, biliary diversion, or vagotomy (Fig. 6). This procedure is performed through a gastrotomy and consists of grasping the pylorus with a Babcock clamp and suturing closed the pylorus with absorbable size 0 polyglycolic acid or polyglactin, Maxon (polyglyconate), or PDS (polydioxanone) suture and construction of loop gastrojejunostomy. Stapling the pylorus closed or using a nonabsorbable suture (e.g., Prolene) should not be done. Although once considered equally effective, the majority of these repairs fail to open, often causing severe complications. The gastrojejunostomy diverts gastric flow away from the duodenum for several weeks while the duodenal and pancreatic injuries heal. The pylorus eventually opens (2 weeks to 2 months) and the gastrojejunostomy functionally closes. In 1993, Asensio and colleagues produced a classical monograph that details all of the surgical techniques in the management of duodenal injuries. Fang and colleagues at Chang-Gung Memorial Hospital in Taiwan have described a technical method of a controlled release of the pyloric exclusion knot and thereby timing the opening of the pyloric occlusion. Marginal ulceration at the site of gastrojejunostomy has been reported in 5% to 33% of patients, prompting some to add truncal vagotomy to the procedure. Most surgeons do not add a truncal vagotomy to pyloric exclusion, however, because nearly all of the pyloric closures open within a few weeks and the occasional marginal ulcer can be medically managed in the interim. The data support the use of pyloric exclusion and gastrojejunostomy in "severe" duodenal injuries or in cases of delayed diagnosis, although no prospective, randomized trial has proved the true benefit of gastric diversion. In addition, the added operating time and the extra anastomosis suggest a good deal of selectivity should be applied to its use.

Recent studies have questioned the utility of pyloric exclusion, clearly the most widely used adjunct to duodenal repair. Nassoura and Ivatury and colleagues reported on 66 patients with penetrating duodenal injuries managed between 1986 and 1992; 7 patients died within 48 hours, and of the 59 survivors, 56 patients had primary repair and only 3 (5%) had a pyloric exclusion as an adjunct to combined duodenal and pancreatic injury. Only 4 patients died, 1 attributable to duodenal mortality (1.7%). These authors recommend use of pyloric exclusion as an adjunct to repair in patients with Penetrating Abdominal Trauma Index greater than 40 or combined pancreatic injury, rather than using the Snyder criteria of Table 1. The presence of a pancreatic injury was present in all 3 patients (2 with primary repair only) in whom a duodenal anastomotic fistula developed, adding to the evidence of the higher risk of complication with associated pancreatic injury. Similar selectivity in the use of pyloric

exclusion is evidenced in data from the National Trauma Data Bank (Dubose et al, 2008). Dubose and colleagues accessed the NTDB 5-year rolling records of over 950,000 patients, and identified 147 patients with severe duodenal injuries (AAST grade $\geq$ 3). Twenty-eight patients (19%) underwent pyloric exclusion compared to 119 patients with primary repair. Although not achieving statistical significance, the 28 patients with pyloric exclusion had a higher mean Injury Severity Score (ISS) (26 vs. 23) and a greater percentage had an ISS higher than 20 (75% vs. 56%). A multivariable analysis showed no statistically significant difference in mortality rate or occurrence of septic abdominal complications between groups. Finally, Velmahos et al reviewed 193 consecutive patients at Los Angeles County Medical Center with duodenal injuries cared for between 1992 and 2004. A total of 50 patients had severe duodenal injuries identified as AAST grade III, IV, or V. Primary repair was performed in 68% and pyloric exclusion as an adjunct in 32%; the pyloric exclusion group had a more severe duodenal injury pattern, more associated pancreatic injuries, and more injuries to the first and second portions of the duodenum. They reported no difference in mortality or morbidity rates between these two groups. It could be that these more recent studies are showing that adjuncts to primary repair, such as pyloric exclusion, are largely unnecessary. Alternatively, these reports could be interpreted as showing the good judgment of the operating surgeons to use pyloric exclusion selectively on the more severely injured patients, and that they are rewarded with no worse outcome. Exactly defining which patients benefit from pyloric exclusion has been hampered by the lack of a prospective randomized trial, which is unlikely to occur given the relative rarity of severe duodenal injuries. However, my practice has been, and continues to be, to use pyloric exclusion in the presence of concomitant pancreatic injury and a severe duodenal injury in which the repair is tenuous

Fatality directly related to the duodenal injury is the result of duodenal dehiscence, uncontrolled sepsis, and subsequent multiple-system organ failure. Knowledge of the lethal nature of duodenal dehiscence and duodenal fistula certainly tempts the operating surgeon to add pyloric exclusion, anastomosis buttressing, and duodenostomy to the repair of grade III or IV duodenal injuries. As noted previously, concomitant pancreatic injury should also be included as a high-risk confounder that might warrant pyloric exclusion added to the duodenal repair. In one report of 40 patients with penetrating duodenal injuries, there were 14 patients with combined duodenal and pancreatic wounds. Five patients with this combination of injuries had primary duodenal repair alone, and two incurred duodenal leaks. Three of the patients with combined injuries had pyloric exclusion as a treatment adjunct, and none had duodenal leaks.

An alternative or addition to gastric diversion is duodenal decompression via retrograde jejunostomy. Stone and Fabian reported a fistula rate of less than 0.5% (1 in 237 patients) in a variety of duodenal injuries all treated by retrograde jejunostomy tube drainage, in contrast to a 19.3% incidence of duodenal complications when decompression was not used. Retrograde duodenodenal drainage is preferred to lateral duodenostomy. Direct drainage with a tube through the suture line results in a high dehiscence or fistula rate of 23%. Hasson and colleagues reviewed the literature up to 1984 on penetrating duodenal trauma and tube duodenostomy, evaluating eight retrospective series and over 550 patients. They reported overall mortality rate of 19.4% and a fistula rate of 11.8% without decompression, compared with 9% mortality rate and 2.3% fistula rate with decompression. They too concluded that tube drainage should be performed either via stomach or retrograde jejunostomy, as these methods had a lower fistula rate and lower overall mortality rate than lateral tube duodenostomy. Nonetheless, as is the case of pyloric exclusion for gastric diversion, there has been no prospective, randomized analysis of the efficacy of tube duodenal drainage techniques, and not all surgeons support use of decompression techniques.

In very massive injuries of the proximal duodenum and head of the pancreas, destruction of the ampulla and proximal pancreatic duct or distal common bile duct may preclude reconstruction. In addition, because the duodenum and the head of the pancreas have a common arterial supply, it is essentially impossible to entirely resect one without making the other ischemic. In this situation, a pancreatoduodenectomy is required, most often representing a completion of a débridement initiated by the injury forces. Between 1961 and 1994, 184 Whipple procedures were reported for trauma, with 26 operative deaths (14%) and 39 delayed deaths, for a 64% overall survival rate. With appropriate selection criteria, pancreatoduodenectomy for injury can be performed with similar morbidity and mortality rates as described in resections done for cancer. Most recently, Asensio and colleagues reported the largest series of pancreaticoduodenectomies or Whipple procedures

for trauma consisting of 18 patients with a reported mortality rate of 33% and reviewed the literature consisting of 247 patients. The authors validated the Facey and Fry criteria for the performance of Whipple procedures in trauma.

DUODENAL HEMATOMA

Duodenal hematoma is generally considered an injury of childhood play or child abuse, but can occur in adults as well. In one report, 50% of the cases of duodenal hematoma in children resulted from child abuse. Remarkably, the duodenum is the fourth most commonly injured intraabdominal organ after blunt abdominal trauma, occurring in 2% to 10% of children. Nearly one third of the patients present with obstruction of insidious onset at least 48 hours after injury, presumably the result of fluid shift into the hyperosmotic duodenal hematoma. Duodenal hematoma in general represents a nonsurgical injury, in that the best results are obtained with conservative or nonsurgical management. It can be diagnosed either by contrast-enhanced CT scan or UGI study (Fig. 7). The initial water-soluble contrast examination (using meglumine diatrizoate) should be followed by barium to provide the greater detail needed to detect the so-called coiled spring or stacked coin sign. Although characteristic of intramural duodenal hematoma, this finding is present in only approximately one quarter of patients with hematoma.

Although the initial treatment is nonoperative, associated injuries should be excluded, particularly pancreatic injury. Desai et al reported that 42% of pediatric patients with a duodenal injury (perforation or hematoma) had a concomitant pancreatic injury, and Jewett et al found a 20% incidence of pancreatic injury in patients with a duodenal hematoma. Continuous nasogastric suction should be employed

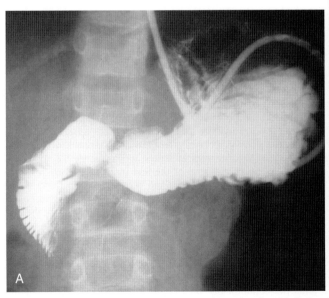
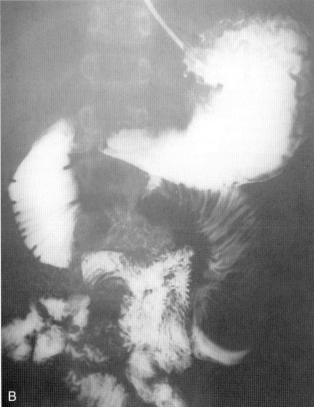

FIGURE 7   Duodenal hematoma. The two images are sequential. **A,** Initial image shows near total duodenal obstruction. **B,** Image portrays contrast passage into the jejunum. The hematoma has infiltrated the wall, producing fold thickening, loop narrowing, and displacement. The mesentery is also involved, and there is a pronounced hematoma component nearly occluding the first jejunal loop. This case shows the characteristic involvement of the duodenum as it traverses the spine, sparing, but obstructing, the proximal duodenal (1 and 2) segments.

and total parenteral nutrition begun. The patient should be reevaluated with UGI contrast studies at 5- to 7-day intervals if signs of obstruction do not spontaneously abate. Ultrasound has also been used to follow a resolving duodenal hematoma. Percutaneous drainage of an unresolving duodenal hematoma has been reported, but operative exploration and evacuation of the hematoma are usually recommended after 2 weeks of conservative therapy to rule out stricture, duodenal perforation, and injury to the head of the pancreas as factors that might be contributing to the obstruction. One review of six cases of duodenal and jejunal hematomas resulting from blunt trauma demonstrated resolution with nonoperative management in five of the six patients, with an average hospital stay of 16 days (range, 10 to 23 days), and total parenteral nutrition of 9 days (range, 4 to 16 days). The sixth case had evidence of complete bowel obstruction on UGI series, which failed to resolve after 18 days of conservative management. Laparotomy revealed jejunal and colonic strictures with fibrosis, which were successfully resected. Another report included 19 cases of duodenal hematoma in children, 17 (89%) managed nonoperatively and 2 patients in whom operative incision and drainage occurred within the first 24 hours and nonoperative management was never attempted. Nasogastric decompression and total parenteral nutrition were employed for an average of 9.3 ($\pm$7.7) days (range, 2 to 29 days), with an average hospital stay of 16.4 ($\pm$17.8) days (range, 2 to 37 days).

If a duodenal hematoma is incidentally found at celiotomy, a thorough inspection must ensue to exclude perforation. This will require an extended Kocher maneuver, which usually successfully drains the subserosal hematoma. It is unclear whether the serosa of the duodenum should intentionally be incised along its extent to "evacuate" the hematoma, or whether this in fact increases the likelihood of converting a partial duodenal wall tear into a complete perforation. Unless my index of suspicion is very high for a full-thickness duodenal wall injury, I generally do not open a duodenal hematoma found incidentally, although I do inspect it carefully. A feeding jejunostomy should be placed, because an extended period of gastric decompression will likely be required.

For the chapter's Suggested Readings list, please visit the book at www.ExpertConsult.inkling.com.

PANCREATIC INJURIES AND PANCREATICODUODENECTOMY

Louis J. Magnotti and Martin A. Croce

The pancreas is relatively protected deep within the confines of the retroperitoneum. As such, injuries to the pancreas are uncommon, but not rare, and can present a diagnostic dilemma. Despite advances in modern trauma care, including damage control surgery and improved imaging techniques, injuries to the pancreas present a continuing challenge to the trauma surgeon. In fact, the morbidity and mortality rates associated with pancreatic injuries have changed little over the past 25 years, with mortality rates ranging from 9% to 34%. Frequent complications are also common following pancreatic injuries, occurring in 30% to 60% of these patients. The high complication rate associated with these injuries is primarily related to diagnostic delays and missed injuries. When identified early, the treatment of most pancreatic injuries is straightforward. It is the delayed recognition and treatment of these injuries that can result in devastating outcomes.

There are few well-documented historical accounts about the management of pancreatic injuries. The first documented case of pancreatic trauma was an autopsy report from St. Thomas Hospital in London in 1827 in which a patient struck by the wheel of a stagecoach suffered a complete pancreatic body transection. Over the next several decades, reports of pancreatic injuries were scattered. In 1903, after extensive review of the literature, only 45 cases of pancreatic trauma, 21 resulting from penetrating injuries and 24 from blunt trauma, could be identified. Mickulicz-Radecki noted that all 20 of the patients observed died and 18 of the 25 (72%) who were operated on survived. With these findings, he recommended a thorough exploration through a midline incision, suture control of hemostasis, and drainage—similar to modern approaches.

Complications following pancreatic injury were also noted early and have continued to be a problem throughout the years. In 1905, Korte reported the first case of a pancreatic fistula following an isolated pancreatic transection. The fistula closed spontaneously and the patient survived. Whipple first described pancreaticoduodenectomy in 1935 and later reported the associated complications of secondary hemorrhage, fistula formation, duodenal leaks, and peritonitis.

This chapter attempts to clarify the anatomic and physiologic basis for the concerns over injuries to the pancreas as well as elucidate specific diagnostic and therapeutic interventions following traumatic injuries to the pancreas.

ANATOMY

A complete understanding of pancreatic relational anatomy is essential for providing appropriate treatment and understanding the potential for associated injuries. The pancreas is about 15 to 20 cm in length, 3.1 cm wide, and 1 to 1.5 cm thick. The average mass is 90 g (ranging from 40 to 180 g). The inferior vena cava, aorta, left kidney, both renal veins, and right renal artery lie posterior to the pancreas. The head of the pancreas is nestled in the duodenal sweep, with the body crossing the spine and the tail resting within the hilum of the spleen. The splenic artery and vein can be found along the superior border of the pancreas. The superior mesenteric artery and vein reside just behind the neck of the pancreas and are enclosed posteriorly by the uncinate process. This process can be absent or can almost completely encircle the superior mesenteric artery and vein.

The head of the pancreas is suspended from the liver by the hepatoduodenal ligament and is firmly fixed to the medial aspect of the second and third portions of the duodenum. A line extending from the portal vein superiorly to the superior mesenteric vein inferiorly marks the division between the head and the neck of the gland. The neck of the pancreas measures approximately 1.5 to 2 cm in length and lies at the level of the first lumbar vertebra. It overlies the superior mesenteric vessels and is fixed between them and the celiac trunk superiorly. The body of the pancreas is technically defined as that portion of the pancreas that lies to the left of the superior mesenteric vessels. There is no true anatomic division between the body and the tail, nor is there any imaginary dividing line as in the case of the head and neck.

The main pancreatic duct of Wirsung originates in the tail of the pancreas and typically traverses the entire length of the gland and joins the common bile duct before emptying into the duodenum. Throughout its course in the tail and body, the duct lies midway between the superior and inferior margins and slightly more posterior. The accessory duct of Santorini usually branches out from the pancreatic duct in the neck of the pancreas and empties separately into the duodenum. A significant number of anatomic variants exist and must be recognized: in 60% of individuals, the ducts open separately into the duodenum; in 30%, the duct of Wirsung carries the entire glandular secretion and the duct of Santorini ends blindly; and in 10%, the duct of Santorini carries the entire secretion of the gland and the duct of Wirsung is either small or absent. In all cases, the ducts lie anterior to the major pancreatic vessels. Regardless, surgeons dealing with pancreatic injuries should be well versed with these anatomic variants.

The arterial and venous blood supply of the pancreas is relatively constant. The arterial blood supply of the pancreas originates from both the celiac trunk and the superior mesenteric artery. The blood supply to the head of the pancreas appears to be the greatest, with less flow to the body and tail and the least to the neck. The veins, like the arteries, are found posterior to the ducts, lie superficial to the arteries, and parallel the arteries for the most part throughout their course. The venous drainage of the pancreas is to the portal, splenic, and superior mesenteric veins.

PHYSIOLOGY

The pancreas is a compound tubuloalveolar gland with both endocrine (insulin, glucagon, somatostatin) and exocrine (digestive enzyme precursors, bicarbonate) function. The endocrine cells are separated histologically into nests of cells known as the islets of Langerhans. There are three predominant subtypes of islet cells: alpha cells (which produce glucagon), beta cells (which produce insulin), and delta cells (which produce somatostatin). Although these cells are distributed throughout the substance of the pancreas, the majority reside primarily within the tail. Consequently, it would seem that a distal pancreatectomy would be poorly tolerated in terms of endocrine function. However, it is well known that resection of more than 90% of the pancreas must occur before endocrine insufficiency develops, provided the remainder of the gland is normal. In fact, partial resection induces hypertrophy and increased activity of the residual islet cells. In animal studies, Dragstedt was the first to show that removal of 80% of the pancreas did not significantly alter carbohydrate and fat metabolism or the digestion and absorption of food, provided that the remaining gland is normal and that pancreatic secretions still have access to the upper digestive tract via the ductal system.

DIAGNOSIS

It is important to remember that whenever there is trauma to the pancreas, particular attention must be given to the possibility of a major ductal injury because this injury is the single most important determinant of outcome following pancreatic injury. In fact, this concept was first recognized as early as 1962. Subsequent investigators have confirmed and reemphasized the necessity of determining the status of the pancreatic duct. In fact, Heitsch et al found that distal resection of ductal injuries significantly lowered postoperative morbidity and mortality rates when compared to drainage alone. This finding was confirmed over a decade later when investigators documented a drop in mortality rate from 19% to 3% following pancreatic resection proximal to the site of ductal injury. Despite improvements in image quality, cross-sectional body imaging techniques in the multitrauma patient do not routinely have adequate sensitivity to accurately assess ductal status. In addition, magnetic resonance imaging is often too unwieldy in the acute trauma setting. Thus, the challenge to make an early, accurate determination of the status of the main pancreatic duct remains.

Successful diagnosis of a pancreatic injury requires a high index of suspicion and underscores the need to limit the time from injury to definitive management. The mechanism of injury, need for laparotomy, and time interval following initial abdominal insult will direct the trauma surgeon to the most appropriate procedures and tests.

Those patients with need for immediate laparotomy require little or no preoperative evaluation as the diagnosis of pancreatic injury can be made at the time of exploration. Conversely, patients without clear need for operative exploration may require extensive efforts to establish the presence of a pancreatic injury. Thus, early identification of a subtle pancreatic injury requires a high index of suspicion coupled with a carefully planned approach and close observation.

Pancreatic injuries typically result from high-energy transfer to the upper abdomen. In adults, motor vehicle accidents are the primary cause of pancreatic injuries, usually secondary to impact of the steering wheel. In children, the typical scenario involves a handle bar injury to the epigastrium. In any case, the energy of impact is directed at the upper abdomen (epigastrium or hypochondrium) resulting in crushing of the retroperitoneal structures. Typical findings suggestive of retroperitoneal injury include contusion/bruising to the upper abdomen with epigastric pain out of proportion to findings on physical examination.

Elevated serum amylase is not a reliable indicator of pancreatic trauma. In one series, only 8% of patients with hyperamylasemia following blunt trauma had a pancreatic injury. In fact, the use of amylase as a screening tool in blunt trauma carries a negative predictive value of 95%. Measurement of the pancreatic isoamylase fraction has failed to substantially improve both the sensitivity and specificity of this value as a marker of pancreatic injury. Nevertheless, the presence of an elevated serum amylase should heighten suspicion for a pancreatic injury.

Asymptomatic patients with elevated serum pancreatic isoamylase require observation and repeat amylase determination. Persistently elevated serum amylase or the development of abdominal symptoms warrants further investigation and may include computed tomography (CT) scan, endoscopic retrograde cholangiopancreatography (ERCP), or operative exploration. Abdominal CT scans have a reported sensitivity and specificity as high as 80% in diagnosing pancreatic injury, although this is largely dependent on interpreter experience, scanner quality, and time from injury. Patton and colleagues reported that in 26 patients who sustained blunt pancreatic trauma, early CT scan was suspicious for injury in 15. CT failed to demonstrate injury in 4 patients (21%), resulting in a delay in operative intervention (mean, 3.8 days). The remaining patients had other indications for exploration.

CT findings diagnostic of pancreatic injury include parenchymal disruption, intrapancreatic hematoma, fluid in the lesser sac or separating the splenic vein and body of the pancreas, peripancreatic edema, thickened left anterior renal fascia, and retroperitoneal hematoma or fluid. Clearly, certain findings are more reliable than others and rarely are all present in one patient. In fact, some of the CT signs of pancreatic injury may not be immediately apparent following injury but rather require time to develop after injury. It is important to remember this when evaluating the patient with worsening abdominal symptoms and an unimpressive initial CT scan.

ERCP can be useful in the diagnosis of pancreatic duct rupture. In addition, it can aid in the diagnosis of and occasionally the management of the complications of missed pancreatic injuries. A report from the University of Louisville documents ERCP as a useful diagnostic tool in the evaluation of the pancreatic duct in the early postinjury period in hemodynamically stable patients with elevated amylase levels, persistent abdominal pain, and abnormal or questionable abdominal CT findings. ERCP is also extremely helpful in the evaluation of those patients in whom the diagnosis of pancreatic injury was missed during the initial evaluation. It is in these patients that ERCP can aid in diagnosing the injury, planning the surgical approach if necessary, internal transpancreatic stent placement, and transductal drainage of a pancreatic abscess. However, ERCP may not always be available and should not delay operation in patients with progressive clinical deterioration, nor does it have a role in the acute evaluation of the hemodynamically unstable trauma patient.

Magnetic resonance imaging, specifically magnetic resonance cholangiopancreatography (MRCP), has emerged as an alternative technique for evaluating the pancreatic duct. Although primarily used in elective circumstances, MRCP has been reported as a viable option for evaluating the status of the duct in those patients with pancreatic injuries. However, it frequently is not practical for use in trauma patients.

In order to successfully diagnose the presence and extent of a potential pancreatic injury, the surgeon must recognize those findings associated with pancreatic injury and adequately visualize the entire gland. In addition, it is also imperative to determine the integrity of the pancreatic parenchyma and status of the major pancreatic duct. Pancreatic injuries are classified based on the status of the duct and the anatomic location of the injury within the gland. Associated injuries often complicate pancreatic evaluation. The presence of a central retroperitoneal hematoma or a hematoma overlying the pancreas, retroperitoneal saponification, or bile staining mandates complete pancreatic exploration.

Once again, it must be stressed that, if possible, it is important to determine the status of the duct at the time of exploration. The majority of these injuries can be diagnosed by local exploration of the pancreas. Injuries to the duct occur in approximately 15% of pancreatic trauma and are generally the result of penetrating injury. Blunt injury can also result in transection of the major duct with or without complete transection of the gland. Minor contusions and lacerations of the pancreatic parenchyma usually do not require further evaluation of the duct. However, an intact pancreatic capsule does not eliminate the possibility of complete transection of the pancreatic duct.

The use of intraoperative observations such as direct visualization of ductal disruption, complete transection of the substance of the gland, free leakage of pancreatic fluid, lacerations involving more than one half of the diameter of the gland, central perforations, and severe lacerations with or without massive tissue disruption can predict the presence of a major ductal injury with a high degree of accuracy. However, in those instances in which the status of the duct is uncertain, intraoperative pancreatography has been used as a technique for visualization of the main pancreatic duct. Although intraoperative pancreatography may sound appealing, it usually is impractical.

Nevertheless, pancreatography can be performed either by directly cannulating the ampulla of Vater through a duodenotomy or the main pancreatic duct through the amputated tail of the pancreas. A 5F pediatric feeding tube is used along with 2 to 5 mL of contrast agent. Cannulating the ampulla of Vater entails creating a duodenotomy unless there is an associated duodenal injury. It should be stressed that identifying the ampulla can be difficult and that resection of the tail does not always ensure visualization of the pancreatic duct.

The simplest technique is a needle cholecystocholangiogram. In this technique, a purse-string suture is placed in the gallbladder just proximal to the cystic duct. An 18-G angiocatheter is then introduced into the gallbladder. The remainder of the gallbladder can be excluded with a bowel clamp. Water-soluble contrast agent is injected into the gallbladder under direct fluoroscopy. A cholecystectomy is not necessary following this procedure. This procedure may or may not visualize the pancreatic duct.

CLASSIFICATION OF PANCREATIC INJURIES

Although a number of classification systems have been devised to categorize pancreatic injuries, the American Association for the Surgery of Trauma (AAST) Committee on Organ Injury Scaling addresses the key issues of treatment of parenchymal disruption and major pancreatic ductal injury by focusing on the anatomic location of the injury (Table 1). Proximal duct injuries require different management than do distal duct and parenchymal injuries. The difficulty arises in those patients with parenchymal disruption and major duct injury. This classification scheme provides a useful management guide by focusing on the anatomic location of the duct and parenchymal injury (proximal vs. distal).

TABLE 1: AAST Pancreatic Organ Injury Scale

Grade	Injury Type	Injury Description
I	Hematoma	Minor contusion without duct injury
	Laceration	Superficial laceration without duct injury
II	Hematoma	Major contusion without duct injury or tissue loss
	Laceration	Major laceration without duct injury or tissue loss
III	Laceration	Distal transection or parenchymal injury with duct injury
IV	Laceration	Proximal (right of superior mesenteric vein) transection or parenchymal injury
V	Laceration	Massive disruption of pancreatic head

AAST, American Association for the Surgery of Trauma.

SURGICAL MANAGEMENT OF PANCREATIC INJURIES

As with any case of abdominal trauma, the primary operative focus is control of ongoing hemorrhage and gastrointestinal contamination. Once these areas have been addressed, systemic abdominal exploration should include recognition and evaluation of the possibility of pancreatic injury.

Proper evaluation of the pancreas requires complete exposure of the gland. Access to the pancreas is best accomplished by opening the lesser sac. That is, by dividing the gastrocolic omentum inferior to the gastroepiploic vessels, the anterior surface and the superior and inferior borders of the body and tail of the pancreas can be visualized. The transverse colon is retracted inferiorly and the stomach superiorly (Fig. 1). Frequently, a few adhesions between the posterior stomach and anterior surface of the pancreatic head need to be incised. The nasogastric tube may be advanced along the greater curvature of

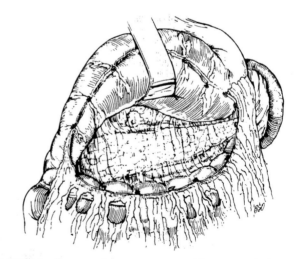

FIGURE 1 Access to the pancreas is gained by opening the lesser sac. Transection of the gastrocolic ligament with superior retraction of the stomach and inferior retraction of the transverse colon allows complete visualization of the body and tail of the pancreas. *(From Asensio JA, Demetriades D, Berne JD, et al: A unified approach to the surgical exposure of pancreatic and duodenal injuries. Am J Surg 174:54–60, 1997.)*

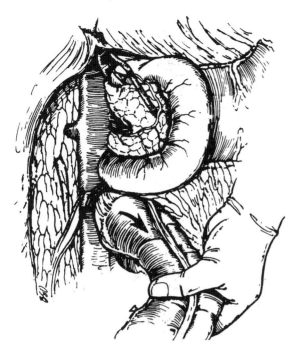

FIGURE 2 The Kocher maneuver is performed by incising the lateral attachments of the duodenum and sweeping the second and third portions of the duodenum medially. *(From Asensio JA, Demetriades D, Berne JD, et al: A unified approach to the surgical exposure of pancreatic and duodenal injuries. Am J Surg 174:54–60, 1997.)*

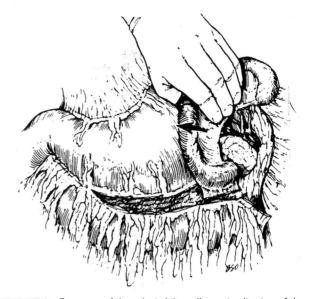

FIGURE 3 Exposure of the splenic hilum allows visualization of the involved pancreatic tail. Mobilization of the spleen from a lateral to a medial position to visualize the spleen and posterior aspects of the tail of the pancreas. *(From Asensio JA, Demetriades D, Berne JD, et al: A unified approach to the surgical exposure of pancreatic and duodenal injuries. Am J Surg 174:54–60, 1997.)*

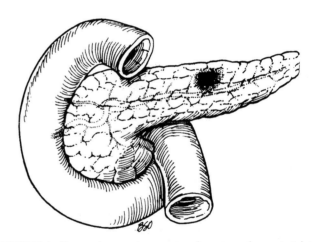

FIGURE 4 Pancreatic contusion or minor hematoma does not violate the capsule. *(From Asensio JA, Demetriades D, Berne TV: Atlas and textbook of techniques in complex trauma surgery, Philadelphia, 2005, Saunders.)*

the stomach and can be used as a handle for retraction of the stomach. An adequate Kocher maneuver will allow complete visualization of the pancreatic head and uncinate process. This is accomplished by incising the lateral peritoneal attachments of the duodenum and sweeping the second and third portions medially with a combination of both blunt and sharp dissection (Fig. 2). If a large retroperitoneal hematoma is encountered, the nasogastric tube should be advanced through the pylorus and used as a palpable guide to avoid iatrogenic injury to the duodenal wall. The Kocher maneuver should be extensive enough that the left renal vein is easily identified. Occasionally, mobilization of the hepatic flexure is necessary to adequately evaluate the pancreatic head. If the tail of the pancreas is involved, exposure of the splenic hilum is necessary. Division of the peritoneal attachments lateral to the spleen and colon facilitate mobilization. A plane is then created between the spleen, colon, and pancreas anteriorly and the kidney posteriorly. This maneuver allows for inspection of the posterior surface of the pancreas (Fig. 3).

Approximately 60% of all pancreatic injuries consist of minor contusions, hematomas, and capsular lacerations (Fig. 4). Lacerations of the pancreatic parenchyma without major ductal disruption or tissue loss account for an additional 20% of pancreatic injuries (Fig. 5). These injuries require only hemostasis and adequate external drainage. The temptation to repair capsular lacerations should be resisted, as this tends to lead to pseudocyst formation, whereas a controlled pancreatic fistula is usually self-limited. Closed-suction drains should be used for drainage of any pancreatic injury. These drains are better tolerated by the patient in terms of decreased intraabdominal abscess formation, more reliable collection of the effluent, and less skin excoriation. Typically, these drains are left in place for a minimum of 10 days, because if a fistula is going to develop, it should be evident by that time.

Nutritional support can be provided via either the oral or gastric route almost immediately. However, with more severe injuries, prolonged gastric ileus and potential pancreatic complications may preclude standard feeding. In addition, the majority of tube feed formulations increase pancreatic stimulation and, in turn, pancreatic

effluent and amylase concentration. Elemental diets (low fat, higher pH) are less stimulating to the pancreas and may be useful in these situations. Intraoperative placement of a feeding jejunostomy at the time of initial exploration should be considered for all patients with grade III to V injuries. These allow for early postoperative enteral feeding and avert the need for total parenteral nutrition in those patients unable to tolerate either oral or gastric feedings.

Distal parenchymal transection, especially with disruption of the main pancreatic duct (Fig. 6), is best treated with distal pancreatectomy. In general, the anatomic distinction between proximal and distal pancreas is defined by the superior mesenteric vessels passing behind the pancreas at the junction of the head and body. Provided that the proximal duct is normal, the transected duct should be closed with either a "U" stitch or a "figure of eight" with direct suture ligation. Although normal endocrine and exocrine function has been reported after 90% pancreatectomy, efforts should be made to leave at least 20% residual pancreatic tissue to minimize postoperative complications.

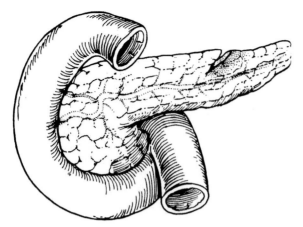

FIGURE 5 Pancreatic parenchymal injury without ductal injury. *(From Asensio JA, Demetriades D, Berne TV: Atlas and textbook of techniques in complex trauma surgery, Philadelphia, 2005, Saunders.)*

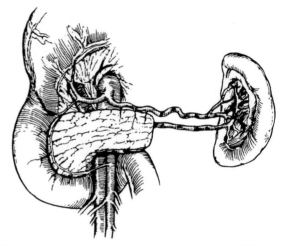

FIGURE 7 Distal pancreas resection with splenic preservation. *(From Asensio JA, Demetriades D, Berne TV: Atlas and textbook of techniques in complex trauma surgery, Philadelphia, 2005, Saunders.)*

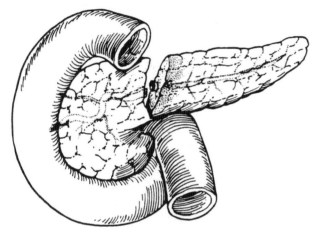

FIGURE 6 Pancreatic parenchymal disruption with ductal injury. *(From Asensio JA, Demetriades D, Berne TV: Atlas and textbook of techniques in complex trauma surgery, Philadelphia, 2005, Saunders.)*

The technique of pancreatic transection depends on individual preference. Interlocking "U" stitches with nonabsorbable sutures placed through the full thickness of the gland from anterior to posterior capsule help minimize potential leak from the transected parenchyma. Others prefer to use stapling devices for closure of the pancreatic parenchyma. Whatever technique is used for resection and closure of the pancreatic parenchyma, the duct itself (if visible) should be identified and individually ligated. If available, a small omental patch can be placed over the area of resection to buttress stump closure, although this is not often necessary. A closed-suction drain should be left near the transection line, similar to injuries undergoing external drainage.

Distal pancreatectomy can be performed with or without splenectomy. The technical challenge in pancreatectomy without splenectomy involves isolating splenic branch vessels and avoiding injury to the splenic hilum (Fig. 7). These, in turn, lead to increased operative time and potential blood loss. Nevertheless, the decision to proceed with splenic salvage requires a completely hemodynamically stable normothermic patient. The risk for postsplenectomy sepsis, albeit small, must also be considered. Generous mobilization of the entire pancreatic gland and spleen must be accomplished prior to even attempting splenic salvage. Transection of the gland just proximal to the point of injury is followed by elevation of the distal body with

meticulous attention to individual ligation of the numerous arterial and venous tributaries found along the superior border of the gland.

The most challenging management problems arise with injuries to the pancreatic head. Although important with all pancreatic injuries, it is essential to define ductal anatomy for all proximal pancreatic injuries. If local inspection and exploration of the defect fails to exclude ductal injury and intraoperative pancreatography is not an option, wide external drainage with postoperative ERCP is an alternative. In fact, because of the high rate of morbidity associated with proximal pancreatic duct injury, closed-suction drainage should be used in virtually all cases of proximal pancreatic injury.

The importance of adequate external drainage cannot be stressed enough. In fact, the pancreas, when injured, can be an unforgiving organ. Uncontrolled leakage of pancreatic secretions (especially pancreatic enzymes) normally used for digestion either into the retroperitoneum or intraperitoneally can cause significant injury to the patient by digesting the retroperitoneum and suture lines used to repair bowel and blood vessels.

Adequate external drainage is effective for injuries to the pancreatic head and neck in the absence of major ductal injury. Similarly, if the patient is hemodynamically unstable and the status of the proximal duct is uncertain, wide external drainage with postoperative ERCP is recommended. Patton and colleagues report the effectiveness of drainage alone for proximal pancreatic injuries. Of the 37 patients with proximal pancreatic injuries managed with closed-suction drainage, only 13.5% developed either a fistula or abscess. Thus, the management of pancreatic injuries becomes relatively straightforward: resection for distal injuries that likely involve the duct or drainage for those without ductal involvement, and drainage for proximal injuries regardless of ductal involvement. This simplified scheme negates the need for intraoperative pancreatography.

In the case of incomplete pancreatic parenchymal transection, some surgeons have described an end jejunum to side pancreas anastomosis. This technique is mentioned for historical interest only and is not recommended because of the difficulty in ensuring the integrity of the anastomosis and potential for a high output pancreatic fistula from the posterior aspect of the injury. Stone has illustrated the high complication rate associated with this dated technique. Of the 7 patients out of 238 patients in whom this technique was used, 5 (71%) developed a fistula and 3 (43%) died.

Fortunately, severe combined pancreatic head and duodenal injuries are rare. These injuries are most commonly caused by penetrating wounds and occur in association with multiple other intra-abdominal injuries. Because of the large number of possible injury patterns, no single therapeutic intervention is right for all patients. The best treatment option is determined by the integrity of the distal common bile duct and ampulla, coupled with the severity of the duodenal injury. For that reason, any patient with a combined injury to the pancreas and duodenum should, at a minimum, have an intraoperative cholangiogram performed before an adequate treatment decision can be made, unless it is obvious that there is no ductal involvement.

The primary cause of fatality in those patients with combined pancreatic and duodenal injuries is secondary to major vascular injury. Once vascular control is obtained, Whipple resection remains the preferred option in that select group of patients with combined massive destruction of the duodenum and pancreatic head. Essentially, in these patients, pancreaticoduodenectomy is the completion of surgical débridement of devitalized tissue. For those patients with hemodynamic instability, hypothermia, coagulopathy, and acidosis, a staged operative approach is often the best course of action. For combined injuries with clear disruption of the common bile duct, following control of hemorrhage, one should proceed with Whipple resection combined with packing, leaving the gallbladder in situ (provided it is uninjured) and plan on definitive reconstruction following correction of hypothermia, coagulopathy, and acidosis (usually within 24 to 48 hours). By leaving the uninjured gallbladder, a cholecystojejunostomy may be performed which is technically easier in patients with a normal common bile duct.

During a 6-year period, 10 of 117 patients at Harborview Medical Center in Seattle underwent Whipple resection for nonreconstructable injury to the ampulla or severe combined pancreaticoduodenal injuries. Postoperative complications included 4 intra-abdominal abscesses, 2 cases of pancreatitis and 1 pancreatic fistula. More importantly, all patients survived. In a review of 129 cases of combined pancreatic-duodenal injuries, 24% were treated with simple repair and drainage, 50% underwent repair with pyloric exclusion, and only 10% required a Whipple procedure. For this reason, every patient with a combined pancreatic-duodenal injury requires a cholangiogram coupled with evaluation of both the ampulla as well as the pancreatic duct. When the common bile duct and ampulla are intact, the duodenum should be repaired and the pancreatic injury treated based on its location and the status of the main pancreatic duct.

PANCREATIC INJURY IN CHILDREN

Fortunately, the majority of pediatric pancreatic injuries are grade I or II, without major ductal injury. In fact, the incidence of major pancreatic duct injury following blunt abdominal trauma in children is only 0.12%. Consequently, several authors have suggested managing all blunt pediatric pancreatic injuries nonoperatively. However, there is a high associated morbidity with pseudocyst formation in 40% to 100% of children with major ductal injury requiring further hospitalization and interventions (i.e., ERCP with stenting, percutaneous drainage), often with atrophy of the distal remnant.

MORBIDITY AND COMPLICATIONS MANAGEMENT

Although the majority of complications related to pancreatic injury are self-limiting or treatable, the possibility of sepsis and multiple-organ failure leading to death is real and results in nearly 30% of the deaths following pancreatic trauma.

A fistula is the most common complication following pancreatic injury, with an incidence of 7% to 20%. In general, a pancreatic fistula is defined as any measureable drain output with an amylase level greater than three times serum level. For the most part, these fistulas are minor (drainage less than 200 mL/day) and resolve spontaneously with adequate external drainage. However, those with output greater than 700 mL/day (high-output fistulas) generally require longer periods of external drainage and may require operative intervention. ERCP can prove helpful for persistent high-output fistulas. In fact, it can be both diagnostic by helping establish the cause of the fistula and therapeutic by enabling stenting of the pancreatic duct (decreases fistula output). During this period, nutritional support is paramount. Low-fat, higher pH elemental formulas result in less pancreatic stimulation and should be tried prior to total parenteral nutrition. Placement of a feeding jejunostomy at the time of initial or subsequent exploration is extremely helpful in those patients with prolonged fistula output in order to provide enteral nutrition.

The use of the long-acting somatostatin analog octreotide acetate has been reported in the management of postoperative complications following elective pancreatic resections. The use of this synthetic analog has been extended to the treatment of posttraumatic pancreatic fistulas, but there are few data in the literature documenting its efficacy. In fact, the reports that do exist are contradictory.

Abscess formation following pancreatic trauma depends on the number and type of associated injuries and ranges from 10% to 25%. The intra-abdominal abscess is often subfascial or peripancreatic. Although a true pancreatic abscess is rare, it is usually the result of inadequate débridement of necrotic tissue or initial drainage and often requires open débridement and drainage. In any case, the mortality rate in this group of patients remains about 25%, underscoring the need for prompt drainage (either percutaneous or open).

Another common complication following operative management of pancreatic trauma is pancreatitis, occurring in 8% to 18% of patients. This type of pancreatitis, characterized by transient abdominal pain and a rise in serum amylase, is amenable to bowel rest, with or without nasogastric decompression and nutritional support. In these cases, the course is usually self-limited and resolves spontaneously. A less common complication is hemorrhagic pancreatitis occurring in fewer than 2% of postoperative patients.

Secondary hemorrhage following operative management of pancreatic trauma may occur in 5% to 10% of patients. This complication is particularly common with inadequate external drainage following pancreatic débridement or in the face of a postoperative intraabdominal abscess. These patients often require reexploration for hemorrhage but angioembolization remains a viable option.

Pseudocyst formation following nonoperative management of unrecognized pancreatic trauma is not uncommon. It is important to remember that, as stated earlier, the major determinant of outcome and primary indicator of optimal treatment following pancreatic trauma is the status of the duct. In fact, if the duct is intact, either watchful waiting or percutaneous drainage is often all that is needed for resolution of a pseudocyst. In contrast, if the duct is injured, percutaneous drainage will not provide definitive therapy but will instead create a fistula. Clearly, if there is any question as to the status of the duct, an endoscopic retrograde pancreatogram should be performed prior to percutaneous drainage.

Neither exocrine nor endocrine insufficiency following pancreatic injury is commonly observed. In fact, in both animal and human studies, it has been shown that only 10% to 20% of normal pancreatic tissue is needed for normal pancreatic function. Thus, distal resection should be well tolerated with little if any physiologic sequelae. This conclusion was confirmed by a multicenter study in which there was only one case of endocrine insufficiency and no exocrine abnormalities identified.

CONCLUSIONS

Injuries to the pancreas following trauma are relatively uncommon. As a result, they are easily missed, even by the experienced surgeon. Consequently, they represent a significant cause of morbidity and mortality relative to their overall incidence. This is primarily related to the accuracy and timing of diagnosis, the completeness of the operative procedure, and the meticulous attention to detail that is required in the postoperative period to identify and treat potential complications associated with pancreatic injury. Prompt diagnosis requires a high index of suspicion (both preoperatively as well as intraoperatively) and appropriate tests performed in a timely fashion. Subsequent operative treatment is dictated by the pattern and severity of injury. In fact, when recognized early, the operative management of the majority of isolated pancreatic injuries is straightforward, with acceptably low morbidity and mortality rates. However, when delayed or missed initially, these injuries result in a protracted, complicated course with often devastating outcome.

For the chapter's Suggested Readings list, please visit the book at www.ExpertConsult.inkling.com.

LIVER INJURY

Manish S. Parikh, Susan I. Brundage, and H. Leon Pachter

The liver is the most commonly injured intraabdominal organ with an incidence of 30% to 40%. The overwhelming majority of liver injuries, however, are minor, with spontaneous cessation of hemorrhage almost always the rule, and operative intervention is rarely required. On the other hand, complex hepatic injuries continue to challenge even the most experienced trauma surgeons. Hepatic injuries have been a fascinating topic since the publication of "Notes on the Arrest of Hepatic Hemorrhage Due to Trauma" in 1908 by J. Hogarth Pringle of the Glasgow Royal Infirmaries who provided the first published scientific foray into the management of severe hepatic trauma and describes one of the operative maneuvers that remains a mainstay in hepatic hemorrhage control to this day.

Perhaps the single greatest advance in the management of hepatic trauma over the past two decades has been advancement and remarkable success of nonoperative management of blunt hepatic injuries. Other advances include the combination of portal triad occlusion, finger-fracture technique (hepatotomy) and omental packing for complex hepatic injuries, and perihepatic packing with planned reexploration in trauma patients demonstrating signs of the "triad of death" (acidosis, coagulopathy, and hypothermia) as well as evolving transfusion strategies stressing 1:1:1 ratio of packed red blood cells (PRBCs), fresh frozen plasma (FFP), and platelets with the goal of prevention of intraoperative coagulopathy.

In the new millennium, a "multidisciplinary approach" concept has evolved as the standard of care in the treatment of complex hepatic trauma. In addition to prompt surgical intervention, when indicated, adjunctive interventional techniques such as hepatic angiography, endoscopic retrograde cholangiopancreatography (ERCP), biliary stenting, and percutaneous computed tomography (CT)–guided drainage have become a part of the trauma surgeon's armamentarium.

INCIDENCE

Hepatic injury occurs in approximately 5% of all trauma admissions. Nationwide, there has been a steady decline in the incidence of penetrating liver injuries. However, blunt injuries seem to be on the rise predominantly because their presence has been more readily detected by the almost routine use of CT scanning in patients sustaining blunt trauma. The incidence of complex hepatic injuries, however, has remained relatively stable over the past 25 years, ranging from 12% to 15%. Motor vehicle crashes (MVCs) continue to account for most blunt hepatic injuries (approximately 80%), followed by pedestrian and car collisions, falls, assaults, and motorcycle crashes.

Most patients with blunt hepatic trauma have associated injuries, both intra-abdominal and extraabdominal. Concomitant chest trauma is the most common associated injury encountered with blunt hepatic trauma, occurring in over 50% of patients. Patients with right-sided lower rib fractures, particularly ribs 9 to 11, have at least a 20% chance of sustaining an underlying hepatic injury. In spite of the high aforementioned incidence of associated chest trauma, injury to the brain remains the single most significant determinant in overall survival outcome. In the era of nonoperative management of blunt trauma, the risk of a missed injury, especially to the diaphragm or small bowel, is of major concern. Adherence to meticulous interpretation on imaging studies by experienced personnel should limit this pitfall to 1% to 2%.

Penetrating thoracoabdominal trauma has been noted to be associated with injuries to the liver in 30% to 40% of such injuries. The extent of the injury is directly related to the type of weapon used. Associated intra-abdominal injuries (e.g., stomach, duodenum, colon, and pancreas) are common but rarely detected preoperatively.

MECHANISM OF INJURY

Blunt Hepatic Injury

In MVCs, those most susceptible to hepatic injury are unrestrained front-seat passengers. These passengers are particularly vulnerable to a compression injury especially during periods of rapid deceleration. Although the anterior abdominal wall stops, the posterior abdominal wall continues to move forward, and the intra-abdominal organs are "trapped" and compressed, resulting in stretching/tearing of the liver at its vascular and structural attachments. As the liver is only partially protected by the rib cage, liver injury from steering wheel contact is one of the most important contributing factors to driver injury.

In lateral impact (broadside or "T-bone") collisions, the target vehicle is hit on its side and accelerated rapidly at 90 degrees to its previous direction of travel. The unrestrained passenger is subject to both compression and shear injuries that cause stretching and tearing and at times result in avulsion of the liver. Furthermore, in lateral impact injuries, because the spine and posterior abdominal wall are not in the line of impact, in contrast to frontal impact injuries, more relative motion of the intraabdominal organs ensues, resulting in a greater likelihood of injury.

Penetrating Hepatic Injury

Damage caused by a penetrating injury is based on the kinetic energy of the projectile and the density and elasticity of the tissue. Low-energy weapons such as knives only cut and do not create a temporary cavity. Medium-energy and high-energy firearms damage not only the tissue directly in the path of the missile but also the tissue on each side of the missile's path. As a missile passes through the relatively inelastic liver parenchyma, a temporary cavity (three to six times the size of the missile's front surface area, lasting for a fraction of a second) and a permanent cavity (visible to the examiner) are created.

The higher-energy firearms create larger temporary and permanent cavities, resulting in far more extensive tissue damage; the vacuum created by this larger cavity pulls clothing, bacteria, and other debris from the surrounding area into the wound as well.

DIAGNOSIS

Hemodynamically Unstable Patients

Patients who arrive with hemodynamic instability (systolic blood pressure <90 mm Hg) and who do not immediately respond to appropriate fluid resuscitation are expeditiously taken to the operating room without delay, irrespective of mechanism of injury. Further diagnostic evaluation at this point is contraindicated, as unnecessary delays inevitably follow and are often responsible for the ensuing fatalities.

In the hemodynamically unstable patient with pelvic fractures from blunt trauma, diagnostic peritoneal lavage (DPL) which has evolved to a quick screening diagnostic peritoneal aspirate (DPA)—or DPA consisting of the initial aspiration portion of the DPL only and focused assessment with sonography in trauma (FAST) are currently the diagnostic modalities used to detect the presence of intraperitoneal blood. A grossly positive aspiration on DPA (>10 mL of gross blood) mandates immediate operative intervention. In most trauma centers, FAST has replaced DPL/DPA as the preferred diagnostic modality for the determination of hemoperitoneum in the unstable bluntly injured patient. Although FAST has a 97% sensitivity for hemoperitoneum greater than 1 L, the location of the parenchymal injury cannot be reliably identified. The sensitivity of FAST drops precipitously when the quantity of intraperitoneal fluid is less than 400 mL. Kuncir and Velmahos found that the sensitivity and specificity of DPA was 89% and 100%, respectively, whereas for FAST it was significantly less at 50% and 95% in their prospective series of hemodynamically unstable patients with blunt abdominal trauma. If a FAST examination is equivocal in a hemodynamically unstable trauma patient, a rapid DPA should be performed.

Hemodynamically Stable Patients

The hemodynamically stable blunt trauma patient, on the other hand, may undergo further diagnostic studies. Hemodynamic stability, however, should not lull the trauma surgeon into a false sense of security, as significant intra-abdominal injuries may be present despite normal vital signs and a normal abdominal examination. The ability to accurately assess the presence or absence of significant intra-abdominal injuries by physical examination alone in the blunt trauma patient is notoriously poor, as up to 20% to 30% of patients with a benign abdomen on physical examination have been shown to subsequently have significant intra-abdominal injuries on imaging or at laparotomy.

CT scanning is the preferred initial diagnostic modality in the hemodynamically stable patient with blunt abdominal or lower thoracic cage injuries. High-speed resolution scanning with a spiral scanner is employed after the administration of intravenous (IV) contrast agent. In most trauma centers, oral contrast material is no longer routinely given for screening abdominal pelvic CT scan for blunt abdominal trauma. Administration of oral contrast agent is usually reserved for the focused assessment of specific hollow viscus injuries such as identification of a duodenal laceration or delineation of a duodenal hematoma. Five-millimeter cuts are obtained after 120 mL of noniodinated contrast agent (Omnipaque) is injected at a rate of 2 mL/second. Scanning commences 50 seconds after injection, a delay that corresponds to the portal venous phase of liver imaging.

Scans should immediately be interpreted and classified according to the American Association for the Surgery of Trauma Liver Injury Scale (Table 1) by the CT fellow or attending radiologist, always in the presence of the chief trauma resident and trauma attending. As a senior trauma attending usually has more experience than the designated in-house radiology resident, the surgical attending physician's initial impartial review of the CT scan is vital. The senior trauma attending in presence makes the final decision as to the appropriateness of nonoperative therapy. It should be noted that the grade of injury or degree of hemoperitoneum on CT does *not* determine the need for operative intervention, as this decision is based primarily on the patient's hemodynamic stability and the absence of peritoneal

TABLE 1: American Association for the Surgery of Trauma Liver Injury Scale

	Grade*	Injury Description	ICD-9	AIS-90
I	Hematoma	Subcapsular, <10% surface area	864.01–864.11	2
	Laceration	Capsular tear, <1 cm parenchymal depth	864.02–864.12	2
II	Hematoma	Subcapsular, 10%–50% surface area; intraparenchymal, <10 cm in diameter	864.01–864.11	2
	Laceration	1–3 cm parenchymal depth, <10 cm in length	864.03–864.13	2
III	Hematoma	Subcapsular, >50% surface area or expanding; ruptured subcapsular or parenchymal hematoma Intraparenchymal hematoma >10 cm or expanding		3
	Laceration	>3 cm parenchymal depth	864.04–864.14	3
IV	Laceration	Parenchymal disruption involving 25%–75% of hepatic lobe or 1–3 Couinaud segments within a single lobe	864.04–864.14	4
V	Laceration	Parenchymal disruption involving >75% of hepatic lobe or >3 Couinaud segments within a single lobe		5
	Vascular	Juxtahepatic venous injuries, i.e., retrohepatic vena cava/central major hepatic veins		5
VI	Vascular	Hepatic avulsion		6

From Moore E, Cogbill T, Jurkovich G, et al: Organ injury scaling: spleen and liver (1994 revision). *J Trauma* 38:323–324, 1995.
*Advance one grade for multiple injuries, up to grade III.

signs and the absence of need for laparotomy if a concomitant hollow viscus injury is identified. Instead, the CT scan merely provides the surgeon with a general anatomic overview of the injury, identifies associated abdominal injuries requiring operative intervention, and can be used as a base for comparing future healing of the hepatic injury and resorption of intraperitoneal blood. CT can also identify injuries involving the bare area of the liver, which commonly present with minimal intra-abdominal bleeding, a paucity of abdominal signs, and often a negative DPL/DPA.

The role of FAST as a screening examination in hemodynamically stable patients is evolving. Currently, many trauma centers forgo CT scanning in stable patients with negative initial FAST examinations and merely repeat the FAST in 6 hours. However, scanning for only free fluid has its diagnostic limitations because not all blunt hepatic injuries result in hemoperitoneum. In a recent study looking specifically at sonographic detection of blunt hepatic trauma, Richards et al determined the overall sensitivity of FAST for blunt hepatic injuries (all grades) to be 67%, based on the detection of free fluid alone. On the other hand, it is clear that most solid organ injuries without intraperitoneal fluid on FAST are, in general, of minimal clinical significance. At present, most trauma surgeons agree that those patients who are hemodynamically stable and who have either intraperitoneal blood on their initial FAST examination or positive findings on physical examination over the lower chest and upper abdomen should have a CT scan to specifically identify a hepatic or splenic injury that can be managed nonoperatively. Once identified, the hepatic injury may be followed with ultrasound if necessary.

Diagnostic laparoscopy (DL) is a safe procedure that has had a major impact in avoiding unnecessary abdominal explorations in patients with stab wounds or gunshot wounds that may not have penetrated the peritoneal cavity. The role of DL in patients with blunt hepatic injury is less clear. DL should allow for an accurate assessment of most hepatic injuries and, as advances in laparoscopic instrumentation progress, perhaps allow for repair of some liver injuries. However, reports of missed enteric and other intra-abdominal injuries with DL are sufficiently numerous to significantly limit the usefulness of DL.

ANATOMIC LOCATION OF INJURY AND INJURY GRADING

Comprehensive knowledge of hepatic anatomy is essential to the proper management of traumatic liver injuries. Couinaud has described the functional anatomy of the liver, based on the hepatic venous drainage (Fig. 1). The ligamentous attachments of the liver are depicted in Figure 2.

The American Association for the Surgery of Trauma (AAST) created the Organ Injury Scaling (OIS) Committee to standardize injury severity scores for individual organs to facilitate clinical investigation and outcomes research. The liver injury scale devised by the AAST is shown in Table 1.

MANAGEMENT

Nonoperative Management of Blunt Hepatic Trauma

Currently, nonoperative management of adult blunt hepatic injuries is the standard of care. Approximately 85% to 90% of all liver injuries may be successfully managed nonoperatively in both adults and the pediatric population. A recent publication examined the data on 14,919 liver injuries submitted to the National Trauma Data Bank and revealed that only 13.6% of all liver injuries underwent operation. As the grade of liver injury increased so did the likelihood of operative intervention: grades I and II = 8.5% ($n = 10,178$), grade III = 21%

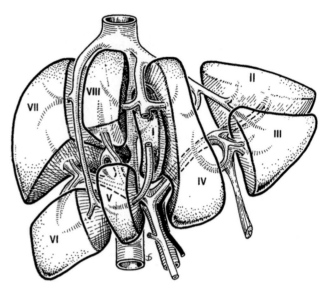

FIGURE I Functional division of the liver, according to Couinaud's nomenclature. *(From Mattox KL, Feliciano DV, Moore EE, editors: Trauma, 4th ed, New York, 1999, McGraw-Hill, Fig. 30-1. Originally appeared in Blumgart LH, editor: Surgery of the liver and biliary tract, New York, 1988, Churchill Livingstone.)*

($n = 2793$), grade IV = 27.2% ($n = 1462$), grade V = 37.4% ($n = 439$), grade VI = 42.6% ($n = 47$). Initial hemodynamic stability or hemodynamic stability achieved and maintained with moderate fluid resuscitation is the single most crucial prerequisite qualifying patients for nonoperative management. Once hemodynamic stability has been ascertained, the following criteria must be met:

- Absence of peritoneal signs
- Precise CT scan delineation and AAST grading (see Table 1)
- Absence of associated intra-abdominal or retroperitoneal injuries on CT scan that require operative intervention
- Avoidance of excessive hepatic-related blood transfusions

Previously cited inclusion criteria such as neurologic integrity are no longer valid, as neurologically impaired patients can be safely managed nonoperatively in a monitored setting. Furthermore, mandatory repeat CT scans to document improvement or stabilization of injury are unnecessary and contribute little to patient outcome. Rather, the patient's clinical course should dictate the need for additional evaluation.

Interestingly, in his landmark 1908 article describing clamping of the portal triad to arrest hepatic hemorrhage, Pringle also alluded to the physiologic tamponade provided by the abdominal wall and the potential advantage of nonoperative management in patients with less severe injuries: "The mere act of opening the abdomen, in some, at any rate, of these cases is, I feel certain, associated with an increase of the amount of blood that is lost to the patient. The blood pressure in the portal vein is not great and as the result of the local injury and the extravasation of blood there is produced reflexly a state of firm contraction of the abdominal muscles. The abdominal wall in these cases becomes absolutely rigid and board-like, the tension in the abdominal cavity thereby brought about must prevent at least a rapid escape of blood and may lead to its arrest altogether."

Today, the majority of blunt hepatic trauma patients can be successfully managed nonoperatively. Although nonoperative management was initially limited to AAST grades I to III injuries, it is now clear that the hemodynamic status of the patient, rather than AAST grade of injury, is the most significant factor in determining the need for operative intervention. Select patients with grades IV and V injuries can be managed nonoperatively. However, many grade

FIGURE 2 Surgical anatomy of the liver. *(From Mattox KL, Feliciano DV, Moore EE, editors: Trauma, 5th ed, New York, 2004, McGraw-Hill, Fig. 30-2.)*

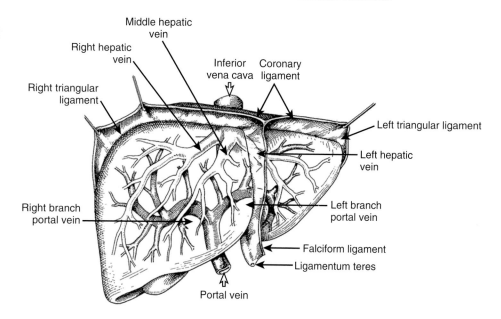

IV and V injuries will usually present with hemodynamic instability or concomitant injuries mandating surgery, thus precluding nonoperative intervention. In a multi-institutional study, grades IV and V injuries were responsible for 67% of all patients who failed nonoperative management and subsequently required operative intervention. Therefore, although hemodynamic stability determines which patients can be managed nonoperatively, the subgroup of patients with complex hepatic injuries (grades IV and V) are at substantially higher risk for treatment failure and should therefore be closely monitored in a critical care unit.

Conversely, the same basic standards apply to patients with lower AAST-grade injuries (i.e., I through III). In these instances, the initial injury may be deemed as "not significant," and thus it becomes tempting to avoid surgical intervention despite hemodynamic instability or a decreasing hematocrit, relying instead on further fluid and blood transfusions. This course of action is fraught with pitfalls and should be avoided to minimize the morbidity and mortality risks of nonoperative management. To summarize, of all the variables monitored, hemodynamic stability appears to be the most crucial and is considered the watershed for nonoperative or operative intervention.

Contrast "Blush" on Computed Tomography

Specific cause for concern is the presence on the initial CT scan, after the administration of IV contrast agent, of a contrast "extravasation," "blush," or "pooling" of contrast material within the hepatic parenchyma. This finding indicates active bleeding. Even in the context of hemodynamic stability and irrespective of AAST grade of injury, preparation for possible surgical intervention should promptly be made, as patients can suddenly and unpredictably decompensate clinically. If the patient remains hemodynamically stable, angiography with the intent of embolizing the lacerated vessel should be attempted (with an operating room on standby secured). An experienced interventional radiologist will usually have little difficulty in selectively catheterizing and embolizing the injured vessel, most often with stainless steel coils rather than Gelfoam to achieve the most dependable and permanent embolization. Successful embolization can then potentially permit further nonoperative management. As the natural history of intrahepatic vessels with evidence of extravasation is unknown, they are best dealt with immediately so that sudden bleeding, false aneurysm formation, and late hemobilia may be avoided.

Persistent and prolonged attempts at controlling the bleeding vessel through angiographic means should be discouraged. In the rare event in which angioembolization (AE) fails to control ongoing bleeding, surgical intervention using the angiogram as an anatomic marker to more rapidly achieve intrahepatic hemostasis should promptly be undertaken.

Operative Management

General Principles

The four basic principles in the management of liver trauma requiring surgery are hemostasis, adequate exposure, prevention of coagulopathy, and consideration of damage control. Débridement and the need for drainage are also important considerations. With hepatic injuries, these objectives can be reached by the use of the finger-fracture technique (hepatotomy) to incise hepatic parenchyma, often combined with temporary occlusion of the portal triad for hemostasis using the Pringle maneuver. Extensive débridement of injured hepatic tissue can then be done, followed by application of a viable pedicled omental pack and closed-suction drainage.

Before the incision is made, the patient should receive a dose of antibiotics to cover aerobic and anaerobic microbes and is placed on a warming blanket. The surgeon must keep in mind that hypothermia is a frequent complication of resuscitation and operation in patients with major hepatic injuries. Appropriate maneuvers to decrease hypothermia are shown in Table 2. Adherence to these maneuvers will usually prevent the development of intraoperative coagulopathies, excessive hemorrhage, and fatal arrhythmias secondary to hypothermia.

The skin is prepped from the chin to the knees and a standard midline incision is made. The midline incision not only affords excellent exposure of the entire liver but also provides wide access to all peritoneal and retroperitoneal structures. The combination of a long midline incision and the use of large "upper-hand" retractors have, for the most part, eliminated the need for thoracic extension of the abdominal exposure. It should be kept in mind that extending the midline incision to the sternal notch (i.e., completing a median sternotomy) exposes the patient to two open cavities with the attendant increased risks of hypothermia and coagulopathy.

Exsanguinating hemorrhage continues to remain the most immediate cause of death in patients sustaining hepatic trauma. The initial

TABLE 2: Maneuvers to Prevent/Decrease Hypothermia in Patients with Major Hepatic Injuries

Resuscitation with warm (37°–40° C) crystalloid solutions

Resuscitation with high-flow blood warmers

Covering the patient's head with plastic bags

Placing the patient on a heating blanket

Use of a Bair Hugger on the lower extremities and on chest if thoracotomy is not needed

Irrigation of open body cavities with warm saline

Use of heating cascade on anesthesia machine

Modified from Pachter H, Liang H, Hofstetter S: Liver and biliary tract trauma. In Feliciano DV, Moore EE, Mattox KL, editors: *Trauma*, 4th ed, Stamford, 2000, Appleton & Lange, p 637.

incision into the peritoneal cavity can be accompanied by profuse hemorrhage once the tamponading effect has been lost. At this time, all efforts should be directed toward intraoperative resuscitation and consideration for utilizing the technique of damage control, temporary packing of the liver, and attendant correction of coagulopathy and hypothermia in the intensive care unit (ICU) with delayed laparotomy as an adjunct. Attempts at definitive surgical hemostasis without proper intraoperative resuscitation usually results in systemic hypothermia and profound coagulation defects with their dire consequences. This fundamental pitfall should be avoided at all costs.

Irrespective of the severity of hepatic injury, almost all liver injuries can be initially managed by manually compressing the injury with lap pads (Fig. 3), while hemodynamic and metabolic stability are restored by the anesthesia team. Failure to correct hypovolemia and acidosis before attempts at surgical control will likely lead to cardiac arrest and subsequent death. Once intraoperative resuscitation has been achieved, manual compression of the liver is slowly released so that a more accurate assessment of the injury can be made.

Division of the falciform ligament allows for placement of an "upper-hand" self-retaining retractor in the incision. In order to better visualize injuries on the superior or lateral aspects of an injured hepatic lobe, it is often necessary to mobilize the liver into the midline wound. Once this is done, careful traction on its hepatic end can aid in exposing the dome of the liver and the suprahepatic inferior

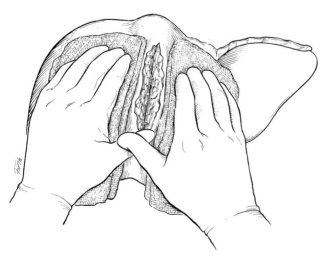

FIGURE 3 Manual compression of a severe liver injury overlap pads.

vena cava. Additional exposure is obtained by placing laparotomy pads behind the posterior surface of the liver. Mobilization of the right and left lobes proceeds with division of the triangular ligaments (Fig. 4). If there is a hematoma within the leaves of the triangular ligament, a hepatic vein or venal caval injury is most likely. If the hematoma is not expanding and there is no immediate active hemorrhage requiring control, entering a stable retrohepatic hematoma is not advised. Extreme caution must be taken even during traction as this may disrupt a stable hematoma and can create massive bleeding.

Minor Injuries (Grades I and II)

Simple techniques of controlling hemorrhage include a 5- to 10-minute period of compression, application of topical agents including fibrin glue, electrocautery/argon beam electrocoagulation, and suture hepatorrhaphy (Fig. 5). In many patients with superficial lacerations of the capsule, a 5- to 10-minute period of compression will frequently control any hemorrhage. If there is no visible leakage of bile, no further therapy is indicated. Topical agents, such as fibrin glue, Surgicel, and Avitene, are useful when avulsion of Glisson's capsule is present. Five minutes of compression with lap pads is performed after the application of a topical agent to the raw surface. After releasing compression, the electrocautery can be used for any remaining bleeders. Fibrin glue or the other hemostatic agents may be overlaid with a large Gelfoam pad creating a nonadherent surface to compress a gauze laparotomy pad against. Drainage is not necessary in the absence of obvious bile leakage.

Suture hepatorrhaphy has historically been the mainstay of hepatic hemostasis in grade II and some grade III injuries. It is important to first enter the hepatic wound and selectively ligate any open or avulsed bile ducts or blood vessels. Figure-of-eight 2-0 or 3-0 Prolene sutures are usually employed. Alternatively, 2-0 or 3-0 chronic sutures or hemoclips can also be used. Small defects in the hepatic parenchyma can be closed with simple interrupted 0-chromic or 2-0 chromic liver sutures either with regular or blunt-nosed needles (Fig. 6). For deeper lacerations, attempts at primary closure of the hepatic defect should not be undertaken. Instead, a flap of omentum on a pedicle is placed within the hepatic parenchymal defect and is then held in place with interrupted liver sutures (Fig. 7). It is important to loosely approximate the edges because portions of the liver beneath can become necrotic in the postoperative period if the sutures are tied too tightly.

Complex Injuries (Grades III and V)

If significant hemorrhage continues after the release of manual compression of the liver, the portal triad should be occluded with an atraumatic vascular clamp (the Pringle maneuver; Fig. 8). In over 85% of patients with complex hepatic injuries, occlusion of the portal triad will temporarily stop the bleeding. This maneuver, coupled with the finger-fracture technique to expose lacerated blood vessels for direct repair, is responsible for the dramatic decrease in deaths from exsanguination.

Complex hepatic injuries (grades III to V) can best be managed by adhering to several sequential crucial steps:

1. Portal triad occlusion (Pringle maneuver)
2. Finger fracture of the hepatic parenchyma (hepatotomy), exposing lacerated vessels and bile ducts for direct ligation/repair
3. Consideration of temporary packing with laparotomy pads to allow appropriate intraoperative resuscitation
4. Consideration of temporary intrahepatic packing with hemostatic agents such as surgical Nu-Knit
5. Débridement of nonviable hepatic tissue
6. Placement of an omental pedicle, with its blood supply intact, into the injury site
7. Closed-suction drainage

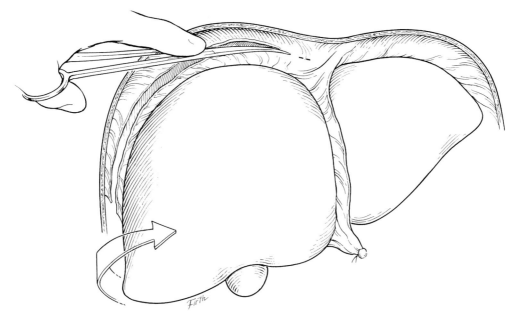

FIGURE 4 Mobilization of right triangular ligament.

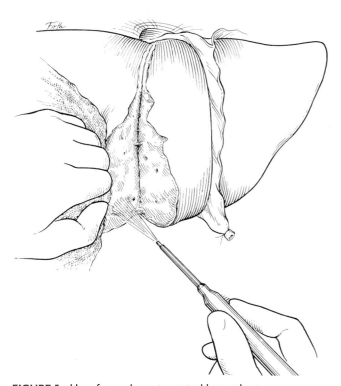

FIGURE 5 Use of argon beam to control hemorrhage.

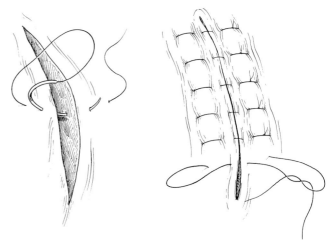

FIGURE 6 Suture hepatorrhaphy.

Much controversy has surrounded the normothermic ischemic time produced by the Pringle maneuver. The data are clear that complex hepatic injuries can be managed with continuous cross-clamping of the porta hepatis for up to 75 minutes without adverse sequelae. With portal triad occlusion achieved by an atraumatic vascular clamp, the surgeon then opens the liver parenchyma (hepatotomy) in the direction of the injury (Fig. 9). Although it initially seems crude, the finger-fracture technique constitutes the benchmark of obtaining rapid, adequate exposure. Specifically, using the electrocautery, Glisson's capsule is incised in the direction of the injury. Normal hepatic parenchyma is then crushed between the surgeon's thumb and index

finger (or a neurosurgical suction device), thereby rapidly exposing injured blood vessels and bile ducts, which are repaired or ligated under direct vision. Narrow Deaver or malleable retractors can be inserted into the hepatotomy tract for better intrahepatic exposure (Fig. 10). Large lacerated intralobar branches of the portal vein or hepatic veins can be repaired in a lateral fashion using 5-0 Prolene sutures (Fig. 11).

After intrahepatic hemostasis has been achieved, thorough débridement of devascularized hepatic tissue is essential to avoid postoperative septic complications. The use of omentum is extremely beneficial in the management of complex hepatic injuries, as it provides viable tissue to fill dead space, tamponades minor venous oozing, and provides a rich source of macrophages that may help combat infection.

The choice to drain a liver injury is controversial and debatable. If bile is noted intraoperatively, drainage is not controversial and is mandatory. The preferred method of drainage is with closed-suction Jackson-Pratt (JP) drains anterior and posterior to the injury. The data rendering drains unnecessary in elective hepatic resection cannot be applied to complex hepatic trauma, in which blood loss,

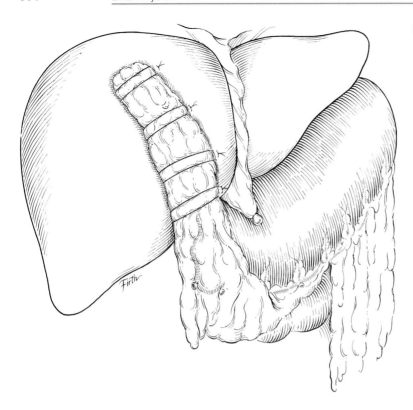

FIGURE 7   Omental packing.

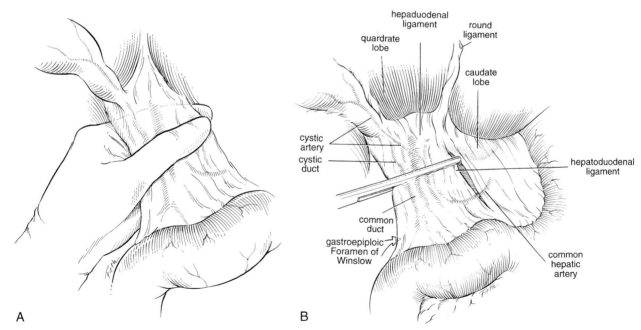

A   B

FIGURE 8   A and **B,** Pringle maneuver.

hypotension, and the frequent need to terminate surgery are the usual order of the day. In addition, the "zone" of injury may extend centimeters beyond what appears to be normal hepatic parenchyma, leading to eventual necrosis and abscess formation. Although routine drainage after elective hepatic resection may be superfluous, enough variables exist in the trauma setting to merit consideration of the use of closed-suction drains for complex hepatic injuries.

Data supporting a clear choice of drains can be found in a noteworthy publication by McSwain et al who reviewed 164 cases of liver trauma with 12 subsequent intra-abdominal abscesses at Charity Hospital and characterized the infection rates associated with various types of drainage catheters in these traumatic liver injuries. Thirty-four percent of the patients had no peritoneal drainage and an abscess rate of 1.8%. Closed-suction drains of the JP variety had the lowest associated infection rate: 18% of patients with a 0% abscess rate. Fourteen percent of patients had open Penrose drains with an infectious complication rate of 8.7%. Nineteen percent of patients had the combination of a Penrose and a sump type of drainage with the highest associated complication rate of 22.5%. Closed JP circuits are the drains of choice for hepatic trauma. Use of open drains such as

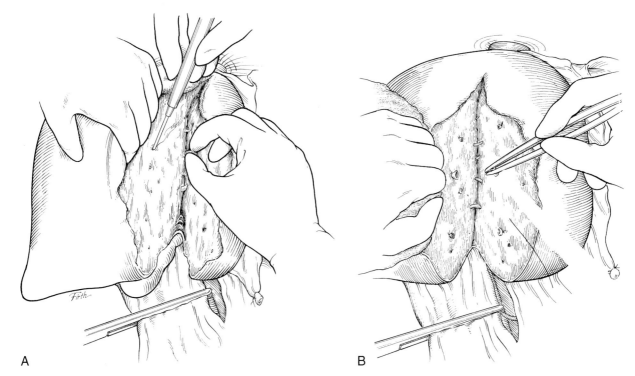

FIGURE 9 **A** and **B,** Finger-fracture technique.

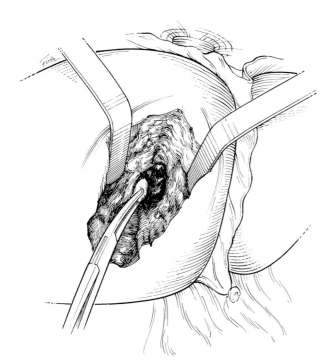

FIGURE 10 Placing Deaver retractors for better exposure.

Penrose or sump drains should be discouraged secondary to their association with unacceptably high rates of abscess formation.

Damage Control: Perihepatic Packing and Planned Reexploration

Perihepatic packing has emerged as an essential lifesaving maneuver in patients with complex injuries refractory to conventional methods of treatment and usually complicated by brisk bleeding, hypothermia (less than 34° C), acidosis (pH <7.2), and coagulation defects from massive transfusion (over 10 units PRBCs). The effectiveness of perihepatic packing is directly related to the tamponading effect of the packs on the hepatic injury. Specifically, the packs raise intraabdominal pressure (IAP), causing tamponade of low-pressure venous and nonmechanical capillary bleeding. The key to the success of perihepatic packing is to insert the packs early in the course of the operation before the onset of repeated episodes of hypotension.

Primary indications for perihepatic packing follow:

- Onset of intraoperative coagulopathy
- Extensive bilobar injuries in which bleeding cannot be controlled
- Large, expanding subcapsular hematomas or ruptured hematomas
- The necessity to terminate surgery as a result of profound hypothermia, which usually results in hemodynamic instability
- Failure of other maneuvers to control hemorrhage
- Patients who require transfer to Level I trauma centers
- Juxtahepatic venous injuries

As a general rule, the liver should be mobilized before packing to help establish a tamponading effect. If, however, a significant hematoma is encountered in the triangular ligament (indicative of a vena caval or hepatic vein injury), further mobilization is contraindicated as massive and uncontrollable bleeding may follow. Most often, dry multiple-lap pads are placed on top of the injured liver until the ipsilateral hemidiaphragm is reached (Fig. 12). In order to lessen the degree of bleeding when lap pads are peeled off the raw liver surface, an option is to routinely place a Steri-Drape (3 M, St. Paul, Minn.) directly upon the liver surface to serve as an interface between the injured liver and the lap pads. Another alternative is to place large noncompressed sheets of Gelfoam over the raw liver surface as a hemostatic adjunct which additionally provides a layer of protection preventing bleeding when the laparotomy packs are removed.

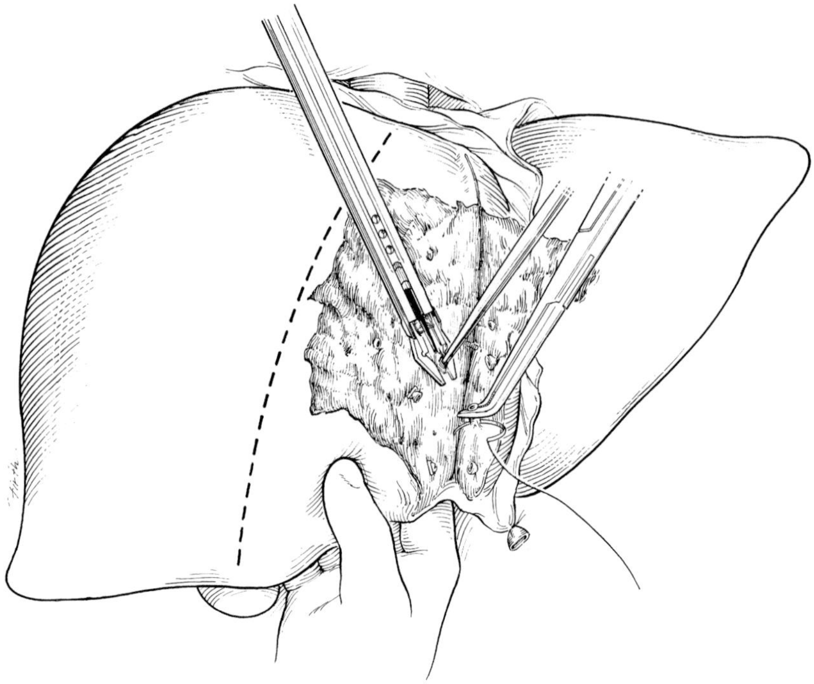

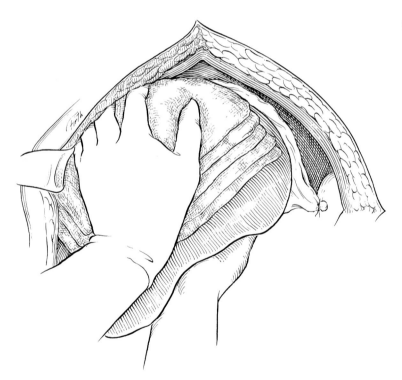

FIGURE 11   Ligating large branches with Prolene sutures or clips.

FIGURE 12   Perihepatic packing.

Resorting to packing is usually synonymous with a dire situation. Under these circumstances, rapid closure of the abdomen with towel clips can be undertaken. Several large Steri-Drapes impregnated with Betadine cover the entire incision, encompassing all towel clips. Towel-clip closure takes minutes to perform and facilitates rapid patient transfer to a critical care setting where the patient's metabolic status can be optimized. Alternatively, prosthetic abdominal wall closure with a sterilized IV bag, commonly known as a Bogata bag, can also be employed. Commercially designed wound VAC (vacuum-assisted closure) systems are also available and extremely useful with both the wound VAC and the latest version of this system—the ABThera Open Abdomen Negative Pressure Therapy System device (KCI, San Antonio, Tex.), which is now being used most of the time.

Because perihepatic packing raises IAP, monitoring IAP in the perioperative period is critical to avoid the development of an abdominal compartment syndrome (ACS). Pack removal should be dictated by the reversal of the patient's hypothermia, acidosis, and coagulopathy. These goals can usually be achieved within 36 to 48 hours. Packing has been historically associated with a 20% to 30% incidence of perihepatic sepsis. However, early pack removal, the evacuation of intraperitoneal clots, and the thorough débridement of necrotic hepatic tissue have lessened the incidence of this complication.

Juxtahepatic Venous Injuries (Grade V)

Juxtahepatic venous injuries, especially from blunt trauma, are often fatal, with mortality rates up to 50%. Failure to control hemorrhage from a deep laceration, missile tract, or stab wound with a Pringle maneuver still in place strongly suggests the presence of a juxtahepatic venous injury. Regardless of the technique used to manage these devastating injuries, early recognition is essential because prompt modification of the surgical approach is necessary.

In the past, in order to try to salvage these patients, trauma surgeons inserted an atriocaval shunt with a resultant prohibitively high mortality rate (60% to 100%). Currently, the use of atriocaval shunting has been virtually abandoned, and these difficult injuries have been, at times, successfully managed using a variety of approaches.

At present, there is a general consensus among trauma surgeons that if a retrohepatic caval injury or a hepatic venous injury (grade V) can be adequately controlled with perihepatic packing, no attempts at further repair should be initiated. When adequate resuscitation has been accomplished, there may be a role for endovascular stenting of the injury before pack removal. Even without endovascular stenting, when planned reexploration is undertaken, no further bleeding is often noted. If bleeding occurs after pack removal, definitive treatment can then be undertaken with the knowledge that the patient's hemodynamic status has been optimized and that adequate personnel are available if a vascular shunt is necessary.

Another approach is direct hepatotomy through Cantlie line to reach the injured retrohepatic cava or hepatic veins. After manual compression, vigorous resuscitation, and prolonged portal triad occlusion, mobilization of the liver is performed with medial rotation, thus providing access to the retrohepatic cava and hepatic veins. Rapid and extensive finger fracture should be directed toward the site of injury until the lacerated retrohepatic cava or hepatic vein is found and repaired under direct vision. The surgeon must be prepared to finger fracture the hepatic parenchyma through normal and frequently nonanatomic planes. Because these patients usually have injured hepatic parenchyma as well, portal triad occlusion serves two purposes: it contributes to controlling hemorrhage from intrahepatic branches of the hepatic artery and portal vein, and it decreases the inflow to the liver, thereby aiding finger fracture and minimizing blood loss.

A third approach comprises venovenous bypass, vascular exclusion, and primary repair. Total vascular isolation of the liver via venovenous bypass (combined with the Pringle maneuver and clamping of the suprarenal and suprahepatic cava) permits direct suture repair of the venous injury. The advantage here is that vascular isolation with venovenous bypass obviates the need for an intracaval shunt. Cannulation for bypass can be done peripherally via saphenous vein and axillary vein cutdowns. Venovenous bypass has been used in a small number of severe retrohepatic liver injuries with an overall survival rate of 88%.

Next is total hepatic resection and delayed liver transplantation. Total hepatectomy and second-stage hepatic transplantation can be a drastic yet lifesaving maneuver for devastating liver injuries that have failed all conventional treatments. Perihepatic packing and total hepatectomy with portacaval shunting can be performed in the primary hospital; the anhepatic patient can then be transferred to a transplant center for eventual liver transplant. Although this radical maneuver can be associated with high morbidity and mortality rates, the prognosis is better if the decision to proceed with total hepatectomy and portacaval shunting is made before the development of intractable multiorgan failure.

Portal Triad Injuries

As exsanguination is the most common (85%) cause of death in these highly lethal and complex injuries, the first priority in portal triad trauma is hemorrhage control, specifically manual compression followed by the Pringle maneuver. A wide Kocher maneuver and mobilization of the hepatic flexure will allow medial rotation of the ascending colon to better expose the portal structures. Exposure of a retropancreatic portal vein injury may require pancreatic transection with distal pancreatectomy after the vascular repair is complete. Although portal vein ligation can be used to expeditiously manage portal vein injuries, the preferred treatment is lateral venorrhaphy, as most series report a 51% to 60% survival rate with this approach.

Hepatic artery injuries should generally be managed with ligation. However, the hepatic parenchyma must be evaluated for ischemia after ligation, especially in the presence of portal vein injury or shock. In addition, the gallbladder should be removed if the hepatic artery is ligated. Partial extrahepatic bile duct injuries (less than 50% circumference) may be primarily repaired, with or without stenting. However, complete or complex bile duct injuries are best managed by Roux-en-Y biliary-enteric anastomosis. For the unstable patient, ligation with external drainage and delayed reconstruction is a reasonable approach.

Adjuncts to Operative Management

The original description of the multidisciplinary approach to the management of complex hepatic injuries by Asensio and colleagues described an approach consisting in immediate surgical intervention utilizing the most complex techniques in the surgical armamentarium including extensive hepatotomy, hepatography and selective deep vessel ligation, nonanatomic resection and débridement, and even hepatectomy along with packing temporary abdominal closure followed by immediate angiography and AE ligation with the ICU team present in the angiography suite to continue the resuscitation process. Afterward, patients were returned to the operating room after their physiologic defects were corrected for unpacking, further hepatic débridement, and nonanatomic or anatomic resection, drainage, and abdominal wall closure. Postoperative complications were treated with the use of percutaneous CT-guided drainage of hepatic collections and ERCP and stenting of major biliary leaks that were detected.

Subsequently, Asensio et al separated their results on 103 patients with AAST-OIS grade IV to V injuries in which they advocated early hepatic angiography and AE in all patients with grades IV and V hepatic injuries. Improved survival was associated with immediate surgery to control life-threatening hemorrhage, the institution of early hepatic packing when necessary, and subsequent patient transport directly from the operating room to the angiography suite for immediate hepatic AE. Clearly, AE is essential in the management of complex hepatic injuries, whether they arise from blunt or penetrating mechanisms.

In the only prospective study in the literature Asensio et al used their multidisciplinary approach in the management of 75 AASI-OIS grades IV and V complex hepatic injuries and confirmed the value of this approach as well as the value of angiography and AE and reported significant improvements in the survival rates for these injuries; 81% for grades IV and 43% for grade V.

Early AE may also be useful in the multiply injured patient whose hepatic injury is being managed nonoperatively but whose serial hematocrits are noted to be dropping. Under these circumstances, the patient should immediately undergo repeat CT scanning, rather than arbitrarily receive incremental blood transfusions. If the repeat CT scan confirms that the liver injury has deteriorated and the patient remains hemodynamically stable, then AE should be attempted. Failure of AE to arrest ongoing hemorrhage or hemodynamic instability at any given time should prompt immediate laparotomy.

Late angiography is therapeutic in the presence of hemobilia, bleeding emanating from abdominal drains in the postoperative period, and vascular abnormalities noted when follow-up CT scan is indicated.

An interesting recent publication by the Western Trauma Association provides an overview of the critical decisions in operative management of blunt hepatic trauma and a suggested treatment algorithm. These recommendations are based on available published prospective, observational, and retrospective data and expert opinion of Western Trauma Association members in an effort to disseminate the expertise of this consortium of senior trauma surgeons. Interestingly, given the success of nonoperative management of hepatic trauma over the last few decades, the surgical resident finishing in the current era has little experience in managing hepatic injuries in the operating room. In their recent publication "The academic challenge of teaching psychomotor skills for hemostasis of solid organ injury," Lucas and Ledgerwood report that on average a graduating resident will perform an operative hemostatic technique only 1.2 times during the course of an entire surgical residency. As operating on liver injuries becomes less and less common, detailed illustrations such as those provided in this chapter become more important in providing training and education, as do hands-on and interactive courses such as the American College of Surgeons Advanced Trauma Operative Management (ATOM) Course.

Nonoperative Management of Penetrating Hepatic Trauma

Most penetrating civilian injuries to the liver result in a lesser degree of parenchymal damage than do those incurred by blunt trauma, at least by AAST criteria. Therefore, it seems logical that nonoperative management of a penetrating isolated hepatic injury would be successful in hemodynamically stable patients without evidence of peritonitis.

Renz and Feliciano nonoperatively managed 13 patients with penetrating right thoracoabdominal gunshot wounds. The authors stressed the importance of serial abdominal examinations and contrast-enhanced CT scanning in their successful nonoperative management. Demetriades et al substantiated this concept with their successful management of select patients with isolated gunshot injuries to the liver. These authors concluded that hemodynamically stable patients with grades I and II liver injuries and no evidence of peritonitis can be safely managed nonoperatively. However, it should be noted that this approach failed in nearly one third (5 of 16) of the patients in the "observed group" who eventually required delayed laparotomy.

Omoshoro-Jones et al described successful nonoperative management in 31 of 33 patients with gunshot wounds to the liver, including grades III to V injuries. Although the higher grade injuries were associated with more complications (most of which were managed nonoperatively), the overall success of nonoperative management did not depend on the AAST grade of liver injury. Most recently, the same group from USC/LAC describes their experience from 2005 to 2007 when 178 patients with penetrating liver injuries were assessed. Overall, 142 (79.8%) patients had associated intra-abdominal injuries, with the diaphragm being the most commonly injured organ (39.3%), followed by the stomach (30.9%), and the colon/rectum (29.2%). Fifty-five of 178 (30.9%) patients were hemodynamically stable and without signs of peritonitis on admission permitting a CT scan evaluation. On the basis of these CT findings, 30 (54.5%) were considered isolated liver injuries and were selected for a nonoperative management (two patients in this group underwent AE), and 25 (45.5%) subsequently underwent laparotomy. Of the 30 patients selected for nonoperative management, one (3.3%) patient with a grade II liver injury failed nonoperative management due to a missed small colon injury after a gunshot wound (false-negative CT finding). The patient underwent primary repair 9 hours after admission and was subsequently discharged without any postoperative complication. Overall, 16.2% (29 of 178) of all penetrating liver injuries, including six cases with grades III to V, or 80.6% (29 of 36), patients with isolated liver injuries were successfully managed nonoperatively. Three patients with high-grade injuries were treated successfully nonoperatively.

The authors concluded that two thirds of patients with penetrating liver injuries require emergent laparotomy due to hemodynamic instability, peritonitis, or inability to evaluate an abdomen and therefore are not amenable for consideration of CT scan evaluation. One third of patients with penetrating liver injuries were amenable for CT evaluation, which reliably predicted successful nonoperative management. However, the authors warn that hollow viscus injuries may remain undetected, and suggest that a high index of suspicion and that serial examinations of the abdomen and monitoring of white blood cell count are critical in all patients selected for nonoperative management, irrespective of the initial clinical examination and CT scan findings.

Clearly, the most difficult aspect in the nonoperative management of penetrating hepatic trauma is patient selection, as only up to 30% of those with gunshot wounds to the liver are eligible for nonoperative management to begin with. Also, given the majority of the nonoperative experience published hails from a single high-volume center, the risks of a missed concurrent injury in this patient population must be weighed against those of a nontherapeutic laparotomy for their liver injury. At the very least, hemodynamic stability, an intact level of consciousness to allow serial abdominal examinations, absence of peritoneal signs, and no evidence of active bleeding on CT are required for successful nonoperative management.

MORBIDITY AND COMPLICATIONS MANAGEMENT

Failure of Nonoperative Management

Nonoperative management of adult blunt hepatic injuries has resulted in a survival rate approaching 100%. Overall complication rates in most series range from 0% to 13%. As the mortality rate associated with nonoperative management essentially is 0%, focus has shifted to the delineating and managing the associated morbidity. Primary hepatic morbid conditions include bleeding, biliary complications, ACS, and infection complications.

In a recent large multicenter study reported by Kozar et al, early risk factors for hepatic related morbid conditions associated with attempted nonoperative management were identified. In their series of 699 patients, 453 (65%) were treated nonoperatively; 13% developed complications. Most common hepatic complications included bleeding (35 patients with 38 bleeding complications; 8%), biliary complications (17 patients with 29 biliary complications; 6.5%), ACS (5 patients; 1%), and infectious complications (15 patients; 3%). Bleeding and ACS tended to develop early—within 3 days after injury; but biliary and infectious complications tended to develop late—greater than 3 days after injury. Hepatic complications developed in 5% (13 of 264) of patients with grade III injuries, 22% (36 of 166) of patients with grade IV injuries, and 52% (12 of 23) of patients with grade V injuries. Univariate analysis revealed the following significant variables associated with development of a complication: 24-hour crystalloid, total and first 24-hour PRBCs, FFP, platelet, and cryoprecipitate requirements and liver injury grade. When subjected to multivariate analysis; liver injury grade (grade IV odds ratio, 4.439; grade V odds ratio, 12.001) and 24-hour transfusion requirements (odds ratio, 6.446) predicted complications associated with nonoperative management.

Early Complications: Hemorrhage and Abdominal Compartment Syndrome

Hemorrhage

Hemorrhage complicating the nonoperative management of hemodynamically stable patients with blunt injuries occurs at a frequency of 5% to 10%. Rates of bleeding are particularly low when a helical contrast-enhanced CT scan fails to show an active blush. Active blush on CT scan mandates AE even when a patient's physiology does not show any current signs of decompensated shock in a preemptive measure to ensure that the patient maintains an acceptable state of hemodynamics. For the most part, failed nonoperative management follows a predictable pattern of ongoing hemorrhage, rather than sudden decompensation. Most failures of nonoperative management secondary to bleeding occur within the first 24 hours. The reported incidence of delayed hemorrhage requiring laparotomy is well under 2% to 3%.

Bleeding after operative management of hepatic injuries is usually not subtle as evidenced by hemodynamic instability that can also be accompanied by brisk bleeding from operatively placed intraperitoneal drains. However, a more subtle presentation is the hemodynamically stable patient with a partially distended abdomen accompanied by a decreasing hematocrit. In the past, reoperation to control bleeding from within the injured liver was promptly undertaken after correction of acidosis, hypothermia, and coagulation defects. Currently, in the absence of hemodynamic instability, AE is the preferred treatment.

In the hemodynamically unstable postoperative patient, reexploration is warranted. The same techniques apply, namely manual compression of the liver with concomitant intraoperative resuscitation, the Pringle maneuver, and finger fracture, if necessary, through the repaired area. If there is a concern that extensive hepatotomy may sever major vascular structures or hepatic bile ducts, persistent bleeding may be controlled by extralobar hepatic arterial ligation or balloon tamponade with Penrose and red rubber catheters. If a diligent search has failed to reveal a mechanical source of bleeding, a transfusion-related coagulopathy is the most likely culprit. Under these circumstances, packing of the injured liver should be undertaken rapidly, following the guidelines for packing removal as described earlier.

Findings from recent military data have revolutionized transfusion practices and contribute to a higher likelihood of prevention of coagulopathy and thus cessation and prevention of hemorrhage. Current transfusion practices of a ratio of 1:1 of FFP to PRBCs have shown to significantly decrease coagulopathy and have had a remarkable impact on overall mortality rate. Although the prior practices of PRBCs to FFP ratios of 4:1 having an overall mortality rate of greater than 65% the single variable of decreasing the ratio of PRBCs to FFP to 1:1.8 was associated with an overall mortality rate of 19%. The goal target ratio of PRBCs to FFP is now agreed upon to be 1:1 with an ideal range of 1:1 to 1:1.8. More frequent platelet administration is also warranted, although the ideal ratio has not yet been identified. These changes in transfusion practices have had a marked impact upon controlling coagulation defects and managing hemorrhage from hepatic injuries, although the specific effects of this new approach in transfusion practices on outcomes in higher grade hepatic injuries has yet to be delineated.

Abdominal Compartment Syndrome

ACS secondary to hepatic injury is a relatively uncommon complication of nonoperative management of liver injuries developing at a rate of approximately 1% and tends to declare itself within 1 to 3 days after injury. More likely, the patient would require operative intervention for hemodynamic instability secondary to ongoing hemorrhage into the peritoneal cavity rather than develop an ACS. The most common cause of ACS secondary to hepatic trauma is patients who have their hemorrhage controlled by AE but who in the course of resuscitation receive a significant amount of blood products. Patients undergoing resuscitation for significant hepatic injuries should have their bladder pressures measured as a matter of routine protocol. Just as patients undergoing hepatic packing are at risk for increased IAPs and ACS, the nonoperatively managed patient is also at risk for ACS and must be closely monitored with a high index of suspicion. The appropriate treatment for most cases of ACS is decompressive laparotomy.

Late Complications: Biliary and Infectious

Looking at all the studies to date; biliary and infectious complications run neck in neck, with rates averaging 3% to 6% for both, depending on the series. Interestingly, the recent multicenter trial evaluating the morbidity associated with nonoperative management of hepatic injuries found that both complications can develop quite late in the patient's course. Biliary complications developed at a mean of 12 days after injury with a range of 2 to 38 days. Infectious complications on average developed on postinjury day 15 with a range of 1 to 90 days.

Bile Collections/Biliary Fistula

Nonoperative management of blunt hepatic injuries can be associated with the development of a collection of bile (biloma) or the formation of a biliary fistula. Although leakage of bile from lacerated biliary radicals after hepatic injuries occurs commonly, the reported incidence of clinically significant bile leaks is low (2%–3%). Extravasation of bile demonstrated on nuclear imaging (hepatobiliary iminodiacetic acid [HIDA] scan) rarely requires operative intervention, as percutaneous drainage is usually successful. The key to the management of bile leaks is adequate closed-suction drainage. Even a biliary fistula (>50 mL/day over 14 days) that is adequately drained usually closes spontaneously. When biliary fistulas fail to resolve, ERCP with stent or sphincterotomy should be performed. A recent series from Anand et al describes their experience with 26 patients who underwent ERCP for the management of biliary fistula as result of severe hepatic trauma. They report a 100% success rate for controlling bile leaks. Fifty-four percent of the injuries were secondary to blunt abdominal trauma; the remainder were due to a penetrating mechanism. ERCP combined with sphinterotomy was used to treat biliary fistula in association with CT or ultrasound-guided drainage of bilomas or other perihepatic fluid collections. ERCP resulted in an average decrease of 72% in bilious drainage within 2 days. No patients suffered a complication as a result of the ERCP. This study is the largest to date supporting ERCP and sphincterotomy as a useful therapeutic intervention resulting in the highly successful management of biliary fistula.

Thoracobiliary fistula is a rare complication of penetrating thoracoabdominal trauma. The responsible mechanism is usually a missed or deliberate nonrepair of small diaphragmatic lesion. Percutaneous drainage of the chest collection combined with endoscopic sphincterotomy is almost always curative. It should be stressed, however, that early diagnosis is critical to avoid the corrosive effect of bile on the lungs and pleural space.

Hemobilia

Hemobilia is an uncommon complication of hepatic trauma, occurring at most in 1%. Hemobilia may result from blunt or penetrating trauma or iatrogenically induced by deep suture hepatorrhaphy. Signs and symptoms of gastrointestinal hemorrhage, right upper quadrant pain, and jaundice (Sandblom triad) may occur 4 days to 1 month after injury. Repeat endoscopy is usually unrevealing. In this setting, a history of trauma mandates celiac angiography. If hemobilia is the cause of the bleeding, angiography will demonstrate a hepatic artery pseudoaneurysm that can be embolized with steel coils, Gelfoam, or acrylate glue. Coils form the most permanent embolization when other methods may recannulize and present a risk of rebleeding. Surgical intervention is rarely necessary and not necessarily advisable secondary to the difficulty associated with anatomically accessing the bleeding vessel, which is often deep within the hepatic parenchyma, unless hemobilia is either associated with a large intrahepatic cavity or angiography is not available. If surgery is required, the optimal treatment is hepatic resection encompassing the large cavity and the pseudoaneurysm. Vascular control (by intraoperative Pringle maneuver or direct ligation of the hepatic artery) is essential before attempting to débride or resect large intrahepatic cavities associated with hepatic artery pseudoaneurysms.

Injury to the Intrahepatic Bile Ducts and Late Stricture

Injuries to the intrahepatic bile ducts are rare. The long-term sequelae of spontaneous healing of the injured hepatic parenchyma surrounding both normal and disrupted intrahepatic bile ducts are presently unknown. Although disruption of secondary and tertiary biliary radicals within the liver occurs often, late intrahepatic bile duct stricture formation is an exceedingly rare occurrence.

Perihepatic Sepsis/Abscess

Perihepatic sepsis/abscess associated with complex hepatic injuries is a late complication and develops at a rate of 3% to 6%. Perihepatic sepsis, especially in the multiply injured patient, can lead to septic shock formation, systemic inflammatory response syndrome, and multiple organ failure, placing the patient at risk for a late death in the final classic trimodal trauma fatalities as described by Baker and Trunkey. Noninfectious factors can also initiate severe inflammatory responses that may culminate in multiple organ failure and death.

A variety of risk factors for postoperative abscesses after hepatic trauma have been identified, including associated enteric injuries, extent of parenchymal damage, transfusion requirements, and inadequate débridement/drainage at the initial operation. For the most part, the rate of hepatic abscess formation in operatively managed hepatic trauma can be significantly reduced with meticulous hemostasis, adequate débridement of nonviable hepatic parenchyma, and avoiding open-suction drainage.

Most abscesses can be drained percutaneously. Failure of the septic patient to improve within 24 to 36 hours after percutaneous drainage is a compelling reason to repeat the CT scan to determine if the catheter needs to be readjusted or whether operative intervention is needed. If surgery is required, the abscess cavity should be unroofed, devitalized tissue débrided, and closed-suction drainage established. Rarely, resectional débridement or frank lobectomy may be required to eradicate either an infected biloma or abscess cavity.

Postobservational Computed Tomography Scanning

The physiology of hepatic repair after blunt injury progresses in a predictable fashion that results in virtually complete restoration of hepatic integrity at the end of 3 months. There is general agreement that postobservational scanning in patients with grades I and II injuries contributes little to the clinical management of asymptomatic patients. In patients with grades III to V injuries, repeat CT scan or ultrasound, showing resolution of the injury, can serve as an invaluable guide in identifying patients for whom critical care monitoring may no longer be necessary. The optimal time frame for follow-up CT scan in these patients, if necessary, is 7 to 10 days after the original injury.

Resumption of Normal Activities

Dulchavsky et al demonstrated in experimental models that hepatic wound bursting strength at 3 weeks after injury was comparable and often exceeded wound bursting strength of normal hepatic parenchyma. Moreover, healing by secondary intention resulted in wound bursting strength equal or greater than hepatorrhaphy or hepatorrhaphy and omental packing at 3 and 6 weeks. The healing mechanism responsible for the increased wound bursting strengths appears to be the proliferative fibrosis throughout the injured hepatic parenchyma and the overlying Glisson's capsule. Hepatic parenchymal healing appears to be virtually complete at 6 to 8 weeks after injury. A reasonable and safe approach to pursue would be to allow patients with grade III or greater injury to resume normal activities after CT scan documentation, at 3 months, of major injury resolution.

MORTALITY

The overall liver-related mortality rate in most large series of nonoperatively managed blunt hepatic injuries is 0.5%. When blunt hepatic injuries are stratified by severity, it is clear that with the exception of grades IV and V injuries, it is the associated organ injuries, specifically brain and cardiopulmonary injury, which ultimately affect mortality rates. In most large series of blunt hepatic injuries, associated brain injuries account for most (60% to 70%) of the deaths.

Most liver-related fatalities result from complex hepatic trauma (grades IV and V), especially juxtahepatic venous injuries and portal triad injuries, which often result in prohibitively high mortality rates. Over the past 2 decades, the mortality rate of complex hepatic injuries has decreased, predominantly because of a reduction in deaths from liver hemorrhage. Responsible contributing factors include prolonged inflow occlusion times, hepatotomy with selective vascular ligation, early packing and reexploration, and adjunctive interventional procedures, especially hepatic artery AE.

CONCLUSIONS AND MANAGEMENT ALGORITHM

Nonoperative management can be used to successfully manage most blunt hepatic trauma patients and a select group of penetrating hepatic trauma patients. The cornerstone of nonoperative management is hemodynamic stability. An active "blush" on contrast-enhanced CT mandates immediate angiography, irrespective of CT grade of injury. Successful embolization of the lesion usually permits continued nonoperative management. Should the patient under observation become hemodynamically unstable or develop peritoneal signs, operative intervention should be undertaken without the slightest hesitation.

When the liver injury requires operative intervention, four essential maneuvers should be kept in mind: (1) manual compression of the injury, (2) resuscitation, (3) assessment of the injury, and (4) the Pringle maneuver (inflow occlusion). These maneuvers can be lifesaving, even in the hands of those with limited experience in this area. Complex hepatic injuries (grades IV and V) continue to challenge trauma surgeons and tax the resources of trauma centers. Most of these patients are hemodynamically unstable, have multiple associated injuries, require massive blood transfusions, and have a significant mortality rate. Nevertheless, surgeons should be familiar with five critical approaches if patients are to be salvaged:

- Hepatotomy and hepatorrhaphy
- Packing and planned reexploration
- Nonanatomic and anatomic resection
- AE
- Endoscopic retrograde cholangiography, papillotomy, and endostenting

Algorithms for the management of hepatic injuries are shown in Figures 13 and 14.

For the chapter's Suggested Readings list, please visit the book at www.ExpertConsult.inkling.com.

FIGURE 13   Algorithm for management of blunt hepatic injury. CT, Computed tomography; ICU, intensive care unit. *(Modified from Feliciano DV, Moore EE, Mattox KL, editors: Trauma, 3rd ed, Stamford, Conn., 1996, Appleton & Lange, p 643.)*

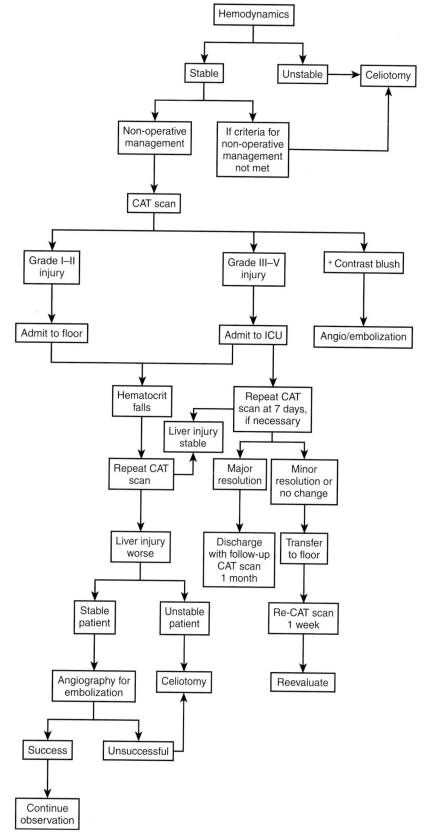

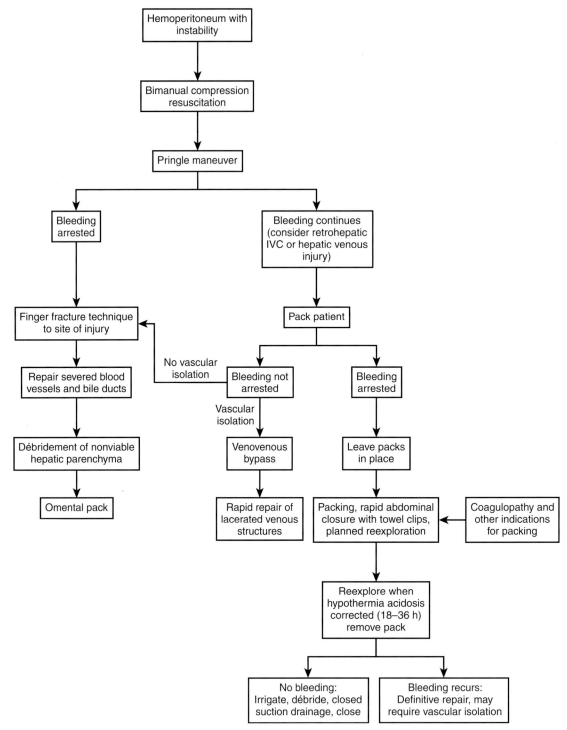

FIGURE 14 Algorithm for the intraoperative management of complex hepatic injuries. IVC, Inferior vena cava.

Splenic Injuries

Joseph M. Galante and David H. Wisner

The spleen has had a prominent role in medical theory and practice throughout history. The Greeks and Romans believed that the spleen played a role in filtering the humors of the body, mirroring some of our modern concepts. During the middle of the last millennium, the Thuggee cult, who worshipped Kali, a Hindu goddess of destruction, were professional assassins, and the act of murder for hire was an act of worship for their goddess. They were most famous for their use of the noose, but also targeted the left upper quadrant where the spleen, often fragile and swollen from malaria, lay. A well-placed blow leading to splenic rupture in the absence of transfusions and modern surgery often proved fatal.

As our understanding of splenic injury has increased, our management of splenic injuries has evolved. Thus, we have steadily moved away from routine aggressive operative management toward nonoperative management. With this evolution, it is still important to keep in mind that splenic injuries can be deadly and patients with damage to the spleen can bleed to death just as they did in the time of the Thuggee.

INCIDENCE AND MECHANISM OF INJURY

The spleen is frequently listed, as either the first or second most commonly injured solid viscus in the abdomen after blunt trauma. Before the advent of computed tomography (CT) scanning, splenic injury was listed as the most commonly injured intra-abdominal solid viscus. As CT scanning became commonplace, it was apparent that the liver is also commonly injured and some series now list hepatic injuries as more common than splenic injuries. Regardless, there needs to remain a high index of suspicion for splenic injuries. One large, multi-institutional study showed a 2.6% incidence of splenic injuries (6308 of 227,656 patients) for all patients evaluated for trauma, with splenic injury confirmed by either laparotomy or CT.

Splenic injuries occur via three mechanisms: penetrating, blunt, and indirect trauma. For penetrating trauma, retrospective reviews of two large centers, Grady Memorial Hospital and Ben Taub General Hospital, showed the incidence of splenic injury from abdominal gunshot wounds to be 7% to 9%, far less than for the hollow organs and the liver. Injuries to the spleen from stab wounds are even less frequent.

Blunt splenic injuries can bleed either immediately or on a delayed basis, a phenomenon of obvious importance in patients treated nonoperatively. The incidence of delayed bleeding, leading to failure of nonoperative therapy, varies depending on the grade of the injury. One hypothesis for the pathophysiology leading to delayed bleeding is that as subcapsular clot breaks down several days after injury into its component parts, the number of osmotically active particles in the area increases and draws more fluid into the area of injury. The resultant increase in size of the area then exceeds the tensile strength of the capsule, leading to rupture and renewed bleeding. Even without being trapped under the capsule of the spleen, the inflammation and fibrinolysis in and around the healing injury and clot may weaken the clot enough to result in renewed hemorrhage.

A third mechanism of injury to the spleen is indirect trauma, specifically during colonoscopy. This is a subtle, frequently unrecognized and underreported complication of routine colonoscopy. Traction on the splenocolic ligament causes a tear in the splenic capsule. Although this is a rare injury mechanism, it has a reported mortality rate of 5%

and requires the same management algorithm used in other types of splenic trauma.

DIAGNOSIS

As with any other trauma patient, the initial management of the patient with splenic injury should follow the ABCs (airway, breathing, and circulation) of trauma resuscitation. A particularly important general comment relative to initial resuscitation is that it is important to recognize refractory shock early and treat it with an appropriate operative response.

In the initial history taking, it is important to note any previous operations the patient has undergone, especially a history of splenectomy. History of direct blows to the lower left chest or left upper abdomen, with concomitant pain, may engender suspicion for splenic injury. Any preexisting conditions that might predispose the spleen to enlargement or other abnormalities also should be ascertained if possible. The patient or significant others should be asked about the presence of liver or portal venous disease, ongoing anticoagulation, propensity for bleeding, or a recent history of aspirin or nonsteroidal antiinflammatory drug use.

On physical examination, it is important to determine if the patient has left rib pain or tenderness. The left lower ribs are particularly important in that they overlie the spleen, especially posteriorly. In children, the plasticity of the chest wall allows for severe underlying injury to the spleen without the presence of overlying rib fractures. Older patients may not report lower rib pain and may not have particularly noteworthy findings on physical examination in spite of severe chest wall trauma and an underlying splenic injury. Examination of the abdomen can demonstrate localized tenderness in the left upper quadrant or generalized abdominal tenderness, but not all patients with splenic injury will reliably manifest peritoneal or other findings on physical examination. Bleeding without clot formation may not generate peritonitis that can be easily elicited. The unreliability of the physical examination is obvious in patients with altered mental status. As a consequence, imaging of the abdomen in hemodynamically stable patients has become an important element of diagnosis and management.

Diagnostic peritoneal lavage (DPL), once a mainstay diagnostic technique after abdominal trauma, is much less frequently used now. Its role as an initial diagnostic maneuver to dictate subsequent testing or operative intervention has been supplanted in many institutions by ultrasonography and CT scanning of the abdomen. Peritoneal lavage remains useful when ultrasonography is not available or reliable, in that it is a quick way of determining whether a hemodynamically unstable patient is bleeding intraperitoneally.

Ultrasound of the abdomen for free fluid, the FAST (focused assessment with sonography in trauma) examination is used frequently as a means of diagnosing hemoperitoneum in blunt trauma patients. Like DPL, it is most useful in unstable patients. As with peritoneal lavage, the ability of ultrasound to determine exactly what is bleeding in the peritoneal cavity is limited. Attempts to image specific organ injuries using ultrasound have met with limited success. The most common method of using FAST is for detection of intraperitoneal fluid and as a determinant of the need for either further imaging of the abdomen or emergency surgery (Fig. 1).

CT of the abdomen is the dominant means of nonoperative diagnosis of splenic injury (Figs. 2 to 4). Patients are sent either directly for abdominal CT scanning after initial resuscitation or are screened by abdominal ultrasonography as reasonable candidates for subsequent CT. When abdominal CT scanning is done, intravenous contrast is quite helpful in diagnosis; oral contrast is less helpful and does not measurably increase the sensitivity of CT for splenic injury detection.

A CT finding in the spleen that has received a great deal of attention is the presence in the disrupted splenic parenchyma of a "blush," or hyperdense area with a collection of contrast agent in it. When

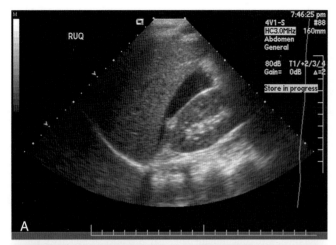

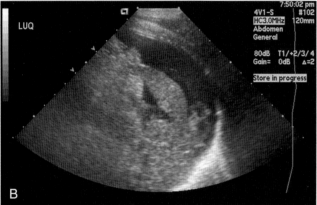

FIGURE 1 Focused assessment with sonography in trauma (FAST). Fluid in Morison pouch. The fluid is the dark area between the posteriorly located kidney and the anteriorly located liver (**A**). Fluid is around the spleen in the left upper quadrant. The fluid is the dark area located laterally (**B**).

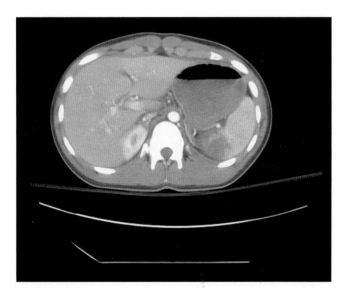

FIGURE 2 Computed tomography findings in blunt splenic injury, grade III. The posterior and inferior aspect of the splenic parenchyma is disrupted with the formation of a subcapsular hematoma.

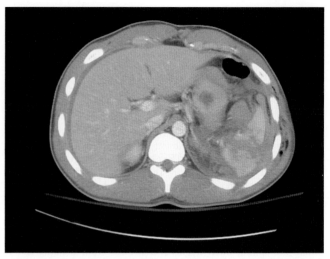

FIGURE 3 Computed tomography findings in blunt splenic injury, grade IV, show a laceration through the parenchyma of the spleen with disruption of the capsule.

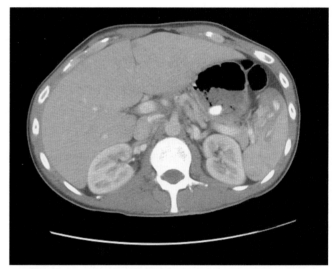

FIGURE 4 Computed tomography findings in blunt splenic injury, grade III, show a laceration through the anterior portion of the spleen with a "blush" in the parenchyma.

present, a blush is thought to represent ongoing bleeding with active extravasation of contrast material. There is some evidence that the presence of a blush correlates with an increased likelihood of continued or delayed bleeding from the splenic parenchyma and the risk of failing nonoperative management when this finding is present has been reported to be higher than when a blush is not present. Such a finding does not mandate altering the initial management of the hemodynamically stable patient, however, especially in the pediatric population, but it should heighten concerns about failure of nonoperative management (Fig. 5).

Anatomic Location of Injury and Injury Grading: American Association for the Surgery of Trauma Organ Injury Scale

Histologically, the spleen is divided into what has been termed *red pulp* and *white pulp*. The red pulp is a series of large passageways that filter old red blood cells and also catch bacteria. The filtering of

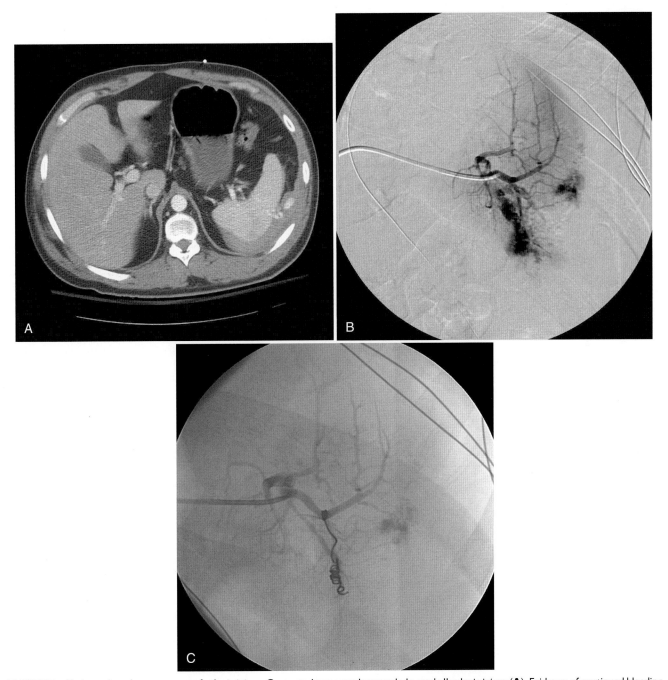

FIGURE 5 Catheter-based management of splenic injury. Computed tomography revealed a grade II splenic injury (**A**). Evidence of continued bleeding led to angiography. The angiogram demonstrated active extravasation (**B**), and the injured area was treated with embolization (**C**).

bacteria in the interstices of the red pulp allows the antigens of the bacterial walls to be presented to lymphocytes in the adjacent white pulp. The white pulp is filled largely with lymphocytes located such that they can be exposed to antigens either on microorganisms or moving freely in the circulation. Lymphocyte exposure to antigens results in the production of immunoglobulins, the most common of which is IgM.

The spleen develops initially as a bulge on the left side of the dorsal mesogastrium and begins a gradual leftward migration to the left upper quadrant. It changes in relative size during maturation. As the child's bone marrow matures, the spleen becomes relatively less important and diminishes in size relative to the rest of the body. There are also some important differences between pediatric and adult spleens with respect to the splenic capsule and the consistency of the splenic parenchyma. The capsule in children is relatively thicker than it is in adults, and there is also some evidence that the parenchyma is firmer in consistency in children than it is in adults. These two differences have implications for the success of nonoperative management; pediatric patients are more likely to succeed with nonoperative therapy.

It is perhaps not intuitive from the anteroposterior views depicted in anatomy textbooks, but the spleen is normally located quite posteriorly in the upper abdomen. It is covered by the peritoneum except at the hilum. Posteriorly and laterally, the spleen is related to the left hemidiaphragm and the left posterior and posterolateral lower ribs. The lateral aspect of the spleen is attached to the posterior and lateral abdominal wall and the left hemidiaphragm (splenophrenic ligament) with a variable number of attachments; these require division during mobilization of the spleen. Posteriorly, the spleen is related to the left iliopsoas muscle and the left adrenal gland. Posteriorly and medially, the spleen is related to the body and tail of the pancreas, and it is quite helpful to mobilize the tail and body of the pancreas along with the spleen when elevating the spleen out of the left upper quadrant. Medially and to some extent anteriorly, the spleen is related to the greater curvature of the stomach. Posteriorly and inferiorly, the spleen is related to the left kidney. There are attachments between the spleen and left kidney (splenorenal ligament) that require division during mobilization. Finally, the spleen is related inferiorly to the distal transverse colon and splenic flexure. The lower pole of the spleen is attached to the colon (splenocolic ligament), and these attachments require division during splenic mobilization. The main arterial blood supply emanates from the celiac axis through the splenic artery, the course which can be somewhat variable along the upper border of the body and tail of the pancreas. The branch points of the splenic artery in the hilum as well as the number of splenic artery branches are also variable. The other sources of arterial blood supply for the spleen are the short gastric vessels that connect the left gastroepiploic artery and the splenic circulation along the greater curvature of the stomach. The venous drainage of the spleen is through the splenic vein and the short gastric veins.

A number of different grading systems have been devised to quantify the degree of injury to the spleen. These systems have been created based both on the computed tomographic appearance of ruptured spleens as well as the intraoperative appearance of the spleen. The best known splenic grading system is the one created by the American Association for the Surgery of Trauma (AAST) (Table 1). Implicit

in the AAST grading system are the perhaps fairly obvious concepts that grade increases with an increase in either the length or depth of parenchymal injury, injury to the hilum, or injuries to multiple areas of the spleen.

The CT and intraoperative appearances of a splenic injury are often different from one another. Some of these differences might be because of evolution of the injury between the time of CT scanning and operation, but it is also likely that CT scanning is imperfect in describing the pathologic anatomy of a splenic rupture. Splenic injury scores based on CT scans can both overestimate and underestimate the degree of splenic injury seen at surgery. It is possible to have a CT appearance of fairly trivial injury but at surgery find significant splenic disruption. Conversely, it is possible to see what looks like a major disruption of the spleen on CT scanning and not see the same kind of severity of injury at surgery. In general, the CT scan and associated scores tend, if anything, to underestimate the degree of splenic injury compared with what is seen at surgery.

An important point about CT-based grading systems is that clinical outcome does not tightly correlate with the degree of injury seen on CT. Although there is a rough correlation between the grade of splenic injury seen on CT scanning and the frequency of operative intervention or rates of nonoperative management failure, exceptions are common. Probably the major usefulness of splenic organ injury grading, particularly when the AAST Organ Injury Scale is used, is to allow for objective standardization of terminology and to ensure that individual injuries are described in precise terms understandable to others. Standardized organ injury scaling is also useful for describing populations of splenic injury patients and for construction of treatment algorithms.

TABLE 1: AAST-OIS: Splenic Injury Grading

Grade*	Injury Type	Description of Injury
I	Hematoma	Subcapsular, <10% surface area
	Laceration	Capsular tear, <1 cm parenchymal depth
II	Hematoma	Subcapsular, 10%–50% surface area
	Laceration	Capsular tear, 1–3 cm parenchymal depth that does not involve a trabecular vessel
III	Hematoma	Subcapsular, >50% surface area or expanding; ruptured subcapsular or parenchymal hematoma; intraparenchymal hematoma 5 cm or expanding
	Laceration	>3-cm parenchymal depth or involving trabecular vessels
IV	Laceration	Laceration involving segmental or hilar vessels producing major devascularization (>25% of spleen)
V	Laceration	Completely shattered spleen
	Vascular	Hilar vascular injury which devascularizes spleen

Modified from Moore EE, Cogbill TH, Jurkovich GJ, et al: Organ injury scaling: spleen and liver. *J Trauma* 38:323, 1995.

AAST-OIS, American Association for the Surgery of Trauma Organ Injury Scaling.

*Advance one grade for multiple injuries, up to grade III.

MANAGEMENT

Nonoperative Management

Although nonoperative management is possible in a large number of patients with splenic injury, appropriate patient selection is the most important element of nonoperative management. Of paramount importance in the determination of the suitability of nonoperative management is the hemodynamic stability of the patient. *Hemodynamic stability* can be a somewhat illusory concept and one for which there is no consensus definition, but hypotension (systolic blood pressure <90 mm Hg in an adult or even higher in elderly patients) is generally considered worthy of concern. Prehospital or emergency department hypotension is worrisome, and a high index of suspicion for ongoing hemorrhage should be maintained when either is present. In most instances, those patients that remain hemodynamically unstable are not candidates for abdominal CT scanning. In addition to resuscitation, they require either a direct trip to the operating room or, more commonly, abdominal ultrasonography or DPL to determine the presence or absence of intraperitoneal fluid and help guide the initial decision-making process.

Assuming hemodynamic stability, the other important prerequisite for consideration of nonoperative management is the patient's abdominal examination. In patients who are alert and can provide feedback on physical examination, it is important that they not have diffuse, persistent peritonitis. Although patients with splenic injury may have abdominal findings secondary to intraperitoneal blood, and localized pain and tenderness in the left upper quadrant are common, obvious diffuse peritoneal signs can be a sign of intestinal injury and warrant abdominal exploration.

If a patient with splenic injury is selected for CT scanning and subsequent nonoperative management, it is important to continue to follow the physical examination. If the examination worsens, the possibility of a blunt intestinal injury should be increasingly considered. The most common CT finding in patients with blunt intestinal injury is free fluid in the peritoneal cavity. In patients with damage to the spleen, the free fluid can be mistakenly attributed solely to the splenic injury, and the presence of an associated bowel injury can be missed; the physical examination becomes of even greater importance in such circumstances.

Reported success rates for nonoperative management are 95% or higher for pediatric patients and approximately 80% or higher in adults. These high success rates can be misleading, however, in that they apply only to the group of patients in whom nonoperative management was chosen rather than all patients with splenic injury. When immediate splenectomy patients are included, the overall nonoperative management rates tend to be around 50% to 60% in adult patients. It is also important to remember that these series generally do not include patients in whom the initial impetus was for nonoperative management but in whom emergency surgery was necessary when the patient got into trouble either in the emergency department or during the acquisition of CT scans. The published series of nonoperatively managed spleens generally include only patients who were stable enough to undergo CT scanning and in whom the scan showed a ruptured spleen.

Beyond hemodynamic stability and abdominal findings in the determination of the appropriateness of nonoperative management, other important considerations are the medical environment and some specific characteristics of the patient. Nonoperative management should only be undertaken if it will be possible to closely follow the patient. If close in patient follow-up is simply not possible, abdominal exploration may be appropriate. Similarly, if rapid mobilization of the operating room and quick operative intervention in the case of ongoing or delayed bleeding is impossible, initial operative intervention may be appropriate.

For patients who are stable enough to undergo CT scanning and in whom a ruptured spleen is seen, nonoperative management is reasonable if they continue to remain stable. In addition to vital signs, one of the other commonly followed parameters in such patients is the hematocrit. A common practice is to determine a cutoff value below which the hematocrit will not be allowed to fall. If the hematocrit drops to that level or below, operative intervention is undertaken. Such an approach works best if there are no associated injuries or no embolization has been performed. When other injuries are present, it can be difficult to know if the spleen is continuing to bleed or if the fall in hematocrit is secondary to bleeding from sites other than the spleen. When contemplating transfusion in patients with splenic injury who are being managed nonoperatively, it should be kept in mind that there is increasingly convincing evidence that transfusion has harmful immunologic effects and is an independent predictor of poor outcome after trauma. There is some evidence older patients (>55 years old) might have a worse prognosis with respect to nonoperative management than do younger patients, but there are other reports concluding that outcomes are the same in older versus younger patients. Although the evidence in this area is mixed, a relatively recent large multicenter study showed older patients are more likely to fail nonoperative management, and older patients undergoing nonoperative therapy would likely benefit from earlier conversion to invasive therapy if their condition worsens. This may be related to the density of splenic architecture in younger spleens that creates a more stable platform for the clot.

The presence of severe associated injuries, particularly head injury, has been suggested as another relative contraindication to nonoperative management of splenic injury. As previously noted, following the hematocrit in a patient with multiple severe injuries can be problematic. Furthermore, there are concerns about the effects of ongoing or delayed splenic bleeding on the prognosis of a severe head injury. Although these factors do not mandate operative intervention in all patients who fall into these groups, they should lower the threshold for operative intervention on an individual basis.

There is little scientific evidence to dictate the specifics of how nonoperative management of splenic injury should be done, and most recommendations are simply matters of common sense and opinion. Most patients should be admitted to an intensive care unit setting for their initial course, including those with grade II or above splenic

injuries and patients with multiple associated injuries that make following serial hematocrit levels and physical examinations difficult.

Patients should initially be kept with nothing by mouth in case nonoperative management fails, which is more likely to occur in the early postinjury period. Nasogastric suction is not necessary unless needed for other reasons. Bed rest had been advocated by many in their nonoperative management protocols, but a recent study showed early mobilization did not contribute to failed nonoperative management, and trauma patients generally benefit from early mobilization. Patients should be followed closely hemodynamically, and the urine output should be monitored. Serial hematocrits should be obtained and compared with each other as well as with the admission hematocrit.

Vaccines for *Haemophilus influenzae*, meningococcal, and streptococcal infection should be given. Although it is agreed that splenectomized patients require vaccination in the perioperative period, the exact timing of the vaccinations remains a matter of debate. Elective splenectomy patients are vaccinated prior to their operations. This practice led to advocating for immediate vaccination, even in patients managed nonoperatively. There are some theoretical reasons to believe vaccinations are more effective if given before splenectomy, and some studies show postoperative pneumococcal vaccinations are effective.

The appropriate length of stay in the intensive care unit is not clearly defined. Most centers keep patients with splenic injury in the intensive care unit for 24 to 72 hours and then transfer them to a ward bed if they have been stable and other injuries permit. At this point, patients are allowed to eat unless other injuries preclude oral intake. Blood count monitoring should continue but can decrease in frequency.

The optimal hospital length of stay is also poorly defined, and there is a variety of practice in this regard. A large multiinstitutional study showed most failures of nonoperative management occur within the first 6 to 8 days after injury. The reason for keeping patients in the hospital is to minimize the potential deadly consequences of delayed splenic rupture. This is especially true in rural areas where immediate operative care is not readily available. Our institutional approach is to keep patients in the hospital for an arbitrary 7 days, picking up the vast majority of delayed bleeding episodes during the in patient stay.

The issue of follow-up CT scans in patients with nonoperatively managed splenic injuries is also controversial. Most series indicate that either they are not necessary or the frequency with which they alter management is extremely low, and further CT scanning does expose the patient to further radiation, a particular concern in pediatric patients. Our policy is to study only patients who have persistent abdominal signs and symptoms after a week of observation. On occasion such patients have developed pseudoaneurysms of the spleen, even if the initial CT did not demonstrate a blush. It is difficult to know exactly what the natural history of these pseudoaneurysms would be if left untreated, but they can be impressive in appearance and are amenable to angiographic embolization.

When patients are discharged to home, they should be counseled not to engage in contact sports or other activities in which they might suffer a blow to the torso. The best length of time to maintain this admonition is unknown, but typical recommendations range from 2 to 6 months. There is experimental evidence most injured spleens have not recovered their normal integrity and strength until at least 6 to 8 weeks after injury, so the recommendation to avoid contact sports for 2 to 6 months seems reasonable.

Transcatheter Embolization

Embolization of bleeding areas in a ruptured spleen can be an important adjunct to successful nonoperative management There are no consensus guidelines at present for when angiography and embolization are indicated, but current trends generally reserve catheter-based interventions for higher grade injuries as well as those with CT evidence of a contrast blush, pseudoaneurysm, arteriovenous fistula, or active extravasation, regardless of the grade of injury. The theoretical basis for splenic embolization is self-apparent, but true prospective and controlled data demonstrating its effectiveness is lacking and reported results of embolization vary.

Operative Management

The best incision for splenic injury, as well as for most trauma operations on the abdomen, is through the midline. Such an approach is versatile, can be extended easily both superiorly and inferiorly, and is also the quickest incision if speed of intervention is important. For operations on an injured spleen, it is often helpful to extend the incision superiorly and to the left of the xiphoid process. This maneuver improves exposure of the left upper quadrant, particularly in large patients and those with a narrow costal angle.

As with all trauma celiotomies, it is important to rapidly examine and pack all four quadrants of the abdomen in patients who are grossly unstable. The initial investigation of the abdomen should not be definitive and should be used only for a quick look at all four quadrants and for packing. While the quadrants are being packed, it is helpful to look for clotting. Clotting tends to localize to the site of injury, whereas defibrinated blood will spread diffusely in the abdomen.

Once attention has been directed to the left upper quadrant, all of the structures in that quadrant should be inspected. There should be an initial look at the greater curvature of the stomach and the left hemidiaphragm. The left hemidiaphragm should be inspected again once the spleen is mobilized if mobilization is necessary. The left lobe of the liver and left kidney should be looked at as well, as should the tail of the pancreas. If the spleen is to be mobilized, inspection of the tail of the pancreas is easier after mobilization has been accomplished.

Splenic mobilization should be done in a stepwise fashion, and the stepwise approach helps in providing adequate mobilization and minimizing the chance of iatrogenic splenic or pancreatic injury. The sequence of splenic mobilization is also important in that it allows for splenic salvage and splenorrhaphy up until the final step of hilar ligation. In hemodynamically unstable patients or patients with other life-threatening injuries the mobilization can be performed quite rapidly with an experienced hand, thereby removing the spleen in an expedited manner.

The first step in mobilization of the spleen is to cut the lateral attachments of the spleen, the splenophrenic and splenorenal ligaments. This step should be started with sharp dissection and can then be continued with a combination of blunt and sharp dissection. The lateral and superior attachments should be cut to near the level of the esophageal hiatus. Cutting the lateral attachments is sometimes facilitated by putting a finger or clamp underneath them and then bluntly developing the underlying plane before dividing the peritoneum. In large patients and in those with a spleen that is very posterior, it may be necessary to do some of the sharp dissection by feel.

After the lateral attachments have been divided, the next step is to mobilize the spleen and tail of the pancreas as a unit from lateral to medial. One of the easier ways to do this is to place the back of the fingernails of the right hand underneath the spleen and tail of the pancreas so that they are adjacent to the underlying left kidney. The kidney can be palpated easily because it is firm and provides an excellent landmark for the proper plane of dissection. Two common errors at this point are trying to mobilize the spleen alone without the adjacent pancreas or entering Gerota's fascia and mobilizing the left kidney. Both of these limit the degree of splenic mobility and make it more difficult to avoid iatrogenic injury to the spleen, kidney, and pancreatic tail. The splenic hilum can be injured during mobilization from lateral to medial; the pancreatic tail can be inadvertently included in the hilar clamping of the spleen. These problems are minimized with optimal mobilization and visualization.

After the spleen and pancreas have been mobilized as a unit to the midline, it is generally apparent that the next constraining attachments of the spleen are the short gastric vessels. Because of the dual blood supply of the spleen though its hilum and also through the short gastric vessels, it is possible to divide the short gastric vessels without compromising splenic viability. The best way to divide the short gastric vessels is to have an assistant elevate the spleen and tail of the pancreas into the operative field and then to securely clamp the vessels starting proximally on the greater curvature of the stomach. A well-placed nasogastric tube along the greater curvature of the stomach can provide a handle upon which to retract the stomach, thereby improving visualization of the short gastric vessels. The short gastric vessels, as the name implies, are short. It is therefore not uncommon to be concerned about a clamp on the gastric portion of a short gastric vessel having included a small portion of stomach. In such cases, the tie on the short gastric vessels and nubbin of stomach can necrose the stomach, leading to a delayed gastric leak. This concern can be addressed by oversewing any gastric areas in question.

The final step necessary for full mobilization of the spleen is division of the splenocolic ligamentous attachment between the lower pole of the spleen and the distal transverse colon and splenic flexure (Fig. 6). During division of both the short gastric vessels and the splenocolic ligament, bleeding from the spleen can be controlled using digital compression of the hilum. If the patient is exsanguinating and the bleeding is massive, a clamp can be placed on the hilum during the later steps of mobilization. Mass clamping should only be done in extreme circumstances, however, because it increases the chances of injury to the tail of the pancreas (Fig. 7).

After the spleen has been fully mobilized, it is possible to inspect it in its entirety. It is also possible to examine the posterior aspect of the body and tail of the pancreas. It is helpful after mobilization to pack

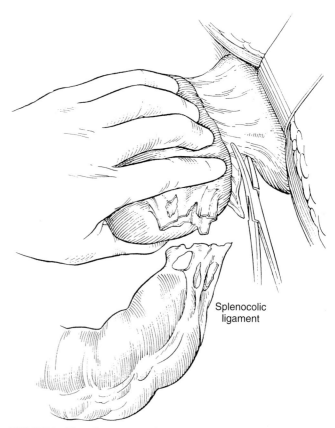

FIGURE 6   The spleen is grasped and the lateral peritoneal ligaments are divided. The splenocolic ligaments have been divided to release the splenic flexure. *(From Khatri V, Asensio JA: Operative surgery manual, Philadelphia, 2002, Saunders, p 189.)*

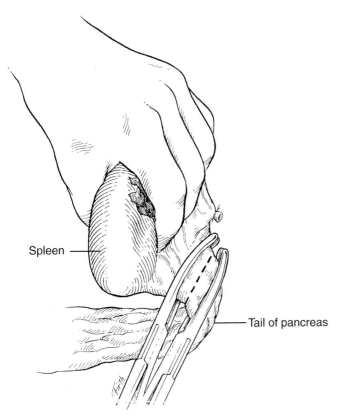

Spleen

Tail of pancreas

FIGURE 7 After complete mobilization of the spleen, the vessels at the hilum are clamped and divided, avoiding injury to the tail of the pancreas. *(From Khatri V, Asensio JA: Operative surgery manual, Philadelphia, 2002, Saunders, p 189.)*

the splenic fossa to tamponade any minor bleeding and also to help keep the spleen and distal pancreas elevated into the field. During this packing maneuver, the left adrenal gland can be inspected and the left hemidiaphragm reexamined.

If the injury is small and bleeding minimally, topical hemostatic agents can be used and the spleen returned to its normal position. Electrocautery is rarely helpful. Argon beam coagulators have shown promise in animal models of splenic injury. If the injury is minor and the patient's overall condition is not too serious, splenorrhaphy can be done, although with the advent of nonoperative management the number of splenic injuries found at surgical intervention that are amenable to repair has decreased. Another factor to consider is that intraparenchymal injury may be more severe than what is observed in the operating room.

If splenorrhaphy is undertaken, the spleen can be sutured, especially when the capsule is intact, but it does not hold sutures particularly well, so it is advisable to use pledgets. Wrapping of either all or part of an injured spleen with absorbable mesh can also be done, but these techniques are moderately time consuming. Partial splenectomy has been described and is possible because of the segmental nature of the splenic blood supply. The blood supply to the damaged portion can be ligated and the spleen observed for its demarcation. The nonviable portion is removed with the exposed parenchyma made hemostatic either with suture or mesh wrapping. There is a higher complication rate associated with splenorrhaphy than with splenectomy and this factor should be kept in mind when deciding in the operating room what to do with an injured spleen. Further, because most patients with splenic injury are treated with nonoperative management, patients who do undergo surgery for their splenic injury have in many cases already been selected out as patients likely to need splenectomy.

Splenectomy should be done in patients who are unstable or who have serious associated injuries. It should also generally be done for the highest grades of splenic injury (IV to V) if operative management has been chosen. The hilar structures should be addressed with serial dissection and division. Suture ligation should be used for large vessels.

After the spleen is removed careful examination of the splenic bed should be performed. This is done by folding a laparotomy pad into thirds and using it to roll from lateral to medial and posterior to anterior in the retroperitoneum and the splenic bed. Although this maneuver is used to visualize the entire operative field, the primary focus of this examination are the gastric ends of the short gastric vessels, which may have gone unligated during mobilization and removal of the spleen or may have been inadequately ligated. Bleeding from the divided short gastric vessels is the most common cause of postoperative bleeding after splenectomy.

Drains should not be routinely placed after either splenectomy or splenorrhaphy and may actually increase the rate of postoperative complications. Drainage is reasonable if there is associated pancreatic injury or an associated renal injury when there is concern about postoperative urine leak.

MORBIDITY AND COMPLICATIONS OF MANAGEMENT

The most common complication of nonoperative management of the spleen is continued bleeding and the rate of failure increases with higher grades of injury. Another potential complication is delayed diagnosis of an associated intra-abdominal injury that requires operative intervention, most commonly an injury to the bowel or pancreas. The frequency with which serious associated injuries are present in patients who are good candidates for nonoperative management is fairly low, at most in the 5% to 10% range, but the possibility of an injury to either the bowel or the pancreas should always be kept in mind when the decision is made to treat a splenic injury nonoperatively. The physical examination of the abdomen is essential in the diagnosis of an initially missed injury.

Even when nonoperative management is augmented by transcatheter embolization, there are risks of failure and complication. Embolization is associated with complications, and several studies have reported failure/major complication rates greater than 20%. Complications include splenic abscess, splenic infarct, and missed injuries. If embolization is employed, there should be a high index of suspicion for the need of operative intervention.

As with any intervention, there is also a risk of bleeding after splenectomy or splenorrhaphy. The source may be from the splenic parenchyma after repair, the splenic bed, the short gastric vessels, or the hilar vessels. Coagulopathy should be addressed, but the possibility of surgical bleeding in the postoperative period should always be entertained when the patient is not doing well, especially when the spleen was not removed. As described previously, short gastric ligatures can result in necrosis of a portion of the greater curvature of the stomach, leading to leakage. Gastric distention may occur after splenectomy and is easily treated with nasogastric decompression if the diagnosis is entertained. Pancreatic injury may be the result of operative dissection or initial injury.

Venous thromboembolic complications are always a concern after trauma, and may be worsened with a splenic injury. Timely anticoagulation or mobilization can be hampered by nonoperative management or splenorrhaphy. Our practice has been to anticoagulate patients after their hematocrit levels have been stable for 24 hours. Splenectomy can cause thrombocytosis, but there is no definitive evidence that postsplenectomy thrombocytosis leads to an increased incidence of deep venous thrombosis.

Although commonly mentioned, overwhelming postsplenectomy sepsis is a rare entity. The actual rate at which overwhelming sepsis in asplenic patients occurs is unknown, but one estimate is a 0.026%

lifetime risk for adults and a 0.052% lifetime risk for children. Pneumococcus and meningococcus are the most common pathogens, and protection against *H. influenzae* may also be helpful. Given the extremely low incidence of overwhelming postsplenectomy sepsis, it is difficult to prove the efficacy of vaccination. Nevertheless, vaccination has become the standard of care in patients who have had splenectomy.

MORTALITY

Mortality risk from splenic injury alone should be fairly low given careful selection and monitoring of nonoperative management and the definitively curative nature of splenectomy. In a study of a national database involving nearly 15,000 patients with splenic injury, the mortality rate was approximately 1% to 3%. Much of the mortality risk in patients with splenic injury results from associated injuries, especially head injury.

CONCLUSIONS AND ALGORITHM

Patients with abdominal trauma and possible splenic injury should be managed initially with the ABCs of initial trauma resuscitation (Fig. 8). If hemodynamically unstable and ultrasound or DPL shows there is intraperitoneal hemorrhage, urgent operative exploration is mandated. If splenic injury is found, splenectomy should be done, especially if the patient has severe associated injuries or hemodynamic instability (Fig. 9).

If the patient on initial presentation is hemodynamically stable, abdominal CT scanning should be done. If there is an injury with no blush and the patient remains hemodynamically stable, a course of nonoperative management should be undertaken. If the patient develops diffuse or worsening peritonitis or shows signs of ongoing bleeding (falling hematocrit, hemodynamic instability), abdominal exploration should be done and the splenic injury managed operatively (Fig. 10).

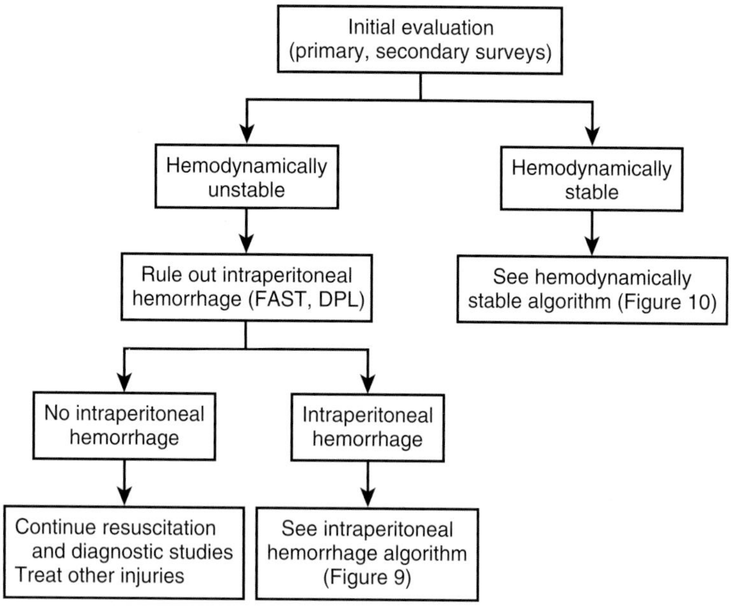

FIGURE 8 Algorithm for initial evaluation of patients with abdominal trauma and possible splenic injury. DPL, Diagnostic peritoneal lavage; FAST, focused assessment with sonography in trauma.

FIGURE 9 Algorithm for management of hemodynamically unstable patients with intraperitoneal hemorrhage.

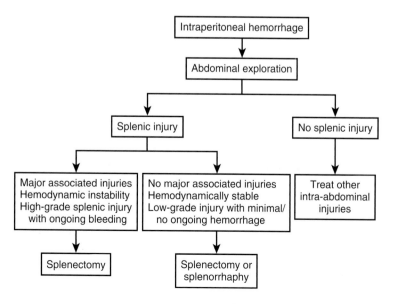

FIGURE 10 Algorithm for management of hemodynamically stable patients. CT, Computed tomography.

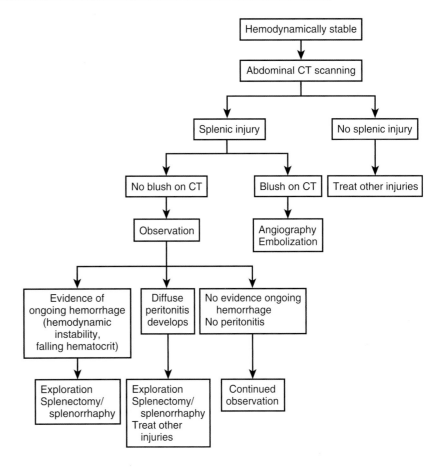

Throughout the management of patients with splenic injury, from the initial resuscitation in the emergency department through the subsequent course of operative or nonoperative management, it should always be borne in mind that splenic injuries can bleed significantly and can lead to major morbidity and even fatality if they are not handled appropriately.

ACKNOWLEDGMENT

We would like to thank Dr. Glenn Tse for his contribution to the previous edition of this chapter.

For the chapter's Suggested Readings list, please visit the book at www.ExpertConsult.inkling.com.

ABDOMINAL VASCULAR INJURY

Christopher J. Dente and David V. Feliciano

Injury to a major abdominal vascular structure, termed *abdominal vascular injury (AVI)*, is associated with significant morbidity and mortality after blunt or penetrating trauma. Because these injuries may be rapidly lethal and the vessels involved are large, it is important to have a thorough understanding of the operative maneuvers used to rapidly expose them.

Although rare in military conflicts, AVIs are much more commonly seen in civilian centers. In the 1970s and 1980s, AVIs accounted for between 18.5% and 33.8% of all cardiovascular injuries in several series. In the modern era, even with the decrease in penetrating trauma, AVI continues to be a significant problem with several reviews by Feliciano, Mattox, and Asensio in the late 1990s documenting the treatment of over 300 patients each. The significantly higher number of AVIs treated in civilian practice likely reflects the more modest wounding capacity of handguns when compared to military ordnance, as well as the shorter prehospital transit times in most urban areas of the United States. Also, advances in military armor have led to a shift in injuries to the extremities rather than the torso, although noncompressible (torso) hemorrhage remained the leading cause of combatant death from hemorrhage in a recent review.

PATHOPHYSIOLOGY

Blunt Trauma

Rapid deceleration in motor vehicle crashes may cause avulsion of small branches from major vessels with subsequent hemorrhage or intimal tears with secondary thrombosis. Crush injuries to the abdomen, such as by a lap seat belt or by a posterior blow to the spine may cause secondary thrombosis of an overlying vessel, also. Direct blows can completely disrupt exposed vessels such as the superior mesenteric artery or vein at the base of the mesentery, leading to massive intraperitoneal hemorrhage, or even partly disrupt the infrarenal abdominal aorta, leading to the formation of a false aneurysm.

Penetrating Trauma

In contrast, penetrating injuries create the same kinds of abdominal vascular injuries that are seen in the vessels of the extremities. They include blast effects with intimal flaps and secondary thrombosis, lateral-wall defects with hemorrhage or pulsatile hematomas, and complete transection with either free bleeding or thrombosis. On rare occasions, a penetrating injury may produce an arteriovenous fistula, most commonly involving the portal vein and hepatic artery, renal vessels, or iliac vessels. In addition, iatrogenic injuries remain a persistent problem in many centers.

DIAGNOSIS

History and Physical Examination

As previously mentioned, an AVI may present with free intraperitoneal hemorrhage, a contained hematoma, or thrombosis of the vessel. Therefore, the presenting signs and symptoms are variable based on both the involved vessel and the presence or absence of active hemorrhage. Active intraperitoneal hemorrhage from a major abdominal arterial structure will generally lead to unrelenting hemorrhagic shock, with the patient described as a "nonresponder" in the Advanced Trauma Life Support course. Conversely, patients with a contained hematoma, especially with a venous injury, may be remarkably stable, or present as a transient responder, and only decompensate once the hematoma is opened in the operating room. Finally, patients with blunt thrombosis of a major vascular structure will generally be hemodynamically normal, but will often complain of severe pain or will have a pulse deficit in a lower extremity.

Imaging

In both stable and unstable patients, a rapid surgeon-performed ultrasound focused assessment with sonography in trauma (FAST) is useful in determining the presence of intraabdominal, intrapleural, or intrapericardial hemorrhage. In a stable patient with an abdominal gunshot wound, a routine plain film of the abdomen is of diagnostic value so that the track of the missile can be predicted from markers placed over the wounds or from the position of a retained missile.

Preoperative abdominal aortography should not be routinely performed to document intra-abdominal vascular injuries after penetrating wounds. Indeed, most patients with such wounds are not stable enough to undergo the manipulation required for appropriate studies of large vessels in an angiographic suite. In patients with blunt trauma, aortography is used to diagnose and treat deep pelvic arterial bleeding associated with fractures and to diagnose unusual injuries such as the previously mentioned intimal tears with thrombosis in the infrarenal aorta, the iliac artery, or the renal artery. An occasional patient is a candidate for endovascular therapy, and this will be discussed later.

As the technology of computed tomography (CT) scanning has advanced, many surgeons and radiologists are comfortable making therapeutic decisions based on data acquired from multiplanar scanning and formal CT angiography. Extensive literature exists on the diagnosis of traumatic thoracic aortic disruption with CT and at least one small prospective study has shown acceptable accuracy of CT angiography in extremity trauma. Conversely, data on the use of CT angiography as a method of diagnosis of AVI remain preliminary. Indeed, in one recent study, contrast-enhanced CT alone had a 94% sensitivity and 89% specificity for the diagnosis of active hemorrhage when compared to angiography.

INITIAL MANAGEMENT AND RESUSCITATION

Resuscitation in the field in patients with possible blunt or penetrating abdominal vascular injuries should be restricted to basic airway maneuvers with insertion of intravenous lines for infusing crystalloid solutions being best attempted during transport to the hospital. There is no consistent evidence to support either the aggressive administration of crystalloid solutions during the short prehospital times in urban environments versus the withholding of similar solutions in patients with penetrating abdominal vascular injuries. Current damage control resuscitation practices, which espouse limiting crystalloid resuscitation, have become the standard in care in many trauma centers and are discussed later.

In the emergency department, the extent of resuscitation clearly depends on the patient's condition at the time of arrival. In the agonal patient with a rigid abdomen after a gunshot wound, emergency department thoracotomy with cross-clamping of the descending thoracic aorta may be necessary to maintain cerebral and coronary arterial flow. This is indicated if the trauma operating room is geographically distant from the emergency department. Unfortunately, survival after emergency department thoracotomy for major AVI is rare. Indeed, in the large series by Feliciano et al, only 1 of 59 patients with isolated penetrating wounds to the abdomen survived after undergoing a preliminary thoracotomy in the emergency department.

In the patient arriving with blunt abdominal trauma, hypotension, and a positive surgeon-performed FAST or penetrating abdominal trauma and hypotension or peritonitis, a time limit of less than 5 minutes in the emergency department is mandatory. As is now recognized, control of hemorrhage is the most effective first step in resuscitation, and for these potentially lethal injuries, this control can be obtained only in the operating room.

Damage Control Resuscitation and Massive Transfusion

In the last 7 years, based mostly on the military experience in Iraq, there has been a dramatic change in the resuscitation philosophy of critically injured patients in many centers. The military resuscitation philosophy of "damage control resuscitation" is seen as an extension of the concepts of "damage control surgery," a term coined in the early 1990s by Rotondo et al. In most civilian centers, where fresh whole blood is unavailable, the central tenet of damage control resuscitation is the early and aggressive use of blood components (fresh frozen plasma and platelets) in high, fixed ratios to packed red blood cells. In most centers, this practice requires the support of the blood bank and a highly organized massive transfusion protocol (MTP). Indeed, there are now multiple published series using institution-specific MTPs, generally with significant improvements in patient outcome. As many patients with AVI will require massive transfusion, the treating surgeons should be familiar with the design and implementation of any MTP that exists in their institution.

OPERATION

Operative Preparations

In the operating room, the entire trunk from the chin to the knees is prepared and draped in the usual manner. Maneuvers to prevent hypothermia should include warming the operating room; covering the patient's head; covering the upper and lower extremities with a heating unit; and the use of a heating cascade on the anesthesia machine.

General Principles

A preliminary operating room thoracotomy with cross-clamping of the descending thoracic aorta is used in some centers when the patient's blood pressure on arrival is less than 70 mm Hg. This may maintain cerebral and coronary arterial flow if the heart is still beating and may prevent sudden cardiac arrest when abdominal tamponade is released. Unfortunately, it has little effect on intra-abdominal vascular injuries because of persistent bleeding from backflow.

A midline abdominal incision is made, and all clots and free blood are manually evacuated or removed with suction. A rapid inspection is performed to visualize contained hematomas or areas of hemorrhage. If active hemorrhage from a major intra-abdominal artery is encountered, a variety of techniques from simple digital pressure to formal proximal and distal control may be required to temporarily arrest the hemorrhage. Generally, further dissection with full exposure and control of the injured vessel proximal and distal to the injury is required for repair. Conversely, venous injuries may be managed very effectively with a series of Judd-Allis clamps applied to the edges of the perforation without the need for formal proximal and distal control. Once hemorrhage from the vascular injuries is temporarily controlled in patients with penetrating wounds, it may be worthwhile to rapidly isolate as many gastrointestinal perforations as possible to avoid further contamination of the abdomen during the period of vascular repair. Once this is accomplished the abdomen is irrigated and the vascular repair is performed, with a soft tissue cover applied over the repair.

Conversely, if the patient has a contained retroperitoneal hematoma at the time of laparotomy, the surgeon occasionally has time to first perform necessary gastrointestinal repairs in the free peritoneal cavity, change gloves, and irrigate prior to opening the retroperitoneum expose the underlying AVI.

Hematomas or hemorrhage associated with abdominal vascular injuries generally occur in zone I, the midline retroperitoneum; zone II, the upper lateral retroperitoneum; zone III, the pelvic retroperitoneum; or in the portal-retrohepatic area of the right upper quadrant, as previously described. The magnitude of injury is best described using the Organ Injury Scale of the American Association for the Surgery of Trauma (AAST), which is included as Table 1.

EXPOSURE OF ABDOMINAL VASCULAR INJURY BY ZONE

Both the size of the vessels and their posterior location make the operative management of AVI one of the most difficult tasks a trauma surgeon may encounter. Conversely, once exposure has been obtained, the actual vascular repair is more straightforward, as these vessels in young, healthy patients are free of atherosclerotic disease, although many may be vasoconstricted or relatively small. Therefore, a trauma surgeon should be very familiar with each of the techniques described here, as well as the thought process associated with choosing the correct maneuver in each situation.

As previously described, the retroperitoneum may be divided into zones and each zone may be exposed by one or more operative maneuvers. These appropriate maneuvers are summarized both in Table 2 and in the algorithm shown later in this chapter (see Fig. 3).

Zone I, Supramesocolic Region

If a hematoma or hemorrhage is encountered in this region, there are several techniques for obtaining proximal vascular control of the aorta at the hiatus of the diaphragm. When a contained hematoma is present, the surgeon usually has time to reflect all left-sided intra-abdominal viscera, including the colon, kidney, spleen, tail of the pancreas, and fundus of the stomach to the midline (left-sided medial visceral rotation (Fig. 1). Because of the dense nature of the celiac plexus of nerves as well as the copious lymphatics that surround the supraceliac aorta, it is frequently helpful to transect the left crus of the aortic hiatus of the diaphragm at the 2 o'clock position to allow for exposure of the distal descending thoracic aorta above the hiatus. This allows for the extra few centimeters of exposure that is essential for complex repair of the vessels within this tightly confined anatomic area. Although this maneuver takes several minutes to perform and risks damage to the spleen, kidney, and left colon, it allows for extensive exposure of the entire length of the abdominal aorta.

Conversely, if active hemorrhage is coming from this area, the surgeon may attempt to control it manually or with one of the aortic compression devices. Failing this, an alternative approach is to divide

TABLE 1: Abdominal Vascular Injury Scale

Grade*	Description of Injury	ICD-9 Code	AIS-90 Score
I	Non-named superior mesenteric artery or superior mesenteric vein branches	902.20/.39	NS
	Non-named inferior mesenteric artery or inferior mesenteric vein branches	902.27/.32	NS
	Phrenic artery or vein	902.89	NS
	Lumbar artery or vein	902.89	NS
	Gonadal artery or vein	902.89	NS
	Ovarian artery or vein	902.81/.82	NS
	Other non-named small arterial or venous structures requiring ligation	902.90	NS
II	Right, left, or common hepatic artery	902.22	3
	Splenic artery or vein	902.23/.34	3
	Right or left gastric arteries	902.21	3
	Gastroduodenal artery	902.24	3
	Inferior mesenteric artery, or inferior mesenteric vein, trunk	902.27/.32	3

Continued

TABLE 1: Abdominal Vascular Injury Scale—cont'd

Grade	Description of Injury	ICD-9 Code	AIS-90 Score
	Primary named branches of mesenteric artery (e.g., ileocolic artery) or mesenteric vein	902.26/.31	3
	Other named abdominal vessels requiring ligation or repair	902.89	3
III	Superior mesenteric vein, trunk	902.31	3
	Renal artery or vein	902.41/.42	3
	Iliac artery or vein	902.53/.54	3
	Hypogastric artery or vein	902.51/.52	3
	Vena cava, infrarenal	902.10	3
IV	Superior mesenteric artery, trunk	902.25	3
	Celiac axis proper	902.24	3
	Vena cava, suprarenal and infrahepatic	902.10	3
	Aorta, infrarenal	902.00	4
V	Portal vein	902.33	3
	Extraparenchymal hepatic vein	902.11	3 (hepatic vein), 5 (liver + veins)
	Vena cava, retrohepatic or suprahepatic	902.19	5
	Aorta suprarenal, subdiaphragmatic	902.00	4

From Moore EE, et al: Organ injury scaling. III: chest wall, abdominal vascular, ureter, bladder, and urethra. *J Trauma* 33:337–339, 1992.
AIS, Abbreviated Injury Scale; ICD, International Classification of Diseases; NS, not scored.
*This classification system is applicable to extraparenchymal vascular injuries. If the vessel injury is within 2 cm of the organ parenchyma, refer to specific organ injury scale. Increase one grade for multiple grade III or IV injuries involving more than 50% vessel circumference. Downgrade one grade if less than 25% vessel circumference laceration for grades IV or V.

TABLE 2: Operative Maneuvers by Zones of the Retroperitoneum

Zone	Operative Maneuvers
I (Supramesocolic)	Left medial visceral rotation Midline suprarenal aortic exposure
I (Inframesocolic)	Right medial visceral rotation Midline infrarenal aortoiliac exposure
II	Midline exposure of the renal hilum Lateral exposure of the renal hilum
III	Midline infrarenal aortoiliac exposure Exposure of right common iliac vein/vena caval confluence Total pelvic isolation
Porta hepatis	Porta exposure Retropancreatic exposure of the portal vein

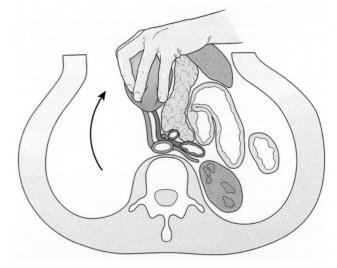

FIGURE 1 Left medial visceral rotation performed with sharp and blunt dissection to elevate the left colon, left kidney, spleen, tail of the pancreas, and gastric fundus. *(From Feliciano DV: Injuries to the great vessels of the abdomen. In Ashley SW, Cance WG, editors: ACS surgery: principles and practice, 7th ed, Canada, 2014, BC Decker, Inc, Fig. 3, p. 3.)*

the lesser omentum manually, retract the stomach and esophagus hard to the left, and digitally separate the muscle fibers of the aortic hiatus to obtain quicker and similar, if more limited, exposure as described previously.

Distal control of the aorta in this location is awkward because of the presence of the celiac axis and superior mesenteric artery. In some patients, the celiac axis may have to be divided and ligated to allow for more space for the distal aortic clamp and subsequent vascular repair. Necrosis of the gallbladder is a likely sequela, and cholecystectomy is generally warranted, although this may be done at repeat laparotomy if need be.

Zone I, Inframesocolic Region

Exposure of an inframesocolic injury to the aorta is obtained by duplicating the maneuvers used to gain proximal aortic control during the elective resection of an abdominal aortic aneurysm. The transverse mesocolon is pulled up toward the patient's head, and the small bowel is eviscerated toward the right side of the table. The midline retroperitoneum is then opened until the left renal vein is exposed and a proximal aortic clamp can then be placed immediately inferior to this vessel. Exposure to allow for application of the distal vascular clamp is obtained by dividing the midline retroperitoneum to the aortic bifurcation, avoiding the left-sided origin of the inferior mesenteric artery (which may be sacrificed whenever necessary for exposure).

If the aorta is intact or if there is active hemorrhage coming through the base of the mesentery of the ascending colon or hepatic flexure of the colon, injury to the infrarenal or juxtarenal inferior vena cava should be suspected. Although it is possible to visualize the vena cava through the midline retroperitoneal incision previously described, more extensive exposure of the vena cava is attained by mobilizing the right half of the colon and C-loop of the duodenum and leaving the right kidney in situ (right medial visceral rotation) (Fig. 2). This permits the entire vena caval system from the confluence of the iliac veins to the suprahepatic vena cava below the liver to be visualized. It is often difficult to define precisely where a hole is in a large vein of the abdomen until much of the loose retroperitoneal fatty tissue is stripped away from the wall of the vessel. Once this is done, the site of hemorrhage can be localized and generally easily controlled.

The two areas in which proximal and distal control of the inferior vena cava below the liver are especially difficult to obtain are at the

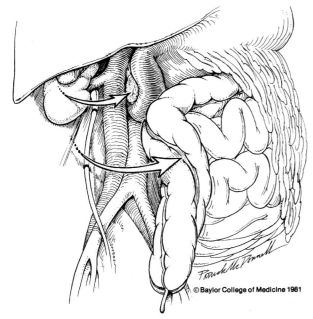

FIGURE 2 Right medial visceral rotation. Medial rotation of the right-sided abdominal viscera (except the kidney) allows for visualization of the entire infrahepatic inferior vena cava. *(From Feliciano DV: Abdominal vascular injury. In Moore EE, Feliciano DV, Mattox KL, editors:* Trauma, *5th ed, New York, 2004, McGraw-Hill, Fig. 36-5, p 765. Copyright 1981 Baylor College of Medicine.)*

confluence of the common iliac veins and at the caval junction with the renal veins. Although sponge-stick compression of the common iliac veins and the vena cava superiorly may control hemorrhage at the confluence, visualization of perforating wounds in this area is compromised by the overlying aortic bifurcation. In the case of difficult exposure, one technique is to divide and ligate the right internal iliac artery, which may allow for lateral and cephalad retraction of the right common iliac artery to expose the venous injury. An alternative and interesting approach, but one that is rarely necessary, is the temporary division of the overlying right common iliac artery itself, with mobilization of the aortic bifurcation to the left. This technique provides wide exposure of the confluence of the common iliac veins and the distal vena cava. The right common iliac artery is then reconstituted by an end-to-end anastomosis. When the perforation occurs at the junction of the renal veins and the inferior vena cava, it should be directly compressed with either sponge sticks or digitally. An assistant then clamps or compresses the infrarenal vena cava and the suprarenal infrahepatic vena cava and loops both renal veins individually with vascular tapes to allow for the direct application of angled vascular clamps.

Zone II

If a hematoma or hemorrhage is present in the upper lateral retroperitoneum, injury to the renal artery, renal vein, and the kidney should be suspected. Patients found to have a perirenal hematoma at the time of exploration for a penetrating abdominal wound should undergo exploration of the wound track. If the hematoma is not rapidly expanding and there is no free intraabdominal bleeding, some surgeons will loop the ipsilateral renal artery with a vessel loop in the midline at the base of the mesocolon. The left renal vein can also be looped with a vascular tape in the same location; however, vascular control of the proximal right renal vein will have to wait for mobilization of the C-loop of the duodenum and unroofing of the vena cava at its junction with the renal veins. It should be noted that obtaining proximal vascular control prior to exploration of a perirenal hematoma is controversial. Indeed, in one study, preliminary vascular control of the renal hilum had no impact on nephrectomy rate, transfusion requirements, or blood loss. Most surgeons take a more direct approach by simply opening the retroperitoneum lateral to the injured kidney and manually elevating the kidney directly into the wound. A large vascular clamp can be applied proximal to the hilum either at the midline on the left or just lateral to the inferior vena cava on the right to control any further bleeding.

Patients who present after blunt trauma may have either a renovascular or renal parenchymal injury, also. Patients in the former group, however, generally present with renovascular occlusion, which will be discussed later. In patients who have suffered blunt abdominal trauma and have undergone imaging that has demonstrated flow to the kidney, there is no justification for exploring the perirenal hematoma should an emergency laparotomy be indicated for other reasons.

Zone III

The fourth major area of hematoma or hemorrhage is the pelvic retroperitoneum. If a hematoma or hemorrhage is present after penetrating trauma, compression with a laparotomy pad or finger or simply grabbing the bleeding vessels with a hand should be performed as proximal and distal vascular control is attained. The proximal common iliac arteries are exposed by eviscerating the small bowel to the right and dividing the midline retroperitoneum over the aortic bifurcation. In young trauma patients, there is usually no adherence between the common iliac artery and vein in this location, and vessel loops can be passed rapidly around the proximal arteries. Distal vascular control is obtained at the point at which the external iliac artery comes out of the pelvis proximal to the inguinal ligament. The major problem in this area is continued backbleeding from the internal iliac artery. This artery can be exposed by further opening the retroperitoneum on the side of the pelvis, elevating the vascular tapes on the proximal common iliac and distal external iliac arteries, and clamping or ligating and dividing the large branch of the iliac artery that descends into the pelvis. When bilateral iliac vascular injuries are present, the technique of total pelvic isolation, which includes cross-clamping of the aorta and inferior vena cava just above their bifurcations and distal cross-clamping of the external iliac vessels, will significantly decrease backbleeding from the internal iliac vessels.

Injuries to the iliac veins are exposed through a technique similar to that described for injuries to the iliac arteries. It is not usually necessary to pass vessel loops around these vessels, however, because they are readily compressible. As previously noted, the somewhat inaccessible location of the right common iliac vein has led to the suggested temporary transection of the right common iliac artery or ligation of the ipsilateral internal iliac artery in order to improve exposure at this location.

Porta Hepatis

A vascular injury in the porta may be in combination with an injury to the common bile duct, so some care must be taken with exposures in this area. When a hematoma is present, the proximal hepatoduodenal ligament should be looped with a vascular tape or a noncrushing vascular clamp should be applied (the Pringle maneuver) before the hematoma is entered. If hemorrhage is occurring, finger compression of the bleeding vessels will suffice until the vascular clamp is in place. The Pringle maneuver clamps the distal common bile duct as well as

the bleeding vessels, but led to only one stricture of the common bile duct in one older series of hepatic injuries from the Ben Taub General Hospital in Houston, Texas. Because of the short length of the porta in many patients, it may be difficult to place a distal vascular clamp right at the edge of the liver and manual pressure generally suffices.

Injuries to the portal vein in the hepatoduodenal ligament are isolated in much the same fashion as injuries to the hepatic artery. The posterior position of the vein, however, makes the exposure of these injuries more difficult. Mobilization of the common bile duct to the left, coupled with an extensive Kocher maneuver, will usually allow for excellent visualization of any suprapancreatic injury. As with proximal wounds to the superior mesenteric artery or vein, division of the neck of the pancreas between noncrushing intestinal clamps or with a stapler is necessary on rare occasions to visualize perforations in the retropancreatic portion of the portal vein. Exposure of the portal vein in this location will require division of the gastroduodenal artery also, as with an elective pancreaticoduodenectomy. Exposure and management of the retrohepatic and supradiaphgramatic inferior vena cava are covered elsewhere in this text.

OPERATIVE MANAGEMENT OF INJURIES BY ZONE (FIG. 3)

As previously mentioned, the management of the vascular injury, once it has been adequately exposed, is relatively straightforward. In addition to the standard techniques of primary repair, end-to-end

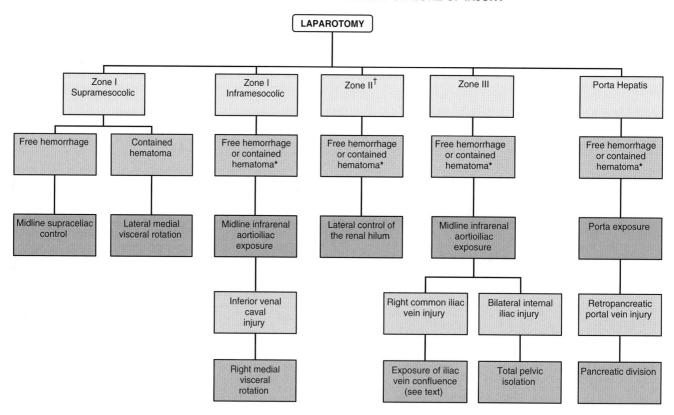

CHOICE OF OPERATIVE MANEUVER BASED ON ZONE OF INJURY

*If hematoma is contained, control of bowel contamination may precede hematoma exploration.

†Zone II: midline control of the renal hilum can be considered if there is a contained hematoma, but has not been shown to improve patient survival or renal salvage rates (see text).

FIGURE 3   Algorithm: choice of operative maneuver based on zone of injury.

anastomosis, and interposition grafting, a surgeon should remember that in a damage control setting, many vessels may be managed with ligation, also. This is true of even many of the important named vessels in the abdomen as discussed next. Ligation of major vascular structures, although occasionally necessary, should not be done without some consideration because this decision may greatly complicate the patient's postoperative course.

Zone I, Supramesocolic Region

Suprarenal Aorta

With small perforating wounds to the aorta at this level, lateral aortorrhaphy with 3-0 or 4-0 polypropylene suture is preferred. When closure of the perforations result in significant narrowing, or if a portion of the aortic wall is missing, patch aortoplasty with polytetrafluoroethylene (PTFE) is indicated. The other option is to resect a short segment of the injured aorta and attempt to perform an end-to-end anastomosis. Unfortunately, this is often impossible because of the limited mobility of both ends of the aorta at this level. Many of these patients have associated enteric injuries, and much concern has been expressed about placing a synthetic conduit in the abdominal aorta, however, the data in the American literature describing these injuries do not support the concern about potential infection of synthetic grafts.

The survival rate of patients with penetrating injuries to the suprarenal abdominal aorta series from the 1970s and 1980s averaged about 35%. More recent reviews have documented a significant decline in survival rate for injuries to the abdominal aorta (suprarenal and infrarenal) ranging from 21.1% to 50%, even when patients with exsanguination before repair or those treated with ligation only were excluded. The reasons for this decrease in survival rate are not defined in the reviews described, though a likely cause is the shorter prehospital times for exsanguinated patients arriving in a pre–cardiopulmonary arrest phase of profound or irreversible shock that have been realized with improvements in emergency medical services.

Blunt injury to the suprarenal aorta is extraordinarily rare. Although blunt injury to the descending thoracic aorta is well described throughout the trauma literature, only 62 cases of blunt trauma to the abdominal aorta were found by Roth et al in a literature review in 1997. Of these, only one case was noted to be in the suprarenal aorta. These injuries generally present with signs and symptoms of aortic thrombosis, rather than hemorrhage, and management is discussed more extensively in the section on infrarenal aortic injuries.

Celiac Axis

Injury to the celiac axis is rare. One of the largest series in the literature, reported by Asensio, documented the treatment of 13 patients with this uncommon injury. Penetrating injuries were the cause in 12 patients, and overall mortality rate was 62%. Eleven patients were treated with ligation and one with primary repair, with the final patient exsanguinating prior to therapy. An extensive literature review could only document 33 previously reported cases, all the result of penetrating trauma. Furthermore, there was no survivor treated with any sort of complex repair. One case of injury to the celiac artery after blunt trauma was reported by Schreiber et al and occurred in a patient with preexisting median arcuate ligament syndrome. Given these results, patients with injuries to the celiac axis that are not amenable to simple arteriorrhaphy should undergo ligation, which should not cause any short-term morbidity other than the aforementioned risk of gallbladder necrosis. Major branches of the celiac axis can also be ligated proximally with minimal sequelae related to the extensive collateral flow of the foregut and midgut.

Superior Mesenteric Artery

Injuries to the superior mesenteric artery are managed based on the level of injury. In 1972, Fullen and coworkers described an anatomic classification of injuries to the superior mesenteric artery that has been used intermittently by subsequent authors in the trauma literature. If the injury to the superior mesenteric artery is beneath the pancreas (Fullen zone I), the pancreas may have to be transected between noncrushing intestinal clamps to access the bleeding point. Because the superior mesenteric artery has few branches at this level, proximal and distal vascular control is relatively easy to obtain once the overlying pancreas has been divided.

Injuries to the superior mesenteric artery also occur beyond the pancreas at the base of the transverse mesocolon (Fullen zone II, between the pancreaticoduodenal and middle colic branches of the artery). Although there is certainly more space in which to work in this area, the proximity of the pancreas and the potential for pancreatic leaks near the arterial repair make injuries in this location almost as difficult to handle as the more proximal injuries. Unfortunately, although ligation of the proximal superior mesenteric artery is theoretically possible, the collateral flow in a hemodynamically unstable patient is generally inadequate to prevent bowel ischemia. So, rather than ligation in the damage control setting, a surgeon may insert a temporary intraluminal shunt into the débrided ends of the superior mesenteric artery. If replacement of the proximal superior mesenteric artery is necessary in a more stable patient, it is safest to place the origin of the saphenous vein or prosthetic graft on the distal infrarenal aorta, away from the pancreas and other upper abdominal injuries (Fig. 4). A graft in this location should be tailored so that it will pass through the posterior aspect of the mesentery of the small bowel and then be sutured to the superior mesenteric artery in an end-to-side fashion without significant tension. It is mandatory to cover the aortic suture line with retroperitoneal fat or a viable omental pedicle to avoid an aortoduodenal or aortoenteric fistula at a later time.

Injuries to the more distal superior mesenteric artery (Fullen zone III, beyond the middle colic branch), and at the level of the enteric branches (zone IV) should be repaired, because ligation in this area is distal to the connection to collateral vessels from the foregut and the hindgut. If repair cannot be accomplished because of the small size of the vessel, ligation may mandate extensive resection of the ileum and right colon.

The survival rate of patients with penetrating injuries to the superior mesenteric artery has remained between 55% and 60% in older and more modern series by both Feliciano and Asensio.

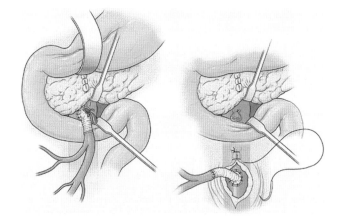

FIGURE 4 Superior mesenteric artery (SMA) reconstruction. **A,** When complete grafting procedures to the SMA are necessary, it may be dangerous to place the proximal suture line near an associated pancreatic injury. **B,** The proximal suture line should be in the lower aorta, away from the upper abdominal injuries, and should be covered with retroperitoneal tissue. *(From Feliciano DV: Injuries to the great vessels of the abdomen. In Ashley SW, Cance WG, editors: ACS surgery: principles and practice, 7th ed, Canada, 2014, BC Decker, Inc, Fig. 3, p. 3.)*

Superior Mesenteric Vein

One other major abdominal vessel, the proximal superior mesenteric vein, lying to the right of the superior mesenteric artery, may be injured at the base of the mesocolon. Injury to the most proximal aspect of this vessel near its junction with the splenic vein is difficult to access, and as described earlier, the neck of the pancreas may have to be transected to gain exposure. Often, the vein can be compressed manually or squeezed between the surgeon's fingers as an assistant places a continuous row of 5-0 polypropylene sutures into the edges of the perforation. If a posterior perforation is present, multiple collaterals entering the vein at this point will have to be ligated to roll the perforation into view. Occasionally, the vein will be nearly transected and both ends will have to be controlled with vascular clamps. With an assistant pushing the small bowel and its mesentery back toward the pancreas, the surgeon can reapproximate the ends of the vein without tension.

When multiple vascular and visceral injuries are present in the upper abdomen and the superior mesenteric vein has been severely injured, ligation can be performed in the young trauma patient. Stone et al have emphasized the need for vigorous postoperative fluid resuscitation in these patients as splanchnic hypervolemia leads to peripheral hypovolemia for at least 3 days after ligation of the superior mesenteric vein. The survival rate of patients with injuries to the superior mesenteric vein in older series was approximately 70% and has dropped to under 60% in more recent reviews.

Zone I, Inframesocolic Region

Infrarenal Aorta

As with injuries to the suprarenal aorta, penetrating or blunt injuries in the infrarenal abdominal aorta are repaired primarily with 3-0 or 4-0 polypropylene sutures or by patch aortoplasty, end-to-end anastomosis, or insertion of an interposition graft. Because the retroperitoneal tissue is often thin in young patients, it may be worthwhile to cover an extensive aortic repair or the suture line of an anastomosis with mobilized omentum before closure of the retroperitoneum.

Although the vast majority of injuries to the infrarenal aorta are penetrating in nature, a small number occur after blunt trauma. In the aforementioned review of 62 cases of blunt aortic trauma prior to 1997 reported by Roth motor vehicle collisions accounted for 57% of the cases and 47% of the total were directly attributed to lap belts. The patients generally present with symptoms of acute arterial insufficiency as stated previously, though a small number present in a delayed fashion with claudication, impotence, or rarely, delayed rupture.

The survival rate of patients with injuries to the infrarenal abdominal aorta in older studies averaged about 45%, although a more recent series noted a survival rate of infrarenal aortic injuries of 34.2%.

Infrahepatic Inferior Vena Cava

Anterior perforations of the inferior vena cava are best repaired in a transverse fashion using a continuous suture of 4-0 or 5-0 polypropylene. If vascular control is satisfactory and a posterior perforation can be visualized adequately by extending the anterior perforation, the posterior perforation can be repaired from inside the vena cava, with the first suture knot outside the lumen. Extensive repairs may lead to a "hour-glassing" effect on the vein, and in the unstable patient who has developed a coagulopathy, no further attempt should be made to modify the repair. In the stable patient, however, there may be some justification for applying a venous patch taken either from the inferior mesenteric vein or an ovarian vein or applying a thin-walled PTFE patch.

In the young patient who is exsanguinating and in whom extensive repair of the infrarenal inferior vena cava appears to be necessary, ligation of this vessel is usually well tolerated as long as certain precautions are taken. The first of these precautions is to measure the pressures in the anterior compartments of the legs and to perform bilateral below-knee four-compartment fasciotomies at the first operation if the pressure is 30 to 35 mm Hg. Bilateral thigh fasciotomies may be necessary, as well, within the first 48 hours The patient may require significant fluid resuscitation and should have the lower extremities elevated with compression wraps in the early postoperative period, also. In addition, patients should wear elastic wraps when they start to ambulate. If there is some residual edema even with the wraps in place at the time of hospital discharge, the patient should be fitted with full-length, custom-made support hose. In a recent review of 100 patients with injuries to the inferior vena cava, 25 had ligation, including 22 with injuries to the infrarenal vena cava. Survival to hospital discharge rate was 41%, and 1-year follow-up was available in seven of nine survivors. Of interest, no patient had more than trace lower extremity edema. Although the majority of patients, therefore, seem to have no or minimal long-term edema, there have been occasional reports of severe edema that occurred in the postoperative period and required later interposition grafting.

Survival rates for patients with injuries to the inferior vena cava obviously depend on the location of injury. If one eliminates injuries to the supradiaphragmatic and retrohepatic vena cava from series published from 1970s and 1980s, the average survival rate was around 75%. The two more recent series, in which injuries are stratified by location, show lower overall survival rates (40% to 60%). Finally, short-term patency after repair of the inferior vena cava has been studied. In 28 patients with prior lateral venorrhaphy of the inferior vena cava, patency of the cava was documented in 86%.

Zone II

Renovascular Injuries: Renal Artery

The renal artery is an extraordinarily small vessel that is deeply embedded in the retroperitoneum. Occasionally, small perforations can be repaired by lateral arteriorrhaphy or resection with an end-to-end anastomosis. Interposition grafting using either a saphenous vein or PTFE graft for extensive injuries is indicated only when there appears to be a reasonable hope for salvage of the kidney. In patients with multiple intra-abdominal injuries or a long preoperative period of ischemia, nephrectomy may be a better choice, as long as intraoperative palpation has confirmed a normal contralateral kidney. The survival rate of patients with injuries to the renal arteries from penetrating trauma in two older studies was approximately 87%, with renal salvage in only 30% to 40%. In three more recent series, the survival rate was 65.1%.

Diagnosis of patients with blunt injury to the renal artery is more difficult. Intimal tears in the renal arteries may result from a variety of mechanisms and usually leads to secondary thrombosis of the vessel and complaints of upper abdominal and flank pain. If a screening CT scan documents occlusion of a renal artery, the surgeon must decide on the need for either operation or endovascular intervention. The time interval from the episode of trauma appears to be the most critical factor in saving the affected kidney. In one study, there was an 80% chance of restoring some renal function at 12 hours, but this dropped to 57% at 18 hours after the onset of occlusion. If surgery is performed, extensive mobilization of the injured renal artery will usually allow a limited resection of the area of the intimal tear 2 to 3 cm from the abdominal aorta, with an end-to-end anastomosis for reconstruction. More commonly, endovascular techniques are used to revascularize the kidneys after renal artery injury and are discussed later.

Renovascular Injuries: Renal Vein

The renal vein is somewhat larger than the artery and either compression with a finger or the direct application of vascular clamps can be used to control bleeding from this vessel. Lateral venorrhaphy remains the preferred technique of repair. If ligation of the right renal vein is necessary to control hemorrhage, nephrectomy should be performed either at the initial operation or at the reoperation if damage control has been necessary. The medial left renal vein, however, can be ligated as long as the left adrenal and gonadal veins are intact. Repair is preferable however, as a greater frequency of postoperative renal complications was noted in older series when ligation was performed. The survival rate for patients with penetrating injuries to the renal veins has ranged from 42% to 88% in the older literature, with the difference presumably due to the magnitude and number of associated visceral and vascular injuries. In three recent reviews, survival rate ranged from 44.2% to 70% with a mean of 60.4%.

Injuries to the renal parenchyma are covered elsewhere.

Zone III

Common, External, and Internal Iliac Arteries

Injuries to the common or external iliac artery should be repaired or temporarily shunted because ligation of either vessel in the hypotensive patient will lead to progressive ischemia of the lower extremity and the need for a high-level amputation. In contrast, one or both internal iliac arteries can be ligated with impunity.

Options in the management of more stable patients with injuries to the common or external iliac artery include the following: lateral arteriorrhaphy; completion of a partial transection and end-to-end anastomosis; resection of the injured area and insertion of a saphenous vein or PTFE graft; mobilization of the ipsilateral internal iliac artery to serve as a replacement for the external iliac artery; or transposition of one iliac artery to the side of the contralateral iliac artery for wounds at the bifurcation.

It should be noted that complex reconstructions of the common or external iliac artery in the presence of significant enteric or fecal contamination in the pelvis remain a serious problem. Both end-to-end repairs and interposition grafts in this location have developed postoperative pseudoaneurysms and blowouts secondary to pelvic infection from the original contamination. Therefore, a surgeon should consider an extra-anatomic bypass such as a femorofemoral crossover in these situations. This would require ligation of the iliac stump with a double-running row of 4-0 or 5-0 polypropylene sutures, followed by coverage with noninjured retroperitoneum or a vascularized pedicle of omentum. If the surgeon chooses not to perform a femorofemoral crossover graft until the patient's condition has been stabilized in the surgical intensive care unit, an ipsilateral four-compartment below-knee fasciotomy should be performed, because ischemic edema below the knee will often lead to a compartment syndrome.

Blunt trauma to the iliac arteries is less common as they are protected by the bony pelvis and lie deep in the retroperitoneum. Partial transections, avulsions, or intimal injuries with secondary thrombosis have all been reported in association with pelvic fractures. Of the 10 patients with blunt thromboses reported in the literature through 1997, most were treated with insertion of a prosthetic graft, although several underwent primary repairs. Only one patient needed an amputation. As noted earlier, the recent study of patients in the National Trauma Data Bank documented a 7.7% amputation rate in patients with pelvic fractures and an associated injury to the iliac artery.

The survival rate among patients with injuries to the iliac arteries will vary with the number of associated injuries to the iliac vein, aorta, and vena cava, but ranged from 45% to 81% in older series and 45% to 55% in more recent series.

Common, External, and Internal Iliac Veins

Injuries to the common or external iliac vein are treated either with lateral repair using 4-0 or 5-0 polypropylene suture or with ligation. Ligation in the young patient is generally well tolerated if the same precautions used after ligation of the inferior vena cava are applied;

however, some centers strongly recommend repair rather than ligation for injuries of these vessels. When significant narrowing of the common or external iliac vein results from a lateral repair, postoperative anticoagulation is appropriate to lessen the risk of thrombosis and/or pulmonary embolism.

The survival rate of patients with injuries to the iliac veins is variable, but was higher than 70% in most older series and approximately 65% in more recent series.

Porta Hepatis

Hepatic Artery

Due to its short course, injury to any portion of the hepatic artery is rare. Replacement of the injured common hepatic artery with a substitute vascular conduit is rarely indicated because most patients with a portal hematoma or hemorrhage have significant associated injuries to the liver, right kidney, or inferior vena cava. Indeed, ligation of the proper or common hepatic artery appears to be well tolerated in the young trauma patient, even when performed beyond the origin of the gastroduodenal artery, owing to the extensive collateral arterial flow to the liver. Because of the small size of the right or left hepatic artery, lateral repairs are often difficult and will frequently be followed by occlusion of the vessel in the postoperative period.

A relatively large multicenter experience was published in 1995 by Jurkovich, which documented the course of 99 patients with injury to the portal triad. Of this group, 28 patients had 29 injuries to segments of the hepatic artery; 19 patients underwent ligation, and there were 8 survivors. Only one patient developed hepatic necrosis requiring débridement, and this patient had an associated extensive injury to that lobe. Seven patients had attempts at repair with only one survivor, and two other patients exsanguinated prior to therapy. Obviously, selective ligation of the right hepatic artery warrants a cholecystectomy.

Portal Vein

As noted earlier, injuries to any portion of the portal vein are more difficult to manage than are injuries to the hepatic artery, owing to the posterior location of the vein, the friability of its wall, and the greater blood flow through it. Techniques for repair of the vein are varied, but lateral venorrhaphy with a 4-0 or 5-0 polypropylene suture is preferred. More extensive maneuvers that have occasionally been used with success include the following: resection with an end-to-end anastomosis, interposition grafting, transposition of the splenic vein down to the superior mesenteric vein to replace the proximal portal vein, an end-to-side portacaval shunt, or a venovenous shunt from the superior mesenteric vein to the distal portal vein or inferior vena cava. Such vigorous attempts at restoration of blood flow have resulted from the concern about viability of the midgut if the portal vein is ligated. However, ligation of the vein is compatible with survival, as both Pachter and Stone have emphasized. In the 1979 review of the literature on this subject by Pachter, 1 of 6 survivors of ligation of the portal vein developed portal hypertension. The 1982 series by Stone et al included 9 survivors among 18 patients who underwent ligation of the portal vein. In essence, ligation of the portal vein should be performed if an extensive injury is present and the patient requires a damage control operation. The surgeon must then be prepared to infuse significant amounts of fluids to reverse the transient peripheral hypovolemia secondary to splanchnic hypervolemia.

More recently, Ivatury et al reported on 14 patients with injuries to the portal vein, among whom exsanguination occurred in 3, venorrhaphy was performed in 10 (of whom 6 survived), and ligation was done in 1 (who survived). Finally, Jurkovich reported on 56 injuries to the portal vein with 33 patients undergoing primary repair (42% mortality rate), 1 undergoing complex repair (died), and 10 undergoing ligation (90% mortality rate). An additional 11 patients died before therapy.

Wounds of the retrohepatic and supradiaphragmatic vena cava are discussed elsewhere in this text.

ENDOVASCULAR INTERVENTION

Although patients with AVI who present with active hemorrhage generally require immediate open exploration, a smaller subset who present with contained hemorrhage or thrombosis may be candidates for endovascular techniques. Although endovascular grafts are now well accepted for contained disruptions of the thoracic aorta and angioembolization has been a very successful adjunct to nonoperative management of solid organ injuries, the role of these types of interventions in true AVI is not as well established. Indeed, the literature describing endovascular techniques in these potentially devastating injuries comprises mostly case reports and small case series and has been reviewed elsewhere.

Endovascular therapy has a longstanding and well-established role in the management of renovascular injury and bleeding from pelvic fractures. As previously mentioned, renovascular injuries are difficult to manage operatively, especially when the renal artery is involved. As the diagnosis is often somewhat delayed and because of the relatively poor function of kidneys revascularized with open surgery, enthusiasm for attempts at open repair has waned. Multiple authors have described endovascular management of injuries to the renal vasculature. Renal arteries and major branches have been embolized in series back into the 1980s with good renal preservation. For example, Sclafani reported on eight patients with renal injuries who were treated with angiographic embolization. Of interest, seven of eight patients had successful procedures, and all seven had preservation of the kidney, with one nephrectomy performed for persistent hematuria. A more recent study reported on the treatment of eight patients, seven of whom were successfully treated with angiographic embolization, obviating the need for open surgery. At discharge, all survivors had normal renal function and all patients were normotensive. Thus, in the hemodynamically normal patient, transcatheter embolization has been used successfully to manage a variety of renovascular injuries and allow for organ preservation. In more recent years with improving technology, there has been an increased interest in preserving blood flow to the renal parenchyma with the use of expandable stents rather than transcatheter embolization. At least three case reports document the successful use of various stents to obliterate intimal flaps in patients with renal artery injuries with preservation of renal function and no short-term complications.

One of the largest series of nonthoracic vascular injuries managed with covered stents in the literature was published in 2006. In this multicenter trial, 62 patients were managed with Wallgraft endoprosthesis grafts over 6 years. This group included 33 patients with injuries to the iliac vessels, most of which were iatrogenic in nature, and included 27 perforations, 4 arteriovenous fistulas, 1 pseudoaneurysm, and 1 dissection. Technical success, as defined by total postprocedure exclusion, was achieved in all but one patient with an injury to the iliac artery and primary patency at 1 year was 76% for these patients. Early adverse events occurred in 14% of patients, mostly related to puncture site complications, and a late adverse event occurred in another 6.5% of patients with one systemic infection, one occlusion, and three stenoses of the repair. All-cause mortality rate was 6.5% in the early postprocedure period and 17.7% in later follow-up. None of the deaths was thought to be the result of the stent graft.

OUTCOMES

The complications of vascular repairs in the abdomen are much the same as those seen in the extremities. They include such problems as thrombosis, dehiscence of a suture line, and infection. Occlusion is not uncommon when small, vasoconstricted vessels, such as the renal artery or superior mesenteric artery, undergo lateral arteriorrhaphy. In such patients, it may be valuable to perform a second-look operation within 12 to 24 hours after the patient's temperature, coagulation abnormalities, and blood pressure have returned to normal. When this is done, correction of a vascular thrombosis may be successful.

Dehiscence of vascular suture lines in the abdomen occurs with some frequency in two locations, and both have been previously discussed. First, a substitute vascular conduit inserted in the superior mesenteric artery near a pancreatic injury may be disrupted if a small pancreatic leak occurs in the postoperative period. Second, the dehiscence of end-to-end anastomoses and conduit suture lines in the iliac arteries can be avoided by limiting the extent of repair if there is significant enteric or fecal contamination in the pelvis and considering early extra-anatomic bypass if the patient's limb is threatened.

Finally, a vascular complication unique to the abdomen is the postoperative development of vascular-enteric fistulas. This complication will occur most commonly in patients who have anterior aortic repairs, aortic grafts, or grafts to the superior mesenteric artery from the aorta. Again, this problem can be avoided by proper coverage of suture lines on the aorta with retroperitoneal tissue or a viable omental pedicle and on the recipient vessel with mesentery.

SUMMARY

Abdominal vascular injuries are commonly seen in patients with penetrating wounds to the abdomen. They present with either a contained retroperitoneal, mesenteric, or portal hematoma or with active hemorrhage. When tamponade is present, proximal and distal vascular control should be obtained before opening the hematoma causing the tamponade. If active hemorrhage is present, direct compression of the bleeding vessels with a finger, hand, laparotomy pad, or spongestick at the site of injury is necessary until proximal and distal vascular control can be attained. Vascular repairs are generally performed with polypropylene sutures and can range from simple arteriorrhaphy or venorrhaphy to the insertion of substitute vascular conduits, much as in vascular injuries in the extremities. Also, in the occasional patient who presents with normal hemodynamics, thrombotic sequelae, or in a delayed fashion after AVI, endovascular techniques may have a role in management. Overall, if hemorrhage can be rapidly controlled and distal perfusion restored, many patients with major abdominal vascular injuries can be saved.

For the chapter's Suggested Readings list, please visit the book at www.ExpertConsult.inkling.com.

COLON AND RECTAL INJURIES

David J. Ciesla

S urgical management of colon and rectal injuries has evolved dramatically since World War II. Accepted treatment at that time generally consisted of resection and end colostomy based on experience with battlefield casualties. Although a difference between civilian and military injuries was recognized, the treatment by civilian trauma surgeons paralleled that of their military counterparts. In the ensuing decades following the Korean and Vietnam wars, primary repair began to replace the "colostomy only" approach in the nonmilitary setting. Numerous prospective randomized trials in civilian centers have since established primary repair as the preferred treatment for most colon and rectal injuries.

INCIDENCE AND MECHANISM OF INJURY

Mechanisms of colon and rectal injuries can be classified as direct penetration of the bowel wall by a foreign body as with stab or gunshot wounds, high-pressure blowout of the bowel wall as occurs in blunt trauma, or devascularization injury secondary to avulsion of the supporting mesentery. The vast majority of colon injuries are caused by penetrating trauma. Firearms account for 75% to 90% of penetrating colon injuries. The colon is second only to the small bowel in the frequency of organs injured in penetrating trauma. The high incidence of colon injuries in penetrating trauma relative to other organs is a reflection of the size and distribution of the colon within the abdominal cavity. In contrast, blunt colon injuries are rare, occurring in less than 5% of patients with abdominal injuries. Most occur following high-energy motor vehicle crashes and present as blowout disruptions of colonic wall or mesenteric avulsions. Approximately 80% of rectal injuries are caused by firearms, 10% by blunt trauma, 6% by transanal or impalement injuries, and 3% by transabdominal stab wounds.

DIAGNOSIS

Colon injuries are most often diagnosed during operative exploration. Although it is rare to make an organ-specific diagnosis preoperatively, free intraperitoneal air may occasionally be seen on chest radiograph or abdominal computed tomography (CT) scan. Blood or a positive occult hemoglobin test on digital rectal examination may also be seen. Suspicion of enteric injury should be raised in all patients with evidence of fever, tachycardia, peritonitis, and leukocytosis. CT scan evidence of intra-abdominal fluid in the absence of solid organ injury warrants further investigation, usually by diagnostic peritoneal lavage. A triple-contrast CT scan may be helpful in patients who have penetrating flank injuries with no clear evidence of intraperitoneal injury.

Blunt colonic injuries are evenly distributed around the colon and usually present as large blowout disruptions of the colon wall or avulsion injuries in which the mesocolon is stripped from the adjacent colon. Although penetrating colon injuries are usually obvious, missed injuries are often the result of small-caliber gunshot wounds or stab wounds to areas that are difficult to examine, such as the splenic flexure and rectosigmoid junction. If a perforation is not obvious, feculent odor, hematoma, or mesenteric staining may suggest an area that requires further evaluation. The suspicious area should be completely mobilized. Division of one or two terminal mesenteric vessels may be necessary to adequately evaluate potential injuries at the mesenteric border. A final diagnostic maneuver is to create a closed loop of colon by proximal and distal manual compression and gently milk the bowel contents toward the suspected injury. The extrusion of fecal material or gas is diagnostic, and its absence effectively rules out colonic injury.

All patients with truncal stab and gunshot wounds; impalements of the lower abdomen, buttocks, perineum, or upper thighs; and any history of anal manipulation and lower abdominal or pelvic pain should be suspected of having a rectal injury. Evaluation begins with a digital rectal examination, in which the presence of gross or occult blood should trigger further investigation. However, it is important to note that a negative digital rectal examination does not rule out a rectal injury. Rigid proctoscopy should be performed in all patients with suspected rectal injury. Unstable patients who have undergone laparotomy for hemorrhage control should have the abdomen temporarily closed and should be repositioned for proctoscopy. Palpation or visualization of a perforation is definitive evidence of an injury. However, intraluminal blood or a submucosal hematoma is often the only evidence of rectal injury. In such cases with distal rectal injuries, transabdominal exploration and rectal mobilization does not improve the chance of definitive diagnosis and may increase the chance of iatrogenic vascular, urologic, or neurologic injury. Therefore, these patients should be treated in the same manner as patients with confirmed rectal injuries.

ANATOMIC LOCATION OF INJURY AND INJURY GRADING

The colon begins at the ileocecal valve and continues to the rectosigmoid junction. Blood is supplied via the ileocolic, right, and middle colic branches of the superior mesenteric artery and the left colic and sigmoidal branches of the inferior mesenteric artery. Venous drainage is via the mesenteric plexus to the superior and inferior mesenteric veins that empty into the portal vein. The rectum begins at the rectosigmoid junction and ends at the dentate line in the anal canal. Blood is supplied by the superior hemorrhoidal branch of the inferior mesenteric artery and the middle and inferior hemorrhoidal branches of the internal iliac or internal pudendal arteries. Venous drainage of the rectum follows the arteries with the superior hemorrhoidal vein draining into the portal system and the middle and inferior hemorrhoidal veins draining via the internal iliac veins.

The Organ Injury Scaling (OIS) Committee of the American Association of the Surgery of Trauma (AAST) has developed colon and rectal injury scales that facilitate comparison of injuries between patients and facilities and helps identify patients at high risk for postoperative complications (Tables 1 and 2). The rectum can be further divided into intraperitoneal and extraperitoneal zones that help guide surgical decision making (Fig. 1).

SURGICAL MANAGEMENT

The current management strategies for colon and rectal injuries have been scientifically established in recent decades in civilian trauma centers where operations are generally performed shortly after injury in patients who have been resuscitated and treated with antibiotics. There are two generally accepted surgical options for contemporary management of colon injuries: primary repair and colostomy. Primary repair, whether direct closure of a defect or segmental resection and primary anastomosis, implies that the initial surgical intervention is definitive and no further treatment is necessary. Colostomy options include proximal end colostomy or ileostomy with distal mucous fistula or distal closure (Hartmann procedure), loop colostomy

TABLE 1: AAST Colon Injury Grading

Grade*	Type	Injury Description
I	Hematoma	Contusion or hematoma without devascularization
	Laceration	Partial thickness, no perforation
II	Laceration	Laceration <50% of circumference
III	Laceration	Laceration >50% of circumference
IV	Laceration	Transection of colon
V	Laceration	Transection with segmental tissue loss

Modified from Organ Injury Scaling Committee of the American Association of the Surgery of Trauma, Moore EE, Cogbill TH, Malangoni MA, et al: Organ injury scaling II: pancreas, doudenum, small bowel, colon and rectum. *J Trauma* 30:1427, 1990.
AAST, American Association of the Surgery of Trauma.
*Advance one grade for multiple injuries up to grade III.

TABLE 2: AAST Rectal Injury Grading

Grade*	Type	Injury Description
I	Hematoma	Contusion or hematoma without devascularization
	Laceration	Partial thickness, no perforation
II	Laceration	Laceration <50% of circumference
III	Laceration	Laceration >50% of circumference
IV	Laceration	Full-thickness laceration with extension into perineum
V	Vascular	Devascularized segment

Modified from Organ Injury Scaling Committee of the American Association of the Surgery of Trauma, Moore EE, Cogbill TH, Malangoni MA, et al: Organ injury scaling II: pancreas, doudenum, small bowel, colon and rectum. *J Trauma* 30:1427, 1990.
AAST, American Association of the Surgery of Trauma.
*Advance one grade for multiple injuries to the same organ.

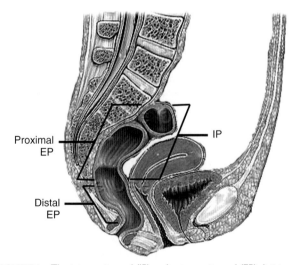

FIGURE 1   The intraperitoneal (IP) and extraperitoneal (EP) divisions of the rectum. *(From Weinberg JA, Fabian TC, Magnotti LJ, et al: Penetrating rectal trauma: management by anatomic distinction improves outcome.* J Trauma 60:508–514, 2006.)

(exteriorization) of the injured segment without repair, and diverting colostomy proximal to suture repair.

Most authorities would agree that modern treatment of colon injuries is either by primary repair or colostomy. Although primary repair of all colon injuries in the nonmilitary setting is a desirable goal, it is not always possible. The key to successful management is patient selection based on the location and degree of injury and the physiologic state of the patient at the time of repair. For simple nondestructive injuries that do not require segmental resection (AAST-OIS grades I–III), the treatment of choice is primary suture repair. Débridement is kept to a minimum except to remove grossly contaminated or ischemic tissue. We employ a single transverse closure using absorbable monofilament suture beginning a few millimeters from each end of the colotomy. Sutures are placed to gently oppose the seromuscular layer in a continuous Lembert fashion (Fig. 2). Alternatively, many surgeons will perform primary repair using two layers, an inner layer encompassing the entire wall of the colon using absorbable sutures and an outer sermomuscular layer with nonabsorbable sutures in the Lembert fashion.

The choice between primary anastomosis and colostomy is more complex for destructive colon injuries. The first consideration is the physiologic state of the patient. A damage control approach should be strongly considered for patients with significant metabolic compromise. Critically injured patients with evidence of acidosis, coagulopathy, and hypothermia are at imminent risk of death. The damage control approach is founded on the principle that the metabolic status of the patient does not allow sufficient time to definitively repair all injuries. The immediate priority is to control bleeding and abdominal contamination, temporarily close the abdomen, and transport the patient to the intensive care unit for vigorous metabolic resuscitation, correction of coagulopathy, and rewarming. The most expeditious method to control fecal contamination is to resect the injured segment of colon using a gastrointestinal anastomosis (GIA) stapler and close the abdomen with an adhesive plastic sheet. Definitive management of the injury is then performed once the patient has been adequately resuscitated, usually within 24 hours.

Primary repair has been established as the optimal treatment of destructive colon injuries. Destructive injuries proximal to the middle colic artery are generally treated with a right colectomy and ileocolostomy. Ileocolostomy has proved to be a robust anastomosis under emergent conditions and the low associated leak rate justifies its use for almost all injuries proximal to the middle colic artery. Lateral suture repair or segmental resection and colocolostomy is also the procedure of choice for destructive injuries distal to the middle colic artery. Several contemporary retrospective and prospective

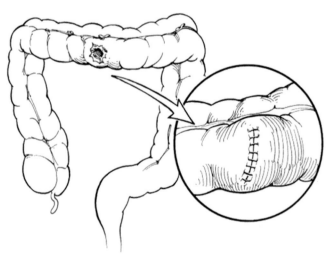

FIGURE 2   Primary repair of a nondestructive colon injury using a single-layer continuous suture. *(Courtesy of Baylor College of Medicine.)*

randomized studies have demonstrated that the results following primary repair are as good as or better than routine colostomy with respect to postoperative complications. These studies have also identified a number of risk factors for suture line failure that include blood loss, concomitant solid organ injury, fecal contamination, mechanism of injury, delayed repair, and patient age. An additional consideration is the subjective evaluation of the degree of bowel edema present at the time of anastomosis. The visceral edema that occurs in the setting of large-volume resuscitation makes the placement and tension of anastomotic sutures uncertain and healing unpredictable. Therefore, colostomy should be considered for injuries distal to the middle colic artery in the presence of significant bowel edema.

Although several methods have been described for creation of ileocolostomy and colocolostomy, we prefer the end-to-end, single-layer technique using absorbable monofilament suture (Fig. 3). The suture line is started at the mesenteric border using a double-armed 3-0 polydioxanone suture. Sutures are then placed 3 to 4 mm from the cut edge of the bowel to include all layers but the mucosa. Each arm is advanced around the bowel and tied at the antimesenteric border resembling a vascular anastomosis. Disparity in bowel caliber can be solved by extension of the enterotomy on the smaller end along the antimesenteric border. The mesenteric defect is then closed with a continuous absorbable suture. Alternatively, a two-layer technique is also used.

Destructive colon injuries distal to the middle colic artery in patients with multiple risk factors for suture line failure should be treated with colostomy. The damaged section of the colon is resected using a GIA stapler and the proximal end of the colon is used for the colostomy. The key technical aspects of colostomy are to ensure that the clamped end of the colon reaches the skin level with no tension, that the end of the colon has an adequate blood supply, and that the colostomy is immediately matured with sutures between the mucosa and the skin without tension. The distal end of the defunctionalized colon is left closed with staples. Treatment of the distal colon segment with mucous fistula is avoided because it is time consuming, is of no additional benefit, adds the potential complications of a second stoma, and adds difficulty to subsequent colostomy closure.

The anatomic level governs the surgical treatment of rectal injuries. As noted previously, the only indication of a rectal injury may be the presence of intraluminal blood or a submucosal hematoma observed during rigid proctoscopy. Nondestructive injuries to the proximal intraperitoneal and extraperitoneal rectum that do not require resection based on intraoperative evaluation (AAST-OIS grades I–III) are repaired primarily. These injuries are generally lacerations with minimal surrounding tissue destruction that are easily exposed after mobilization of the proximal rectum and sutured. The technique is the same as that used for primary repair of colon injuries using a running single layer of 3-0 polydioxanone suture. Placement of drains in the pelvis is not necessary and may increase the risk of fistula. Injuries with extensive loss of the rectal wall or devascularization (AAST-OIS grades IV and V) are best treated by resection distal to the injury and proximal end colostomy. The rectum can be divided within a few centimeters of the anal verge with the aid of a TA stapler after mobilization of the distal rectum. In addition, the advent of the end-to-end circular stapling device has facilitated elective colostomy closure. This has proved to be a much safer approach to destructive colon injuries than primary repair.

FIGURE 3 Resection and primary repair of a destructive colon injury using a single layer continuous suture to create an end-to-end anastomosis. *(Courtesy of Baylor College of Medicine.)*

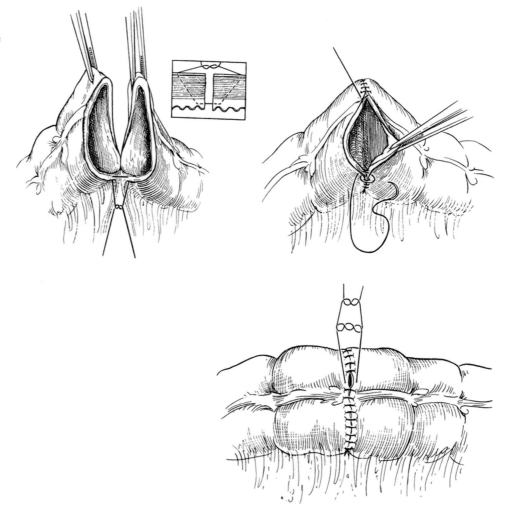

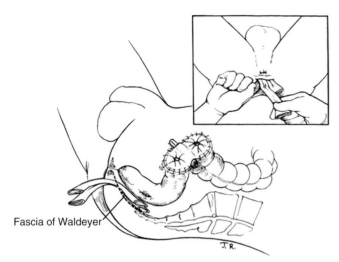

Fascia of Waldeyer

FIGURE 4   Technique for presacral drainage and proximal diversion for treatment of occult or unrepaired distal colon injuries. *(Courtesy of Baylor College of Medicine.)*

Wounds to the distal extraperitoneal rectum should be treated with colostomy. Extensive dissection to definitively visualize distal rectal injuries should be avoided because of the potential for vascular, urologic, neurologic, or iatrogenic rectal injury. In such cases, the patient is treated as if a rectal injury is present with proximal diversion (Fig. 4). Although several methods for proximal diversion are described, it is essential that the chosen technique must completely divert the fecal stream from the rectal injury. We employ a loop colostomy located in the patient's left lower quadrant using the sigmoid colon. The critical technical elements to ensure complete diversion are creating a longitudinal colotomy, maintaining the common wall or spur between the afferent and efferent limbs above the level of the skin, and maturing the stoma to the skin immediately. A loop colostomy created in this manner completely diverts the fecal stream.

Although presacral drainage has long been considered an integral component to treatment of distal rectal injures, its utility has been questioned in some reports. Nonetheless, many still advocate its use to minimize the risk of infectious complications such as pelvic sepsis. A curved incision is made posterior to the anus and the presacral space developed bluntly to the level of the sacrum. Ideally, Penrose drains are placed in proximity but not in contact with the injury. The drains are secured to the skin with silk sutures for better patient comfort and are usually removed between 4 and 7 days after injury.

MORBIDITY AND COMPLICATIONS MANAGEMENT

Intra-abdominal abscess is the most frequent septic complication following colon repair, occurring in 5% to 15% of patients. Small abscesses of less than 2 cm often respond to intravenous antibiotic therapy and do not require drainage. Many intra-abdominal abscesses can be managed by image-guided percutaneous drainage. Occasionally, percutaneous drainage reveals an underlying fistula. In such cases when the patient has no evidence of sepsis, the percutaneous drain is left in place until follow-up imaging demonstrates obliteration of the abscess cavity. Once this occurs, the drain is slowly removed. Larger intra-abdominal abscesses that are inaccessible to percutaneous drainage and those associated with sepsis require operative drainage.

Suture line failure and fecal fistula may occur regardless of the treatment method chosen and have been observed in 1% to 8% of

patients. Fistulas that extend to the incision are often associated with intra-abdominal abscesses and evidence of sepsis. A fistulogram should also be performed to determine if there is diffuse leakage throughout the abdominal cavity and an abdominal CT obtained to look for intra-abdominal abscesses. Controlled fistulas can be managed nonoperatively but the wound must be carefully inspected for evidence of necrotizing fasciitis. Uncontrolled fistulas require operative intervention and are usually treated by resection of the fistula and leaking segment of colon followed by proximal diversion with an end colostomy.

Stoma complications including stomal necrosis, obstruction, peristomal evisceration, and subcutaneous abscess occur in 3% to 14% of patients. Most stomal complications require operative intervention.

Wound infections occur in up to 50% of patients with colon or rectal injuries but should not be considered a complication of the repair. Virtually all wound infections can be avoided by leaving the wound open at the time of abdominal closure. Closure of the wound during the initial operation should be reserved for the patient who has few associated injuries, minimal subcutaneous fat, and little contamination and who has not suffered prolonged shock.

Stab wound and missile tract infections occur frequently and must be considered in any patient with evidence of systemic sepsis. A reasonable effort should be made to remove missiles and material that have traversed the colon and lodged in the soft tissue to avoid soft tissue infection and possible necrotizing fasciitis.

MORTALITY

Early death in the multiply injured patient with colon and rectal injuries is most often a result of exsanguination from associated injuries. The late mortality rate associated with colon injuries in contemporary studies ranges from 1% to 4%, most often a result of sepsis or multiple-organ failure. Death occurs more often in the patients treated with colostomy, but this may be a reflection of injury severity rather than treatment method.

CONCLUSIONS AND MANAGEMENT ALGORITHM

Despite the evolution in management of colon and rectal injuries in the recent past, the key elements to treatment have remained the same. Prompt recognition, hemorrhage control, and control of enteric spillage are the immediate management priorities followed by reconstruction or diversion. Although treatment must be individualized based on each injury, the constellation of associated injuries, and the physiologic state of the patient, it is important to have a generalized institutional approach to assess treatment outcomes.

With these considerations, we have adopted an approach to colon and rectal injuries outlined in Figure 5. The critical decision-making points for colon injuries are the metabolic status of the patient, the need for segmental resection, the location of the injury, and the condition of the bowel at the time of repair. Adherence to this approach enables primary repair in 70% to 90% of patients. The first consideration in rectal injuries is whether the injury is identified and repaired. Nondestructive injuries to the proximal rectum are repaired primarily but those requiring segmental resection are best treated with colostomy rather than primary anastomosis during the initial operation. Distal rectal injuries that are not directly identified or not repaired because of anatomic location are treated with proximal diversion and consideration of presacral drainage.

For the chapter's Suggested Readings list, please visit the book at www.ExpertConsult.inkling.com.

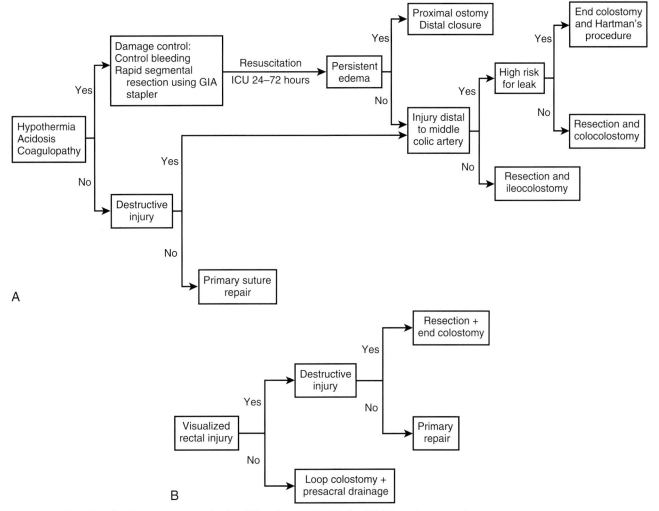

FIGURE 5 Algorithms for the management of colon (**A**) and rectal (**B**) injuries. ICU, Intensive care unit.

GENITOURINARY TRACT INJURIES

Lucas R. Wiegand and Steven B. Brandes

KIDNEY TRAUMA

Incidence and Mechanisms of Injury

At most urban trauma centers, mechanisms of kidney injuries are predominantly blunt (80–90%) and uncommonly penetrating (10–20%). The kidney is injured in up to 5% of all trauma cases. Children are more likely to sustain a blunt renal injury owing to the relatively large size of the kidney, scant perirenal fat, and incomplete rib ossification. The majority of renal injuries are minor and heal spontaneously. Significant kidney injuries occur in only 4% of blunt trauma yet up to 70% of penetrating renal injuries.

Diagnosis

Signs and Symptoms

Hematuria is the hallmark of renal injury. The degree of hematuria often does not correspond or predict the extent of renal injury. Up to 40% of renal pedicle injuries present with no hematuria. A history is obtained to quantify the forces involved in the renal injury. Falls from a height and injuries due to high-speed motor vehicle crashes imply deceleration injury and require evaluation of the renal pedicle and ureteropelvic junction (UPJ). Patients with trauma to the flank, abdomen, or lower chest; flank ecchymosis or tenderness; low posterior rib fractures; or lumbar transverse process fractures should be suspected of having a renal injury—and thus should undergo imaging. A major renal injury that results from a minor mechanism usually occurs in a congenitally abnormal kidney (such as UPJ obstruction).

For gunshot wounds (GSWs) to the kidney, it is important to determine if the injury is due to a high- or low-velocity missile. High-velocity missiles usually cause extensive kidney injury and delayed necrosis. The entrance and exit wounds should be marked with radiopaque markers. Stab wound (SW) entrance sites posterior to the anterior axillary line and above the nipple line are less likely to have associated intraperitoneal organ injury or warrant abdominal exploration.

Imaging

Indications for imaging a suspected kidney injury are as follows:

1. Blunt trauma and gross hematuria
2. Blunt trauma, microscopic hematuria (>5 red blood cells/high-power field [RBCs/HPF]), and shock (systolic blood pressure <90 mm Hg)
3. Major acceleration or deceleration injury
4. Microscopic or gross hematuria after penetrating flank, back, or abdominal trauma; or when the missile path is in line with the kidney
5. Pediatric trauma patient with any degree of hematuria
6. Associated injuries/physical signs suggesting underlying renal injury

Intravenous urography (IVU) for potential kidney injuries in stable trauma patients has been replaced by abdominal computed tomography. In unstable patients who require abdominal exploration, a one-shot IVU study is commonly advocated by urologists, prior to any exploration of a retroperitoneal (perirenal) hematoma. Intravenous contrast agent, at 2 mL per kilogram of body weight, is generally given, followed by a single abdominal radiograph at 10 minutes. The one-shot IVU is performed to determine the function of the contralateral kidney, in order to avoid removing a solitary kidney. Practically, the one-shot IVU is often "fuzzy" and difficult to interpret. Most trauma surgeons do not use the one-shot IVU, but rather palpate the contralateral side for kidney presence or administer intravenous methylene blue or indigo carmine and temporarily occlude the ipsilateral ureter. Blue urine in the Foley bag indicates a functional contralateral kidney.

Computed tomography (CT) is the imaging study of choice for demonstrating renal parenchymal injury, perirenal or retroperitoneal hematomas, urinary extravasation, injuries to the renal hilum and great vessels, and associated intra-abdominal organ injuries. Renal artery occlusion and renal infarct are noted by lack of parenchymal enhancement or by a "cortical rim sign." An arteriographic phase (to assess major vessel injury) and a delayed nephrographic phase (to assess for contrast extravasation) are essential to accurately stage the kidney injury.

Ultrasonography (US) is primarily used in Europe for evaluating renal trauma but is of limited value. US can be useful for demonstrating perirenal fluid collections, but cannot distinguish fresh blood from extravasated urine. *Arteriography* and superselective embolization have important roles in the evaluation and treatment of a contrast "blush" noted on CT, or delayed renal bleeding (pseudoaneurysms). In select cases, arteriography and endoluminal stent placement have also been successful in managing renal artery intimal tears and thrombosis from blunt trauma.

Stage of Injury

Detailed Injury Scoring Scales for genitourinary trauma can be found at http://www.aast.org/library/traumatools/injuryscoringscales.aspx.

Management

Figure 1 offers a treatment algorithm for renal trauma. Blunt renal injuries are almost all managed conservatively. Only with shattered kidneys or renal pedicle avulsion injuries, when there is a potential

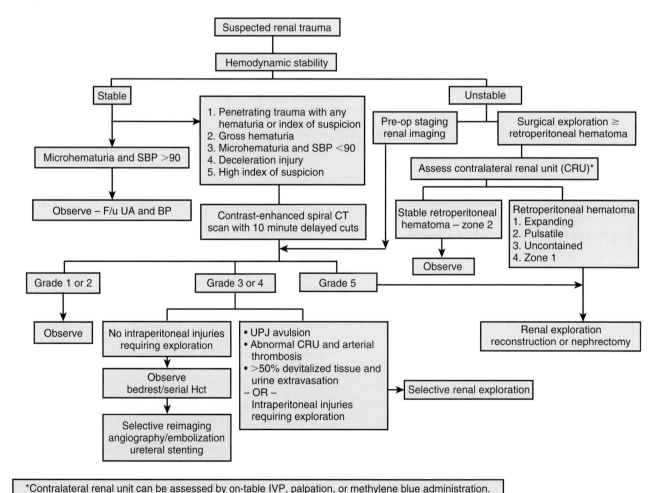

FIGURE 1 Algorithm for renal trauma. BP, Blood pressure; CT, computed tomography; F/u, follow-up; Hct, hematocrit; IVP, intravenous pyelogram; SBP, systolic blood pressure; UA, urinalysis; UPJ, ureteropelvic junction.

for exsanguination, is exploration required. Unless the UPJ is completely disrupted, urine extravasation from the kidney will usually resolve spontaneously. In order to select nonoperative management, the renal injury needs to be imaged and accurately staged. Conservative management of renal injuries requires strict bed rest until the urine visibly clears, frequent hematocrit blood draws, and reimaging after 2 to 3 days for major renal injuries with noted urine (contrast) extravasation. Persistent bleeding demands repeat imaging, arteriography, or surgical exploration. Worsening or symptomatic urinary leaks require ureteral stenting. Most penetrating kidney traumas demand exploration because the injuries are usually high grade and are associated with other major organ damage. Roughly 75% of renal GSWs and 50% of renal SWs demand exploration. Grade 3 and 4 penetrating injuries can be managed by observation, yet roughly 25% require subsequent angioembolization.

Surgery

Absolute indications for exploration are persistent and potentially life-threatening renal bleeding. Such bleeding usually occurs with avulsion of the renal pedicle or a shattered kidney. The primary sign of continued renal bleeding is a pulsatile, expanding, or unconfined retroperitoneal hematoma. *Relative indications* for kidney exploration are as follows:

1. Devitalized renal parenchyma that is greater than 50%.
2. Urinary extravasation in itself does not demand surgical exploration. The majority of such cases resolve spontaneously (usually within 72 hours), except for UPJ avulsion injuries, which are best managed by prompt surgical repair.
3. Incomplete staging demands either further imaging or renal exploration.
4. In patients with two normal kidneys, isolated renal artery thrombosis that is not associated with extensive bleeding or urinary extravasation is best managed conservatively, because revascularization rarely preserves significant renal function. Revascularization should be reserved only for bilateral renal artery occlusion or unilateral occlusion in a solitary kidney.
5. High-grade renal injuries need surgical exploration when abdominal exploration is performed for an associated intra-abdominal injury. Exploring a high-grade blunt kidney injury is controversial and should be attempted only by an experienced urologic surgeon.
6. High-grade penetrating renal injuries generally should be managed surgically because of high rates of delayed bleeding.

The injured kidney is best exposed through a midline transperitoneal incision. Classic teaching dictates that, for zone 1 hematomas, proximal vascular control takes place before renal exploration. Without control of the hilar vessels, exploration can risk releasing the tamponade effect and thus cause massive bleeding. Uncontrolled bleeding results in a nephrectomy. Consistent proximal vascular control of the renal pedicle for zone 2 hematomas is controversial, as kidney bleeding can typically be controlled by hilar clamping or manual compression. Briefly, repair of the damaged kidney requires broad exposure of the kidney and injured area, temporary vascular occlusion for brisk renal bleeding, sharp excision of all nonviable parenchyma, meticulous hemostasis, water-tight closure of the collecting system, and parenchymal defect suture closure over a bolster.

Complications

Complications after renal trauma are most commonly prolonged urinary extravasation, delayed bleeding, arterial pseudoaneurysm, abscess, urinary fistula, and hydronephrosis. Renal vascular hypertension after renal trauma is almost always transient. Very rarely, sustained hypertension is seen with subcapsular hematomas that cause parenchymal compression (Page kidney).

URETERAL TRAUMA

Incidence and Mechanism

External Trauma

Ureteral injuries from external trauma are very rare. The mechanism of ureteral injuries is 95% penetrating and 5% blunt. GSWs in proximity to the ureter can cause severe ureteral contusion due to a blast-effect. After a deceleration injury, the kidney is often dislocated, and tears typically occur at the fixation point of the UPJ and hilar vasculature. Another mechanism for injury is hyperextension of the back, when the ureter is avulsed, stretched by the lumbar and lower thoracic vertebral bodies. This classically occurs in limber children with a pedestrian versus motor vehicle crash.

Iatrogenic Trauma

Iatrogenic ureteral injuries usually occur during difficult or bloody pelvic operations. Overall, the ureter is injured in only 0.5% to 1.0% of pelvic operations. Iatrogenic ureteral injury most commonly occurs during transabdominal hysterectomy. Injuries can also occur during urologic, colorectal (abdominal perineal or low anterior resections), and vascular surgeries.

Diagnosis

Signs and Symptoms

Successful surgical management of ureteral injuries requires a high index of suspicion, early diagnosis (and thus a low threshold for urinary tract imaging), and an intimate knowledge of ureteral anatomy and blood supply. Hematuria (gross or microscopic) is not a reliable sign and is absent in up to 45% of penetrating and 67% of blunt ureteral injuries. If recognized and repaired intraoperatively, the morbidity of a ureteral injury is usually small. Unrecognized ureteral injuries usually present in a delayed fashion with persistent ileus, fever/sepsis, abdominal/flank pain, leukocytosis, or fistula.

Direct exploration is the most accurate method for diagnosis of ureteral injury. Intravenous or retrograde injection of indigo carmine or methylene blue is also helpful in identifying ureteral injury by extravasation of blue dye from the injury site.

Imaging

Imaging of ureteral injury by one-shot IVU is inconsistent and unreliable and thus not recommended. Retrograde pyelography (RPG) is very accurate in demonstrating presence and location of extravasation, but it is both time consuming and cumbersome. RPG has little role in the acute trauma setting. RPG is helpful in the stable patient with equivocal imaging, providing not only diagnosis, but also treatment with ureteral stent placement. CT has been used with increasing frequency to evaluate ureteral trauma—in particular CT urography with delayed images and fine cuts through the entire course of the ureter. Medial perirenal extravasation of contrast material is the most common finding of UPJ collecting system injury.

Management

Figure 2 shows a treatment algorithm for ureteral trauma. General considerations are the patient's overall physical condition, presence of associated injuries, any delay in diagnosis, and the level and extent of ureteral injury. Promptly diagnosed ureteral injuries should be explored and surgically reconstructed. Ureteral contusions or bruising due to proximity blast injury from GSWs should be stented and drained at minimum. With severe contusions, the ureter should be segmentally resected, débrided to a bleeding edge, reanastomosed tension-free over a stent, isolated from associated injuries, and drained with a Jackson-Pratt drain.

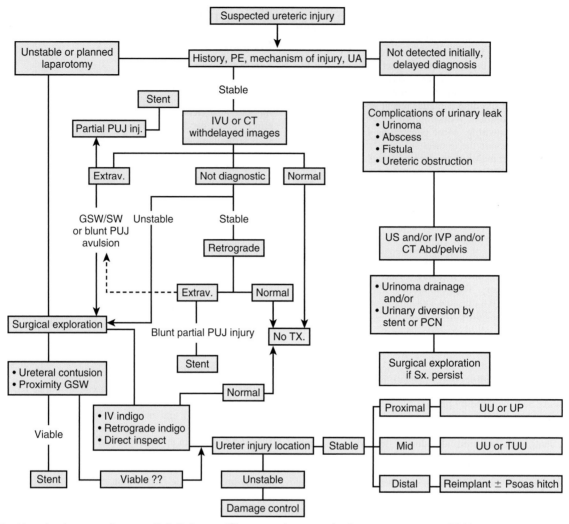

FIGURE 2 Algorithm for ureteral trauma. Abd, Abdomen; CT, computed tomography; Extrav, extravasation; GSW, gunshot wound; Inj, injury; IVP, intravenous pyelogram; IVU, intravenous urogram; PCN, percutaneous nephrostomy; PE, physical examination; PUJ, pelvoureteral junction; SW, stab wound; Sx, signs and symptoms; TUU, transureteroureterostomy; Tx, treatment; UA, urine analysis; UP, ureteropyleostomy; US, ultrasonography; UU, ureteroureterostomy. *(Modified from Brandes SB, Coburn M, Armenakas N, et al: Consensus on genitourinary trauma, diagnosis and management of ureteric injury: an evidence-based approach. BJU Int 94:277–289, 2004.)*

Management of ureteral injuries is dictated mostly by the location of the injury. Distal ureteral injuries (below the iliac vessels) are typically managed by ureteroneocystostomy. With greater distal ureteral loss, a psoas hitch is performed, in which the mobilized bladder is sewn to the ipsilateral psoas minor tendon. This will usually bridge a distal ureteral gap, allowing the ureter to then be reimplanted. A transureteroureterostomy (TUU) is a method of bringing the injured ureter across the midline and sewing it to the side of the contralateral ureter. This is particularly useful when there are associated rectal, pelvic, vascular injuries, or when the bladder is very small and not compliant. There are multiple relative contraindications to a TUU, including recurrent nephrolithiasis, transitional cell carcinoma of the upper tract, and abnormal contralateral kidney, among others. Complex reconstructions like an ileal interposition (small bowel used as a ureteral replacement), Boari flap (bladder tube flap), renal displacement, or autotransplantation into the pelvis are best reserved for delayed settings. The majority of midureteral injuries can be repaired by primary ureteroureterostomy (UU; end-to-end anastomosis). Injuries to the upper third of the ureter are best repaired by UU. Avulsion of the UPJ is the most common blunt ureteral injury seen, and occurs primarily in children. UPJ lacerations can often be successfully managed expectantly, but avulsion

demands acute surgical repair or nephrostomy tube placement and delayed repair.

When the patient is too unstable to undergo lengthy ureteral reconstruction, a "damage control" approach of temporary cutaneous ureterostomy (bringing the ureter to the abdominal wall skin) or ureteral ligation followed by percutaneous nephrostomy should be performed. Definitive reconstruction is delayed until the patient has stabilized.

Complications

Delayed recognition of ureteral injuries is common. However, even with immediate recognition and repair, there is risk of significant morbidity, including sepsis, abscess, hydronephrosis, loss of renal function, ureteral stricture, fistula, and urinoma.

BLADDER TRAUMA

Incidence and Mechanisms of Injury

The majority of bladder injuries are due to blunt abdominal trauma from motor vehicle crashes or crush injuries. Ninety percent of bladder injuries from external trauma are associated with pelvic fractures, and 10% to 15% of pelvic fractures have a ruptured bladder. Bladder ruptures are roughly 60% extraperitoneal, 30% intraperitoneal, and the remaining 10% combined injuries. Iatrogenic bladder injuries typically occur during pelvic surgery, such as a transabdominal hysterectomy.

Intraperitoneal bladder rupture occurs by severe blunt lower abdominal or pelvic trauma to a distended or full bladder. Ruptures are commonly at the dome of the bladder. Empty bladders are seldom injured. High mortality rate is due to associated injuries. Extraperitoneal bladder injuries are nearly always associated with pelvic fracture. Injuries are primarily due to shearing forces, and very rarely from perforation by bony spicules.

Diagnosis

Signs and Symptoms

Nearly all blunt bladder ruptures have gross hematuria (95% to 100%), and the remaining 5%, microhematuria. Penetrating bladder injuries have roughly half microscopic and half gross hematuria. Symptoms of bladder injury are pelvic or lower abdominal pain and inability to urinate. Signs of bladder rupture are suprapubic tenderness, low urine output, and gross hematuria. Intraperitoneal bladder ruptures that are diagnosed late often present with azotemia, acidosis, hypernatremia, hyperkalemia, and elevated serum urea nitrogen. Women need a careful pelvic examination to assess for possible vaginal or urethral tears. Suspected intraoperative bladder injuries are diagnosed by retrograde filling of the bladder with methylene blue–stained saline via a Foley catheter, and looking for any blue staining in the abdomen.

Imaging

Indications for imaging are as follows:

1. Free pelvic fluid noted on FAST (focused assessment with sonography in trauma)

2. Blunt trauma: gross hematuria and pelvic fracture
3. Penetrating trauma: any degree of hematuria or injury tract crosses bladder

Conventional cystography is performed by gravity filling of the bladder with dilute contrast agent, via a Foley, to at least 300 mL or until contrast extravasation is noted under fluoroscopy. Postdrainage films are essential so as not to miss 10% to 15% of injuries. Bladder injuries noted on cystography are typically categorized into bladder contusion, interstitial rupture, intraperitoneal rupture (contrast outlining loops of bowel or filling of the cul-de-sac), extraperitoneal rupture (contrast extravasation in the shape of a flame or star-burst), or pelvic hematoma ("tear-drop" shape). *CT cystography* is typically the imaging modality of choice and is most often used in hospitals today. The bladder is retrograde filled to at least 300 mL or till extravasation is noted by CT. It is as accurate as conventional cystography and has the advantage that no postdrainage imaging is required.

Management

Figure 3 shows a treatment algorithm for bladder trauma. For blunt *intraperitoneal injuries*, the injury to the bladder is typically at the dome and large (centimeters long). Such injuries will not heal spontaneously with Foley catheter drainage and require open repair with absorbable suture. A two-layer closure is preferred. For *penetrating* bladder injuries, surgical exploration is also required—mainly out of concern for associated intra-abdominal injuries and possible injury to the ureters or trigone. The bullet injuries should be explored, debris and devitalized tissue débrided, and injuries closed with absorbable suture. After formal bladder repair, the urine is diverted by large-bore Foley. Suprapubic tube is rarely needed.

In contrast, most blunt *extraperitoneal* bladder injuries can be successfully managed by catheter drainage alone, and do not need to be explored or sutured closed. In nearly 90% of cases, within 2 weeks the bladder will heal spontaneously with adequate Foley catheter drainage. When the abdomen is explored for other associated injuries,

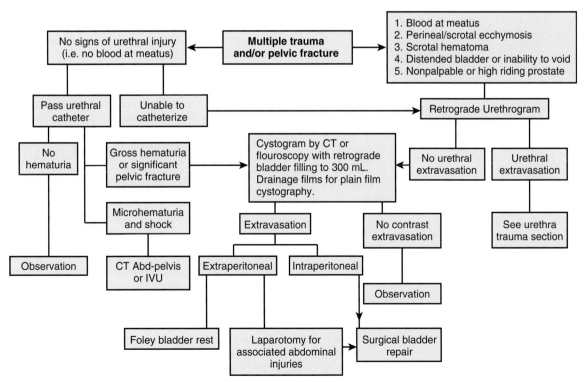

FIGURE 3   Algorithm for bladder trauma. Abd, Abdomen; CT, computed tomography; IVU, intravenous urogram. *(Modified from Brandes SB: Trauma to the genitourinary tract. In Rakel RE, Bope ET, editors:* Conn's current therapy, *57th ed. Philadelphia, 2005, Saunders.)*

extraperitoneal bladder ruptures are commonly repaired at the same time. The bladder should be exposed through a midline abdominal incision and the bladder opened at the dome to avoid the pelvic hematoma. Opening the pelvic hematoma may cause bacterial contamination and can release the tamponade effect and result in brisk bleeding. The bladder neck and ureteral orifices need to be inspected for possible injury at this time. Injuries to the ureteral orifices usually require the ureteral reimplantation. A bladder neck injury needs to be surgically repaired, because unrepaired injuries typically result in significant stress urinary incontinence. Extraperitoneal injuries that require repair are those related to bone fragments, those associated with rectal or vaginal injury, and cases in which bladder drainage is not adequate with a Foley catheter because of severe bleeding/blood clots.

Complications

Delayed recognition of an intraperitoneal bladder injury can result in a critically ill patient. Delayed presentation and diagnosis often result in significant morbidity, including metabolic acidosis, ileus, abdominal/pelvic pain, sepsis, and possibly peritonitis.

URETHRAL TRAUMA

Urethral injuries are relatively uncommon and are usually divided into anterior and posterior injuries. Posterior urethral injuries are due to pelvic fracture and anterior urethral injuries to straddle injury. Penetrating injuries are usually due to a GSW to the anterior urethra. The management goal for urethral injuries is to minimize the chances for the debilitating complications of incontinence, impotence, and urethral stricture.

Posterior Urethral Injuries

Incidence and Mechanism

The posterior urethra is injured in up to 3.5% to 15% of pelvic fractures. Urethral injury is complete in 73% and partial in 27%. Urethral injuries are mainly the result of shearing forces between a fixed prostate and a mobile bladder, resulting in bladder neck injury, and between a fixed membranous urethra and a mobile bulbar urethra, resulting in membranous urethral injury. In contrast to men, injuries to the female urethra and bladder neck are usually due to bony fragments.

Diagnosis

Signs and Symptoms

Symptoms of posterior urethral disruption include inability to void, lower abdominal swelling, and hematuria. Signs of male urethral injury are blood at the meatus (98% sensitive), gross hematuria, perineal ecchymosis/hematoma, scrotal or penile hematoma, difficulty passing a Foley catheter, distended bladder and inability to void, or high-riding prostate. Female urethral injury is suspected when a pelvic fracture presents with vaginal bleeding and laceration, hematuria, labial swelling, or inability to void.

Imaging

On pelvic film, urethral injury is suggested by pelvic ring disruption, and often associated with bilateral pubic rami fractures or vertical shear fractures. Retrograde urethrography (RUG) is the procedure of choice to evaluate for urethral injury. Contrast medium is instilled in small volumes (20 to 30 mL), ideally under fluoroscopy. Grades of injury are determined by RUG. The urogenital diaphragm separates the pelvis from the perineum and is the most important landmark.

Management

Management goals for urethral injuries are preserving continence and potency, and avoiding the pelvic hematoma. Despite previous controversy, it is generally felt that the complications of impotence and incontinence result from the initial injury itself and not the management method. The most traditional treatment method is suprapubic tube urinary diversion, followed by delayed surgical intervention for the urethral obliteration. Placement of a urethrovesical catheter in the setting of urethral disruption is known as primary realignment. This can be done immediately if the patient is stable, or delayed a few days until the orthopedic repair of the pelvic fracture. Primary realignment, when a Foley is placed across the injury under cystoscopy and fluoroscopy, may lead to easier surgical repair or decrease the need for open surgical repair in up to 50%. Incomplete lacerations usually heal with catheter drainage alone.

Anterior Urethral Injuries

Incidence and Mechanism

Blunt anterior urethral injuries are caused by direct injury to the penis and urethra and have few associated injuries and relatively low morbidity rates. Penetrating urethral injuries occur in 18% to 57% of GSWs to the penis and half of perineal GSWs.

Diagnosis

Signs and Symptoms

Symptoms of anterior urethral injury include hematuria or inability to void. Signs of potential anterior urethral injury are history of direct perineal trauma or straddle injury, penetrating wounds to the penis or perineum (i.e., GSW), blood at the meatus (the most important predictor), perineal or scrotal swelling/ecchymosis or tenderness (i.e., classic "butterfly" hematoma), penile "sleevelike" hematoma, or inability to void.

Management

Incomplete blunt injuries are successfully managed with catheter urinary diversion for 2 to 3 weeks. Complete blunt crush injuries are best managed by suprapubic tube and *not* primary realignment or immediate repair. Subsequent stricture rate is high and requires a delayed open surgical repair. For SWs and low-velocity GSWs, treatment is primary repair with primary anastomotic urethroplasty. When the urethral injury defect is extensive, the urethra should be marsupialized, urine diverted, and reconstruction delayed.

Complications

Delay in diagnosis or treatment predisposes the genitalia to abscess formation, sepsis, and fasciitis. Long-term complications are urethral stricture, penile curvature, penile foreshortening, erectile dysfunction, and urinary incontinence.

For the chapter's Suggested Readings list, please visit the book at www.ExpertConsult.inkling.com.

Gynecologic Injuries: Trauma to Gravid and Nongravid Uterus and Female Genitalia

Patrizio Petrone and Areti Tillou

G ynecologic trauma includes a large variety of relatively rare and challenging injuries from blunt and penetrating mechanisms. Although motor vehicle crashes are the leading cause of major injury in pregnant women, penetrating trauma accounts for almost all injuries to the fallopian tubes, ovaries, and nongravid uterus. Pelvic fractures and straddle injuries often result in trauma to perineum, vagina, and less commonly the cervix and uterus. Injuries to the external genitalia are frequently associated with interpersonal violence and should be treated in that context.

TRAUMA DURING PREGNANCY

Trauma has been recognized as the leading cause of death during pregnancy and remains the most common cause of fetal demise. Women between the ages of 10 and 50 years have the potential for pregnancy, and this possibility must be taken into consideration when a female patient is examined in the emergency room after sustaining a traumatic event. Pregnancy produces significant physiologic and anatomic changes that must be recognized and understood by all health care providers treating pregnant trauma patients (Table 1).

Incidence

According to some authors, nearly 50% of maternal deaths are related to trauma. From 6% to 7% of all pregnancies are complicated by trauma, and 0.4% of the patients require hospitalization for treatment of injuries. In 1995, Weiss reported an epidemiologic 1-year study in which all women of childbearing age who required hospitalization for injuries were screened for pregnancy; of 16,722 women, 761 were identified (4.6%) as being pregnant. The actual number of injured pregnant women is underestimated as many of them are unreported, especially with injuries resulting from domestic violence.

In 2011, Petrone et al reported a 155-month study from two Level 1 trauma centers in which 321 pregnant patients were included, of which 291 (91%) sustained a blunt injury, and 30 (9%) were victims of penetrating trauma. One of the conclusions of this study was that fetal mortality rate and overall maternal morbidity rate remain exceedingly high, at 73% and 66%, respectively, following penetrating abdominal injury.

Mechanism of Injury

Motor vehicle collisions are the most common causes of injury during pregnancy. As the pregnancy progresses, the shift in the woman's center of gravity and diminished agility can result in falls and accidental injuries. Other common causes of injury include automobile-pedestrian collisions and firearm injuries. Younger women are at higher risk for injury during pregnancy, with a maternal age ranging from 22 to 25 years.

TABLE 1: Changes in Maternal Physiology during Pregnancy

Change	Consequence
Cardiac output and blood volume increase	Shock after >40% of blood lost
Expansion of plasma volume	Physiologic anemia
Decline in arterial and venous pressure	Vital signs are not reflective of hemodynamic status
Increase of resting pulse	
Chest enlargement	Change in anatomic landmarks Caution during thoracic procedures (e.g., tube thoracostomy)
Diaphragm rise	
Substernal angle increase	
Decrease in functional residual capacity	Rapid decline in Po_2 during apnea or airway obstruction
Increase in oxygen consumption	
Airway closure when supine	
Increase in tidal volume and minute ventilation	Fall in Pco_2 and bicarbonates
Decrease in anesthetic requirements	Need for adjustment of sedative doses
Decreased gastric motility	Risk of aspiration
Relaxation of gastroesophageal sphincter	

Young pregnant women are also at high risk for injuries resulting from battery. It has been reported that 10% to 30% of women are abused during pregnancy, and 5% of cases involving abuse result in fetal death. Of injured pregnant patients, 17% experience intentional trauma and 60% suffer repeated episodes of domestic violence. Physical abuse is suspected when the injuries are located proximally and in the midline, rather than distally, and trauma is evident to the neck, breast, face, upper arms, and lateral thighs, as well as bizarre injuries such as cigarette burns or bites.

Diagnosis

Care is undertaken with attention to both mother and fetus. Uterine blood flow lacks autoregulation and is related directly to maternal blood pressure; consequently, treatment priorities are the same as for the nonpregnant trauma patient, as the best initial treatment for the fetus is the optimal resuscitation of the mother. A thorough physical examination complemented by imaging studies is necessary to identify some of the unique problems that might be present in any pregnant patient, including blunt or penetrating injury to the uterus, placental abruption, amniotic fluid embolism, isoimmunization, and premature rupture of membranes.

Prehospital Care

As a result of significant changes in maternal physiology, supplemental oxygen should be administered to prevent maternal and fetal hypoxia during transport and in the resuscitation room. Fluid resuscitation should be initiated even in the absence of signs of hypovolemia and shock. To avoid supine hypotension associated with the uterine compression of the inferior vena cava (IVC), patients in the second or third trimester of pregnancy should be transported on a backboard tilted to the left, with special attention to immobilization of the cervical spine. If the patient is kept in a supine position, the right hip should be elevated 4 to 6 inches, and the uterus should be displaced manually to the left. This maneuver increases cardiac output by 30% and restores circulating blood volume. Although only about 10% of pregnant patients at term develop symptoms of shock in the supine position, fetal distress may be present even in normotensive mothers; therefore, right hip elevation should be maintained at all times including during operative procedures.

Hospital Care

Primary survey includes assessment of airway, breathing, and circulation (ABC), including volume replacement and hemorrhage control. Secondary survey includes the obstetric history, physical examination, and evaluation and monitoring of the fetus. The history should include the date of the last menstrual cycle, expected date of delivery, and any problems or complications of the current and previous pregnancies such as preterm labor or placental abruption. Comorbid conditions such as pregnancy-induced hypertension and diabetes mellitus should also be documented.

The abdominal examination is critically important, as is a determination of uterine size (Fig. 1), which provides an approximation of gestational age and fetal maturity. A discrepancy between dates and uterine size suggests uterine hemorrhage or rupture. Uterine rupture is suspected with peritoneal signs, abdominal palpation of fetal parts

due to extrauterine location, and inability to palpate the uterine fundus. However, as the uterus enlarges, it displaces the intestines upward and laterally, stretching the peritoneum and making the abdominal physical examination unreliable.

Determination of gestational age is particularly important because this will guide the decision for a premature delivery if indicated. Most institutions will accept a 24- to 26-week pregnancy as viable, with a probability of survival rate ranging from 20% to 70%. Radiographic estimation of gestational age is bound to an error of 1 to 2 weeks. Unless the date of the conception is known exactly, gestational age is particularly difficult to determine. A good rule of thumb is to consider patients with a uterus halfway between the umbilicus and the costal margin as having a viable pregnancy. An algorithm for initial maternal and fetal assessment is presented in Figure 2.

Physical evaluation of the pregnant patient must be directed to the detection of the following six pregnancy-related acute conditions:

- *Vaginal bleeding:* This is an ominous sign that suggests premature cervical dilation, early labor, placental abruption, or placenta previa. Placental abruption after trauma occurs in 2% to 4% of minor accidents and in up to 50% of major injuries. Maternal mortality rate from abruption is less than 1%, but fetal death ranges from 20% to 35%.
- *Ruptured membranes:* In addition to increased risk of infection, prolapse of the umbilical cord can occur, resulting in compression of the umbilical vein and arteries.
- *Bulging perineum:* This is caused most commonly by pressure from extrauterine location of fetal parts.
- *Presence and patterns of contractions:* Direct or indirect trauma to the myometrium may result in release of arachidonic acid that can cause uterine contractions. Although most contractions will cease spontaneously, preparation for a premature delivery should be made.
- *Abnormal fetal heart rate and rhythm:* It may be the first indication of a major disruption in fetal homeostasis. During trauma resuscitation, evaluation of the fetus should begin with auscultation of heart tones and continuous electronic fetal heart rate monitoring (EFM). Any viable fetus of 24 or more weeks' gestation requires monitoring after trauma. Cardiotocographic monitoring should be started in the resuscitation room and continued for a minimum of 4 hours; a minimum of 24 hours is recommended for patients with frequent uterine activity (more than six contractions per hour), abdominal or uterine tenderness, ruptured membranes, vaginal bleeding, or hypotension.
- *Fetomaternal hemorrhage:* Fetomaternal hemorrhage is the transplacental hemorrhage of fetal blood into the normally separate maternal circulation and occurs in 8% to 30% of patients with trauma during pregnancy. The severity of injury and the gestational age have no correlation with the frequency and volume of fetomaternal hemorrhage. The Kleihauer-Betke (KB) test is used after maternal injury to identify fetal blood in the maternal circulation. The ratio of fetal to maternal cells is recorded, allowing calculation of the volume of fetal blood leaked to the maternal circulation. Complications of fetomaternal hemorrhage include Rh sensitization in the mother, fetal anemia, fetal paroxysmal atrial tachycardia, and fetal death from exsanguination. As the volume of fetomaternal hemorrhage sufficient to sensitize most Rh-negative women is well below the 5-mL sensitivity level of the typical laboratory's KB test, all Rh-negative mothers who present with a history of abdominal trauma should receive one 300-µg prophylactic dose of Rh immune globulin (anti-D immunoglobulin; RhoGam) within 72 hours of the traumatic event. An additional 300 µg of Rh immune globulin should be given for every 30 mL of fetal blood found in maternal circulation. Only 3.1% of major trauma cases require more than one 300-µg Rh immune globulin dose. The KB test is probably unnecessary before 16 weeks' gestation because the fetal blood volume is below 30 mL at this gestational age.

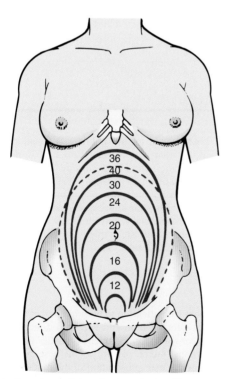

FIGURE I Location and size of uterus during different stages of pregnancy. *(Modified from Wilson SF, editor: Assessment of the pregnant client, Health assessment for nursing practice, ed 4, Mosby, 2009; Original credit Seidel et al, 2006.)*

FIGURE 2 Algorithm for initial maternal and fetal assessment. ABC, Airway, breathing, and circulation; C-section, cesarean section; DPL, diagnostic peritoneal lavage; OB, obstetrics; US, ultrasound. *(Modified from Knudson MM, Rozycki GS, Paquin MM: Reproductive system trauma. In Moore EE, Feliciano DV, Mattox KL, editors: Trauma, 5th ed, New York, 2004, McGraw-Hill, pp 851–875.)*

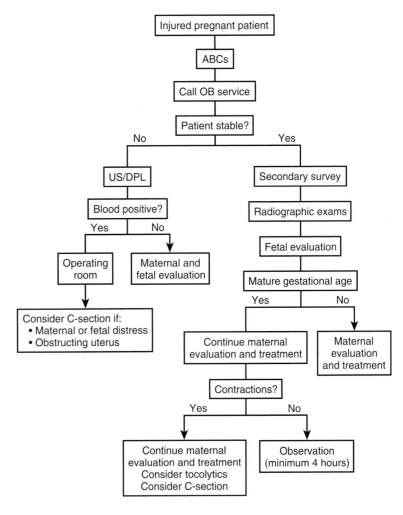

Radiographic Examination

There are three phases of radiation damage related to gestational age of the fetus. Before 3 weeks of gestation, either during preimplantation and early implantation, exposure to radiation can result in death of the embryo. Between 3 and 16 weeks of gestation, during organogenesis, radiation can damage the developing fetal tube, resulting in anomalies in the central nervous system. After 16 weeks, neurologic defects are the most common complication. Prenatal radiation exposure may be associated with certain childhood cancers.

Although there is existing concern about radiation exposure during pregnancy, in most instances the benefits outweigh the risks. It is generally believed that exposure of the fetus to less than 5 to 10 rad causes no significant increase in the risk of congenital malformations, intrauterine growth retardation, or miscarriage. Radiation doses from common imaging studies are shown in Table 2. All indicated radiographic studies should be performed, as for nonpregnant patients (Fig. 3). It is obvious that unnecessary duplication of studies should be avoided.

Abdominal Evaluation

Evaluation of the abdomen in the pregnant patient may be challenging. Superior displacement of the viscera by the expanding uterus changes the anatomic relation of the intra-abdominal organs (Fig. 4). Special attention is needed for patients with rib or pelvic fractures, unexplained hypotension, blood loss, hematuria, or altered sensorium caused by drugs, alcohol, or brain injury.

TABLE 2: Radiation Doses from Plain Radiographs and CT

Plain anteroposterior chest radiograph	<0.005 rad
Pelvic radiograph	<0.4 rad
CT scan of head (1-cm cuts)	0.05 rad
CT scan of upper abdomen (20 1-cm cuts)	3.0 rad
CT scan of lower abdomen (10 1-cm cuts)	3.0–9.0 rad

CT, Computed tomography.

Focused assessment with sonography in trauma (FAST) has a major role in the abdominal evaluation because it provides rapid detection of intra-abdominal and pericardial fluid in the mother as well as quick assessment of fetal condition. In the hemodynamically normal patient, abdominal computed tomography (CT) scanning can also be done safely to evaluate both mother and fetus. If CT scan is necessary, both oral and intravenous contrast media should be administered as needed. The main drawback of a diagnostic peritoneal lavage (DPL) is its invasiveness, and DPL should be performed above the umbilicus using an open technique.

The American Association for the Surgery of Trauma (AAST) Organ Injury Scale for gravid uterus is shown in Table 3.

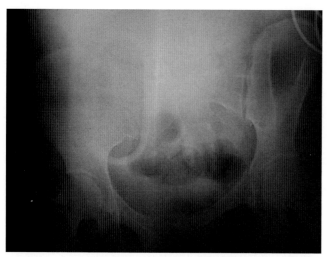

FIGURE 3 Pelvic radiograph of a pregnant patient after blunt trauma. Vertebrae and other parts of the fetus can be seen.

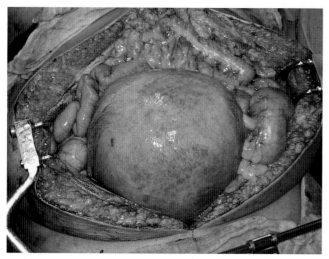

FIGURE 4 Exploratory laparotomy after motor vehicle collision. Gravid uterus displacing viscera.

Surgical Treatment

Blunt Injury

Solid organ injuries may be managed nonoperatively in the hemodynamically stable pregnant patient. In contrast, unstable patients or those with intestinal injury clearly require early operation, as hypotension and infection can be harmful or even lethal for the fetus.

Pelvic fractures represent the most challenging blunt injuries during pregnancy. Hemorrhage from dilated retroperitoneal veins can cause massive and fatal hemorrhagic shock. Maternal pelvic fracture is the most common cause of fetal death, with a fetal mortality rate approaching 25%. In nonpregnant patients, angioembolization is the usual treatment for pelvic hemorrhage, but the radiation dose for the procedure is considered excessive during pregnancy.

The abdominal wall, uterine myometrium, and amniotic fluid act as a cushion to direct forces from blunt trauma. Placental abruption is the most common cause of fetal death, resulting from anoxia, prematurity, or exsanguination. Manifestations include abdominal pain, vaginal bleeding, uterine tenderness, and contractions. One of the most serious complications associated with abruption is disseminated

TABLE 3: AAST-OIS for Gravid Uterus

Grade	Injury Description	AIS-90 Score
I	Hematoma or contusion without placental abruption	2
II	Superficial laceration <1 cm in depth or partial placental abruption <25%	3
III	Deep laceration 1 cm in depth in second trimester or placental abruption 25% but <50%; deep laceration in third trimester	3–4
IV	Laceration extending to the uterine artery; deep laceration 1 cm with 50% placental abruption	4
V	Uterine rupture in second or third trimester; complete placental abruption	4–5

Modified from Moore EE, Jurkovich GJ, Knudson MM, et al: Organ injury scaling VI: extrahepatic biliary, esophagus, stomach, vulva, vagina, uterus (non-pregnant), uterus (pregnant), fallopian tube, and ovary. *J Trauma* 39:1069–1070, 1995.
AAST-OIS, American Association for the Surgery of Trauma Organ Injury Scale; AIS, Abbreviated Injury Scale.

intravascular coagulation (DIC), caused when placental thromboplastin enters maternal circulation.

Penetrating Injury

As the uterus grows and expands out of the pelvis, it becomes an easier target for penetrating trauma. The thick density of its musculature allows the uterus to absorb energy from low-velocity penetrating injuries; maternal death is very uncommon except for injuries in the upper abdomen, which usually produce severe maternal damage. Gunshot wounds cause fetal injuries in 60% to 70% of cases, with fetal death in 40% to 65%. If the bullet has penetrated the uterus and the fetus is viable, cesarean section is indicated (Table 4).

Perimortem cesarean section is indicated in the case of maternal death if the fetus is viable (24–26 weeks). Timing is critical, as the probability of fetal survival is excellent when delivery occurs within 5 minutes or less of maternal demise. As the time increases, the chance of survival diminishes. In the rare situation when the mother is declared brain dead but maintains good vital signs, the fetus can be allowed to mature before delivery (Fig. 5).

TABLE 4: Indications for Cesarean Section for Penetrating Trauma

Maternal shock
Threat to life from exsanguinations from any cause
Mechanical limitation for maternal repair
Irreparable uterine injury
Fetal distress in viable fetus
Unstable thoracolumbar spine injury
Pregnancy near term
Maternal death

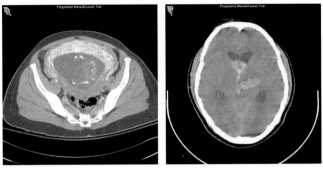

FIGURE 5 Intracranial hemorrhage *(right panel)* in an 18-week pregnant patient declared brain dead. As the fetus was not viable *(left panel)*, the patient's family agreed to organ donation.

TABLE 5: Predictors of Fetal Outcome

Maternal death

Maternal hypotension

Maternal traumatic brain injury

High Injury Severity Score (ISS)

Pelvic fracture

Ejection of pregnant woman from a vehicle

Severe abdominal injury to pregnant woman

When performing an emergency cesarean section on a trauma patient, instead of the commonly used transverse incision, a vertical incision through all the layers into the uterus is safer and faster. This incision avoids injury to the uterine vessels, which enter the uterus from both sides.

Between gestational age 24 to 32 weeks, open cardiopulmonary resuscitation without aortic cross-clamping should be seriously considered before an emergency cesarean section is performed. If open cardiopulmonary resuscitation proves successful, the delivery may be delayed so that chances of postnatal survival improve. A proposed algorithm for emergency cesarean section after trauma is presented in Figure 6.

Morbidity and Mortality

Trauma has become the most frequent cause of maternal death in the United States. Older reports attributed 80% maternal mortality rate to amniotic fluid embolism, which together with pulmonary

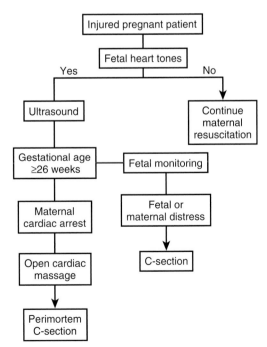

FIGURE 6 Algorithm for emergency cesarean section after trauma. C-section, Cesarean section. *(Modified from Morris JA Jr, Rosenbower TJ, Jurkovich GJ, et al: Infant survival after cesarean section for trauma. Ann Surg 223:481–488, 1996.)*

thromboembolism was cited as the leading cause of maternal fatality. In contrast to declining maternal mortality risks from infection, hemorrhage, hypertension, and thromboembolism, accidental deaths during pregnancy have risen steadily. Although overall maternal mortality rate from abdominal gunshot wounds is around 7%, fetal mortality rate reaches 73%, and overall maternal morbidity rate is 66%. Risk factors associated with poor fetal outcome are listed in Table 5.

Conclusions

Trauma has become the leading cause of death in women aged 34 and younger, including pregnant patients. Assessment of a female trauma patient in the fertile age should always include the possibility of pregnancy. Pathophysiologic changes during pregnancy affect all aspects of traumatic injury and require a detailed and meticulous management.

TRAUMA TO NONGRAVID UTERUS AND FEMALE GENITALIA

Although injuries to the female genitalia are uncommon in the nonpregnant patient, they are more often seen in cases in which there is pathologic enlargement of the internal genitalia or in the early postpartum period. Missed or improperly treated female genital injuries can result in hemorrhage, sepsis, and loss of endocrine and reproductive function.

Incidence

The incidence of injuries to the female genitalia is largely unknown. Most information on the subject comes from isolated case reports or small series of patients. Vaginal lacerations complicate approximately 3.5% of pelvic fractures in female patients. Urethral and bladder injuries are also commonly present.

Mechanism of Injury

Blunt injuries involving the female genitalia are most frequently associated with pelvic fractures. Injuries to the external genitalia can also be the result of straddle injuries or accidental penetration. Water skiing, gymnastics, and bicycling accidents have been reported as the causes of blunt trauma to the lower genitalia. Penetrating injuries are almost exclusively responsible for injuries to the upper genital organs, although several reports of blunt trauma to normal ovaries and uterus have been reported.

Many of the injuries to the external genital organs are the result of violent acts in pregnant as well as nonpregnant women. This possibility should be always be considered, especially when the mechanism of injury is unclear. If sexual assault has occurred, informed consent for the remainder of the assessment must be obtained.

Domestic violence crosses lines of ethnicity and race, age, national origin, sexual orientation, religion, and socioeconomic status, although an overwhelming majority of the victims in heterosexual relationships are women. Typically, battery tends to occur as a pattern of violence rather than a one-time event. Physicians treating trauma victims should be able to recognize the signs of domestic violence, refer patients to appropriate agencies, and provide social support.

Diagnosis

Initial assessment and resuscitation are performed as for any trauma patient. The secondary survey should include a detailed physical examination of the perineum. Examination under anesthesia may be needed for patients with severe pain or active bleeding. A complete examination should include bimanual palpation and speculum examinations of vagina and anorectum. Some authors recommend anesthesia for all patients with perineal trauma in order to evaluate the extent of the injury.

Intra-abdominal genital injuries are usually diagnosed at laparotomy for associated injuries. As blunt injury is more common with pathologically enlarged internal genitalia in the nongravid patient, CT scan of the abdomen or DPL may aid the diagnosis, although the latter is very rarely used. Detailed grading of gynecologic injuries is presented (Tables 6 through 10).

Surgical Management

Isolated perineal lacerations should be repaired after appropriate irrigation and débridement with or without placement of drains. Large perineal hematomas require incision and drainage because of the high associated incidence of infection and sepsis. Vulvar lacerations may be closed primarily with absorbable sutures.

Repair of vaginal and cervical lacerations may be challenging because of the abundant blood supply. Absorbable sutures including the mucosal and submucosal layers are commonly used. These injuries must be diagnosed promptly in patients with pelvic fractures, as any delay can result in sepsis and death.

TABLE 6: AAST-OIS for Gynecologic Injuries: Vagina

Grade	Injury Description	AIS-90 Score
I	Contusion or hematoma	1
II	Superficial laceration involving mucosa	1
III	Deep laceration extending into submucosal fat or muscle	2
IV	Complex laceration extending into the cervix or peritoneum	3
V	Injury to adjacent organs	3

Modified from Moore EE, Jurkovich GJ, Knudson MM, et al: Organ injury scaling VI: extrahepatic biliary, esophagus, stomach, vulva, vagina, uterus (non-pregnant), uterus (pregnant), fallopian tube, and ovary. *J Trauma* 39:1069–1070, 1995.
AAST-OIS, American Association for the Surgery of Trauma Organ Injury Scale; AIS, Abbreviated Injury Scale.

TABLE 7: AAST-OIS for Gynecologic Injuries: Vulva

Grade	Injury Description	AIS-90 Score
I	Hematoma or contusion	1
II	Superficial laceration involving skin only	1
III	Deep laceration extending into subcutaneous fat or muscle	2
IV	Avulsion of skin, fat, or muscle	3
V	Injury to adjacent organs	3

Modified from Moore EE, Jurkovich GJ, Knudson MM, et al: Organ injury scaling VI: extrahepatic biliary, esophagus, stomach, vulva, vagina, uterus (non-pregnant), uterus (pregnant), fallopian tube, and ovary. *J Trauma* 39:1069–1070, 1995.
AAST-OIS, American Association for the Surgery of Trauma Organ Injury Scale; AIS, Abbreviated Injury Scale.

TABLE 8: AAST-OIS for Gynecologic Injuries: Nongravid Uterus

Grade	Injury Description	AIS-90 Score
I	Hematoma or contusion	2
II	Superficial laceration <1 cm in depth	2
III	Deep laceration 1 cm in depth	3
IV	Laceration extending to uterine artery	3
V	Devascularization or avulsion	3

Modified from Moore EE, Jurkovich GJ, Knudson MM, et al: Organ injury scaling VI: extrahepatic biliary, esophagus, stomach, vulva, vagina, uterus (non-pregnant), uterus (pregnant), fallopian tube, and ovary. *J Trauma* 39:1069–1070, 1995.
AAST-OIS, American Association for the Surgery of Trauma Organ Injury Scale; AIS, Abbreviated Injury Scale.

TABLE 9: AAST-OIS for Gynecologic Injuries: Fallopian Tube

Grade	Injury Description	AIS-90 Score
I	Hematoma or contusion	2
II	Laceration involving <50% of circumference	2
III	Laceration involving 50% of circumference	2
IV	Complete transection	2
V	Devascularized segment	2

Modified from Moore EE, Jurkovich GJ, Knudson MM, et al: Organ injury scaling VI: extrahepatic biliary, esophagus, stomach, vulva, vagina, uterus (non-pregnant), uterus (pregnant), fallopian tube, and ovary. *J Trauma* 39:1069–1070, 1995.
AAST-OIS, American Association for the Surgery of Trauma Organ Injury Scale; AIS, Abbreviated Injury Scale.

TABLE 10: AAST-OIS for Gynecologic Injuries: Ovary

Grade	Injury Description	AIS-90 Score
I	Contusion or hematoma	1
II	Superficial laceration <0.5 cm in depth	2
III	Deep laceration 0.5 cm in depth	3
IV	Partial disruption of blood supply	3
V	Complete parenchymal disruption or avulsion	3

Modified from Moore EE, Jurkovich GJ, Knudson MM, et al: Organ injury scaling VI: extrahepatic biliary, esophagus, stomach, vulva, vagina, uterus (non-pregnant), uterus (pregnant), fallopian tube, and ovary. *J Trauma* 39:1069–1070, 1995.
AAST-OIS, American Association for the Surgery of Trauma Organ Injury Scale; AIS, Abbreviated Injury Scale.

Injuries to the uterus are repaired in two layers using slowly absorbable running or interrupted figure-of-eight sutures. Hysterectomy for trauma is extremely rare and is needed only in extreme cases of massive destruction or exsanguinating hemorrhage. Injuries to the fallopian tubes and ovaries are also managed by either primary repair or excision according to injury severity. Vaginal packing with antibiotics is frequently used for 24 hours after procedures involving the vagina, cervix, or uterus.

Morbidity and Mortality

Morbidity is primarily determined by the associated injuries. Profuse bleeding from the perineal wounds as well as vagina, cervix, and uterus may be the cause of hemorrhagic shock. These wounds may be difficult to control. Missed perineal injuries in association with pelvic fracture may be fatal. Long-term complications include sexual dysfunction and infertility.

CONCLUSIONS

Injuries to the nongravid uterus as well as female genital organs are rare and should be suspected in all assault victims and all patients with direct perineal trauma, pelvic fractures, or penetrating injury to the pelvis. Thorough physical examination, preferably in the operating room, with prompt surgical treatment improves the outcome of these potentially challenging injuries.

For the chapter's Suggested Readings list, please visit the book at www.ExpertConsult.inkling.com.

MULTIDISCIPLINARY MANAGEMENT OF PELVIC FRACTURES: OPERATIVE AND NONOPERATIVE MANAGEMENT

Thomas M. Scalea and Deborah M. Stein

Very few injuries are as complicated as multisystem trauma and pelvic fracture. The pelvis is a complex anatomic region. The bony pelvis affords great protection to the structures it contains. Within the pelvis are important gastrointestinal, genitourinary, vascular, and neurologic structures. The force necessary to fracture a pelvis is extreme. Therefore, every pelvic fracture must be assumed to be a high-energy injury. The proximity of the pelvis to the abdomen makes combined injuries common. Patients with pelvic fracture often have other associated injuries as well. Over 50% will have either traumatic brain injury or associated long-bone fracture.

Optimal management of multiply injured patients with pelvic fractures is perhaps the best example of true multidisciplinary care. This is especially true in patients who are hemodynamically unstable. Emergency physicians, trauma surgeons, orthopedic surgeons, urologists, and interventional radiologists all have key roles in managing these patients. A multiplicity of treatment options exists. The correct option for an individual patient is a function of the anatomy of the bony injury, the hemodynamic status of the patient, the presence or absence of other associated injuries, and local expertise within each individual institution.

It is vital to have a management strategy for the patient with a significant pelvic fracture prior to patient presentation. Each institution should have an algorithm available that plays to that individual institution's strengths. Expertise and institutional resources must be instantly available 24 hours a day, 7 days a week, to care for these complicated patients. In this chapter, we will attempt to delineate all options available and discuss individual advantages and disadvantages. It is our hope that the reader will gain an understanding of this complex disease and that this work may serve as background for development for institutional guidelines.

INCIDENCE

Pelvic fractures following blunt trauma are reported to be between 2% and 8% of all bony injuries. In patients with polytrauma, up to 20% of patients sustain pelvic fractures. In one series, the incidence of pelvic fractures was reported to be 37 per 100,000 person-years and in another; the incidence was 24 per 100,000 person-years. There is a bimodal peak in the incidence of pelvic fractures, with high-energy unstable fractures occurring in teens and young adults, and low-energy fractures occurring most commonly in the elderly patient populations.

MECHANISM OF INJURY

The bony pelvis is held together by the strongest ligaments in the body. Thus, the force required to fracture the pelvis and to produce pelvic ligamentous stability is significant. A ring of bone consisting of two innominate bones and the sacrum forms the pelvis, but there is no inherent stability to the bones of the pelvis. The innominate bones and the sacrum are held in a structural unit primarily by the ligaments of the pelvis. These ligamentous complexes provide stability for the articulations of the pelvis.

Because of the anatomy of the pelvis, some mechanisms are much more likely to produce pelvic fractures than are others. Vehicular crashes are the most common cause of pelvic injury in most environments. They are followed in order of frequency by automobile-pedestrian collisions, falls from a height, motorcycle crashes, and crush injuries. Owing to a variety of age-related changes in the pelvis, lower energy mechanisms such as minor motor vehicle crashes and mechanical falls are frequently seen as the source of pelvic fractures in geriatric patients. Although typically not associated with the degree of bony instability seen with high-energy fracture patterns, these fractures may be associated with significant hemorrhage and hemodynamic instability.

DIAGNOSIS

There are five areas into which a patient can exsanguinate: thorax, abdomen, retroperitoneum, muscle compartments, and externally. In the patient presenting with polytrauma, identification of the source of bleeding is of the greatest importance. Up to 20% of patients with pelvic fractures will have concomitant thoracic injuries. The diagnosis of intrathoracic bleeding can be made with a combination of physical examination and a chest radiograph or ultrasound examination. Tension pneumothorax and massive hemothorax can be identified rapidly and treated with tube thoracostomy. Muscle compartment bleeding should be readily identifiable on physical examination, and external blood loss can generally be diagnosed by history from prehospital providers and physical examination. One should keep in mind that external blood loss may become much more apparent once the hypotensive patient is resuscitated and blood pressure increases. The distinction between intra-abdominal and retroperitoneal bleeding can be most difficult. Combined abdominal and pelvic injuries are extremely common. Physical findings such as abdominal pain, distention, or tenderness do not differentiate between intra-abdominal and retroperitoneal bleeding. In addition, physical findings can be quite nonspecific. Patients can bleed a large volume of blood into the abdomen and retroperitoneum with minimal physical findings. In the past, the diagnosis of intra-abdominal injury was generally made by diagnostic peritoneal lavage (DPL) in patients who were hemodynamically labile. The advent of the focused ultrasound examination, however, has revolutionized the early diagnosis of intra-abdominal injury. The focused assessment with sonography in trauma (FAST) is a rapid bedside technique that can make the diagnosis of intra-abdominal injury in several minutes. FAST is portable and can be repeated easily if results are equivocal. Although FAST is rapid and can be performed readily during ongoing resuscitation, it is nonspecific. It can identify the presence of blood but is not an organ-specific test. Computed tomography (CT) scanning allows imaging of both the intra-abdominal as well as retroperitoneal structures. It can identify blood loss into both compartments. Approximately 25% of patients with pelvic fractures will have intra-abdominal injuries despite having a true negative FAST. Thus, CT scanning should be performed in all patients with pelvic fractures at some time in the evaluation process, but CT scanning requires transport from the resuscitation unit and is relatively time consuming, and therefore, it is of limited utility in patients who are hemodynamically unstable.

The presence of retroperitoneal hemorrhage should be suspected in any patient with a pelvic fracture. A pelvic radiograph is a rapid screening test that should alert the clinician to the possibility of pelvic hemorrhage. This is usually performed as a screening radiograph with a chest radiograph as part of the initial assessment. Although a pelvic radiograph is a good screening test, it only describes pelvic anatomy in two dimensions and can vastly underestimate the degree of a pelvic bony injury posteriorly. However, radiographic injury patterns

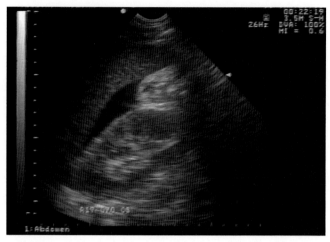

FIGURE 1 Fluid in the abdomen can signal a positive focused assessment with sonography in trauma (FAST), pelvic fracture, and hemodynamic instability. Such patients are almost certainly best served by an immediate laparotomy.

identified in the pelvic film such as widened symphysis pubis diastasis, sacroiliac (SI) joint widening, and "butterfly fracture" in which all four pubic rami are fractured indicate a severe injury pattern and usually mandate pelvic angiography, as these fractures are usually associated with severe pelvic bleeding.

Initial physical examination of the pelvis can be helpful in determining skeletal stability even before a radiograph is taken. Although some advocate rocking the pelvis vigorously, we believe that this is a potentially dangerous maneuver. In patients with unstable pelvic fractures, this produces excruciating pain; in addition, displacement of the fracture fragment may exacerbate bleeding that had previously been attenuated. Instead, we encourage clinicians to gently compress the pelvis inward at the level of the iliac crest. If the pelvis is skeletally stable, no motion is detected. If there is "give" in the pelvis, the patient almost certainly has a skeletally unstable pelvic fracture.

It is important to distinguish between patients with *skeletally unstable* pelvic fractures and patients who are *hemodynamically unstable*. Skeletal stability describes the bony architecture of the pelvic fracture. Hemodynamic stability describes the patient's physiologic response. Not all patients with skeletally unstable pelvic fractures are hemodynamically unstable. In addition, patients who have skeletally stable fractures can still lose a substantial amount of blood into their retroperitoneum.

Patients with a pelvic fracture, positive FAST, and hemodynamic instability are almost certainly best served by an immediate laparotomy. In many patients, the hemoperitonuem can be detected on FAST with 400 mL of fluid in the abdomen (Fig. 1). Although free fluid could certainly be from a relatively minor intraabdominal injury or a ruptured hollow viscus such as the bladder, diagnostic laparotomy is probably the most rapid and definitive test in patients who are hemodynamically unstable. If minor injury is found and bleeding is thought to be coming from the pelvis, abbreviated laparotomy should be performed and other plans made to control the pelvic bleeding.

ANATOMIC LOCATION OF INJURY AND INJURY GRADING

A number of classification schemes are available that describe the bony architecture of pelvic fractures. Probably the most commonly used scheme was described by Young et al in 1986 and classifies pelvic fractures by their vector of force (Table 1). Each classification is subdivided to describe the degree of pelvic instability, which is quite useful in describing fracture anatomy and guiding initial attempts at

TABLE 1: Classification of Pelvic Fractures

Type of Fracture	Description
Anteroposterior Compression	
Type I	Disruption of pubic symphysis of <2.5 cm of diastasis; no significant posterior pelvic injury
Type II	Disruption of pubic symphysis of >2.5 cm, with tearing of anterior sacroiliac and sacrospinous and sacrotuberous ligaments
Type III	Complete disruption of pubic symphysis and posterior ligament complexes, with hemipelvic displacement
Lateral Compression	
Type I	Posterior compression of sacroiliac joint without ligament disruption; oblique pubic ramus fracture
Type II	Rupture of posterior sacroiliac ligament; pivotal internal rotation of hemipelvis on anterior sacroiliac joint with a crush injury of sacrum and an oblique public ramus fracture
Type III	Findings in type II injury with evidence of an anteroposterior compression injury to contralateral hemipelvis

Data from Young JWR, Burgess AR, Brumback RJ, et al: Pelvic fractures: value of plain radiography in early assessment and management. *Radiology* 160:445, 1986.

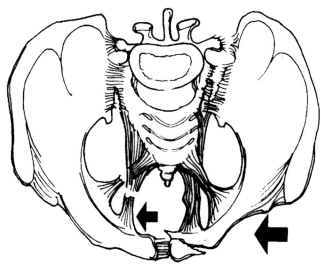

Lateral compression type III

FIGURE 2   Lateral compression pelvic fracture. *(From Moore EE, Feliciano DV, Mattox KL: Trauma, 5th ed, New York, 2003, McGraw-Hill.)*

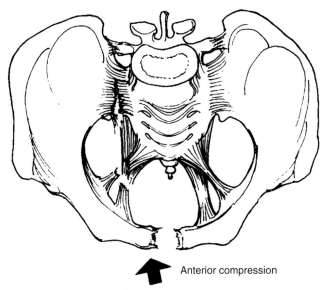

Anterior compression

FIGURE 3   Anterior/posterior compression fracture. *(From Moore EE, Feliciano DV, Mattox KL: Trauma, 5th ed, New York, 2003, McGraw-Hill.)*

hemostasis. The notion that fracture anatomy could predict bleeding has been debated, however. One study from Wake Forest reported on the use of angiography and embolization for pelvic hemostasis and in this series, low-grade anteroposterior (AP) compression fractures required angiography most often. In one study from our institution, the Young et al classification was found to predict transfusion requirements.

Lateral compression (LC) pelvic fractures caused by side impact generally occur after broadside (T-bone) vehicular crashes or car-pedestrian collisions (Fig. 2). LC fractures cause an acute shortening of the pelvic diameter. The pelvic ring does not open but rather "closes down." The pelvic ligaments generally stay intact. Thus, these fractures classically do not bleed. Hemodynamic instability after an LC fracture more likely results from torso injuries such as intra-abdominal bleeding or intrathoracic bleeding. The exception to this occurs in geriatric patients who have a substantial risk of hemorrhage despite a relatively benign-appearing fracture pattern. We demonstrated that LC fractures occurred more commonly in patients over the age of 55 and that these patients were two times more likely to require transfusion than younger patients and required more blood transfusions (7.5 vs. 5 units). These LC fractures were minor, yet still bled substantially. Not surprisingly, overall mortality rate was higher in the older patients.

AP compression fractures generally occur after frontal vehicular crashes or may occur after pelvic crush injuries with the force occurring in the anteroposterior direction (Fig. 3). With this mechanism, pelvic diameter widens and the pelvis opens. The injuries can be purely ligamentous if the SI joints rupture, even in the absence of significant bony injury. Pelvic vascular injuries are quite common. AP compression fractures have the highest associated rate of hemorrhage, and transfusion requirements are the greatest in patients with these fractures.

Vertical shear (VS) injuries occur when patients land on an outstretched foot, which generally occurs after falling from a height or in motorcycle crashes, particularly if patients are riding with their legs outstretched (Fig. 4). In VS fractures, the force is transmitted up the axial skeleton through the posterior pelvis. Posterior fractures and ligamentous ruptures are quite common. If there is a complete disruption of both the anterior and posterior elements (Malgaigne fracture), the psoas muscle pulls the hemipelvis cephalad without opposition. This may be visualized on a pelvic radiograph. VS injuries have an intermediate risk of bleeding in the Young and Burgess classification of pelvic fractures.

Pelvic fractures do not always occur in pure form, such as when a pedestrian is struck obliquely. Thus, a clear classification may not be obvious. The site of bleeding often correlates with pelvic fracture anatomy. AP compression fractures generally bleed from either the pudendal or obturator artery. VS fractures most often bleed from the superior gluteal artery. If LC fractures bleed, they can bleed from virtually any vascular structure.

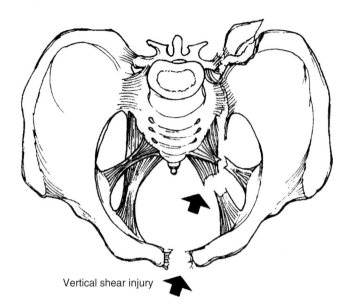

Vertical shear injury

FIGURE 4   Vertical shear fracture. *(From Moore EE, Feliciano DV, Mattox KL: Trauma, 5th ed, New York, 2003, McGraw-Hill.)*

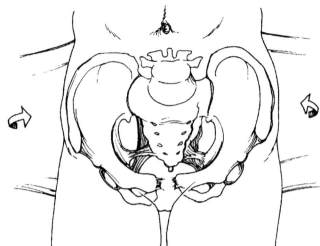

FIGURE 5   Achieving external compression by wrapping a bed sheet around the patient, crisscrossing anteriorly across the pelvis. *(From Moore EE, Feliciano DV, Mattox KL: Trauma, 5th ed, New York, 2003, McGraw-Hill.)*

Although fracture anatomy may be able to predict both the likelihood and location of bleeding, clearly it is far from perfect. The astute clinician will recognize that any patient with a pelvic fracture can bleed. Patients with evidence of ongoing blood loss should obviously have a search for blood loss in other cavities. If none is found, it should be assumed that the patient is probably bleeding from the pelvis. Regardless of the pelvic fracture anatomy, action should be taken to obtain hemostasis.

MANAGEMENT

A number of techniques are available to stop bleeding from the bony pelvis. Bleeding from the pelvis can stem from several sources. The vast majority of bleeding is venous and, although it can be of significant volume, bleeding tends to be relatively self-limited as the pelvic hematoma tamponades this low-pressure vascular injury. Patients can also bleed from fracture fragments themselves as well as smaller pelvic arterial injuries. Larger arteries such as major branches of the hypogastric distribution (pudendal, obturator, or superior gluteal artery) are often the source of large-volume pelvic hemorrhage. Major vascular structures, such as the proximal hypogastric artery or the external or common iliac artery, are rarely the source of major hemorrhage in a typical pelvic fracture, but when these vessels are injured, bleeding is typically massive and the patients are almost uniformly hemodynamically unstable.

Hemostatic techniques for pelvic fracture bleeding can include external compressive devices, fracture fixation, angiographic embolization, and intraoperative control. External compressive devices reduce the pelvic volume, helping to reduce venous bleeding. External compression can help "stabilize the clot" that has formed. Additionally, reducing the fracture fragments limits direct bony bleeding. Stabilizing the fracture fragments also limits recurrent fracture motion and should help prevent recurrent bleeding. A number of devices are available to help achieve external compression.

Perhaps the simplest is using a bed sheet. Ideally, the sheet is placed on the stretcher, even before the patient arrives. Alternatively, the patient can be gently lifted and the bed sheet placed underneath the patient. The bed sheet is then crisscrossed across the pelvis anteriorly and tied down (Fig. 5). This low-tech practice has proved to be extraordinarily helpful. It can be especially helpful in small community emergency departments (EDs) that have limited resources and

may not have sophisticated technology. We generally advise the emergency physician to tie the bed sheet down snugly but not excessively tight. Patients can then be transported within the hospital or to a higher level of care.

The military antishock garment (MAST) was originally used as a resuscitative technique in the prehospital phase. The MAST was originally thought to autotransfuse blood from the capacitance vessels of the lower extremities. It is now clear that increases in blood pressure are caused by increases in systemic vascular resistance, not increases in cardiac preload. The MAST can, however, be an effective pelvic and lower extremity splint and can keep pelvic fractures reduced, much like the bed sheet. The lower extremity portion must be inflated if the abdominal and pelvic portion is inflated. If the pressure on the MAST is set too high, increases in intra-abdominal pressure can occur, leading to abdominal compartment syndrome. Patients must be carefully monitored for this complication. Use of the MAST has largely been abandoned as it has been demonstrated to be of little value in treating hypotension in the prehospital setting.

The posterior pelvic C clamp is another option for external pelvic compression. The C clamp is inserted posteriorly to reduce the posterior fracture fragments. This is placed percutaneously in the ED in many European trauma centers. In most American trauma centers, fluoroscopic guidance in the operating room is used, which limits its effectiveness as an acute resuscitation tool. The anterior portion of the C clamp can be rotated out of the way to provide access for angiography or laparotomy. Clearly, if the pins are poorly placed, complications including gastrointestinal perforation or iatrogenic nerve injury can occur.

In the past, external fixation was very commonly used as a compressive device for pelvic hemostasis. External fixation is the most rigid of the external devices and closes the pelvis down definitively (Fig. 6). In centers with expertise, external fixators can be applied rapidly in the ED. In other centers, they are often placed in the operating room similar to the C clamp. In some cases, external fixation may provide definitive fracture fixation. The anterior portion of the frame can be rotated similar to the C clamp to allow access for angiography or laparotomy. Use of external fixation during the resuscitative phase requires that these resources be immediately available. External fixation may degrade CT images and may interfere with patient motion through the CT gantry. The pins for external fixation are placed in the iliac crest and the frame is then applied anteriorly. In patients with badly displaced posterior element pelvic fractures, the inward motion

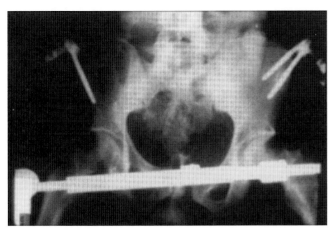

FIGURE 6 External fixation, commonly used in the past as a compressive device for pelvic hemostasis. External fixation is the most rigid of the external devices and closes the pelvis down definitively. *(From Moore EE, Feliciano DV, Mattox KL: Trauma, 5th ed, New York, 2003, McGraw-Hill.)*

produced by tightening down the frame can cause further displacement of the posterior fracture fragments and increase blood loss.

Many American trauma centers have abandoned virtually all other external compressive devices and exclusively use a commercially available pelvic binder. The pelvic binder is a Velcro device that applies even, direct pressure on the pelvis. The pressure is set by the Velcro and lace system on the anterior portion of the binder. The binders can be applied rapidly and require a minimum of expertise. The commercially available binders have been shown to reduce pubic diastasis in AP fracture types (Fig. 7). The binder should be applied across the femoral greater trochanters, not across the lower abdomen. Correct placement of the binder can limit access to the groins for angiography, however. If angiography is required, a hole can be cut in the binder or the binder can be placed slightly higher or lower across the upper thigh. Deciding whether external compression would be helpful is a function of pelvic fracture anatomy. A wide open, AP III pelvic fracture is ideally treated with external compression. An LC pelvic fracture in which the pelvis has imploded—not exploded—is unlikely to be helped by external compression. VS injuries may respond in an intermittent manner. In the days of using external fixators, this discussion was quite germane. The advent of the pelvic binder has obviated many of these discussions. Although a pelvic binder is unlikely to help an LC pelvic fracture, it can be applied quickly and almost certainly will not exacerbate bleeding. The pelvic binder can act as a pelvic splint and limit fracture fragment motion during transport to the CT scanner, the operating room, or the angiography suite. Thus, we have become quite liberal in the use of the pelvic binder, and place it on virtually any patient with a pelvic fracture who is hemodynamically unstable.

Angiographic embolization for pelvic hemostasis has been used for over 30 years. Diagnostic pelvic angiography should be able to identify all sites of pelvic arterial injury. Indications for angiography in patients with pelvic fractures include hemodynamic instability, large pelvic or retroperitoneal hematoma, and pseudoaneurysm or contrast extravasation on CT. Transfusion triggers such as more than 4 units in 24 hours or 6 units in 48 hours have also been advocated (Table 2). Embolization with Gelfoam, stainless steel coils, or both can be quite effective in achieving pelvic hemostasis. A number of angiographic techniques are available. One would like to be as selective as possible with pelvic embolization to limit potential complications such as impotence or distal ischemia resulting in pelvic or gluteal necrosis. The more selective technique, however, requires a greater amount of time and expertise to use. An alternative to selective embolization is blind proximal hypogastric embolization with stainless

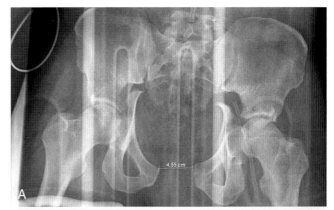

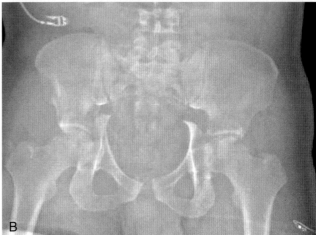

FIGURE 7 An anteroposterior pelvic fracture before (**A**) and after (**B**) application of the pelvic binder, a Velcro device that applies even, direct pressure on the pelvis.

TABLE 2: Indication for Angiography

4 units of blood in 24 hours
6 units of blood in 48 hours
Hypotension with negative focused assessment with sonography in trauma (FAST)/diagnostic peritoneal lavage
Large pelvic hematoma on computed tomography (CT) or in operating room
Pseudoaneurysm on CT

Data from Moore EE, Feliciano DV, Mattox KL: *Trauma*, 5th ed, New York, 2003, McGraw-Hill.

steel coils. This is intended to reduce perfusion pressure within the hypogastric distribution and allow spontaneous hemostasis to occur. This could produce suboptimal hemostasis, as there is a rich collateral circulation within the pelvic vasculature. With the proximal hypogastric artery embolized, the angiographic window to achieve hemostasis is now closed if recurrent bleeding occurs. Alternatively, blind hypogastric embolization with particulate Gelfoam may achieve the same purpose as coil embolization.

Operative approaches to achieve hemostasis have generally been discouraged. Laparotomy does not allow the surgeon to directly visualize the injured blood vessel. Opening the retroperitoneum releases tamponade and can restart bleeding that had been attenuated, especially venous bleeding. The main hypogastric artery is a very short structure. In most patients, it is only several inches long and then quickly branches into a large number of much smaller vessels that disappear deep into the pelvis. Identifying the injured blood vessel is extraordinarily difficult, and attempts to do this typically make a bad situation worse. Empiric hypogastric ligation is an option similar to proximal hypogastric embolization. It does carry risks of unroofing the pelvic hematoma, as well as risks of bleeding from collateral flow. In many centers, hypogastric embolization can be accomplished in approximately the same amount of time that it takes to achieve hypogastric ligation. However, if angiographic embolization is not immediately available and patients are exsanguinating, hypogastric ligation remains an option. Intraoperative hypogastric embolization is another option for patients in extremis. The proximal hypogastric artery is isolated with a vessel loop. The surgeon then mixes a slurry of hemostatic agents, which could include fresh frozen plasma and small-particulate Gelfoam. The hypogastric artery is accessed with an angiocatheter and blind embolization performed. There is limited experience in the literature with hypogastric embolization. This course should be avoided unless no other options exist.

Some patients almost certainly benefit from an attempt at direct operative hemostasis. Patients who present in hemorrhagic shock and have a unilateral absence of a femoral pulse likely have injury to either the common or external iliac artery. Typically, these patients have a traumatic hemipelvectomy (Fig. 8). An extreme amount of force is necessary to produce this injury, and these patients usually are in refractory shock. A direct operative approach using medial visceral rotation, combined with a direct approach to the iliac arteries is potentially lifesaving for these patients. Injuries can be treated with ligation or simple repair. Those who have injuries not amenable to a simple technique should generally undergo shunting in a damage-control fashion.

Most recently, the notion of extraperitoneal packing has again gained significant popularity. The patient is approached via a lower midline or a Pfannenstiel incision. The lower abdominal muscles are split in the midline and the pelvic hematoma entered directly. The pelvic hematoma is evacuated and the pelvis then packed (Fig. 9). It is important to stay extraperitoneal. When the packs are applied up against the peritoneum, the peritoneum increases the tamponade effect. The retroperitoneal fascia can be closed to increase tamponade or the patient can be temporized with a vacuum dressing. Occasionally, pelvic packing is used in concert with a laparotomy. In that case, we generally use a transverse incision to avoid having the

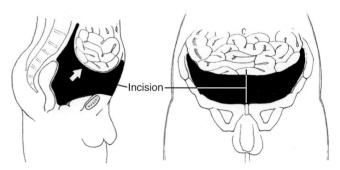

FIGURE 9   Low midline incision to approach pelvic hematoma. *(From Moore EE, Feliciano DV, Mattox KL: Trauma, 5th ed, New York, 2003, McGraw-Hill.)*

abdominal and retroperitoneal incisions meet. The muscles can be split and the pelvic packed in the same manner. Retroperitoneal packing is most successful when used in concert with some sort of bony pelvic stabilization. External fixation or a C clamp can be placed at the time of pelvic packing. Alternatively, the pelvic binder can simple be replaced. This technique can also be used in conjunction with more formal pelvic fracture fixation such as pelvic plating or placement of percutaneous SI screws, depending on the patient's clinical status.

Early rigid fixation in patients with significant pelvic fractures is ideal. Definitive reduction of the fracture fragments can be quite helpful in achieving hemostasis. However, early open reduction and internal fixation risks significant blood loss. Percutaneous SI screw fixation can reduce the posterior pelvis with minimal blood loss. These percutaneous screws are threaded under fluoroscopic guidance and rigidly reduce the pelvis (Fig. 10). We typically use this technique with AP II or AP III fractures. The patients must be hemodynamically stable enough to undergo the operative procedure, though, as this technique is not recommended for patients in profound shock. Percutaneous SI screws allow for good reduction of the pelvic fracture, reduction of pelvic volume, and clot stabilization. Once the fracture is definitively fixed in this manner, the patients can be mobilized out of bed, minimizing the risk of pulmonary complications.

Anterior pelvic fixation can also be accomplished at the time of concomitant trauma laparotomy in the hemodynamically stable patient. In this scenario, patients undergo laparotomy and treatment for intra-abdominal injuries. When the abdominal portion is finished, the incision can be lengthened or a separate Pfannenstiel incision can be performed. The anterior fracture fragments are manually reduced and then an anterior pelvic plate placed. Again, this provides definitive anterior fracture fixation that obviates the need for other techniques such as external fixation or a binder.

Open pelvic fractures represent a distinct problem. They can be the source of torrential external blood loss. As the blood loss in these cases is external, there is often not a large component of retroperitoneal hemorrhage. The diagnosis should be made on physical examination. As patients typically present in the supine position, it is important to examine the perineum. It may be necessary to do a vaginal or rectal examination to appreciate the laceration. The abdomen should then be evaluated using a FAST. Patients with a positive FAST should proceed to laparotomy, and those with a negative FAST should undergo further diagnostic evaluations.

Bleeding from open pelvic fractures can be controlled initially with packing. If the opening to the outside is small, it may be necessary to widen the external opening in order to get the packs deep into the pelvis. It is important to characterize the anatomy of the pelvic fracture. This can generally be accomplished with a combination of physical examination and pelvic radiograph. The pelvic fracture should be reduced using any of the compressive devices discussed previously. The entire multidisciplinary team should be alerted, including the

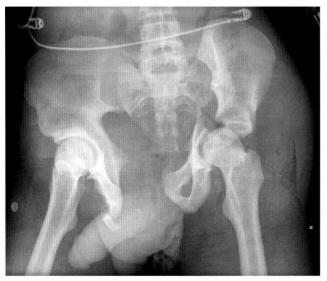

FIGURE 8   Traumatic internal hemipelvectomy.

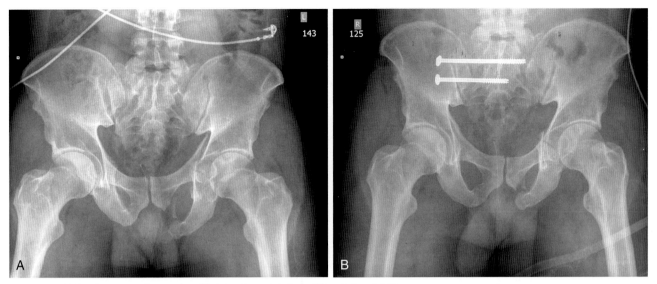

FIGURE 10 Pelvic fracture with sacroiliac (SI) joint diastasis before (**A**) and after (**B**) SI percutaneous screw placement.

operating room, the orthopedic service, and the angiography suite. Even if the bleeding looks venous and is controlled with packing, we advocate angiography for these patients. The patient should go to the operating room for local exploration, repacking, and whatever hemostasis can be achieved via local control. This can be performed as the angiography team is setting up the angiography suite. If there is torrential bleeding when the patient is unpacked and explored, simply repacking the patient is the wisest course. Once hemostasis is achieved, the patient should undergo operative débridement of non-viable soft tissue and muscle. Fecal diversion is often required in patients with perirectal involvement but is not an emergency and can be deferred until the patient is hemodynamically stable and bleeding has been controlled.

MORBIDITY AND COMPLICATIONS MANAGEMENT

The mortality rate for patients with pelvic fractures has been reported to be approximately 6% in pooled series. Historically, most deaths were due to pelvic hemorrhage, but more recently an increasing number of deaths have been caused by hemorrhage from concomitant injuries. Presumably, earlier recognition of the pelvis as a potential source of blood loss has resulted in fewer people dying from pelvic hemorrhage. Other common causes of major morbidity and fatality include traumatic brain injury, sepsis, and multiple-organ failure.

In the short term, patients with pelvic fractures are at high risk for a number of complications directly relatable to the pelvic fracture itself. Soft tissue injury can be exacerbated by hemostatic procedures leading to skin, subcutaneous tissue, and muscle ischemia. Operative débridement is indicated for patients with soft tissue necrosis. Deep pelvic infections, particularly in patients with open fractures, also occur and may contribute to multiple-organ dysfunction and failure and death. These infections should be aggressively treated with culture targeted antibiotics and drainage. Hardware removal may be required, resulting in prolonged immobilization.

Patients with pelvic fractures are also at exceptionally high risk for many of the common complications that affect multiply injured and immobilized patients. Pelvic fractures increase the risk of deep vein thrombosis (DVT). Patients with pelvic fractures are at particular risk for thromboembolism, because they all have some degree of pelvic venous injury and are immobilized for some time. The best treatment strategy is an aggressive program of prevention with early fracture fixation and mobilization, which are also probably the best way to prevent DVT. Respiratory failure occurs commonly owing to high risk of atelectasis, pneumonia, fat embolism, pulmonary embolism, and aspiration. Nosocomial infections, such as urinary tract infections and ventilator-associated pneumonia, should be aggressively diagnosed and treated to prevent the development of sepsis and multiple-organ failure.

Unfortunately, patients surviving major pelvic fractures often have significant long-term morbidity. Historically, nearly 50% of these patients may have serious pain and disability. The adequacy of pelvic reduction and degree of residual displacement may play a significant role. The functional results with newer combined operative approaches are likely to be better than historically reported, with a few newer studies reporting over two thirds of patients with overall good functional status following major pelvic ring disruption. Open fractures, in particular, are associated with poor functional outcome. Other long-term complications in patients with pelvic fractures include problems with sexual function, impotence, and dyspareunia.

CONCLUSIONS AND ALGORITHM (FIG. 11)

The multiply injured patient with pelvic fractures represents one of the greatest challenges to the trauma service. Diagnosing sources of hemorrhage and efficiently performing resuscitation and appropriate treatments are critical. Various techniques are available to evaluate the patient and help achieve hemostasis. It is important that an institutional algorithm that is tailored to an organization's expertise and resources be devised that will allow efficient, rapid, coordinated, and effective care for these badly injured patients.

For the chapter's Suggested Readings list, please visit the book at www.ExpertConsult.inkling.com.

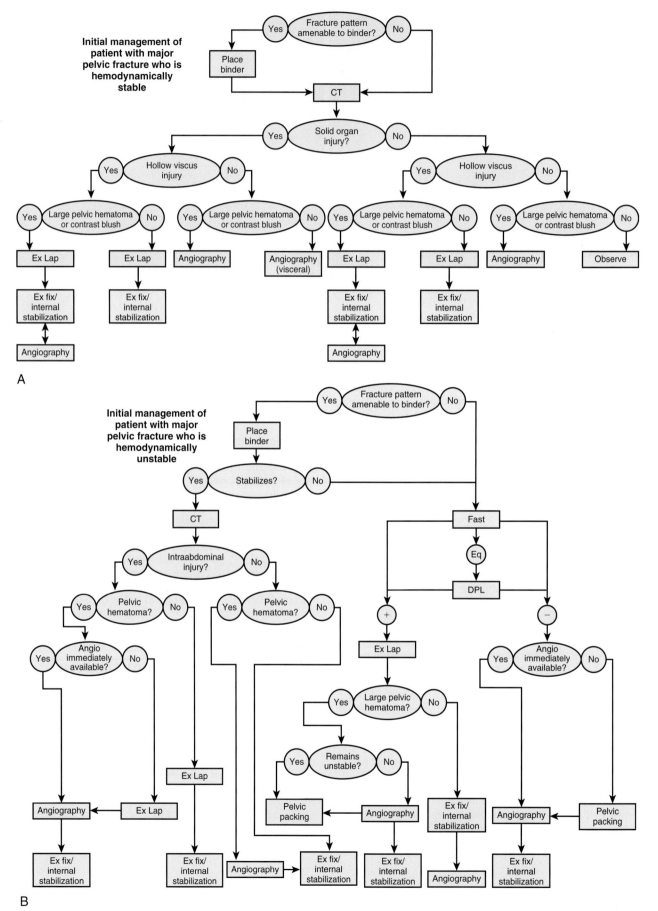

FIGURE 11   A, Algorithm for initial management of patient with major pelvic fracture who is hemodynamically stable. **B,** Algorithm for initial management of patient with major pelvic fracture who is hemodynamically unstable. Angio, Biplanar angiography; CT, computed tomography; DPL, diagnostic peritoneal lavage; Ex fix, external fixator; Ex lap, exploratory laparotomy; Eq, equivocal; FAST, focused assessment with sonography in trauma.

SPECIAL ISSUES IN MAJOR TORSO TRAUMA

CURRENT CONCEPTS IN THE DIAGNOSIS AND MANAGEMENT OF HEMORRHAGIC SHOCK

Juan Carlos Puyana, Samuel Tisherman, and Andrew B. Peitzman

The precipitating single common factor of hemorrhagic shock is severe acute blood loss, yet the clinical syndrome of hemorrhagic shock is heterogeneous. The diagnosis and management of this condition at first would appear to be simple. However, the very nature of how shock occurs and how the individual compensatory mechanisms respond to both the injury itself and the resuscitative interventions translate into a complex spectrum of diseases. This disease spectrum extends from immediate circulatory collapse to total body ischemia reperfusion injury with associated complex inflammatory and anti-inflammatory responses that in many instances evolve into multiple organ dysfunction. The purpose of this chapter is to provide a review of the current issues and a clinical perspective regarding the diagnosis and management of shock.

EPIDEMIOLOGY OF SEVERE HEMORRHAGIC SHOCK

Injuries are the second leading cause of death worldwide, and the leading cause of years of life lost in the United Sates. Trauma-induced severe hemorrhage is the leading cause of potentially preventable deaths. Overall, trauma results in approximately 150,000 deaths per year, and severe hypovolemia due to hemorrhage is a major factor in nearly half of those deaths. The leading causes of death remain head injury and hemorrhage. These findings have been reported both in the civilian literature and military experiences, including the Vietnam conflict, and most recently in Iraq and Afghanistan. Approximately one third of trauma deaths occur out of hospital; exsanguination is a major cause of deaths occurring within 4 hours of injury. The distribution of battlefield injuries in the Vietnam War showed that 25% of the deaths occurred as a result of massive exsanguination and were not salvageable. An additional 19% of deaths were deemed salvageable, and these deaths were the result of torso exsanguination (10%) and peripheral exsanguination

(19%). Recent data on the indications for early use of transfusions in civilian trauma showed that 58% of all deaths were due to hemorrhage and the majority (66%) occur within 3 hours of admission; brain injury and multiple organ failure were the leading causes of death 24 hours after admission.

THE CLINICAL PERSPECTIVE: CHANGING CONCEPTS ON RESUSCITATION

Severe hemorrhagic shock is characterized by cool, moist, pallid, or cyanotic skin. The patient is tachycardic and hypotensive and the severity of these clinical manifestations may vary from patient to patient depending on age, underlying cardiovascular disease, and the presence of medications or associated toxic compounds such as drugs or alcohol. Hypotension is the hallmark of shock, it is easily measured, and its presence is always a predictor of poor outcome. The severity of shock, however, can only be partially quantified by the presence of hypotension. Obviously, patients with rapid and massive blood loss will manifest low blood pressure shortly after the injury. Sophisticated devices or monitoring techniques are not required to establish that such patients are close to dying. Prompt and efficient interventions must be instituted immediately, aimed at control of hemorrhage and replacement of the blood volume. Unfortunately, the absence of hypotension after injury does not rule out the presence of shock. In fact, it may mislead the inexperienced clinician to a false sense of security about the need for aggressive resuscitation.

Injured patients arriving to the trauma center with hypotension or a history of transient hypotension account for only 6% to 9% of the total number of trauma patients. From a practical viewpoint, patients with hemorrhagic shock can be stratified into three groups. Group 1 are those patients with exsanguinating hemorrhage. They generally have significant chest injuries to the heart or great vessels, massively disruptive abdominal visceral injury, or significant retroperitoneal bleeding such as pelvic fractures. This group represents one third of the total number of hypotensive patients or 2% of the total trauma patient population. They arrive alive to our trauma centers only as a direct result of well-organized prehospital and trauma systems. The response to fluid administration in this group is minimal or completely absent and these patients are termed *nonresponders*.

Another one third of hypotensive patients (2% of the total trauma population) constitute group 2 with moderate to severe hemorrhage, bleeding at a slower rate than group 1. Group 2 patients can die within 6 to 12 hours if adequate and timely therapy and hemorrhage control are not provided. They respond to the initial resuscitation and may do so transiently. Even if managed appropriately they may develop organ failure or infection.

The third group is also 2% of the total trauma population and comprises those patients with transient hypotension whose compensatory response is sufficient to achieve spontaneous stabilization of their vital signs. The final outcome of these patients is better but the onset of complications or organ dysfunction may result from the net time spent in a state of underresuscitation, better described as unrecognized hypoperfusion or compensated shock.

Increased understanding of the causes of death after injury suggests that truncal hemorrhage represents a major cause of potentially preventable death. Patients suffering from severe penetrating trauma to the chest or abdomen, with major injuries to the thoracic or intraabdominal vessels, who arrive alive to the trauma center, will require aggressive interventions that could include an emergency thoracotomy and massive transfusion (MT). A better understanding regarding the use of crystalloids, blood products, and the management of trauma-induced coagulopathy has been generated over the last 10 years prompted by the war experiences in the Middle East. Traditional resuscitation strategies taught by Advanced Trauma Life Support (ATLS) courses are now being reexamined as new findings indicating the deleterious effects of excessive use of crystalloids and the true incidence of trauma-induced coagulopathy in patients with hemorrhagic shock continue to emerge. These patients are severely coagulopathic upon admission to the emergency department and carry an increased risk of fatality.

This new knowledge has challenged the dogma that dates back to the 1970s regarding fluid resuscitation when separation of donated whole blood into its component parts was implemented. Patients who require an MT are now being managed differently by providing increased ratios of plasma and platelets; however, there is still no broad consensus on the optimal blood products ratios for civilian trauma patients. Clearly, a change from the classic resuscitation approach is needed, especially for those patients who present in shock and are predicted to require MT.

MT patients usually require damage control interventions, and manifest severe hypothermia and coagulopathy as well as circulatory failure even after their hemorrhage has been controlled. Because the spectrum of hypoperfusion, ischemia, and total body reperfusion may differ significantly from one clinical scenario to the next one, it is obvious then that future therapeutic interventions will need to be more sophisticated and specifically targeted. Fluid resuscitation and specifically blood products replacement ratios and proactive management of coagulopathy will evolve further and other specific interventions will be needed as increased understanding of this complicated pathophysiologic process continues to improve.

The potential enhancement of early recognition of progressive or refractory shock and reducing the onset of circulatory collapse early in the management of the patient with hemorrhage offers the opportunity of redefining the "golden hour" (i.e., the window of opportunity for efficacious resuscitation).

The Discrepancies between the Clinical Syndrome of Shock and the Animal Models Used to Study It

When devising models of hemorrhagic shock, investigators in this field are challenged by two sometimes mutually incompatible goals. First, researchers desire to minimize animal-to-animal variability. Second, researchers seek to achieve a model with clinical relevance. Bleeding in the clinical environment is typically uncontrolled. As hemorrhage continues and arterial pressure decreases, the rate of bleeding tends to slow. Hemostatic mechanisms may come into play when blood pressure is low enough so that bleeding ceases entirely. Resuscitation can actually dislodge the nascent clot by raising blood pressure, and thereby precipitate recurrent hemorrhage. Numerous animal models of uncontrolled bleeding have been described. These models are generally useful for studying novel approaches to achieve hemostasis, for determining the optimal timing of resuscitation, or for determining the optimal parameters/end points for resuscitation.

However, uncontrolled hemorrhage models, although attractive because of their clinical relevance, suffer from a high degree of animal-to-animal variability. Therefore, the use of these models for preclinical efficacy studies of new therapeutic agents requires relatively large sample sizes to obtain statistically meaningful data.

On the other hand, controlled hypotension, as originally described by Wiggers, allows a more standardized grading of injury. When hemorrhagic shock is induced using the Wiggers model, it is initially necessary to periodically withdraw additional aliquots of blood to maintain the target blood pressure because of the body's normal compensatory responses to acute hypovolemia. However, after the shock state has persisted for a period of time, it is no longer possible to withdraw blood to maintain the target blood pressure. On the contrary, it now becomes necessary to reinfuse aliquots of the shed blood to maintain the target blood pressure. This phase has little resemblance to what happens in clinical practice, but in the laboratory it is used to delineate what is known as the "decompensation end point," defined as the transition point from withdrawal to reinfusion of blood. This transition point typically occurs after 90 to 120 minutes of shock, depending on the species. This model is imperfect as well because variability occurs as to the time of the decompensation end point from one animal to the next one. Obviously the Wiggers model allows for a more reproducible injury, one that has little resemblance to the clinical scenario but one that facilitates mechanistic or cause/effect studies and that has been used extensively to delineate many of the cellular and molecular events described after hemorrhage that are beyond the scope of this chapter.

New models of bleeding have been developed in mice that allow for sophisticated analyses of the many cascades of detrimental signaling events that may play a role in hemorrhage-induced fatality. Advances in the assessment of biologic systems (i.e., systems biology) have enabled the scientific community to further understand complex physiologic networks and cellular communication patterns that underline the pathologic bases of shock.

DIAGNOSIS OF SHOCK

Measurement of blood pressure may not always be feasible and it is not a necessary requirement to initiate therapy during the primary survey. In fact, a quick global assessment of adequacy of perfusion can rapidly be obtained by examining the characteristics of the pulse. Obvious signs of shock are sufficient to establish the diagnoses and determine the severity of blood volume loss. Additional information such as blood pressure measurement, electrocardiogram, pulse oximeter, and capnography may be useful. Adequate intravenous (IV) access for infusion of normothermic fluids is the next priority but other causes of severe hypotension and shock are being ruled out, such as tension pneumothorax, pericardial tamponade, or neurogenic shock.

Ideally, any fluid therapy must be accompanied with control of bleeding. An estimate of blood volume deficit after trauma may be calculated at the bedside by estimating blood losses associated with specific injuries. A unilateral hemothorax may contain 3000 mL of blood, the abdomen can hold 2000 to 5000 mL, and abdominal distention may not be apparent. Other injuries that may precipitate massive hemorrhage include pelvic fracture, associated with blood losses of 1500 to 2000 mL in the retroperitoneum without any external signs of trauma. A femur fracture may bleed between 800 to 1200 mL, and a tibia fracture 350 to 650 mL.

The early diagnosis of trauma-induced coagulopathy and the ability to quantify the severity of the coagulation dysfunction using point of care thromboelastography (TEG) is a promising new approach to the management of severe shock. Advances on more practical techniques for the use of TEG in the trauma bay may aid in targeting specific coagulation disorders early in the course of hemorrhage with a more rational use of blood products, coagulation factors, and antifibrinolytic therapy.

The phenomenon of ischemia and reperfusion has been extensively studied. Shock and resuscitation are functionally a total body ischemia/reperfusion injury. SIRS (systemic inflammatory response syndrome) and MODS (multiple organ dysfunction syndrome) are the expressions of a conglomerate of events associated with ischemia and reperfusion. Unfortunately, we rely on nonspecific global methods to provide indirect information regarding tissue perfusion. The current challenge is to identify innovative methods for quantifying the magnitude of shock. Questions that should guide future research in this field include consideration into how the interaction between the patient's physiologic reserve, compensatory responses, and the individual organs' endurance/response to ischemia may ultimately manifest, and determining the best methods to accurately measure each of these components. Presently, we scarcely understand these issues and use rather crude methods to quantify the insult. The term *tissue perfusion* is used liberally to refer to an entity not readily quantifiable. In practical terms, we rely on base deficit (BD) and lactate as the global parameters used to gauge tissue perfusion. In the intensive care unit (ICU), we add to the interpretation of these values by hemodynamic parameters that are commonly obtained only after invasive monitoring techniques can be implemented, such as thermodilution cardiac output or continuous $S\overline{V}O_2$ from either the central or the mixed venous circulation.

Assessment of Tissue Perfusion

BD and lactic acid provide information about the degree of anaerobic metabolism. Lactate is an indirect measure of oxygen debt. BD is defined as the amount of buffer necessary to bring the pH back to 7.40 with P_{CO_2} of 40 mm Hg. Davis et al stratified patients by BD as mild (2–5), moderate (6–14), and severe (>15). The magnitude of the initial BD was found to directly correlate with hypotension and further need for fluid resuscitation. In addition, 65% of patients who had a worsening BD despite resuscitation had ongoing hemorrhage. BD is considered a reliable marker for shock and the need for transfusion in multiple trauma patients. Davis et al also demonstrated that BD could remain abnormal despite improvements in mean arterial pressure, cardiac output, mixed venous O_2 saturation, and oxygen extraction in an animal model of hemorrhagic shock. Rutherford et al found that BD, age, and head injury had an additive effect on the incidence of fatality. BD is an expedient and sensitive measure of both the degree and the duration of inadequate perfusion. It is useful as a clinical tool and enhances the predictive ability of other trauma scores.

Lactate is the end product of anaerobic glycolysis. As a more direct measurement of tissue hypoxia-induced acidosis, it has been shown to have strong prognostic value. Normalization of serum lactate below 2 mmol/L or less within the first 24 hours is associated with 100% survival rate. Only 78% of patients survived when lactate levels remained elevated during the period of 24 to 48 hours after shock. The mortality rate is greater than 85% if lactate remains elevated at 48 hours after shock. Sauaia et al demonstrated an association between an early (12 hour) rise in serum lactate above 2.5 mmol/L and multiorgan failure. Manikis et al further found that initial and peak lactate levels, as well as the duration of hyperlactatemia, correlated with the development of MODS after trauma. Recent data from the Inflammation and Host Response to Injury large-scale collaborative project (Glue Grant) corroborated the predictive value of BD and lactate in a cohort of severely injured blunt trauma patients. Early elevated lactate levels and continued evidence of shock measured by elevated BD for 12 to 24 hours after injury were found to be independent predictors of multiple organ failure.

In summary, the initial lactate level and time to normalization of lactate correlate with risk of MODS and death. However, improved survival rate using lactate or BD as end points for resuscitation has not been shown.

MANAGEMENT OF SHOCK

Management priorities in the bleeding trauma patient include airway control, ventilation, and oxygenation. The goal of resuscitation is to stop the bleeding and replete intravascular blood volume to maximize tissue oxygen delivery. Cardiac output, blood pressure, and oxygenated blood flow to vital organs are important determinants of outcome.

Shock may be managed by different strategies along the continuum of care from the moment of the insult to the time of stabilization in the ICU. Prehospital interventions may be lifesaving, but may be limited by the specific environment in the field, for example, an urban inner city, a rural setting, the battlefield, or after a mass casualty scenario. During the hospital phase, more definitive therapies may be implemented with the level of care, depending upon the capabilities of the receiving hospital. When this is not the case, transfer to a Level I or II trauma center may be necessary. Therefore, the actual care that a patient may receive for a similar magnitude of injury may vary significantly depending on the variables listed previously, the state of the regionalization of the trauma system, and the maturity of the trauma center.

The key for success in treating patients with life-threatening hemorrhage is based on expedited surgical control of bleeding. A skilled full operation and a thorough knowledge of the vascular anatomy will continue to be the cornerstone of lifesaving interventions. Yet, interventional radiologists and vascular surgeons in the angiogram room are now managing an increasing variety of trauma-related vascular injuries. In this chapter, however, we will focus on describing therapeutic strategies according to the physiologic opportunities or therapeutic windows that may be available. These interventions may range from adjunct measures to control hemorrhage, enhancement of the compensatory response, replacement of blood volume lost, and support of the organs during the spectrum of hypoperfusion inherent to a particular clinical scenario. Prompt airway control and expedient control of bleeding are obviously fundamental tenets.

Vascular Access for Patients with Severe Hemorrhage

Vascular access is essential to restore circulatory volume rapidly. The most important factor in considering the procedure for procuring vascular access is the anatomic location and magnitude of the injuries and the level of skill and expertise of the care provider. Venous access should be avoided in an injured limb. In patients with injuries below the diaphragm, at least one IV line should be placed in a tributary of the superior vena cava, as there may be vascular disruption of the inferior vena cava. For rapid administration of large amounts of IV fluids, short, large-bore catheters should be used. Doubling the internal diameter of the venous cannula increases the flow through the catheter 16-fold. A 14-G, 5-cm catheter in a peripheral vein will infuse fluid twice as fast as a 16-G, 20-cm catheter passed centrally. When using 8.5F pulmonary catheter introducers, the side port should be removed, as this increases the resistance roughly fourfold.

ATLS guidelines recommend rapid placement of two large-bore (16-G or larger) IV catheters in the patient with serious injuries and hemorrhagic shock. The first choice for IV insertion should be a peripheral extremity vein. The most suitable veins are at the wrist, the dorsum of the hand, the antecubital fossa in the arm, and the saphenous vein in the leg. These sites can be followed by the external jugular vein and femoral vein. The complication rate of properly placed IV catheters is low. Intravascular placement of a large-bore IV catheter should be verified by checking for backflow of blood. An IV site should infuse easily without added pressure. IV fluids can extravasate into soft tissues when pumped under pressure through an infiltrated IV line, and may create a compartment syndrome. A patient in extremis who loses pulses in the trauma bay needs a cutdown in the femoral vein.

Subclavian and internal jugular (IJ) catheterization should not be used routinely in hypovolemic trauma patients. The incidence of complications is higher and the rate of success is lower due to venous collapse. Rapid peripheral percutaneous IV access may be difficult to achieve in patients with hypovolemia and venous collapse, edema, obesity, scar tissue, history of IV drug abuse, or burns. Under such circumstances, central access with wide-bore catheters may be attempted by percutaneous femoral puncture or cutdown. Subclavian catheterization provides rapid venous access in experienced hands. The most frequent complication of subclavian venipuncture is pneumothorax. Pneumothorax is more likely to occur on the left side because the left pleural dome is anatomically higher. Subclavian and IJ catheters should be inserted on the side of injury in patients with chest wounds, reducing the chances of collapse of the uninjured lung, especially if a thoracostomy tube is already in place. A simple pneumothorax may result in respiratory compromise in individuals with pulmonary contusions or a pneumothorax in the contralateral hemithorax. Venous air embolism is another complication of central line insertion.

Although percutaneous placement of IJ catheters is an excellent means of attaining rapid large-bore catheter access, this is an unusual site for IV insertion in trauma patients because of the possibility of cervical trauma and the need for cervical collar immobilization.

Femoral vein cannulation is another alternative for line placement and is associated with fewer acute complications. Bowel perforation may occur, especially in patients with femoral hernia. Penetration of the hip may result in septic arthritis. Thrombophlebitis occurs more often with femoral than with IJ or subclavian catheters; however, thrombophlebitis is most likely with prolonged use of catheters.

Venous cutdowns can be performed when rapid, secure, large-bore venous cannulation is desirable, when percutaneous peripheral or central access is either contraindicated or impossible to achieve. Strict aseptic technique should be used. Surgical masks and caps should be worn. Venous cutdown has a low potential for anatomic damage. Cutaneous nerve injury is the most common problem. The infection rate is relatively low when used acutely but increases over time. Therefore, it is recommended that venous cutdown catheters be removed as soon as it is possible to achieve IV access through standard percutaneous IV catheters or a central venous catheter. In addition, any lines placed during resuscitation of a trauma patient without strict aseptic technique should be removed as soon as the patient's condition allows.

ADJUNCT MEASURES TO CONTROL HEMORRHAGE

Local Hemorrhage Control

A number of agents are being used to achieve local hemostasis. Such agents may be used topically or systemically. Topical hemostatic agents include vasoconstrictive agents such as epinephrine and procoagulant agents such as thrombin, "hemostatic fibrin," gelatin, and cellulose material.

QuikClot is a new agent designed to induce local hemostasis of large wounds associated with vascular lesions. It is a zeolite mineral granular powder that increases the concentration of clotting factors in the wound. It has been used in models of extremity arterial injury and hepatic laceration with good results. QuikClot has been deployed with the United States military forces. In a recent study, Rhee et al reported on 103 cases of QuikClot use: 69 by the U.S. military in Iraq, 20 by civilian trauma surgeons, and 14 by civilian first responders. There were 83 cases involving application to external wounds and 20 cases of intracorporeal use by military and civilian surgeons. The overall efficacy rate was 92%. Failures were seen in patients with massive injuries when used as a last resort and in cases in which it was not possible to deliver the agent directly to the source of hemorrhage. Patients did experience mild to severe pain and discomfort due to the exothermic reaction caused when the QuikClot was applied.

Systemic Hemorrhage Control

Tranexamic Acid

Tranexamic acid inhibits plasmin generation, it is distributed throughout all tissues in the body, and it has a plasma half-life of 120 minutes. Its use has been recommended on the basis of its antifibrinolytic effect that can potentially reduce bleeding and the need for transfusions. Evidence that the use of tranexamic acid improves the outcome of trauma patients comes from the recently published CRASH-2 trial. This study includes more than 20,000 trauma patients with or at risk for substantial bleeding who were randomly assigned to a tranexamic acid treatment group or to placebo. Tranexamic acid was administered as a bolus of 1 g followed by another 1 g over 8 hours.

The mortality rate in the tranexamic acid treated group was 14.5% compared to 16% in the placebo group, relative risk 0.91 (95% confidence interval [CI] 0.85 – 0.97; $p = 0.0035$). Bleeding-related mortality rate in the tranexamic group was 4.95% versus 5.7% in the placebo group. There was no increase in the number of fatal or nonfatal vascular thrombotic events. It is recommended that patients presenting with a high risk of TIC should receive a bolus of 1 g tranexamic acid upon admission to the trauma unit followed by continuous infusion of 1 g over 8 hours. In patients showing laboratory evidence of hyperfibrinolysis, the continuous infusion of tranexamic acid should be increased to 20 mg/kg/hour. Tranexamic acid treatment should be continued once bleeding has been adequately controlled.

Factor VIIa

Factor VIIa (FVIIa) was approved in 1999 by the Food and Drug Administration (FDA) for the treatment of bleeding in hemophiliacs and in patients with inhibitors to factor VIII or factor IX. Unlike hemophiliacs however, trauma patients suffer from a global deficiency of all clotting factors, along with hemoglobin and platelets, yet off-label use of FVIIa in trauma patients showed hopeful results when given in patients undergoing damage control. In 2005 a randomized clinical study including patients with blunt and penetrating trauma patients indicated that although recombinant factor VIIa (rFVIIa) significantly reduced the need for transfusion requirements and the incidence of acute respiratory distress syndrome (ARDS), it had no effect on the overall mortality rates. A follow-up phase III randomized trial was stopped ahead of schedule (573 of 1502 patients enrolled) for futility.

Probably the greatest experience using FVIIa outside these trials come from the U.S. troops who used it aggressively during the Middle East conflicts. Despite anecdotal success stories, a critical analyses performed in 506 patients treated with rFVIIa compared to matched control subjects ($n = 266$ per group), the drug was not found to be associated with an improvement in survival or a decrease in need for MT. Other findings also reported increased risk of thrombotic complications following the unlabeled use of rFVIIa.

Prothrombin Complex Concentrates

Promising results using prothrombin complex concentrates (PCCs) in trauma patients who use warfarin suggest that PCCs may be an important adjunct therapy to reverse the coagulopathy associated to vitamin K–dependent clotting factors, especially in elderly patients with traumatic brain injury (TBI). Randomized clinical trials (RCTs) are ongoing in patients who require correction of coagulopathy for surgery or for TBI, when PCCs are being compared to standard treatment (fresh frozen plasma [FFP] or vitamin K).

TIMING AND VOLUME OF RESUSCITATION FLUID THERAPY

The optimal volume of IV fluid administered to patients with uncontrolled hemorrhage is a balance between improvements in tissue oxygen delivery against increase in the blood loss by raising blood pressure. Aggressive fluid resuscitation in an attempt to achieve normal systemic pressure prior to hemostasis and control of the bleeding may exacerbate blood loss and thereby potentially increase mortality risk. The knowledge regarding the best time to infuse fluids to patients with hemorrhagic shock dates from almost a century ago, yet studies addressing the effects of massive resuscitation and best fluid management strategies during the prehospital phase have created controversy. Nevertheless, this work has demonstrated that withholding fluid resuscitation until hemorrhage control does not increase mortality risk. The Cochrane Database of Systematic Reviews also addressed the issue of timing and volume of fluid resuscitation in bleeding patients. They found only six RCTs in which a careful review failed to provide any evidence in support of (or against) early or large volume IV fluid administration in uncontrolled hemorrhage. Based on all this information, it is reasonable to recommend that patients with penetrating injuries and without evidence of TBI be resuscitated to a lower admissible blood pressure (hypotensive resuscitation) to prevent "popping the clot" until surgical or local control of the hemorrhage can be obtained. The effects of this strategy and the associated hypoperfusion on organs such an injured brain suggest that patients with central nervous system (CNS) injuries should be managed with a higher blood pressure end point.

Type of Fluid

Crystalloids

Shires' original studies of crystalloid volume replacement showed such an impressive improvement in survival compared to blood alone or plasma that these data were promptly translated into clinical practice. It is remarkable, however, that after having used Ringer's lactate as a volume expander and resuscitation fluid for more than half a century, only recently have investigators described the deleterious effects of crystalloid resuscitation. These effects include impaired immunologic function and increased proinflammatory effects on neutrophils and other cells involved in host defense mechanisms. Furthermore, evidence appeared over the last 3 decades indicating that exaggerated use of crystalloids has been also associated with ARDS, increased gut and heart interstitial fluid, and abdominal and extremity compartment syndrome. A recent review summarized not only these deleterious clinical effects of aggressive resuscitation but also the derangements in cellular, metabolic, and immune function underlying these effects. The use of crystalloids is now being reexamined, and like any other drug, fluids need to be prescribed based on appropriate indications, correct doses, and knowledge regarding their side effects and possible complications. Current trends point toward a more selective and more restricted use of crystalloids, limiting the total volume by providing earlier replacement of blood and blood products. A simplified approach toward measuring end points of resuscitation based on adequate pulse and mentation rather than a targeted blood pressure has also had an impact in restricting the total amount of fluid. Limiting the rate and volume of fluid resuscitation before hemorrhage control should become a standard practice in large trauma centers. Interestingly, not all crystalloids are equal, in an RCT comparing Ringer's lactate versus normal saline (NS), Waters et al showed that NS was associated with increased bleeding. Patients treated with NS required a larger volume of platelet transfusion (478 ± 302 mL in the NS group versus 223 ± 24 mL in the Ringer's lactate group; mean $\pm$ SD). The NS treated group received significantly more blood products ($P = 0.02$).

Colloids

Albumin

The use of albumin in critically ill patients has been analyzed in a Cochrane report. The authors carried out a systematic review of RCTs comparing administration of albumin or plasma protein fraction versus no fluid or administration of crystalloid solution in critically ill patients with hypovolemia, burns, or hypoalbuminemia. A total of 1419 patients from 30 separate trials were studied. For each patient category, the risk of death in the albumin-treated group was higher than in the comparison group. For hypovolemia, the relative risk of death after albumin administration was 1.46 (95% confidence interval 0.97 to 2.22), for burns the relative risk was 2.40 (1.11 to 5.19), and for hypoalbuminemia it was 1.69 (1.07 to 2.67). This review, however, was based on relatively small trials in which there were only a small number of deaths. Therefore, these results must be interpreted with caution. Finally, the Saline versus Albumin Fluid Evaluation (SAFE) trial carried out in Australian and New Zealand (the SAFE study is a collaboration of the Australian and New Zealand Intensive Care Society Clinical Trials Group) indicated there is no difference in mortality rate or incidence of organ failure between albumin and saline in a double-blind randomized population of 7000 patients. When treating patients with hypoalbuminemia, efforts must be centered upon correction of the underlying disorder, rather than attempting to reverse primarily the hypoalbuminemia. In trauma patients with severe hypovolemia, rapid correction using human albumin is not practical. The use of albumin to correct hypovolemia in trauma patients has not been shown to have a significant benefit in survival when compared with other plasma substitutes. In contrast, in patients with TBI, a post hoc follow-up analysis of the data from the SAFE study showed a significantly increased mortality rate for the group treated with albumin as opposed to the non-albumin-treated group.

Hextend

Hextend (Abbott Laboratories, North Chicago, Ill.) is a modified, physiologically "balanced" first-generation high-molecular-weight hydroxyethyl starch (HES) preparation (average molecular weight, approximately 670 kDa; MW, 550 kDa). HES contains balanced electrolytes (Na, 143 mmol/L; Cl, 124 mmol/L; lactate, 28 mmol/L; Ca^{2+}, 2.5 mmol/L; potassium [K], 3 mmol/L; Mg^{2+}, 0.45 mmol/L; glucose, 5 mmol/L). Hextend is currently being used as the fluid of choice for resuscitation in battlefield casualties because of its greater effect on intravascular volume compared to Ringer's lactate. Unlike previously used preparations of starch such as Dextran or Hespan, Hextend may have less effect on coagulation parameters, but even this observation is debatable. Animal studies have shown that Hextend is an efficient volume expander in models of hemorrhage and in models of combined hemorrhage and head injury. In addition, Hextend may be a more effective volume expander than smaller starches. A clinical study demonstrated that Hextend, with its novel buffered, balanced electrolyte formulation, is as effective as 6% hetastarch in saline for the treatment of hypovolemia. The Fluids in Resuscitation of Severe Trauma (FIRST) study compared Hextend (HES) against 0.9% saline in the resuscitation of 115 patients with severe blunt or penetrating trauma at a single center in South Africa. No differences were found between the two groups of patients with blunt trauma. In penetrating trauma, HES 130/0.4 reduced fluid requirement significantly but less than generally expected and showed no effect on normalization of gastrointestinal function. FIRST investigators reported improvement in renal function and lactate clearance among patients with penetrating trauma receiving HES. Interestingly, however, they observed an increase in transfusion of blood products among HES recipients with blunt trauma. Blunt trauma patients required a mean transfusion of packed red blood cells (PRBCs) twice as great in the HES as the 0.9% saline group, FFP three times as great, and platelets five times as great.

Unfortunately, this study was found to have several discrepancies between prespecified and actually evaluated end points. Furthermore, the poor matching at baseline of the study groups, the small sample size, the failure to report key data, and some deficits in the statistical analysis make it difficult to draw firm conclusions about the efficacy and safety of HES in trauma.

Hypertonic Saline

Hypertonic saline is characterized by its osmotic properties that attract fluid into the intravascular compartment when the addition of a dextran, or hetastarch, helps to prolong its effects through binding of the recruited water. The concept of resuscitation using hypertonic solutions entails rapid infusion of a 4 mL/kg body weight dose of 7.2% to 7.5% sodium chloride (NaCl), which corresponds to a 250 mL bolus in an adult patient. This is given in combination with a colloid solution. This mode of therapy has been shown to have a rapid effect in the circulation. Studies suggest that hypertonic saline seems to be superior to conventional volume therapy with faster normalization of microvascular perfusion during shock phases and early resumption of organ function. Patients with head trauma in association with systemic hypotension particularly appear to benefit.

The Resuscitation Outcomes Consortium (ROC), a network of nine major regional clinical research centers in the United States and Canada, conducted two separated trials to study the effect of hypertonic saline in patients with shock and in patients with TBI. The study on blunt or penetrating trauma patients in hypovolemic shock was stopped in February 2009. The shock study sought to determine the impact of hypertonic resuscitation on survival in trauma patients in hypovolemic shock. The trial was stopped because patients who received the concentrated saline solutions were no more likely to survive than those who received an NS solution and had earlier, although not increased, fatality. A parallel study using the same intervention for TBI study was stopped in May 2009. This study sought to determine the impact of hypertonic resuscitation on long-term (6-month) neurologic outcome and survival. The study was stopped because it was determined that the hypertonic saline solutions were no better than the standard treatment of NS and that it was unlikely that continuing to enroll new patients would change the outcome of the study.

Red Blood Cell Transfusion

The decision to initiate blood transfusion during resuscitation is based on a clinical assessment, which can be aided by estimating the mechanism of injury, the rate and magnitude of blood loss, the degree of cardiopulmonary reserve, and the overall oxygen consumption of the patient. Any storage of blood products outside a blood bank is difficult and may not be possible in many institutions. Thus, blood products are ordered at the physician's discretion with the inherent risk of underestimating blood transfusion requirements.

Transfusion therapy for the massively bleeding trauma patients evolved significantly over the last 40 years. Shires and Carrico's last contribution to the literature on the management of shock was published in 1976. At that time they recommended moderation in the use of crystalloids (no more than 2 L) while whole blood could be obtained. At that same time, blood component therapy was introduced and blood banks begin to separate all components from blood. No clinical trials were performed, and little evidence-based medicine emerged while a transition from whole blood toward the use of PRBCs took place in most emergency departments in the United States. Three clinical studies totaling less than 80 patients were published regarding the role of blood products in trauma patients over these many years. ATLS recommendations on the use of plasma in trauma patients refer to the study published in 1985 by Lucas et al suggesting the ratio of 1:3 for FFP and PRBCs. Studies describing the limitations and disadvantages of PRBCs began to appear describing diminished O_2 transport efficiency in PRBCs after 24 hours of storage, increased incidence of MODS per unit of PRBCs transfused, and elevated K and interleukin 8 concentrations in aging blood as well as absence of clotting factors.

Looking back, it is possible to suggest that inadvertent hemodilution, exaggerated crystalloid use, and overresuscitation leading to ARDS and abdominal compartment syndrome may have all been temporally related to all these changes in transfusion therapy that occurred while whole blood became no longer available.

Understanding the true incidence of trauma-induced coagulopathy and the introduction of the concept of "damage control resuscitation" have completely changed how severe hemorrhage is now treated not only in trauma patients but in many other settings of acute severe bleeding. Experienced gained in Iraq and Afghanistan promulgate the following basic tenets: (1) avoid crystalloid resuscitation; (2) aim for permissive hypotension whenever possible; (3) prevent coagulopathy through early use of blood products; and (4) aggressively break the vicious cycle of acidosis, coagulopathy, and hypothermia.

Based on the battlefield experience, the U.S. Army has now instituted a policy of using a 1:1:1 ratio of PRBC:FFP:platelets in the battlefield for those who are expected to receive more than 10 units of PRBCs (MT). However, no well-designed RCT has conclusively identified the optimal ratios of blood components.

In 2006 a review of transfusion practices around the world identified only 10 publications describing the use of MT protocols. Since that time many studies verifying the efficacy of introducing MT protocols have appeared. A historical control study published by Cotton compared mortality rate in 94 patients over an 18-month period after the introduction of the protocol against a matched cohort of similar patients during the prior 18 months. The study found that implementation of the protocol reduced 30-day mortality rate (51% vs. 66%, $P < 0.03$), decreased intraoperative crystalloid administration (4.9 L vs. 6.7 L, $P = 0.002$), and reduced postoperative blood product use (2.8 units PRBCs vs. 8.7 units RBCs; 1.7 units FFP vs. 7.9 units FFP; 0.9 unit platelets vs. 5.7 units platelets).

Although further prospective research is needed to specify the exact ratios, there is convincing evidence that implementation of standardized protocols for blood component transfusion improves processes of care, reduces overall use of blood components, and improves outcomes.

Blood Substitutes

Only administration of PRBCs restores oxygen-carrying capacity, but their supply is limited and their use is associated with a wide range of adverse effects, including immunomodulation. Attempts at developing artificial oxygen carriers began in the 1930s. The greatest obstacle has been related to the toxic effect of stromal contamination. The hemoglobin molecule in hemoglobin-based artificial O_2 carriers needs to be stabilized to prevent dissociation of the α2β2-hemoglobin tetramer. By doing so, intravascular retention is prolonged and nephrotoxicity is eliminated.

Early agents designed as blood substitutes were found to be of limited value. Serious adverse effects including profound hypertension, myocardial damage, and vascular complications were described. Several products have been developed including Diaspirin cross-linked hemoglobin (HemAssist), human recombinant hemoglobin (rHb1.1 and rHb2.0), polymerized bovine hemoglobin-based O_2 carrier (HBOC-201), human polymerized hemoglobin (PolyHeme), hemoglobin raffimer (Hemolink), maleimide-activated polyethylene glycol-modified hemoglobin (MP4).

The most recent experience with PolyHeme showed an increased incidence of myocardial infarction in the PolyHem treated group. A blinded post hoc committee convened to objectively determine if each patient truly suffered myocardial infarction found no association between PolyHeme and myocardial infarction. However, because of the trend toward greater adverse events, after publication of this trial,

PolyHeme failed to attain FDA approval. Northfield Laboratories subsequently declared bankruptcy, halting production and testing of PolyHeme.

The development of blood substitutes designed to overcome these limitations is ongoing. MP4 studies completed in Europe in elective arthroplasty patients showed a similar rate of adverse events in the MP4 group compared to a control group; however, there are no current studies of MP4 use in trauma patients with severe hemorrhage.

PHARMACOTHERAPY

Vasopressin

Vasopressin is emerging as a potentially major advance in the treatment of a variety of shock states. Increasing interest in the clinical use of vasopressin has resulted from the recognition of its importance in the endogenous response to shock and from advances in understanding its mechanism of action. Vasopressin has been shown to produce greater blood flow diversion from nonvital to vital organ beds when compared to epinephrine during vasodilatory shock. Under normal conditions, the doses of vasopressin used have little or no pressor action, and significant elevation of plasma vasopressin due to unregulated release of hormone (i.e., the syndrome of inappropriate secretion of antidiuretic hormone) does not cause hypertension.

The likely effect of vasopressin in shock may be related to its effect on vascular smooth muscle. Vasopressin can inhibit both adenosine triphosphate (ATP)-sensitive potassium (K^+ATP) channels and nitric oxide (NO)-induced accumulation of cyclic guanosine monophosphate (cGMP). Landry et al have shown that activation of the K^+ATP channels contributes to the hypotension of several types of shock, including hemorrhagic shock. Furthermore, activation of NO synthesis also contributes to the hypotension of this condition. Thus, vasopressin inhibits vasodilator mechanisms that contribute to both hypotension and vascular hyporeactivity in the late phase of hemorrhagic shock. Arterial hypotension is the principal stimulus for vasopressin secretion via arterial baroreceptors located in the aortic arch and the carotid sinus. If central venous pressure diminishes, then these receptors first stimulate secretion of natriuretic factor, the sympathetic system, and renin secretion. Vasopressin is secreted when arterial pressure falls to the point that it can no longer be compensated for by the predominant action of the vascular baroreceptors. Vasopressin potentiates the vasopressor efficacy of catecholamines. However, it has the further advantage of eliciting less pronounced vasoconstriction in the coronary and cerebral vascular regions. It benefits renal function, although these data should be confirmed. The effects on other regional circulations remain to be determined in humans.

NEW THERAPEUTIC POSSIBILITIES: HYPOTHERMIA AND HEMORRHAGIC SHOCK

Hypothermia during hemorrhagic shock appears to be a double-edged sword. Laboratory studies have consistently found that mild (33–36° C) to moderate (28–32° C) hypothermia improves survival following hemorrhagic shock. In contrast, retrospective clinical trials have suggested that trauma patients who become hypothermic are generally more severely injured and have higher mortality rates than those patients who remain normothermic.

Laboratory studies have demonstrated beneficial effects of hypothermia during hemorrhagic shock on individual organs and the entire organism. As an example, Mizushima et al found that mild hypothermia during hemorrhagic shock in rats with rewarming during resuscitation produced the best left ventricular performance and cardiac output, compared to normothermia throughout or prolonged hypothermia. Meyer and Horton similarly found better cardiac performance with hypothermia compared to normothermia during hemorrhagic shock in dogs. They also demonstrated improved survival. Studies by Wu et al in rats have demonstrated benefit of continued hypothermia after cooling during hemorrhagic shock, mimicking exposure hypothermia as in patients, compared to active rewarming during resuscitation. Mild hypothermia is also beneficial during very prolonged hemorrhagic shock.

Clinically, retrospective studies by Luna et al and Jurkovich et al suggested that trauma patients who become hypothermic have increased mortality risk compared to those who remain normothermic. Because the more severely injured patients are more likely to become hypothermic, it has been difficult to separate the effects of hypothermia from those of confounding factors such as degree of shock, injury severity, volume of fluid and blood products infused, and need for operation. A more recent retrospective analysis from a large statewide database by Wang et al demonstrated that a body temperature of 35° C or lower upon admission was independently associated with an increased risk of death (odds ratio 3).

The only prospective trial of temperature management in trauma patients was that of Gentilello et al. Hypothermic trauma victims were randomized in the ICU to standard rewarming versus more active rewarming via continuous arteriovenous rewarming (CAVR) using a counter-current heat exchanger (Level I Technologies, Rockland, Mass.). The CAVR group rewarmed faster and required less fluids but had similar hospital mortality rate compared to the standard treatment group.

To understand this dichotomy between the laboratory studies of hemorrhagic shock and the clinical findings with trauma victims, we must consider that uncontrolled, exposure hypothermia, which is common in trauma patients, is physiologically different from controlled, therapeutic hypothermia, during which shivering and the sympathetic response are blocked. Another issue is potential coagulopathy from hypothermia, although clinically significant changes do not seem to occur unless the temperature is lower than 34° C.

SUMMARY

Shock after hemorrhage is a complex syndrome that may have a diverse clinical manifestation associated with the magnitude of injury and the type of resuscitation or lack thereof. Innovative interventions targeting many of the therapeutic windows within the spectrum from injury to definitive resuscitation are available and have been discussed. Active research in this area will bring new contributions and better understanding of the complex disease.

For the chapter's Suggested Readings list, please visit the book at www.ExpertConsult.inkling.com.

THE SYNDROME OF EXSANGUINATION: RELIABLE MODELS TO INDICATE DAMAGE CONTROL

Juan A. Asensio, Robert Bertelotti, Federico N. Mazzini, José Ceballos Esparragon, Chris Okwuosa, Steven Cheung, Riaan Pretorius, Luis Manuel García-Núñez, and Alicia M. Mohr

Exsanguination has been defined as an extreme form of hemorrhage with ongoing bleeding that, if not surgically controlled, will lead to death. Exsanguination is second only to neurologic injury among causes of fatality after trauma. Therefore, the speed by which the exsanguinating trauma patient moves through the prehospital phase, emergency department, operating room, and intensive care unit (ICU) is important to survival. The syndrome of exsanguination was described by Asensio. Certain conditions and complexes of injuries require damage control to prevent exsanguination. This chapter will describe validated indicators that can be used both preoperatively and intraoperatively to improve outcomes. This chapter will also outline current guidelines for the institution of damage control in trauma patients. Emphasis is placed on the current indications for damage control as defined by key studies. Awareness of these guidelines can improve outcomes after major intraabdominal injuries and hemorrhage and also assist in the management of one of the well-known sequelae of damage control, the posttraumatic open abdomen.

HISTORY

Bailout/damage control surgery following trauma has developed as a major advance in surgical practice since the early 1980s. The principles of damage control surgery defied the traditional surgical teaching of definitive operative intervention and were slow to be adopted. Currently, damage control techniques developed by trauma surgeons have been used successfully to manage traumatic thoracic, abdominal, extremity, and peripheral vascular injuries. In addition, damage control surgery has been extrapolated for use in general, vascular, cardiac, urologic, and orthopedic surgery.

In 1983, Stone and associates were first to describe the "bailout" approach of staged surgical procedures for severely injured patients. This approach emerged after their observation that early death following trauma was associated with severe metabolic and physiologic derangements following severe exsanguinating injuries. Following massive transfusion (MT) exceeding two blood volumes in trauma and emergency surgery, severe physiologic derangement ensued and mortality rate was found to be greater than 60%. Profound shock along with major blood loss initiates the cycle of hypothermia, acidosis, and coagulopathy. It was at this time that hypothermia, acidosis, and coagulopathy were described as the "trauma triangle of death" or the "bloody vicious cycle." A fourth component, dysrhythmia, which usually heralded the patient's death, was later added by Asensio. Coagulopathy, acidosis, and hypothermia make the prolonged and definitive operative management of trauma patients dangerous. This new approach, now called "damage control," describes the operative phase as multiphasic, in which reoperation occurs after correcting physiologic abnormalities.

METABOLIC FAILURE

Hypothermia is a consequence of severe exsanguinating injury and subsequent resuscitative efforts. Severe hemorrhage leads to tissue hypoperfusion and diminished oxygen delivery, which leads to reduced heat generation. Clinically significant hypothermia is important if the body temperature drops to less than 36° C for more than 4 hours. Hypothermia can lead to cardiac arrhythmias, decreased cardiac output, increased systemic vascular resistance, and left shift of the oxygen-hemoglobin dissociation curve. Hypothermia exerts a negative inotropic effect on the myocardium with depression of left ventricular contractility. The initial electrocardiographic change seen with hypothermia is sinus tachycardia, but as the core temperature decreases, progressive bradycardia ensues. The cardiac response to catecholamines may also be blunted in hypothermic hearts, and cold cardiac tissue poorly tolerates hypervolemia and hypovolemia. Hypothermia can also induce coagulopathy by inhibition of the coagulation cascade, of platelet activation, and of platelet function. Low temperature also impairs the host's immunologic function. Hypothermia is aggravated by further heat loss resulting from either environmental factors or surgical interventions. The multidisciplinary team caring for trauma patients must make every effort to prevent heat loss and help to correct hypothermia.

More than 25% of trauma patients exhibit overt coagulopathy at the time of admission and it is associated with a threefold increase in mortality risk. The causes of coagulopathy in patients with severe trauma are multifactorial, including consumption and dilution of platelets and coagulation factors, as well as dysfunction of platelets and the coagulation system. Clinical coagulopathy occurs because of hypothermia, platelet and coagulation factor dysfunction that occurs at low temperatures, activation of the fibrinolytic system, and hemodilution following massive resuscitation. Platelet dysfunction is secondary to the imbalance between thromboxane and prostacyclin that occurs in a hypothermic state. Hypothermia and hemodilution produce an additive effect on coagulopathy. After replacement of one blood volume (5000 mL or 15 units of packed red blood cells [PRBCs]), only 30% to 40% of platelets remain in circulation. The prothrombin time (PT), partial thromboplastin time (PTT), fibrinogen levels, and lactate levels are therefore not predictive of the severe coagulopathic state.

The predominant physiologic defect resulting from repetitive and persistent bouts of hypoperfusion is metabolic acidosis. Anaerobic metabolism starts when the shock stage of hypoperfusion is prolonged, leading to the production of lactate. Acidosis decreases myocardial contractility, cardiac output, functional clotting, and clot strength. Acidosis also worsens as a result of multiple transfusions, the use of vasopressors, aortic cross-clamping, and impaired myocardial performance. It is clear that a complex relationship exists among acidosis, hypothermia, and coagulopathy, and each factor compounds the other, leading to a high mortality rate once this cycle ensues and cannot be interrupted.

MODELS FOR DAMAGE CONTROL

Stone and associates' original work in 1983 only provided the intraoperative observation of coagulopathy as an indication for bailout. In this study, 17 patients underwent the bailout procedure, which included an initial laparotomy, followed by packing in patients with an observed clinical coagulopathy, and then completion of the surgical procedure once the coagulopathy was improved. This resulted in 11 survivors with a mortality rate of 35%. Subsequently, Rotondo et al described the multiphase approach to the management of exsanguinating patients sustaining abdominal injury, but did not define any objective parameters during the intraoperative phase of damage control. The authors reported a survival rate of 77% in a very small subgroup of patients with major vascular injury and two or more physical injuries. Burch et al proposed a model based on core temperature 32° C or less, pH 7.09 or less, and PRBC transfusion of more than 22 units that could predict 48-hour survival; the authors also described the "lethal triad." In a study based on 39 patients, Sharp defined a temperature 33° C or less, pH 7.18 or less, PT 16 seconds or longer, PTT 50 seconds or longer, and more than 10 units of PRBCs transfused as objective parameters to indicate the need for early packing.

Morris et al described 107 patients who underwent staged laparotomy and abdominal packing. They proposed proceeding with damage control early in the course of operation based on patient's temperature of less than 35° C, a BD greater than 14 mEq/L, and the presence of coagulopathic bleeding. Similarly, Moore described a progressive coagulopathy as the most compelling reason for staged laparotomy. A severe coagulopathic state was described as PT and PTT greater than two times normal, massive and rapid blood transfusion exceeding 10 units in 4 hours, persistent shock defined as oxygen consumption less than 110 mL/minute/m^2, lactic acid level greater than 5 mmol/L, pH under 7.2, BD higher than 14 mEq/L, and core hypothermia less than 34° C. It was postulated that the ability to predict the onset of coagulopathy would have significant implications for instituting damage control. Another predictive model for life-threatening coagulopathy included systolic blood pressure less than 70 mm Hg, temperature higher than 34° C, pH less than 7.10, and Injury Severity Score (ISS) of 25 or higher.

No single model has been able to accurately predict the timing for institution of damage control. A pH less than 7.1 or a core temperature of less than 33° C may indicate that the "bloody vicious cycle" is too far advanced and cannot be interrupted. Similarly, it is difficult to obtain intraoperative results for PT, PTT, fibrinogen, and lactate levels at all hospitals, or to place a Swan-Ganz catheter in the operating room.

To define the patient at greatest risk for exsanguination and death, one must determine the threshold levels of pH, temperature, and highest estimated level of blood loss. Therefore, in an attempt to institute the development of intraoperative guidelines for "damage control/bailout," Asensio first retrospectively evaluated 548 patients over 6 years who were admitted to a large urban trauma center with the diagnosis of exsanguination. Inclusion criteria were intraoperative blood loss of 2000 mL or more, minimum transfusion requirement of 1500 mL PRBCs or greater during the initial resuscitation, and diagnosis of exsanguination. Data collected included demographics, prehospital and admission vital signs and physiologic predictors of outcome, Revised Trauma Score (RTS), Glasgow Coma Scale (GCS) score, ISS, volume of resuscitative fluids, need for thoracotomy in the emergency department (EDT), volume of fluids in the operating room, need for thoracotomy in the operating room (ORT), and intraoperative complications. In this patient population, the RTS was 4.38 and the mean ISS was 32, denoting a physiologically compromised and severely injured patient population. There were 180 patients who underwent EDT with aortic cross-clamping and open cardiopulmonary resuscitation (CPR); 99 (55%) succumbed in the emergency department. In addition to the 81 patients who survived EDT, 117 required ORT for a total of 198 EDT and ORT, of which 56 (28%) survived to leave the operating room and the hospital. In this series, mean admission pH was 7.15 and mean temperature was 34.3° C in the operating room, and these patients received an average of 14,165 mL of crystalloid, blood, and blood products. Overall, 449 patients survived to arrive in the operating room with some signs of life, and 281 patients died; 37% of these patients survived damage control. Table 1 shows the objective intraoperative parameters developed to predict outcome and provide guidelines on when to institute damage control based on these findings. This series also provided independent risk factors for survival, which included an ISS less than 20, spontaneous ventilation in the emergency room, no EDT or ORT, and the absence of abdominal vascular injury. This paper fully

TABLE I: Physiologic Guidelines That Predict Need for Damage Control

Hypothermia 34° C
Acidosis pH 7.2
Serum bicarbonate 15 mEq/l
Transfusion of 4000 mL blood (packed red blood cells)
Transfusion of 5000 mL blood and blood products
Intraoperative volume replacement 12,000 mL
Clinical evidence of intraoperative coagulopathy

describes the syndrome of exsanguination as well as the indicators to invasive damage. These views have been subsequently validated by others.

One of the natural sequelae in patients surviving damage control is an open abdomen. These guidelines were prospectively validated in a series of 139 patients who underwent damage control and had posttraumatic open abdomen. This study consisted of two groups of patients: 86 patients studied retrospectively prior to instituting the guidelines, and 53 patients studied prospectively after instituting the guidelines. The groups were comparable in all relevant parameters. Although there was no difference in the mortality rate between the two groups (24% for each), there were statistically significant differences in the number of intraoperative transfusions, less hypothermia and bowel edema, less postoperative infections and gastrointestinal complications, and shorter ICU and hospital length of stay for the prospective group. Another significant finding in this study was that 93% of patients were able to undergo definitive abdominal closure in their hospital stay as compared with the historic 22%.

Awareness of potential triggers to initiate damage control is vital. A study of 68 patients who underwent damage control surgery found that the inability to correct pH greater than 7.21 and PTT greater than 78.7 seconds was predictive of 100% mortality rate. In addition, a temperature less than 32° C and increasing age can independently predict mortality rate following damage control. In an attempt to predict the outcome following damage control, Karirinos developed the following damage control equation:

$$x = (0.012)Age - (0.707)pH - (0.032)Temperature + 6.002.$$

If x is greater than 0.5, then death is more likely. Similarly, Ordonez developed a clinical predictive model for mortality rate that uses a combination of ICU admission pH, hypothermia, the number of PRBC units transfused in first 24 hours, and age. Delayed recognition of the need for damage control as well as poor communication with the anesthesia and nursing team are deleterious to the care of the multiply injured patient.

PATIENT SELECTION

Not all trauma patients require damage control measures. In addition to the physiologic guidelines for the institution of damage control (Table 2), certain conditions and complexes of injuries assessed both preoperatively and intraoperatively require damage control (see Table 2). Multiple mass casualties and the need for EDT predict the need for damage control. In the multiply injured trauma patient sustaining major abdominal injury, the need to evaluate for other extra-abdominal injuries in a timely fashion may also indicate damage control. The preoperative duration of hypotension (systolic blood pressure <90 mm Hg) was significantly different in those patients who exsanguinated as compared with survivors (45 minutes vs.

TABLE 2: Preoperative and Intraoperative States That Suggest Need for Damage Control

Preoperative	Intraoperative
Multiple mass casualties	Need for intraoperative thoracotomy
Multisystem trauma with major abdominal injury	Major abdominal vascular injuries
Open pelvic fracture with major abdominal injury	Major thoracic vascular injuries
Major abdominal injury with need to evaluate extra-abdominal injury	Severe complex hepatic injuries
Traumatic amputation with major abdominal injury	Presence of sustained hypotension
Need for emergency department thoracotomy	Presence of coagulopathy
Presence of sustained hypotension	Presence of hypothermia
Presence of coagulopathy	
Presence of hypothermia	
Need for adjunctive use of angioembolization	

85 minutes). Therefore, in addition to other factors such as the preoperative assessment of hypothermia and coagulopathy, a period of sustained hypotension greater than 60 minutes would predict the need for damage control. Intraoperatively, certain complexes of injuries also predict the need for this technique. These injuries include major abdominal vascular, complex hepatic, and major thoracic vascular injuries and the need for intraoperative thoracotomy.

Patients with exsanguination are perhaps the best candidates to undergo damage control. Asensio has described an algorithm for the management of exsanguination that involves three phases (Fig. 1). First, the patient is classified as exsanguinating; and second, resuscitation under the Advanced Trauma Life Support protocols is begun (see Fig. 1). In patients who require surgical hemorrhage control, damage control resuscitation begins and MT protocols are initiated. This is a three-part damage control resuscitation that combines high plasma and platelet ratios, permissive hypotension, and limited crystalloid, which combined have been shown to increase survival in select trauma patients. The third phase requires rapid transport to the operating room (exsanguination from penetrating injuries is a dramatic ill-defined entity that requires leadership, fast thinking, aggressive surgical intervention, and a well-thought-out plan). Rapid damage control surgery along with damage control resuscitation can lead to effective management of exsanguination and improved survival.

TECHNIQUE OF DAMAGE CONTROL

The most important goal of early institution of damage control is patient survival. A four-stage damage control approach has been recently defined by Johnson et al in a study of 24 patients who underwent damage control and were retrospectively compared with patients who underwent damage control a decade earlier as described by Rotondo et al (Fig. 2). The "ground-zero" stage includes the prehospital phase as well as early resuscitation in the emergency room.

 PHASE 1
CLASSIFY PATIENT AS EXSANGUINATING
Hemodynamic instability
Initial blood loss >40%
Massive ongoing blood loss
Injuries prone to exsanguination

 PHASE 2
RESUSCITATE PER ATLS PROTOCOLS
Crystalloids 2–3 L (Ringer's lactate)
Blood (uncrossmatched, type specific, or crossmatched)
Rapid infusion of warm fluids
Determine need for ED thoracotomy and thoracic aortic cross-clamping

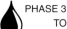 PHASE 3
TO OR EXPEDIENTLY
Determine need for OR thoracotomy and aortic cross-clamping
Control bleeding source or sources
Use adjunct techniques
Rapid volume infusers
Autotransfusion
Packing
Shunts
Damage control
Prevent hypothermia and coagulopathy
Proper replacement of blood and blood products

FIGURE 1 Algorithm for the management of exsanguination. ATLS, Advance Trauma Life Support; ED, emergency department; OR, operating room.

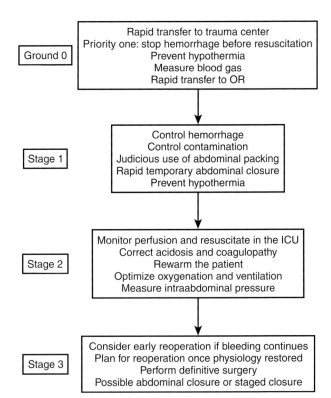

FIGURE 2 Four stages of damage control. ICU, Intensive care unit; OR, operating room.

This ground-zero phase includes short paramedic scene times and identification of injury patterns in the emergency department who require damage control, as well as damage control resuscitation along with rewarming maneuvers that begin in the trauma bay.

Damage control implies immediate control of life-threatening hemorrhage, control of gastrointestinal contamination with rapid resections or closures, the use of intraluminal shunts, and judicious abdominal packing with temporary abdominal wall closures. Specifically, for chest injuries, one should repair cardiovascular injuries, perform stapled pulmonary tractotomy as described by Asensio, pack if needed, place chest tubes, and close the skin. For abdominal injuries, damage control can involve control of major hemorrhage, hepatic packing, pancreatic drainage, temporary hollow viscus closures, rapid stapled resections, splenectomy, nephrectomy, vascular pedicle clamping in situ, and the use of intraabdominal vascular shunts. Frequently, these patients experience abdominal compartment syndrome. Therefore, the posttraumatic open abdomen with temporary abdominal wall closure is used as an extension of damage control. Minimal time in the operating room is essential, and staged operations are performed.

The second stage begins in the ICU where the metabolic disorder is corrected. Rewarming the patient is a high priority, as coagulopathy and acidosis can only be corrected and maintained once the body temperature returns to normal. Damage control resuscitation continues and crystalloids are used judiciously. Further inspections are then made to identify injuries that may not have been detected in the initial survey. Twenty-four to 72 hours may be needed to correct metabolic derangements.

The last stage of damage control involves the timing of reoperation when definitive procedures are performed. Reoperation is considered early if major blood losses continue. Usually, there is a window of 36 to 48 hours after the initial injury between the correction of the metabolic disorder and the onset of the systemic inflammatory response syndrome or multiple organ failure. In this phase, definitive procedures are undertaken. Thorough reexploration is made for any additional injuries, and restoration of gastrointestinal continuity and vascular repair are done. Provisional feeding access may be placed, followed by washout of the abdominal cavity and attempts at definitive closure. The patient then returns to the ICU for further care.

CONCLUSIONS

The management of exsanguination requires leadership, prompt thinking, aggressive surgical intervention, and a well-conceived plan. The exsanguinating trauma patient who requires MT incurs the greatest risk for the multifactorial interactions among acidosis, hypothermia, and coagulopathy. The ultimate goal is the prompt and effective control of the exsanguinating source; delays in the decision to perform damage control contribute to higher rates of morbidity and mortality. Therefore, damage control is a vital part of the management of the multiply injured patient and should be performed before metabolic exhaustion.

For the chapter's Suggested Readings list, please visit the book at www.ExpertConsult.inkling.com.

DAMAGE CONTROL RESUSCITATION: AN EVIDENCE-BASED REPORT

Juan C. Duchesne, Chrissy Guidry, Louis A. Aliperti, Lance E. Stuke, and Norman E. McSwain, Jr.

Damage control resuscitation (DCR) has become a topic of increasing relevance and popularity over the past several years. Hemorrhage secondary to trauma accounts for 40% of trauma fatalities and is the leading cause of preventable death in trauma. Research in military and civilian populations regarding DCR have focused on ways to improve survival in patients with severe hemorrhage. It should be mentioned that the majority of trauma patients do not require DCR and its techniques should be reserved for those who are the most severely injured. For these patients the rapid and effective use of techniques to control bleeding and correct acute coagulopathy of trauma shock (ACoTS) is essential.

Once massive transfusion protocol (MTP) is initiated, the target is to achieve a close ratio for resuscitation of 1:1:1 using fresh frozen plasma (FFP), platelets (Plts), and packed red blood cells (PRBCs). The rationale behind early and sustained administration of FFP involves the replacement of fibrinogen and clotting factors. In mathematical studies, Hirshberg et al noted that resuscitation with more than 5 units of PRBCs will lead to a dilutional coagulopathy, and the ideal manner to correct for this coagulopathy would be to add FFP to PRBCs in a 2:3 FFP:PRBC ratio. Another study by Ho et al noted that once excessive deficiency of factors has developed, 1 to 1.5 units of FFP must be given for every unit of PRBCs transfused.

It should be emphasized that FFP replacement alone does not address the coagulopathy seen in trauma patients with severe hemorrhage. A quantitative and qualitative platelet dysfunction has been shown to play a role as well in the mechanism of coagulation. Although not as extensively as FFP, platelet replacement as a part of transfusion protocols has been studied to determine the most effective ratio of platelets to PRBCs. Hirshberg et al suggest a ratio of Plt:PRBC of 8:10 is effective in preventing dilution of platelets below the hemostatic threshold. It should be noted, however, that both studies were theoretical models and did not take into the account factors such as hypothermia, acidosis, thrombocytopenia, and ACoTS. These mathematical models for FFP and platelets set forth by Hirschberg et al and Ho et al have helped modify ratios used for MTPs throughout the world.

Historically, transfusion protocols have been cultivated throughout the years from early observations to studies on smaller and limited patient populations. More extensive, original evidence evolved from military experience, specifically from increased combat activity associated with Operation Iraqi Freedom and Operation Enduring Freedom. In addition, many civilian populations have begun to adopt the use of DCR into their MTPs. However, there still exits variability among MTPs throughout civilian institutions. The difference may ultimately stem from the variability of patient populations, especially with regard to the mechanism complexity of injuries.

Blood transfusions in trauma patients have been identified as an independent predictor of multiple organ failure (MOF), systemic inflammatory response syndrome, increased postinjury infection, and increased fatality. However, complications related to aggressive crystalloid resuscitation in this specific group of patients cannot be discarded and include cardiac and pulmonary complications, abdominal compartment syndrome, coagulation disturbances, and immunologic and inflammatory mediator dysfunction. By providing an evidence-based appraisal of available literature regarding blood product transfusions, this analysis attempts to reconcile some of the more recent observations, including complications, mortality, specific optimal resuscitation ratios, timing of transfusions, and effect on total transfusions.

EVIDENCE CLASSIFICATION

Fifty-seven articles from 1985 to 2011 were retrieved and stratified into three classes according to the quality assessment instrument developed by the Brain and Trauma Foundation and adopted by the Eastern Association for the Surgery of Trauma (www.east.org). Classes ranging from I to III were assigned according to the strength of scientific evidence. Articles are summarized in the Appendix that accompanies this chapter and can be found online. The evidence that was evaluated included topics in ratios of transfused products, quantity transfused, timing of transfusion, morbidity and mortality rates associated with transfusions, MTPs, and survival bias. Following the analysis, recommendations were grouped into three levels based on the quality assessment instrument developed by the Brain and Trauma Foundation and adopted by the Eastern Association for the Surgery of Trauma.

Class I: Prospective randomized controlled trials, which are the gold standard of clinical trials. Some prospective randomized controlled trials, however, suffer from poor design, inadequate numbers, or methodologic inadequacies that are not clinically significant. There was one class I study identified.

Class II: Prospective and retrospective analyses that were based on clearly reliable data. These types of studies include observational studies, cohort studies, prevalence studies, and case control studies. There were 17 studies within this category, of which 10 involved a retrospective review of prospectively collected data and 7 were prospective studies.

Class III: Mostly retrospectively collected data trials. Evidence used in this class includes clinical series, databases or registries, case reviews, case reports, and expert opinion. There were 41 studies identified within this category.

EVIDENCE REPORT

Ratios of Fresh Frozen Plasma to Packed Red Blood Cells

The determination of optimal FFP:PRBC ratios has been a controversial discussion in the field of massive transfusion and DCR. Mathematical models have determined optimal FFP:PRBC ratios to be between 1:1 and 2:3. These mathematical models are classified as class III evidence and serve as a guide to understanding how optimal plasma ratios work.

Human studies comparing different FFP:PRBC ratios have varied in approach. Sperry et al's patients were classified into two groups (both of which patients required >8 units of PRBCs), either receiving more than 1:1.5 FFP:PRBCs or less than 1.1.5 FFP:PRBCs. Those with FFP:PRBC ratio of 1:1.5 or greater had significantly lower risk of fatality, with the highest risk reduction coming within the first 48 hours from the time of injury. Gunter et al performed a retrospective observational study involving 259 patients that compared cohorts receiving high ratio and low ratio FFP:PRBC, finding improvement in mortality rate with ratios of 2:3 or greater (41% vs. 62%, $P = .008$, 30-day mortality rate). Shaz et al demonstrated an improvement in survival in high FFP:PRBC ratio with a 30-day survival rate of 59% versus 44% for patients with a low FFP:PRBC transfused ratio ($P = .03$).

Eighteen class III studies were found that address FFP:PRBC ratios. Kashuk et al compare the probability of death for differing ratios of FFP:PRBCs (1:1, 1:2, 1:3, 1:4, and >1:5) and discovered the lowest predicted mortality probability correlated with transfusion ratios in the range of 1:2 to 1:3. Other trials on civilian populations grouped patients into those receiving a low ratio versus a high ratio and demonstrated a lower risk of fatality and higher survival rate in patients who received a high FFP:PRBC ratio. Holcomb et al compared patients receiving high ratio to low ratio FFP:PRBC and Plt:

PRBC and found that patients receiving high ratios had a significantly improved 30-day survival rate of 59.6% versus 40.4% ($P < .01$). A longitudinal study by Duchesne et al examined the role of hemostatic resuscitation in trauma-induced coagulopathy. A significant difference in mortality rate was found in patients who received more than 10 units of PRBCs when FFP:PRBC ratio was 1:1 versus 1:4 (28.2% vs. 51.1%; $P = .03$). Additionally, time in intensive care unit (TICU) length of stay (LOS) was shorter (10 days vs. 23 days, $P < .01$) in patients who received FFP:PRBC ratio of 1:1 versus 1:4. A total of six other class III studies compared the effects of transfusion for three or more FFP:PRBC ratios. These studies showed that mortality rate improved with a high ratio, although one study by Teixeira et al showed that there did not seem to be a survival advantage for any FFP:PRBC ratio higher than 1:3.

Ratios of Platelets and Packed Red Blood Cells

Differences also vary in the use of platelets and PRBCs in trauma patients. Hirshberg et al address Plt:PRBC ratios in their previously mentioned mathematical model and find optimal Plt:PRBC ratios to be 8:10. Gunter et al classified patients into two groups, either receiving a ratio more than 1:5 or less than 1:5, and noted a decreased 30-day mortality rate in those receiving a ratio of 1:5 or greater as compared to those who received a ratio less than 1:5 of Plt:PRBC. The authors demonstrated high ratio attainment as an independent predictor for survival.

Four class III studies were identified that evaluated the ratio of Plts:PRBCs. Shaz et al classified patients into two groups: (1) those who received ratios higher than 1:2 and (2) those who received ratios lower than 1:2. The high versus low ratios were associated with improved 30-day survival rate of 63% versus 33% ($P < .01$). A second class III study, Perkins et al, classified patients into three categories: (1) those with a ratio higher than 1:8, (2) those between 1:16 and 1:8, and (3) those lower than 1:16. They demonstrated a higher survival rate at 24 hours for patients receiving a high ratio of platelets (>1:8) as compared to those receiving a medium (1:16 to <1:8) or low (<1:16) ratio (95% vs. 87% vs. 64%, $P < .001$). In addition, those receiving either high or medium ratios continued to have a survival benefit at 30 days over the low ratio group (75% and 60% vs. 43%, $P < .001$). In a more extensive study by Holcomb et al involving 16 Level I trauma centers and 466 massively transfused patients, FFP: PRBC and Plt:PRBC ratios were studied. They found patients treated with high Plt:PRBC ratio had a higher 30-day survival rate compared to patients treated with low Plt:PRBC ratio (59.9% vs. 40.1%, $P < .01$, respectively). They then looked at four groups consisting of patients administered: (1) high FFP and high platelet ratios, (2) high FFP and low platelet ratios, (3) low FFP and high platelet ratios, and (4) low FFP and low platelet ratios. They noted the high FFP and high platelet group had significantly increased survival rates at 6 hours, 24 hours, and 30 days compared to the other groups. Interestingly, there was found to be no difference between the high FFP and high platelet group to the low FFP and high platelet group at 30 days. Inaba et al found a stepwise improvement in survival with increasing Plt: PRBC ratios. A high Plt:PRBC ratio was independently associated with improved survival at 24 hours.

Quantity of Units Transfused

Several studies demonstrate an increased risk of complications with every unit of PRBCs transfused. One justification for increased FFP:PRBC and Plt:PRBC ratios is to decrease the total number of PRBC units transfused with the hopes of decreasing nosocomial complication rates. Four of the 57 studies were able to demonstrate a decreased requirement for blood transfusions in massively transfused patients who were administered higher ratios of FFP:PRBC. Cotton et al demonstrated a reduced 24-hour blood product use in patients who were transfused according to a trauma exsanguination protocol that included 6 units of PRBCs, 4 units of thawed plasma, and 2 units of single donor platelets when compared to patients transfused before the protocol was in place (39 ± 29 vs. 31.8 ± 19, $P < .017$). Sperry et al, in their class II study, showed significantly decreased transfusion requirements at 24 hours (16 ± 9 units vs. 22 ± 17 units, $P = .001$) in patients who received an FFP:PRBC ratio more than 1:1.5 versus patients receiving an FFP:PRBC ratio of less than 1:1.5. A previously described class III study by Zink et al showed that patients receiving FFP:PRBC ratio of less than 1:1 in the first 6 hours required a median of 18 units of PRBCs over the first 24 hours, whereas those with a ratio more than 1:1 required a median of 13 units of PRBCs ($P < .001$). Arulselvi et al looked at the percentage of trauma patients who underwent transfusion (94%), the ratio of transfusion used (3 PRBC:2 FFP:1 Plt), and the calculated crossmatch to transfusion ratio (C:T ratio). In regard to the PRBC C:T ratio, in 206 blunt trauma patients, 953 total units of PRBCs were crossmatched and only 450 units were transfused (C:T ratio = 2.1). For 146 penetrating trauma patients, 612 units of PRBCs were crossmatched and 248 units were transfused, equaling a 2.4 C:T ratio. Therefore, at least 2 units of PRBCs are crossmatched and only 1 unit of PRBCs are actually transfused in both blunt and penetrating trauma patients at this institution.

Utilization of Platelets, Fibrinogen, and Antifribrinolytics

Out of the 57 papers, there is one class III study involving massively transfused combat patients retrospectively observing fibrinogen: PRBC ratio. Stinger et al found that a high fibrinogen:PRBC ratio (0.48 g/unit ± 0.2 vs. 0.1 g/unit ± 0.06) was independently associated with decreased fatality, primarily by decreasing death from hemorrhage. Schoechl et al published two studies demonstrating an improvement in mortality rate in trauma patients treated with fibrinogen concentrate or prothrombin concentrate. Their studies did not necessarily confine themselves to massive transfusion patients but rather to trauma patients receiving 5 units of PRBCs or more. In one paper, Schoechl et al compared the observed mortality rate with Trauma Injury Severity Score (TRISS) versus the treatment group and saw a comparable mortality rate difference of 24.4% versus 33.7% ($P = .032$), and after excluding patients with traumatic brain injury (TBI) the observed mortality rate was 14% versus 27.8% TRISS ($P = .0018$). In his other study, Schoechl showed coagulopathic patients treated with either fibrinogen or FFP had comparable outcomes, with those in the fibrinogen cohort having a statistically lower hospital LOS (23 days vs. 32 days, $P = .005$).

With regard to platelet use and mortality, several class III studies have been published. Inaba et al, a class III study, showed a stepwise improvement in survival as the ratio of platelets to PRBCs increased. The relative risk (RR) of death increased from 1.67 (high ratio group) to 2.28 (medium ratio) to 5.51 (low ratio). Perkins et al describe a retrospective chart review in which their group found that high Plt: PRBC ratios were independently associated with improved survival. The study groups were split into those receiving high, medium, or low Plt:PRBC ratios. They found the 24-hour survival rate to be 95%, 87%, and 64%, respectively ($P < .001$). Holcomb et al demonstrated an increased 30-day survival rate (59.6% vs. 40.4%, $P < .01$) in patients treated with high plasma:PRBC ratio ($\geq 1:2$) relative to low plasma:PRBC ratio ($< 1:2$). Also observed was an increase in 30-day survival rate (59.9% vs. 40.1%, $P < 0.01$) in patients with high Plt:PRBC ratio ($\geq 1:2$) relative to those with low Plt:PRBC ratio ($< 1:2$).

Antifibrinolytics have taken a major spotlight in the recent past. The multicenter class I CRASH-2 study, the only known randomized placebo-controlled trial to address the use of antifibrinolytics, demonstrates an improvement in mortality rate through a well-designed study. The CRASH-2 trial involved 20,000 patients in 40 countries, with 10,115 patients receiving placebo and the 10,096 patients receiving tranexamic acid, an antifibrinolytic. All-cause mortality rate in the tranexamic acid cohort was 14.5% versus 16.0% in the placebo cohort (RR 0.91, 95% confidence interval [CI] 0.85–0.97; $P = .0035$). The risk of death from massive hemorrhage was also reduced significantly with an RR in the treatment cohort 4.9% versus 5.7% in the placebo cohort (RR 0.85, 95% CI 0.76–0.96; $P = .0077$). This trial demonstrates potential for this type of therapy in hemorrhagic trauma requiring massive transfusions.

Three class III studies were found focusing on the use of fibrinogen in coagulopathic trauma patients. A combat-related coagulopathy study by Stinger et al demonstrated that using a high fibrinogen:PRBC ratio is independently associated with improved mortality rate with a lower incidence of death in high fibrinogen: PRBC ratios compared to low ratios (24% vs. 85%, $P < .001$). Schoechel et al compare the use of fibrinogen-prothrombin complex concentrate (PCC) and FFP in coagulopathic trauma victims. They demonstrated the use of fibrinogen can avert the use of large quantities of PRBCs and may be more effective than FFP in decreasing the amount of PRBCs transfused. By using fibrinogen and PCC, PRBC transfusion was averted in 29% of cases as opposed to only 3% with FFP. Furthermore, platelet transfusion was avoided in 91% of cases when fibrinogen-PCC was used as compared to only 56% of cases with FFP. There was no statistically significant difference in mortality rate between the two groups. In another study by Schoechl et al, fibrinogen use demonstrated an improvement in mortality rate in patients treated with fibrinogen concentrate, prothrombin concentrate, FFP, or all three. The directed retrospective therapy was based on thromboelastometry.

Timing of Transfusions

None of the trials directly studied the effect of the timing of the transfusion of FFP with PRBCs. However, in many settings early initiation of plasma therapy is often delayed by limited immediate availability in the trauma center, despite the evidence that the pathologic changes of coagulopathy occur much earlier in the resuscitation process than previously thought. A class III study showed that uncorrected coagulopathy at ICU admission (to include emergency department resuscitation) is associated with ongoing transfusion requirements and therefore ongoing coagulopathy. Zink et al showed the largest difference in mortality rate occurs during the first 6 hours after admission, suggesting the early administration of FFP and platelets is critical. Magnotti et al demonstrate that 6-hour mortality rate is correlated with achieving a high FFP:PRBC ratio early. Moore et al examined patients who died early in the resuscitation effort and found those dying early were coagulopathic (mean international normalized ratio [INR] 2.4) yet received a mean of 26.4 units of PRBCs and a mean of 6.5 units of FFP with 12% receiving no FFP and concluded the coagulopathy of those dying early was inadequately corrected.

Establishment and Effectiveness of Massive Transfusion Protocols

The concept of MTP is a rapidly developing one that has seen an increase in implementation in the past decade. A 2006 article by Malone et al found a paucity of MTPs in the United States and abroad. The implementation of MTPs has increased dramatically in the past several years. A 2008 survey by Hoyt et al revealed only 45% of respondents worldwide followed MTPs consistently with 19% admitting inconsistent protocol adherence and 34% of respondents not having an MTP. A 2010 paper by Schuster et al polled trauma centers and directors around the United States (186 surgeons and 59 center directors responded) and found 85% of respondents had MTPs in place and that 65% of these MTPs had been established in the past 5 years. The authors note protocols varied widely by institution both in method of activation and in component ratios and timing.

Núñez et al describes the development of a protocol at a large Level I trauma center that involves a team approach with an aim to eventually improve clinical survival and decrease the overall blood use, decreasing wastage. They described a method of identification, ABCs (airway, breathing, and circulation), and a scoring method based on four parameters: (1) penetrating mechanism, (2) positive focused assessment with sonography in trauma, (3) systolic blood pressure (SBP) less than or equal to 90 mm Hg on arrival, and (4) heart rate greater than or equal to 120 beats per minute on arrival. In this scoring method, a score of 2 or greater is 75% sensitive and 86% specific for predicting massive transfusion.

MTPs have attempted to resolve the user variability of transfusion practices. Several trials have examined the effectiveness of these protocols. One retrospective cohort at Parkland Hospital showed significant decrease in blood component use, faster turnaround, and lower costs per patient after the implementation of an MTP. By using fewer overall blood products, MTPs expose patients to fewer of the complications associated with blood product transfusions. Cotton et al demonstrated that full compliance with their institution's MTP was independently associated with improved survival rate (86.7% vs. 45.0%, $P < .001$). Failure to comply with the established MTP was an independent predictor of wasted blood products. The authors note that their institution's compliance was 27%. Another study by Cotton et al demonstrated a lower incidence of severe sepsis/septic shock and multiorgan failure in patients transfused according to an MTP. Gunter et al demonstrated patients receiving transfused blood products according to an MTP experienced a significant reduction in 30-day mortality rate compared with those transfused before the inception of the protocol (41% vs. 62%, $P < .008$). Dente et al demonstrated a marked improvement in risk-adjusted 30-day mortality rate (34% vs. 55%, $P < .04$) in addition to overall mortality rate (36% vs. 17%, $P < .008$) in patients transfused according to an MTP. Importantly, Riskin et al demonstrated that an implementation of MTP is associated with mortality rate reductions despite the unchanged ratio used pre-MTP and post-MTP. Their data underscores the importance of expeditious delivery of products when the MTP is initiated. Some conflicting evidence suggests MTP may not have an effect on mortality in severe hemorrhage. Simmons et al investigated mortality before and after the establishment of MTP during Operation Iraqi Freedom/Enduring Freedom and revealed no change in mortality rate.

Transfusion Complications

Mortality

Twenty-four of the 57 studies specifically address the effect of transfusion of FFP on mortality. Class II evidence for the use of high ratio of FFP:PRBC is overwhelming; however, there is a lack of prospective randomized controlled studies to support the results. Eight class II studies were found, most showing reduction in mortality rate with increased FFP:PRBC ratios. Cotton et al showed a 74% reduction in the odds of mortality rate ($P < .001$) after risk adjustment among patients treated according to an MTP consisting of 10 units PRBCs, 4 units of thawed plasma, and 2 units of platelets. Dente et al showed lower 30-day and overall mortality rates after the institution of an MTP incorporating a 1:1 FFP:PRBC ratio. They note an improvement in 24-hour mortality rate from 36% to 17% ($P = .008$) and 30-day mortality rate of 55% versus 34% ($P = .04$). Sperry et al compared mortality rate among patients who were transfused with an FFP:PRBC ratio more than 1:1.5 with those receiving an FFP:PRBC ratio less than 1:1.5 and found a significant difference in early (24-hour) mortality rate (3.9% vs. 12.8%, $P < .012$), yet no statistically significant difference in overall crude mortality rate. Gunter et al demonstrate that the implementation of an MTP requiring high FFP:PBRC ratio of 2:3 or more resulted in improved 30-day mortality rate (41% vs. 62%, $P = .008$). Additionally, comparing Plt:PRBC ratio of 1:5 or greater had lower 30-day mortality rate (38% vs. 61%, $P = .001$)

(not using DCR). Bochicchio et al demonstrates a dose-dependent correlation between increased ratios of blood products and adverse outcomes. This study compared trauma cohorts treated without blood products compared those treated with blood products and demonstrated a statistically significant increase in adverse events, specifically infection increased in the blood product group (34% vs. 9.4%, $P < .001$). Mortality rate also increased in the cohort receiving blood products (21.4% vs. 6.5%). The authors acknowledge, however, patients treated with blood product transfusion had a statistically significant increased ISS (27 ± 13 vs. 19 ± 11, $P < .001$) and INR (1.8 ± 1 vs. 1.1 ± 0.09, $P < .001$) and were therefore more likely to succumb to their injuries and coagulopathy. Simmons et al compared matched military cohorts after implementation of the Clinical Practice Guideline (CPG). They found that the post-CPG cohort did receive a higher FFP:PRBC ratio and patients were presenting normothermic with higher hemoglobin levels. However, overall mortality rate (not a specific outcome study variable in their study) was not statistically different between the two groups (24% vs. 19%, $P = .115$). Scalea et al were unable to find a significant difference in mortality rate for the FFP:PRBC ratio as a continuous variable (odds ratio [OR] 1.49, $P = .37$) or 1:1 ratio as a binary variable (OR 0.60, $P = .35$). However, the patient population used in this study was limited to 250 of 806 enrolled that actually received more than 1 unit of both RBCs and FFP within 24 hours, highlighting the variability of resuscitation efforts to exclusively include only DCR. Magnotti et al attempt to challenge DCR principles, which include high ratios of FFP:RBC used in traumatic hemorrhage. The postulated challenge suggests a survival bias in the trauma patient skewed the results of improvement in survival in patients that were able to reach a high ratio of FFP:PRBC early. However, this study lacks support for survival bias. They noted that patients reaching a high ratio had a lower severity of shock. Also, their results revealed that the 6-hour mortality rate was less in the high group (10% vs. 48%, $P < .002$).

The majority of the class III studies were able to demonstrate a significant improvement in mortality rate among patients who were resuscitated with higher FFP:PRBC ratios. Six studies, including one multicenter clinical analysis, were able to show an improved mortality rate with higher ratios of FFP:PRBCs when compared to lower ratios previously administered. Five studies were able to independently demonstrate an improved survival rate with high FFP:PRBC ratio. A study by Mitra et al concluded that a higher FFP:PRBC ratio is associated with an increased initial survival, but when deaths in the first 24 hours were excluded, the FFP:PRBC ratio had no association with mortality. Mitra et al concludes that further trials are needed to determine the optimal ratio. In a study of massively transfused TBI patients, Peiniger et al found mortality rate to be statistically lower in high ratio versus low ratio groups independent of time, and the presence/absence of TBI. A military study comparing military resuscitations among patients receiving an FFP:PRBC ratio of 1:1.4 vs. 1:1.7 showed no significant difference in mortality rate, with no deaths in either cohort.

Inaba et al addressed the use of unmatched blood during acute resuscitation as a source of variability affecting outcome, showing patients receiving unmatched blood had a higher mortality rate than patients receiving matched blood (39.6% vs. 11.9%, $P < .001$), therefore indicating the use of uncrossmatched blood represented an independent predictor of mortality rate. Interestingly, a different military study comparing the effects of whole blood versus component therapy was able to demonstrate increased 24-hour and 30-day survival rate in those transfused with whole blood compared with component therapy.

Morbidity

A multitude of studies have demonstrated a dose-dependent relationship between in-hospital complications and blood product transfusion. Silverboard et al demonstrate in a class II study an increasing incidence of acute respiratory distress syndrome (ARDS) in patients transfused with greater quantities of PRBCs. In this study, patients were separated into three groups requiring 0 to 5 units of PRBCs, 6–10 units, and greater than 10 units with 21%, 31%, and 57% of patients developing ARDS, respectively. A prospective class II study by Bochicchio et al demonstrated by risk-adjusted, multivariate analysis that every unit of PRBCs administered increased the risk of infection by 5%, and hospital LOS, TICU, and ventilator days increased by 0.64, 0.42, and 0.47 days, respectively. A class II study by Sadjadi et al showed an observed infection rate of 61% versus 20% ($P < .01$) in transfused patients versus nontransfused patients with similar ISS and an eightfold greater chance of infection in the transfused cohort (OR, 7.97; 95% CI, 2.3 to 27.5; $P < .001$). Another class II study conducted based on military data by Dunne et al showed patients receiving greater than 4 units of blood had impaired wound healing rate (54% vs. 9%, $P < .05$), higher ICU admission rate (78% vs. 9%, $P < .01$), increased perioperative infection rate (89% vs. 27%, $P < .01$), a longer hospital LOS, and increased serum inflammatory markers.

Several studies have addressed complications associated with FFP and transfusion ratios with PRBCs. Sperry et al showed, in a class II study, that patients transfused with a higher FFP:PRBC ratio required significantly less blood, experienced a lower mortality rate, and showed no difference in organ failure or nosocomial infection, but did have a twofold higher risk of ARDS. These conclusions were echoed by another retrospective study by Chaiwat et al, which demonstrated patients receiving at least 5 units of PRBCs had a 2.5 times greater chance of developing ARDS. Each additional unit of PRBCs transfused conferred a 6% higher risk of ARDS with an adjusted OR of 1.06 (95% CI 1.03–1.10). Watson et al concluded that FFP was associated with a 2.9% decreased risk of mortality per unit transfused but a 2.1% increased risk of MOF (hazard ratio [HR] 1.021; $P = .029$; 95% CI 1.002–1.04) and 2.5% increased risk of ARDS per unit transfused (HR 1.025; $P = .038$; 95% CI 1.001–1.049). Cotton et al, comparing the effect of implementing an early, predefined transfusion protocol, including a 3:2 FFP:PRBC ratio, showed no difference in renal failure or systemic inflammatory response syndrome, and a lower incidence of pneumonia, pulmonary failure, open abdomens, and abdominal compartment syndrome in the protocol group. They discovered a lower incidence of severe sepsis/septic shock (9% vs. 20%, $P = .011$) and multiorgan failure (16% vs. 37%, $P < .001$).

Many class III studies demonstrate conflicting results with regard to complications and the use of FFP transfusions. Peiniger et al demonstrate patients transfused with a higher FFP:PRBC ratio did not have a higher incidence of sepsis and MOF. Zink et al showed that patients who received higher ratios of FFP:PRBCs as part of an MTP had a similar number of ventilator-free days as those with low ratios. Holcomb et al showed that high FFP with high platelet ratios were associated with improved 30-day survival rate, no change in multiorgan failure deaths, yet longer ICU stays and more days on a ventilator. Fox et al demonstrated a lower amputation rate and better physiologic recovery among military patients transfused with a higher FFP:PRBC ratio. Mahambrey et al demonstrated a 48 hour increased organ dysfunction but no increase in hospital mortality rate in patients transfused with high volumes of RBCs. Khan et al demonstrate acutely medically ill patients having an increased risk of ALI and ARDS receiving FFP and with or without other blood components as an adjusted risk ratio of 2.48 (95% CI 1.29–4.74) versus patients receiving any amount of PRBCs with or without other blood components of 1.39 (95% CI 0.79–2.43). Sarani et al showed an OR of infection of 1.039 (1.013–1.067) for every unit of FFP transfused. The authors also demonstrate an RR for all types of infection in FFP transfusions of 2.99 (95% CI 2.28–3.93). A large, class III European study by Maegele et al showed improved 30-day mortality rate but increased ventilator days and ICU stay among patients who received a high ratio of FFP.

Although platelets are thought to have fewer complications than FFP, they are not without risk of allergic reaction, transfusion-associated acute lung injury (TRALI), ARDS, and bacterial infection. In a class III study, Khan et al demonstrate an increase in risk of acute lung infection and ARDS in their small retrospective cohort study with an adjusted risk of 3.89 (5% CI 1.36–11.52) in patients receiving any proportion of platelets versus 1.39 (95% CI 0.79–2.43) in medically ill patients receiving PRBCs with or without other blood product transfusion. However, a class II study by Watson et al performed on a multicenter prospective cohort of blunt trauma patients with hemorrhagic shock demonstrated in patients who survived the initial traumatic event, FFP was independently associated with a greater risk of MOF and ARDS, whereas cryoprecipitate was associated with lower risk MOF.

Survival Bias

Three of the 57 studies, all class III studies, address FFP:PRBC ratio after adjusting for survival bias in the analysis. Snyder et al found an association between higher FFP:PRBC ratios at 24 hours and improved survival rates. However, after adjusting for survival bias in the analysis, the association was no longer statistically significant. Rajasekhar et al looked at survival advantage in 11 different studies on 1:1 FFP:PRBC ratio. They conclude survival bias, and heterogeneity between studies, prevent statistical comparisons concerning FFP:PRBC ratio, and that there is insufficient evidence to support a survival advantage with a high FFP:PRBC ratio. The third study by Magnotti et al concluded improved survival was observed in patients receiving a higher plasma ratio over the first 24 hours. They proposed patients do not die *because* of a low FFP:PRBC ratio but rather *with* a low FFP:PRBC ratio.

RECOMMENDATIONS

Stratification Scheme and Level Definitions

Level I Recommendations

This recommendation is convincingly justifiable based on the available scientific information alone. It is usually based on class I data; however, strong class II evidence may form the basis for a level I recommendation, especially if the issue does not lend itself to testing in a randomized format. Conversely, weak or contradictory class I data may not be able to support a level I recommendation.

1. An FFP:PRBC ratio of 1:1 is associated with less transfusions. Sufficient evidence does exist for showing transfusion with FFP will decrease the number of transfusions needed. It should be noted there are no randomized, prospective class I trials. Conducting such trials in the future will be essential to continuing to understand the ideal manner to transfuse during trauma.
2. Class I evidence supports use of antifibrinolytics in massive transfusion. The recently completed CRASH-2 trials demonstrate improved all-cause mortality rate as well as mortality due to hemorrhage. Further class I, II, and III studies should be performed to further support these findings.

Level II Recommendations

This recommendation is reasonably justifiable by available scientific evidence and strongly supported by expert critical care opinion. It is usually supported by class II data or a preponderance of class III evidence.

1. An MTP will improve outcomes for trauma resuscitations. There are many logistic challenges associated with this strategy. Many civilian institutions, even Level I trauma centers, have yet to adopt an MTP. However, simple ratios such as 1:1 FFP:PRBC have the benefit of ease of use and the relatively higher plasma doses appear to be associated with improved outcome.

Such a standard protocol can foster multicenter research on resuscitation and hemorrhage control.

2. High FFP:PRBC ratio is supported by class II and class III evidence and should be considered in the treatment of massively transfused coagulopathic trauma patients. Class II and class III data demonstrate the potential for severe complications such as ARDS/ALI, increased hospital and TICU LOS, and increased ventilator time; however, most studies demonstrate improved mortality rate, suggesting an overall improvement in the use of these therapies.

Level III Recommendations

These recommendations are supported by available data but adequate scientific evidence is lacking. They are generally supported by class III data. This type of recommendation is useful for educational purposes and in guiding future studies.

1. Increased FFP:PRBC ratio leads to improved outcomes in massive transfusion with the potential for severe complication. MTP implementation and adherence yield improved results with decreases in mortality and complication rates.
2. The use of high Plt:PRBC ratio is supported by some class II studies and several class III studies. Increased Plt:PRBC ratio has become an integral part of DCR in recent years.
3. Several class III studies demonstrate mortality rate improvement with the use of fibrinogen concentrate. The use of fibrinogen in the trauma-induced coagulopathy and DCR should be studied further in class I and class II trials.
4. Increased FFP:PRBC ratio administered early leads to improved outcomes in massive hemorrhage. This benefit is believed to be extended to patients undergoing transfusion with increased FFP:PRBC ratios due to lower transfusion requirements, lower risk of complications secondary to the transfusions, and better ability to compensate for the coagulopathy

of trauma. Although there is not yet a consensus regarding fatality reduction from increased FFP:PRBC ratios, there does appear to be a trend toward decreased mortality rate. It is likely that optimized protocol guidelines will contribute to standardizing variations among current practices.

CONCLUSION

There remains a need for further examination of the role of transfusion ratios in trauma. Sufficient evidence does exist to demonstrate that an FFP:PRBC ratio of 1:1 is associated with the need for less transfusions. In addition, the evidence so far indicates the incorporation of these principles into an MTP will also contribute to less transfused units by minimizing variability of transfusion practices. Importantly, fewer units transfused will contribute to fewer complications associated with transfusions. These conclusions will need to be verified, especially with regard to the effect of MTPs incorporating higher ratios of FFP:PRBC on varying mechanism of injury, the timing of transfusions, and the number of units actually transfused.

In the setting of DCR, the focus remains on prolonging life in the initial stages of the resuscitation. Uncertainty still exists regarding the association of higher ratios of FFP:PRBC and Plt:PRBC with improved outcomes, including improved mortality rate. Several class III trials noted improved mortality rate but increased complications. Also, many of the class II studies have attempted to account for the wide variability, which exists in trauma patients by risk-adjusting conclusions for mechanism of injury, patient demographics, and severity of injury. However, although this does lend some degree of evidence to the conclusions concerning the ideal ratios for FFP, platelets, and PRBCs, definitive conclusions can only be made with randomized, prospective trials in the future.

Please visit the book online at www.ExpertConsult.com for Suggested Readings and an online chapter Appendix.

SURGICAL TECHNIQUES FOR THORACIC, ABDOMINAL, PELVIC, AND EXTREMITY DAMAGE CONTROL

Greta L. Piper, Kimberly A. Davis, and Fred A. Luchette

INTRODUCTION

Injury severity and spectrums of injury have continually evolved, resulting in greater and different challenges for the modern trauma surgeon. High-energy blunt trauma with multisystem organ injury, as well as increasingly sophisticated firearms with greater wounding capacity, has produced greater severity of injury. Despite the fact that these injury patterns are more likely to result in the death of a patient, improvements in prehospital transport and trauma resuscitation have allowed an increasing number of moribund patients to reach the hospital alive but in extremis. Damage control surgery, addressing the life-threatening injuries immediately but delaying definitive repair until the metabolic and physiologic perturbations have been corrected, has evolved to address this population of patients.

Damage control has three separate and distinct phases of management. The first phase includes aggressive volume expansion, rapid control of hemorrhage, and the minimization of contamination from hollow viscus injuries. Packing is frequently left in place to tamponade bleeding, and temporary wound management strategies are employed. The second phase, which occurs in the intensive care unit (ICU), involves the aggressive rewarming of the hypothermic patient, with correction of coagulopathy and ongoing resuscitation with crystalloids and blood products. Once normal physiology has been reestablished, the third phase involves definitive operative management of the patient's injuries.

The goal of the damage control procedure is to preserve life in the face of devastating injuries with profound hemorrhagic shock. As described by Moore et al, indications for a damage control strategy include an inability to achieve hemostasis due to ongoing coagulopathy, a technically difficult or inaccessible major venous injury, a time-consuming procedure in the face of underresuscitated shock, and a need to address other life-threatening injuries. These indications have been expanded to include hemodynamically unstable patients with either high-energy blunt torso trauma or multiple penetrating injuries, or any trauma patient presenting in shock with hypothermia and coagulopathy (Box 1). Most commonly applied to the abdomen, damage control approaches have also been applied successfully to devastating thoracic and orthopedic injuries.

The Lethal Triad

Damage control procedures attempt to truncate surgical intervention prior to the development of irreversible physiologic derangement. Uncontrolled hemorrhage results in global ischemic injury, but

Hemodynamic instability due to hemorrhagic shock
Presenting coagulopathy or hypothermia
Major abdominal vascular injury with or without associated visceral injury
Complex hepatic injuries with or without associated visceral injury
Multicavitary injuries with hemorrhagic shock
Multisystem trauma with competing management priorities
Metabolic acidosis with pH <7.3
Massive transfusion requirements

Modified from Rotondo MF, Zonies DH: The damage control sequence and underlying logic. *Surg Clin North Am* 77:761–777, 1997.

resuscitation subjects the patient to further injury during the period of reperfusion. Inevitably the lethal triad of hypothermia, coagulopathy, and acidosis develops. Although each of these individual complications is potentially life threatening, the combination of all three results in an exponential increase in morbidity, contributing to a downward spiral that eventually results in the patient's demise if not corrected. Damage control surgery, by abbreviating surgical intervention and returning the patient to the ICU for correction of the lethal triad, has resulted in improved survival over time.

Hypothermia is defined as a core temperature of less than 35° C. Cooling of the core temperature by radiant heat loss begins in the prehospital setting and continues after arrival to the emergency department (ED) during the primary and secondary surveys. Aggressive resuscitation with unwarmed fluids and evaporative loss from exposed peritoneal and pleural surfaces in the operating room contribute to continued loss of body temperature. The incidence of clinical hypothermia after trauma laparotomy is 57%. Hypothermia has clearly been shown to increase risk of mortality, increasing significantly in patients with a core temperature less than 34° C, and is uniformly fatal in injured patients with a core temperature less than 32° C.

Hypothermia has systemic effects, including a negative impact on hemodynamics (decreased heart rate and cardiac output, increased systemic vascular resistance), renal function (decreased glomerular filtration rates), and the central nervous system (depressed mental status). Reduction of body temperature also independently affects the coagulation cascade, as clot formation relies on a series of temperature-dependent enzymatic reactions. Studies have demonstrated hypothermia-related increases in prothrombin time (PT), thrombin time, and partial thromboplastin time (PTT). Hypothermia also affects platelet function, leading to sequestration in the portal circulation and prolonged bleeding times.

Metabolic acidosis occurs after hemorrhagic shock due to the switch from aerobic to anaerobic metabolism during periods of hypoperfusion. The detrimental effects of acidosis include depressed myocardial contractility and a diminished response to inotropic medications. Acidosis predisposes the myocardium to ventricular dysrhythmias. It can also worsen intracranial hypertension. Finally, acidosis has been shown to worsen coagulopathy by independently prolonging PTT and decreasing factor V activity. Coagulopathy is exacerbated by acidosis, which also contributes to the development of disseminated intravascular coagulation (DIC).

Even in the absence of hypothermia and acidosis, coagulopathy develops secondary to dilutional effects when massive resuscitation is composed of crystalloid and packed red blood cells without clotting factor replacements. Exposed tissue factor secondary to tissue injury also contributes to the development of coagulopathy through the activation of the clotting cascade and the resultant consumption of clotting factors.

Initial Resuscitation Concerns

A systematic approach to the initial management of the injured patient has been promulgated by the Advanced Trauma Life Support course of the American College of Surgeons Committee on Trauma. The primary and secondary surveys as described in this course allow the rapid identification of life-threatening injuries and enable the surgeon to prioritize subsequent operative management of the unstable trauma patient. Patients with exsanguinating hemorrhage should be expeditiously transported to the operating room, where a decision regarding the initiation of damage control strategies should be made early in the operative course based on the patient's physiologic parameters, body temperature, and intravascular volume status (see Box 1). In patients with obvious ongoing resuscitation requirements, a central venous catheter should be placed for aggressive volume resuscitation. Given the multiple factors that predispose these patients to coagulopathy, early consideration should be given to the initiation of damage control resuscitation as described in a later chapter (Torso Trauma on the Modern Battlefield), with a focus on the early administration of coagulation factors (fresh frozen plasma and cryoprecipitate) and platelets in addition to the standard crystalloid and packed red blood cell resuscitation. Recent literature supports the administration of blood and blood products in the ratio of one unit of packed red blood cells to one unit of fresh frozen plasma to one unit of platelets, and an attempt to minimize crystalloid resuscitation.

PHASE I: THE DAMAGE CONTROL OPERATION

The Damage Control Laparotomy

Most damage control procedures are performed in the abdomen. The earliest descriptions of what subsequently became known as damage control surgery involved patients with major hepatic injuries, in whom the placement of perihepatic packing and staged operative management resulted in decreased morbidity and mortality rates. The most common injuries that trigger a damage control approach are major liver injuries and major vascular injuries.

The primary method of controlling hepatic hemorrhage is packing. The technique of pack placement is of the utmost importance, and depends on the anatomic nature of the liver injury. Major hepatic lacerations require complete mobilization of the liver, and inflow occlusion at the porta hepatis (the Pringle maneuver) to minimize blood loss. Direct ligation of bleeding vessels in the depth of the laceration is necessary to obtain surgical hemostasis. Once major vessel bleeding has been controlled, perihepatic packs should be placed anteriorly and posteriorly, compressing the liver between the two beds of packs and providing tamponade similar to that which occurs with bimanual compression of the injured liver. Patients should be considered for angiography with embolization of bleeding hepatic artery branches prior to reexploration with pack removal to aid in hemostasis (phase 3). In penetrating injuries, balloon tamponade of the missile tract, in conjunction with perihepatic packing, can be lifesaving.

There are several options available for the management of major vascular injuries. Some venous injuries will respond to packing. Ongoing bleeding, however, requires direct surgical intervention. Many abdominal vascular injuries can be managed with simple ligation of the bleeding vessel (Table 1). Ligation, however, is not tolerated in aortic or proximal superior mesenteric artery injuries, and is not technically feasible in retrohepatic caval injuries. These injuries are typically initially approached by an attempt at repair, or the placement of a temporary intraluminal shunt, with planned repair at a second operation (phase 3). Commonly, Argyle carotid shunts and Javid shunts have been used for this purpose. Chest tubes may be used when larger conduits are necessary. The shunts should be secured using umbilical tapes, vessel loops, or suture and do not require anticoagulation to maintain patency. Another technique for the management of exsanguinating vascular injury is the use of endoluminal balloon catheters to obtain proximal and distal control of the hemorrhage. The catheters are inserted into the vessel at the site of injury,

TABLE 1: Abdominal Vessel Ligation and Expected Complications

Vessel	Complication	Recommendations
Celiac axis	None	
Splenic artery	None if the short gastric vessels are intact	
Common hepatic artery	None if the portal vein is intact, possible gallbladder ischemia	Cholecystectomy (may be done at second-look procedure)
Superior mesenteric artery	Bowel ischemia	Second-look procedure
Superior mesenteric vein	Bowel ischemia	Second-look procedure
Portal vein	Bowel ischemia	Second-look procedure
Suprarenal inferior vena cava	Possible renal failure	Wrap and elevate legs, assess for compartment syndrome
Infrarenal inferior vena cava	Lower extremity edema	Wrap and elevate legs, assess for compartment syndrome
Left renal vein (proximal)	None	
Right renal vein	Renal ischemia	Nephrectomy
Common and external iliac artery	Lower extremity ischemia	Ipsilateral calf fasciotomies or extra-anatomic bypass
Common and external iliac vein	Lower extremity edema	Wrap and elevate legs
Internal iliac artery	None	
Internal iliac vein	None	

Modified from Shapiro MB, Jenkins DH, Schwab CW, Rotondo MF: Damage control: collective review. *J Trauma* 49:969–978, 2000.

and the balloon inflated. This technique allows repair of the injured vessel in a relatively dry operative field. Finally, in rare cases in which retrohepatic vena caval bleeding can be controlled with packing, venography with endoluminal stenting remains an option.

Candidates for damage control surgery often have associated hollow viscus injury. The goal in management of these injuries is to control contamination. Intestinal lacerations may be controlled by suture or linear stapling or may be stapled closed. If enterectomy is necessary, the gastrointestinal tract is left in discontinuity, and the decision to perform an anastomosis or stoma is postponed until the patient has been stabilized and can return to the operating room for definitive management (phase 3). Associated biliary or pancreatic injuries can often be managed with judicious placement of closed suction drains, with plans to address the injury at the second procedure (phase 3).

Hemodynamic instability due to splenic lacerations should be managed with expeditious splenectomy. Similarly, hemorrhagic shock due to extensive renal lacerations (grade IV) or pedicle injuries (grade V) should be managed by nephrectomy, especially if attempts at perinephric packing have failed. Ureteral injuries diagnosed during the damage control procedure should be stented, ligated, or drained with a percutaneous urostomy. Intraperitoneal bladder injuries should be rapidly oversewn with definitive management delayed until the second operation.

Given the volume of resuscitation to restore tissue perfusion after a damage control procedure, and the edema that results from reperfusion of previously ischemic tissue, primary closure of the abdominal wall is associated with a prohibitively high risk of developing recurrent abdominal compartment syndrome (ACS), acute respiratory distress syndrome (ARDS), and multisystem organ failure (MSOF). Multiple options exist for the temporary closure of the abdomen. The goals of temporary closure should be containment of the abdominal viscera, control of abdominal ascites, maintenance of tamponade on areas that have been packed, and preservation of fascial integrity to aid in later closure.

Simple techniques for temporary abdominal closure (TAC) of the abdomen involve closure of only the skin, either with suture or with towel clips. This technique will facilitate the tamponade of bleeding while coagulopathy, acidosis, and hypothermia are corrected. However, it does not expand abdominal volumes significantly and may set the stage for development of recurrent ACS. When this occurs, the ACS can be easily decompressed in the ICU by simply reopening the skin with application of one of the following TACs. Techniques that expand the abdominal volume include coverage of the viscera with a Bogota bag, a 3-L urologic bag that is sewn to the skin. The benefit of the Bogota bag over the vacuum-assisted techniques described next is that it allows visualization of the underlying viscera and assessment of viability, which may be important after the use of shunting or ligation for a major vascular injury.

Vacuum-assisted techniques for TAC have been well described. The vacuum-assisted wound coverage is constructed beginning with a nonadherent fenestrated drape placed over the viscera, followed by the application of a sterile surgical towel. Following placement of two closed suction drains, the wound is sealed with an adhesive plastic sheet applied to the skin. The benefits of this technique include maintenance of some tension on the abdominal wall fascia to minimize the risk of loss of domain and to facilitate subsequent delayed fascial closure. There are several commercially available devices capable of providing similar function. Another potential technique for temporary closure involves the use of a Velcro patch, which is sutured to the fascia and sequentially tightened. In the acute setting, there is little role for prosthetic material for temporary closure of the abdomen. As there are no prospective trials comparing methods of TAC, the method used is at the discretion of the trauma surgeon and is often institution specific. However, retrospective data suggest that the use of vacuum-assisted closure at the time of initial exploration facilitates fascial closure when compared to other options.

The Damage Control Thoracotomy

Trauma patients with penetrating thoracic injuries who present in extremis should undergo ED thoracotomy. ED thoracotomy is rarely successful in patients with blunt trauma or with extrathoracic penetrating injury and should therefore be avoided in those situations.

ED thoracotomy is classically performed though a left anterolateral thoracotomy at the level of the fourth or fifth intercostal space. This exposure permits rapid evacuation of the thoracic cavity as well as inspection of the pericardial sac to rule out tamponade. On entering the chest, any hemothorax is evacuated, and the pericardium is inspected. If tamponade is present, a longitudinal pericardotomy is performed in a cephalad to caudad direction, avoiding the phrenic nerve. In the patient in extremis, the inferior pulmonary ligament is divided, allowing access to the posterior mediastinum, where the aorta can be cross-clamped.

Cardiac lacerations may be temporarily controlled using a number of methods. Digital pressure over the laceration or perforation is often quite effective, although the finger should not be inserted into the laceration or perforation as this may inadvertently extend its size. A Foley catheter can be carefully passed through the injury into the ventricle and gentle traction applied after inflating the balloon to control hemorrhage. Finally, simple cardiac injuries can be repaired in the ED using a skin stapler to reapproximate the lacerated myocardium.

Exsanguination from pulmonary injuries may be controlled in several ways, including direct pressure, packing, hilar cross-clamping, or lung torsion at the hilar axis. Once in the operating room, penetrating pulmonary injuries are often amenable to a technique known as pulmonary tractotomy, described by Asensio. A linear stapler is placed into the missile tract, allowing the tract to be opened with good hemostasis. With serial applications of the stapler, the base of the tract is exposed, permitting direct ligation of bleeding sites. Air leaks can be selectively oversewn. Bleeding controlled using the tractotomy technique is associated with a significantly lower mortality rate when compared to formal lobar resection.

Following damage control thoracotomy, it is not always possible to formally close the chest without increasing the intrathoracic pressure, which increases alveolar pressure and airway pressure, which compromise the ability of the ventilator to deliver adequate tidal volumes. Temporary closure of the thoracic cavity can be accomplished should packing be necessary for control of medical bleeding. Following insertion of a chest tube, a skin-only closure may be fashioned to provide adequate tamponade. Routine closure of the incision can be accomplished in a delayed fashion at 48 to 72 hours (phase 3).

Damage Control Orthopedics

Damage control orthopedics is characterized by rapid, temporary fracture stabilization. This concept applies particularly to femoral shaft fractures and pelvic fractures, which have an increased risk of adverse outcome related to significant soft tissue injury and blood loss. The impetus for the development of damage control orthopedics was the observation that patients with severe thoracic, abdominal, and head injuries had worse outcomes when subjected to extended operative procedures for definitive fracture stabilization with ongoing evidence of hypothermia, coagulopathy, and acidosis.

The most common technique for lower extremity fractures is the application of an external fixator device to provide temporary fracture stabilization. External fixation is quick and can be performed safely either in the operating room or even at the bedside in the ICU. The surgeon then places two pins above and two pins below the fracture site, avoiding neurovascular structures. Fluoroscopy is used to reduce the fracture with alignment. The external fixator bars are then applied to the pins, spanning the fracture and providing stability. Although concerns have been raised over the increased risk for deep tissue infection due to pin site sepsis, no significant increase in local infection has been reported.

Pelvic ring disruptions continue to be a significant source of both morbidity and fatality after trauma. Pelvic fractures account for 3% to 8% of all skeletal fractures and are most commonly due to high-energy trauma, with motor vehicle collisions the predominant

mechanism of injury. During the acute phase, the goal of treatment should be the control of hemorrhage. The intact retroperitoneum can contain up to 4 L of blood, and bleeding from the associated vascular injuries will continue until physiologic tamponade is obtained. If the retroperitoneal space or skin (open fracture) is disrupted, there is no ability for tamponade and the hemorrhage is uncontrolled until the wound is packed with sterile gauze so as to reestablish a closed retroperitoneum and pelvic space.

Decreasing the intrapelvic volume by restoring the normal pelvic anatomy remains the first step in the damage control management of the bleeding associated with pelvic fractures. This can be accomplished by multiple methods, including tying a bed sheet around the pelvis or using several commercially available pelvic slings and belts. External fixators and pelvic C clamps may also be used for this purpose and are ideal for "open book" disruptions of the pelvic ring. The external fixator involves placement of two percutaneous pins on each iliac crest. The pins are then connected with rods after manually reapproximating the edges of the pubic symphysis. The external fixator maintains reduction of the disrupted symphysis and decreases the pelvic volume. The C clamp consists of two pins applied on the posterior ilium in the region of the sacroiliac joints. The application of this device is relatively contraindicated in patients with fractures of the ilium and transiliac fracture dislocations.

If the patient remains hemodynamically labile after the application of an external stabilization device for a pelvic fracture, ongoing bleeding from branches of the internal iliac arteries must be considered as the source of hemorrhage. Arterial bleeding occurs in only 10% of patients with unstable pelvic fractures. In this patient population, pelvic arteriography with embolization of the bleeding vessel and collaterals is the optimal method of management. In situations in which interventional radiology is not available, exploratory laparotomy with ligation of the ipsilateral internal iliac artery and pelvic packing is a viable alternative, although this procedure has a reported mortality rate of 25%. Given the high mortality rate associated with intraperitoneal pelvic packing, Cothren described the technique of extraperitoneal pelvic packing, illustrating the placement of six laparotomy packs in adults and four in children (Fig. 1). In a recent review of pelvic ring injuries associated with hemodynamic instability, Papakostidis determined that a combined approach of early pelvic ring stabilization and tamponade of pelvic bleeding with extraperitoneal packing, followed by selective angioembolization when necessary, may provide the best survival advantage.

PHASE 2: RESUSCITATION IN THE INTENSIVE CARE UNIT

Following damage control procedures, patients are returned to the ICU for correction of their physiologic abnormalities, including hypothermia, acidosis, and coagulopathy. Aggressive correction of hypothermia is of paramount importance. External rewarming techniques include warming of the room and ventilator circuits and application of a Bair Hugger. All fluids and blood products should be given through a level I fluid warmer. In patients with severe hypothermia, defined as a temperature less than 32° C, consideration should be given to the use of body cavity lavage via a nasogastric tube, thoracostomy tubes, peritoneal lavage, or a Foley catheter. Recently, several external devices as well as indwelling catheters have been developed to facilitate systemic rewarming. Extracorporeal bypass is the most invasive and efficient rewarming technique that also provides circulatory support in patients with profound exposure-related hypothermia who are prone to cardiac dysrhythmias and cardiac arrest.

Patients who are acidotic after damage control procedures are most likely underresuscitated, and they require optimization of oxygen delivery for correction. Invasive monitoring, including central venous pressure monitoring or Swan-Ganz monitoring, may be necessary in the immediate postoperative period to guide resuscitative efforts. Alternatively, noninvasive measures of cardiac output may be used to guide resuscitative measures. Persistent acidosis in a

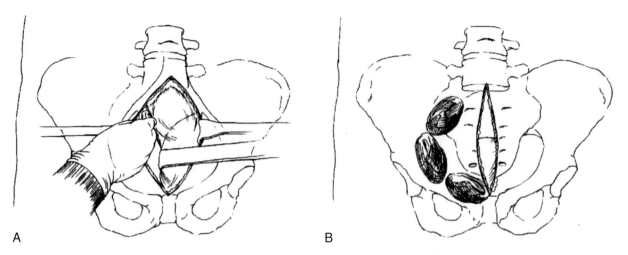

A   B

FIGURE I   A and **B,** Extraperitoneal pelvic packing. *(From Cothren CC, Osborn PM, Moore EE, et al: Preperitoneal pelvic packing for hemodynamically unstable pelvic fractures: a paradigm shift.* J Trauma *62:834–839, discussion 839–842, 2007.)*

patient felt to be adequately resuscitated may be due to a hyperchloremic acidosis following aggressive resuscitation with normal saline. An anion gap can be used to differentiate lactic acidosis from hyperchloremic acidosis. Hyperchloremic acidosis results in a narrowed anion gap, and lactic acidosis results in a widened anion gap.

Although correction of acidosis and hypothermia will aid in the correction of the coagulopathy seen after damage control procedures, these patients will require ongoing transfusion of fresh frozen plasma, cryoprecipitate, and platelets, or ongoing damage control resuscitation. All products should be delivered through fluid warmers to minimize the time to rewarming. Recombinant human factor VII has also been shown to be useful in this population, as it corrects coagulation defects rapidly, although its use has not been shown to decrease mortality risk.

PHASE 3: DEFINITIVE OPERATIVE MANAGEMENT

Following normalization of physiologic parameters, with particular attention to the correction of the lethal triad of hypothermia, acidosis, and coagulopathy, the patient should be returned to the operating room for definitive management of the previously temporized repairs. The timing of reoperation has not been standardized, but most trauma surgeons will return to the operating room within 48 to 72 hours, as reexploration prior to 72 hours is associated with decreased rates of morbidity and mortality.

During reexploration, a formal exploration is performed to identify any injuries that may have been missed during the damage control procedure. Previously placed packing is removed, and bleeding sites controlled. Intestinal continuity is reestablished. Small bowel injures may be safely managed with anastomosis, and colon injuries may be anastomosed or exteriorized, depending on the extent of the injury and the surgeon's level of concern. Consideration should be given to delayed primary closure of the abdominal wall fascia, although this may not be feasible if significant edema persists. Most patients (80%) can have their fascia primarily closed within 5 to 7 days of injury. Velcro closure devices may also be employed and can result in primary fascial closure up to 21 days following injury. Those who cannot are candidates for split thickness skin grafting of their open abdominal wound, after closure of the fascial defect with either a spanning vicryl or biologic mesh. Delayed repair of this planned ventral hernia can then occur after 6 to 12 months.

Following damage control thoracotomy, the patient may safely be returned to the operating room after correction of all physiologic derangements. Chest drainage (tube thoracostomy) and definitive thoracic closure are possible after removal of packing and control of bleeding or air leaks.

There is extensive literature indicating that the timing of definitive orthopedic stabilization should be delayed longer than 72 hours. It has been shown that days 2 to 4 after the initial damage control procedure are not optimal for definitive stabilization of orthopedic injuries, as this period is marked by ongoing systemic inflammatory response and generalized edema. A statistically significant increase in multisystem organ dysfunction has been reported in patients undergoing stabilization at 2 to 4 days compared to those patients who had their fractures stabilized at 6 to 8 days.

COMPLICATIONS FOLLOWING DAMAGE CONTROL SURGERY

Immediate Complications

The most common complication after damage control laparotomy is ACS. Despite liberal use of TAC methods, intraabdominal hypertension may occur due to increased visceral swelling, ongoing bleeding, and the mechanical effects of intraabdominal packing. Signs of ACS include a distended abdomen, increasing peak airway pressures, worsening acidosis, oliguria progressing to anuria, and decreased cardiac output with resultant systemic hypotension. The onset of ACS may be insidious or acute. Measurement of intravesical bladder pressure via a Foley catheter can be used as a surrogate for the intraabdominal pressure. A pressure greater than 25 mm Hg with evidence of physiologic compromise mandates abdominal decompression. Alternatively, an abdominal perfusion pressure may be determined (mean arterial pressure minus intraabdominal pressure); decompression should be performed for abdominal perfusion pressures less than 60 mm Hg. Decompression is accomplished by either reopening the previous laparotomy incision or adjusting the TAC. Primary ACS requires performing a midline laparotomy incision, which can be done in the ICU with conscious sedation. After decompressing the abdomen, there should be an immediate improvement in visceral perfusion, renal perfusion, cardiac function, and ventilatory mechanics.

Unplanned reoperation may be necessary in the patient with ongoing postoperative hemorrhage despite aggressive resuscitation and correction of the lethal triad. Indications for return to the operating room within the first 24 hours after a damage control procedure are listed in Box 2.

Continued bleeding and coagulopathy in the face of normothermia (>6–10 units of packed red blood cells within 12 hours)
Abdominal compartment syndrome
Ischemic tissue causing metabolic derangement
Gastrointestinal soilage of the abdomen after failed repair, missed injury, or staple line disruption

Modified with from Martin RR, Byrne M: Postoperative care and complications of damage control surgery. *Surg Clin North Am* 77:929–942, 1997.

Delayed Complications

Patients who undergo damage control procedures are at high risk of developing ARDS, MSOF, and death. The presence of sepsis, transfusion requirements of greater than 15 U of packed red blood cells, pulmonary injury, and long-bone fractures have been shown to be independent risk factors for posttraumatic ARDS. Shock, infections, multiple transfusions, and severe injury are all associated with late MSOF. Mortality rate following damage control surgery ranges from 20% to 67%. When formal closure of the abdominal wound is not accomplished within the first week after injury, the presence of an open abdomen increases the risk of fistula formation. These patients will require abdominal wall reconstruction at the time of fistula takedown.

SUMMARY

Damage control procedures are lifesaving in the multiply injured patient. Damage control allows life-threatening issues to be addressed expeditiously during truncated operative procedures. Normal physiology is then restored in the ICU. The ability to stage the definitive surgery allows correction of the lethal triad of hypothermia, coagulopathy, and acidosis and results in improved survival in patients who previously would have died of their injuries.

For the chapter's Suggested Readings list, please visit the book at www.ExpertConsult.inkling.com.

ABDOMINAL COMPARTMENT SYNDROME, DAMAGE CONTROL, AND THE OPEN ABDOMEN

Oliver L. Gunter, Jr., Nathan J. Powell, and Richard S. Miller

Current critical care supportive measures make it possible for patients with severe injuries and physiologic impairment to survive what otherwise might have been lethal conditions. One of the major surgical consequences of extensive resuscitation efforts regards the condition of the abdominal wall. Although the objective should be to always close the abdomen following laparotomy, primary closure may be technically impossible or deleterious owing to any number of conditions. In this chapter, we will discuss the management of the posttraumatic abdominal wall, beginning with a discussion of abdominal compartment syndrome (ACS). This will be followed by a review of damage control principles and temporary abdominal closure (TAC). The chapter will conclude with a discussion of special considerations of the open abdomen, including abdominal wall reconstruction, nutritional support, and outcomes.

ABDOMINAL COMPARTMENT SYNDROME

The effects of intraabdominal hypertension (IAH) were first described in 19th century by Marey and Burt, who identified the relationship between intrathoracic pressure and elevated intraabdominal pressure (IAP). The term "abdominal compartment syndrome" was popularized over a century later when Kron and associates and Richards and colleagues reported separate series of patients who developed tense abdominal distention with elevated pulmonary pressures and increased IAPs postoperatively despite normal mean arterial blood pressure and cardiac performance. All of these patients improved with abdominal decompression. Although primary compartment syndrome may develop as a direct result of intraabdominal injuries, ACS has also been shown to develop as a consequence of resuscitation in the absence of abdominal injuries and thus should be considered potentially preventable (Fig. 1).

Owing to the wide variety of proposed definitions, the World Congress on Abdominal Compartment Syndrome (WCACS) was established and has endorsed a definitive classification system. IAH is defined as IAP higher than 12 mm Hg and is further graded from I to IV (Box 1).

Generically, a compartment syndrome is a condition in which increased pressure in a confined space adversely effects the circulation and threatens the function and viability of the tissue within the space. Compartment syndromes may occur in the extremities, orbital globe, cranium, and abdominal cavity. ACS refers to a clinical entity in which IAH reduces blood flow to abdominal organs and impairs pulmonary, cardiovascular, renal, and gastrointestinal (GI) function. The development of ACS is dependent on both the degree of IAH as well as the rate of pressure increase. The definition of ACS according to the WCACS is IAP higher than 20 mm Hg with new onset of multiple organ failure (Fig. 2).

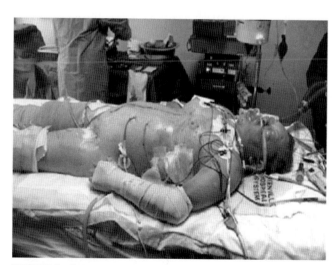

FIGURE I Postoperative trauma patient at high risk for abdominal compartment syndrome.

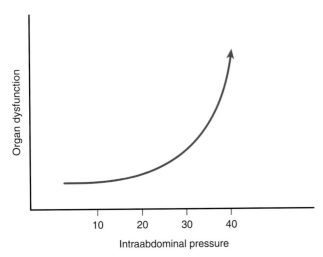

FIGURE 2 Progressive organ dysfunction with worsening intraabdominal pressure.

ACS may be further characterized as follows:

1. *Primary/acute*: Intraabdominal injury is directly and proximally responsible for the compartment syndrome.
2. *Secondary*: No visible intraabdominal injury is present but injuries outside the abdomen cause fluid accumulation. (Differentiation between the primary and secondary ACS may be important as secondary ACS has been shown to have a worse outcome.)
3. *Chronic*: ACS occurs in the presence of cirrhosis and ascites, often in the later stages of the disease.

Worsening compartment syndrome leads to fulminant multiple organ dysfunction, and if left untreated, it is typically fatal. Critical care management in severely injured patients at risk for developing ACS should center on prevention as well as early recognition of signs and symptoms of IAH.

Although the cause of ACS is poorly understood, it represents a hyperinflammatory response and response to shock (Fig. 3). The anatomic effects of ACS begin with the direct compression of intra- and retroperitoneal structures. Especially affected are low-pressure systems such as the intestinal tract and venous systems, which collapse.

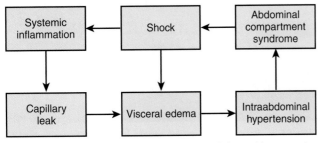

FIGURE 3 A cycle of ischemia producing intraabdominal hypertension and the abdominal compartment syndrome.

TABLE 1: Effects of Intraabdominal Hypertension on Organ Systems

Organ or Structure	Effect
Head	↑ Intracranial pressure
	↓ Cerebral perfusion pressure
Heart	↓ Cardiac output
	↓ Venous return
	↑ Pulmonary artery occlusion pressure and central venous pressure
	↑ Systemic vascular resistance
Lungs	↑ Peak inspiratory pressure
	↑ Pulmonary artery wedge pressure
	↓ Dynamic compliance (Cdyn)
	↑ Arterial oxygen pressure (Pao_2)
	↑ Arterial carbon dioxide pressure ($Paco_2$)
	↑ Intrapulmonary shunt (Qsp/Qt)
	↑ Fraction of dead space to total expired tidal volume (V_D/V_T)
Liver	↓ Portal flow
	↓ Mitochondria
	↑ Lactate
Kidney	↓ Urine output
	↓ Renal flow
	↓ Glomerular filtration rate (GFR)
Intestines	↓ Celiac flow
	↓ Superior mesenteric arterial (SMA) flow
	↓ Mucosal flow
Abdominal wall	↓ Compliance
	↓ Rectus flow

Immediate effects such as thrombosis or bowel wall edema may be accompanied by translocation of bacterial products leading to additional fluid accumulation, further increasing IAP (Table 1). At the cellular level, oxygen delivery is impaired leading to ischemia and anaerobic metabolism. Vasoactive substances such as histamine and serotonin increase endothelial permeability, and further capillary leakage impairs red blood cell transport, and ischemia worsens. Although current practice management guidelines come as a result of experiences with the development of ACS in the trauma setting, it is important to recognize that the role for damage control laparotomy and open abdomen management is not exclusive to the trauma population. Various medical and surgical conditions including diffuse peritonitis, acute pancreatitis, and mesenteric ischemia may potentially expose the patient to an increased risk of developing IAH and ACS (Box 2).

Other risk factors for the development of ACS include ascites or intraabdominal fluid accumulation, intra- or retroperitoneal hemorrhage/hematoma, requirement of renal replacement therapy, pregnancy, abdominal burns, massive volume resuscitation, abdominal packing for control of hemorrhage, reperfusion injury following bowel ischemia, ileus and bowel obstruction, intraabdominal masses, and closure of the abdomen under undue tension.

The most practical and reliable method of measuring IAPs is through the urinary bladder, which acts as a passive conduit. The urinary bladder transmits IAPs without imparting any additional pressures from its own musculature. Saline is injected into the fully drained bladder. A Foley catheter is clamped distal to the aspiration port and a 16-G needle is inserted into this port, which is then attached to a transducer system with the iliac crest used as the zero reference point. Commercial kits are also available for measuring bladder pressures.

Prevention of ACS requires identification of an at-risk patient, timely surgical intervention for the primary problem (e.g., hemorrhage), and judicious fluid management. Medical management is limited to sedation/chemical paralysis, gastric and bladder decompression, reduced tidal volume ventilator strategies, fluid restriction, and diuresis. However, more severe forms of compartment syndrome necessitate surgical intervention, including early decompressive laparotomy. Although decompression can be performed safely as a bedside procedure in the intensive care unit (ICU), hemorrhagic sources of ACS may be best managed in the operating room (Fig. 4). Once completed, decompressive laparotomy often rapidly reverses adverse effects of ACS and improves oxygenation and pulmonary compliance, returning peak inspiratory pressures toward normal and promptly reversing the oliguria with brisk diuresis. Before decompression, attempts to correct acid-base and electrolyte disturbances (including potassium, magnesium, and calcium imbalance) may avoid cardiac dysrhythmias after decompression. Maintenance of the open

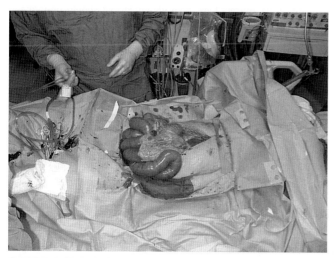

FIGURE 4   Bedside decompressive celiotomy for abdominal compartment syndrome. Note massive small bowel edema.

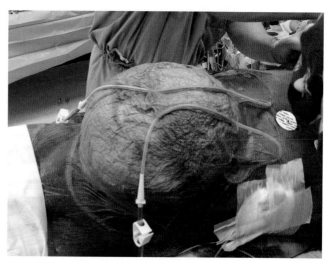

FIGURE 5   Temporary abdominal closure with vacuum pack device.

abdomen after decompression necessitates the maintenance of an open abdomen or laparostomy with TAC (Fig. 5).

Untreated ACS is presumed to be uniformly fatal, although survival rate may be limited to as low as 50% despite abdominal decompression. Although IAH is part of the progression to ACS, IAH alone may not adversely affect outcome such as multiple organ failure and fatality. In terms of prevention of ACS, identification of IAH is essential so that medical or surgical measures may be undertaken to halt the progression of the syndrome.

DAMAGE CONTROL

Damage control surgery represents one of the major advances in the surgical management of patients in extremis over the past 20 years. Traditionally, damage control has been defined as follows:

1. Rapid control of bleeding and contamination
2. TAC
3. Physiologic resuscitation of metabolic failure
4. Delayed definitive operation

This paradigm shift in the surgical management of the multi-injured trauma patient evolved with the recognition that patients in extremis were more likely to die from their intraoperative metabolic failure than from a failure to complete operative repairs. Characterized in part by the "lethal triad" of coagulopathy, hypothermia, and metabolic acidosis, metabolic failure frequently results in death. The impetus is on the operating surgeon to recognize this physiology and anticipate the need to perform damage control based on a rapid initial injury inventory because a failure to do so may increase risk for fatality.

However, in an effort to solve one problem, another has been created: the posttraumatic open abdomen, defined as a large postoperative ventral hernia with the abdominal viscera covered by a temporary dressing or closure. Many lessons have been learned in managing the complications associated with these critically ill patients and through these lessons, four essential principles in the management of the open abdomen have evolved:

1. Protection of the bowel
2. Preservation of the fascia to prevent domain loss
3. Early fascial closure if at all possible
4. Minimizing planned ventral hernia and delayed reconstruction

One of the earliest descriptions of damage control techniques was by Pringle in 1908 who described the use of gauze packs for hemorrhage control in the setting of hepatic trauma. Although these techniques were later discouraged based on wartime experience, interest in an abbreviated abdominal operation for severe trauma was rekindled toward the latter half of the 20th century. With the first description of the "bail out" technique in Harlan Stone's seminal paper, the era of abbreviated laparotomy and damage control was initiated. Rotondo and colleagues' description of improved survival when "damage control" techniques were applied to patients with severe abdominal vascular injuries helped fuel the paradigm shift away from the surgical dictum that a trauma patient's first operation must be definitive. The current management scheme of damage control has been revised to include four stages (Fig. 6).

The initial preoperative assessment and resuscitation of a patient with massive hemorrhage in the emergency department can be considered as a preface to the damage control continuum (DC0). The highest priorities during DC0 are (1) identification of an exsanguinating patient and (2) initiation of blood and coagulation factor therapy while (3) preparing for definitive hemorrhage control. Resuscitation must be provided judiciously as high-volume resuscitation of blood products, coagulation factors, and crystalloid solutions may be associated with the development of ACS. Large-volume crystalloid-based resuscitation should be discouraged as this not only increases IAH but also contributes to worsening of bleeding and coagulopathy in the setting of hemorrhage. Early hemostatic resuscitation is preferred with whole blood or component therapy to reverse the effects of trauma-induced coagulopathy and shock. There is growing evidence to support hypotensive resuscitation which centers on maintenance of circulation and hemostasis irrespective of normalization of hemodynamic parameters particularly in the setting of vascular injuries. Despite some controversy in the literature, numerous reports have shown that massive transfusion with a high ratio of plasma and platelets to red blood cells improves survival an exsanguinating patients and may decrease overall transfusion requirements.

During the initial trauma celiotomy (DC1), it is important to estimate each patient's physiologic reserve in order to make appropriate

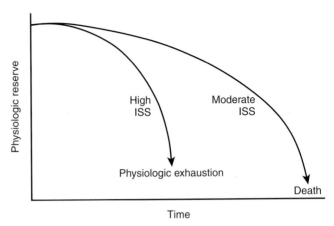

FIGURE 7 Depletion of physiologic reserve as a consequence of injury severity. ISS, Injury Severity Score.

operative decisions. Physiologic reserve is defined as an individual's unique ability to tolerate injury and is a function of several host factors including age, gender, preexisting disease, genetics, and immunocompetence. This is best performed by assessing the inventory of injuries in the context of each individual patient's physiology and estimated reserve. Accordingly, the extent of injury severity determines the slope leading to physiologic exhaustion (Fig. 7). As physiologic reserve becomes depleted during hemorrhagic shock, regional and then global malperfusion occur, leading to physiologic exhaustion and subsequent death.

Perioperative communication with the anesthesia team enhances survival and reduces complications. This communication includes maintaining the operating room as warm as possible, advising the anesthesia personnel of anticipated blood loss, and avoiding overresuscitation before surgical control of hemorrhage.

During the initial trauma celiotomy, the surgeon must recognize the need for immediate control of major hemorrhage and contamination with maximum replacement of coagulation factors including platelets, fresh frozen plasma, and cryoprecipitate, and in certain circumstances factor VIIa for microvascular bleeding. Intraoperative monitoring of temperature, arterial blood gases, and volume of resuscitation are important in determining whether a patient is descending down the physiologic curve toward physiologic exhaustion. In addition, for patients suffering hollow viscus injuries, contamination is controlled with linear staples to transect the bowel ends and leave them in discontinuity until the patient can physiologically tolerate definitive reconstruction.

Clinical parameters have been identified that should prompt the surgical team to initiate damage control maneuvers, abort the operation, and return to the ICU for resuscitation and restoration of reserve (DC2) (Table 2). Damage control should be instituted early, well before reaching the upper limits of physiologic exhaustion. Using these intraoperative predictors of the need for damage control, Asensio and associates, in a follow-up study, proved that patients with posttraumatic open abdomen incurred less hypothermia and fewer postoperative complications including intraabdominal abscess and fistula formation. Patients with early damage control were also subjectively noted to have less bowel edema and were more likely to undergo definitive abdominal wall closure during their initial hospitalization.

Asensio and colleagues, in a hallmark study involving 548 patients who exsanguinated and required damage control, described and statistically validated criteria to enable the early institution of damage control. These criteria include pH lower than 7.2, HCO_3^- 15 mEq/L or less; temperature 34° C or lower, $\geq$12 XXX volume replaced, and up to 4000 mL (10 to 12 units) of packed red blood cells (PRBCs).

Once a patient fulfills the requirements for damage control or is decompressed for signs and symptoms of ACS, the surgeon must commit the patient to the posttraumatic open abdomen and a TAC (Box 3).

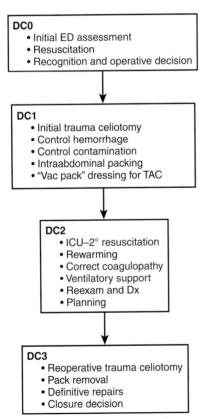

DC0
- Initial ED assessment
- Resuscitation
- Recognition and operative decision

DC1
- Initial trauma celiotomy
- Control hemorrhage
- Control contamination
- Intraabdominal packing
- "Vac pack" dressing for TAC

DC2
- ICU–2° resuscitation
- Rewarming
- Correct coagulopathy
- Ventilatory support
- Reexam and Dx
- Planning

DC3
- Reoperative trauma celiotomy
- Pack removal
- Definitive repairs
- Closure decision

FIGURE 6 Algorithm for damage control. DC, Damage control; Dx, diagnosis; ED, emergency department; ICU, intensive care unit; TAC, temporary abdominal closure.

TABLE 2: Clinical Guidelines to Abort Initial Trauma Celiotomy and Initiate Damage Control Maneuvers

Problem	Description
Hypothermia	<35° C
Acidosis	pH <7.2
	Base deficit (BD) ≥ –8 mEq/L
	Lactate ≥4
Coagulopathy	Activated partial thromboplastin time (aPTT) >60
	International normalized ratio (INR) >1.6
Ongoing resuscitation	Persistent shock systolic blood pressure <90 mm Hg
	>10 L crystalloid
	>10 units packed red blood cells
Operative time	>60–90 minutes with abdominal cavity opened

BOX 3 Indications for Temporary Abdominal Closure

Depletion of physiologic reserve
Unable to close fascia without undue tension secondary to bowel edema
To avoid development of abdominal compartment syndrome after large fluid resuscitation
Planned return to operating room
Unpacking
Reestablish bowel continuity
Enteral access
Thorough exploration to reevaluate known injuries and identify missed injuries
Associated need for management of extraabdominal life-threatening injuries (e.g., major pelvic fracture, severe closed head injury)

Temporary Abdominal Closure

TAC is defined as any technique that contains the abdominal viscera during the acute phase of care. Historically, a wide variety of techniques for TAC have been used to contain the abdominal viscera during the acute phase of care (Box 4). Despite multiple options for TAC, our opinion is that the "vacuum pack" technique best fulfills the first two principles in the management of the posttraumatic open abdomen: (1) protecting the bowel and (2) preserving the fascia. This method, as described by Barker and associates, protects the bowel and abdominal viscera by placing a perforated, nonadherent material plastic material over the abdominal contents placed in a subfascial position. This is followed by placement of a surgical towel with two large drains which are brought out through the superior portion

BOX 4 Options for Temporary Abdominal Closure

Bogota bag
Towel clips
Zipper
Wittman patch
Skin-only closure
Barker vacuum pack
Negative pressure wound systems
Prosthetic mesh
Gauze packs

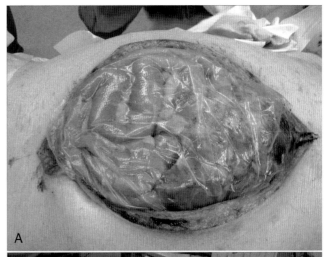

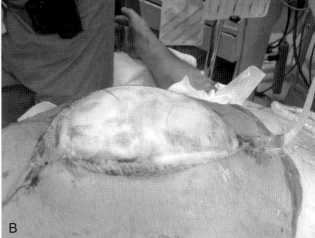

FIGURE 8 Vacuum pack temporary abdominal closure. **A,** Bowel isolation bag. **B,** Sterile surgical towel with large drains and adhesive barrier.

of the wound (Fig. 8). The entire abdominal defect is covered with a large adhesive dressing and the drains are attached to wall suction to create continuous negative pressure. This technique also counteracts the lateral retraction of the fascial edges and preserves the rectus musculofascial complex for subsequent closure (Box 5).

The ultimate goal in the management of the open abdomen is to achieve delayed primary fascial closure. However, certain clinical scenarios preclude closure or present technical challenges to successful primary fascial closure, and continued open abdomen management may be necessary. These patients may demonstrate ongoing contamination and physiologic insult, a prolonged inflammatory response with grossly distended viscera, an anticipated need for reoperation in 12 to 96 hours, or loss of abdominal domain. In these patients, serial TAC is indicated while strategies for a delayed primary closure versus abdominal wall reconstruction are made.

BOX 5 Advantages of Vacuum Pack Technique

Protects bowel and keeps it below fascia
Preserves fascia and prevents loss of domain
Readily available, rapidly applied, easily removed
Keeps patient dry and maintains hygiene
Quantifies fluid loss
Prevents intraabdominal hypertension/abdominal compartment syndrome
Simple, atraumatic, and inexpensive

Definitive Reconstruction and Closure (DC3)

Three potential stages follow TAC:

1. Resuscitation in the ICU until physiologic end points of resuscitation are met
2. Restoration, or reoperation and attempts at early fascial closure (days to weeks)
3. Reconstruction, or planned ventral hernia and delayed fascia closure

Resuscitation

The goals of the resuscitation in the ICU after damage control or decompressive celiotomy for ACS are repayment of the sustained oxygen debt, restoration of adequate perfusion to meet metabolic needs, and reversal of hemorrhagic shock. This includes coagulopathy correction, clearance of lactic acidosis, correcting electrolyte disturbances, and rewarming (Box 6). Serial monitoring of abdominal pressure should be considered as the risk of ACS is high in this patient population. For patients exhibit ongoing blood transfusion requirement despite normalization of temperature, acid-base status, and coagulopathy, prompt surgical reexploration should be considered as this would indicate inadequate hemorrhage control.

Additional resuscitative measures during ICU management also include the use of arteriography and embolization, especially for severe pelvic arterial hemorrhage and extensive hepatic vascular injuries. Extremity and pelvic fractures can also be temporarily realigned with the use of external fixators, deferring complex orthopedic reconstruction until later stages in the patient's course when the inflammatory response has dissipated.

Restoration

After ICU resuscitation and correction of physiologic and hemodynamic derangements that occurred during the initial trauma celiotomy or after decompression for ACS, patients with a TAC are returned to the operating room for further evaluation. During this reexploration, the surgeon must once again make important clinical and technical decisions. All retained perihepatic and intraabdominal lap pads are carefully removed, preventing dislodgement of clot over liver injuries and avoiding serosal tears from lap pads that are adherent to the bowel. A reevaluation of the known injuries and a thorough exploration to identify missed injuries are undertaken. If bowel resection was necessary during the initial damage control celiotomy, establishment of GI continuity is performed and enteral access is established. It is important to protect suture or staple lines and place them deep within the peritoneal cavity and attempt to cover the anastomosis with unaffected bowel loops or omentum. If ostomy creation is necessary, placement should keep subsequent restorative procedures and possible abdominal wall reconstruction in mind. The risk of anastomotic failure is increased after damage control laparotomy, despite physiologic restoration in the ICU. Careful consideration of intestinal diversion should be undertaken in this setting.

Nasoenteric feeding tubes or surgical placed enteral access procedures should be performed during the reconstructive phase. Either a nasoenteric feeding tube placed past the ligament of Treitz with nasogastric decompression or an open gastrojejunostomy feeding tube are options for long-term enteral access and supplemental nutrition.

Washout and evacuation of any further hematoma is performed, and a plan on definitive closure is made. If bowel edema is minimal or completely resolved and the fascial edges can be easily approximated without undue tension, then a primary fascial closure can be performed. Communication with the anesthesia team is essential during closure, particularly with regard to ventilation pressures. If the peak inspiratory pressures rise higher than 10 mm Hg from baseline during fascial approximation, attempts at primary fascial closure should be abandoned. Closure under excessive tension can result in abdominal wall necrosis, recurrent ACS, serious infectious complications, and respiratory insufficiency. Routine postoperative radiologic evaluation of the abdominal cavity on all patients must be obtained if the fascia is successfully closed at this stage to ensure that no unplanned retained foreign body remains.

BOX 6 Intensive Care Unit Resuscitation Checklist

Rewarming/Correct Hypothermia
Cordis introducer central line
Rapid infuser (level I) with heat exchanger set at 40° C
Infuse warm intravenous (IV) fluids, blood, blood products
Humidifier on vent set at 40° C
Convection air warmer (Bair Hugger)
Placed over entire torso
Cover hands, feet, head
Prevent insensible heat loss
Keep ambient temperature >85° F

Correct Coagulopathy, Acidosis, Electrolyte Imbalance
Measure hemoglobin and hematocrit, prothrombin time, partial prothrombin time, international normalized ratio (INR), platelet count, fibrinogen
Replace with packed red blood cells, fresh frozen plasma, platelets, cryoprecipitate, ± factor VIIa
Normalize arterial lactate, base deficit, correct K^+, Mg^+, Ca^+ deficiency

Monitoring
Insert oximetric pulmonary artery catheter to maintain oxygen delivery and obtain end points of resuscitation
Do_2I (oxygen delivery index) 500 mL/minute
Cardiac index (CI) >3 L/minute
End-diastolic volume index (EDVI) 120–140 mL
Arterial oxygen saturation (Sao_2) >95%
Venous oxygen saturation (Svo_2) >65%
Temperature >36.5° C

Hematocrit >21%
Check for adrenal insufficiency if not responding to resuscitation
Random cortisol level
Adrenocorticotropic hormone (ACTH) stimulation test

Medications
Peptic ulcer prophylaxis
H_2 blockers or proton pump inhibitor
Deep venous thrombosis (DVT) prophylaxis
Low-molecular-weight heparin
Sequential compression devices
Insulin drip
Maintain blood glucose 80–110 mg/dL
IV analgesia and sedation
Continuous drips
Broad-spectrum antibiotics × 24 hours or until intraabdominal packs out
Cover gram-negative organisms and anaerobes

Nursing
Elevate head of bed (HOB) 30 degrees
Thoracic, lumbar, and sacral spine cleared
Frequent tracheal suctioning and oral hygiene
Functioning nasogastric tube
Wall suction for vacuum-pack sump drains
Foley catheter
Check hourly urine output
Check bladder pressures
Pad pressure points to reduce incidence decubiti (occiput, chin, scapulas, sacrum, heels)

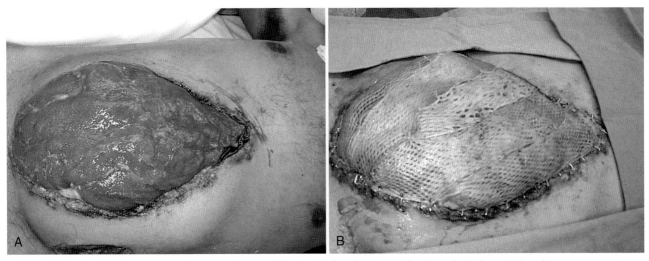

FIGURE 9   **A** and **B,** Mature granulation tissue in an open abdomen, which is then covered with a split-thickness skin graft.

If the abdomen cannot be closed by the end of the first week, granulation tissue may start to develop, and a "frozen abdomen" is evident by the end of the second week. This creates a hostile environment for early fascial closure and thus necessitates a planned ventral hernia with a delayed reconstruction. Because of the concern for increased morbidity when definitive closure is significantly delayed, we have advocated attempting definitive closure by the eighth postoperative day. In the setting of absorbable mesh with development of granulation tissue, split-thickness skin graft (STSG) maybe applied over the granulation bed, and the patient then requires a 6- to 12-month recovery period for protein and calorie stores to be replenished before successful abdominal wall reconstruction can be performed (Fig. 9). This decision, although lifesaving, is very costly and is associated with a loss of productive lifestyle and an inability to return to the workforce.

Although absorbable mesh implantation had been routine practice in many centers, the complexities associated with the development of "enteroatmospheric" fistulas in the wound bed have prompted investigation into alternative techniques. Polyglactin mesh has been widely used because of its absorbability and promotion of the development of granulation tissue even when used in a contaminated field. Despite these advantages, incidence of enterocutaneous fistula has been shown to be as high as 21% to 25% of patients closed with polyglactin mesh. Because of the high complication rate under these circumstances, an aggressive approach to obtaining primary fascial closure or closure with the use of biologic material in the posttraumatic open abdomen has been described. Alternative approaches use a combination of the vacuum pack, negative pressure wound devices, and bioprosthetic materials to bridge the gap in the abdominal fascia, even up to 3 weeks after initial damage control procedures or decompressive celiotomy.

Similar to the vacuum pack, there are multiple negative-pressure wound vacuum systems available on the market that use sponge-like material enclosed within an adhesive barrier (Fig. 10). These devices serve the goals of protecting the bowel and preserving the fascia while recapturing loss of abdominal domain (Box 7).

Unlike synthetic prosthetic materials, which the body recognizes as foreign and leads to encapsulation, bioprosthetic materials support cellular growth and integration with rapid revascularization and transition to the patient's own tissue. These materials serve as a bioscaffold for the native autologous tissue (Fig. 11). The tissue used for these implants may be obtained from bovine, porcine, or human sources following chemical treatment to render them biocompatible and minimize immunogenicity. Bioprosthetic materials are tolerant of contamination and can be used for closure in situations in which synthetic material is contraindicated (Fig. 12). On a cellular level, biologic mesh implants may have higher initial strength when chemically cross-linked; however, native tissue ingrowth is impaired, resulting in encapsulation that is akin to reaction seen with nonbiologic prosthetic implants.

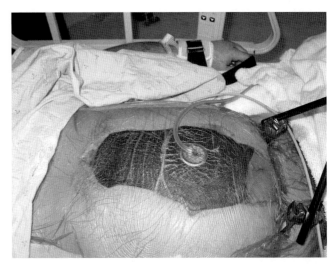

FIGURE 10   Vacuum-assisted wound device. Note external fixator from damage control orthopedic procedure.

BOX 7   Advantages of Negative-Pressure Wound Systems

Reduced need for frequent dressing changes
Removes excess interstitial fluid
Increases vascularity of wound
Decreased bacterial counts
Improves wound contraction
Delays onset of "frozen abdomen"—prevents granulation tissue adhering to fascia
Extends window of opportunity for definitive fascial closure

Even though long-term results regarding recurrence rates and the development of abdominal wall laxity are not yet available, this method of fascial approximation certainly has significant advantages over the planned ventral hernia method of management with its inherent high risk of wound complications as mentioned previously. The combination of negative-pressure wound dressings and adjunct use of bioprosthetic mesh fulfills the final essential principle with posttraumatic open abdomen: early abdominal wall closure.

Reconstruction

Once the window of opportunity for early primary fascial closure has passed secondary to an ongoing inflammatory response and bowel

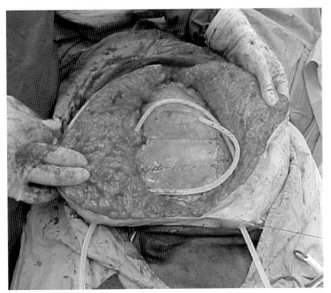

FIGURE 11   Biologic prosthetic implant with overlying skin flaps for abdominal wall reconstruction.

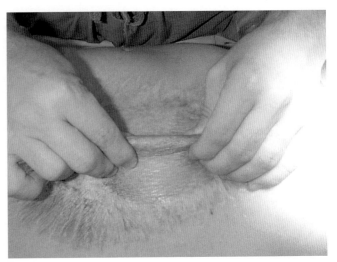

FIGURE 13   Pinch test.

edema, a delayed staged closure of the abdominal wall is necessary. Because the open abdomen group remains at high risk for infectious complications, the use of synthetic prosthetic material for reconstruction is not recommended for definitive reconstruction, although staged repair with eventual prosthetic explanation has been described. Once the STSG can be elevated from the underlying intestines, the inflammatory response can be assumed to have resolved and the underlying viscera are typically mobile (Fig. 13). This tissue separation usually requires 6 to 12 months to occur and is essential to prevent bowel injury during reconstruction. The STSG is removed and the fascia is mobilized from the surrounding tissue. The skin and subcutaneous tissue are then raised as lateral flaps circumferentially (Fig. 14). Options for bridging the fascial gap at this point include the component separation technique and closure with bioprosthetic material.

The component separation technique reconstructs the fascial defect with advancement flaps by transecting the external oblique just lateral to its insertion into the rectus sheath and separating it from the internal oblique. The rectus muscle can then be advanced medially and sutured in the midline to close the defect (Fig. 15). This technique can approximate a 10-cm defect without undo tension. Using the modified component separation technique several more centimeters of mobility can be obtained by separating the rectus muscle from the posterior rectus sheath. The recurrence rate with unreinforced component separation alone is 22% to 32%. Therefore, our current practice is to complement this procedure with the use of bioprosthetic implant.

Damage control techniques and preventive measures to avoid the development of ACS are now the standards of care in the management

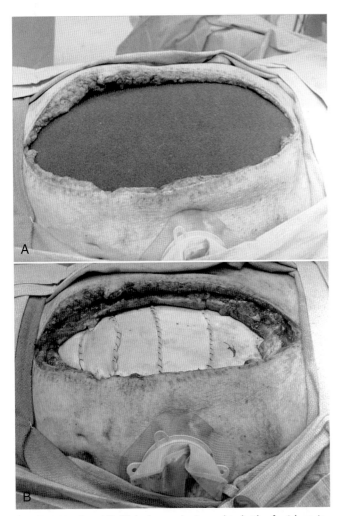

FIGURE 12   **A** and **B,** Biologic prosthetic used to bridge fascial gap in contaminated open abdomen wound with negative-pressure wound system placed over the biologic fascial replacement.

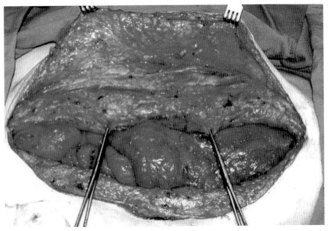

FIGURE 14   Fascial edges freed from surrounding tissue and skin flaps raised past lateral edge of the rectus muscle.

COMPONENT SEPARATION CLOSURE

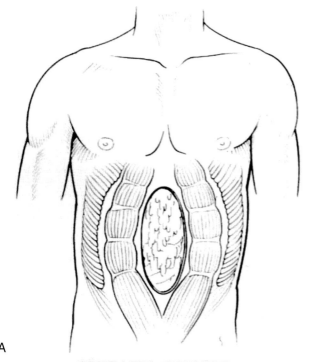

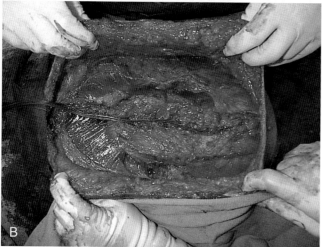

FIGURE 15   A and **B,** Component separation technique.

of traumatic shock. Using a vacuum pack for TAC during the early stages of resuscitation protects the bowel and preserves the fascia. Complications can then be avoided by not attempting to close the fascia under great tension and maintaining abdominal domain during the recovery phase with the use of the KCI VAC. Multiple attempts at fascial closure can then be safely performed either primarily or with the use of biologic material to bridge the fascial gap during initial hospitalization.

It is no longer desirable to commit the posttrauma open abdomen patient to a large ventral hernia and delayed reconstruction except for unusual circumstances when a prolonged inflammatory response precludes early fascial approximation.

▌ SPECIAL CONSIDERATIONS: NUTRITION SUPPORT

After damage control surgery, a large abdominal wound defect is created during the period of greatest physiologic stress with ongoing metabolic demands and catabolism. Therefore, close attention to nutritional support and caloric needs is essential to reduce both early and late complications. Ideally, nutritional support in the open abdomen should be initiated during the restoration phase, after intraabdominal packing is removed, GI continuity reestablished, and coagulopathy, acidosis, and hypothermia are corrected.

Superiority of enteral versus parenteral nutrition in those trauma patients without an open abdomen has been repeatedly demonstrated in the literature over the past decade. Benefits of nutrition via enteral route include improved wound healing, decreased infection risk, reduced length of stay, and improved survival from injury and illness.

During hemorrhagic shock and multitrauma, gut mucosal blood flow is decreased and remains below normal levels despite volume resuscitation. This decreased blood flow is associated with microbe translocation, ischemic bowel, and eventual multiorgan failure. Enteral feeding has been shown to improve gut mucosal integrity by preventing atrophy and abnormal permeability. Some studies have suggested immune benefits from "early" initiation of enteral nutrition (within 24–48 hours). Despite these findings, there continues to be reluctance and uncertainty about the use, safety, and timing of enteral nutrition in the critically ill and patients with laparostomy. Reasons cited for withholding enteral feeds in those patients with open abdomen include fear of intolerance, development of intestinal ileus and bowel edema, potential for aspiration, risk of small bowel necrosis and poor absorption with vasopressor use, fear of difficulties with glucose control, and contraindication of enteral feeds with the presence of bowel discontinuity following damage control surgery (Box 8). Parenteral nutrition, when compared to enteral nutrition, is considerably more expensive to manufacture and administer, requires frequent monitoring of electrolytes, and may be associated with significant complications such as central-line complications, central-line associated bloodstream infections, intestinal villous atrophy with possible bacterial translocation, metabolic disorders, and biliary stasis.

Tsuei demonstrated the feasibility of enteral nutrition in open abdomen patients, with the majority of patients being fed postpylorically (75%), achieving 77% of caloric needs. Early enteral nutrition (i.e., within 36 hours) may not also lead to a substantial reduction in incidence of ventilator-associated pneumonia with no adverse effect on abdominal closure rate after damage control. More recent studies have suggested that early enteral nutrition may be associated with earlier fascial closure along with a decrease in the rate of enterocutaneous fistula formation.

Our current recommendation is to initiate enteral nutrition in the early postresuscitation phase of care provided the bowel is in continuity regardless of the status of the abdominal wall. Obtaining enteral access should be considered a high priority in damage control patients, particularly for those in whom a protracted course is predicted. In these circumstances, early enteral nutrition should be supplemented with parenteral nutrition to reach acceptable protein and calorie goals. In addition, enteral nutrition can continue safely during other extra-abdominal operations and procedures.

BOX 8 Reasons for Withholding Enteral Nutrition

Concern for intolerance
Adynamic ileus
Bowel edema
Aspiration risk
Concern for small bowel necrosis in the setting of pressors
Poor absorption
Difficulties with insulin and glucose management
Bowel discontinuity after damage control
Clinician preference/discomfort

OUTCOMES AND COMPLICATIONS OF OPEN ABDOMEN

Multiple studies have validated the use of open abdomen in those patients with DCC and ACS, citing improved survival decreased morbidity, and improved long-term outcomes. Although maintaining an open abdomen is a potentially lifesaving maneuver in patients with ACS or those trauma patients necessitating damage control laparotomy, this management strategy places the patient at risk for potentially devastating complications. Mortality rate associated with damage control after trauma has been estimated as high as 31%, commonly attributed to the consequences of multiple organ system failure.

Other complications include increased transfusion requirements, increased ICU use and hospital charges, fistula formation, abdominal hernia, and significant fluid, electrolyte, and protein losses from the exposed viscera. Health care–associated infections such as surgical site infections, bloodstream infections, and ventilator-associated pneumonias have also been shown to be increased in those patients with persistent open abdomens (Table 3).

In 2005, Miller et al published their experience of 344 patients with open abdomen; morbidity associated with the open abdomen was quoted as 25%, with achievement of primary fascial closure in 65%. Primary fascial closure within the first week after the initial celiotomy was associated with a very low complication rate (9%). However, the complication rate increased significantly with three circumstances:

1. Attempts at closing the fascia primarily under too much tension
2. Awaiting the formation of granulation tissue before applying a STSG
3. Using nonbiologic prosthetic material for closure

Complications from delay in abdominal closure include wound infection, abscess, and wound dehiscence, the incidence of which increases significantly after 8 days from the initial intervention (Fig. 16). It should also be noted that although we would advocate primary abdominal wall closure when feasible, the long-term outcomes of primary closure in the setting of damage control/open abdomen remains unknown. Vogel et al substantiated these conclusions by associating higher incidences of surgical site infections, bloodstream infections, and ventilator-associated pneumonias in those patients with persistent open abdomens.

Mortality rate associated with damage control has been estimated as high as 31%, commonly attributed to the consequences of multiple organ system failure.

Arguably, one of the most devastating complication from persistent open abdomen is fistula formation, an expensive, labor-intensive, and morbid complication. The cause of fistula formation is multifactorial and includes the presence of abdominal infection, bowel ischemia and obstruction, inadvertent enterotomy, exposure of the bowel to atmospheric air for prolonged periods (causing desiccation), and the use of packs, dressings, or prosthetic materials that adhere to the serosa of the intestines (Fig. 17). Protecting the exposed abdominal viscera

TABLE 3: Complications Associated with Open Abdomen

Abdominal	Extra-abdominal
Wound infection	Ventilator-associated pneumonia
Wound dehiscence	Aspiration pneumonitis
Abdominal wall fasciitis/necrosis	Bloodstream infection
Intraabdominal abscess/sepsis	Urinary tract infection
Enteroatmospheric fistula	Deep venous thrombosis/pulmonary embolism
	Pressure ulcers (occiput, scapulas, sacrum, heels)
	Multiple organ dysfunction syndrome/ multiple organ system failure

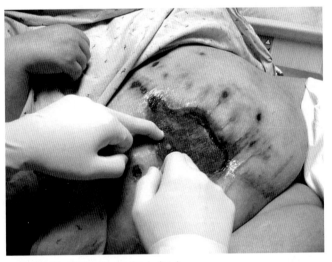

FIGURE 17 Enteroatmospheric fistula.

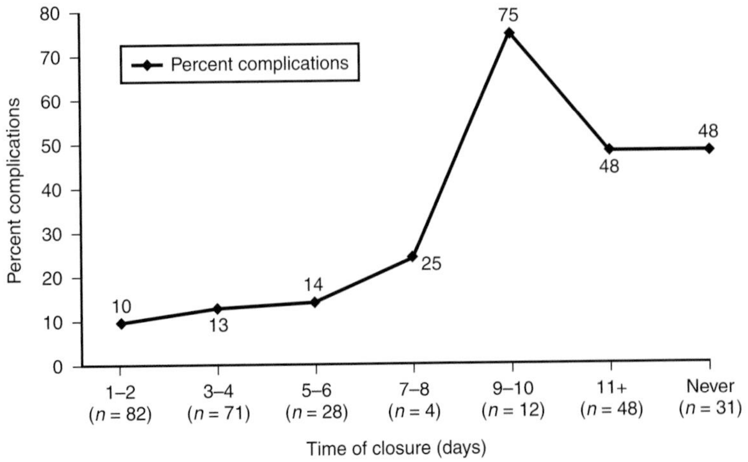

FIGURE 16 Percentage of patients with wound complications versus days to fascial closure.

Percent complications graph:

- 1–2 (n = 82): 10
- 3–4 (n = 71): 13
- 5–6 (n = 28): 14
- 7–8 (n = 4): 25
- 9–10 (n = 12): 75
- 11+ (n = 48): 48
- Never (n = 31): 48

Time of closure (days)

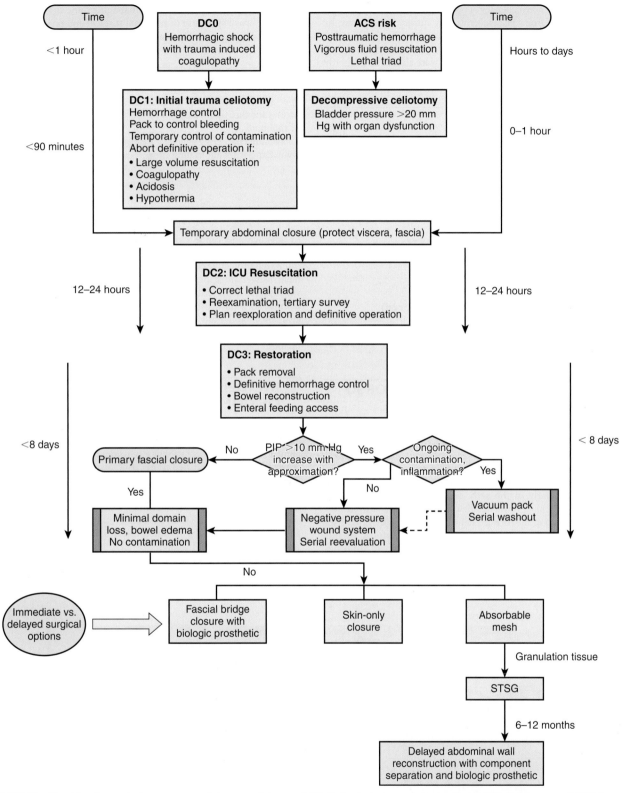

FIGURE 18 Algorithm for surgical management of the open abdomen. ACS, Abdominal compartment syndrome; DC, damage control; ICU, intensive care unit; PIP, peak inspiratory pressure; STSG, split-thickness skin graft.

from injury and desiccation using the vacuum pack, appropriate nutritional support, and early tension-free closure of the abdominal wall are all good preventive measures. However, once a fistula forms, the adjacent viscera must be protected, and the effluent from the fistula controlled. Early repair of the fistula is typically not feasible due to the inflammatory changes and anatomic disturbances. Complex wound

management systems are required to control the fistula egress and allow granulation of the bowel. STSG coverage is sometimes necessary to heal the wound while awaiting a delayed abdominal wall reconstruction and fistula resection/closure. Fistula rates are minimized by early abdominal wall closure either with primary repair of the rectus defect, skin-only closure, or using biologic prosthetic implants.

The psychosocial consequences of open abdomen on each individual patient are far from insignificant, and quality of life may be adversely affected even years later. There are data that suggest that long-term outcomes of patients who were left open with a planned ventral hernia approaches that of patients who were able to be primarily closed, especially when the hernia patients undergo reconstruction.

CONCLUSION

The application of damage control techniques to injured and critically ill patients may be lifesaving. Surgeons who treat this patient population must be experienced in managing these conditions, which require a broad spectrum of potential surgical and physiologic interventions. See algorithm for damage control (Fig. 18).

ACKNOWLEDGMENT

Special acknowledgment is given to Drs. Richard Miller and John Morris for their contributions to this chapter in the previous edition of this book.

For the chapter's Suggested Readings list, please visit the book at www.ExpertConsult.inkling.com.

TORSO TRAUMA ON THE MODERN BATTLEFIELD

Colonel Matthew J. Martin and Colonel (retired) Brian Eastridge

INTRODUCTION TO COMBAT TORSO TRAUMA

In the modern era, combat trauma care frequently involves the management of major torso injuries that would have been rapidly fatal in previous conflicts. In addition to the severe wounds and altered physiology, surgeons may be required to operate in a variety of austere forward settings with significant limitations in personnel and equipment, particularly in the early or "immature" phases of any combat action (Fig. 1). A more detailed overview of the current military medical system in the forward deployed setting is provided elsewhere (Field Triage in the Military Arena). The purpose of this chapter is to focus on the unique issues and management strategies for patients with major torso trauma (chest, abdomen, or combined thoracoabdominal) in a combat environment. Throughout history, lessons learned from the treatment of wartime wounds have helped to advance and refine global trauma care, with a resultant major decline in the risk of death from battlefield torso injuries. However, improved protective equipment, prehospital care, and transport times have resulted in an increase in the number of severely injured patients who survive to presentation at a forward medical facility. The modern combat surgeon must have a rapid and organized approach to the evaluation and early management of patients with major torso trauma, as any delays or errors can result in major morbidity or fatality.

INCIDENCE AND EPIDEMIOLOGY OF COMBAT TORSO TRAUMA

The true incidence of traumatic injuries during wartime is difficult to ascertain due to the complexities of collecting robust and complete clinical data in the operational environment. Most of what is currently known and published comes from analysis limited to U.S. facilities and military personnel, and does not account for the massive numbers of nonmilitary personnel injured and often treated at local national or coalition medical facilities. Data from an analysis of 3102 combat casualties in the Joint Theater Trauma Registry (JTTR) found an incidence of 6% for thoracic injuries and 11% for abdominal wounds. A subsequent analysis of all injuries from 2001 through 2009 in the JTTR (unpublished data) has demonstrated an overall 15% incidence of truncal wounds. Table 1 demonstrates the percentage of wounds by body region with comparison to previous conflicts.

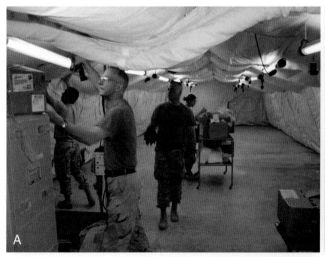

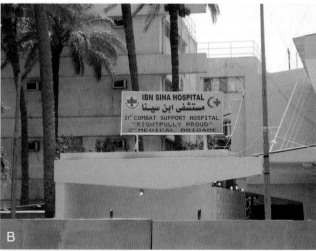

FIGURE 1   Conditions and capabilities of forward deployed facilities may vary widely. **A,** Trauma operating room being set up in a tent in Tikrit, Iraq. **B,** Fully equipped and relatively modern Ibn Sina Hospital in Baghdad, Iraq.

TABLE 1: Distribution of Combat Wounds by Body Region since World War II

Body Region	World War II	Vietnam	OIF and OEF
Head and neck	21%	16%	30%
Thorax	14%	13%	6%
Abdomen	8%	9%	9%
Extremities	58%	61%	55%

From Owens BD, Kragh JF Jr, Wenke JC, et al: Combat wounds in operation Iraqi Freedom and operation Enduring Freedom. *J Trauma* 64:295–299, 2008.
OEF, Operation Enduring Freedom; OIF, Operation Iraqi Freedom.

The significant decline in major thoracic wounds in the current conflicts is likely attributable to improved personal protective equipment and vehicles. Despite the decline in incidence, the importance of rapid treatment of these injuries is highlighted by data indicating that approximately 50% of all deaths among patients with potentially survivable wounds are attributable to noncompressible hemorrhage from torso wounds. It is also important to remember that although the incidence of torso injuries has declined among wounded soldiers, it will remain significantly higher among civilian casualties or combatants who do not possess body armor or other protective gear. The unique severity and nature of combat wounds, particularly torso wounds, has prompted current efforts to develop a military-specific version of the widely used Injury Severity Score (ISS).

NONCOMPRESSIBLE TORSO HEMORRHAGE: DEFINING THE PROBLEM

Active bleeding from abdominal or thoracic structures carries a high associated mortality rate, accounting for 60% to 70% of potentially preventable deaths in the civilian setting and 80% in the combat setting. Although the problem of "noncompressible" hemorrhage has long been recognized in combat settings, detailed study of the problem has been limited by the lack of any widely accepted definition or classification/scoring system. However, a recently published analysis that focused on hemorrhage and combat torso injuries describes the development of a set of diagnostic and classification criteria for noncompressible torso hemorrhage (NCTH) that are shown in Table 2. Using these definitions, 13% of battlefield casualties met anatomic criteria and 2% were identified as having NCTH. The most lethal

TABLE 2: Criteria and Epidemiology of Noncompressible Torso Hemorrhage

Anatomic	Physiologic	Relative Incidence	Odds Ratio for Mortality
Thoracic cavity	SBP < 90 mm or need for emergent surgery	32%	1.9
Solid organ injury > grade 3		20%	1.0
Named axial torso vessel		20%	3.4
Pelvic ring disruption		15%	0.80

Modified from Morrison JJ, Rasmussen TE: Noncompressible torso hemorrhage: a review with contemporary definitions and management strategies. *Surg Clin North Am* 92:843–858, 2012.
SBP, Systolic blood pressure.

of these patterns was injury to a named torso vessel (odds ratio for death of 3.4), which was present in 20% of NCTH cases. A similar incidence of NCTH of around 2% has been demonstrated in civilian trauma, but with a higher prevalence of blunt traumatic mechanisms. Similar to combat statistics, NCTH accounts for a large percentage (45% to 85%) of potentially preventable deaths from bleeding in civilian trauma centers. Unlike peripheral or junctional vascular trauma, these injuries are not amenable to direct compression or simple inflow occlusion (tourniquet) in the prehospital or emergency department (ED) phase, and thus have been a focus of great interest and innovation. Critical concepts or interventions for patients with NCTH are: (1) minimizing delays in transfer from ED to operating room (OR) (or direct to OR resuscitation), (2) permissive hypotension until vascular control is obtained, (3) balanced or "hemostatic" resuscitation with early use of plasma, (4) procoagulant adjuncts such as tranexamic acid (TXA), and (5) use of damage control surgery techniques and intravascular shunts when indicated. Innovative work that could directly impact survival from NCTH is being done and includes the use of endovascular techniques such as aortic balloon occlusion for temporary vascular control and the development of pharmacologic metabolic or hormonal agents to induce a "prosurvival" phenotype that is more tolerant to severe hemorrhage.

MECHANISMS OF COMBAT TORSO INJURIES

Modern warfare is characterized by an ever-increasing array of sophisticated and lethal weaponry that can create wounds that are unlike anything that is seen in civilian trauma centers. Although penetrating missile wounds may be commonly seen at many urban trauma centers, the resultant injuries from these primarily low velocity weapons often pale in comparison to the devastating tissue destruction associated with high-velocity military projectiles. However, the most striking difference is encountered when dealing with blast and explosive injuries in a combat setting. The resultant combination of blast injury, penetrating fragment wounds, blunt trauma (such as vehicular rollover), and thermal injury frequently results in severe multisystem wounds including multiple amputations or mangled extremities, head and neck wounds, and major torso injuries (Fig. 2). In previous conflicts, these types of injuries were mainly seen with military explosive devices such as mortars, rockets, and landmines. The current conflicts in Iraq and Afghanistan have been marked by insurgent type warfare, with the improvised explosive

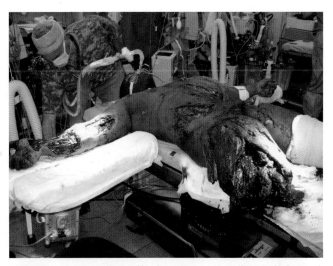

FIGURE 2 Injuries sustained by the passenger in a military vehicle struck by an improvised explosive device, including mangled/amputated extremities, penetrating hollow viscus injuries, pelvic fracture, brachial artery laceration, and pulmonary contusions.

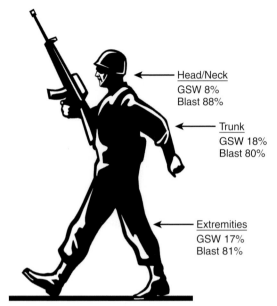

FIGURE 3 Predominant combat wounding mechanisms by anatomic area of injury. GSW, Gunshot wound. *(Data from Owens BD, Kragh JF Jr, Wenke JC, et al: Combat wounds in Operation Iraqi Freedom and Operation Enduring Freedom. J Trauma 64:295–299, 2008.)*

device (IED) evolving as the enemy forces' weapon of choice. The predominant wounding mechanisms by anatomic area are shown in Figure 3. This is in striking contrast to prior conflicts, when gunshot wounds played a much more significant role. However, high-velocity military weaponry also continues to play a major role and can result in devastating and challenging wounds (Fig. 4).

Two of the most important responses of the U.S. military to the IED threat have been: (1) the development of hardened vehicles resistant to explosives and (2) improvements and widespread distribution of personal protective equipment that includes torso body armor, helmets, gloves, and eye protection. The most notable impact of these improvements has been on the incidence of truncal trauma, with a 50% reduction seen in the incidence of thoracic injuries compared to previous conflicts. In the authors' experience with multiple deployments to both Iraq and Afghanistan, this protective gear has frequently converted a fatal wounding mechanism to relatively minor and non-life-threatening injuries such as chest wall contusions or rib fractures (Fig. 5).

INITIAL EVALUATION

Initial evaluation of the combat casualty with truncal wounds must proceed in a rapid and orderly manner, often made difficult by the chaotic setting and severity of injuries. It is easy to become distracted by the presence of drastic-appearing (but non-life-threatening) extremity wounds; these should be ignored initially as long as they are hemostatic. Pneumothorax and noncompressible internal hemorrhage should be assumed in all patients until ruled out and must take priority. The combination of physical examination, chest radiograph, and focused sonography can be performed in minutes and should identify any sources of major bleeding. Figure 6 shows an algorithm for truncal evaluation in these patients. One of the most critical aspects of the early evaluation in these patients is avoiding any delay or unnecessary imaging in the unstable patient, or the patient with clear indication for operative intervention. Much more liberal use of true "exploratory" operations is made in combat situations due to decreased availability of high-resolution imaging, higher likelihood of intracavitary injuries, and lack of ability to perform serial examinations and monitoring due to multiple casualties and the need for rapid evacuation to another facility. Although many of the forward deployed medical units do not have computed tomography (CT) scan capability, high-quality portable ultrasound devices are universally available and should be used liberally. With little additional training, a physician operator can reliably and rapidly evaluate for pneumothorax or hemothorax, tamponade, gross cardiac contractility, and volume status (vena cava size and respiratory variation). This technology has even been extended to the prehospital combat environment and may augment the rapid identification and treatment of potentially fatal injury, particularly pneumothoraces.

OPERATIVE INTERVENTION

A description of operative interventions for the wide variety of truncal injuries seen in the combat setting is beyond the scope of this chapter, and there are now several excellent combat trauma guides available that cover this topic in detail. Most of the technical aspects of combat surgery for truncal injury do not differ from civilian trauma as covered elsewhere in this book. However, optimal outcomes are obtained only by understanding the important areas of difference from civilian trauma and adherence to several basic principles of combat surgery. First and foremost is that the severely injured and hypotensive patient with truncal wounds should be moved immediately to the OR with simultaneous initiation of blood product resuscitation and

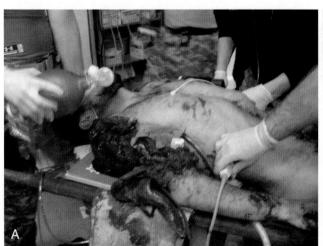
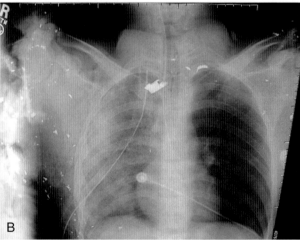

FIGURE 4 Single high-velocity gunshot wound to right shoulder results in devastating soft tissue injury with near-amputation (**A**) and the corresponding radiograph demonstrates the bony injury and fragmentation of the missile (**B**).

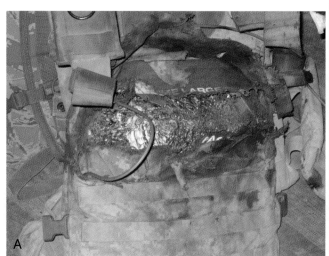
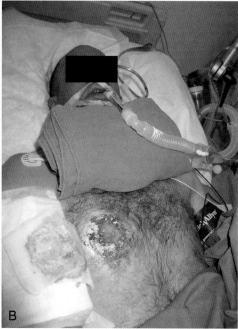

FIGURE 5   A, Body armor of soldier struck in the chest by a rocket-propelled missile. The soldier suffered no significant truncal injury. **B,** Wounded soldier with a chest wall contusion where a missile struck his body armor.

Chest
- Chest Xray
- Ultrasound (pericardial and pleural)
- Bilateral chest tubes or needle aspiration

Abdomen
- FAST exam
- Bedside diagnostic peritoneal aspiration (DPA)

Pelvis
- Physical exam (instability, scrotal/perineal hematoma)
- Pelvis Xray
- FAST exam

Extremity
- Exam (hemorrhage, thigh swelling)

Other
- External survey (scalp, neck, back, perineum)
- Blood loss in field
- Spinal cord injury (neurogenic shock)

Unidentified
- Laparotomy (fully examine retroperitoneum)
- Pericardial window

FIGURE 6   Algorithm for rapid evaluation and search for hemorrhage in the combat trauma patient. FAST, Focused assessment with sonography for trauma. *(From Martin M, Beekley A, editors:* Front line surgery: a practical approach. *New York, 2010, Springer.)*

preparation for operative intervention. The entire body with all injured areas (including injured extremities) should be prepped and draped into one operative field, and head/neck or extremity injuries should be addressed simultaneously by a separate team whenever possible. As resources permit, all emergent operative procedures, particularly in the chest or abdomen, should be staffed by at least two surgeons working together in order to maximize exposure and thoroughness while minimizing operative time. Emergency department thoracotomy (EDT) should be performed selectively for patients arriving in extremis with truncal or major extremity injuries and has been associated with an 11% survival rate. However, EDT should not be performed during MASCAL (mass casualties) situations and consideration must always be given to the expected consumption of limited resources such as blood products. The following sections outline some specific principles and approaches for several common combat truncal injury scenarios.

Choice of Incision

Inexperienced trauma surgeons use "elective" surgical approaches aimed at maximizing ease and exposure at the expense of flexibility and options. A good combat surgeon will accept less than perfect (although always adequate) exposure to maintain the maximal amount of flexibility and options. A typical example of this is positioning a patient in lateral decubitus to explore the hemithorax for bleeding or other injuries. This is a potentially disastrous situation when the bleeding is actually found to be coming from the abdomen, the mediastinum, or the other side of the chest. Exploratory operations on the trunk should almost always be performed in the supine position, thus preserving your options to access the neck, both sides of the chest, and the mediastinum, abdomen, and groin. Avoid mini-incisions and extend incisions liberally if there is any difficulty with exposure. For an anterolateral thoracotomy one of the best and most underused maneuvers to improve exposure is to extend the skin incision medially for 5 to 10 cm onto the opposite side of the chest and divide the sternum. Completely adequate exposure for all immediately life-threatening thoracic injuries can be obtained with either an anterolateral thoracotomy or median sternotomy instead of the posterolateral thoracotomy approach that is preferred for elective surgery.

Damage Control in the Chest

Thoracic damage control follows the same principles as abdominal damage control surgery but is markedly different in practice because of differences in anatomy and the often decreased comfort level of the trauma surgeon. Although the only true immediately life-threatening issue in the abdomen is hemorrhage, in the chest there are multiple issues: tension physiology, tamponade, refractory hypoxia/hypercarbia, arrhythmia, and air emboli. Single-lung ventilation will often not be readily available, but the exposed lung can be deflated with manual compression and packing during exhalation. For bleeding, the first maneuver should be manual clot evacuation and then either direct hemorrhage control or packing. In some cases with communicating thoracoabdominal wounds and ongoing hemorrhage it may be difficult to sort out whether the ongoing bleeding is from the chest or abdomen. Rapid temporary closure of any large diaphragm defect to reestablish separation of the cavities can greatly assist in identifying and treating the source of bleeding. Most diaphragm repairs will develop an associated postoperative effusion, so always leave a chest tube above the repair. Close communication with the anesthesia provider and coordination of ventilation parameters is of key importance to avoid severe hypoxia or respiratory acidosis, and serial point of care blood gas measurements should be followed during the procedure. Finally, a temporary closure in the chest is an option similar to that in the abdomen but must maintain some degree of normal respiratory or chest wall mechanics while avoiding creation of a tension pneumothorax or tamponade by closing the cavity without adequate drainage. The authors prefer placement of two large-bore chest tubes for adequate drainage, and an en masse single layer running suture temporary closure incorporating muscle, fascia, and skin.

Operative Lung Injury

Penetrating combat wounds to the chest are much more likely to require operative intervention than their civilian counterparts. Data from the Croatian conflicts demonstrated that 63% of war-related thoracic wounds required surgery, with 34% requiring lung repair or resection. Standard lung injury techniques apply, with the caveat that the simple through-and-through injury often seen with low-velocity civilian gunshot wounds is extremely rare. The involved lung tissue is often macerated and bleeding, and often is not amenable to the usual stapled tractotomy that is touted for civilian penetrating lung injuries (Fig. 7). A stapled wedge resection or formal lobectomy, depending on the extent of involved lung parenchyma, should be performed. The possibility of air embolus must always be considered and can be prevented by rapid control of the injury, hilar clamping until local control is obtained, or flooding the area with saline to submerge the injured area. Finally, attempts at prolonged pulmonary vascular repairs or extensive subtotal resections in an unstable or deteriorating patient should be avoided. Damage control with hilar clamping and temporary closure or stapled pneumonectomy can be performed in minutes, but immediate intraoperative and postoperative planning for the resultant cardiac and pulmonary dysfunction must be initiated (Fig. 8).

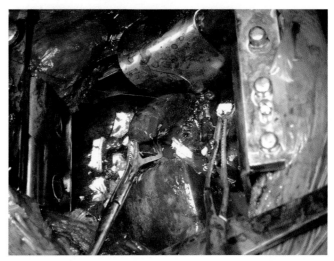

FIGURE 7 High-velocity penetrating injury to lung required wedge resection and then pledgeted repair of disrupted parenchyma to control bleeding and air leak.

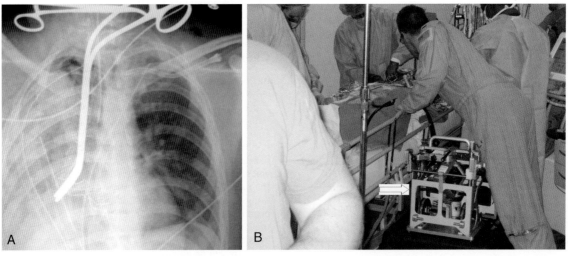

FIGURE 8 A, Postoperative chest radiograph in a soldier with a destructive lung injury who underwent damage control thoracic procedure and closure with vascular clamp on the right pulmonary hilum. **B,** Same patient being placed on portable extracorporeal membrane oxygenation for transfer from Afghanistan to Germany. *(Courtesy of CDR Rodd Benfield and CDR Eric Elster, U.S. Navy.)*

Large Hemothorax

Although immediate tube thoracostomy (in the ED) is the standard treatment, large hemothoraces in the combat setting more often require immediate intervention for ongoing bleeding or delayed intervention for retained hemothorax. An excellent option is to take these patients to the OR (if available) and perform the procedure as follows: prep and drape the entire chest with the patient supine and the affected side slightly elevated with a towel roll, make a 2-cm tube thoracostomy incision and insert a Poole suction into the chest to remove all liquid blood, lavage the chest copiously to remove any formed clot, and then place a large-bore chest tube through the incision. If there is initial large output or ongoing bleeding, then an anterolateral thoracotomy or median sternotomy is easily performed. In the authors' experience, this approach has minimized delays to operative intervention and decreased the incidence of retained hemothorax and the need for subsequent thoracotomy or thoracoscopy.

Multiple Truncal Fragment Wounds

It is not uncommon to have patients wounded by explosive devices present with innumerable small truncal fragment wounds, somewhat similar to civilian shotgun injuries but typically covering a larger surface area (Fig. 9). It is often difficult to ascertain if they are entirely superficial or have penetrated any major intracavitary structures. A lateral radiograph, in addition to standard anteroposterior views, is often helpful for determining the depth and position of fragments. It may also be difficult to identify vascular injuries because the fragments can produce small holes in the vessels that immediately seal. Unless there is ongoing hemorrhage or ischemia this is not an emergent issue, but there should be a low threshold for performing standard or CT angiography for any fragments in proximity to major vascular structures. CT or digital fluoroscopy will often not be available in many far-forward facilities, and surgical exploration for concerning proximity wounds should be liberally used in this setting. Another not-uncommon finding is embolization of fragments that have entered a peripheral artery or vein. Chest radiograph and distal imaging as needed should be performed to rule this out. A subxiphoid

or transdiaphragmatic pericardial window should be performed if there is any suspicion of cardiac injury based on the cardiac ultrasound windows, the location of fragments on chest radiograph, or unexplained hemodynamic decline.

Patients with hemodynamics or physical examination findings indicating an intracavitary injury should proceed immediately to the OR for exploratory surgery. Even with a normal initial chest radiograph, there should be a low threshold for tube thoracostomy placement for chest fragments, particularly for patients placed on positive-pressure ventilation or immediately placed into the evacuation system. Nonoperative management of truncal fragment wounds will depend on the setting and resources available. At far-forward Level II facilities without CT scan or holding capability, operative exploration should be performed unless the wounds are clearly superficial. At more robust Level III facilities, selective nonoperative management of truncal fragment wounds using physical examination combined with CT imaging has been shown to be safe and effective (98% sensitivity).

Abdominal Solid Organ Injury

Although isolated abdominal solid organ injuries (SOIs) are typically associated with civilian blunt trauma, they may be seen in the combat setting as a result of either missile or fragment wounds, blast effects, or vehicular accidents. Unlike the civilian setting, where nonoperative management of both blunt and penetrating SOI has been highly successful, operative management for most identified SOI is the treatment of choice on the battlefield. In addition to the increased average severity and presence of associated injuries with combat SOI, there is typically a limited (or nonexistent) capability to observe and closely monitor patients for a prolonged period of time. Therefore, the majority of patients with abdominal trauma and either a positive focused assessment with sonography for trauma (FAST) examination or a significant SOI (grade 2 or higher) identified on CT scan should undergo operative exploration, unless the resources and personnel are available to perform adequate nonoperative management. Another significant difference seen with combat SOI, particularly with blast or high-velocity missile injuries, is the larger

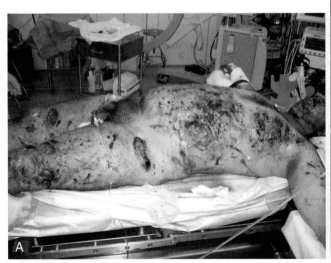
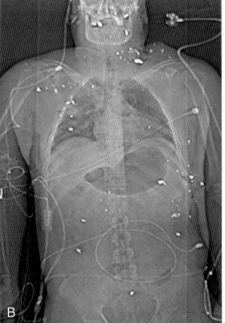

FIGURE 9 Patient injured in an improvised explosive device blast. **A,** Head to toe fragment wounds of varying size and depth. **B,** Radiograph showing diffuse truncal fragments.

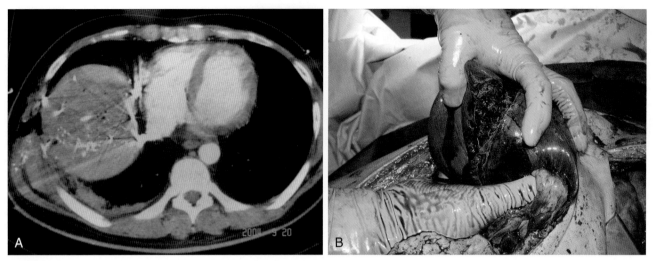

FIGURE 10 **A,** Computed tomography scan showing blast/fragment wound to right hepatic lobe. **B,** Intraoperative findings of major parenchymal liver injury that required resectional débridement.

area of tissue shredding and destruction that is often present. Combat liver injuries may be particularly more challenging and often require more formal débridement or resectional procedures (Fig. 10). In addition to consideration of the individual SOI, management decisions should also take into account the presence and severity of associated injuries, the resuscitation requirements, and the potential subsequent development of coagulopathy and severe hemorrhage from even minor SOIs that appear relatively innocuous at initial exploration.

Bowel Injuries

The debate about optimal management of bowel injuries has been particularly keen in the military setting, and has evolved from mandatory colostomy or exteriorization for all colon wounds in WWII to the current selective policy. At the time of initial surgery this is usually not a concern, as most bowel injuries are managed with a damage control approach, and decisions about reconstruction versus ostomy are made at a later time. Combat large and small bowel wounds are usually better managed by stapled resection, with a higher failure rate for primary repair than is seen in the civilian setting. High-velocity

projectiles create destructive bowel injuries (Fig. 11A) and fragment wounds typically create smaller holes, and careful meticulous inspection must be performed in order to avoid missed injuries. A unique finding that is rarely seen in civilian trauma is the presence of a significant thermal injury to the bowel wall surrounding the fragment wound (Fig. 11B). Although the actual defect is small, the entire burned area must be completely excised. Large mesenteric rents with intact bowel wall may also be seen and should prompt resection of the involved segment owing to the degree of devascularization and risk for subsequent necrosis (Fig. 12). Decisions about proximal diversion versus primary repair must consider not only the standard patient factors but also the battlefield realities of multiple casualties waiting for surgery and the need to immediately evacuate the patient with limited ability to closely observe for an anastomotic leak. Although colostomy is certainly not mandatory for most colon wounds, it should be used more liberally than in the civilian setting, and particularly with associated high-risk abdominal injuries such as pancreas or duodenum. If an ostomy is felt to be needed, a loop or "end-loop" ostomy is preferred as it provides adequate fecal diversion and is much easier to subsequently reverse (frequently without the need for full laparotomy).

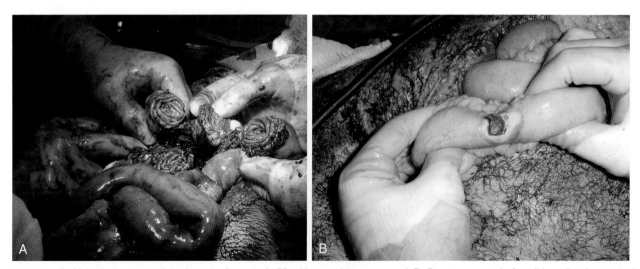

FIGURE 11 **A,** Multiple destructive bowel injuries from single 50-caliber machine-gun round. **B,** Fragment wound of small bowel with surrounding thermal injury. *(From Martin M, Beekley A, editors:* Front line surgery: a practical approach. *New York, 2010, Springer.)*

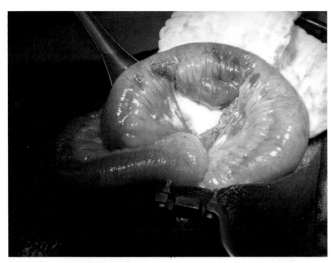

FIGURE 12 Significant small bowel mesenteric tear. Although there is no bowel wall disruption, this area should be resected due devascularization of the involved segment.

Massive Abdominal Wall and Perineal/Pelvic Wounds

The increase in explosive mechanisms in current combat operations has resulted in an increased incidence of massive wounds to the abdominal wall or pelvis/perineum, usually associated with significant skin and subcutaneous tissue loss that makes primary closure impossible. Full-thickness loss of sections of the abdominal wall with associated evisceration is not uncommon, and exploratory laparotomy should be immediately performed because of the near universal presence of hollow viscus injury (Fig. 13). Management of massive abdominal wall defects can be extremely challenging and may require complex flap coverage, but the initial management has been greatly simplified with the widespread availability of vacuum-assisted closure devices (Fig. 14). One of the most challenging and unfortunately common wounds associated with IED blasts is the massive perineal/pelvic wound. These devastating injuries are often coupled with mangled or amputated lower extremities that add additional complexity and significant morbidity (Fig. 15). These wounds are particularly difficult to deal with due to the typical associated severe hemorrhage, contamination, and associated injuries (major vascular, bony pelvis, bowel, bladder, rectum). These patients truly belong in the OR as soon as possible, and often are best served by bypassing the ED phase completely. Damage control resuscitation should be begun immediately as they invariably arrive in some degree of shock. Initial operative intervention typically consists of two phases: (1) a supine approach to control hemorrhage and address gastrointestinal or bladder injuries and (2) a lateral or prone approach for débridement and local hemorrhage control. Diverting colostomy should be performed for most of these wounds regardless of anorectal involvement, but is not a priority at the initial operation.

One of the most difficult aspects of managing these massive perineal/pelvic wounds and proximal thigh amputations is controlling the exsanguinating hemorrhage that is frequently present. Although the fractures and soft tissue injuries may be dramatic, attention should always be focused initially on obtaining adequate vascular control. Direct vascular control of the femoral vessels in the wounded area may be rapidly obtained in some cases, but prolonged attempts at direct exposure in an actively bleeding and distorted field should be abandoned in favor of an alternative approach. There is often significant combined arterial and venous bleeding from these high groin vascular injuries, and in these cases it is usually preferable to obtain proximal aortoiliac control via laparotomy or an extraperitoneal abdominal vascular exposure versus attempts at direct femoral exposure and control (Fig. 16A). Once proximal control is obtained, direct exposure of the thigh/groin vasculature is facilitated and all efforts should be made to repair major arterial injuries rather than ligate. Temporary shunts can be rapidly replaced to restore flow and delay definitive repair until the patient is more stable and resuscitated (Fig. 16B). Even in the face of a proximal amputation, repair of the femoral vasculature may significantly improve the final amputation level and preserve as much muscle function as possible. The entire torso and the injured extremities should all be prepped into the surgical field to allow for abdominal or thoracic exposure and proximal vascular control, as well as simultaneous truncal and extremity surgery by multiple teams. Once proximal control is obtained, then a more direct wound exploration can be performed. The extent of tissue injury and the involvement of the proximal arterial and venous supply with these high thigh or groin wounds may ultimately necessitate a hip-disarticulation procedure.

FUTURE DIRECTIONS

Although tremendous strides have been made in the understanding and management of combat truncal injuries, there remain multiple areas that are ripe for improvement and innovation. Arguably the most important of these are initiatives aimed at improving survival

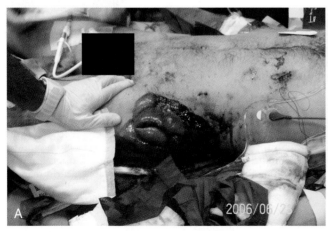
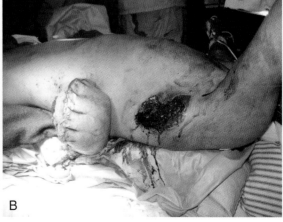

FIGURE 13 Blast injuries involving the abdominal wall and fascia. **A,** Evisceration of small intestine. **B,** Flank injury with large gastric evisceration.

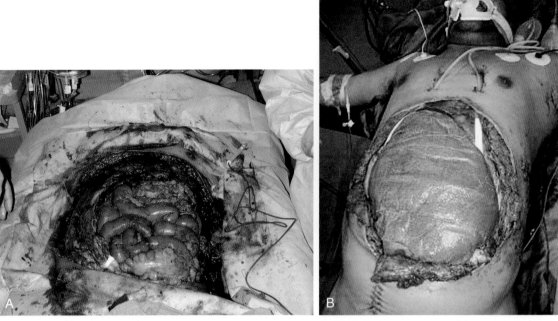

FIGURE 14   A, Near-complete loss of entire anterior abdominal wall due to blast injury. **B,** Early management of this complex wound is greatly simplified by application of a vacuum-assisted temporary closure device.

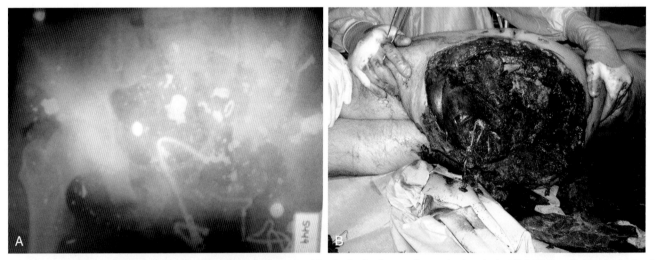

FIGURE 15   A, Pelvis radiograph demonstrating multiple fragments and foreign bodies from an improvised explosive device injury. **B,** Massive perineal wound that includes destruction of the anorectal complex and requiring extensive débridement and diverting colostomy.

and outcomes among patients with noncompressible hemorrhage, typically in the chest or abdomen. These are not only focusing on improved fluids and resuscitation strategies, but on novel therapeutic interventions with the potential to induce cellular tolerance to shock states. This "demand side" approach to hemorrhage is in its infancy and holds great promise to achieve the "holy grail" of trauma—induction of a temporary suspended animation-like state after severe injury. A number of promising compounds such as valproic acid, hydrogen sulfide, estradiol, and others have shown benefit in animal models of hemorrhagic shock, and could potentially evolve into therapies available to forward trauma surgeons or even front-line medics.

Additional promising avenues of investigation include pushing more advanced diagnostic and therapeutic capabilities closer to the battlefield and during the evacuation process. Portable ultrasound for use by forward medics and flight crews has shown promise in limited initial trials in diagnosing life-threatening truncal injuries and directing interventions. Current prehospital battlefield fluid resuscitation is limited to cold crystalloid or colloid solutions, but the ongoing development of freeze-dried or lyophilized blood products is expected to make plasma and other blood products available outside fixed medical facilities. Finally, there is a renewed interest in augmenting prehospital MEDEVAC (medical evacuation) crews with advanced providers such as intensive care nurses or trauma

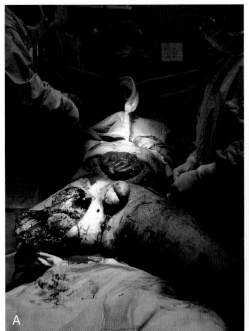 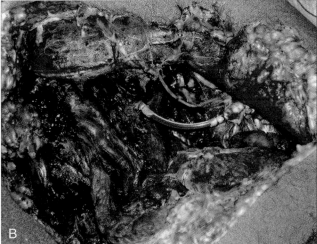

FIGURE 16   A, Significant combined arterial and venous bleeding from high groin vascular injury. **B,** Temporary thigh shunts.

physicians. This model has been used by some allied forces, such as the British Medical Emergency Response Team (MERT), and allows for the delivery of advanced interventions and initiation of blood product resuscitation at the point of injury and during helicopter or ground transport. A recently published analysis from the combat experience in Afghanistan demonstrated a reduction in mortality rate among moderately injured patients that were transported by the MERT advanced provider model compared to those evacuated by traditional medic-led prehospital teams (12% vs. 18%, $P = .035$). Further studies will be needed to better clarify the composition of these advanced prehospital transport teams, as well as the optimal patient populations and triage criteria to positively impact outcomes and resource use. A number of other truly innovative and groundbreaking advances in combat trauma care are in various stages of

development and are a testament to the dedication and vision of both military medical professionals and a wide network of civilian collaborators. In addition, the past decade of combat operations in Iraq and Afghanistan have resulted in the development of extensive collaborative efforts and networks of support from the civilian surgical community and professional organizations. These have greatly helped to foster open communication and exchange of ideas, rapid dissemination of battlefield lessons and advances, and application of cutting-edge research and technology to the far-forward environment. It has been said that "the only winner in any war is medicine," and we must remember that these lessons have come at too high a price to waste any opportunity for advancement or improvement.

For the chapter's Suggested Readings list, please visit the book at www.ExpertConsult.inkling.com.

PERIPHERAL VASCULAR INJURY

VASCULAR ANATOMY OF THE EXTREMITIES

Norman M. Rich and David R. Welling

From Egyptian, Greek, and Roman battlefields centuries ago, extremity vascular injuries were identified and treated. Subsequently, knowledge regarding the management of vascular trauma has also been gained from more modern military conflicts. Napoleon's surgeon Larrey was an expert with rapid amputations, having documented 200 amputations in 24 hours during the Battle of Borodino in 1812. During the American War between the States, amputation was the known treatment for extremity injuries, including vascular injuries. Historians debate even today whether amputation was overused; however, it was, "life over limb." Although there was knowledge both experimentally and clinically regarding repair of injured arteries and veins in the first half of the 20th century, amputation was still lifesaving. DeBakey and Simeone reported a 49% amputation rate in World War II following vascular trauma. During the Korean Conflict (1950–1953), Hughes, Spencer and others demonstrated that repair of both injured arteries and veins could be successful, even under less than ideal circumstances. In the last half of the 20th century, surgical advances lowered the amputation rate to approximately 13%, both during the Korean Conflict and in the Vietnam War. There have been further improvements in the early 21st century in managing American casualties in both Afghanistan and Iraq. Civilian management of vascular trauma in the last 50 years has led to even improved results over those from the battlefield. Battlefield wounding agents frequently cause much more extensive damage than low-velocity civilian wounds.

Pulsatile bright red bleeding, absence of distal pulses, a distal cool extremity, a pale distal extremity, neurologic deficits, and expanding or pulsatile hematomas all can be associated with arterial trauma. Presence of a thrill or a bruit at the injured site should alert one to the presence of an arteriovenous fistula. An injured vein can result in extensive hemorrhage, and the blood is dark, because it is less oxygenated. Proximity of a penetrating wound, previous hemorrhage that has stopped, osseous injury, hematoma, and neurologic deficit are all suspicious for vascular trauma. Further diagnostic studies can be helpful. Basic care for vascular trauma injuries should follow the precepts of the Advanced Trauma Life Support (ATLS). A thorough knowledge of anatomy is very important; today gross anatomy is not taught to the extent that would be desirable in most medical schools. Distortion and destruction of tissue planes by hemorrhage occurs, challenging the vascular surgeon. Perineural hemorrhage in a nerve can look like a thrombosed artery in a massive wound, making it increasingly confusing and difficult to manage the patient.

VASCULAR ANATOMY OF THE UPPER EXTREMITY

Axillary Artery and Vein

The axillary artery begins at the lateral border of the first rib as a direct continuation of the subclavian artery. It enters the axilla at the apex and crosses the first intercostal space to run along the lateral wall of the axilla. As the artery emerges from beneath the costoclavicular area, it becomes closely related to the brachial plexus. These nerves surround the axillary artery to eventually become the median, ulnar, and radial nerves at the distal portion of the axillary artery. This neurovascular bundle is enclosed in the axillary sheath, which separates it from the axillary vein. The axillary vein lies inferior to the axillary artery. The close proximity of the vein to the artery often results in the occurrence of traumatic arteriovenous fistulas.

The axillary artery continues as the brachial artery distally at the lateral edge of the teres major muscle. The axillary artery goes behind the pectoralis minor muscle, which originates on the chest wall and inserts into the coracoid process. The muscle divides the artery into three anatomic portions. The first portion runs from the later edge of the first rib to the upper border of the pectoralis minor muscle behind the clavipectoral fascia and the clavicular head of the pectoralis major muscle. The supreme thoracic artery is the only branch at this level. The second portion lies behind the pectoralis minor muscle, being the shortest portion, and it has two branches of clinical significance, the thoracoacromial artery and the lateral thoracic artery. The cords of the brachial plexus surround the axillary artery at this section. The third portion starts at the lateral border of the pectoralis minor muscle to the lateral border of the teres major muscle. There are three branches—the subscapular artery, the anterior circumflex humeral artery, and the posterior circumflex humeral artery—at this portion of the axillary artery.

Brachial Artery and Veins

The continuation of the axillary artery at the lower quarter of the teres major muscle becomes the brachial artery. The brachial artery lies along the side of the median nerve. At the elbow, it bifurcates into the radial and ulnar arteries, opposite the neck of the radius. There is a rich network of collateral arteries around the elbow joint, important in keeping the forearm and hand perfused when the brachial artery is occluded.

Radial and Ulnar Arteries and Veins

The radial artery is usually the smaller branch of the brachial artery. The radial artery gives rise to two major branches, the radial recurrent branch near its origin and the superficial palmar branch, which takes part in the formation of the superficial palmar arch. The main radial artery goes on to form the deep palmar arch of the wrist. The ulnar artery is the larger of the two terminal branches of the brachial artery. Near the origin of the ulnar artery is found the anterior and posterior ulnar recurrent arteries, which arise from the common interosseous artery. The distal ulnar artery terminates as the superficial palmar branch. Accompanying veins are small and inconsequential.

VASCULAR ANATOMY OF THE LOWER EXTREMITY

The Femoral Arteries and Veins

The common femoral artery is a direct continuation of the external iliac artery, entering the femoral triangle behind the inguinal ligament, midway between the anterior superior iliac spine and the symphysis pubis. Within the femoral triangle, the common femoral artery is medial to the femoral nerve, and the femoral vein is medial to the femoral artery. Posteriorly, one finds the psoas and pectineus muscles. Near the origin of the common femoral artery arises the superficial epigastric, superficial circumflex iliac, and superficial and deep external pudendal arteries. After traveling about 4 to 6 cm, the artery bifurcates in the distal femoral triangle into the superficial femoral artery and the profunda femoris artery.

The superficial femoral artery is usually the larger of the two terminating branches. It descends through the thigh with the sartorius muscle medially, the vastus medialis anterolaterally, and the adductor longus and magnus muscles posteriorly. The saphenous nerve lies anterior to the artery. The artery pierces the adductor magnus at the adductor hiatus to become the popliteal artery, giving off the superior geniculate artery branches, medial and lateral. The superficial femoral vein accompanies closely the superficial femoral artery. It is not unusual for the superficial vein to have duplication and even multiple veins.

The profunda femoris artery provides the main blood supply to the thigh. It arises from the posterior lateral aspect of the common femoral artery and descends laterally and posteriorly to the superficial femoral artery. Consequently, it runs deep in the thigh to the adductor longus. The medial and lateral circumflex femoral arteries arise soon after the origin of the profunda femoris artery. These important branches serve as collaterals around the hip. Three perforating arteries arise during the course of the profunda femoris arteries to supply the muscle of the thigh. They are connected with a rich anastomotic network. Veins accompany the arteries.

Popliteal Artery and Vein

The popliteal artery is the direct continuation of the superficial femoral artery beginning at the adductor hiatus. It travels slightly laterally to go behind the distal femur as it descends to enter the popliteal fossa. This is an important anatomic area because all neurovascular structures pass from the thigh to the leg through this space. The fossa is diamond-shaped behind the knee. The popliteal artery runs on the floor of the popliteal fossa between the condyles of the femur until it reaches the distal border of the popliteus muscle where it terminates into the anterior tibial artery and the tibioperoneal trunk. Three pairs of branches form important collaterals about the knee. The popliteal vein accompanies the artery and it can be bifid.

Tibial Arteries and Veins

The anterior tibial artery is the smaller terminating branch of the popliteal artery that arises from the lower border of the popliteus muscle. It passes through the interosseous membrane into the anterior compartment of the leg. At the ankle, the artery continues as the dorsalis pedis. Throughout its length it is surrounded by two interlacing venae comitantes and the deep fibular nerve. The tibioperoneal artery is the larger terminating branch of the popliteal artery. It originates and descends just behind the soleal arch. A network of complex and thin-walled venous vessels surround the artery. The tibial nerve accompanies the artery. The tibioperoneal artery is of variable length, extending up to 5 cm before bifurcating into the posterior tibial and fibular (peroneal) arteries. In a small percentage of patients, there can be a true trifurcation of all three distal tibial vessels from the popliteal artery. Posterior tibial artery is the direct continuation of the tibioperoneal trunk. It descends in the posterior compartment, becoming more superficial in the distal third of its course. At its termination it lies midway between the medial malleolus and the medial tubercle of the calcaneus. A pair of deep veins accompany the artery as venae comitantes. Throughout the course the tibial nerve runs alongside the artery. The fibular artery descends laterally toward the fibula after branching off from the tibioperoneal trunk. At the ankle the artery gives off a branch that perforates the interosseous membrane, forming an anastomotic network around the malleolus with the lateral and posterior malleolar branches of the fibular artery. A pair of deep veins accompanies the artery; however, no major nerve travels with the artery.

Saphenous Veins

Saphenous veins in the lower extremities have no associated arteries. The long saphenous vein is the longest vein in the body, beginning as the medial marginal vein of the dorsum of the foot. The vein runs the length of the leg in relationship with the saphenous nerve. The vein enters the femoral triangle, being joined by other collateral veins to enter the common femoral vein. The short saphenous vein begins behind the lateral malleolus as a continuation of the lateral marginal vein of the foot. It ascends to end in the popliteal vein between the heads of the gastrocnemius muscle. In the lower third of the leg it is in close relation with the sural nerve and in the upper two thirds with the medial sural cutaneous nerve.

For the chapter's Suggested Readings list, please visit the book at www.ExpertConsult.inkling.com.

DIAGNOSIS OF VASCULAR TRAUMA

John T. Anderson and F. William Blaisdell

The diagnosis of vascular trauma is usually not a problem, as most injuries manifest overt blood loss, shock, or loss of critical pulses. However, in certain instances, the lesion may not be recognized initially, only to manifest itself later by sudden secondary hemorrhage or the development of critical organ or extremity ischemia.

Most of the vascular injuries of immediate concern to the clinician are those related to arteries. The reason for this is that venous hemorrhage is usually well controlled by the adjacent soft tissues, and excellent collateral flow compensates for occlusive lesions. Late progression of thrombosis and pulmonary embolism are the primary complications related to venous injury.

DIAGNOSIS

The first priority should be to identify and manage life-threatening injuries and treat shock. Except for head injuries, nearly all injuries associated with immediate fatality are related to the cardiovascular system.

Advanced Trauma Life Support (ATLS) guidelines should be followed while proceeding with evaluation and treatment simultaneously. Shock from internal hemorrhage can be differentiated from cardiac compression or injury by a quick glance at neck veins. If neck veins are full, the presumption is cardiac compression from tamponade, tension pneumothorax, or cardiac failure. Collapsed neck veins indicate hypovolemia, and failure of response to fluid therapy dictates immediate operative intervention involving the most likely body cavity. This is usually dictated by an emergency chest radiograph. External hemorrhage is usually obvious, and immediate control is essential. Generally, direct pressure is effective for temporary control.

The presence of shock may lead to diminished pulses in the extremities and confusion about the location of vascular injury. Associated fractures and dislocations may compromise vascular patency and should be reduced before any decision about vascular injury is reached.

Prompt resuscitation and identification and management of vascular injuries should be the goals in order to minimize mortality risk and prevent permanent extremity ischemic damage.

History

Prehospital personnel should be questioned about bleeding at the scene and the presence or absence of shock. The need for resuscitation and the volume of fluid administered should be solicited. The use and duration of application of a tourniquet should be determined, and the amount and character of blood loss at the accident scene ascertained. A history of bright red pulsatile bleeding suggests arterial injury, but dark blood suggests venous origin. In many instances, bleeding may have ceased by the time the patient reaches the emergency room, leading to a false sense of security. In this type of patient, particularly one with an arterial injury, secondary hemorrhage is possible at any time.

Both the patient and prehospital personnel should be questioned about the mechanism of injury. Most civilian penetrating trauma results from low-velocity mechanisms such as knives or handguns. Arterial injuries in these cases are typically the result of direct injury, that is, from the knife or bullet. Information should be collected to aid in determining the trajectory of injury and potential structures injured. This could include the knife type and length, the number and direction of bullets, and the body position at the time of injury. Vascular injury from blunt mechanisms is often the result of stretching or compression from associated fractures or dislocations. Evidence of extremity fracture, dislocation, or altered perfusion should be elucidated. Additionally, specific mechanisms such as "car bumper" injuries or posterior knee dislocations are often associated with vascular injury and should be sought as appropriate.

Information about neurologic symptoms including sensory and motor deficits should be obtained. Potential confounding factors such as preexisting peripheral vascular disease, diabetes, or neuropathies should be elicited.

Physical Examination

The patient should be undressed and thoroughly examined. The skin folds of the axilla or perineum and buttocks should not be neglected, as wounds resulting from penetrating trauma may be missed in these areas. Deformity resulting from fracture or dislocation should be identified. In the case of penetrating trauma, the location and number of wounds should be noted in an attempt to identify the trajectory of the wounding object (particularly with reference to major arteries).

Evidence of active bleeding or hematoma formation should be sought. The character of the bleeding, pulsatile bright red blood, or a steady ooze of dark blood should be noted. A tense or expanding hematoma indicates the presence of an arterial injury with bleeding contained by surrounding soft tissues. The opposite uninjured extremity should be evaluated as a comparison. Chronic peripheral vascular disease is generally symmetrical. Absent pulses in the noninjured leg would support a diagnosis of preexisting peripheral vascular disease.

The examination should include palpation of pulses proximal and distal to the injury. Perfusion and tissue viability can be further assessed with skin temperature and capillary refill distal to the injury and determination of motor function. Alterations in any of these parameters warrant further assessment. Conversely, an apparent "normal" pulse does not exclude the possibility of vascular injury. Pulses may be palpable and assessed as normal in up to 30% to 33% of patients with later proven vascular injury. Again, the opposite noninjured extremity serves as a useful comparison.

Arteriovenous (AV) fistulas may occasionally be identified by auscultation of a bruit over the involved arterial segment. Generally the AV fistulas progress over time—often a bruit is not apparent early after injury. A glove should be placed over the bell of the stethoscope to keep the stethoscope free of blood when there is an open injury.

A thorough neurologic examination should be documented. Anatomically, the blood vessels and nerves are located in close proximity to each other. A neurologic deficit may hint toward the presence of an associated vascular injury. Further, the examination is of prognostic importance, as functional outcome is very dependent on intact sensation and motor function. A "stocking glove" deficit frequently indicates neurologic dysfunction resulting from ischemia—peripheral nerves are susceptible to ischemia because of a high metabolic rate and low glycogen stores. Blood flow should promptly be reestablished to prevent development of muscle death and gangrene.

HARD AND SOFT SIGNS OF VASCULAR INJURY

On the basis of history and physical examination, manifestations of vascular injury can be classified into two general prognostic categories, hard signs and soft signs (Table 1).

TABLE 1: Hard Versus Soft Signs of Vascular Injury

Hard Signs	Soft Signs
Active arterial bleeding	Neurologic injury in proximity to vessel
Pulselessness/evidence of ischemia	Small- to moderate-sized hematoma
Expanding pulsatile hematoma	Unexplained hypotension
Bruit or thrill	Large blood loss at scene
Arterial pressure index <0.90 pulse deficit	Injury (due to penetrating mechanism, fracture, or dislocation) in proximity to major vessel

From Anderson JT, Blaisdell FW: Diagnosis of vascular trauma. In Rich N, Mattox KL, Hirshberg A, editors: *Vascular trauma*, 2nd ed, Philadelphia, Saunders, 2004.

Hard signs are strong predictors of the presence of an arterial injury and the need for urgent operative intervention. Obvious examples include bright red pulsatile bleeding or a rapidly expanding hematoma. Evidence of extremity ischemia (manifested by the six Ps—pulselessness, pallor, pain, paralysis, paresthesia, and poikilothermia) and a bruit or thrill are additional examples. For extremity trauma, we also consider an arterial pressure index (API), also known as the ankle-brachial index, of less than 0.90 to be a hard sign. The API is determined by dividing the systolic pressure of the injured limb by the systolic pressure of the noninjured limb. Johansen and colleagues demonstrated 95% sensitivity and 97% specificity for identification of occult arterial injury with an API of less than 0.90. An API of more than 0.90 had a 99% negative predictive value for the presence of an arterial injury. The API is readily determined at bedside, and should be considered an extension of the physical examination. An important caveat is that the API may be normal in nonconduit vessels such as the profunda femoris.

Soft signs are those suggestive of an arterial injury, although with a much decreased likelihood than hard signs (see Table 1). These consist of mild pulse deficits, soft bruits, nonexpanding hematomas, and fractures or wounds in close proximity to major vessels. The actual incidence of arterial injury with these findings varies. For instance, patients with injury in proximity to a major vessel as the only finding are found to have an identifiable injury in less than 10% of cases; further, many of these injuries do not require additional treatment beyond simple observation. Most of the controversy of vascular trauma evaluation revolves around the assessment of patients with soft signs.

ADDITIONAL ANCILLARY TESTS

Ancillary imaging includes plain films, duplex scanning, computed tomography (CT) angiography, and formal arteriography. A chest radiograph and plain film imaging of the site of suspected vascular injury are warranted in essentially all patients. The utility of the remaining modalities are most beneficial when dealing with patients with soft signs, when the location of arterial injury is not obvious, or for assorted injuries (e.g., thoracic aorta) when information gained may greatly impact subsequent management. In many patients, the presence of an arterial injury is obvious and the need for surgical intervention clear; these patients are generally best served by prompt operation without additional tests.

A chest radiograph and plain films are readily obtained in the emergency room and should be a part of the initial screening of the injured patient. Radiopaque markers should be placed on all open wounds suspected to have resulted from a penetrating mechanism. Radiographs should completely cover the injured areas; often this requires imaging overlapping areas of the torso to ensure adequate coverage. Films should be scrutinized for foreign bodies, fractures, and dislocations. The trajectory of the injury is assessed as possible. The number of bullets identified and the number of wounds should sum to an even number. If not, the patient should be evaluated for additional unidentified wounds and films should be obtained to locate additional bullets. An important caveat is the possibility of a foreign body from a prior injury. At times, the bullet may travel as a missile embolism in the vascular system to a site distant from the site of entry. Occasionally, fluoroscopy (or the scout film of the CT scan) will assist in localizing additional bullets. A note should be made if the foreign body appears blurred, as this implies motion and the possibility of close contact with, or location within, a vascular structure.

Duplex ultrasonographic scanning combines two-dimensional imaging to assess anatomic detail and Doppler insonation to assess flow characteristics. Several investigators have demonstrated high sensitivity and specificity in the detection of vascular injury in various anatomic locations. Duplex ultrasonography is more sensitive to the presence of vascular injury than the API. Importantly, duplex ultrasonography can identify arterial injuries in nonconduit vessels such as the profunda femoris (the API will remain normal). However, duplex ultrasonography is limited, as it is technician dependent and in most centers is not readily available after hours.

Recently, there has been a groundswell of interest in the use of CT angiography as a diagnostic modality for vascular injury in multiple anatomic locations. Major advantages include almost universal availability and three-dimensional (3D) detail. Compared with formal angiography, an interventional radiologist does not need to be in attendance at the time of the examination. In general, the examination can be obtained more expeditiously than formal angiography, particularly after hours. Technological advancements in imaging resolution and software have been significant. Arterial anatomy can be reconstructed in 3D detail for easy evaluation. However, the modality is diagnostic only. A subsequent angiogram may be required for therapeutic embolization. Notably, the combined contrast load from both a CT angiogram and a subsequent angiogram can be significant. An additional technical limitation is that CT angiography is compromised by scatter from metallic fragments much more than formal angiography. CT angiography is of particular value when thoracic vascular injury is suspected, and it has proved to be a highly sensitive screening test. However, mediastinal hematoma alone, without evidence of arterial disruption, may still require arteriography to confirm large-vessel injury.

Arteriography has long been regarded the gold standard for assessment of arterial injury. It is well tolerated and has a low complication rate. Major complications such as iatrogenic pseudoaneurysm or AV fistulas are very uncommon in the young population typical of most trauma centers. A major advantage of arteriography is the availability of therapeutic options (such as embolization). Further, compared with CT angiography, formal arteriography is not prone to scatter from the presence of metallic fragments. Even in centers that rely on CT imaging as the predominant diagnostic study, formal arteriography still has a diagnostic role in confirming or further delineating the presence of equivocal CT findings. This latter point is particularly applicable in the assessment of carotid injuries in which even minor injuries may be of importance. An occasional patient requires urgent operation before availability of formal arteriography or CT angiography. In these patients, an on-table, surgeon-performed arteriogram can be obtained in the operating room. For instance, a femoral artery can be cannulated with an arterial catheter and injected with a contrast agent, and images can be obtained either with plain films or fluoroscopy. O'Gorman and colleagues have demonstrated that the axillary artery can be visualized by injection of contrast agent into the brachial artery with distal outflow occlusion with a blood pressure cuff inflated to a level well beyond the systolic arterial blood pressure. A benefit of the recent popularity of endovascular techniques has been increased availability of formal arteriography in the operating room. In fact, some centers have the capability of embolization of pelvic or visceral vessels in the operating room, thereby precluding the need to transport an unstable patient to a radiology suite that may not have the resources of the operating room.

SPECIFIC AREAS OF INJURY

Each of the major anatomic areas presents some unique symptoms or requirements for diagnostic screening for vascular injury. These areas are the neck, chest, abdomen, and extremities.

Cervical vascular trauma may be manifested by initial signs of external hemorrhage, expanding hematoma, or ipsilateral hemispheric ischemic symptoms, including hemiplegia, hemiparesis, or monocular blindness. The latter neurologic symptoms must be assumed to result from carotid artery interruption or thrombosis until proven otherwise. Deficits resulting from cranial nerves IX, X, XI, and XII suggest the possibility of vascular injury because of their immediate proximity to the carotid artery and the jugular vein. Penetrating trauma is associated with hemorrhage or false aneurysms, whereas blunt trauma invariably produces symptoms through thrombosis. This can be either immediate or delayed. In cases of major neck trauma, duplex scanning has greatly facilitated screening for intimal disruption or dissection, and some institutions use it liberally. CT angiography has recently been established as a viable alternative to formal angiography in the screening of blunt carotid injury as well as in the assessment of penetrating neck injury. Formal angiography should still be considered the gold standard, and is required in equivocal cases as well as the occasional patient who requires embolization of a disrupted vertebral artery.

Thoracic great vessel injuries are those to the arteries at the base of the neck and the thoracic aorta. As is true of all penetrating trauma, massive hemorrhage is the usual manifestation of injury to any one or more of these vessels. In this instance, immediate operation is indicated, with location based on the presumed path of the missile, location of the stab wound, and chest radiograph. Because of the significance of delayed diagnosis, most patients who are stable and have penetrating injuries of the base of the neck should be evaluated with arteriography. CT angiography is an appropriate alternative in centers with late-generation multidetector/high-resolution CT scanners, and when appropriate radiologic expertise is readily available. Blunt trauma, particularly from deceleration injuries, is associated with traumatic rupture. As opposed to smaller vessels, subclavian, innominate, and aortic injuries are rarely associated with thrombotic symptoms, even though there has been intimal disruption. The primary problem relates to gross vessel disruption. Complete separation is rarely if ever a clinical problem, as death is usually instantaneous. Surviving patients manifest vascular injury by the presence of false aneurysms, mediastinal or cervical hematomas, or apical capping. CT scanning has been an excellent screening tool for these injuries. However, unless vessel disruption is demonstrated, arteriography should follow the demonstration of hematomas, as many of these are associated with small vessel disruption that does not require surgery.

Abdominal vascular injuries after penetrating trauma invariably are associated with hemorrhage. Because laparotomy is indicated for almost all gunshot wounds of the lower chest and abdomen and all stab wounds associated with blood loss, the diagnosis of arterial or venous injury is usually made at the time of operation. Because of the relatively protected nature of the abdominal great vessels, blunt traumatic injuries are quite rare, and when present are manifested by weak or absent femoral pulses. For the reasons given previously, special diagnostic studies are rarely necessary when dealing with abdominal vascular trauma. CT scanning is used frequently to assess the source of ongoing hemorrhage but is of greater value in identifying specific organ injury rather than major vascular injury. Notable exceptions that may require arteriography are unstable pelvic fractures with evidence of ongoing bleeding. Arteriography may be indicated to assess the internal iliac vessels and treat the bleeding embolically. There may be a role for CT angiography in patients with unstable pelvic fractures from blunt trauma to identify suspect areas to target for subsequent embolization; often the CT scan can be obtained while awaiting setup of the angiography suite. Further, additional intra-abdominal and pelvic injuries may be delineated and 3D information obtained regarding the pelvic fracture pattern.

Extremity vascular injuries lend themselves to the diagnostic and screening maneuvers described in the previous sections. These patients fall into three general categories: (1) patients with evidence of pulselessness/ischemia, active bleeding, or a pulsatile hematoma; (2) patients with hard signs and a palpable pulse; and (3) patients with soft signs or an injury known to be associated with vascular injury. Initially, all patients should be adequately resuscitated and undergo reduction and stabilization of associated dislocations and fractures. Perfusion should be reassessed after these initial measures. In some cases, perfusion normalizes, and subsequent workup can proceed more deliberately. Ongoing assessment of patients with suspected extremity vascular injuries is outlined in Figure 1 and in the following discussion.

In the first category, patients with evidence of pulselessness/ischemia, active bleeding, or a pulsatile hematoma, urgent attention is required to prevent exsanguination or tissue necrosis from ischemia. Generally, these patients should be taken promptly to the operating room. If ischemia is complete, such as with a tourniquet, muscle necrosis will result from 4 hours of ischemia; fortunately, there is often some collateral flow that extends this critical time period. In most cases, the location of injury is apparent from the history, physical examination, and preliminary plain films; operative intervention can proceed accordingly. In other situations, the exact location and degree of injury are not apparent (Table 2). To minimize the duration of warm ischemia, on-table angiography can be performed. In some centers, formal angiography is available in the operating room.

Patients in the second category manifest hard signs, but do not demonstrate evidence of active bleeding or absence of perfusion. These patients can undergo a more deliberate, albeit expedient, assessment. Often the location and extent of injury are delineated with formal angiography. More recently, enthusiasm for CT angiography has grown. An advantage of formal angiography is the ability to perform therapeutic endovascular interventions such as embolization of muscular bleeders, or to control pseudoaneurysms or AV fistulas. As mentioned, in some cases associated injuries warrant urgent operative intervention before angiography can be obtained. In these cases, on-table angiography or formal angiography in the operating room are viable alternatives.

The final category involves patients with suspected extremity vascular injuries who present with soft signs only. Much of the controversy regarding evaluation of vascular trauma concerns this category. In patients with an injury in proximity to a major artery (although without hard signs), radiologic abnormalities may be present in as many as 10% of patients who undergo arteriography. However, a much smaller proportion of patients require operative intervention—several series indicate a range of 0.6% to 4.4% of patients. Dennis and colleagues have made a cogent argument in support of physical examination alone in this patient population. They argue that patients requiring operative intervention will be identified from subsequent development of hard signs. Typically, patients are admitted for a short period of observation. Concerns regarding poor patient compliance for follow-up and a push to expeditiously identify significant injuries early (ideally, shortly after presentation to the emergency room to guide appropriate disposition) have led many others to use alternative protocols involving ultrasonography or CT imaging. Ultimately, the choice is often determined by cost, availability of modalities, center volume/resources, and local expertise.

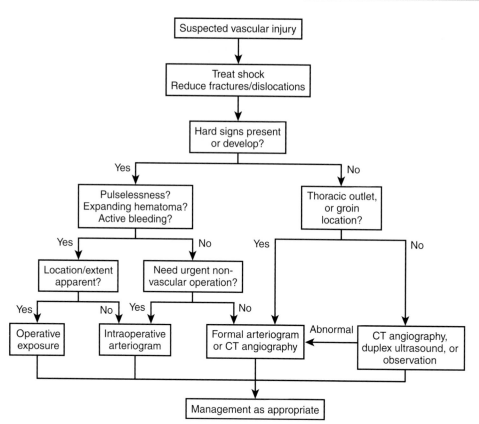

FIGURE 1 *Algorithm: evaluation of extremity trauma. CT, Computed tomography. (Modified from Anderson JT, Blaisdell FW: Diagnosis of vascular trauma. In Rich N, Mattox KL, Hirshberg A, editors: Vascular trauma, 2nd ed, Philadelphia, Saunders, 2004.)*

TABLE 2: Indications for Arteriography: Extremity Trauma

Unclear location or extent of vascular injury
Extensive soft tissue injury
Fracture or dislocation
Trajectory parallel to an artery
Multiple wounds
Gunshot injuries
Peripheral vascular disease

From Anderson JT, Blaisdell FW: Diagnosis of vascular trauma. In Rich N, Mattox KL, Hirshberg A, editors: *Vascular trauma*, 2nd ed, Philadelphia, Saunders, 2004.

Although injuries to any of the two lower arm vessels or three lower leg vessels can result in bleeding that requires treatment, for the most part, unless clinical symptoms point to the need for intervention, operation is rarely indicated and screening for injury is not indicated. These vessels have abundant collateral flow, so injury that results in occlusion to any one of them is rarely symptomatic, and hemorrhage from a disrupted vessel usually stops spontaneously.

Two scenarios that require mention are patients with a posterior knee dislocation and patients with an injury in the region of the groin or thoracic outlet. Unrecognized popliteal injuries can lead to delayed thrombosis and severe distal ischemia because of poor collateral flow about the knee. For this reason dislocations of the knee and major fractures of the supracondylar and proximal tibial areas should have vascular screening. The minimal screening comprises duplex assessment or vigilant observation/examination, and the more optimal uses angiographic imaging. An additional critical area relates to the profunda femoral artery that is buried deep in the thigh, and may be responsible for deep hemorrhage and hematomas that require intervention. When there is any question regarding injury, femoral arteriography is the best screening method and lends itself to embolic treatment of distal bleeding (proximal injuries are best exposed and repaired). In the absence of hard signs of vascular injury, patients with injuries in the region of the groin, thoracic outlet, or neck generally should be evaluated with either formal angiography or CT angiography. Duplex ultrasonography of the subclavian and iliac vessels is generally limited. Prompt evaluation is mandatory, as missed vascular injuries in these regions may lead to exsanguination into the intrapleural or retroperitoneal space.

For the chapter's Suggested Readings list, please visit the book at www.ExpertConsult.inkling.com.

PENETRATING CAROTID ARTERY: UNCOMMON COMPLEX AND LETHAL INJURIES

Juan A. Asensio, Patrizio Petrone, Alejandro Perez-Alonso, Joe DuBose, Irony C. Sade, Erin Hale, Peter Collister, Thomas P. Brush, and Frank Plani

Carotid arterial injuries are the most difficult and certainly the most immediate life-threatening injuries found in penetrating neck trauma. Their propensity to bleed actively and potentially occlude the airway makes surgical intervention very challenging. Their potential for causing fatal neurologic outcomes demands that trauma surgeons exercise excellent judgment in the approach to their definitive management (Fig. 1). Frequently, the rapidity with which these injuries bleed causes early airway occlusion from the extensive hemorrhage contained within the fascial planes of the neck, often necessitating the immediate achievement of an airway either by intubation an occasionally via surgical cricothyroidotomy. Establishing a surgical airway can be a difficult procedure, given the distortion of anatomic landmarks by hemorrhage. It is also fraught with danger, as the incision may release the contained hematoma resulting in torrential bleeding that can obscure the operative site and place the patient at risk for aspiration. These injuries incur high morbidity and mortality rates. Their neurologic sequelae can be devastating. Fortunately, they are not common.

HISTORICAL PERSPECTIVE

The first documented case of the treatment of a cervical vascular injury is attributed to the French surgeon Ambroise Paré (1510–1590), who was able to ligate the lacerated carotid artery and a jugular vein of a wounded soldier. The patient's survival was complicated by the development of a profound neurologic defect consisting of

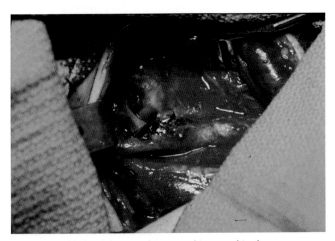

FIGURE I   High-velocity gunshot wound impacted in the common carotid artery below the bifurcation.

aphasia and left-sided hemiplegia. In 1803, Fleming ligated the lacerated common carotid artery of a sailor with a successful outcome. In 1811, Abernathy ligated the lacerated left common and internal carotid arteries in a patient who had been gored by a bull. This patient developed profound hemiplegia and subsequently died from this injury. During World War I, Makins reported 128 patients of which 30% underwent carotid artery ligation with subsequent neurologic deficits. These complications prompted a conservative approach to the treatment of the acutely injured carotid arteries reserving operative intervention for complications. During World War II Lawrence reported only two attempts at repair of a carotid artery injury; and only four repairs were reported from the Korean conflict by Hughes. Both Cohen and Rich reported 50 carotid artery injuries from the Vietnam conflict for an incidence of 5%. Thirty-eight were common injuries and 12 were internal carotid artery injuries. It wasn't until the 1970s that significant civilian series emerged in the literature incorporating knowledge derived from military experiences (Table 1).

INCIDENCE AND MECHANISM OF INJURY

Carotid artery injuries are estimated to be present in 6% to 13% of all penetrating injuries to the neck. Asensio has reported an incidence of 11% to 13% carotid arterial injuries for all penetrating neck injuries. According to Demetriades carotid artery injuries are present in 6% of all penetrating injuries to the neck and account for 22% of all cervical vascular injuries. Weaver estimates that cervical vessels are involved in 25% of penetrating head and neck trauma and that carotid artery injuries account for 5% to 10% of all arterial injuries. In 1970, Rich reported a 5% incidence in his hallmark series of 1000 arterial injuries reported from Vietnam. Penetrating mechanisms of injury are responsible for the vast majority of carotid artery injuries. Gunshot wounds, rarely shotgun wounds, and occasionally lacerations by jagged and cutting objects such as glass often produce these injuries.

ANATOMY

The anatomy of the neck is unique. In no part of the body are there so many vital structures located within such tight confines, nor is there any other area of the body that includes representative structures of so many different systems—the cardiovascular, respiratory, digestive, endocrine, and central nervous systems. All neck structures are invested by two fascial layers: the superficial fascia that encompasses the platysma, and the deep cervical fascia that encompasses the sternocleidomastoid muscle. The pretracheal fascia attaches to the thyroid and cricoid cartilages and blends with the pericardium in the thoracic cavity. The prevertebral fascia encompasses the prevertebral muscles and blends with the axillary sheath, which houses the subclavian vessels. The carotid sheath is formed by all three components of the deep cervical fascia. Such tight fascial compartmentalization of the neck structures limits external bleeding from vascular injuries, thus minimizing the chance of exsanguination.

The neck is divided into three anatomic zones: zone I extends from the clavicle to the cricoid cartilage, zone II extends from the cricoid to the angle of the mandible, and zone III extends from the angle of the mandible to the base of the skull. These zones are used to describe the location of injury in the neck. The origin of the common carotid arteries differs on the two sides. On the left the common carotid artery originates from the aortic arch whereas the right common carotid artery arises from the brachiocephalic artery. However, in the neck the anatomy is the same.

The common carotid artery originates in the neck behind the sternoclavicular joint. Each artery courses obliquely upward from beneath this joint and terminates at the level of the upper border

TABLE 1: Anatomic Location of Carotid Arterial Injuries

Authors (Year)	Number of Patients	Number of Injuries	Common Carotid Artery	Internal Carotid Artery	External Carotid Artery
Cohen et al (1970)	85	85	66	19	0
Bradley (1973)	24	26	17	7	2
Rubio et al (1974)	72	81	61	10	10
Thal et al (1974)	60	60	48	12	0
Liekweg et al (1978)	18	19	17	2	0
Ledgerwood et al (1980)	33	33	23	10	0
Unger et al (1980)	564	564	415	49	0
Brown et al (1982)	129	143	103	20	20
Demetriades et al (1989)	124	124	104	10	10
Ditmars et al (1997)	13	15	0	11	4
Mittal et al (2000)	18	18	9	7	2
Navasaria et al (2002)	32	34	24	4	6
Ferguson et al (2005)	6	6	0	3	3
Totals	1160	1189	870 (73%)	262(22%)	57 (5%)

of the thyroid cartilage, where it divides into the external and internal carotid arteries. The common carotid artery is the largest artery in the neck. It has a widened portion known as the carotid bulb at its bifurcation, which is innervated by the nerve of Hering, a branch of the glossopharyngeal nerve. The carotid bulb contains a specialized sensory organ, known as the carotid body, which is a vascular chemoreceptor located at the bifurcation on the posteromedial side. The common carotid artery, internal jugular vein, and vagus nerve are contained within the carotid sheath. There are no branches from the common carotid artery prior to its bifurcation. The external carotid artery is the smaller of the two terminal branches of the common carotid artery and extends from the upper portion of the thyroid cartilage to the angle of the mandible. The internal carotid artery ascends into the skull, piercing the skull via the foramen lacerum as it passes into the carotid canal of the temporal bone from its origin at the upper border of the thyroid cartilage, terminating intracranially by dividing into the anterior and middle cerebral arteries.

At the upper border of zone II the surgeon will often encounter the common facial vein, which is often ligated or retracted when exposing carotid artery injuries. The hypoglossal nerve crosses anteriorly to the internal carotid artery at the upper borders of zone II of the neck. The marginal mandibular branch of the facial nerve is located directly under the inferior border of the mandible.

DIAGNOSIS

Physical findings serving as reliable indicators of the presence of injuries to the vascular structures in the neck include pulsatile or expanding hematomas, the absence of pulse, the presence of bruits, and active external hemorrhage. A global neurologic defect associated with aphasia or hemiplegia likewise signals an underlying vascular injury. However, a thorough neurologic examination cannot often be performed, as many patients are admitted in shock and are thus unable to cooperate with such an examination. Establishing a diagnosis of vascular injury has been greatly facilitated by the reliability of the available diagnostic tools. Some surgeons believe that physical

examination is a very safe and reliable mode for detecting significant vascular injuries requiring treatment. Demetriades in a prospective study of 335 patients with penetrating neck injuries evaluated vascular structures on the basis of a detailed written protocol and reduced the incidence of angiography. Demetriades and Asensio reported another prospective study consisting of 223 patients who underwent a clinical examination according to a written protocol. Forty-seven patients did not undergo angiographic evaluation because of life-threatening problems that required an emergency operation (19 patients) or because they refused angiography (28 patients). The remaining 176 patients underwent four-vessel angiography. Abnormal angiographic findings were identified in 34 of these 176 patients (19.3%), but only 14 of the patients (8.0%) required treatment of the vascular lesions. The remaining 20 patients were successfully managed nonoperatively. Altogether 160 patients (71.7%) had no clinical signs suggestive of vascular injury, and none of them required operation or any other form of treatment (specificity and negative predictive value were both 100%). Angiography was performed on 127 of these 160 patients, and another 5 patients were operated on because of other associated injuries requiring surgery. None of the 5 patients who underwent neck exploration had vascular injuries. Angiography revealed 11 vascular injuries (8.3%), none of which required any type of treatment. This study supports the use of physical examination to exclude patients requiring four-vessel angiography.

Although angiography remains the gold standard for evaluation and diagnosis of cervical vascular injury, it should be reserved for injuries to zone I and III and for confirming injuries detected by color flow Doppler (CFD), which has become the technique of choice for the investigation of zone II injuries. Numerous studies by several authors consistently report sensitivities, specificities, and accuracies of greater than 95% for CFD in establishing the diagnosis of carotid arterial injuries.

We currently recommend a thorough and meticulous physical examination for all patients suspected of harboring carotid artery injuries. Those who present with clinical signs associated with cervical vascular injuries or who are hemodynamically unstable should be immediately transported to the operating room. Patients who are hemodynamically stable may be clinically observed or examined using CFD or angiography. Nemzek et al in 1996 suggested that CT angiography (CTA) could replace routine conventional angiography as a screening test in trauma. Munera et al in a study comparing CTA and angiography in the diagnosis of penetrating trauma to the arteries of the neck demonstrated favorable results for CTA with 90% sensitivity, 100% specificity, 100% positive predictive value, and 98% negative predictive value. Any injuries requiring further definition should be investigated with angiography. Angiography should be reserved for the evaluation of patients that are hemodynamically stable and may be thought of harboring injuries to vascular structures in zones I and III.

ANATOMIC LOCATION OF INJURY

The majority of carotid arterial injuries are confined to the common carotid artery. We reviewed 1160 patients who incurred 1189 carotid artery injuries. Of these patients 870 (73%) had common carotid artery injuries, 262 (22%) had internal carotid artery injuries, and 57 (5%) had external carotid artery injuries (see Table 1).

SURGICAL MANAGEMENT

In the operating room, the patient is placed supine on the operating table with the head extended and rotated to the side opposite to the area to be explored. Placement of a towel roll under the shoulders is very helpful. The face, neck, supraclavicular, and thoracic areas are included in the operating fields should an extension of the incision high in the angle of the mandible or a thoracotomy be necessary for exposure and the management of zone I and III injuries involving the very proximal and very distal carotid artery. The contralateral groin is prepared and draped separately should a segment of a saphenous vein be needed as an autogenous graft for the repair of carotid injuries.

The neck is explored though a standard incision in the anterior border of the sternocleidomastoid muscle extending from the angle of the mandible to the sternoclavicular junction (Fig. 2). An extension of the incision toward the origin of the sternocleidomastoid may be made. For injuries located in zone III, additional exposure may be obtained by division of the digastric muscle. Access to the internal carotid artery above the digastric muscle may also be facilitated by anterior subluxation of the mandible. Fixation of the subluxed

mandible can be accomplished by using arch bars, or more simply by securing the lower teeth to a wire passed transnasally. This converts the narrow triangular field at the junction of zones II and III into a much wider rectangular opening, thus allowing further exposure of the internal carotid artery up to the base of the skull. Further exposure can be obtained by extending the skin incisions circumferentially around the lobe of the ear and elevating the lower lobe. This exposure has been described by Fisher and Dossa (Fig. 3).

In the lower aspect at the junction of zones II and I, the omohyoid muscle is usually transected to obtain greater exposure. If exposure is necessary to deal with the origin of the carotid arteries in zone I, a median sternotomy is the incision of choice. This will allow for dissection of the origin of the carotid arteries off the arch of the aorta and in the case of a right common carotid artery, off the brachiocephalic trunk. Rarely, in the presence of an associated subclavian vessel injury a clavicular incision can be made for the exposure and control of these vessels. When bilateral neck explorations are needed, the incisions on the anterior borders of the sternocleidomastoid muscle may be connected by transverse incision, which will allow the trauma surgeon to elevate a flap in a cephalad direction thus exposing all structures in the midline of the neck.

Once exposure has been obtained, the first priority is to secure immediate control of life-threatening hemorrhage. Digital control of the bleeding site is maintained while dissection is carried out to obtain both proximal and distal control of the carotid artery and its branches. Rapid but meticulous dissection of the carotid sheath with meticulous attention to the preservation of the structures contained in it is of the utmost importance. It is always easier to locate the common carotid artery at the base of the neck. This is facilitated by transection of the omohyoid. This maneuver will provide for rapid proximal vascular control. A 45-degree angled DeBakey vascular clamp should be used to obtain proximal control. Alternatively, a 60-degree angled DeBakey or a Castaneda clamp (Fig. 4) can also be used. These same clamps can be used to obtain proximal control of the internal carotid artery and control of the external carotid artery. Total control of these three vessels is very important. Right or left Kitzmiller clamps are optimal to obtain very high proximal control of the internal carotid artery (Fig. 5).

Routine techniques for vascular surgical repair should be employed to deal with carotid arterial injuries. Lateral arteriorrhaphy for injuries amenable to primary repair should be employed. However, injuries that have caused significant destruction to the wall of the carotid vessels should be excised and débrided meticulously with

FIGURE 2 Exposures for zones I and II injuries.

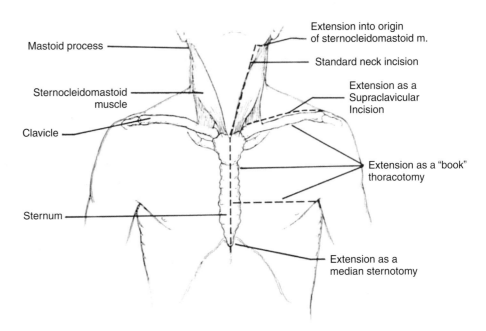

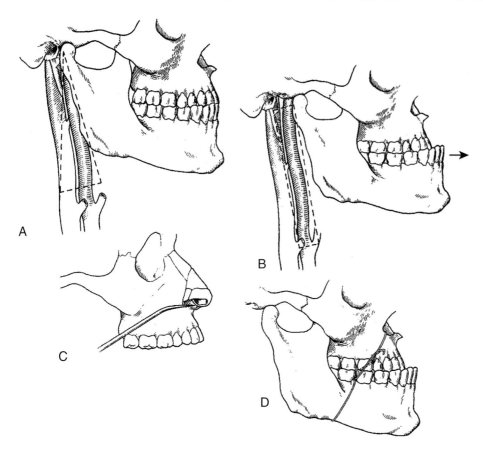

FIGURE 3 Exposure for zone III injuries.

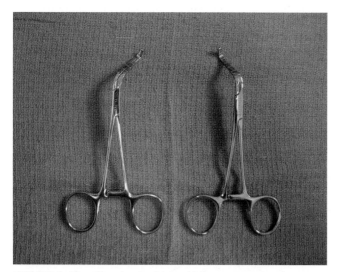

FIGURE 4 Kitzmiller clamps, right and left.

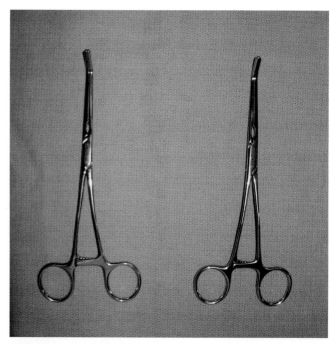

FIGURE 5 Castaneda clamps.

Potts scissors. If there are jagged edges of the intima present, they should be meticulously elevated using either a Penfield or a Freer dissector and the feathered edges should be tacked down with monofilament sutures of 6-0, 7-0, or 8-0 polypropylene. The presence of backflow from the proximal carotid artery should be observed. The presence of excellent backflow signifies adequate cross cerebral perfusion via the circle of Willis. The trauma surgeon must be cognizant of the fact that an intact circle of Willis is present in only 20% of the population. Some surgeons prefer to measure stump pressures as an objective indicator for when to use shunts. If a stump pressure is measured, a pressure of 40 to 50 mm Hg is stated to be a safe pressure indicating that no shunt needs to be used. However, our group is a proponent of using carotid artery shunts for any complex internal carotid or common carotid artery injury that would require extensive reconstruction with either an autogenous or prosthetic graft or if the patient has experienced any period of hypotension (Figs. 6 to 8).

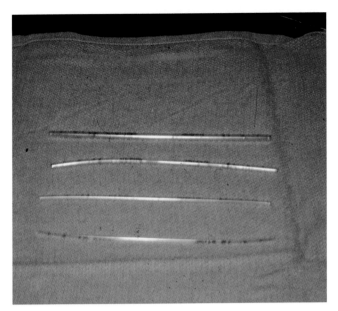

FIGURE 6 Argyle shunts.

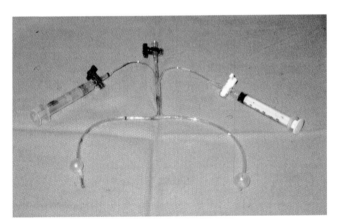

FIGURE 7 Pruitt-Inahara shunts.

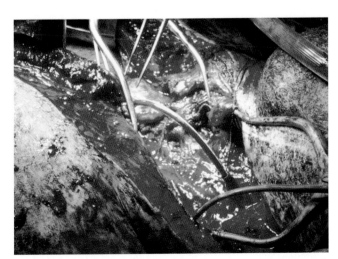

FIGURE 8 Argyle shunt placed in left carotid artery prior to bypass with nonreversed autogenous saphenous vein graft.

The passage of Fogarty catheters into a proximal injury of the internal carotid artery to reestablish blood flow is a decision that needs to be made by the attending trauma surgeon with full knowledge that this is one particular area where the creation of an iatrogenic injury with such catheter can have devastating circumstances. Although some authors prefer not to systemically heparinize patients with carotid artery injuries, serious consideration must be given by the attending trauma surgeon for using heparin as a very valuable adjunct when completing these repairs. We prefer to use 5000 U of heparin systemically in the presence of any carotid artery injury.

Common carotid artery injuries can be primarily repaired if they are tangential injuries. Occasionally, a primary end-to-end anastomosis of the vessel can be carried out if the vessel is not under tension. It is best to use an interposition graft if any degree of tension is present. It is preferable to use an autogenous saphenous vein graft for the repair of all carotid artery injuries; however, if such conduit is not available for common carotid artery injuries, then polytetrafluoroethylene (PTFE) may be used. For internal carotid artery injuries every effort should be made to secure an autogenous saphenous vein (Figs. 9 to 14). When a carotid artery injury repair is completed, release of the proximal clamps should be carried out first so that any debris or clots are flushed out prior to the completion of the anastomosis. The distal clamp is then replaced and the proximal clamp released to also flush out any debris or clot. The external carotid artery is then released, and the proximal clamp is again released so that if there is any debris or clots it may preferentially flush into the external carotid artery. After this is done and if a shunt has been placed, it is

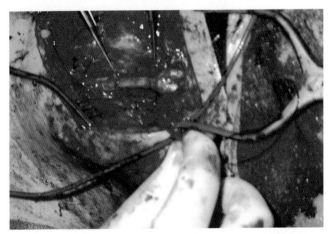

FIGURE 9 Nonreversed autogenous saphenous vein graft used to repair a common carotid artery below the bifurcation.

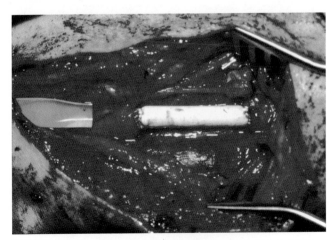

FIGURE 10 Polytetrafluoroethylene graft used to repair a common carotid artery.

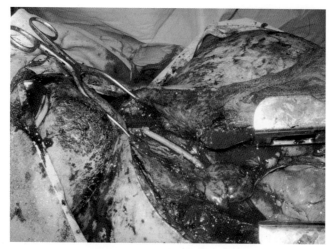

FIGURE 11 Autogenous nonreversed saphenous vein graft used to repair a common carotid artery at its origin, approximately 3 cm from the aortic arch. Patient required a median sternotomy as the injury was intrathoracic.

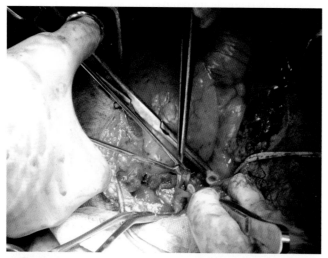

FIGURE 12 Gunshot wound to intrathoracic left common carotid artery. Note proximal and distal control. The artery is being débrided with Potts scissors.

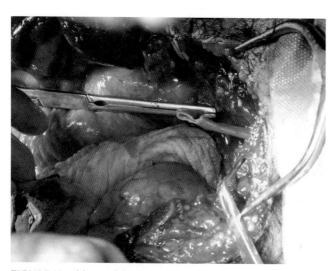

FIGURE 13 After mobilization, repair is by end-to-end primary anastomosis.

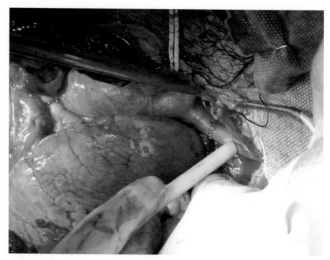

FIGURE 14 Repair completed, approximately 2 cm from the arch of the aorta. Doppler probe is used to detect triphasic flow signal.

then removed and the anastomosis is completed by placement of the last sutures. It is extremely important that systemic heparinization be used always when a shunt has been placed. We generally use 6-0 polypropylene sutures.

Asensio has recently reviewed several series describing the management of carotid arterial injuries. A total of 433 patients who incurred 456 injuries were examined; 392 (86%) of these patients underwent primary repair and 64 (14%) of these patients underwent ligation. Every conceivable attempt must be made to repair carotid artery injuries, as outcomes are much better with primary repair. Ligation for carotid artery injuries should be reserved for injuries when hemorrhage is life threatening and cannot be controlled by any other means. Ligation should also be employed for distal thrombosed or nonreconstructible internal carotid artery injuries or for patients who have fixed and profound neurologic deficits prior to exploration (Table 2).

TABLE 2: Operative Management of Carotid Arterial Injuries

Authors (Year)	Number of Cases Under Operative Repair	Number of Injuries	Repaired	Ligated
Cohen, 1970	85	85	78	7
Bradley, 1973	22	22	20	2
Rubio, 1974	72	81	69	12
Liekweg, 1978	18	19	15	4
Ledgerwood, 1980	36	36	31	5
Fry, 1980	54	54	42	12
Brown, 1982	125	139	115	24
Richardson, 1988	39	39	37	2
Ditmars, 1997	3	5	2	3
Mittal, 2000	18	18	16	2
Navsaria, 2002	32	34	28	6
Ferguson, 2005	6	6	3	3
Totals	492	519	441 (85%)	78 (15%)

TABLE 3: Mortality Rates of Carotid Artery Injuries

Authors (Year)	Number of Cases*	Mortality Rates (%)[†]
Cohen et al (1970)	85	15.0
Bradley (1973)	24	33.0
Rubio et al (1974)	72	23.4
Thal et al (1974)	60	8.3
Liekweg and Greenfield (1978)	233	10.0
Ledgerwood et al (1980)	36	16.0
Fry and Fry (1980)	54	10.0
Unger et al (1980)	722	21.0[‡]
Brown et al (1982)	129	20.9
Richardson et al (1989)	45	6.6
Demetriades et al (1989)	124	22.0
Ditmars et al (1997)	13	0
Mittal et al (2000)	18	16.6
Navasaria et al (2002)	32	6.3

*Total = 1647.
[†]Average calculated mortality rate = 15%.
[‡]Defined for only 513 cases.

OUTCOMES AND MORTALITY

Numerous reports by Liekweg and Greenfield, Fry, Ledgerwood, and Weaver confirm that outcomes are much improved if primary repair of the carotid can be carried out. Unger analyzed 722 patients who sustained carotid artery injuries. Of the 186 patients presenting with severe neurologic deficit, 34% improved if they underwent primary repair in contrast to only 14% of those who underwent ligation or were not treated surgically. We reviewed 1647 patients who sustained carotid artery injuries. Mortality rate in all of these reviewed series ranged from 0% to 33%. The average mortality rate for carotid artery injuries is 15% (Table 3).

MORBIDITY

Short-term complication from carotid arterial repairs include acute thrombosis, distal embolization, propagation of cerebral infarction, hemorrhage wound hematomas, wound infections, and nerve injury either to the hypoglossal or marginal mandibular nerve. The most devastating complication is massive cerebral infarction leading to cerebral death or a permanent vegetative state.

CONCLUSIONS

Carotid artery injuries are uncommon but extremely challenging. Their repair requires excellent and meticulous surgical techniques to avoid devastating consequences. They incur high rates of morbidity and mortality. Every conceivable attempt must be made to repair these injuries as outcomes are much better with primary repair versus ligation.

For the chapter's Suggested Readings list, please visit the book at www.ExpertConsult.inkling.com.

SUBCLAVIAN VESSEL INJURIES: DIFFICULT ANATOMY AND DIFFICULT TERRITORY

Juan A. Asensio, Patrizio Petrone, Alejandro Perez-Alonso, Mamoun Nabri, Gerald Gracia, Michael Ksycki, Paul W. White, and Robert F. Wilson

Thoracic and thoracic-related vascular injuries represent complex challenges for the trauma surgeon. Subclavian vessel injuries, in particular, are uncommon and highly lethal. Regardless of the mechanism, such injuries can result in significant morbidity and frequent fatality. Subclavian vessel injuries are generally associated with multiple life-threatening injuries. Over the years, the overall mortality rate has continued to improve as a result of significant advancements in resuscitation, emergency medical transport systems, and increased development of regionalized systems of trauma.

HISTORICAL PERSPECTIVE

Halsted in 1892 performed the first successful subclavian aneurysmal ligation. Given the infrequent occurrence of subclavian vessel injuries,

surgeons had minimal experience in their management prior to wartime. Commonly the general practice was simple ligation. During World War I, the American and British surgeons estimated the overall rate of vascular injury to range from 0.4% to 1.3%. In 1919, Makins reported 45 subclavian artery injuries among British casualties during World War I. A landmark study from DeBakey and Simeone in 1946 reported an incidence of less than 1%, accounting for 21 patients of 2471 arterial injuries sustained by American soldiers during World War II. During the Korean Conflict, Hughes's study of 304 major arterial vessel injuries reported only 3 subclavian artery cases. The relatively few cases throughout the history of war may account for exsanguination on the battlefield. Penetrating subclavian injuries accounted for less than 1% of all vascular injuries reported during the Vietnam conflict. During this time, 48 different surgeons treated this injury; only two encountered this injury more than once, for a total of 68 reported cases. Rich reported a total of 63 subclavian artery injuries in the original report of the Vietnam Vascular Registry for acute arterial vascular injuries during the Vietnam War.

During the recent conflicts of Iraq and Afghanistan, the overall rate of vascular injury was reported to be greater than in previously reported conflicts. This increase in rate may be related to improved hemorrhage control, shorter evacuation times, and improved survivability. High-velocity injuries from explosives and gunshot wounds accounted the majority of these injuries. Interestingly, the incidence of vascular injury was higher in Iraq than in Afghanistan, 12.5% and 9%, respectively. White et al identified 1570 U.S. troops, in both Iraq and Afghanistan, who presented with war-related vascular injuries. Of these, 12% resulted in vascular injuries of the torso, with subclavian vessel injuries accounting for 2.3%. Over a 24-month period, Clouse et al identified 301 arterial vascular injuries, of which 3.7%

TABLE I: Military Experience with Subclavian Vessel Injuries

Conflict	Authors (Year)	Total Arteries	Subclavian	Percentage of Total
WWI	Makins (1919)	1191	45	3.8
WWII	DeBakey and Simeone (1946)	2471	21	0.9
Korea	Hughes (1958)	304	3	1
Vietnam	Rich (1970)	1000	8	0.8
Afghanistan	Sherif (1992)	224	Combined w/axillary	N/A

were due to subclavian-axillary vessel injury. Nevertheless, both the management and treatment strategies have evolved from the various wars and battlefields over the course of time (Table 1).

ANATOMY

The subclavian arteries have different origins according to their right and left anatomic locations. On the right, the subclavian artery arises from the innominate artery behind the right sternoclavicular articulation; on the left side, it originates directly from the arch of the aorta. The subclavian artery is divided into three portions. The first portion courses from the origin to the medial border of the scalenus anterior. The second portion lies behind this muscle, and the third portion courses from the lateral border of the scalenus anterior up to the lateral border of the first rib (Fig. 1).

The first portion of the right subclavian artery arises behind the upper part of the right sternoclavicular articulation, and passes upward and laterally to the medial margin of the scalenus anterior. It ascends a little above the clavicle, the extent to which it does varying in different cases. It is crossed by the internal jugular and vertebral veins, by the vagus nerve and the cardiac branches of the vagus nerve, and by the subclavian loop of the sympathetic trunk, which forms a ring around the vessel. The anterior jugular vein is directed lateralward in front of the artery but is separated from it by the sternohyoid and sternothyroid strap muscles.

The first portion of the left subclavian artery arises behind the left common carotid, and at the level of the fourth thoracic vertebra; it ascends in the superior mediastinum to the root of the neck and then arches lateralward to the medial border of the scalenus anterior. Its anatomic relations are as follows: in front, the vagus, cardiac, and phrenic nerves, which lie parallel with it; the left common carotid artery; left internal jugular and vertebral veins; and the commencement of the left innominate vein. It is covered by the sternothyroid, sternohyoid, and sternocleidomastoid muscles. The second portion of the left subclavian artery lies behind the scalenus anterior. It is very short and forms the highest part of the arch described by the vessel.

On the right side of the neck, the phrenic nerve is separated from the second part of the artery by the scalenus anterior, and on the left side it crosses the first part of the artery close to the medial edge of the muscle. Behind the vessel are the pleura and the scalenus medius; above are the brachial plexus of nerves; below, the pleura. The subclavian vein lies below and in front of the artery, separated from it by the scalenus anterior.

The third portion of the left subclavian artery runs downward and lateralward from the lateral margin of the scalenus anterior to the outer border of the first rib, where it becomes the axillary artery. The external jugular vein crosses its medial part and receives the transverse scapular, transverse cervical, and anterior jugular veins, which frequently form a plexus in front of the artery. Behind the veins, the nerve to the subclavius muscle descends in front of the artery. The terminal part of the artery lies behind the clavicle and

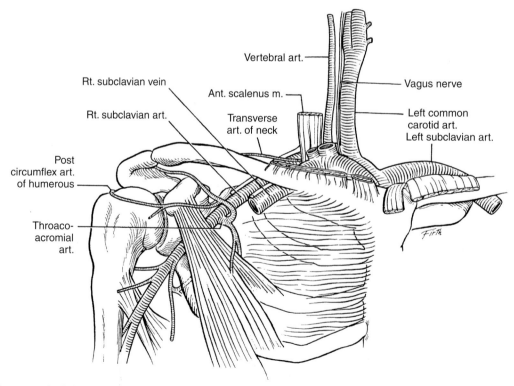

FIGURE I Anatomy of subclavian vessels.

the subclavius muscle and is crossed by the transverse scapular vessels. The subclavian vein is in front of and at a slightly lower level than the artery. Behind, it lies on the lowest trunk of the brachial plexus, which intervenes between it and the scalenus medius. Above and to its lateral side are the upper trunks of the brachial plexus and the omohyoid muscle.

The branches of the subclavian artery are the vertebral, internal mammary, thyrocervical, and costocervical trunks. On the left side, all four branches generally arise from the first portion of the vessel; but on the right side the costocervical trunk usually originates from the second portion of the vessel. On both sides of the neck, the first three branches arise close together at the medial border of the scalenus anterior; in the majority of cases, a free interval of 1.25 to 2.5 cm exists between the commencement of the artery and the origin of the nearest branch.

INCIDENCE

Subclavian vessel injuries account for approximately 5% of all vascular injuries. Busy urban trauma centers report admitting between two and four subclavian vascular injuries per year, although some international trauma centers have reported admitting as many as four patients per month. Subclavian artery injury specifically accounts for 1% to 2% of all acute vascular injuries. Although a majority of these injuries are penetrating, up to 25% are related to blunt mechanism of injury. The low incidence of subclavian artery injury is primarily explained by the anatomic location and the protective barrier provided by the clavicle and thoracic cage. In a study combining both prospective and retrospective reviews Demetriades et al reported that isolated subclavian vein injuries were present in 44% of the patients, isolated subclavian artery involvement in 39%, and combined injuries in approximately 17% of the cases. On the other hand, Lin et al reported that 24 of 54 patients presenting with subclavian artery injuries also sustained associated venous injuries.

The subclavian vessels are relatively well protected by the overlying clavicle and first rib; however, fractures to these and other adjacent osseous structures may lead to serious life-threatening injury. In one of the largest series published, Natali reported a total of 10 patients with clavicle fracture-induced injury. The incidence of clavicular fractures and associated subclavian vessel injury is estimated to be less than 1%. Richardson et al identified first rib fracture as a useful indicator of severe upper thoracic trauma. In this study, 55 patients with first rib fractures were evaluated, of which 5.5% sustained associated blunt subclavian artery injuries. A comparable review by Phillips demonstrated similar findings in the presence of displaced first rib fractures, with 9% presenting with associated blunt subclavian artery injuries.

The majority of subclavian vessel injuries in the civilian population result from penetrating trauma. Over the past several decades, there has been a steady rise in firearm-related injuries in the United States as a result of increased civilian use of weaponry. Several published series observed a similarly low incidence of blunt versus relatively high incidence of penetrating injury across the globe. Graham's largest civilian series reported 93 patients sustaining subclavian artery injuries over a 24-year period. Of these, only two resulted from a nonpenetrating injury. Over a period of 10 years, a retrospective review by Lin identified 54 patients with penetrating subclavian artery injuries, of which 85% resulted from gunshot wounds. Conversely, McKinley reported 82% of subclavian artery injuries resulted from stab wounds and 10% from low-velocity gunshot wounds, a trend not appreciated in U.S. regional trauma centers (Table 2).

On the other hand, blunt subclavian artery injuries occur far less frequently. Urban trauma centers report approximately that 1% to 3% of all traumatic subclavian artery injuries result from blunt trauma. The relatively low incidence of blunt vascular trauma is due to the subclavian vessel's protected anatomic location. Both rapid deceleration injury and bony fractures are responsible for blunt injury of this

TABLE 2: Subclavian Artery Injury: Civilian Reports

Cities	Year	Author	Injuries
Louisville	1962	Cook	3
Memphis	1964	Pate and Wilson	12
Rochester	1968	Matloff and Morton	3
Chicago	1969	Amato	14
Houston	1970	Bricker	14
Baltimore	1970	Brawley	11
Durban	1978	Robbs	24
Johannesburg	1987	Demetriades	127
Johannesburg	1994	Degiannis	56
Houston	1999	Cox	56
Los Angeles	1999	Demetriades and Asensio	79
Durban	2000	McKinley	260
Atlanta	2000	Kalakuntla	25
Chicago	2003	Lin	54
Istanbul	2004	Aksoy	12
Houston	2008	Carrick	15

artery. Not uncommonly, however, the injury remains unrecognized secondary to normal physical examination findings. In other cases, patients experience a delay in symptoms after their initial injury, thereby postponing treatment.

CLINICAL PRESENTATION

Patients sustaining penetrating thoracic inlet injuries presenting with hemodynamically instability should undergo early intubation, judicious fluid resuscitation, and immediate treatment of life-threatening injuries upon presentation. Contralateral upper extremity or lower extremity intravenous access and orotracheal intubation should be carried out in cases in which cervical or mediastinal swelling is present, resulting from expanding hematomas caused by subclavian vessel injury

In a retrospective study of subclavian vessel injury, DeGiannis et al reported that 50% of the patients in their series presented with an initial systolic blood pressure lower than 100 mm Hg. Several published series confirm similar hemodynamic findings consistent with hypovolemic shock upon presentation. In Agarwal's experience, profound shock was present in 80% of those who sustained injury to both the subclavian artery and vein. The unstable patient in hypovolemic shock unresponsive to resuscitation should be transported immediately to the operating room.

Any penetrating injury to subclavian artery with pulsatile bleeding should be controlled with direct external compression. When possible, manual compression should be continued until primary vascular control in the operating room is achieved. In cases of penetrating retroclavicular injuries, direct pressure may not be effective, and thus balloon tamponade may be a lifesaving option. In a combined retrospective and prospective study, Demetriades et al reported active bleeding from the wound in 65% of the patients upon initial evaluation, along with findings of shock in 72%. More than 20% of patients with subclavian or axillary vascular injuries reach the hospital with no vital signs or with imminent cardiac arrest as a result of exanguinating blood loss. Of note, associated intrathoracic injuries are also found in about 28% of these patients. Once the airway is secured, these patients should undergo immediate emergency department thoracotomy (EDT) on the side of injury; if necessary, the incision may be extended to the opposite side.

In McKinley et al's prospective study of 260 patients, approximately 25% of subclavian artery injuries had minimal symptoms and delayed complications, prompting patients to seek medical advice. In a series reported by Lim et al, only 24% of the patients had a pulse deficit. Apparent soft tissue ecchymosis and hematoma at the base of neck and upper chest can be a diagnostic clue on physical examination. Other characteristic findings of brachial plexus palsy, arm swelling, pulsatile hematomas, or bruit may indicate traumatic arteriovenous fistula.

DIAGNOSIS

Early diagnosis of subclavian vessel injury is essential. Physical examination findings of subclavian arterial injury may be more subtle than obvious pulsatile bleeding as seen with penetrating wounds. Other concomitant injuries adjacent to the subclavian vessels are highly suspicious for a neurovascular injury. Neurologic deficits of the upper extremity; overlying bruits; decreased or absent pulses in the brachial, radial, or ulnar arteries; and ipsilateral clavicle or rib fracture are diagnostic clues. The clinical diagnosis may be obvious with a comprehensive vascular examination revealing a cool, pulseless, and pale upper extremity. Specific signs of subclavian artery injury may also include expanding or pulsatile hematomas in the supraclavicular space or the axilla, as the hematoma dissects along the neurovascular sheath. Brachial plexopathy can also be a reliable predictor of underlying subclavian injury.

Radiographic investigations should only be performed in hemodynamically stable patients. In these cases, an initial plain chest radiograph is completed without delay. Graham et al reported that 16% of their 93 patients with penetrating subclavian injuries had radiographic evidence of mediastinal widening. Injuries to the proximal portions of the subclavian vessels may present with massive hemothorax and mediastinal widening on chest radiograph. Other diagnostic investigations include obtaining a simple ankle brachial index (ABI) in patients who are hemodynamically stable; an ABI of less than 0.9 is considered abnormal and believed diagnostic or suspicious for underlying arterial injury. However, normal ABIs may result even in the presence of a subclavian arterial injury owing to the rich collateral circulation from this vessel.

Color flow Doppler (CFD) studies are an additional noninvasive technique in assessing subclavian vessel injury. Unfortunately, CFD studies can be suboptimal in those with a large body habitus and are limited in the views of the aortic arch, innominate vessels, and left subclavian artery. Readily available spiral computed tomography (CT) scans with intravenous contrast have become a favorable option in identifying vascular injuries. CT angiography is a potential alternative in selected cases, avoiding conventional angiography in 85% of the cases.

The value of emergent angiography is restricted and should be entertained only for hemodynamically stable patients after appropriate resuscitation. Ideally, the surgeon should accompany the patient to the angiography suite. If acute decompensation occurs, the angiogram should be aborted, and the patient transferred to the operating room. Positive studies without clinical examination findings may warrant surgical exploration of the affected segment, as in cases of intimal dissection, pseudoaneurysm, and contained transection. Many advocate the routine use of angiography with subclavian artery injuries. Precise surgical planning and the identification of additional arterial injuries support these views.

In Graham's series, 20% of concomitant arterial injures were identified by angiography. Nevertheless, CFD and CT angiography are now used more frequently than conventional angiography. Angiography, however, remains the "gold standard" and should be reserved for those without any evidence of hemodynamic compromise.

SURGICAL MANAGEMENT

The operative approach of subclavian vessel injury requires great familiarity with local anatomy. The basic vascular surgical principles of proximal and distal control are imperative. Historically, a variety of classical operative exposures have been described for the management of subclavian artery injuries. The surgical approach is dictated by the clinical presentation and site of injury. The patient is initially placed in supine position with the ipsilateral arm abducted at 30 degrees and the head turned away from injury. A clavicular incision is planned, with the initial incision in the region of the sternoclavicular junction with extension over the medial half of the clavicle, and if necessary, continued onto the deltopectoral groove (Figs. 2 to 5). Adjacent muscle attachments are stripped off the clavicle to better facilitate upward retraction. Clavicular resection and disarticulation of the sternoclavicular joint are surgical techniques that offer additional exposure to proximal injuries. Henly subclavian clamps are useful in providing proximal and distal control (Fig. 6).

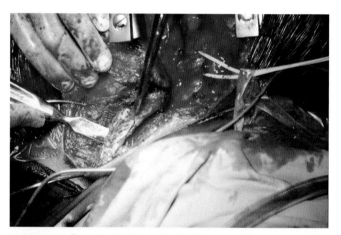

FIGURE 2 Clavicular incision with clavicle removal for exposure of subclavian vessels for gunshot wound.

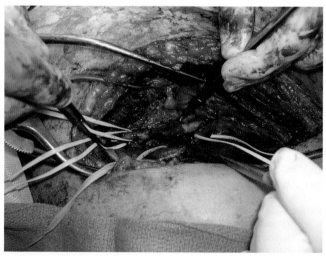

FIGURE 3 Thrombosed right subclavian artery after gunshot wound.

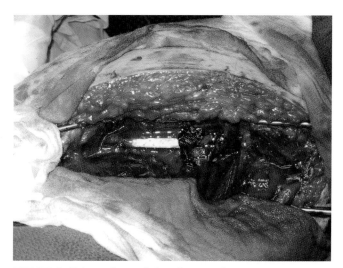

FIGURE 4 Polytetrafluoroethylene 8-mm graft.

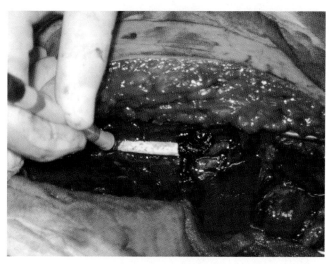

FIGURE 5 Doppler probe being used to ascertain flow and velocity post repair.

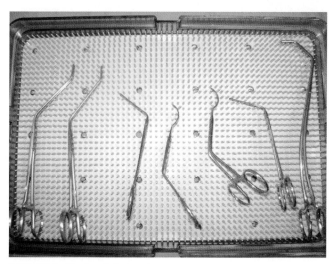

FIGURE 6 Henly subclavian clamps.

A median sternotomy with cervical extension also provides optimal control of proximal right subclavian injuries. Well described but neither recommended nor used often nowadays is the "trapdoor" incision, which allows for exposure to the first and second parts of the left subclavian artery. The components of this approach include a clavicular incision, limited median sternotomy, and an anterolateral thoracotomy. This exposure is advantageous only for left subclavian injuries, not right, because of the vessel's posterior location. These described surgical approaches are selected individually on a case-by-case basis and according to each surgeon's overall experience.

Traditionally, the operative management of subclavian artery injury includes ligation, primary repair, or interposition graft. The vascular repair chosen is influenced by the degree and level of injury. Ligation should be reserved for those who are unstable with multiple life-threatening associated injuries, extensive shoulder trauma, or infected or ruptured aneurysm. Anatomically, extensive collateral flow through the thyrocervical trunk permits safe ligation of the subclavian arteries. Arterial reconstruction should, however, be attempted whenever feasible. Occasionally temporary shunting can be used with the intention of arterial repair at a later stage.

Stab wounds sometimes can be managed appropriately with débridement and repair (Figs. 7 and 8). Simple lateral arteriorrhaphy

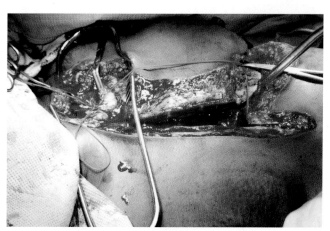

FIGURE 7 Young female who sustained a stab wound to the left thoracic inlet arrived in cardiopulmonary arrest. She required left anterolateral thoracotomy and open cardiopulmonary resuscitation. In the operating room she required median sternotomy and supraclavicular incision for the control of a left subclavian arterial injury. Clamps are providing proximal and distal control.

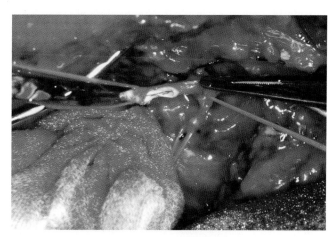

FIGURE 8 Partial transection of the left subclavian artery in the previous patient. Required resection and interposition graft with autogenous reversed saphenous vein graft.

is the preferred technique in the appropriate setting, but this method is able to be used only 20% of the time (Figs. 9 to 11). Ligating multiple arterial branches may provide additional length during primary repair, but considerable mobilization should be performed cautiously, as these branches provide an extensive collateral network to the upper extremity. On the other hand, gunshot wounds generally cause significant blast injury and usually require an interposition graft (Figs. 12 and 13). Autogenous reverse saphenous vein or prosthetic grafts with end-to-end anastomosis following débridement is one of the conventional methods used with arterial injury. Prosthetic grafts can be

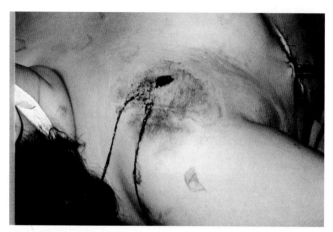

FIGURE 9 Gunshot wound in right infraclavicular area.

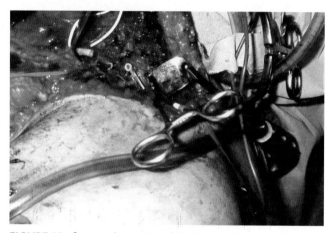

FIGURE 10 Segmental resection of the injured right subclavian artery

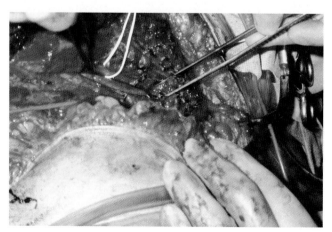

FIGURE 11 Repaired with an autogenous reverse saphenous vein graft.

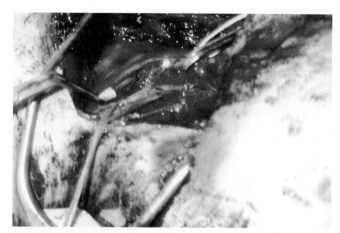

FIGURE 12 Gunshot wound right subclavian artery. Vessel débridment and resection.

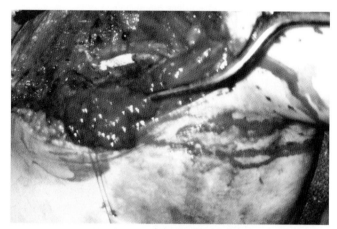

FIGURE 13 Polytetrafluoroethylene 6-mm graft inserted.

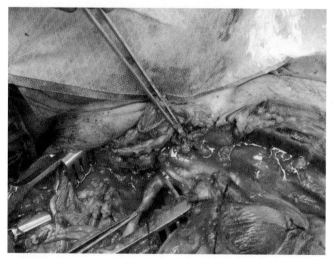

FIGURE 14 Blunt injury right subclavian artery at take-off of brachiocephalic trunk. Origin of the right common carotid artery.

safely used with acceptable outcomes due to their reported low incidence of graft infection (Figs. 14 to 16). At the same time, prosthetic grafts offer expedient repair compared to the delay associated with autologous vein harvesting. Lateral venorrhaphy in subclavian venous injuries should be attempted if it does not cause significant luminal narrowing (Fig. 17). If not feasible, then simple ligation is acceptable with little morbidity.

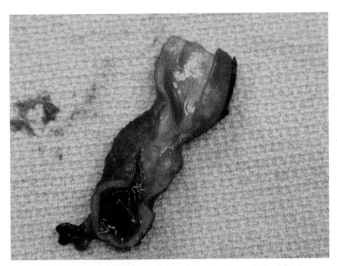

FIGURE 15   Resected segment of the subclavian artery. Intimal flap is seen.

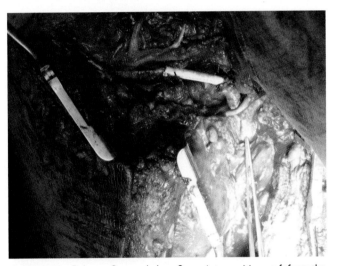

FIGURE 16   Polytetrafluoroethylene 8-mm interposition graft from the origin of the right subclavian artery. Brachiocephalic trunk.

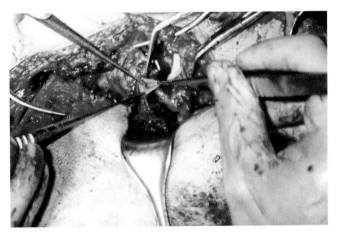

FIGURE 17   Lacerated left subclavian vein.

Recent advancements in endovascular techniques have provided another viable option to those who are poor surgical candidates and those who meet strict select criteria. Minimally invasive approaches to subclavian artery injuries are well documented and are promising alternatives in the management of these injuries.

Carefully selected patients, such as those with arterial stenosis, false aneurysms, or arteriovenous fistulas, may be managed with catheter-based stent grafts by interventional services. Definitive catheter-based repair by stent grafts are, unfortunately, not without consequence. At this time, however, endovascular repair does not appear to be superior to traditional surgical therapy but does remain an alternative option for very carefully selected patients. Similarly, there are no data available reporting on their long-term outcome (Table 3).

MORBIDITY

Delay in diagnosis, complicated operative exposure, and associated injuries are all contributing factors influencing the patient's overall morbidity at the time of admission. Hemodynamic compromise on arrival to the hospital also corresponds to higher morbidity and longer hospitalizations, as demonstrated in Kalakuntla's 6-year retrospective review in managing subclavian artery injuries. The morbidity and mortality risks with subclavian artery injuries are greatly influenced by the number of concomitant injuries. In penetrating wounds the severity of injury correlates to the location and, for cases of gunshot wounds, the velocity of the missile. Neighboring structures, particularly the subclavian vein, brachial plexus, lung, clavicle, and first rib, are most susceptible to injury.

Generally the long-term morbidity of subclavian artery injury is closely linked to the presence of associated brachial plexus injuries. Brachial plexus symptoms have resulted in debilitating ipsilateral neurosensory deficits from contusion or crush (direct trauma) and traction injury. In Graham's series of 65 patients, associated brachial plexus injury were observed in 35% of the patients. Similar findings of 43% were reported by Johnson. In this series they identified 83% of partial brachial plexus injury on follow-up, demonstrating some functional improvement, indicating neuropraxia as the initial deficit. Unfortunately, cases of complete brachial plexus transection and secondary nerve repair may only return minimal functional improvement and render the patient with permanent functional disability.

Known vascular complications such as thrombosis, graft infection, and aneurysm formation are familiar postoperative drawbacks. At the same time, postponement of medical attention following injury with symptoms of arm paralysis may occur from large false aneurysms compressing brachial plexus. These patients, despite intervention, met with poor outcomes. In cases of venous ligation, Demetriades and Asensio observed transient swelling of the upper extremity but no significant venous-related complication. Elevation of the affected extremity over a course of several days results in considerable improvement. Clavicular division also has the potential for debilitating consequences such as osseous malunion, pseudoarthrosis, and osteomyelitis.

Other complications in the management of subclavian vessel injury may predispose the patient to local surgical wound infections, coagulopathy, massive transfusions, thoracic duct injury, and air embolism. The risk of prosthetic graft infection also exists, but remains low with graft long-term patency rates of 94%. Scapulothoracic dissociation, although rare, is without question a devastating injury that results from high-energy trauma. A constellation of injuries includes clavicular fracture or dislocation, avulsed shoulder muscles, and neurovascular damage. In cases of absent brachial plexus function, vascular reconstruction should not be attempted, and the arm should be amputated below the shoulder.

OUTCOMES AND MORTALITY

Both penetrating trauma and occasionally blunt trauma to the subclavian vessels can result in significant blood loss and hemorrhagic shock prior to presentation. Select patients who have short transport times and hemorrhage control by contained hematoma or thrombosis experience improved hemodynamic status upon arrival and thus have

TABLE 3: Results of Subclavian Artery Repair

Author	Year	Injuries	Repairs	Complications	Amputations	Deaths
Amato	1969	14	13	0	0	0
Bricker	1970	14	11	0	0	3
Rich	1970	8	7	1	0	0
Drapanas	1970	16	0	0	1	4
Perry	1971	23	0	0	0	1

better survival rates. In-hospital mortality rate ranges from 5% to 35% with penetrating injuries, which is higher than in blunt trauma. The reported overall mortality rate ranges from 39% to 80%, with the majority succumbing prior to arrival to the hospital. This unfortunate statistic is directly related to exsanguination or associated head trauma in cases of blunt injury. McKinley et al's series confirms these findings and also details postmortem evaluation on violent deaths over 4 years, documenting 135 deaths as a result of isolated injury to the subclavian artery and exsanguination.

The reported operative mortality rate in published civilian series ranges from 4.7% to 30%, with higher mortality rates seen with combined subclavian artery and vein injuries. In a large series of 228 penetrating subclavian vessel injury, 61% of these patients were dead on arrival. In these series venous injuries experienced higher mortality rate than arterial injuries, 82% and 60%, respectively. Similar findings were found in another published series of 20 patients in which isolated subclavian vein injuries resulted in a mortality rate of 50%. This high rate may be due to possible venous embolus or ongoing bleeding from venous injury without the vasocontrictive effects of arterial injuries.

The morbidity and mortality risks with subclavian artery injuries are greatly influenced by the number of associated injuries. Lin reported that patients with three or more associated injuries incurred a mortality rate of 83% versus 17% for those with isolated subclavian artery injury. At the same time, those presenting with hypotension had a much higher mortality rate of 57% versus 18% for nonhypotensive patients.

CONCLUSIONS

The rarity of traumatic subclavian vessel injuries prevents many trauma surgeons or trauma centers from developing a substantial experience in their management. These injuries are associated with significant morbidity and mortality rates. Patients who survive transport are subject to potentially debilitating injury and possibly death. Management of these injuries varies, depending on hemodynamic stability, mechanism of injury, and associated injuries. Despite significant advancements the mortality rate for subclavian vessel injury remains high.

For the chapter's Suggested Readings list, please visit the book at www.ExpertConsult.inkling.com.

OPERATIVE EXPOSURE AND MANAGEMENT OF AXILLARY VESSEL INJURIES

Juan A. Asensio, Patrizio Petrone, Alejandro Perez-Alonso, Angela Osmolak, Jason Loden, Gerald Gracia, Michael Ksycki, D'Andrea Joseph, Takashi Fujita, and Yasuhiro Otomo

Axillary vessel injuries are uncommon and challenging injuries encountered by trauma surgeons. Proximity of this vessel to other adjacent veins including the axillary vein, brachial plexus, and the osseous structures of the shoulder and upper arm account for a large number of associated injuries. Hemorrhage from the axillary vessels and particularly from the axillary artery can be torrential and may lead to exsanguination if uncontrolled. This vessel is always difficult to expose and control, especially when it sustains penetrating injury. Injury to the axillary vessels may lead to severe disability, limb loss, and even death.

HISTORICAL PERSPECTIVE

In 1920 Makins described the WWI British experience with penetrating vascular injuries. He reviewed a total of 1191 arterial injuries of which 108 were axillary artery injuries and calculated a 9.0% incidence; however, none underwent repair. In 1946, DeBakey and Simeone published the WWII American experience. In this series they reported a total of 2471 vascular injuries, of which 74 were axillary artery injuries, for an incidence of 2.9% and a high rate of limb loss of 43.2%. During the Korean Conflict, Hughes reported a total of 304 arterial injuries, of which 20 were axillary artery injuries, for an incidence of 6.5%. Rich, in 1970, reported 1000 cases from the Vietnam War sustaining vascular injuries, of which there were 59 axillary injuries for an incidence of 2.6% (Table 1).

INCIDENCE AND MECHANISM OF INJURY

Reports of the military experience from the major conflicts reveals an incidence of axillary injuries ranging from 2.9% to 9% of all arterial injuries sustained in combat. This incidence is remarkably similar to that reported from the civilian experience, which ranges from 1.5% to 8.6%. A review of recent civilian series reveals that axillary arterial injuries account from 4.7% to 42.9% of all upper extremity vascular injuries (Table 2).

TABLE 1: Incidence of Axillary Artery Injury in Military Experiences

Conflict	Authors	Total Arteries	Axillary	Incidence
WWI	Makins	1191	108	9.0%
WWII	DeBakey and Simeone	2471	74	2.9%
Korean	Hughes	304	20	6.6%
Vietnam	Rich	1000	59	5.9%
Iraq	Clouse	163	10	6.1%

TABLE 2: Incidence of Axillary Artery Injury in Civilian Upper Extremity Vascular Injuries

Authors (Year)	Total Upper Extremity Arteries	Axillary	Percentage
Orcutt, 1986	150	20	13.3%
Oller, 1992	361	17	4.7%
Andreev, 1992	50	6	12.0%
Pillai, 1997	21	5	23.8%
Sriussadaporn, 1997	28	12	42.9%
Prichayudh, 2009	52	3	5.8%
Franz, 2009	30	3	10.0%

Penetrating mechanisms account for the majority of all axillary vascular injuries. Graham recently reported 65 patients with axillary vascular injuries; 95% were due to penetrating trauma but only 5% were due to blunt trauma. Similarly, the experience from the Vietnam War revealed that 98% of all axillary arterial injuries resulted from gunshots and fragment injuries (i.e., grenades or shrapnel) and only 2% were caused by blunt trauma.

ANATOMY

The axillary artery measures approximately 15 cm in length. It is the natural continuation of the subclavian artery. It begins at the lateral border of the first rib and ends at the inferior border of the teres major muscle, where it transitions to become the brachial artery.

The pectoralis minor muscle divides the axillary artery into three parts. The first part is proximal to the muscle and gives rise to one branch, the superior thoracic artery, which courses medially to supply the muscles of the first two intercostal spaces. The second part courses under the muscle and gives rise to two branches, the thoracoacromial and lateral thoracic arteries. The thoracoacromial artery is an important branch contributing to a very rich collateral circulation. It arises as a short trunk, and divides into four branches to supply the deltoid and pectoral muscles as well as the acromioclavicular region. The lateral thoracic artery travels along the lower border of the pectoralis minor muscle to supply the chest wall.

The third part lies lateral to the muscle and gives rise to three branches: the subscapular artery and the anterior and posterior circumflex humeral arteries. The subscapular artery is the largest branch. It originates from the axillary artery at the level of glenoid

fossa and descends along the lower border of the scapula to the muscles of the posterior axillary wall. It anastomoses with the descending branch of the profunda brachii artery beneath the triceps and contributes to the collateral blood supply of this area. The anterior and posterior circumflex arteries form a ring around the neck of the humerus. Anastomosis of the posterior circumflex humeral artery with the ascending branch of the profunda brachii artery provide another important contribution to the collateral circulation.

The axillary vein is formed by the joining of the two venae comitantes of the brachial artery, the brachial veins, and the basilic vein. It courses into the axilla and becomes the subclavian vein once it travels underneath the clavicle, entering the thoracic cavity by the ligament of Halsted. The axillary vein covers the axillary artery when the arm is abducted. This relationship may contribute to arteriovenous fistula formation following penetrating injuries.

The brachial plexus also lies in close proximity to the axillary artery; as a matter of fact they are invested in a common fascial sheath. The three major cords of the plexus (medial, lateral, and posterior) surround the axillary artery in its proximal portion. The major peripheral nerves of the upper extremity derive directly from these cords. The median nerve lies anteriorly, the ulnar nerve lies medially, and the radial nerve lies posteriorly to the axillary artery.

DIAGNOSIS

All patients with periclavicular or axillary trauma should be evaluated for the presence of vascular trauma. Hard signs classically diagnostic of vascular injury include significant hemorrhage, large expanding hematoma, absent or diminished peripheral pulses, and bruits on auscultation. Soft signs indicative of vascular trauma include stable hematomas, slow continuous bleeding, and associated nerve injures as well as proximity injury. The presence of peripheral pulses distally does not reliably exclude significant proximal arterial injuries given the excellent collateral circulation prevalent for this vessel.

The brachial plexus should always be evaluated. Associated injuries occur in approximately 33% of patients presenting with axillary vascular injuries. Attention should also be given to identifying associated thoracic injuries, such as pneumothoraces or hemothoraces secondary to associated pulmonary injuries, which are present in 28% to 30% of patients.

In the presence of severe hypotension, major active bleeding, or a threatened limb, the patient should be rapidly transported to the operating room. Chest radiograph should be obtained if the hemodynamic condition of the patient allows it because it may reveal an associated hemothorax, missiles, or a mediastinal hematoma that will need to be addressed.

The ankle brachial index and the brachiobrachial index (i.e., the ratio of systolic blood pressure of an injured limb to that of an uninjured limb) are useful measurements and should be obtained in all stable patients. An abnormal index (less than 0.9) is diagnostic or highly suspicious for the presence of an arterial injury. However, significant axillary arterial injuries may be associated with a normal index given the rich collateral circulation of this vessel.

Angiography should be reserved for stable patients presenting with soft signs of vascular trauma and rarely for the stable patient who presents with hard signs but the site of injury is uncertain, such as those sustaining multiple gunshot wounds, shotgun wounds, or multiple fractures (Figs. 1 to 3). Patients with proximity injury to the axillary artery without completely defined indications for operative exploration should also undergo angiography because significant injuries can be present and can thus be identified in asymptomatic patients. False aneurysms, arteriovenous fistulas, and intimal disruption of the axillary artery have been managed successfully with endovascular stenting, but this experience remains quite limited.

Computed tomography angiography (CTA) is another promising diagnostic modality that may eventually replace or become complementary to angiography. The adoption of helical multidetector CT

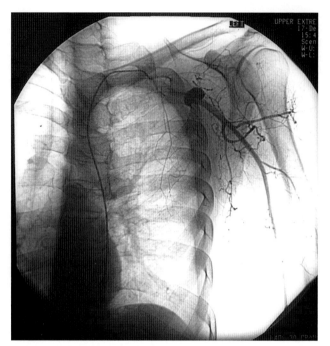

FIGURE 1 Gunshot wound, left axillary artery. Angiogram reveals injury to the second portion of the axillary artery.

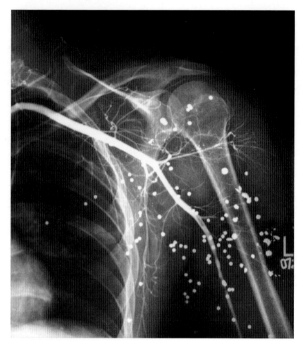

FIGURE 3 Angiogram revealing segmental injury to the left axillary artery.

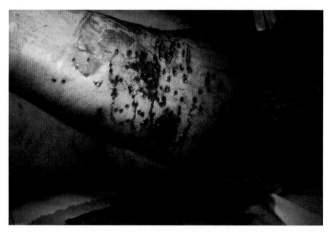

FIGURE 2 Intermediate range shotgun injury to the left arm and axilla.

scanners (64 sections) and three-dimensional reconstruction has increased the resolution and decreased scanning time. Studies investigating CTA in upper and lower extremity injuries have demonstrated sensitivity and specificity of CTA to be 95% to 100% and 87%, respectively. Limitations of CTA include difficulty differentiating spasm from occlusion and the presence of artifacts from high-attenuation structures such as missile fragments or other foreign matter which at times may prove rendering a definitive diagnosis difficult.

SURGICAL MANAGEMENT

Basic Principles for the Management of Vascular Injuries

A number of critical surgical maneuvers are standard in the management of all vascular injuries and are applicable to the management of axillary vessels injuries:

1. Apply direct pressure for control of active bleeding.
2. Prep the person holding pressure into the operative field.
3. Choose the appropriate surgical exposure and plan to expose the injured vessel widely.
4. Obtain proximal and distal control of both arteries and veins, as combined injuries are common.
5. Isolate the injured vessels with meticulous dissection.
6. Retraction of injured or uninjured vessels can be carried out by looping them with vessel loops or Cushing vein retractors.
7. To retract nerves, use gentle dissection and place two vessel loops at distal points for retraction to distribute the pressure required to retract the nerve evenly.
8. Identify the injury and approach directly after proximal and distal control have been obtained.
9. Expose the injured vessel widely with meticulous surgical dissection. This maneuver may require taking down some of their branches and collaterals; however, care must be exercised to preserve as many as possible.
10. Except for some stab wounds and lacerations in which the vessel can be directly repaired or anastomosed, resect appropriate length of the injured vessel until normal proximal and distal vessel is obtained. In the case of arteries, resection should avoid raising intimal flaps.
11. Inspect the transected edges of the artery. If there are intimal flaps, reresect. In cases in which there is an extensive flap and further resection is not possible, tack the intimal flap with internal horizontal mattress sutures of Halsted, placing the sutures from the inside of the vessel lumen and tying the knots outside the vessel. Use the finest monofilament polypropylene sutures.
12. Flush the proximal and distal ends of the transected vessel with heparinized saline. Check for distal back-bleeding. Flush frequently and gently.
13. If there is no distal back-bleeding, pass Fogarty catheters of the appropriate size and length gently and, if possible, under direct vision of the vessels being thrombectomized. Do not hyperinflate the balloon and do not pass the catheter more than necessary to achieve good back-bleeding as this will increase the risk of intimal damage. If there is no arterial flow return, papaverine may be instilled to break vasospasm.

14. Arterial injuries may be repaired by primary arteriorrhaphy or by end-to-end anastomosis. They may also require a bypass or interposition graft either with an autogenous reverse saphenous vein graft or with a prosthetic graft. Repairs and bypasses should never be under tension. They also should not be excessively long in order to prevent kinking. Bypasses placed across a joint must have their length properly selected with consideration of the range of motion (flexion) of the joint to prevent kinking or graft occlusion. All anastomoses should be performed end to end with double-armed polypropylene sutures, preferably in a running fashion. Although it has been commonly thought that straight anastomosis might eventually develop stenosis, this is not the case.

15. Vessel discrepancies may be addressed by spatulating or "fish-mouthing" the graft. For small end-to-end vessel anastomoses simple interrupted sutures of polypropylene may be used circumferentially and for difficult anastomoses the tripartite suture technique of Carrel may be used.

16. Bypasses performed to smaller vessels such as distal radial and ulnar arteries may require their distal anastomosis to be end to side, which increases both the size of the anastomosis as well as its flow characteristics.

17. Venous injuries may be ligated or primarily repaired. Double ligation with silk sutures is preferred for all veins. Primary venorrhaphy should be carried out with fine monofilament polypropylene sutures preventing narrowing of the repaired vein. Very rarely venovenous bypass may be required.

18. Fasciotomies should be performed early, expediently, and when indicated. The more soft tissue injury there is, the shorter amount of ischemic time is tolerated. We recommend using cadaveric skin grafts as biologic dressings.

19. At the completion of the arterial repair or bypass, pulses should be checked by digital palpation and interrogated by a handheld Doppler probe including the proximal and distal anastomosis of the bypass, the bypass itself, and all distal vessels.

20. The use of completion angiography should be individualized; however, it is highly recommended to detect correctable defects intraoperatively, which will prevent a vessel and bypass failure.

Specific Management of Axillary Vessels Injuries

Preoperatively, external bleeding is controlled by direct pressure over the wound; however, bleeding from vessels behind the clavicle is difficult if not impossible to control by direct compression. In these patients balloon tamponade with a Foley catheter may be effective.

In the operating room the patient should be placed in the supine position with the arm abducted at 90 degrees and the head turned to the opposite side. Excessive abduction should be avoided, as it distorts the anatomy and makes the exposure more difficult. The entire anterior chest, abdomen, and neck should be prepped and draped within the operative field to allow for possible thoracic and cervical exploration. The whole arm should also be prepared to allow for repositioning, extension of the incision, and palpation of brachial, radial, and ulnar pulses.

Exposure of the axillary artery via an infraclavicular approach provides an excellent exposure (Fig. 4). The incision begins inferior to the middle of the clavicle and is carried laterally to the deltopectoral groove. This incision can be extended onto the proximal arm into the medial bicipital sulcus to obtain additional exposure of the distal axillary and brachial artery. If exposure of the subclavian artery or proximal axillary artery is required to obtain proximal control, an incision can be made at the sternoclavicular junction, extending it over the medial half of the clavicle at the middle of clavicle where it curves downward over the deltopectoral groove to join the infraclavicular incision. Furthermore, the medial half of the clavicle may be divided and excised to gain exposure to the proximal axillary and the subclavian artery, especially in bleeding patients.

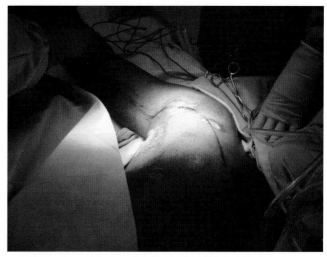

FIGURE 4   Incision for the exposure of axillary vessel injuries.

The exposure of the axillary vessels requires separation of the pectoralis major muscle fibers and retraction of the underlying pectoralis minor muscle. In the presence of active bleeding and when rapid and extensive exposure is required, the muscles should be divided. The pectoralis major is divided about 2 cm from its attachment to the humerus and retracted inferomedially. The underlying pectoralis minor then is divided near its insertion on the coracoid process and retracted inferiorly. The axillary vessels are thus exposed fully. During dissection, all efforts should be made to preserve collateral branches and avoid iatrogenic brachial plexus injury.

After obtaining proximal and distal control, the injured segment of the artery should be carefully examined to delineate the extent of the injury. Simple arteriorrhaphy may be performed if the injury allows for approximation without tension. However, the injured segments usually require resection and débridement before operative repair. Thrombectomy with a Fogarty catheter should be gently performed with the end point of obtaining good inflow and back-bleeding before repairing the injured vessels. End-to-end anastomosis may be possible in some injuries; however, in most gunshot wounds, an interposition graft is usually required. The choice of graft—autogenous vein versus prosthetic graft—is a matter of personal preference, availability, and general condition of the patient (Figs. 5 to 7). There is no evidence of superiority for any of them. In critically ill patients who cannot tolerate definitive repair, ligation and temporary intravascular shunting with an Argyle shunt are viable damage control options; however, ligation of the acutely injured axillary artery has been associated with an amputation rate ranging from 9.0% to 43.2%.

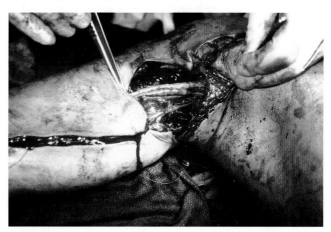

FIGURE 5   Autogenous reverse saphenous vein bypass graft.

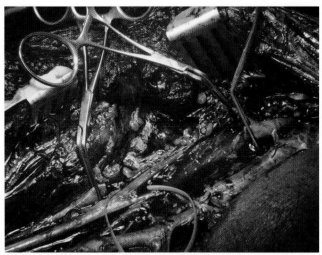

FIGURE 6 Resected right axillary artery after gunshot wound in anticipation of bypass. Please note axillary vein.

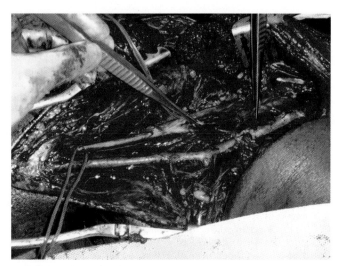

FIGURE 8 Ligated axillary vein.

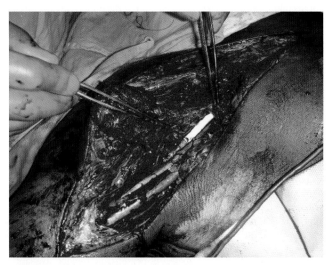

FIGURE 7 Polytetrafluoroethylene 6-mm bypass graft.

Axillary venous injuries can be repaired by simple venorraphy; more complex repairs including vein-vein bypass or using grafts should not be attempted as ligation of the vein is well tolerated by almost all patients (Fig. 8). Furthermore, there is no evidence suggesting that complex reconstruction has superior outcome. Following axillary vein ligation, the patient may develop transient edema that subsides within a few days. Close observation and fasciotomy of the upper arm when indicated may provide a safe approach.

OUTCOMES AND MORTALITY

Amputation rates for axillary artery injuries in recent civilian series have ranged from 0% to 3%, which is much lower when compared to 8.5% to 43.2%, which is the incidence reported during early military experiences. Associated brachial plexus injury remains the major determinant of long-term functional outcome. These injuries are present between 30.4% and 35.4%. Thrombosis after arterial repair has been reported to range from 1.5% to 10%, and infectious complications have been reported to range from 0% to 21%. Mortality rate in recent civilian series has ranged from 3% to 14.8% (Table 3).

TABLE 3: Outcomes of Axillary Artery Injuries in Recent Civilian Series

Authors (Year)	Number of Patients	Treatments	Amputation (%)	Brachial Plexus Injury (%)	Deaths (Mortality Rate)
Graham, 1982	65 (31 arteries, 14 veins, 20 combined)	Arterial ligation, 0 Venous ligation, 9 Arterial repair, 51 Venous repair, 25	2 (3%)	23 (35.4%)	2 (3%)
Degiannis, 1995	32 (penetrating axillary artery injuries)	Repair, 31 (died before repair, 1)	0 (0%)	11 (34.4%)	2 (6.3%)
Demetriades and Asensio, 1999	79 (penetrating subclavian and axillary; 39 arteries, 20 veins, 20 combined)	Arterial ligation, 0 Venous ligation, 26 Arterial repair, 59 (endovascular repair, 1) Venous repair, 14 ED thoracotomy, 18 (all expired)	N/A	26 (32.9%)	27 (34.2%) Excluding ED thoracotomy 9 (14.8%)

TABLE 3: Outcomes of Axillary Artery Injuries in Recent Civilian Series—cont'd

Authors (Year)	Number of Patients	Treatments	Amputation (%)	Brachial Plexus Injury (%)	Deaths (Mortality Rate)
McKinley, 2000	260 (proximal axillary and subclavian artery injuries)	Repair, 236 Ligation, 5 No surgery, 19	N/A	79 (30.4%)	10 (11.5%)
Aksoy, 2005	38 (axillary and subclavian artery injuries)	Repair, 33 Ligation, 5	1 (2.6%)	12 (31.5%)	2 (5.2%)

ED, Emergency department.

CONCLUSIONS

Although uncommon, axillary arterial injuries can result in significant morbidity, limb loss, and fatality. Early diagnosis and timely repair of the artery lead to good outcomes. Selection of an appropriate extensile incision and adequate exposure of the artery are of paramount importance in the surgical management of axillary vessel injuries.

For the chapter's Suggested Readings list, please visit the book at www.ExpertConsult.inkling.com.

Brachial Vessel Injuries: High Morbidity and Low Mortality Injuries

Juan A. Asensio, Patrizio Petrone, Alejandro Perez-Alonso, Parth Shah, Austin Person, Anthony M. Udekwu, John K. Bini, and Ari Leppäniemi

Reports of arterial injuries from both the civilian and military arenas report the brachial artery as the most frequently injured vessel, accounting for approximately 25% to 33% of all peripheral arterial injuries. The frequency of injury is similar in some reports to that of the superficial femoral artery as both arteries are long and located in vulnerable positions in their respective extremities. Experiences from both the Korean and Vietnam conflicts have also revealed that nearly 30% of all arterial injuries involve the brachial injury.

Certain anatomic characteristics are particularly important with regard to brachial arterial injuries. There is a marked difference in the degree of ischemia resulting from injuries proximal and distal to the profunda brachii branch. Accordingly, the risk of gangrene is approximately twice as great following ligation of the common brachial artery as compared to the superficial brachial artery.

The brachial artery is surrounded by important peripheral nerves—the median, ulnar, and radial—and also parallels the humerus and associated veins. Because of its close proximity to these structures, associated nerve and osseous injuries are frequent, with residual neuropathy from such nerve injuries often the main source of permanent disability. In the lower extremity, weight bearing is the principal consideration in rehabilitation; however, in the upper extremity functional use of the hand remains the most important outcome.

HISTORICAL PERSPECTIVE

Hallowell, in 1759, was first to repair a brachial artery injury using the "veterinarian's or Farrier's stitch," supplanting the original technique of ligation and thus providing the founding step for the management of vascular trauma. Torrance, in 1903, performed a successful suture repair of a brachial artery injury following a blunt trauma, and Jones, in 1919, reported two cases of brachial artery ligation following gunshot wounds with a 1-year follow-up reporting that both patients had extensive residual disability of the affected arm. Since that time there have been many evolutionary and revolutionary advances. Even with these early reported cases, ligation remained the primary treatment during both World War I and World War II, especially in combat situations. Long transport times to definitive care, lack of antibiotics, and inadequate fluid resuscitation necessitated amputation for other than technical reasons. The results were far from desirable, with amputation rates of nearly 50% for these patients (Table 1).

INCIDENCE AND MECHANISM OF INJURY

Brachial artery injuries are the most commonly reported arterial injury of the upper extremity. In large military and civilian series, brachial artery injury accounts for 15% to 30% of all peripheral arterial injuries. The reason for this relatively high frequency is that the brachial artery is relatively long, superficial, and exposed when compared to other peripheral arteries. Furthermore, the upper extremity is often used as a lever, hammer, and weapon, as well

TABLE 1: Military Experience with Brachial Artery Injuries

Conflict	Authors (Year)	Total Arteries	Brachial	Percentage
WWI	Makins (1919)	1191	200	16.8
WWII	DeBakey and Simeone (1946)	2471	601	24.3
Korea	Hughes (1958)	304	89	29.3
Vietnam	Rich (1970)	1000	283	28.3

TABLE 2: Civilian Experience with Brachial Artery Injuries

City	Authors (Year)	Total Arteries	Brachial	Percentage
Houston	Morris (1960)	220	55	25.0
Atlanta	Ferguson (1961)	200	29	14.5
Denver	Owens (1963)	70	14	20.0
Detroit	Smith (1963)	61	13	21.3
Dallas	Patman (1964)*	271	46	17.0
St. Louis	Dillard (1968)	85	26	30.6
New Orleans	Drapanas (1970)	226	39	17.3
Dallas	Perry (1971)	508	78	15.4
Memphis	Cheek (1975)	155	21	13.5
Denver	Kelly and Eiseman (1975)	116	37	31.9
Jackson	Hardy (1975)	360	75	20.8
New York	Bole (1976)	126	14	11.1
Indianapolis	Cikrit (1990)	101	23	22.7
Johannesburg	Degiannis (1995)	170	37	21.8
Cape Town (SA)	Zellweger (2004)†	N/A	124	N/A
Izmir (Turkey)	Ergunes (2006)†	N/A	58	N/A
Tehran (Iran)	Rasouli (2009)	130	18	13.8
Chicago	Kim (2009)†	N/A	139	N/A

*Continuing series.
†Only brachial artery injuries included in series.

as a protective or restraining device for the torso, all of which place the brachial artery at risk for injury.

Overall vascular injuries of the extremities are infrequently reported. A recent review of the National Trauma Database (NTDB) medical records of 1,861,779 patients revealed that 1.6% of all patients sustained vascular injuries, 0.3% of all patients had upper extremity vascular injuries, and 0.1% of all patients sustained brachial arterial injuries. Brachial artery injury composed 28% of all upper extremities injury and 15.5% of all peripheral vascular injures. Ninety-seven percent of brachial artery injuries were due to penetrating trauma. Some reports showed great differences in the rate of reported brachial injuries ranging from 14% to 50%.

Data from the military setting revealed that between 3.8% and 6.6% injuries were vascular related. Brachial artery injuries accounted for 23% of all extremity vascular injures and as much as 58% of all upper extremity vascular injuries. The mean age of injury has been reported to be from 27 to 31 years of age in both civilian and military populations; males represent about 90% of the injuries in civilian series and nearly 100% in all military series.

There was a preponderance of males versus females in the civilian population, almost 90% being male and nearly 100% of military brachial artery injuries were male. Of these injuries the vast majority were penetrating (94%) versus blunt (6%).

Penetrating trauma remains the most common cause of brachial artery injury. Most injuries are caused by gunshot wounds, stab wounds, or lacerations from broken glass or other jagged objects, especially in civilian trauma. Rich in 1970 reported a large series from the Vietnam conflict consisting of 283 patients with brachial artery injuries; 250 of these patients sustained injuries from either fragments or shrapnel. Over 50% of the brachial artery injuries occurred secondary to fragments from various exploding devices and, approximately 40% of the patients sustained gunshot wounds.

Recently, the increase in the number of diagnostic cardiac catheterizations has resulted in a concomitant increase in the number of brachial artery injuries, often followed by thrombosis, that are seen at most tertiary medical centers. In contrast to the civilian experience, in the military setting, thrombosis of either the axillary or brachial arteries occurs infrequently, occurring in less than 1%. With penetrating trauma being the most common mechanism of injury, the majority of brachial artery injuries found at the time of surgery are transections (60–84%) followed by lacerations (13%), thrombosis (5–16%), intimal flaps (3%), and pseudoaneurysms (15.3%), yet arteriovenous (AV) fistulas are uncommon (3%). Interestingly enough isolated brachial arterial injuries occur, with a frequency of 22%.

Blunt injury of the brachial artery occurs with a lesser frequency but deserves emphasis, as its diagnosis may be easily overlooked. Supracondylar fracture of the humerus, particularly with anterior displacement or elbow dislocation, should alert the trauma surgeon to the possibility of an underlying brachial artery injury. This has resulted in the ischemic syndrome of Volkmann's contracture. Fortunately, this is now a rare occurrence due to awareness and monitoring of high-risk injuries and immediate vascular repair and decompression if symptoms of a compartment syndrome are present (Table 2).

ANATOMY

The brachial artery is a continuation of the axillary artery and begins at the lower border of the teres major muscle. Exiting the axilla, the brachial artery is a relatively superficial structure covered only by skin, subcutaneous tissue, and deep fascia. Proximally, it lies medial to the humerus and is accompanied by the median nerve (superiorly and laterally) and the ulnar and radial nerves (medially). Distally, it lies anterior to the elbow and is crossed by the median nerve, which then lies medial to the artery. Just proximal to the elbow, the ulnar nerve is posterior to the artery as it goes behind the medial epicondyle of the ulna. The brachial artery terminates approximately 3 to 5 cm below the elbow skin crease, where it divides into the radial and ulnar arteries.

The brachial artery has three main branches. The first (most proximal) is the profunda brachii, which is accompanied by the radial nerve and passes posteriorly between the medial and long head of the triceps muscle. The profunda brachii provides an important collateral anastomosis with the axillary artery through its posterior circumflex humeral branch. The profunda also has a collateral anastomosis with the radial recurrent artery. The profunda brachii artery has two branches: the anterior branch, which anastomoses with the radial recurrent artery, and the posterior interosseus recurrent artery. Both branches form additional important collateral pathways. The second main branch of the brachial artery is the superior ulnar collateral, which accompanied by the ulnar nerve passes behind the medial epicondyle to provide a collateral anastomosis with the posterior ulnar recurrent. The third (most distal) main branch is the inferior ulnar collateral, which provides a rich anastomotic collateral network around the elbow with the ulnar artery through its anterior recurrent branch.

DIAGNOSIS

The diagnosis of brachial arterial injuries is often made clinically. Hard signs of injury include absent/diminished pulses, active (pulsatile) bleeding, distal ischemia, expanding or pulsatile hematoma, and presence of a thrill or bruit. Hard signs of injury mandate immediate surgical exploration of the vessel unless the patient harbors multisystemic injuries that are life threatening.

The use of hard signs as an indication for surgery in patients with gunshot wounds has resulted in 100% therapeutic exploration rate. Soft signs of injury include associated osseous injuries, proximity of a penetrating wound, significant hemorrhage that has ceased or hemorrhagic shock, neurologic deficit and hematomas. Confirmation of arterial injury in this setting requires radiologic evaluation. Pulse deficit is the most common finding occurring in 43% to 89% with brachial arterial injures.

Brachial-brachial indices (assuming the other extremity is uninjured) must always be obtained. A threshold of less than 0.9 is an indication for invasive studies or operative exploration. Additional modalities useful in making a diagnosis include noninvasive studies such as Doppler ultrasound (Figs. 1 and 2). Angiography remains the gold standard for the diagnosis of vascular injuries (Fig. 3); however, considerable advances in computed tomography angiography (CTA) are quickly overtaking standard angiography. CTA has the advantage of being quicker, more operator-independent, and more readily available than standard angiography. Approximately 10% of patients may require an angiogram. Common angiographic findings of brachial arterial injury are arterial occlusion, intimal tears, and presence of pseudoaneurysm.

ANATOMIC LOCATION OF INJURY

The brachial artery has an almost equal distribution of injury throughout its course with proximal, middle, and distal being each injured about one third of the time.

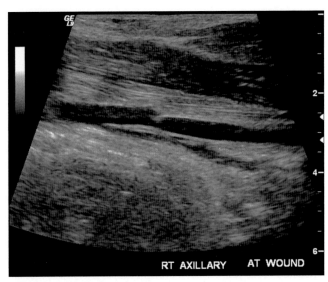

FIGURE 1 A 26-year-old man with a right brachial artery injury resulting from a gunshot wound to the right axillary region. Gray scale ultrasound images demonstrate an intimal flap along the proximal third of the brachial artery.

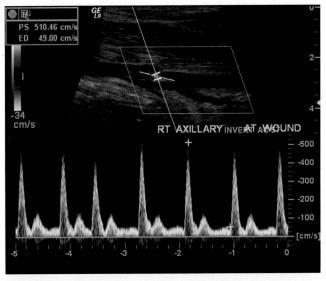

FIGURE 2 A 26-year-old man with a right brachial artery injury resulting from a gunshot wound to the right axillary region. Color flow Doppler and spectral waveforms show focal high peak systolic velocities indicating high-grade stenosis along the injury.

SURGICAL MANAGEMENT

Hemorrhage can be controlled by direct pressure over an open wound. Blindly attempting to clamp bleeding vessels in the upper extremity is never necessary and is fraught with the hazard of significant injury to the accompanying median, radial, or ulnar nerves. For suspected proximal injury, the patient should be prepped and draped in a fashion similar to that used to manage an axillary artery injury. For injuries that are more distal, prepare the arm and hand to the fingertips to allow intraoperative palpation of the radial and ulnar pulses, and prepare the contralateral leg for possible harvesting of a conduit. The arm should be supported on a board but be mobile. The draping should allow space for one operator to be positioned cephalad and another to be positioned caudad to the arm support.

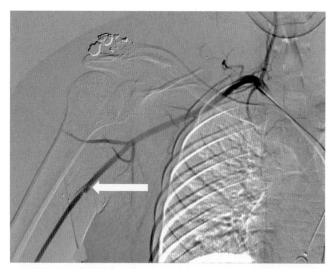

FIGURE 3 A 26-year-old man with a right brachial artery injury resulting from a gunshot wound to the right axillary region. Angiogram confirms a brachial injury *(arrow)* and shows the bullet fragments overlying the acromioclavicular joint.

As with most arteries in the upper extremity, exposure is best obtained by making a longitudinal incision over the bicipital sulcus between the biceps and triceps, which is easily identified by abduction of the biceps muscle from the arm. Care must be exercised in avoiding injury to the superficial basilic vein, which is easily retracted once identified. Distally, the artery dives below the bicipital aponeurosis, which should be divided to obtain maximal exposure of the artery. At the level of the antecubital fossa, the incision should make a laterally oriented S curve to allow access to the bifurcation and to avoid joint contracture.

General principals of vascular exploration are applicable in the management of brachial arterial injuries. They include proximal/distal control, exploration of injured arterial segment, débridement of nonviable vessel, and identification of associated injures (Fig. 4). When possible, the brachial artery should be repaired. The exact method of repair is determined by the extent of the injury, the amount of damage to the surrounding tissues and the length of arterial segment damaged.

Interposition grafts using reversed autogenous saphenous vein are the standard for repair of long segmental injury (Fig. 5). Its use has been well documented for repair of a variety of different mechanisms

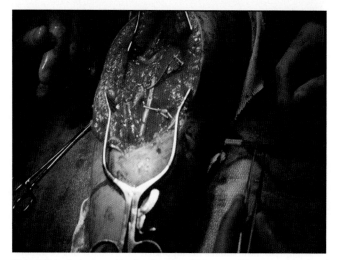

FIGURE 4 Stab wound in the distal brachial artery. Notice proximal and distal control with Dietrich bulldog clamps.

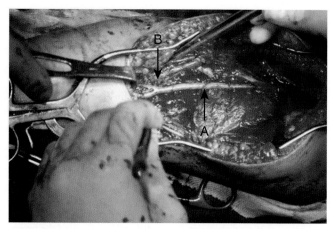

FIGURE 5 Gunshot wound in the distal brachial artery. Repaired with autogenous reversed saphenous vein graft. Distal anastomosis (**A**) is close to origin of the bifurcation of the brachial artery (**B**).

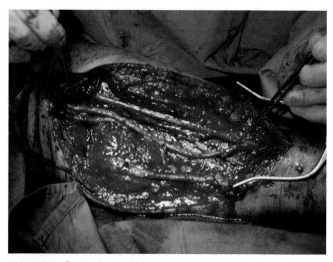

FIGURE 6 Brachiobrachial bypass with autogenous reversed saphenous vein graft after segmental resection of brachial artery secondary to gunshot wound. Gerald forceps point to proximal and distal anastomosis.

of injury in both military and civil studies. Simultaneous harvesting of an autogenous saphenous vein after obtaining proximal and distal control of the vessel is followed by débridement of the injured vessel and end-to-end bypass with either vein and polytetrafluoroethylene (PTFE) grafts (Figs. 6 and 7).

Smaller injuries may be treated with débridement followed by end-to-end anastomosis or simple arteriorraphy if the defect is small. Care must be taken, as with all vascular repair procedures to ensure that there is no undue tension on the artery.

Successful use of temporary vascular shunts has been reported in both the military and civilian arenas. Temporary shunts may be used in the setting of damage control surgery, or in some instances of more complex injury and with associated fractures of the upper arm (Figs. 8 to 11). In a review of shunt usage in severely traumatized patients, there was an 88% limb salvage rate. If associated orthopedic injuries are present, the most popular technique is to place an indwelling temporary shunt to restore arterial flow while the orthopedic surgeons achieve length and stability of the arm before attempting definitive vascular repair. Ligation should rarely be a consideration as it carries a significant risk for limb loss. If the patient is in extremis from other associated injuries, surgical exposure of the brachial artery is rapidly obtained by a longitudinal incision along the course of the artery with

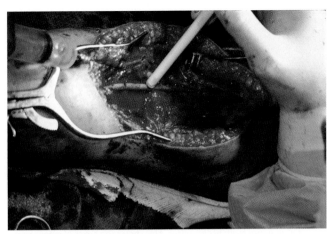

FIGURE 7 The assessment of triphasic flow signals as well as flow velocities should always be carried out after repair with a Doppler probe.

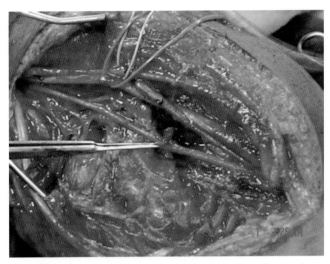

FIGURE 9 Segment of thrombosed left brachial artery after gunshot wound. Jerrel forceps point to the thrombosed segment in this very small vessel. Red vessel loop is retracting the contused left median nerve.

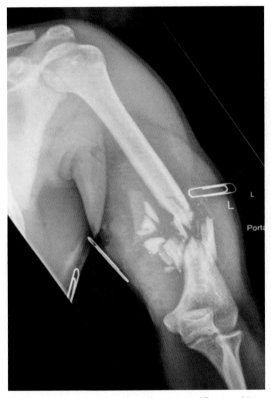

FIGURE 8 Gunshot wound to the left arm in a 15-year-old man resulting in a complex humeral fracture and associated brachial artery injury.

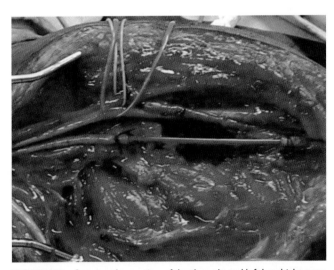

FIGURE 10 Segmental resection of the thrombosed left brachial artery. The patient experienced significant vasospasm requiring intra-arterial papaverine and the use of a 3.5 coronary probe in order to dilate the vessel prior to placement of a No. 8 Argyle shunt to restore blood flow in anticipation of open reduction and internal fixation prior to definitive vascular repair.

an extension as an S curve either across the axilla proximally or across the antecubital fossa distally as needed. The median nerve and basilic veins are in close proximity to the artery. A temporary shunt can be placed quickly and left in place for several days without systemic heparinization.

Ligation should be reserved for life-threatening situations, overwhelming damage, or inability to repair. In the absence of ischemic signs prior to ligation, there is often a significant chance for limb survival and preservation of function.

Fasciotomies, if not performed initially are often required in up to 30% of cases (Figs. 12 to 15). Intraoperative blood loss, combined arterial and venous injury, and open fractures have been found to be independent risk factors for development of compartment syndrome (Table 3).

OUTCOMES AND MORTALITY

Since the early days of military operations when the primary techniques included ligation and subsequent amputation, most patients today can expect excellent outcomes if their injuries do not involve massive tissue destruction and can be repaired promptly. Large series have reported successful brachial artery repair with primary patency rates of 92% to 98%.

Kim reported repair failures diagnosed intraoperatively in 7.2% of patients, and Padayachy reported 4.4% of repair failures diagnosed immediately postoperatively. Klocker and Kim reported repair failures within a few days after surgery. Up to 10% of war-related injuries required a secondary surgical procedure. Graft replacement, thrombectomy, fasciotomy, ligation of the artery, and rarely amputation are the surgical options in this situation. Fatality in this kind of injury is extremely rare and usually is related either to immediate or late complications of associated injures.

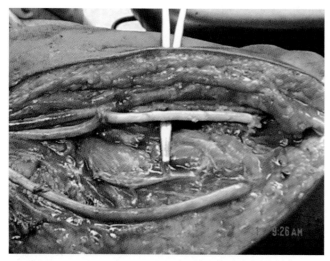

FIGURE 11 Definitive vascular repair with autogenous reversed saphenous vein graft. Vessel was quite small and required 6-0 polypropylene single interrupted sutures using the tripartite suture technique of Carrel. Notice the fish-mouth incisions in both the proximal and distal anastomosis in order to increase the luminal size. Clamp is placed through the entrance wound. Median nerve is visualized at the bottom of the figure.

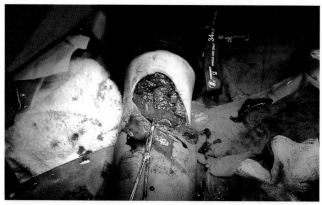

FIGURE 12 A 28-year-old man sustained a self-inflicted brachial transection injury from broken glass. Tourniquet was applied to control life-threatening hemorrhage. Transected basilic vein was clamped.

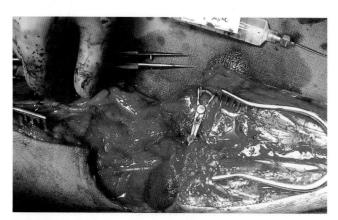

FIGURE 13 A 28-year-old man sustained a self-inflicted brachial transection injury from broken glass. This shows the proximal and distal segment of the transected brachial artery. The distal segment is located approximately 3 cm above the bifurcation. Vessel controlled with Dietrich bulldog clamps. Notice syringe with heparinized saline.

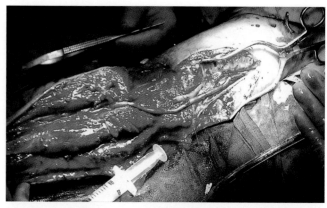

FIGURE 14 A 28-year-old man sustained a self-inflicted brachial transection injury from broken glass. This shows the brachial artery repair with end-to-end bypass with autogenous reversed saphenous vein graft extended distally to the bifurcation. The patient also had a transected proximal radial artery. Notice titanium Castroviejo forceps used for the creation of the anastomosis with 6-0 polypropylene sutures. Patient required extensive fasciotomies and carpal tunnel release.

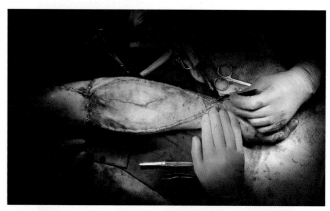

FIGURE 15 A 28-year-old man sustained a self-inflicted brachial transection injury from broken glass. Following bypass repair of the brachial artery with autogenous reversed saphenous vein graft, fasciotomy was performed and covered with cadaveric skin graft in anticipation of definitive reconstruction with autogenous skin graft 5 days after the injury.

MORBIDITY

Commonly associated injuries are nerve injuries (62%); stratified according to the major nerves, we find 79% of median nerve followed by the ulnar nerve (23%), radial (12%), and musculocutaneous nerve injuries (4%), with multiple nerve injuries occurring in a little over 10%. Approximately 13% of explorations will not yield evidence of injury and should not be seen as unnecessary or not indicated. Much like a negative exploratory laparotomy in trauma, the threshold to take the patient to the operating room must be low to avoid missed injuries.

Neurologic injury continues to impair the function of the upper extremity even after a successful arterial repair. Major venous injuries, fractures, and widespread tissue destruction may also influence the long-term function of the extremity. Whether primary and secondary nerve repair procedures are helpful is a point of controversy. The rate of functional disability ranges from 27% to 44% when injury to the upper extremity includes nerve injuries.

TABLE 3: Surgical Techniques Used for Management of Brachial Artery Injuries: Civilian Experience

Author (Year)	Number of Cases	No repair	Primary Repair	Saphenous Vein Interposition	Prosthetic Graft Interposition	Ligation
Combined Series (1984–1994)	223	5 (2.2%)	121 (54.2%)	87 (39.0%)	0 (0%)	3 (1.3%)
Degiannis (1995)	37	0 (0%)	13 (35.1%)	24 (64.8%)	0 (0%)	0 (0%)
Zellweger (2004)	124	0 (0%)	47 (21.1%)	74 (59.7%)	2 (1.6%)	2 (1.6%)
Ergunes (2006)	58	0 (0%)	40 (70%)	18 (30%)	0 (0%)	0 (0%)
Kim (2009)	139	0 (0%)	46 (33.1%)	82 (60.0%)	8 (57.6%)	1 (0.7%)

CONCLUSIONS

The morbidity and mortality rates associated with brachial artery injuries depend on the cause of the injury itself, which vein or tendon is injured, and whether musculoskeletal and nerve injuries are also present. During the last 20 years, amputation associated with upper extremity arterial injuries has decreased to a rate of 3% because of advances in the treatment of shock, the use of antibiotic therapy, and increased surgical experience.

For the chapter's Suggested Readings list, please visit the book at www.ExpertConsult.inkling.com.

Iliac Vessel Injuries: Difficult Injuries and Difficult Management Problems

Juan A. Asensio, Patrizio Petrone, Alejandro Perez-Alonso, Richard Denney, Gerald Gracia, Michael Ksycki, Bradley S. Putty, James B. Sampson, and Robert F. Wilson

Injury to the iliac vessels poses a serious and frustrating treatment dilemma for all trauma surgeons. Throughout both civilian and military history injuries to the iliac vessels have been devastating, due to the often uncontrollable hemorrhage and severe associated injuries that accompany them. Generally, patients present in profound shock secondary to severe hemorrhage from either iliac arterial, venous, or combined injuries. The associated problems and injuries that further complicate management include spillage and contamination from associated small and large bowel and genitourinary tract injuries. Pelvic fractures are more commonly present in blunt trauma and are associated with blunt injury of the internal iliac artery and vein and their branches. Even after struggling to obtain proximal and distal control of the vessels, the majority of patients will succumb to the deadly effects of acidosis, hypothermia, and coagulopathy as well as the sequelae of reperfusion injury. Despite improvements in our emergency medical services (EMS), rapid transport, standard training of trauma surgeons, and improved technology, the morbidity and mortality rates of iliac vessel injuries still remain high, ranging from 25% to 40%.

HISTORICAL PERSPECTIVE

Significant advances in the field of trauma surgery have emerged from both military and civilian arenas of warfare. The earliest known documents concerning vascular trauma date from 1600 BC The Ebers papyrus reported the Egyptians use of styptics consisting of vegetable matter, lead sulfate, and copper sulfate to stanch hemorrhage. The Chinese in the year 1000 BC were first to use tight bandaging to control hemorrhage from wounds in conjunction with the use of styptics for hemorrhage. The treatment of choice for vascular injuries throughout the Middle Ages consisted of cautery with boiling oil. In 1497, Jerome of Brunswick published his work on ligatures as treatment for bleeding gunshot wounds. Ambroise Paré was first to report the use of ligatures to control hemorrhage from vessels during amputation. Paré was also credited with the development of the first hemostat "le bec de corbin (crow's beak)." The first attempt at vascular reconstruction was attempted by Hallowell in 1759 when he reported the repair of a brachial artery with the Farrier's or veterinarian's stitch. Some 127 years would pass until vascular repair was again attempted.

The latter part of the 19th century saw such pioneers as Jassinowsky and Postemski revive the idea of direct vascular repair. Isreal, in 1883, described the first successful primary repair of a laceration to the iliac artery. In 1897 Murphy of Chicago completed the first successful end-to-end anastomosis of a femoral artery, and Goyanes of Spain in 1906 was first to report the use of a saphenous vein graft to repair a popliteal artery.

Attempts at vascular repair emerged during the Balkan Wars (1912–1913) when Soubbotitch reported a series of 77 false aneurysms and arteriovenous fistulas from penetrating injuries which were managed with ligation (45), arteriorrhaphies (19), venorrhaphies (13), and 11 with end-to-end arterial anastomosis and 4 with end-to-end venous anastomoses. In this series there were few repair failures reported and infection was avoided in almost all of the procedures. Further advances and refinements in the technique of vascular anastomosis were reported by Carrel in 1902 with the tripartite suture and by Frouin in 1908 with his quadrangulation method.

During World War I vascular repair saw a promising emergence with German surgeons attempting and successfully treating more than 100 arterial injuries in multiple vessels. However, the face of this conflict was about to change with the introduction of high explosive ordnance into the battlefields of World War I. The increase in the numbers of wounded at a single time added to the poor evacuation process and, accompanied by a high rate of gangrene, curbed the initial experiences of German military surgeons. By the same token the poor follow-up of those who were successfully treated led many to question the long-term patency of those repairs.

Despite these setbacks there were those who proceeded with promising results. Weglowski presented a series consisting of over 600 patients during his service in the Russian army and subsequently as the surgeon general of the Polish army. In his 1919 report, he recommended all arterial injuries and associated posttraumatic aneurysms be repaired immediately after the injury or, if not feasible, 1 month later for any pulsatile masses. This included all extremity injuries as well as injuries to carotid, aortic, subclavian, and iliac arteries. In 1924 he reported his personal experience with 193 vascular repairs, including 46 lateral repairs, 12 end-to-end anastomoses, and 56 venous grafts. Wound infection forced him to revert to ligation for the remaining 79 patients. His results and data were surprisingly good and have been unfortunately overlooked.

During World War II DeBakey and Simeone reported results that were not as promising when compared to WWI results. A total of 2471 arterial injuries were collected; nearly all were treated with ligation resulting in an amputation rate of 49%. There were only 81 attempts at repair of which 78 required lateral suture repair and only 3 end-to-end anastomoses were performed. The authors summarized their findings by pronouncing that ligation of the damaged artery was applicable and no other procedure should be attempted. "It is not a procedure of choice. It is a procedure of stern necessity, for the basic purpose of controlling hemorrhage."

Despite these findings there were isolated attempts from both sides of the conflict that reported some success with arterial repair. Possible reasons for such poor results included irreparable injuries from multiple types of high-velocity weaponry; increased destructive power of ordnance, resulting in higher numbers of casualities; and significant delays in transport, resulting in irreversible ischemia. Inadequate timely evacuation to higher echelons of surgical care along with understaffed and poorly supplied field hospitals added to the high incidence of ligation rates and high rate of amputations.

The Korean conflict saw greater success in arterial repairs based not only on the advances made in the surgical techniques of the past wars; other factors such as improvements in anesthesia, the advent of antibiotics, and the development of blood transfusions were responsible for improving the success rate of vascular repairs. Perhaps the single greatest factor was the development of forward aid stations accompanied by rapid evacuation of the wounded by helicopter. Wound infection was less rampant due to acceptance and practice of débridement of dead tissue, delayed primary closure, and

antibiotics. The U.S. Army established specialized research groups to improve treatment of vascular injuries in 1952. There were significant contributions from Jahnke in 1953, followed by Hughes in 1955 and 1958. During the Korean conflict a series by Hughes reported 304 arterial injuries of which 269 were repaired and 35 ligated. The overall amputation rate was significantly reduced from the WWII rate of 49% to 13%.

During the Vietnam conflict advances in evacuation and transport along with a higher number of surgeons trained to perform vascular repairs resulted in improved outcomes along with the creation of the Vietnam Vascular Registry at Walter Reed Army Medical Center to provide follow-up for the wounded sustaining vascular injuries starting with the first 500 patients who had sustained 718 vascular injuries, including injury to carotid, subclavian, axillary, brachial, aorta, renal, iliac, femoral, and popliteal vessels. Rich, in 1969, reported the amputation rate during the Vietnam conflict at approximately 8%; this number was subsequently revised by Rich and Hughes to 13%, who included amputations performed within the first month following injury. During the initial report; 126 end-to-end anastomoses, 127 vein grafts, 29 lateral sutures, and 2 prosthetic grafts were recorded. The registry was expanded several times to include many patients treated by other branches of the military, becoming an invaluable resource to the development of vascular surgery.

INCIDENCE

DeBakey and Simeone reported a total 43 iliac artery injuries out of 2471 patients for an incidence of 1.7%. The incidence of iliac injury was similar for both the Korean and Vietnam Wars. Hughes in 1958 reported an incidence of 2.3% for the Korean conflict and Rich in 1970 reported an incidence of 2.6% for the Vietnam War. Interestingly enough, a number of different institutions have reported their own experiences with iliac vessel injuries over the past several decades with surprisingly similar incidence, morbidity, and mortality rates (Tables 1 and 2).

The incidence of iliac vessel injuries has increased in the civilian arena secondary to increases in violence seen in urban trauma centers. Overall, the incidence of iliac vessel injury has been reported at approximately 10% for penetrating injury and gunshot wounds. Stab wounds and impalement account for 2% of iliac vessel injuries. The most infrequent injuries are those due to blunt trauma, accounting for 5% of injuries in Asensio's series consisting of 185 iliac vessel injuries. The internal iliac vessels were most commonly injured from blunt trauma; the mechanism of injury results in stretching of the vessel over the bony pelvis resulting in intimal tears and thrombosis.

The incidence of iliac vessel injuries during major military conflicts has remained the same. DeBakey reported an incidence of 1.7% of iliac vessel injuries in World War II. Hughes reported an incidence of 2.3% for the Korean conflict, and Rich reported an incidence of iliac vessel injury of 2.6% for the Vietnam War.

TABLE 1: Wartime Incidence of Iliac Vessel Injuries

Conflict	Author(s)	Year	Total Vascular Injuries	Iliac Vessel Injuries	Incidence (%)
WWI	Makins	1919	1191 (isolated arteries)	6	0.5
WWII	DeBakey and Simeone	1946	2471 (isolated arteries)	44	1.7
Korea	Hughes	1958	304 (isolated arteries)	7	2.3
Vietnam	Rich	1970	1000 (isolated arteries)	26	2.6
Iraq	Clouse	2007	408 (301 arteries and 107 veins)	14	3.4
Iraq-Afghanistan	White	2011	1570 (arteries and veins)	61	3.8

TABLE 2: Civilian Incidence of Iliac Vessel Injuries

| Author(s) | Year | Total Injuries | ILIAC INJURIES | | | Incidence (%) |
			Artery	Vein	Total	
Mattox[†]	1989	5760	232	289	521	9.0
Bongard[†]	1990	478				10–15
Asensio*	2000	504	60	52	112	23.4
Davis*	2001	489	72	100	172	35.2
Tyburski*	2001	731	118	104	222	30.4
Paul*	2010	167	24	32	56	33.5
Clouse[†]	2007	408	9	5	14	3.4
White[†]	2011	1570	19	17	61 (25 combined injuries)	3.8

*Series reporting abdominal vascular injuries.
[†]Series reporting cardiovascular injuries.

ANATOMY

The retroperitoneum is divided into three anatomic zones. Zone I is the central retroperitoneum, from the diaphragm all the way down to the bifurcation of the aorta and the cava. Zone II includes the lateral and superior aspect of the retroperitoneum. Zone III involves the medial and lateral portions of the lower retroperitoneum and the pelvis. The abdominal aorta divides, on the left side of the body at the fourth lumbar vertebra, into the two common iliac arteries. Each is about 5 cm in length. They diverge from the termination of the aorta, travel down and lateralward, and divide, opposite the intervertebral fibrocartilage between the last lumbar vertebra and the sacrum, into two branches, the external iliac and internal iliac—the former supplies the lower extremity; the latter, the viscera and parietes of the pelvis.

The right common iliac artery is somewhat longer than the left, and passes more obliquely across the body of the last lumbar vertebra. In front of it are the peritoneum, the intestines, branches of the sympathetic nerves, and, at its point of division, the ureter. Behind, it is separated from the bodies of the fourth and fifth lumbar vertebrae, and the intervening fibrocartilage, the termination of the two common iliac veins, and the commencement of the inferior vena cava. Laterally, its relations are as follows: above, with the inferior vena cava and the right common iliac vein; below, with the psoas major. Medial to it, above, is the left common iliac vein.

The left common iliac artery is in relation, in front, with the peritoneum, the intestines, branches of the sympathetic nerves, and the superior hemorrhoidal artery; and it is crossed at its point of bifurcation by the ureter. It rests on the bodies of the fourth and fifth lumbar vertebrae and the intervening fibrocartilage. The left common iliac vein lies partly medial to and partly behind the artery; laterally, the artery is in relation with the psoas major.

The common iliac arteries supply small branches to the peritoneum, psoas major, ureters, and the surrounding loose areolar tissue, and occasionally give rise to the iliolumbar, or accessory, renal arteries. Their point of origin varies according to the bifurcation of the aorta. In three fourths of cases, the aorta bifurcates either upon the fourth lumbar vertebra, or upon the fibrocartilage between it and the fifth lumbar vertebra; the bifurcation being, in 1 case out of 9, below, and in 1 out of 11, above this point. In about 80% of the cases the aorta bifurcated within 1.25 cm above or below the level of the crest of the ilium, more frequently below than above.

The point of division is subject to great variety. In two thirds of a large number of cases it was between the last lumbar vertebra and the upper border of the sacrum, being above that point in 1 case out of 8,

and below it in 1 case out of 6. The left common iliac artery divides lower down more frequently than the right.

The relative lengths, also, of the two common iliac arteries vary. The right common iliac was the longer in 63 cases, the left was longer in 52, and they were equal in 53. The length of the arteries varied, in 5 out of 7 cases examined, from 3.5 to 7.5 cm; in about half of the remaining cases the artery was longer, and in the other half, shorter; the minimum length being less than 1.25 cm, the maximum 11 cm. In rare instances, the right common iliac has been found wanting, the external iliac and internal iliac arising directly from the aorta.

Collateral circulation of the common iliac artery include the anastomoses of the hemorrhoidal branches of the internal iliac with the superior hemorrhoidals from the inferior mesenteric; of the uterine, ovarian, and vesical arteries of the opposite sides; of the lateral sacral with the middle sacral artery; of the inferior epigastric with the internal mammary, inferior intercostal, and lumbar arteries; of the deep iliac circumflex with the lumbar arteries; of the iliolumbar with the last lumbar artery; of the obturator artery, by means of its pubic branch, with the vessel of the opposite side; and with the inferior epigastric.

CLINICAL PESENTATION

Abdominal vascular injury should always be suspected in the presence of penetrating injuries to the abdomen, pelvis, and buttocks, either from gunshot or stab wounds or impalements. The presence of a distended abdomen, hemorrhagic shock, or diminished or absent pulses in the lower extremities is virtually pathognomonic. Associated injuries may also indicate potential iliac vessel injuries. Gross hematuria suggests renal or bladder injury, which may place the iliac vessel within the path of injury. Bright red blood on rectal examination or gross spillage of stool indicates an injury to the colon or rectum and places the iliac vessel in proximity to the potential area of injury.

Blunt trauma to the iliac vessels is usually associated with fractures to the pelvis. The loss or decreases of lower extremity pulses in the presence of an unstable pelvis is highly suggestive of an iliac injury. Patients who present in shock after sustaining blunt pelvic trauma must be evaluated for the presence of intraperitoneal hemorrhage. Continued hemorrhage from the internal iliac vessels or branches is a common cause of persistent hypotension and shock in blunt pelvic trauma. These patients may harbor an unstable pelvis on physical examination, which is suspicious for fractures as well as a sacroiliac joint disruption, which should be confirmed immediately by radiographic examination. Temporary pelvic volume reduction with a pelvic binder will reduce pelvic hemorrhage by tamponade and slow the expansion of the hematoma. These patients, in the absence of other sources of intraperitoneal hemorrhage, should undergo angiography for evaluation and possible embolization of bleeding vessels. Regardless of the mechanism of injury, stabilization and resuscitation must be immediate and the need for operative intervention determined quickly to affect a positive outcome.

DIAGNOSIS

Patients who present with penetrating abdominal injury and suspected of harboring abdominal vascular injury require no other intervention than resuscitation and immediate transport to the operating room (OR) for exploration. Diagnostic examinations and radiographic evaluation should not delay transporting an unstable patient to the OR. Hemodynamically stable patients with penetrating trauma may benefit from a cross-table lateral radiograph of the chest and abdomen to better identify the path and location of the projectile, which may predict iliac vessel involvement.

The focused assessment with sonography in trauma (FAST) examination may also suggest an iliac injury with positive findings in the pelvis consistent with the path of injury. Blunt injuries in the hemodynamically stable patient may require a more in-depth workup starting with radiographic study of the chest, pelvis, and involved lower extremities. Orthopedic findings associated with iliac vessel injury include sacroiliac joint disruption, bilateral superior and inferior pubic rami fractures ("butterfly fracture"), and symphysis pubis diastasis greater than 2.5 cm.

These above-mentioned radiologic findings should prompt use of angiography and external fixation. Computed tomography (CT) scan of the abdomen and pelvis with arterial contrast has become a viable part of the diagnostic workup in hemodynamically stable patients. This is most beneficial in patients with pelvic fractures diagnosed on baseline pelvic films. A contrast blush demonstrates an area of arterial injury and suspected bleed for which angiography followed by embolization provides the definitive treatment. However, there are limitations to its use. Blunt trauma resulting in pelvic fractures benefits from its diagnostic ability and the ability to angioembolize and stop extravasation from the internal iliac artery and branches. There is some benefit to addressing intimal tears and occlusions of the external or common iliac arteries and temporizing any active bleeding with balloon occlusion until surgical intervention is available.

SURGICAL MANAGEMENT

Prior to exploratory laparotomy for a suspected iliac vessel injury, arrangements should be made for blood to be available in the OR; in addition, consideration should be given to activate the institution's massive transfusion protocol. In addition, all possible efforts should be made to maintain the patient normothermic. Broad-spectrum antibiotics should be administered prior to incision, and the patient should be prepped and draped under the usual sterile conditions from the sternal notch and axilla bilaterally to the knees. If a zone III hematoma is encountered secondary to penetrating trauma, it must be explored.

Initial control of an exsanguinating vessel is achieved by direct compression and subsequently by obtaining proximal and distal control. This may be obtained by one of two ways; direct dissection down onto the vessel or by transection of the avascular line of Toldt paracolic peritoneum and medial rotation of the descending colon and sigmoid on the left, or ascending colon on the right. Care must be taken on either side during dissection not to injure the ureters as they cross over the common iliac artery at the bifurcation as well as the iliac vein coursing beneath the artery.

The level at which cross-clamping for both proximal and distal control will vary depending on the area of injury; injuries to the

common iliac near or at the bifurcation can be proximally controlled by aortic cross-clamping. Distal control can be obtained by progressive dissection along the artery or if involving the distal external artery, a groin incision may be needed to obtain control at the proximal common femoral artery or distal external iliac and thus can be obtained by transecting the inguinal ligament. Vascular clamps and alternatively vessel loops may be used to occlude flow. An alternative method for proximal and distal vessel control may include endoluminal blockade using large-bore Fogarty catheters, small Foley catheters, or an aortic occlusion balloon. This is very infrequently feasible as most patients sustaining iliac vessel injuries arrive in shock, with multiple other associated injuries that require immediate control. Similarly, the vast majority of America's busiest trauma centers lack hybrid ORs.

Lacerations or partial transections to the common or external iliac arteries may be repaired primarily with a 4-0 or 5-0 Prolene suture in either interrupted or running fashion. Whichever method is chosen, great care must be taken to avoid narrowing the artery or causing stenosis. Fogarty catheters should be sized appropriately and used to clear distal and proximal arteries of potential clot; this should be performed prior to completion of the repair or anastomosis. As with any injury, damaged or devitalized tissue must be débrided, even if this renders primary repair no longer a feasible option. End-to-end anastomosis is an option following proper débridement as long as there is adequate length to perform the repair without any tension. Patch repair with either polytetrafluoroethylene (PTFE) or vein may be appropriate in very selective semicircumferential injuries. Again, care must be demonstrated in order not to create stenosis of the artery or cause aneurysmal dilation with a poorly sized patch.

Interposition grafts are indicated when there has been significant vessel destruction and primary end-to-end anastomosis is not feasible. PTFE is an excellent choice for conduit; it is available in variable sizes and shows moderate resistance to contaminated fields. Saphenous vein is very rarely adequate in size, and spiraling a vein graft is too time consuming in a hypotensive patient and is thus not recommended.

Extra-anatomic bypass including the classic axillofemoral bypass has been used as an option for patients who have sustained significant associated colonic injuries with massive contamination. Several forms of internal iliac artery interposition bypasses have been described in the literature but all are time consuming and are technically difficult, especially in hypotensive, acidotic, and coagulopathic patients. For these patients and those with multiple injuries, damage control should be instituted early. Vascular shunting should be used early. Temporary Argyle vascular shunts, pediatric chest tubes, and even nasogastric tubes provide for temporizing and lifesaving measures and may be placed in both artery and vein. In the face of prolonged ischemic time or shunting for damage control, it is advisable to perform lower extremity fasciotomies on both the lower and upper leg.

The controversy of PTFE grafts versus extra-anatomic bypass in contaminated fields has been the subject of much debate; Burch reviewed 233 penetrating iliac artery injuries. Some of these injuries had associated gastrointestinal and urologic injuries. He stated the presence of contamination did not impact the operative decision or outcome of graft repair. However, with severe contamination, extra-anatomic bypasses, or the more complicated iliac artery transpositions should be considered. This becomes more complicated in the face of multiple injuries and hemorrhagic shock. Similarly, finding the appropriate size autogenous vein for a vessel this size is almost impossible.

Blunt arterial injuries are caused by compression of the iliac vessels between the pelvic girdle and the vertebral column during blunt trauma. Motor vehicle collision and direct application of blunt forces to the pelvic girdle are often at fault. The result is usually an intimal disruption with thrombus formation. Surgical repair demands resection and débridement of the injured section of artery. Repair with interposition grafting, usually PTFE, will suffice.

TABLE 3: Management of Iliac Vessel Injuries

Author		Total Iliac Vessel Injuries	Arteriorraphy	Ligation	Ligation and EAB	End-to-End	PTFE	Other	None
Wilson (1990)	Artery								
	Vein	49	18 (36.7%)	31 (63.3%)					
Cushman (1997)	Artery	36	7 (19.4%)	12 (33.3%)	1 (2.8%)	7 (19.4%)	3 (8.3%)	2 (5.6%)	5 (13.9%)
	Vein	56	17 (30.3%)	33 (58.9%)					5 (8.9%)
Davis (2001)	Artery	72	29 (40.3%)	25 (34.7%)				10 (13.9%)	8 (11.1%)
	Vein	100	35 (35%)	59 (59%)					6 (6%)
Asensio (2003)	Artery	72	57 (79.2%)	1 (1.4%)		14 (19.4%)			
	Vein	113	12 (10.6%)	101 (89.4%)					
Haan (2003)	Artery	48	17 (35.4%)	17 (35.4%)	10 (20.9%)			4 (8.3%)	
	Vein	49	19 (38.8%)	27 (55.1%)				3 (6.1)	
Clouse (2007)	Artery	9	2 (22.2%)	1 (11.2%)			2 (22.2%)	4 (44.4%)	
	Vein	5	3 (60%)					2 (40%)	

EAB, Extraanatomic bypass; PTFE, polytetrafluoroethylene.

Repair of venous injuries are dependent on several factors such as location, exposure and size of disruption, and patient stability. The best results are obtained with primary repairs with 4-0 or 5-0 Prolene vascular sutures with great care taken not to restrict or narrow the vessel lumen. A saphenous vein patch can rarely be attempted with a segment of vein harvested and sutured in place with 4-0 or 5-0 Prolene sutures. If destruction of the vessel is severe and primary repair is not feasible, ligation is warranted due to the reported poor patency rates of PTFE in vein injury. Several more time-consuming and technically difficult variations exist including jugular vein interposition and panel grafting from saphenous vein, which have been anecdotally reported but are not recommended. Again, in the unstable patient with multiple injuries, ligation may be the lifesaving option (Table 3) (Figs. 1 to 12).

Although biologic patches such as bovine pericardium or other antibiotic impregnated grafts may be available, experienced trauma

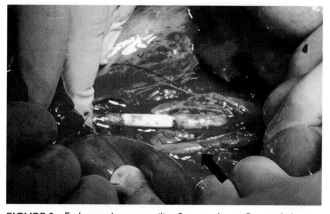

FIGURE 2 End-to-end common iliac 8-mm polytetrafluoroethylene graft replacing the injured right common iliac artery. Note the right ureter *(arrow)*.

surgeons such as Asensio, Burch, Mattox, Bongard, and Feliciano do not recommend them in their respective series. Asensio and Burch have reported the largest series in the world's literature. Similarly, Mattox and Feliciano have described the resistance of PTFE to infection.

Options for endovascular treatment are very limited, as the vast majority of these patients have sustained penetrating injuries and arrive in shock, as described in Asensio's series, and are thus hemodynamically unstable, preventing their transportation to an angiographic suite. Coil embolization is not a suitable option as vessels of this size cannot be completely occluded without ischemic consequences. Blunt injuries to the iliac arteries are very rare, result in immediate ischemia, and the extent of their thrombosis is significant, thus precluding stent grafts. Supporting statements can be found in Asensio's series that reported eight blunt iliac artery injuries, all requiring interposition grafting. Although these eight patients were reported within the group of 185 iliac vessel injuries, to our knowledge this is the largest group of blunt iliac vessel injuries in the literature. Most other series report one and two.

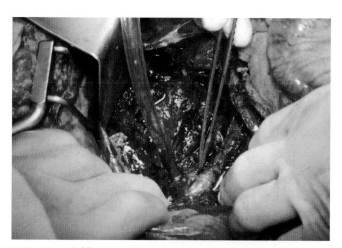

FIGURE 1 A 37-year-old man who sustained a gunshot wound to the pelvis. He sustained a transected right common iliac artery and a thrombosed right common iliac vein. The forceps are holding the transected right common iliac vein, which was subsequently ligated.

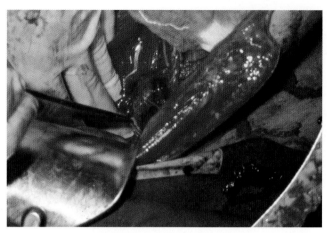

FIGURE 3 A 27-year-old man who sustained a transpelvic gunshot wound arrived in shock. He sustained a left external iliac artery injury, which has been ligated to control the exsanguinating hemorrhage. The patient also sustained a sigmoid colon destructive injury along with massive fecal contamination as well as an associated bladder injury with large urinary spillage. The forceps is holding the proximal end of the ligated left external iliac artery.

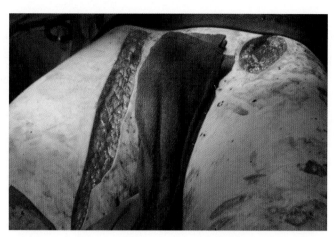

FIGURE 6 Left groin incision with the tunnel beneath the left inguinal ligament in anticipation of vascular reconstruction with a primary distal left external iliac to proximal left common femoral reverse saphenous vein interposition graft. The right groin depicts the site of harvesting of the saphenous vein. In the senior author's extensive experience in the management of vascular injuries, this is the only patient who had a large suitable greater saphenous vein of sufficient size to perform this interposition graft.

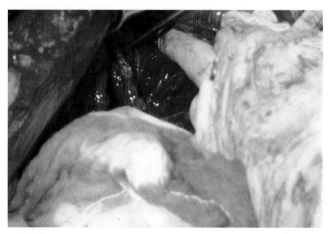

FIGURE 4 Ligated left distal external iliac artery as it is about to become the common femoral artery.

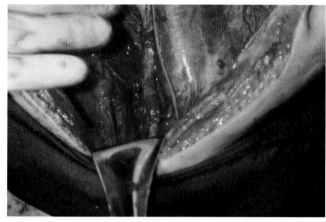

FIGURE 7 The proximal anastomosis between the left distal external iliac artery prior its entrance into the left inguinal canal. Notice the ilioinguinal nerve.

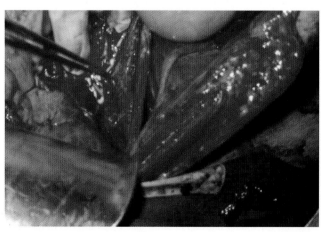

FIGURE 5 Preserved left ureter.

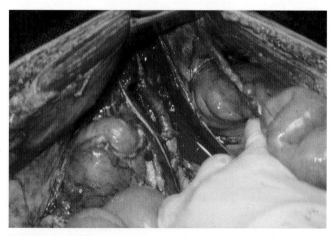

FIGURE 8 A different view showing the interposition graft passing through the left inguinal canal. Notice the ilioinguinal nerve.

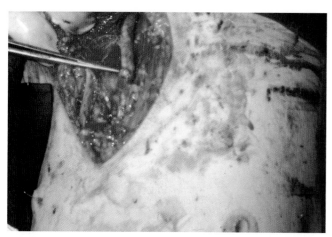

FIGURE 9   The distal anastomosis to the proximal left common femoral artery.

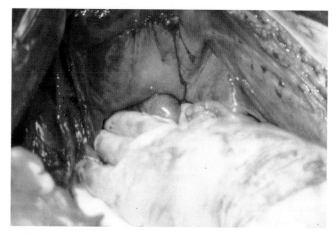

FIGURE 11   Primary repair of the bladder.

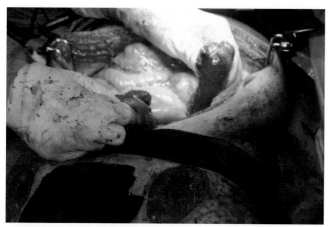

FIGURE 10   Partial resection of the sigmoid colon secondary to a destructive injury. The distal segment was left as a Hartmann pouch and the proximal segment was matured as a left end colon colostomy.

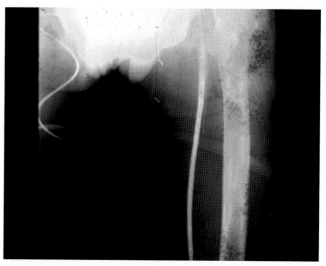

FIGURE 12   The completion angiogram and the distal anastomosis at the level of the common femoral artery.

Anticoagulation is not warranted in high-flow, larger-diameter vessels and is thus not warranted in iliac repairs. When the accompanying vein of an arterial injury is ligated, fasciotomies of the extremity should be considered to avoid postoperative compartment syndrome.

MORBIDITY AND MORTALITY

Carrillo et al in 1997 evaluated their institutional results with iliac vessel injury and found a mortality rate of 23%, consistent with the present literature. Several key points included the use of damage control and poststabilization extra-anatomic bypass to maintain extremity survival, fasciotomies and deep venous thrombosis (DVT) prophylaxis for limb preservation after vein ligation, and the use of PTFE grafts in the face of bowel contamination. Haan described his institutional experience and found a mortality rate of 25% with a bypassed single vessel injury versus 83% mortality rate with both injured vessels. They concluded that shock was the most significant prognostic factor for mortality rate.

Lee and Bongard reported a mortality rate ranging between 24% and 40% with iliac vessel injuries accounting for 10% of all abdominal vascular injuries and 2% of all vascular injures at their center. Paul et al in 2010 evaluated their previous work on abdominal vascular injuries and compared it with their most recent experience. Their original series for the time period of 1970 to 1981 included 112 patients who sustained abdominal vascular injuries, of which there were 17 iliac artery and 14 iliac vein injuries; the overall mortality rate was 32%. When compared with data from their January 1996 through June 2007 period, 242 patients were identified with abdominal vascular injuries including 24 iliac artery and 32 iliac vein injuries with an overall mortality rate of 28%. The most common injured arteries were iliac artery, aorta, and superior mesenteric artery, with the most common injured veins being the inferior vena cava, iliac vein, and portal vein. They showed that despite improvements in prehospital care and EMS training and better staffed Level I trauma centers, there was no real improvement in the mortality rate of intra-abdominal vascular injures of all types.

Despite the advances made in vascular repair, the use of damage control, and improvements in critical care, iliac vessel morbidity and mortality rates have not changed much over the years. The most common quoted mortality rates range from 24% to upward of 40%, with morbidity ranging from 8% to 15%. For patients arriving in cardiopulmonary arrest and requiring an emergency department thoracotomy (EDT), mortality rate approaches 100%. In a series of 185 iliac vessel injures reported over an 8-year period, Asensio reported a 57% survival rate for arteries and 55% for veins and an overall survival rate of 51%. In this series the mean Injury Severity Score (ISS) was 20 with 95% of injuries resulting from penetrating injuries and 5% from blunt trauma. Paul found that despite great improvements in the EMS and the increased presence of well-staffed Level I trauma centers, the morbidity and

TABLE 4: Survival Data for Injuries to the Iliac Artery and Vein

Author	Year	ILIAC ARTERY			ILIAC VEIN		
		Number of Patients	Number of Survivors	Survival Rate (%)	Number of Patients	Number of Survivors	Survival Rate (%)
Millikan	1981	19 (6)*	9 (5)*	47.4 (83.3)*	16 (8)†	11 (8)†	68.8 (100.0)†
Ryan	1982	66 (17)*	41 (15)*	62.1 (88.2)*	97 (48)†	71 (45)†	73.2 (93.8)†
Sirinek	1983	21	15	71.4	28	23	82.1
Burch	1990	130 (34)	80 (26)*	61.5 (76.5)*	214 (81)†	153 (70)†	71.5 (86.4)†
Wilson	1990				49	24	48.9
Davis	2001	55	35	63.6	76	58	76.3
Tybusrki	2001	70	37	52.9	73	40	54.8
Asensio	2001				37 (22)†	23 (18)†	62.2 (81.8)†
Jasmeet	2009	39	11	71.8	36	8	77.8
White	2011	19			17		
Overall		361 (57)*	217 (46)*	60.1 (80.7)*	590 (159)†	403 (141)†	68.3 (88.7)†

*Isolated injury to iliac artery.
†Isolated injury to iliac vein.

mortality rates of abdominal vascular injuries remained overall 28% with iliac artery mortality rate at 28% and iliac vein at 22% (Table 4).

CONCLUSIONS

Injuries to the iliac vessel remain a daunting task even after great advances in anatomic injury grading, damage control, and advancements in surgical techniques and critical care. The establishment of EMS and rapid transportation has not drastically changed the overall morbidity and mortality rates of iliac vessel injuries. Advances in vascular grafts and surgical equipment have made the repair of these injuries easier and faster, but the rapid deterioration of these patients and large number of associated injuries have led to the incorporation of damage control practices in the majority of abdominal vascular injuries. Established Level I trauma centers with fellowship-trained trauma surgeons and well-equipped staff have fared no better over several decades of emergency vascular treatment. As before, a high suspicion for the presence of iliac vessel injuries and rapid transport together with rapid surgical control of hemorrhage and contamination remain the mainstay of their treatment. When damage control is initiated, shunted vessels should be accompanied by fasciotomies of the associated lower extremity and adequate DVT prophylaxis. Despite all the advances in treatment and appropriate management strategies, morbidity and mortality rates of iliac vessel injury remain high, demonstrating the complex challenge their treatment presents to even the modern day trauma surgeon.

For the chapter's Suggested Readings list, please visit the book at www.ExpertConsult.inkling.com.

FEMORAL VESSEL INJURIES: HIGH MORTALITY AND LOW MORBIDITY INJURIES

Juan A. Asensio, Patrizio Petrone, Alejandro Perez-Alonso, Kulsoom Laeeq, Abhishek Sundaram, Mamoun Nabri, Brandon Propper, and William G. Cioffi

Femoral vessel injuries are among the most common vascular injuries admitted in busy trauma centers. The evolution of violence and the increase in penetrating trauma from the urban battlefields of city streets has raised the incidence of femoral vessel injuries, which account for approximately 70% of all peripheral vascular injuries. Despite the relatively low mortality rate associated with these injuries, there is a high level of technical complexity required for the performance of these repairs. Thus, they incur low mortality rate but are associated with significantly high morbidity. Prompt diagnosis and treatment are the keys to achieve successful outcomes with the main goals of managing ischemia time, restoring limb perfusion, accomplishing limb salvage, and instituting rehabilitation as soon as possible.

ANATOMY

The femoral artery is a direct continuation of the external iliac artery, in the femoral triangle, posterior to the inguinal ligament. Its most proximal portion, known as the common femoral artery, courses deep to the sartorius muscle coursing together with the femoral vein contained within a fibrous sheath. The femoral sheath contains three compartments: the lateral compartment contains the femoral artery, the middle (intermediate) contains the femoral vein, and the most medial compartment is the femoral canal. After a short course, the common femoral artery, which can be palpated through the skin on the proximal aspect of the inner thigh midway between the anterior superior iliac spine and the symphysis pubis, divides into a deep (profunda femoris artery) and the superficial femoral artery. The profunda femoris artery traverses deep into the thigh muscles and is the main contributor of blood flow to this area. The superficial femoral artery traverses almost the entire length of the femur and ends at the opening of the adductor magnus, also known as Hunter's canal, where it becomes the popliteal artery. The main branches of the femoral artery are the pudendal, the superficial epigastric, the circumflex iliac, and both the greater and lesser saphenous arteries.

The femoral vein is a continuation of the popliteal vein. It accompanies the femoral artery and receives drainage both from the profunda femoris vein and the greater saphenous vein, which pierces the femoral sheath on its anterior aspect before passing under the inguinal ligament where it becomes the external iliac vein.

INCIDENCE

Traumatic injury to the femoral vessels accounts for approximately 67% of all vascular injuries in the military setting. Recently, the incidence of femoral vessel injury in the civilian arena has increased secondary to an increase in urban violence. Penetrating injuries are reported in approximately 88% of the cases and are usually secondary to gunshot or stab wounds due to knife or impalement. Less common are blunt injuries, which account for approximately 12% of all injuries.

The incidence of injuries differs during the major military conflicts of the past century and has increased slightly with each conflict. During World War I, Makin's (1919) classical textbook detailed a 31% incidence reported by British surgeons, whereas the incidence of femoral vessel injury reported by American surgeons was lower at 22%. DeBakey and Simeone (1946) reported a total of 517 femoral arterial injuries for an incidence of 21% during World War II with a very high 53% amputation rate. Hughes (1958) reported a slightly higher incidence of 31% for the Korean conflict, and Rich (1970), reported a 35% incidence of femoral vessel injuries during the Vietnam War.

HISTORICAL PERSPECTIVE AND WARTIME EXPERIENCES

The earliest documents reporting vascular injuries date from 1600 BC. Egyptians were known to use styptics consisting of vegetable matter, lead sulfate, and copper sulfate to control hemorrhage, as reported in the Ebers Papyrus. The Chinese, in 1000 BC, were first to use tight bandaging to control bleeding in the affected limb as well as styptics for the control of hemorrhage.

However, the treatment of choice for vascular injuries throughout the Middle Ages consisted mainly of cautery. In 1497, Hieronymus Brunschwig, also known as Jerome of Brunswick, published his work on ligatures as treatment for injuries secondary to gunshot wounds. His work was further refined in 1552 by Ambroise Paré, who promoted the use of ligatures to control hemorrhage. Paré also recommended amputation above the line of demarcation to achieve better outcomes and developed the first hemostat, le bec de corbin (crow's beak). However, Hallowell was first to attempt a vascular reconstruction in 1759, when he repaired a brachial artery with a suture known as the Farrier's stitch or veterinarian's stitch.

Some 127 years would pass until vascular repair was again attempted. During the latter part of the 19th century pioneers such as Jassinowsky and Postemski promoted the concept of direct vascular repair. Isreal, in 1883, described the first successful primary repair

of a laceration to an iliac artery, and John B. Murphy from Rush Medical College in Chicago, completed the first successful end-to-end anastomosis of a femoral artery in 1897. This was later followed by the first autogenous reverse saphenous vein graft to repair a popliteal aneurysm in 1906 by Goyanes of Spain. Despite these advances made at the end of the 19th century, it would take almost 3 decades before vascular repairs were again systematically used.

World War I

During the first part of World War I, vascular injuries were limited secondary to the low-velocity projectiles used; however, the second half saw the introduction of high explosive artillery with improved, high-velocity munitions. The change in the destructive power of ordnance saw an increase in mass casualties and a decrease in the number of wounded evacuated. The time between injury and definitive surgical treatment drastically increased and vascular repair became impractical. Although the chance for immediate repair was lost, vascular repair was attempted to manage false aneurysms and arteriovenous (AV) fistulas on a delayed basis.

Limited attempts at repair of femoral vessel injuries were made during World War I. Makins reported the British experience of femoral artery injuries consisting of 366 arterial injuries in 1202 patients for an incidence of 31%. American surgeons also reported 78 femoral injuries in 344 patients for an incidence of 22%.

World War II

The years between World Wars I and II showed an uneven advance between the instruments of destruction and the advent of surgical interventions. Vascular surgery again seemed to take a step backward despite an increase in the severity of injuries. DeBakey and Simeone reported a total of 2471 arterial injuries from the European theater of war; unfortunately, nearly all were treated with ligation, resulting in a very high amputation rate of 49%. In this study, DeBakey and Simeone reported only 81 attempts at repair, of which 78 were lateral suture repairs/arteriorrhaphies with only 3 end-to-end anastomoses performed. Of 2471 cases of vascular injuries reported, 517 were femoral vessel injuries for an incidence of 21%.

The main factors contributing to this low number of vascular repairs included delays in transport time, lack of training in vascular trauma for military surgeons, and relative lack of access to antibiotics; although penicillin and sulfa had been introduced during this conflict, they were available only in very limited supply. Other factors included the absence of appropriate suture material, and unavailability of vascular instruments. Interestingly enough, the first vascular clamp was created by Victor Satinsky precisely during World War II.

Korean Conflict

Vascular surgery advanced in leaps and bounds during the Korean conflict thanks to several factors. Improvements in anesthesia, the advent of antibiotics, and the development of blood transfusions greatly enhanced the success rate of vascular repairs. Perhaps the single greatest factor was the development of forward aid stations accompanied by rapid evacuation of wounded by helicopter, which significantly improved transport of the wounded. Similarly, surgeons such as Hughes, Jahnke, Spencer, and Howard demonstrated an interest in developing techniques for vascular injury repair.

Several reviews from this time period showed primary vascular repair to be gaining wide acceptance. Jahnke and Seeley reported 14 femoral artery injuries for an incidence of 19%. Hughes subsequently reported 95 femoral vessel injuries out 304 patients for an incidence of 31%. These are among the earliest series in the literature demonstrating a well-defined approach to the management of vascular trauma.

Vietnam Conflict

The Vietnam conflict built on the previous advances in evacuation and faster transport of the wounded and a higher number of surgeons trained in vascular surgical techniques; this combination allowed for improved outcomes and more patients who would now be followed on a long-term basis as the war ended. The Vietnam Vascular Registry created by Dr. Norman Rich and based at Walter Reed Hospital allowed for long-term follow-up and continued evaluation of all vascular injuries from the Vietnam conflict. The landmark report from Rich in 1969 showed 351 femoral artery injuries out of a total 1000 patients for an incidence of 35%. Unfortunately, paucity of data exists for femoral venous injuries from this conflict, with ligation being the standard of care in the wartime literature.

Iraq and Afghanistan

The Iraq and Afghanistan campaigns that have spanned most of the last decade have seen significant improvements in the overall survival of combat casualties. Increases in survival rates can be attributed to the wide use of body armor, which has dramatically decreased torso injuries; the widespread use of prehospital tourniquets; and the use of damage control techniques along with the rapid evacuation for definitive surgery to Landstuhl Regional Medical Center and subsequently to the continental United States (CONUS).

The injury patterns seen in these two conflicts are notably different from those seen in other wars. As a result of the widespread use of body armor, the number of torso injuries has decreased significantly, but there has been a great increase in head injuries and distal extremity vascular injuries. These changes in injury patterns resulted given the departure from regular warfare to counterinsurgency combat, which involves ambush techniques and the use of antipersonnel devices such as improvised explosive devices (IEDs). The use of high explosives in these IEDs has resulted in a very large incidence of very severe extremity injuries and, in some cases, multiple amputations. There have also been a large number of vascular injuries.

Data collected from war registries have shown a general increase in the incidence of all types of vascular injuries, which has accounted from 4% to 9% of the total combat casualties. When accounting for only extremity vascular injuries it appears that most of the injured vessels are located in the lower extremities with a reported incidence of 7% for femoral arteries, 3% for isolated femoral venous injuries, and a combined incidence of femoral vessel injuries accounting for 7% of all cases. The policy of wide use of damage control for the management of vascular injuries consisting of early restoration of vessel flow with temporary vascular shunts, wide use of fasciotomies, external fixation of open fractures, and the rapid transport to Landstuhl Regional Medical Center have resulted in large number of limbs salvaged (senior author's personal experience) (Table 1).

MECHANISM OF INJURY

Penetrating trauma remains the predominant cause for the majority of femoral vessel injuries. This was confirmed in the series by Cargile, who reported an 88% incidence of penetrating injuries and a 12% incidence of blunt trauma. In Feliciano's series, the incidence of penetrating trauma was 81%. Martin reported 104 of 105 femoral arterial injuries were from penetrating trauma. In Asensio's series, 86% of the patients were admitted with penetrating injuries and 28 (14%) sustained blunt injuries.

CIVILIAN EPIDEMIOLOGY

The incidence of femoral vessel injury is well documented in the civilian trauma literature. Feliciano reported a series of 220 lower extremity vascular injuries, of which 142 were femoral artery,

TABLE 1: Military Experience with Femoral Vessel Injuries

Conflict	Authors (Year)	Total Injuries	Femoral Vessels	Incidence (%)
WWI	Makins (1919)	1191	366	30.5
WWII	DeBakey and Simeone (1946)	2471	517	20.9
Korea	Hughes (1958)	304	95	31
Vietnam	Rich (1970)	1000	351	35
Iraq	Michael (2007)	192 (arterial only)	41	21.3
Iraq and Afghanistan	Jasmeet (2011)	1570	268	17

for an incidence of 65%. Martin reported 188 lower extremity injuries with 105 femoral artery injuries for an incidence of 56%. Cargile reported the Parkland Hospital experience consisting of 233 patients who sustained a total of 321 femoral vessel injuries over a 17-year period. In this study he reported a total of 112 isolated femoral artery injuries (48%), 36 isolated femoral vein injuries (15%), and 85 combined injuries for an incidence of 36%. Femoral venous injuries were infrequently reported in Martin's series, in which out of 105 femoral vessel injuries there were only 3 femoral vein injuries.

Asensio reported a series of 204 patients who sustained 298 vessel injuries treated during a 10-year period for an incidence of 26% of all the vascular injuries reported for the same period treated at his institution (Table 2).

CLINICAL PRESENTATION

The clinical presentation of patients sustaining femoral vessel injuries ranges from severe hemodynamic instability and cardiopulmonary arrest requiring emergency department thoracotomy (EDT), aortic cross-clamping, and cardiopulmonary resuscitation to patients who are hemodynamically stable admitted with either the classical hard signs of vascular injury secondary to distal decreased flow and ischemia or those who harbor soft signs of vascular injury.

Cargile reported 87 (37%) patients who presented with a femoral vessel injury and had systolic blood pressures of less than 90 mm Hg, noting that 35 (40%) presented in profound shock.

Degiannis reported 19 patients with femoral vessel injuries who arrived hypotensive, with systolic blood pressures lower than 90 mm Hg, and 37 (46%) of 81 patients with isolated extremity injury who were hypotensive; 4 patients arrived in cardiopulmonary arrest requiring EDT. In Asensio's series, 11 (5%) patients arrived in cardiopulmonary arrest, requiring EDT; 3 (27%) of these patients ultimately survived.

Less commonly, the lacerated or transected femoral artery may retract and thrombose, resulting in distal limb ischemia. Associated muscle and bone injuries are common with penetrating injuries, and therefore, meticulous care should be exercised when reducing long-bone fractures. With large tissue defects resulting from penetrating injuries, actual hemorrhage may be present and requires prompt control with direct pressure or tourniquet application depending on

TABLE 2: Incidence of Femoral Vessel Injuries in Lower Extremity Vascular Injuries

| Author | Year | Total Injuries in Lower Extremities | FEMORAL INJURIES | | | Incidence (%) |
			Artery	Vein	Total	
Feliciano (24)	1988	352	142	93	235	66.7
Timberlake (26)	1990	322		116 (36%)		
Bongard (20)	1990					
Martin (16)	1994	188	105	21	126	67
Clouse (14)	2007	220	74	37	111	50.4
Randall (29)	2010	76	32 (42.1%)			
Jasmeet (18)	2011	94	44 (46.9%)		44	

the location of the injury. However, if the common femoral or very proximal superficial femoral artery is involved, the use of a tourniquet may not be feasible. In this instance, direct pressure on or above the injury with immediate proximal and distal surgical control is mandatory.

With blunt injuries, loss of blood flow is accompanied by ischemic pain and sensory and motor loss, depending on the associated structures involved. Hemorrhage from blunt injury is rare but may occur secondary to associated orthopedic injuries resulting in partial or complete laceration or transection of the vessel.

In Cargile's series, 90 (40%) of 233 patients presented with hard signs of vascular injury requiring immediate surgical intervention. Despite a significant number of these patients presenting with hard signs, preoperative angiography was performed in 106 patients. Degiannis and associates relied more on clinical examination, noting that 70% of their patients presented with an ischemic extremity.

In Asensio's series, the majority of patients presented with hard signs of vascular injury; 48% of his patients presented with distal ischemia, 43% presented with absent or diminished pulses, and 29% presented with an expanding hematoma. In this series, the reliance on clinical examination alone for detection of femoral vessel injuries reduced the incidence of preoperative angiography to 15%. Fewer patients presented with soft signs of vascular injury: peripheral nerve deficits accounted for 10% and proximity injuries for 7%.

DIAGNOSIS

The need for diagnostic workup is limited in penetrating trauma but frequently can clarify a confusing clinical picture with blunt injuries. The bifurcation of the common and superficial femoral artery is superficial enough to allow clinical diagnosis by inspection and palpation. Penetrating injury with tissue destruction and active hemorrhage needs no diagnostic workup. Patients who have sustained blunt trauma or penetrating injury without active bleeding benefit from a thorough clinical examination initially. Changes in the clinical examination of the femoral, popliteal, posterior tibial, or dorsalis pedis arteries and their respective pulses and alterations in the sensory and motor examination may indicate an injured vessel. Tight or painful compartments and associated orthopedic injuries warrant further investigation. The first and easiest diagnostic test to perform is the ankle-brachial index (ABI) examination. This examination is performed by measuring the systolic blood pressure at the ankle, which is then divided by the brachial artery systolic pressure. A difference less than 0.9 is considered suspicious for the presence of vascular injury and warrants further imaging either with computed tomography (CT) angiography or formal angiography (Table 3).

TABLE 3: Hard and Soft Signs of Vascular Injury at Admission

Hard Signs

Signs of distal ischemia

Absent of diminished pulses

Expanding hematoma

Palpable thrill

Pulsatile bleeding

Bruit

Soft Signs

Capillary refill > 3 seconds

Peripheral nerve deficit

Proximity injury

Moderate bleeding (limited)

SURGICAL MANAGEMENT

Prior to admission to the operating room (OR) arrangements for blood to be immediately available are required. Every possible effort should be made to avoid hypothermia. Broad-spectrum antibiotics should be administered prior to the commencement of the procedure. In preparing the patient for surgery, the lower abdomen, both groins, and both lower extremities should be prepared and draped for possible involvement.

Initial control of an exsanguinating vessel is obtained by direct compression followed by obtaining proximal and distal control, which may be accomplished by direct dissection down onto the common femoral artery though a longitudinal incision overlying its course from the inguinal ligament distally to the area of injury. More proximal control may be obtained by gaining control of the external iliac artery either by performing an exploratory laparotomy with cross-clamping of the vessel in the pelvis or by transecting the inguinal ligament through a muscle-splitting lower quadrant incision carried down to the retroperitoneum. With this approach, the vessels can be controlled without entry into the peritoneum. The profunda femoris artery is exposed through the same incision employed to expose the common femoral artery. The superficial femoral artery

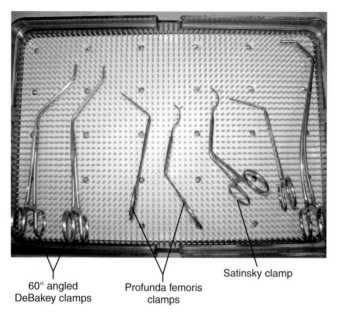

FIGURE 1   One of Professor Asensio's vascular trays. Notice 60-degree angled DeBakey clamps, profunda femoris clamps, and Satinsky clamp.

is dissected proximally and posterolaterally to identify the origin of the profunda femoris artery.

With inflow controlled, a careful dissection along the anatomic path limits secondary injury to the artery and avoids secondary hemorrhage from neighboring vessels. Vascular clamps, Silastic vessel loops, and ocular magnification in the form of loupes are essential tools necessary for obtaining definitive control of the injured vessel. Meticulous dissection of the femoral vessels is the utmost importance, especially the femoral veins, as they tend to be delicate, have a propensity to bleed significantly, and are easily injured iatrogenically. To obtain both proximal and distal control we recommend using 30-, 45- or 60-degree angled DeBakey clamps for both the femoral arteries and veins. If venorrhaphy of the superficial femoral vein is feasible, the use of small partial occlusion Cooley or Satinsky clamps is preferred (Fig. 1). The profunda femoris artery should be controlled with special profunda vascular clamps. Argyle shunts should always be available to temporarily restore perfusion to the common or superficial femoral arteries and as an adjunct to damage control (see Figs. 1 and 2).

Primary Repair

Arteriorrhaphy should be performed with 4-0 or 5-0 polypropylene monofilament sutures in either an interrupted or running fashion. Whichever method chosen, great care must be taken to avoid narrowing the artery, causing stenosis. Fogarty catheters should be sized

appropriately and used to clear the distal and proximal femoral artery of potential clot. This should be performed prior to completion of the repair or anastomosis; as with any injury, damaged or devitalized segments of the vessel must be débrided, even if this renders primary repair no longer a feasible option. End-to-end anastomosis is an option following proper débridement as long as there is adequate length to perform the repair without any undue tension whatsoever (Figs. 3 to 22).

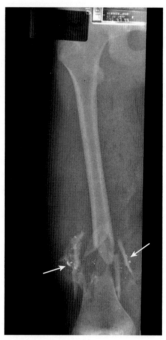

FIGURE 3   Anteroposterior view of an open right femur fracture associated with a distal femoral arterial injury just above Hunter's canal. Note missile fragments within the wound (arrows).

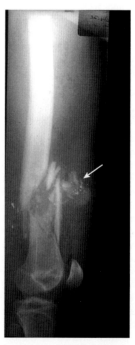

FIGURE 4   Lateral view of an open left femur fracture with associated femoral arterial and venous injury. Note comminuted bone fragments, which often act as secondary missiles (arrow).

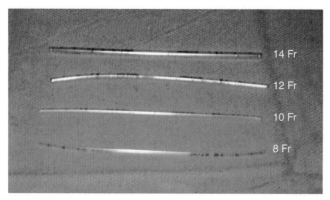

FIGURE 2   Argyle shunts.

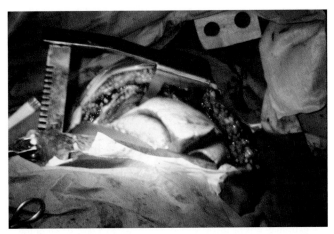

FIGURE 5 Emergency department resuscitative thoracotomy with aortic cross-clamping and open cardiopulmonary resuscitation required in a patient who sustained an exsanguinating combined gunshot wound to the right superficial femoral artery and superficial femoral vein.

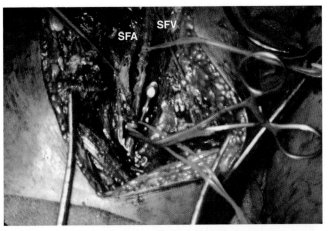

FIGURE 6 After a successful emergency department thoracotomy the patient was transported to the operating room while digital control of the femoral vessels was applied along with simultaneous intravascular volume replacement with crystalloids, blood, and blood products. Figure shows proximal and distal control of a right superficial femoral artery (SFA) and superficial femoral vein (SFV).

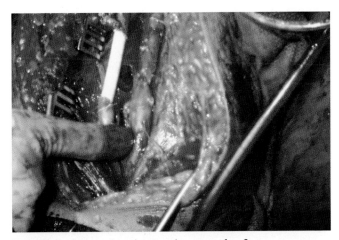

FIGURE 7 Same patient showing placement of an 8-mm polytetrafluoroethylene graft in the right superficial femoral artery and a primary venorrhaphy of the superficial femoral vein. The patient required thigh and foreleg four-compartment fasciotomies, which were initially covered with cadaveric xenografts and subsequently closed on the fifth postoperative day.

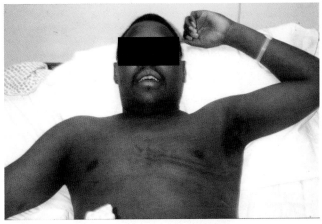

FIGURE 8 Patient after emergency department resuscitative thoracotomy.

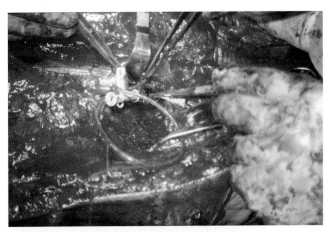

FIGURE 9 Young man who sustained an exsanguinating gunshot wound secondary to a high-velocity handgun missile that lacerated his right superficial femoral artery and right superficial femoral vein. The patient was rapidly transported to the operating room, and a No. 10 Argyle shunt was placed to rapidly restore blood flow. The patient also sustained a comminuted right femur fracture.

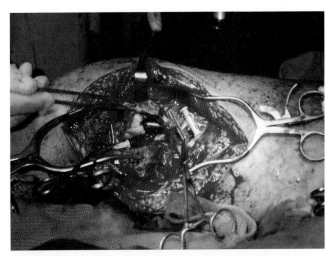

FIGURE 10 The same patient shown in Figure 9 after the shunt has been removed and the orthopedic surgeons have performed an open reduction and internal fixation with a reamed femoral rod. The Fogarty bulldog clamps are controlling the superficial femoral vein while the 45-degree and 60-dgree angled DeBakey clamps are controlling the superficial femoral artery.

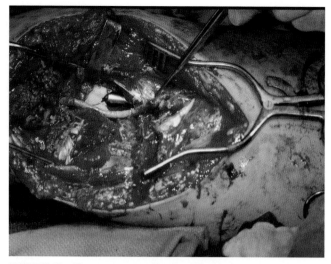

FIGURE 11   The same patient (see Fig. 10) after ligation of the superficial femoral vein. The patient has undergone an end-to-end superficial femoral artery interposition graft with an autogenous reverse saphenous vein graft. Note femoral rod bridging the open femoral fracture.

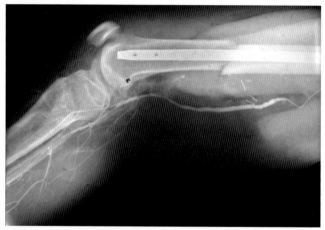

FIGURE 12   The same patient (see Fig. 11). Intraoperative arteriogram demonstrates excellent flow in the interposition graft. Notice the absence of interlocking screw in the distal femoral rod.

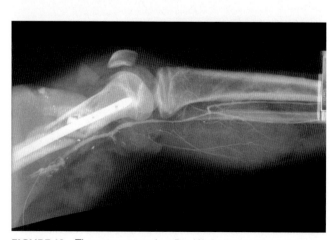

FIGURE 13   The same patient (see Fig. 12). Intraoperative completion arteriogram showing excellent blood flow in the interposition graft as well as in the tibioperoneal trunk and shank vessels. Note absence of interlocking screw in the distal femoral rod.

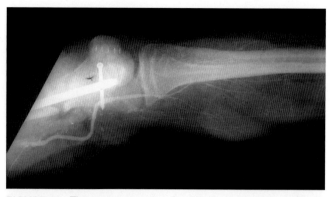

FIGURE 14   The same patient (see Fig. 13) after orthopedic surgeons placed an interlocking screw. Notice a 90-degree angle on the graft after the extremity was properly aligned. This required a take-down of the original interposition graft.

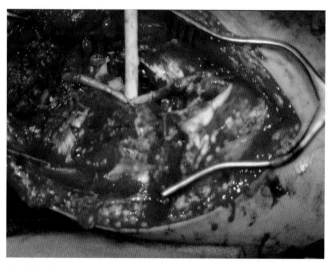

FIGURE 15   Angled interposition graft redone. The Doppler probe is used to detect triphasic flow signals on the actual graft.

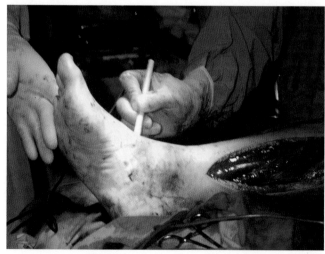

FIGURE 16   The Doppler probe is used to detect triphasic flow signals at the dorsalis pedis pulse after the redo graft. Notice four-compartment fasciotomies at the foreleg.

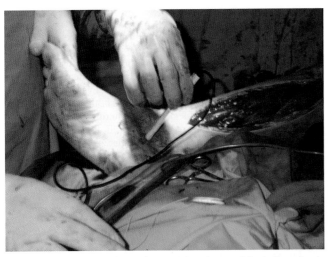

FIGURE 17 The Doppler probe is used to detect triphasic flow signals in the posterior tibialis pulse after the interposition graft has been redone. Notice four-compartment fasciotomies of the foreleg.

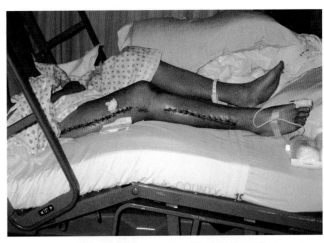

FIGURE 20 The same patient (see Fig. 19) with closed fasciotomies.

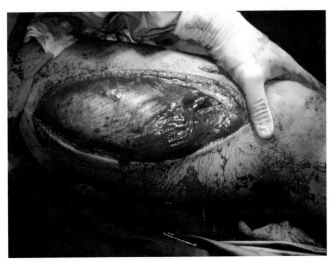

FIGURE 18 The same patient (see Fig. 17) who required both thigh and foreleg four-compartment fasciotomies covered with cadaveric xenografts.

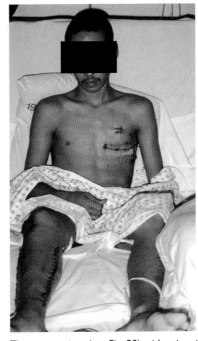

FIGURE 21 The same patient (see Fig. 20) with primarily closed right foreleg fasciotomies and healed left anterolateral thoracotomy incision.

Grafts

Interposition grafts must be used when there has been significant vessel destruction and primary end-to-end anastomosis is thus not possible. Polytetrafluoroethylene (PTFE) is an excellent choice for a replacement conduit, as it is available in various sizes and has moderate resistance to infection in contaminated fields.

Autogenous reverse saphenous vein grafts have been traditionally advocated as the preferred conduit because of their long-term patency and resistance to infection. Feliciano reported on a prospective study the use of PTFE and concluded that it had good long-term patency. Asensio reported on his series that the use of PTFE was associated with increased mortality rate only because it was employed on patients who sustained greater injury severity, suffered multiple associated injuries, and presented in shock. He recommended its

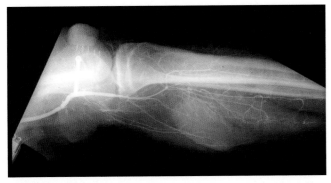

FIGURE 19 The same patient (see Fig. 18) after the correction of his 90-degree angled graft. Intraoperative arteriogram shows flow in the popliteal, tibioperoneal trunk, and shank vessels, but there is significant spasm.

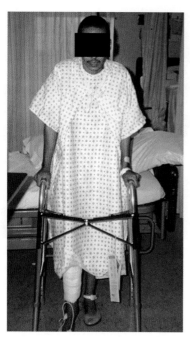

FIGURE 22 The same patient (see Fig. 21) ambulating. Physical therapy is of the utmost importance in these patients.

use in patients in whom hypothermia, coagulopathy, acidosis, and increased requirements of blood and blood products was present, given its availability and because it decreases significantly operative time.

The senior author of this chapter has subsequently evolved toward the use of ringed PTFE grafts (see Figs. 3 to 22).

Fasciotomies and Shunting

Patients sustaining extremity vascular injuries are at risk for the development of compartment syndromes depending on the length of ischemia and associated tissue destruction. The consequences of missing the diagnosis are dire, with the patient often losing entire muscle compartment if not the entire extremity. Even after successful revascularization, the systemic complications of the reperfusion syndrome, its effects on the kidney, and its resulting electrolyte abnormalities and acidosis can result in significant morbidity. The performance of fasciotomies on the revascularized limb allows swelling and edema to occur without vascular compromise, thus ensuring limb salvage. Compartment fasciotomies should be performed via separate incisions (Table 4). They should be complete fasciotomies. Thigh fasciotomies including lateral and medial incisions may also be necessary (see Figs. 3 to 22).

VENOUS INJURIES

Injuries to the femoral vein are life threatening but not to the extent of their arterial counterparts and these veins are usually ligated in the face of associated massive arterial hemorrhage. Ligation, although a reasonable approach, is fraught with the risk for the development of significant complications prevalent with ligation of the major paths of venous return. Venous thrombosis places the patient at risk for clot propagation and potentially the development of pulmonary emboli, requiring long-term anticoagulation if the patient survives. The development of venous insufficiency can be debilitating and leads to disability and increased infectious complications throughout the postoperative course. The resulting lower extremity edema can be devastating for patients who were once physically active. Repair of the femoral vein is encouraged for appropriate situations when the patient's survival is not in question.

Several studies including those by Nypaver, Timberlake, Kerstein, and Zamir agree in major vein repair when feasible. This is also

TABLE 4: Surgical Management of Femoral Vessel Injuries

| Authors (Year) | Vessel | Total Femoral Injuries | PROCEDURE | | | | | | | |
			Lateral Suture	Ligation	End-to-End	Autogenous	PTFE	Vein Patch	Other	Amputation
Phifer (1984)	Artery	25	7 (28%)		8 (32%)	9 (36%)	1 (4%)			
	Vein	25	14 (56%)	6 (24%)	2 (8%)	2 (8%)	1 (4%)			
Feliciano (1988)	Artery	142	10 (7%)	21 (14.8%)	40 (28.2%)		59 (41.5%)		6 (4.2%)	6
	Vein	93	49 (52.7)	19 (20.4%)	7 (7.5%)		18 (19.3%)			
Timberlake (1990)	Artery									
	Vein	116	45 (38.8%)	71 (61.2%)						
Cargile (1992)	Artery	190	34 (17.9%)	2 (1%)	81 (42.6%)	66 (34.7%)	1 (0.5%)	6 (3.2%)		11
	Vein	131	69 (52.7%)	12 (9.2%)	15 (11.4%)	22 (16.8%)	3 (2.3%)	70 (7.6%)		
Martin (1994)	Artery	105	25 (23.8%)			25 (23.8%)	55 (52.4%)			1
	Vein	21	10 (47%)	6 (28.6%)		1 (4.8%)	4 (19%)			
Asensio (2006)	Artery	204	53 (26%)	13 (6.4%)		108 (52.9%)	21 (10.3%)	9 (4.4%)		6
	Vein	94	41 (43.6%)	49 (52.1%)		4 (4.3%)				
Michael (2007)	Artery	44	8 (18.2%)	7 (15.9%)		23 (52.3%)		6 (13.6%)		
	Vein									
Clouse (2007)	Artery	74	14 (18.9%)	9 (12.2%)		46 (62.2%)	4 (5.4%)		1 (1.3%)	
	Vein	37	12 (32.4%)	11 (29.7%)		14 (37.9%)				

recommended by Asensio. The surgical repair of venous injuries is dependent on several factors: limb salvage, patient safety, and associated complications. It is noted that the presence of an associated venous injury in addition to an arterial injury greatly increases limb morbidity. If warranted, the vein should be repaired first, with simple lacerations then repaired with a running technique. If débridement is necessary, a tension-free end-to-end anastomosis is also an option, although this is very rarely performed. If there is extensive damage and a more involved repair is required, especially when there has been extensive destruction of the venous system or for important veins such as the common femoral vein, a shunt can also be placed to temporarily reestablish outflow as a lifesaving measure and in anticipation of performing a vein-vein bypass (Figs. 23 to 26).

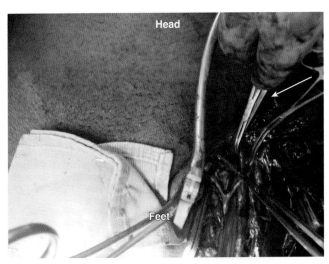

FIGURE 25 A high-velocity gunshot wound caused combined arterial and venous injuries to the left common superficial and profunda femoris arteries and vein. *Arrow* shows both the profunda femoris artery and vein controlled with profunda femoris clamps.

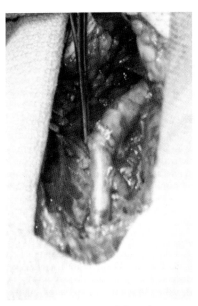

FIGURE 23 A complex venorrhaphy of the right common femoral vein (CFV). The CFV should always be repaired if at all possible. Ligation frequently results in significant complications and possibly limb loss.

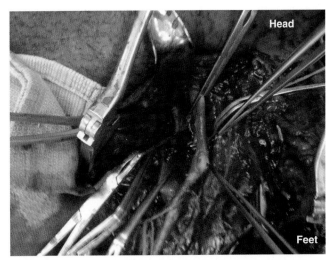

FIGURE 26 Same patient (see Fig. 25) showing the common femoral artery (CFA), superficial femoral artery (SFA), and profunda femoris arteries (PFAs) controlled after massive exsanguinating hemorrhage. Similarly, the left common femoral vein (CFV) and superficial femoral vein (SFV) and profunda femoris vein (PFV) are also controlled. This patient arrived in profound shock with a systolic blood pressure of 60 mm Hg and was rapidly transported to the operating room with digital control. He was acidotic, hypothermic, and coagulopathic. Given his severely compromised hemodynamic status, we initially performed damage control, but were unable to shunt his CFV; he thus required ligation of his CFV, SFV, and PFV as a lifesaving procedure. He also required an 8-mm ringed PTFE CFA to distal femoral SFA interposition graft just above Hunter's canal. Unfortunately the PFA was severely damaged and could not be incorporated as a profundaplasty in the proximal CFA anastomosis. The patient required thigh and foreleg fasciotomies, which were later closed. The patient survived and has resumed work as a senior officer in a counterterrorist team.

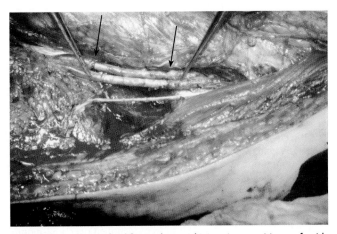

FIGURE 24 A superficial femoral arterial injury interposition graft with an autogenous reverse saphenous vein graft being shown with Gerald forceps. *Arrows* also depict a superficial femoral vein interposition graft with nonreversed autogenous saphenous vein.

OUTCOMES AND MORTALITY

The advances in diagnosis and techniques for injuries to the femoral artery have shown significant improvements in patient survival rates that are close to 95%, as reported by Asensio, with a concomitant decrease in the amount of amputations and a general improvement on the functional outcomes. The morbidity rate has remained high, despite improvement in detection, operative techniques, and follow-up. Asensio, in his study of 298 femoral injuries in the span of more than a decade, identified and statistically validated predictors of outcome. A Glasgow Coma Scale (GCS) score less than 8, the need for emergency intubation as well as the need for EDT, and Injury Severity Score (ISS) more than 25 are significant predictors of fatality. Hypotension, hypothermia, and coagulopathy, as well as the use of PTFE or the presence of an associated abdominal injury or bony fracture, are also associated with high mortality rate and wound sepsis. No other maneuvers other than prompt detection, quick vascular control, and sound surgical technique are likely to decrease the morbidity and mortality rates of femoral vessel injuries.

CONCLUSIONS

Femoral vessel injuries are the most common peripheral vascular injuries encountered in both civilian and military arenas. Throughout history they have evolved from rare and highly lethal to frequent with low mortality but highly morbid injuries.

Clinical evaluation is often sufficient with penetrating injuries; however, blunt injures will require a combined clinical and invasive approach to defining the area and type of injury. Advances in vascular grafts and surgical instruments has made the repair of these injuries easier and faster, but the associated morbidy caused by prolonged ischemia and the complications resulting from ligation of the venous system are still significant. When suspected, rapid transport together with rapid surgical control of hemorrhage and restoration of flow remain the mainstay of femoral vessel injury management. When damage control is initiated, shunted vessels should be accompanied by fasciotomies of the associated lower extremity and adequate deep venous thrombosis (DVT) prophylaxis. With prompt identification and rapid surgical intervention along with aggressive postoperative care, patients should be able to survive with every possible precaution undertaken to minimize the high complication rates resulting from these injuries.

For the chapter's Suggested Readings list, please visit the book at www.ExpertConsult.inkling.com.

POPLITEAL VESSEL INJURIES: COMPLEX ANATOMY AND HIGH AMPUTATION RATES

Juan A. Asensio, Patrizio Petrone, Alejandro Perez-Alonso, Mark Traynham, Ananth Srinivasan, Stephen Serio, Jeremy Cannon, and John T. Owings

Peripheral vascular injuries account for approximately 5% of all major injuries treated at urban trauma centers. Popliteal vessel injuries, in particular, pose a challenge to the trauma surgeon both in the operating room and postoperatively. These injuries may be associated with extensive soft tissue injury, fractures, neurologic deficit, and other life-threatening injuries, depending on the mechanism of injury. In both military and civilian experiences, popliteal vessel injuries are associated with significant rates of morbidity and mortality. Historically, these injuries demonstrated high rates of complications, amputations, and death; however, with improved emergency response systems, aggressive resuscitation, early recognition, and prompt repair, the overall morbidity and survival rates have dramatically improved.

HISTORICAL PERSPECTIVE

In 1906, José Goyanes from Spain first resected a traumatic popliteal artery aneurysm and used the adjacent popliteal vein to reconstruct the popliteal artery with an interposition graft. He is thus credited with the description of the first autogenous reverse saphenous vein graft.

Any further discussion of popliteal vessel injuries should commence by reviewing the knowledge acquired in the management of battlefield injuries. These lessons have proved to be invaluable in the management of these injuries: the overwhelming majority of battlefield injuries involve the lower and upper extremities. These injuries are the consequence of high-velocity missiles, shrapnel, and fragments as well as antipersonnel devices causing considerable soft tissue loss, complex bony fractures, and nerve injuries.

Any time delays between the battlefield and immediate surgical care is always detrimental. At the end of World War II, the time lost with evacuation and surgical preparation was not improved until the surgical support could be moved forward to the front lines of future conflicts. Introducing surgical teams to the battlefield proved to be a valuable lesson with each conflict. However, vascular injuries in the lower extremity were met with higher complications than the upper extremity in early wartime history. In the WWI British experience, Makins observed a 12% incidence of popliteal injuries with an amputation rate of 43%. During World War II, DeBakey and Simeone's review demonstrated 502 popliteal artery injuries, accounting for an overall incidence of 20%. Of those patients, 499 required ligation resulting in an amputation rate of 72.5%. When comparing both World Wars, the higher rates of amputation may correspond to the change in weaponry, notable tissue destruction, disrupted collateral circulation, and ligation as a primary surgical intervention as opposed to repair.

During the Korean War, Hughes reported 79 popliteal artery injury repairs, of which 32.4% required amputations. Approximately 600 popliteal vessel injuries were recorded in the Vietnam Vascular Registry including identification of 300 popliteal artery injuries for an overall incidence of 18.3%. Rich evaluated 150 of these patients who completed comprehensive follow-up and found that 58.7% had concomitant venous injuries. In addition, they identified 110 patients with popliteal venous trauma without any associated arterial trauma. Ligation of the injured vein was also an acceptable practice during in the management of early wartime vascular trauma; however, it was during the Korean War that popliteal vessel repair demonstrated a reduction in the amputation rates compared to ligation, a common practice in both World Wars. When vascular repair was performed during Vietnam and Korean conflicts, amputation rates dropped significantly to 32% and 33%, respectively. These prior wartime endeavors markedly contributed to the advanced practices in vascular trauma for the modern conflicts of the 21st century.

In Woodward et al's analysis of the Balad Vascular Registry database, 9289 battle-related casualties were identified over a 32-month period. Of these, 488 patients were diagnosed with 513 vascular injuries including 45 popliteal vessel injuries. Popliteal artery injury alone accounted for 35.6%, and 62.2% represented combined popliteal

TABLE 1: Wartime Experience with Popliteal Vascular Injuries

Author	Conflict	Year	Total Artery Injuries	Number of Popliteal Artery Injury	Incidence of Popliteal Vascular Injury	Total Amputation	Amputations due to Popliteal Injury
Makins	WWI	1919	1202	144	12%	218 (18%)	62 (43%)
DeBakey and Simeone	WWII	1946	2471	502	20.3%	995 (40.3%)	364 (72.5%)
Hughes	Korea	1958	304	79	26%	53 (17.4%)	30 (38%)
Rich	Vietnam	1970	1000	217	21.7%	128 (13.5%)	64 (29.5%)

venous and arterial injury. Modern wartime trauma presents with other mechanisms of injury compared to previous historical conflicts. The reintroduction and use of improvised explosive devices (IEDs) by Iraqi insurgents accounted for 27 popliteal injuries, and high-velocity gunshot wounds accounted for 18 additional injuries. Regardless of the wounding mechanism, considerable soft tissue loss and orthopedic injury are common components of these traumas, therefore mandating multiple surgical interventions and a multidisciplinary approach.

Unfortunately, the prevalence of vascular injury in Iraq was twice that of Vietnam. Popliteal artery injury accounts for 8.6% of vascular injuries with an early amputation rate of 14.3% in survivors. In a retrospective study by Fox et al, 8618 casualties were admitted to a combat support hospital in Baghdad. All injuries were sustained from gunshot wounds or high-energy explosives. Among those wounded 48 popliteal artery injuries were identified with 37% combined venous and arterial injury. Various surgical therapies were used, including autogenous reversed saphenous vein graft (69%), vein patch (2%), lateral arteriorrhaphy (19%), and end-to-end anastomosis (2%). Any concomitant venous injury identified required management by ligation, repair, or graft. The overall limb salvage failures accounted for 29%; however, complications rates remain high.

Historical outcomes proved high rates of amputations with vessel ligation in vascular trauma. Remarkable improvements, however, were later appreciated with surgical repair. Successful modern wartime vascular surgery evolved from these historical conflicts by reductions in evacuation times, improved resuscitation efforts, and the evolving surgical management practices. Changes in evacuation and development of neighboring surgical care drastically reduced ischemic delays and, when combined with aggressive damage control resuscitation initiatives, contemporary wartime vascular injuries have resulted higher rates of battle casualty survival and improved limb salvage (Table 1).

ANATOMY

The popliteal artery arises from the superficial femoral artery as it travels through the adductor canal, which is enclosed by the sartorius muscle and covered by the semimembranosus and semitendinosus muscles. As it continues coursing posteriorly in the popliteal fossa, the artery and vein, as well as the tibial nerve, become sheltered by superficial subcutaneous tissue. The popliteal artery and vein are positioned anatomically between the medial and lateral heads of the gastrocnemius and popliteus muscle. The floor of the popliteal fossa is formed by the knee joint's capsule, popliteal surface of the femur, and the fascia of the popliteus muscle. It is in this location that the popliteal artery becomes most susceptible to trauma secondary to skeletal injury, such as fractures or dislocations. At this level, a complete collateral network supplied by the popliteal artery gives rise to the geniculate, sural, and muscular branches to join both the profunda femoris proximally and the tibial arteries distally. It is above

the knee joint that the popliteal artery gives rise to the superior lateral and superior medial genicular arteries and below the knee are the inferior lateral and inferior medial genicular arteries. The terminating branch of the popliteal artery begins at the level of its bifurcating branches, the tibioperoneal trunk and the anterior tibial artery (Fig. 1).

Understanding the "traditional" popliteal anatomic description is as important as recognizing that the vascular framework of the adult popliteal artery and vein remains variable regarding the length and branching patterns. The most common terminal branch arrangement of the popliteal artery is the anterior and posterior tibial arteries. This is classically found several centimeters distal to the femoral condyle, followed by a more distal fibular artery arising from the posterior tibial artery. This "normal" popliteal artery pattern has been described as occurring in 92.8% by Bardsley and Staple, with similar findings appreciated in other investigative publications. Complex variability in popliteal venous anatomy is well demonstrated by lower limb dissections as reported by Cross, illustrating distinctive components of interconnecting veins. These anatomic descriptions portray appreciable vessel variation within the popliteal fossa and therefore justify the importance of surgical repair whenever feasible.

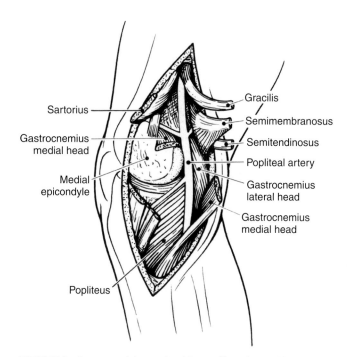

FIGURE 1 Anatomy of the popliteal fossa. *(From Asensio JA, Demetriades D: Atlas of complex trauma surgical techniques, St. Louis, 2014, Elsevier.)*

INCIDENCE

In busy urban trauma centers, management of civilian popliteal vessel injuries remains a daunting task. The majority part of surgical literature consists of institutional retrospective data review; furthermore, traumatic mechanisms and characteristic injuries are fittingly investigated. Mullenix et al's analysis of 1,130,000 patients from the National Trauma Data Bank (NTDB) identified 1395 popliteal injuries for an incidence of less than 0.2%. In Kauvar et al's NTDB review, 651 isolated infrainguinal arterial injuries were identified, the popliteal artery being the most common injured vessel at 35.5%. In South Africa, comparable results reveal a 30.7% incidence reported in the international literature (Table 2).

Lower extremity arterial injury overwhelmingly results from penetrating trauma in high-volume Level I trauma centers. In Fabian's series consisting of 165 popliteal artery injuries, 125 patients' injuries resulted from penetrating trauma. Other trauma centers may observe injuries predominantly associated with blunt mechanism. Harrell et al evaluated 38 popliteal artery injuries, all the direct consequence of blunt mechanisms. On closer evaluation of 24 series by Frykberg, penetrating popliteal artery injury accounted for 56% of the cases. Universally, blunt injury to the popliteal artery varies from 20% to 84% in various urban trauma centers.

Hafez's 10-year review examined 641 lower extremity injuries, of which 30.7% were popliteal arterial injuries. The highest rates of limb loss, approximately 25%, were appreciated in above-knee popliteal artery injuries. Stab injuries were less likely to be associated with amputation. The overall contributing factors to limb loss include nerve injury and compound fractures. The most common associated injury was venous, specifically venous segmental branches. Several review series report an incidence of associated venous injury up to 34%. Franz found a 25% incidence of associated venous injuries with popliteal arterial injuries and Jaggers found that 28% of his patients had combined arteriovenous injuries.

Older series exhibited higher rates of amputation than the last several decades. Limb-threatening vascular injuries can be associated with high-energy blunt mechanisms with resulting knee dislocation and complex orthopedic injury as well as high-velocity gunshot wounds. The incidence of civilian amputation rates from popliteal vessel injury range from 6% to 37%. In selected series various mechanisms of blunt crush injury have been seen amputation rates as high as 52.5%.

Managing limb ischemia represents the highest priority with the most important goal being immediate restoration of circulation. Patterson reported on 18 patients from the Lower Extremity Assessment Project (LEAP) study, a multicenter, prospective longitudinal study. All were due to blunt mechanical forces with associated knee dislocations and popliteal artery injury. Sixteen lower extremities had at least a popliteal injury repair and at final follow-up, 14 knees were successfully salvaged but 4 required amputation. On further review, knee dislocation and associated vascular injury in high-volume trauma centers may result in amputation rates as high as 52%.

Adult traumatic vascular injury constitutes the majority of published reviews, leaving minimal emphasis on pediatric vascular trauma. Most pediatric vascular injuries are due to iatrogenic causes. However, sporadic documented cases and series review articles of penetrating and blunt popliteal injury exist and are still exceptionally rare. Corneille's retrospective review identified 116 pediatric trauma patients sustaining 138 vascular injuries over a 13-year period. In these series, there were 29 patients with lower extremity injuries with a total of 36 vessels injured. The popliteal vein was the most commonly injured vein. The popliteal artery, however, only accounted for 19% of the injuries in comparison to 30.6% of all vessels injured below the knee. Regardless, noniatrogenic vascular injury in the pediatric population is rare and when popliteal vessel injuries present themselves, limb salvage rates are exceptional high with early identification and surgical treatment.

CLINICAL PRESENTATION

Immediate lower limb arterial injuries, whether blunt or penetrating, are considered limb threatening until proved otherwise (Table 3). The primary responsibility of the trauma team is prevention of immediate exsanguination and expeditious surgical management with restoration of limb perfusion. The majority of popliteal artery injuries can be diagnosed by history and physical examination; however, blunt injuries may be difficult to diagnose in the setting of other associated thoracic or abdominal injuries. Miranda's prospective series of 35 knee dislocations reported negative physical examinations and concluded that physical examination can reliably identify patients with vascular

TABLE 2: Incidence of Popliteal Vascular Injury in the Lower Extremity

Author	Year	Lower Extremity Vascular Injuries	Popliteal Vascular Injuries (%)
Zorita	1990	11	45.4% (5)
Berga	1991	32	31.2% (10)
Martin	1994	188	21.2% (40)
Hafez	2001	641	37% (237)
Rozycki	2003	77	16.8% (13)
Yahya	2005	60	31.6% (19)
Tam	2006	57	70% (40)
Mäkitie	2006	38	21% (8)
Degiannis	2007	103	32% (33)
Henry	2010	19	26.3% (5)
Kauvar	2011	651	34.7% (226)
Franz	2011	75	21.3% (16)

TABLE 3: Mechanism of Popliteal Vessel Injury

Author	Year	Number of Popliteal Vascular Injuries	Penetrating Injury	Blunt Injury
Jaggers	1982	61	49 (80%)	12 (20%)
Downs	1986	63	10 (16%)	53 (84%)
Krige	1987	28	16 (57%)	12 (43%)
Martin	1994	40	26 (65%)	14 (35%)
Fainzilber	1995	81	67 (82.7%)	14 (17.3%)
Melton	1997	102	62 (61%)	40 (39%)
Yahya	2005	19	6 (31.6%)	13 (68.4%)
Mullenix	2006	1395	543 (39%)	852 (61%)
Moini	2007	40	8 (20%)	32 (80%)
Callcut	2009	36	34 (94%)	2 (6%)
Franz	2011	16	7 (43.7%)	9 (56.3%)

injury. Also routine arteriography was found not to be necessary in all patients with knee dislocations. On the other hand, Barnes et al performed a meta-analysis to define whether physical examination was sensitive enough to detect injury, and concluded that it was not.

Frank hemorrhage, as well as other classic "hard" signs of vascular injury including a pulsatile bleeding expanding hematoma, loss of pulses, presence of bruit or thrill, and signs of distal ischemia, requires immediate surgical intervention. Clinical signs of ischemia with evidence of cyanosis, neurologic deficit, and temperature change are reliable clues obtained during assessment. Wagner found that 55% of all injured limbs had clinical ischemia detected preoperatively, but capillary refill was considered an unreliable measurement of distal perfusion. Those selected patients with delayed presentation up to 12 to 24 hours after injury and clinical evidence of false aneurysm, gangrene, or arteriovenous fistula will require immediate surgery. In selected cases such as this, vascular mapping by means of angiography is completed preoperatively.

As previously mentioned, popliteal artery injury may be fraught with extensive soft tissue injury and bone destruction. Unfortunately, with these compound injuries, hypovolemic shock may be evident during prehospital transport or on presentation to the emergency department. One may propose the early use of prehospital tourniquets to control hemorrhage, a measure taken to improve chances in any preventable deaths. The rationale behind the use of tourniquets reasons that any death from an isolated lower extremity vascular injury is the result of exsanguination. The use of topical agents with intrinsic hemostatic properties as recently used in military theaters might have some efficacy, if tourniquets are not readily available. The use of temporary arterial shunts in civilian blunt popliteal trauma has been associated with improvement in limb salvage.

Vascular repair will always take precedence; many patients will, however, have significantly complex orthopedic and neurologic injuries. Associated ligamentous injury and soft tissue disruption are responsible for knee stability. Attempts at reduction of a knee dislocation or fracture may be performed on initial examination. The absence of pulses with reduction is a clear sign of vascular injury within the popliteal fossae and should raise immediate concern. Harrell evaluated 38 posterior knee dislocations, of which 90% with associated vascular injuries had an abnormal examination. When presented with traumatic vascular injuries to the lower extremity, one should always anticipate the need for four-compartment fasciotomy. Patients with combined arterial and venous injuries, prolonged ischemic time, associated arterial or venous with fractures, and delayed recognition of compartment syndrome are the most common indications for four-compartment fasciotomies. In Jaggers's review of 56 popliteal artery injuries, 21 required fasciotomies during their first operation and 3 others required delayed fasciotomies.

DIAGNOSIS

The diagnosis of popliteal artery injury is often and reliably made by physical examination alone. The majority of cases will present with clear clinical evidence of vascular injury with the presence of "hard" signs. In the absence of concomitant life-threatening injuries, the presence of one or more of these hard signs mandates immediate surgical exploration in the setting of uncomplicated penetrating trauma to the lower extremity. The use of hard signs present during physical examination as an indication for surgery has proved to be safe and reliable, with therapeutic exploration rates approaching 100%. Any further imaging is unnecessary and may result in delaying definitive repair and prolonging ischemia. Furthermore, asymptomatic vascular injuries, which are nonocclusive, have been shown to be benign and have a self-limited history 95% of the time. Because these occult injuries often spontaneously resolve and do not require repair, they do not require the expenditure of resources for detection. In addition Fryberg showed that those occult injuries that do show progression could be repaired without sequelae. It should be noted, however, that patients require extremely close follow-up.

In certain circumstances arteriography may help in establishing diagnosis of popliteal artery injury. These circumstances include blunt trauma and complex injury to the lower extremity. These injuries can account for substantial skin and muscle loss with destructive orthopedic injury. Hard signs can also potentially develop secondary to extensive damage, even in the absence of vascular injury. The use of arteriography has been recommended to reduce the rate of nontherapeutic exploration in this circumstance. Shotgun blasts are another type of injury in which imaging is of value. These wounds can cause injuries at multiple anatomic levels that may be missed at the time of exploration. In these cases performing arteriography in the operating room can reduce the time to initiating repair after diagnosis and reduce the likelihood of amputation. As previously mentioned, arteriography is also useful in the setting of delayed presentation (>12 hours). When time is not a pressing factor, imaging can help plan definitive management (Figs. 2 to 4).

Some controversy still exists on how to manage patients with "soft" signs. These include an ankle-brachial index of less than 0.9, history of significant bleeding which has ceased, nonexpanding hematoma, and the presence of a bruit. Arteriography has historically proved to be the gold standard to diagnose clinically significant injuries in patients with these findings. The use of computed tomography angiography has been shown to be highly sensitive and specific in detecting clinically significant injuries.

Another noninvasive option for diagnosis is duplex ultrasound. This modality has a reported sensitivity ranging between 50% and 100% with a specificity and accuracy consistently greater than 95%. Problems with this technique include the initial expense of the equipment, potential limited availability of a qualified sonographer on a 24-hour basis, and uncertain accuracy in the setting of vascular injuries in limbs with associated fractures, hematomas, swelling, and bulky dressings.

MANAGEMENT

Once a patient with a popliteal injury has been identified, expeditious transport to the operating room is required. The patient should be prepped and draped including the injured extremity and at least one uninjured extremity for the harvesting of autogenous vein grafts. The foot of the injured extremity should be accessible from the operative field to facilitate the palpation of pulses. With the patient in the supine position, the hip should be abducted and externally rotated with the knee slightly flexed and elevated with folded towels. A medial approach is often more practical and should be used in the setting of acute trauma.

A generous incision longitudinally placed proximally 1 cm posterior to the distal femur, between the vastus medialis and sartorius muscles is required. This incision typically is continued inferiorly, staying 1 cm posterior to the posterior border of the tibia until adequate exposure is achieved. The greater saphenous vein resides within the posterior flap and care should be taken to avoid injury. The greater saphenous vein remains an important outflow vessel to the lower extremity, and every precaution must be undertaken to prevent any damage. The sartorius, semimembranosus, and semitendinous muscles are divided. To minimize postoperative disability, these muscles should be reapproximated at the end of the case (see Fig. 1).

Control of hemorrhage can initially be accomplished with digital pressure until the vessel can be exposed in anticipation of proximal and distal control with clamps or loops. Devitalized segments of the artery should be débrided back to grossly viable-appearing vessel. Primary repair with an end-to-end anastomosis is the preferred method of repair, if it can be done without tension. This method of repair is unlikely to be successful if the span of vessel lost is greater than 2 cm. In the vast majority of cases tension-free anastomosis cannot be achieved, and thus an interposition graft should be used with a reversed autogenous saphenous vein obtained from the contralateral leg. Prosthetic grafts should be avoided across the knee

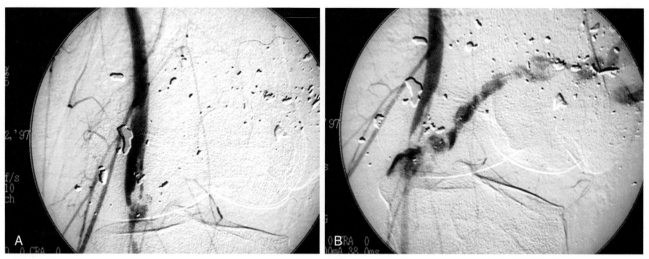

FIGURE 2 **A,** Angiogram of a patient who sustained gunshot wound and arrived with a nontreatened limb. **B,** The same patient demonstrating active bleeding, which began in the angiography suite. Patient was rapidly transported to the operating room.

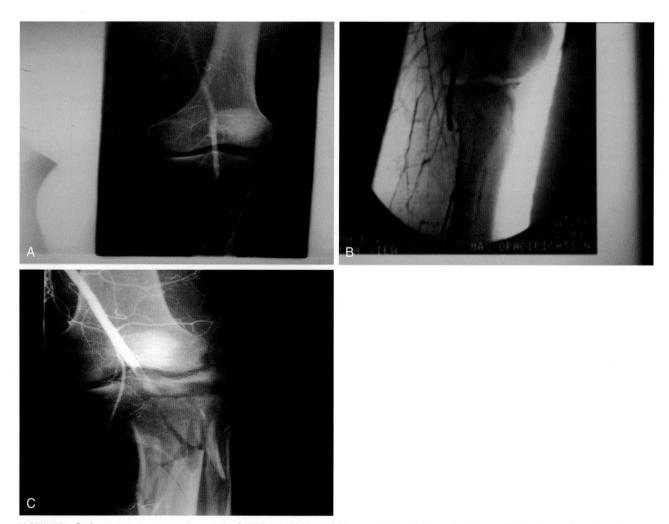

FIGURE 3 **A,** Angiogram in patient who sustained a dislocated knee with blunt occlusion of the popliteal artery. **B,** Angiogram in patient who also sustained a dislocated knee with blunt occlusion of the popliteal artery. Note collaterals. **C,** Angiogram on patient who sustained a high-impact proximal tibial fracture with occluded popliteal artery.

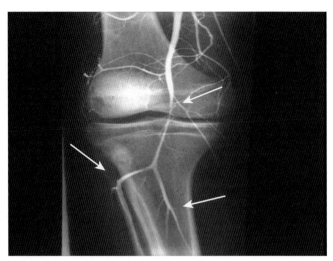

FIGURE 4 Angiogram on patient who sustained gunshot wound to the popliteal fossa and presented with a decreased ankle-brachial index. Note narrowing of the popliteal artery behind the knee. Note sharp take-off of the current tibial artery, tibioperoneal trunk, and its bifurcation giving rise to the posterior tibial and peroneal arteries *(arrows)*.

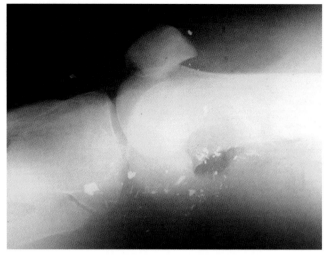

FIGURE 6 Film of the same patient shown in Figure 5. Notice multiple tissue fragments. Patient was transported immediately to the operating room.

because they have a lower rate of patency than vein in this particular situation. If associated injuries allow, systemic heparinization should be considered during the repair and postoperatively. This will help reduce the risk of distal thrombosis and increase the likelihood of successful revascularization. Fogarty embolectomy catheters should be passed distally and proximally to ensure good backward and forward bleeding before repair. Heparinized saline should be injected into the distal artery to help prevent further thrombus formation.

A 5-0 or 6-0 monofilament polypropylene suture, in a running fashion, should be used for repairs of the popliteal artery. A lateral repair should only be attempted if the injury is less than 30% of the vessel's circumference. Care should be taken to avoid stenosis. Another option is to resect the injured section and perform a primary anastomosis. Liberal use of arteriography at the completion will help identify anastomotic problems, which require revision (Figs. 5 to 43).

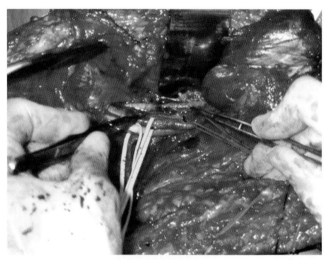

FIGURE 7 Intraoperative picture demonstrating the lacerated popliteal artery. Notice popliteal vein retracted with blue vessel loops and tibial nerve retracted with yellow vessel loops.

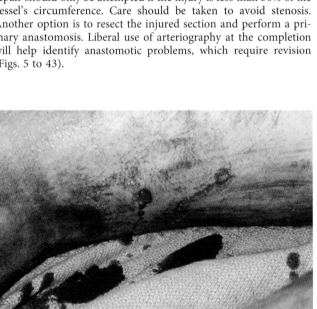

FIGURE 5 Patient admitted with gunshot wound to the popliteal fossa.

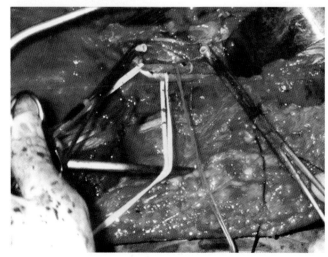

FIGURE 8 Resected popliteal artery.

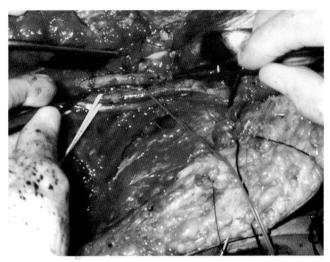

FIGURE 9 Autogenous reverse saphenous vein interposition graft. Notice popliteal vein and posterior tibial nerve.

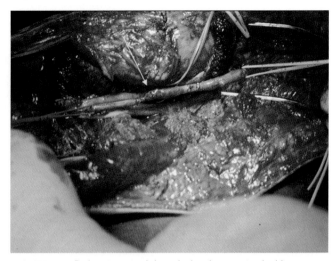

FIGURE 11 Pedestrian struck by vehicle who sustained a blunt occlusion of the popliteal artery with thrombosis *(arrow)*.

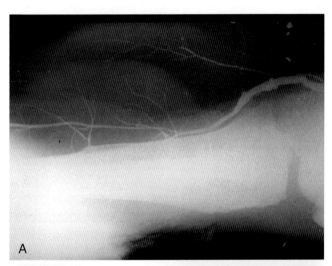

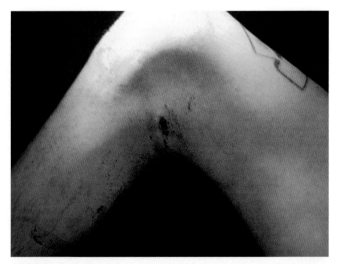

FIGURE 12 Thrombosed popliteal artery resected and repaired with an autogenous reverse saphenous vein graft.

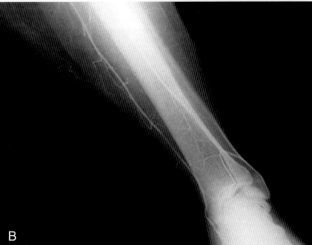

FIGURE 10 **A,** Completion angiogram on the same patient shown in Figure 9 showing excellent flow. **B,** Completion angiogram showing flow distally in both the anterior and posterior tibial arteries.

FIGURE 13 Patient who sustained gunshot wound to popliteal fossa. Doppler interrogation of pulses revealed biphasic flow signals. Ankle-brachial index 0.90. Patient was taken to the operating room.

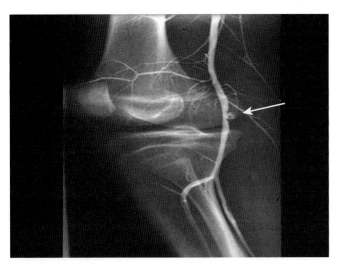

FIGURE 14   Intraoperative angiogram demonstrated small pseudoaneurysm of the popliteal artery *(arrow)*. Notice mild vessel narrowing and excellent distal flow.

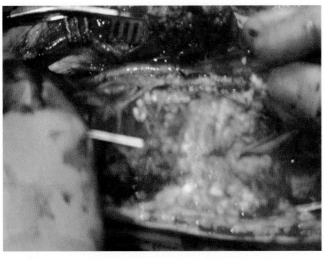

FIGURE 15   Popliteal artery and pseudoaneurysm resected and artery repaired with an autogenous reverse saphenous vein graft.

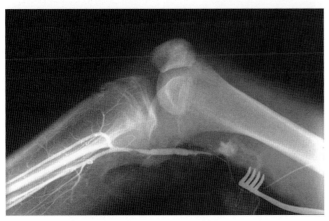

FIGURE 16   Intraoperative completion angiogram showing excellent flow in all shank vessels distally.

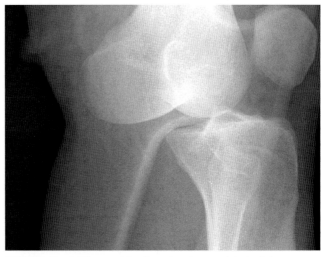

FIGURE 17   A 35-year-old male pedestrian struck in both knees sustained bilateral knee dislocations. The left leg was ischemic, the right was not. The patient also sustained blunt abdominal trauma requiring exploratory laparotomy and extensive segmental small bowel resection.

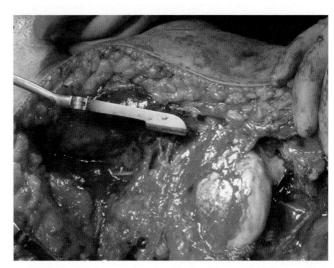

FIGURE 18   Left knee exploration. Notice dislocated and destroyed left knee capsule and ligaments.

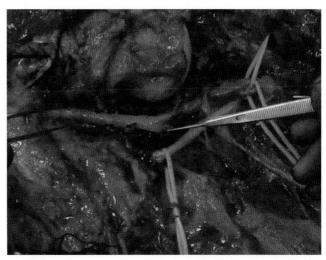

FIGURE 19   Patient sustained complete avulsion of right anterior tibial artery and tibioperoneal trunk. Gerald forceps point to the injury.

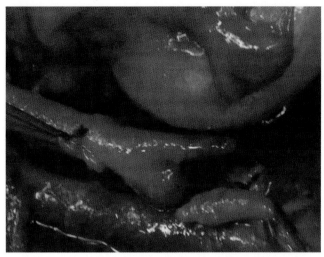

FIGURE 20 Closer view of transected anterior tibial and tibioperoneal artery with proximal and distal thrombosis.

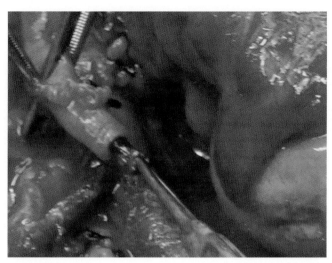

FIGURE 23 Clot being extracted from the proximal popliteal artery.

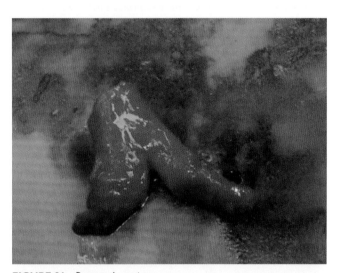

FIGURE 21 Resected specimen.

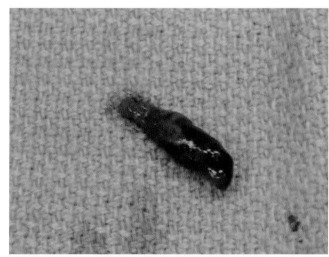

FIGURE 24 Extracted clot that had propagated into the proximal popliteal artery. Extraction prevented further proximal clot propagation.

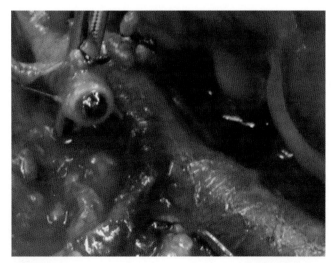

FIGURE 22 Clot present in proximal popliteal artery. Notice popliteal vein.

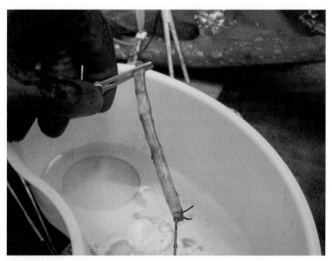

FIGURE 25 Autogenous saphenous vein harvested and being prepared by distention with heparinized saline.

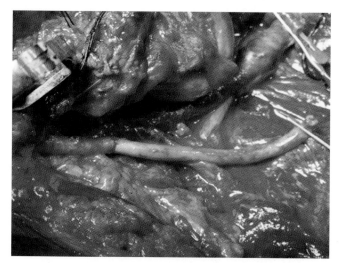

FIGURE 26 Proximal anastomosis completed.

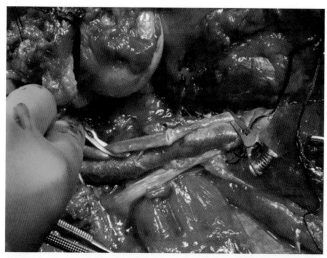

FIGURE 27 Distal anastomosis almost completed. Notice bulldog clamps.

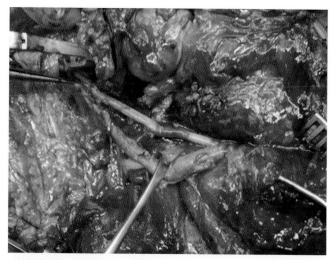

FIGURE 28 Popliteal to tibioperoneal autogenous reversed saphenous vein graft showing both anastomosis. Anterior tibial artery ligated. Notice popliteal vein being retracted with a Cushing vein retractor.

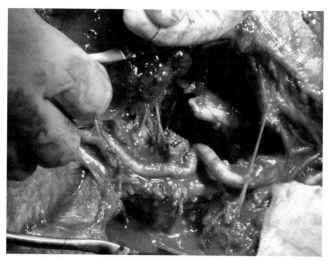

FIGURE 29 A 55-year-old patient involved in a motorcycle collision. Patient sustained a "floating knee" with a comminuted distal femur fracture and a proximal tibiofibular fracture. Notice kinked and thrombosed popliteal artery and disrupted knee joint.

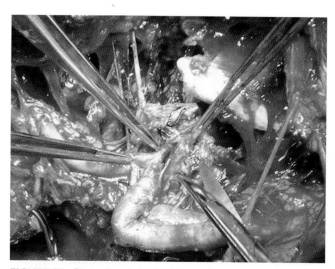

FIGURE 30 Dissection of the distal artery. Notice bone fragments. Forceps point to origin of the anterior tibial and tibioperoneal arteries.

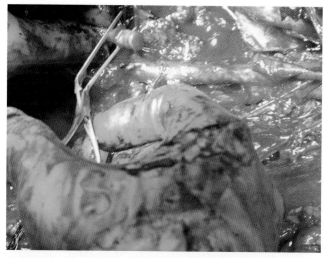

FIGURE 31 Thrombosed popliteal artery resected. Distal popliteal artery unclamped. Notice 60-degree angled DeBakey clamps.

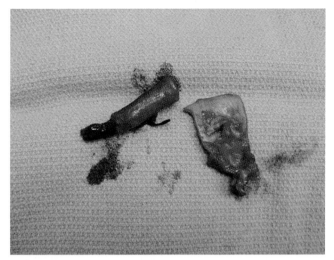

FIGURE 32   Resected thrombosed popliteal artery with intimal flap.

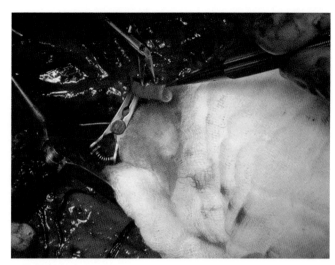

FIGURE 35   Popliteal artery reresected in preparation for anastomosis.

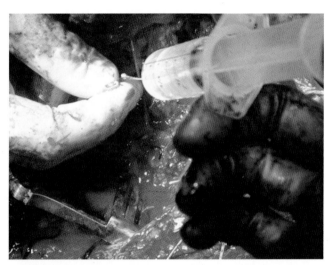

FIGURE 33   Distal popliteal artery irrigated with heparinized saline.

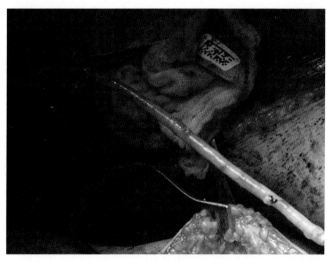

FIGURE 36   Autogenous reversed saphenous vein graft.

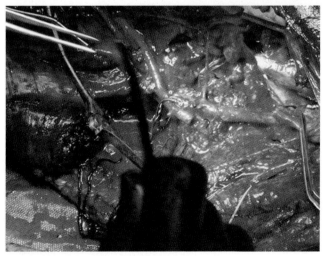

FIGURE 34   Resected popliteal artery.

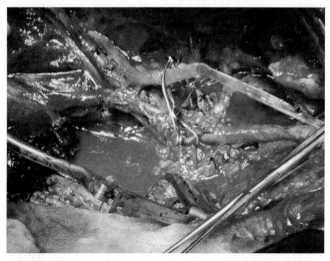

FIGURE 37   Proximal anastomosis almost completed. Notice bulldog clamp, vein marked to maintain orientation.

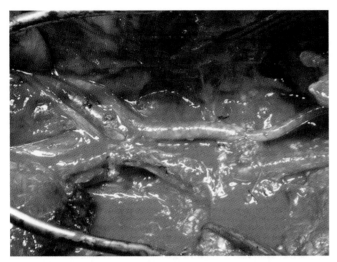

FIGURE 38   Interposition graft completed.

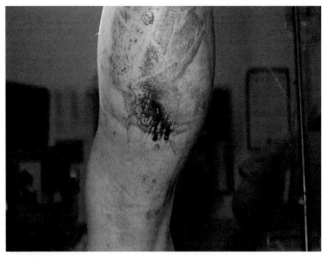

FIGURE 41   Patient who sustained a gunshot wound to the knee. Exit wound sustaining popliteal artery injury.

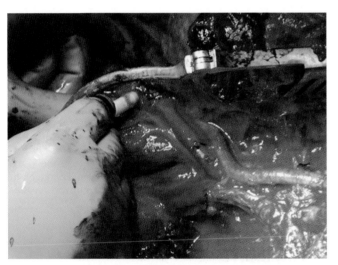

FIGURE 39   Interrogation with Doppler probe.

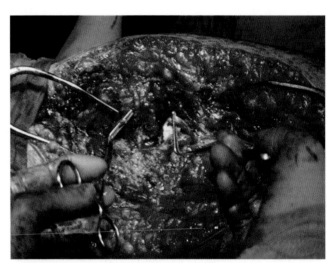

FIGURE 42   Resected popliteal artery.

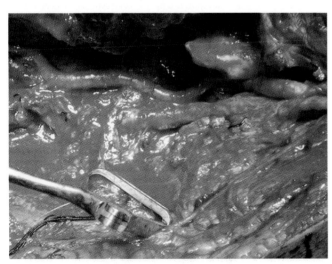

FIGURE 40   Complete graft. Notice bone fragments.

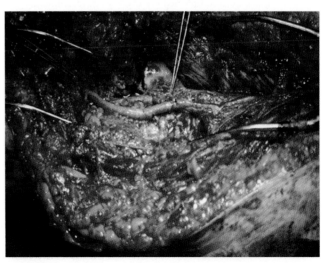

FIGURE 43   Popliteal to popliteal autogenous reversed saphenous interposition graft.

TABLE 4: Surgical Management of Popliteal Arterial and Venous Injuries

Author	Year	POPLITEAL INJURY		GRAFT VEIN		GRAFT SYNTHETIC		PRIMARY REPAIR		LIGATION		OTHER	
		Artery	Vein	Artery	Vein	Artery	Vein	Artery	Vein	Artery	Vein	Artery	Vein
Jaggers	1982	56	29	19.6%	13.8%	39.3%	6.9%	25%	70%		10.3%		
Downs	1986	58	17	60%		5%		34.5%	41.2%				
Krige	1987	28	12	42.8%	25%	14.3%		35.7%	66.7%	1	8.3%		
Martin	1994	40	16	47.5%	56%	12.5%	18.7%	40%	25%				
Fainzilber	1995	73	42	41%	26.2%	15%	9.5%	19%	40.5%		23.8%	25%	
Melton	1997	90	28	51.1%	3.6%	2.2%	4.4%	43.3%	82%				
Hafez	2001	237		55.7%		6%		16.5%					
Yahya	2005	17	4	53%		6%		17.6%	50%				
Degiannis	2007	32				12.5%							
Callcut	2009	33	11	73%				27%					
Franz	2011	12				91.7%		8.3%					

Extra-anatomic bypasses should only be considered in specific circumstances. These include repairs that would be in an infected vascular bed or in areas of extensive soft tissue injury or loss. In these instances an interposition graft can be tunneled through healthy and uncontaminated tissue. The injured vessel, however, should be removed to prevent the formation of pseudoaneurysms, which could expand, rupture, or embolize.

Popliteal vascular injuries are at high risk for the development of lower leg compartment syndrome. Factors that can increase this risk include prolonged ischemia (>4 hours), combined vascular and skeletal injuries, thrombosed repairs, combined arterial and venous injuries, and arterial or venous ligation. The decision to perform four-compartment fasciotomies remains a clinical one and has been recommended liberally by some groups. Injuries that involve concomitant skeletal injuries add a further level of complexity to the management of these already challenging vascular injuries. Priority should be given to revascularization. Temporary reperfusion can be accomplished rapidly with intraluminal Argyle shunts. Definitive repair can then be accomplished after skeletal stabilization. This applies to open reduction and internal fixation of the femur.

The institution of early amputation remains a difficult decision and requires careful judgment. Even with successful limb salvage, the functional outcome may be unsatisfactory secondary to associated nerve injury and significant muscle and osseous tissue loss inclusive of entire compartments. The Mangled Extremity Severity Score (MESS) has been used to select those patients who will require amputation after a lower extremity injury. Scores from 7 to 10 have been used to select patients who will likely require primary amputation. Ultimately the decision to amputate must be considered on an individual basis, keeping in mind the best interests of the patient. The decision to amputate should involve the entire multidisciplinary team and, if possible, the patient.

Controversy remains about how to manage patients with nonocclusive injuries that do not have hard signs. These issues include narrowed vessels, intimal flaps, small pseudoaneurysms, and arteriovenous fistulas. Historically, these injuries were routinely surgically explored. However, Frykberg reported that these clinically occult injuries have a mostly benign natural history and can be safely observed. In the event that these lesions do deteriorate to the point that they require repair, it can be done without any negative sequelae. However, this series has a small number of patients and not a very long follow-up. The senior author of this chapter considers the popliteal artery to be an end artery given its small branches and low flow characteristic of such branches. Furthermore, the tibial vessels as well as peroneal artery are prone to significant spasm, which leads to prolonged ischemia. Therefore, he recommends that all popliteal arteries must be definitively repaired (Table 4).

MORBIDITY

Short-term complications from popliteal artery injuries include acute thrombosis, distal embolization, hemorrhage, neurologic deficits, and wound infections. Acute thrombosis is of clinical importance and, if identified promptly, can potentially be reversed. Technical errors should be suspected in the early postoperative period and must be addressed surgically on an immediate basis. Other extremity complications are also due to nonvascular type injuries. Débridement of devitalized tissue and removal of any foreign material is crucial during initial or subsequent surgeries. Tissue necrosis and adjacent wound infections can lead to fatal hemorrhage secondary to disruption of the vascular repair. Unfortunately, soft tissue coverage can be limited and additional surgical flaps may be necessary for protection of the vascular repair.

Successful limb salvage and long-term follow-up demonstrate the disability associated with popliteal vessel injuries. At the time of discharge, patients having undergone orthopedic repair may require extensive rehabilitation or have the need for mechanical devices when ambulating. Nonunion of fractures, knee instability, and osteomyelitis are also well-known orthopedic complications prevalent in the setting of trauma. Neurologic deficits, such as foot drop secondary to associated perineal nerve injury, either primary or due to an untreated compartment syndrome, do demand the placement of a brace as well as aggressive physical therapy. In Melton's series, 20% of successful limb salvage cases had foot drop

TABLE 5: Amputation Rates Resulting From Popliteal Vessel Injuries

Author	Year	Total	Primary	Secondary	Blunt Injury	Penetrating Injury
Jaggers	1982			14.8%		
Downs	1986	28%	8%	22.4%	23%	20%
Krige	1987	10.7%			25%	0
Martin	1994	15%			43%	0
Fainzilber	1995	16.5%			47%	6.2%
Melton	1997	25%	11%	14%	36%	18%
Hafez	2001	27%	8.5%	18.5%		
Yahya	2005	26.3%	10.5%	15.5%	23%	33.3%
Mullerix	2006	14.5%			18%	9%
Degiannis	2007	18%	3%	15.6%		
Callcut	2009	14%	5.6%	8.3%	11.7%	50%
Kauvar	2011	9.7%				
Franz	2011	18.7%	6.2%	12.5%		

at discharge. In Wagner's retrospective review, findings of temporary or permanent peroneal nerve dysfunction were present in 63% and 37%, respectively.

Previous limb salvage strategies during early wartime proved to be debilitating with high incidence of amputation rates in popliteal vessel injuries. Far better outcomes and lower amputation rates are appreciated in various retrospective reviews over the past several decades. Civilian amputation rates reported in several series are reported to range from 6% to 37%. In blunt or crush type injuries, amputation rates may be as high as 52.5%, as previously mentioned. Extremity compartmental hypertension and limb salvage is a critical concern at time of injury, presentation, and hospitalization. Continued controversy remains regarding the timing of fasciotomies; however, in the setting of compartment syndrome, immediate four-compartment fasciotomy is mandated. The risk of limb loss as a consequence of not promptly performing fasciotomies is stressed in several published reviews. In Fainzilber et al's retrospective series, fasciotomy instituted during initial vascular repair showed a sixfold decrease in the rate of amputations.

Historically, popliteal venous injury demonstrated significant morbidity associated with the lower extremity including profound leg edema, compartment syndrome, thrombophlebitis, chronic venous insufficiency, and concerns of pulmonary embolus. The consequence of acute popliteal venous interruption as a result of ligation and the development of subsequent venous hypertension and leg edema was illustrated by Rich in a series evaluating the Vietnam Vascular Registry. A 51% incidence of significant edema with popliteal vein ligation when compared with 13% with venous repair was appreciated. This observation clearly demonstrates the importance of preserving outflow by performing venous repairs whenever feasible (Table 5).

OUTCOMES AND MORTALITY

In urban trauma centers, the mortality risk associated with lower extremity vascular trauma remains low in patients presenting isolated popliteal vessel injury, excluding patients with associated thoracoabdominal and head injuries. Regarding preventable deaths, prehospital exanguinating arterial hemorrhage remains a factor, but the liberal use of tourniquets in the field and in trauma centers has improved survival. Analysis of NTDB in two series revealed the overall mortality rate was 1.3%; however, Mullenix et al's analysis found the in-hospital mortality rate to be 4.5% and did not significantly differ from the different mechanism of injury. In Fabian's series of 164 popliteal injuries, 13 deaths resulted from several conditions including associated head injury, pulmonary embolism, infection, and postoperative hemorrhage. Several retrospective reviews have shown similar outcomes with multiple traumatic injuries and mortality rates ranging 1% to 6% (Table 6).

TABLE 6: Survival Rates for Popliteal Vessel Injuries

Author	Year	Number of Patients	Number of Deaths	Survival Rate
Jaggers	1982	61	0	100%
Downs	1986	63	4	93.7%
Krige	1987	28	0	100%
Martin	1994	40	1	97.5%
Fainzilber	1995	80	3	96.25%
Melton	1997	102	5	95%
Mullerix	2006	1395	63	95.5%
Callcut	2009	35	0	100%
Kauvar	2011	226	3	98.7%
Franz	2011	16	0	100%

CONCLUSIONS

Popliteal vessel injuries in both civilian and military arenas demonstrate significant morbidity. These injuries present themselves as a difficult challenge from admission until discharge. Although the overall incidence remains low, devastating consequences such as limb loss and permanent disability are a genuine risk. Successful outcomes for limb salvage and survival result from early recognition and rapid surgical intervention. A multidisciplinary approach has proved a greater success with the participation from trauma, orthopedic, and plastic surgical services, and remains a hallmark in the care of popliteal vessel injuries.

For the chapter's Suggested Readings list, please visit the book at www.ExpertConsult.inkling.com.

TEMPORARY VASCULAR SHUNTS

David V. Feliciano

M ost cervical, truncal, and peripheral vascular injuries can be treated using simple techniques of repair performed by general, trauma, or vascular surgeons. Certain locations of injury and complex injuries, however, mandate more advanced techniques of exposure and innovative operative approaches to save the patient's limb and even his or her life. A partial list of complex injuries would include the following: carotid artery at the base of the skull; carotid artery combined with injury to the esophagus or trachea; posterior wound or arteriovenous fistula in the superior mediastinum or thoracic outlet; combined vascular injuries in the abdomen; injury to the retrohepatic vena cava; near-exsanguination from a wound in an extremity; shotgun wound of the groin; loss of soft tissue over a vascular injury in an extremity; or a Gustilo IIIC open fracture in an extremity. Although temporary vascular shunts are occasionally used with selected cervical and truncal vascular injuries, the complex peripheral vascular injuries listed here are when they are most commonly indicated.

DEFINITION

A temporary vascular shunt is defined as an intraluminal plastic conduit for the temporary maintenance of arterial inflow/venous outflow.

HISTORICAL PERSPECTIVE

Alexis Carrel (1873–1944), winner of the 1912 Nobel Prize in Physiology or Medicine, first described the insertion of a glass tube coated with paraffin into the abdominal aorta of a dog in 1911. The early clinical use of vascular shunts following 1911 has been briefly described by Walker et al. Silver tubes as vascular shunts/conduits were used by the French surgeon Professor Theodore Tuffier (1857–1929) during World War I. A comprehensive description of vascular shunts/conduits by George H. Makins, a former President of the Royal College of Surgeons (Eng.), is available in his post-World War I textbook entitled "On gunshot injuries to the blood vessels, founded on experience gained in France during the Great War, 1914–1918."

Plastic shunts/conduits were used by American surgeons in World War II in the hope that collaterals would develop as the shunt/conduit thrombosed. In 1950, Clatworthy and Varco described the use of a "small bore polythene shunt to prevent mechanical shock after prolonged cross-clamping of the thoracic aorta." Two extraordinary laboratory and clinical reports on the use of "polythene shunts" in both trauma and elective vascular surgery were published by Creighton A. Hardin in 1952.

The use of shunts in contemporary times was first described by Eger, Golcman, Goldstein, and Hirsch from Beer-Seba, Israel, in 1971. The authors constructed their own shunt from "regular polyethylene tubing of adequate size and length." Of interest, they placed a three-way adapter in the middle of the tubing and commented that the rubber cap on the adapter allowed for the "injection of heparin." Since the report by Eger et al, there has been a continuing series of papers on the use of temporary vascular shunts in both civilian and military centers.

INDICATIONS FOR TEMPORARY VASCULAR SHUNTS

The seven current indications for temporary vascular shunts are as follows: (1) complex repair of the internal carotid artery in zone III of the neck (from the angle of the mandible to the base of the skull); (2) Gustilo IIIC open fracture of an extremity; (3) need for perfusion as a complex revascularization after trauma is performed; (4) perfusion of an amputated part of an upper extremity prior to replantation; (5) "damage control" for the patient with near-exsanguination from a peripheral vascular injury; (6) "damage control" for the patient with multiple intra-abdominal injuries including an abdominal vascular injury, a complex abdominal vascular injury, or near-exsanguination from a truncal vascular injury; and (7) "damage control" for the patient with a cervical, truncal, or peripheral vascular injury and a surgical team with an overwhelming number of casualties, limited resources, or limited operative experience with vascular injuries (military triage) (Fig. 1).

The need for a complex repair of the internal carotid artery in zone III is uncommon. There are numerous options for controlling hemorrhage from an internal carotid artery secondary to a penetrating wound in zone III or an operative mishap during the resection of a cervical neoplasm. These options include percutaneous passage of a balloon catheter for external tamponade; transcarotid passage of a balloon catheter for internal tamponade; passage of an endovascular stent; operative ligation; and operative repair. Although balloon tamponade or operative ligation is lifesaving, it exposes the patient to cerebral ischemia or a stroke. Endovascular stenting is an appealing option that depends on the ability of the trauma team to temporarily control hemorrhage, the experience of the interventionalist, and the magnitude of the injury to the internal carotid artery. With an inability to fully control hemorrhage with compression or balloon tamponade, operative repair will be necessary. Exposure of the artery will mandate subluxation of the temporomandibular joint with interdental wiring or with monocortical screws and steel wiring or by a vertical ramus osteotomy. Because of the delay in obtaining vascular control, a temporary intraluminal shunt should be inserted before a complex repair (segmental resection and an end-to-end anastomosis or insertion of an interposition graft) is performed if back-bleeding from the distal internal carotid artery is modest.

A Gustilo IIIC open fracture in an extremity is defined as any open fracture with an arterial injury requiring repair for limb salvage. There are numerous scoring systems or algorithms in place to help decide whether attempted limb salvage or immediate amputation is appropriate. When limb salvage is to be attempted, the immediate insertion of a temporary arterial and, if needed, venous shunt to restore inflow

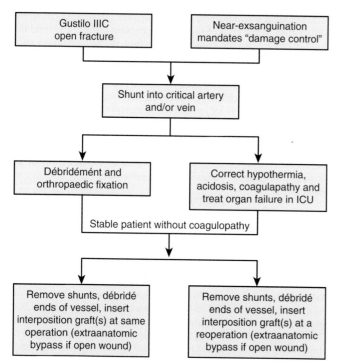

FIGURE 1 Algorithm for use of shunts with complex fractures or need for "damage control." ICU, Intensive care unit.

and outflow to the foot or hand is performed. This allows the orthopedic trauma team to perform soft tissue and bony débridement and stabilize the open fracture without being concerned about continuing ischemia. Following the completion of bony stabilization and depending on the patient's condition, the trauma vascular team scrubs back in, removes the shunt(s), and performs a definitive vascular repair.

When a complex revascularization such as an extra-anatomic bypass is to be performed after trauma to an extremity, the insertion of temporary intraluminal shunts is appropriate to maintain inflow/outflow to the foot or hand. This will allow for proper tunneling of the graft before the proximal and distal anastomoses of the definitive graft are performed.

A "clean" amputation of an upper extremity at the wrist, in the forearm, or in the arm may be treated with replantation. The decision to perform this complex repair will, of course, depend on the patient's overall health, the magnitude of other injuries, hemodynamic status upon presentation, and local expertise. Should replantation be appropriate, the amputated part can be perfused and drained by the use of long temporary shunts connected to the injured extremity as débridement and limb-shortening are performed.

Near-exsanguination from a peripheral vascular injury is accompanied by hypothermia, acidosis, and a transient coagulopathy if a massive transfusion protocol is used for resuscitation. Profound hypothermia ($<35°$ C), a severe metabolic acidosis (arterial pH < 7.2), and the presence of a coagulopathy (coagulation studies $1.5 \times$ normal) should prompt a "damage control" operative procedure. Even with the control of hemorrhage, correction of this metabolic failure may take several hours and the patient's life remains in danger. With either a major arterial or venous injury (common femoral, femoral, popliteal, tibioperoneal), a temporary arterial and/or venous shunt will allow for salvage of the injured extremity as resuscitation (rewarming; transfusion of blood and blood components) continues.

A patient with multiple intra-abdominal injuries including an abdominal vascular injury, a complex abdominal vascular injury (e.g., proximal superior mesenteric artery adjacent to injured pancreas, common or external iliac artery injury adjacent to injury to colon with contamination), or near-exsanguination from a truncal vascular injury should have a temporary arterial shunt inserted

instead of a formal repair. This is a particularly true with injuries to the superior mesenteric artery or common or external iliac artery as mentioned previously, as ligation will often lead to catastrophic complications postoperatively. In DeBakey and Simeone's classic report of arterial ligations in World War II, ligation of the common or external iliac artery resulted in amputation rates of 53.8 and 46.7%, respectively. Following a damage control laparotomy, the patient is, once again, rewarmed and resuscitated in the intensive care unit. During this phase, plans for arterial reconstruction (in situ graft with omental coverage versus extra-anatomic bypass) are made as well.

Forward Surgical Teams at Battalion Aid Stations (Echelon II) in Iraq and Afghanistan have used large numbers of temporary vascular shunts in recent years for the reasons mentioned previously. Once the wounded soldier is transported to the appropriate Combat Support Hospital (Echelon III), the temporary shunt is removed and a formal vascular repair is completed. Temporary vascular shunts are not permitted on the flights from Afghanistan to Landstuhl Regional Medical Center (Echelon IV) near Frankfurt, Germany.

AVAILABLE SHUNTS

Although intravenous tubing can be used as a temporary vascular shunt, a number of shunts historically available for carotid endarterectomy have been the most commonly used in civilian trauma centers. Argyle carotid artery shunts (Kendall, Mansfield, Mass.) are rigid with tapered ends, can be cut to an appropriate length, and are available in 8 to 14F sizes (Fig. 2). Argyle thoracostomy tubes are appropriately sized to be inserted as temporary shunts in the large veins of the extremities, such as the common femoral, femoral, and popliteal. The Javid carotid bypass shunt (Bard Peripheral Vascular, Tempe, Ariz.) is a soft flexible shunt with dilations at either end that allow for Javid clamps to hold the shunt in place. The shunt is 17F in size and is designed to lie outside the operative field during a carotid endarterectomy. The Pruitt-Inahara carotid shunt (LeMaitre Vascular, Inc., Burlington, Mass.) is a soft flexible shunt with inflatable balloons

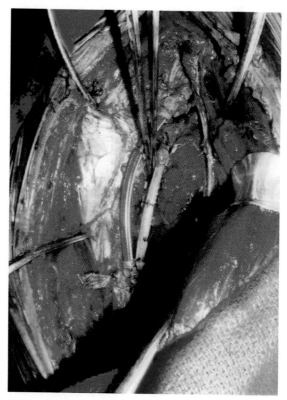

FIGURE 2 Argyle shunts (8 F) in left popliteal artery and vein.

at either end to hold the shunt in place. It is 7F in size and has a T-piece, which will allow for flushes, arteriography, or the injection of anticoagulants. The Sundt internal and external carotid endarterectomy shunts (Integra NeuroSciences, Plainsboro, N.J.) are soft and flexible and reinforced with stainless steel. They have cone-shaped bulbs at either end that prevent leakage and come in 3 × 4 mm up to 4 × 5 mm internal diameters. The temporary limb salvage shunt (TLSS) (Vascutek Ltd., Renfrewshire, Scotland) was approved by the U.S. government Food and Drug Administration (Center for Devices and Radiological Health) on February 9, 2007. This shunt has been used occasionally by U.S. military surgeons, but is currently not available for use in civilian trauma centers in the United States.

OPERATIVE TECHNIQUE

Proximal and distal vascular control is obtained by applying vascular clamps, bulldog clamps, or Silastic vessel loops on the injured vessel. The injured segment of the vessel or the injured ends are débrided back to uninjured intima. If a rigid Argyle shunt or thoracostomy tube is to be inserted, the largest possible size that can fit into the transected ends of the vessel is chosen. The shunt is then trimmed at one end so that the overall length is approximately 4 cm longer than the gap between the two ends of the vessel. A 2-0 silk tie is placed around the midpoint of the tailored shunt for orientation, and a hemostat is placed at the same point to occlude the shunt. The blunt (trimmed) end (larger lumen than tapered end) is then gently advanced into the proximal end of the artery or distal end of the vein for a distance of 1.5 cm. A 2-0 silk tie is passed around the proximal artery or distal vein and tied down to prevent leakage and to fix one end of the shunt in place. The hemostat is opened to verify that arterial or venous flow is adequate and then reapplied. The distal smooth end of the shunt is then gently advanced into the distal end of the artery or proximal end of the vein for a distance of 1.5 cm. Once again, a 2-0 silk tie is used to prevent leakage and to fix the end of the shunt in place. After removal of the hemostat on the mid-aspect of the shunt, arterial pulsations should be readily palpable in the distal artery beyond the shunt or Doppler pulses audible at the ankle or wrist. When a venous shunt has been inserted, dilation of the proximal vein is a sign that the temporary venous shunt is patent. Confirmation of venous return beyond the shunt can be obtained using a handheld Doppler device.

If the Javid shunt is used, Javid clamps are placed adjacent to the dilated areas at the ends of the shunt to prevent leakage and hold the shunt in place. With the Pruitt-Inahara shunt, the balloons at the ends of the shunt are inflated till leakage ceases.

Once the patient and extremity are stable, and the shunt is to be removed, intravenous heparin (if not already administered) is administered at a dose of 100 U/kg body weight. Vascular clamps, bulldog clamps, or vessel loops are applied to the ends of the vessel beyond the shunt, which is then removed. As the Argyle shunts or thoracostomy tubes are held in place by 2-0 crushing silk ties, the ends of the vessel will have to be further débrided to remove the crushed vessel ends. In the authors' experience, this always mandates the insertion of an interposition graft rather than performing an end-to-end anastomosis.

OUTCOMES

In the largest civilian series published in the United States to date, approximately 9% of all patients with vascular injuries treated over a 10-year period at an urban trauma center had insertion of a temporary intravascular shunt. When the seven patients who died on trauma day 0 or who had an amputation of an extremity at the first operation were excluded, data on 66 patients (8.4%) with 119 shunts (72 arterial, 47 venous) were available for review. The mechanism of injury was a gunshot wound in 62%, blunt trauma in 36%, and a stab wound (1) in 2%. Primary indications for the insertion of a shunt were "damage control" in 47% and "nondamage control" in 53% (Gustilo IIIC fracture 42%, need for temporary perfusion 9%, and replant of a limb 2%) (Table 1). As would be expected, the "damage control" group had a worse base deficit on admission (−15.2 vs. −7.2, $p < 0.001$), a greater transfusion requirement (15.2 U vs. 8.0 U, $p = 0.002$), and a higher amputation rate (23 vs. 11%, $p = 0.003$) (see Table 1).

Peripheral vascular shunts were inserted in 60 patients, and truncal or visceral shunts were inserted in 6 (3 external iliac artery, 2 superior mesenteric artery, 1 subclavian artery). In patients with the insertion of peripheral vascular shunts, the most common arterial locations were the superficial femoral (21), popliteal (21), and brachial (10) arteries. The most common venous locations were the popliteal (15) and femoral (12) veins (Table 2). A 14F Argyle shunt was the most commonly used in the series and was placed in

TABLE 1: Indications for Temporary Intravascular Shunts

| | DAMAGE CONTROL GROUP | | | NONDAMAGE CONTROL GROUP | | | | | |
	All Damage Control	Extremity	Truncal	All Nondamage Control	Gustilo IIIc Open Fractures	Perfusion During Prep	Limb Replant	Total	P value
Number of patients (%)	31 (47%)	25 (38%)	6 (9%)	35 (53%)	28 (42%)	6 (9%)	1 (2%)	66 (100%)	-
Mean BD	15.2 + 1.5	15.3 ± 1.7	15.1 ± 2.4	7.2 ± 0.8	6.8 ± 3.5	7.2 ± 9.7	-	10.7 ± 7.8	< .001
Mean ISS	18 ± 1.7	18 ± 2.0	17 ± 3.1	13 ± 1.3	13 ± 1.6	11 ± 1.8	9	15 ± 1.1	.016
Mean PRBCs (units)	15.2 ± 2.2	12.6 ± 1.8	26.0 ± 7.3	7.9 ± 0.7	8.0 ± 4.4	10.7 ± 7.7	18	11.8 ± 9.7	.002
Fasciotomy rate	86%	92%	67%	74%	68%	100%	100%	82%	.19
Mean "dwell" time (h)	23.5 ± 2.8	23.0 ± 3.2	25.7 ± 6.6					23.5 ± 2.8	
Amputation rate	23%	20%	33%	11%	14%	0%	0%	17%	.003
Shunt thrombosis rate	10%	4%	33%	0%	0%	0%	0%	5%	.06
Survival rate	81%	84%	67%	94%	100%	67%	100%	88%	.09

From Subramanian A, Vercruysse G, Dente C, et al: A decade's experience with temporary intravascular shunts at a civilian level I trauma center. *J Trauma* 65:316–326, 2008.
BD, Base deficit; ISS, Injury Severity Score; PRBCs, packed red blood cells; prep, preparation.

TABLE 2: Anatomic Distribution of Temporary Intravascular Shunts

Type of Shunt	*n* (%) SFA (*n* = 21)	POA (*n* = 21)	POV (*n* = 15)	SFV (*n* = 12)	BrA (*n* = 10)
14F Argyle	9 (39%; all males)	7 (33%; 6 males, 1 female)	7 (47%; all males)	5 (42%; all males)	
12F Argyle	5 (22%; 4 males, 1 female)	2 (10%; all females)	3 (20%; 2 males, 1 female)		3 (30%; all males)
10F Argyle		6 (29%; 5 males, 1 female)			3 (30%; all males)
24F CT				2 (17%; all males)	
20F CT			2 (13%; all males)	1 (8%; female)	
18F CT			1 (7%; female)	1 (8%; male)	
16F CT			1 (7%; female)	2 (17%; all males)	
9F P-I	7 (30%; all males)	6 (29%; 1 male, 5 females)	1 (7%; male)		3 (30%; all males)
5F ped FT					1 (30%; male child)

From Subramanian A, Vercruysse G, Dente C, et al: A decade's experience with temporary intravascular shunts at a civilian level I trauma center. *J Trauma* 65:316–326, 2008.
Argyle, Argyle shunt; BrA, brachial artery; CT, chest tube; FT, feeding tube; ped, pediatric; P-I, Pruitt-Inahara shunt; POA, popliteal artery; POV, popliteal vein; SFA, superficial femoral artery; SFV, superficial femoral vein.

TABLE 3: Utilization of the 24F Argyle Shunt

Injured Vessel	Number of Patients (%)
SFA	9 (30)
POA	7 (23)
POV	7 (23)
SFV	5 (17)
EIA	1 (3)
AxA	1 (3)
Total	30 (100)

From Subramanian A, Vercruysse G, Dente C, et al: A decade's experience with temporary intravascular shunts at a civilian level I trauma center. *J Trauma* 65:316–326, 2008.
AxA, Axillary artery; EIA, external iliac artery; POA, popliteal artery; POV, popliteal vein; SFA, superficial femoral artery; SFV, superficial femoral vein.

18 arterial injuries (17 peripheral, 1 truncal) and in 12 peripheral venous injuries (Table 3).

Thirty patients (30/66 = 45%) had two temporary intravascular shunts inserted, and 1 patient had three shunts inserted at the initial operation. In the 31 patients who left the operating room with one or more shunts at the end of the first operation, the mean dwell time was 23.5 ± 15.7 hours. Of interest, the longest period of time that a shunt remained in place and was patent was 71 hours for an arterial shunt and 35 hours for a venous shunt.

Early amputation or resection of an end organ was necessary after shunting of 5 of the 119 injured vessels (4.2%). The indications were an unsalvageable extremity in three instances and a thrombosed shunt in two. After removal of the shunt, the other 114 vascular injuries in the series were treated with 89 interposition grafts (58 greater saphenous vein, 31 polytetrafluoroethylene), 14 end-to-end anastomoses, and 11 ligations. The overall survival rate was 88% in this review, with a limb salvage rate of 74%, and anticoagulation was rarely used. The main conclusions from this study were that temporary intravascular shunts of an adequate caliber stay patent, are difficult to dislodge, and maintain arterial inflow/venous outflow to injured parts. The main indications for shunting in this study were as follows: (1) a need for a "damage control" procedure; (2) a Gustilo IIIC fracture of an extremity; (3) patient with a complex vascular injury requiring reperfusion while preparing for revascularization; and (4) replantation of a hand, forearm, or arm. Finally, another recent study confirms that temporary intravascular shunts are underused in trauma centers in the United States.

PRACTICAL POINTS IN CONCLUSION

1. With the spasm that often accompanies vascular injuries in young patients, it may be necessary to apply topical papaverine and gently dilate the distal end of an injured artery so as to allow for the insertion of the largest possible shunt.
2. The patency of a temporary arterial shunt will be compromised if the adjacent major named vein as been ligated. The tie on the ligated vein should be removed and a temporary venous shunt inserted as well. Thrombosis of an arterial shunt, although uncommon as noted earlier, is inevitably related to overwhelming muscle damage in the distal extremity and lack of adequate venous return.
3. Many seriously injured patients requiring damage control shunting or shunting for a Gustilo IIIC open fractures have some element of an intraoperative and postoperative coagulopathy. With massive transfusion protocols ("damage control resuscitation"), the incidence and magnitude of the coagulopathy are much decreased. Even so, the magnitude of the patient's injury or associated injuries usually precludes the use of heparin for anticoagulation after the insertion of a shunt. And as noted earlier, no prospective data suggest that postoperative heparinization will decrease the modest incidence of shunt thrombosis reported.
4. Shunts in the extremities are usually placed in open wounds that are exposed to contamination from the intensive care unit in the postoperative period. At the time of removal of the shunt, an extra-anatomic vascular bypass is mandatory if there is inadequate healthy muscle to cover an in situ location of an interposition graft.

For the chapter's Suggested Readings list, please visit the book at www.ExpertConsult.inkling.com.

MUSCULOSKELETAL AND PERIPHERAL CENTRAL NERVOUS SYSTEM INJURIES

UPPER EXTREMITY FRACTURES: ORTHOPEDIC MANAGEMENT

Steven Kalandiak and Stephen M. Quinnan

Fractures and dislocations of the upper extremity can vary from benign problems requiring minimal intervention to life- and limb-threatening emergencies. The treatment plan is based on the injury pattern, including location, mechanism, status of the soft tissues, associated neurologic or vascular injury, and other associated injuries. This chapter discusses several key issues in the decision-making process, and follows with descriptions of specific injuries and their treatment.

OPEN FRACTURES

An associated open soft tissue injury adds an element of urgency to the treatment of these fractures. A fracture is classified as "open" if the fracture or fracture hematoma communicates with the environment via a wound in the soft tissues. This can be caused by the bone protruding through the skin from "inside-out," or from a penetrating mechanism causing an injury from the "outside-in." Regardless, the implication is that environmental contamination can increase the incidence of both infection and fracture healing complications. If there is a wound in the same limb segment as the fracture, the fracture should be considered open until proved otherwise. A classification system for open fractures can be seen in Table 1. Infection rates are typically reported as quite low, on the order of a few percent, for type I, type II, and type IIIA fractures, but range from 10% to 50%, and 25% to 50% for type IIIB and IIIC fractures, respectively.

Treatment of these fractures begins with prompt antibiotic therapy, tetanus prophylaxis, and urgent irrigation and débridement of the fracture in the operating room. Although many still adhere to the dictum of proceeding to surgery within 6 to 8 hours, some centers with dedicated orthopedic trauma rooms have found no increase in infection rate when open fractures arriving late at night are held over until the next morning when the full resources of the center are more readily available. True life and limb emergencies, such as vascular injury, compartment syndrome, and severe crush injury are exceptions to this "new rule" and should be taken to the operating room as soon as the patient is adequately stabilized for these emergent surgeries.

In either circumstance, the skin and fascia are further opened until the full internal extent of the injury is revealed. All contamination, dead muscle, and devitalized diaphyseal bone are meticulously removed. Tissue that has not yet declared its viability may be left in situ, and the patient should be returned to the operating room at regular intervals until all tissues have declared themselves and all that is nonviable is removed. Preliminary or definitive stabilization of the fracture and continuation of appropriate antibiotic therapy should follow. It is apparent that short-course, high-dose antibiotic therapy is appropriate for open fractures and need not be continued over the course of the fracture healing process. Recommendations are as follows:

Grade I and II fractures (and closed fractures with soft tissue injury): 1 to 2 g of a cephalosporin on admission followed by 1 g every 6 to 8 hours for 24 to 48 hours.

Grade III fractures: additional therapy to cover both gram-positive and gram-negative organisms is warranted—3 to 5 mg/kg/day in divided doses of an aminoglycoside in addition to the cephalosporin. This dosage may be adjusted for patients with renal failure or substituted with once per day dosing to minimize renal toxicity. Two to 4 million units of penicillin G every 4 hours are added for patients with severe crush, farm injuries, and soil contamination.

DISLOCATIONS

Dislocations also require urgent assessment, diagnosis, and treatment. By definition, a joint is dislocated when the articular surfaces are no longer in contact. The diagnosis of a joint dislocation is often made from the history and physical examination. Acute dislocation is usually very painful, with muscle spasm and limited motion. The limb will usually be held in a somewhat fixed position characteristic of the specific dislocation. For example, an anterior shoulder dislocation will leave the arm in external rotation and slight abduction. Internal rotation and adduction are usually very limited. Loss of the normal contour of the joint can be seen with the humeral head palpable anteriorly and a sulcus sign evident posteriorly beneath the acromion.

Radiographic evaluation is essential in the management of these injuries so that associated fractures are recognized prior to attempt at reduction. Failure to do so may result in further displacement of fractures and significantly worsen the prognosis of the injury.

Joint dislocations are considered emergencies because the risk of neurovascular compromise or progressive worsening of a neurovascular deficit increases with the amount of time the dislocation is present. Prolonged dislocation also increases the chance of osteonecrosis, although this is more commonly a concern in the lower extremity. Osteonecrosis is believed to be due to possible interruption of capsular blood supply from the increased capsular tension caused by the dislocation.

TABLE 1: Classification of Open Fractures

Grade I: Wound <1 cm, low-velocity trauma with minimal contamination or soft tissue damage. Fracture has little or no comminution.

Grade II: Wound >1 cm, without extensive soft tissue damage. Contamination and comminution are moderate.

Grade III: Characterized by extensive soft tissue damage including muscle, skin, and neurovascular structures with a high degree of contamination. Fractures are significantly comminuted.

Grade IIIA: Soft tissue coverage of the bone is adequate despite extensive laceration, flaps, or high-energy trauma. This grade includes severely comminuted or segmental fractures regardless of the wound size.

Grade IIIB: Associated with extensive injury to the soft tissue with periosteal stripping, massive contamination, and severe comminution. After débridement a local or free flap is needed for coverage.

Grade IIIC: Includes any open fracture with an associated arterial injury that must be repaired.

Dislocations and fractures with neurologic or vascular compromise should therefore be reduced as quickly as possible in order to reduce the potential for irreversible injury to the affected structures. Following reduction, a repeat examination is required to determine if the neurovascular compromise has been relieved.

GUNSHOT WOUNDS

Fractures associated with gunshot wounds deserve special mention because they are difficult to classify as either open or closed. Their status as an "open" or "closed" injury is determined by whether the injury was inflicted by a high- or low-velocity weapon. The exact distinction is somewhat cloudy, but according to the Wound Ballistics Manual of the Office of the Surgeon General, muzzle velocity greater than 2500 feet/second constitutes "high velocity." This is important because the kinetic energy of the bullet varies directly with the square of its velocity and only linearly with its mass. Shotgun wounds are generally considered high energy despite a lower muzzle velocity because of the high level of energy imparted by the blast.

The majority of fractures caused by low-velocity weapons can be given antibiotics but otherwise be treated as "closed" fractures, with little to no increased risk of infection. Many may be treated to completion with closed methods, such as functional bracing or casting. If one chooses open management, fracture comminution is often found to be more extensive than can be appreciated on plain radiographs.

In contrast, high-velocity gunshot wound fractures are best treated as "open" injuries. As the high-velocity missile passes through the limb, it not only causes significant fracture comminution but also carries with it a shock wave that passes through the soft tissue and creates a cavitary lesion with severe muscular and neurovascular injury. In this situation, a prompt débridement is necessary to remove devitalized bone and muscle, and additional serial débridements may be required until all tissues have declared themselves as viable or not.

There may also be associated neurologic deficits due to the "blast effect" of the initial injury. When due to a low-velocity gunshot wound, these are usually due to the percussive wave produced by the bullet, which leads to a temporary neuropraxia without laceration of the nerve. These injuries do not warrant immediate exploration as most will resolve with observation alone. If persistent neurologic

deficits occur, an electromyogram (EMG) may be indicated between 3 and 6 weeks to assess the nerve for evidence of recovery. High-velocity gunshot wounds should be treated more aggressively. The cavitary lesion may be so large that the nerve may be disrupted and may even have a segmental defect. Because the cavitary wound itself requires emergent débridement, nerves that are not functioning should be explored simultaneously. If lacerated, the nerve should be repaired, if possible. However, in most cases, the extent of the nerve injury from the blast cannot be determined at the time of the initial exploration, and the patient may require a delayed exploration to determine the size of the nerve defect and to perform a reconstruction by staged nerve grafting.

COMPARTMENT SYNDROME

In 1881, Volkmann first described permanent contracture of the forearm flexors as a result of ischemia. He believed that the pathophysiology was arterial insufficiency and venous stasis resulting from a tight cast or bandage. For nearly the next hundred years, attention primarily focused on the "arterial" problem, with some improvements in clinical results noted when compartments were opened to explore for arterial injury and perform repair.

In the 1970s and 1980s, a better understanding of the pathophysiology of compartment syndrome emerged. Any condition that results in increased tissue pressure within a closed compartment will obstruct venous flow. If the problem continues unabated, pressure will rise until arteriolar pressure is exceeded, at which point flow through the capillary bed ceases. This typically occurs when the pressure within the compartment is within 30 mm Hg of the diastolic blood pressure. If the situation persists, the muscle within the compartment will become ischemic, necrose, and eventually contract. In the upper extremity, this most commonly occurs in the forearm.

Signs of compartment syndrome include marked pain on passive digital motion, a tense or swollen forearm, and either paresthesia or reduced sensation in the hand. Intracompartmental pressure measurements may be helpful in deciding borderline cases, but in general, the diagnosis is made on clinical grounds. Once the diagnosis of acute compartment syndrome is established, an emergent forearm fasciotomy is required to release the pressure in order to prevent muscle necrosis and subsequent late contracture of the fingers due to contracture of the necrotic flexor muscles in the forearm.

Gunshot wounds to the forearm require special attention even if there is no associated fracture due to a high risk for development of forearm compartment syndrome. Patients should be monitored for at least 8 to 12 hours for clinical evidence of increased pressure within the forearm from arterial injury causing bleeding into the relatively confined spaces of the forearm compartments.

In contrast to an acute compartment syndrome, a compartment syndrome diagnosed late or a "crush" syndrome should not be routinely released. Recent examples of this injury would be seen in victims of earthquake disasters such as in Haiti and elsewhere. If an extremity is severely crushed, muscle necrosis occurs immediately, with pressure rising later as a response to, rather than a cause of, the muscle damage. Once muscle necrosis has already occurred, fasciotomy does nothing to prevent it, and it does expose the necrotic muscle to outside contaminants, thus leading to an increased risk of infection and a possible need for amputation.

IMAGING STUDIES

For fractures and dislocations, proper radiographic evaluation is essential before making any decisions regarding treatment of the injury. Ideally, two orthogonal views of the injured extremity should be obtained along with radiographs of the joints adjacent to the injured bone. Injuries to the shoulder girdle should have a minimum of three radiographic views in a standard "trauma series." This series

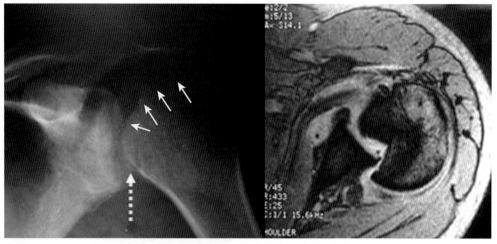

FIGURE 1   Anteroposterior radiograph on the left depicts a missed posterior dislocation. There is overlap of the humerus and glenoid *(white dotted arrow)* and a large impaction fracture of the humeral head *(white arrows)*. Magnetic resonance imaging on the right clearly shows the dislocation and associated humeral head impaction fracture.

includes a true anteroposterior (AP) view (also known as a "Grashey"), a scapular Y view, and an axillary view. Subtle injuries can be missed if adequate radiographs are not obtained. Figure 1 shows a missed posterior dislocation that was not properly diagnosed until a magnetic resonance imaging (MRI) study was obtained 6 months after the initial injury.

INJURIES TO THE SHOULDER GIRDLE AND HUMERUS

Sternoclavicular Dislocation

The sternoclavicular joint has the least bony stability of any major joint in the body. Virtually all of its integrity comes from the surrounding ligaments. Sternoclavicular dislocation is one of the rarest dislocations, representing perhaps 3% of shoulder girdle injuries, but is common enough that most major trauma centers will see

one or two a year. The true ratio of anterior to posterior dislocations is unknown, because most reports concern the more rare posterior type, but anterior dislocations are clearly more common.

Imaging of these injuries is difficult because the sternoclavicluar joint overlies the spine and ribs on standard radiographs. A "serendipity" view, an AP chest film centered on the top of the sternum and aimed 45 degrees cephalic, will occasionally show the dislocation, but a computed tomography (CT) scan will demonstrate the injury most clearly (Fig. 2).

Because of the proximity of the mediastinum and its great vessels to the sternoclavicular joint, we typically recommend treatment in the operating room, with the trauma team on notice nearby if an open procedure is to be performed. Although most anterior dislocations are unstable after closed reduction, we still recommend an attempt to reduce the dislocation closed. Occasionally, the clavicle remains reduced, but if it does not, one usually accepts the deformity, because an anteriorly dislocated sternoclavicular joint typically becomes asymptomatic, and the deformity is less of a problem than the potential complications of operative fixation.

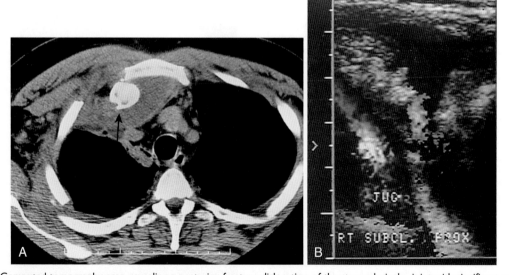

FIGURE 2   **A,** Computed tomography scan revealing a posterior fracture-dislocation of the sternoclavicular joint with significant soft tissue swelling and compromise of the hilar structures. **B,** Duplex ultrasound study revealing a large pseudoaneurysm of the right subclavian artery. Note the large neck of the pseudoaneurysm, which measured approximately 1 cm in diameter *(arrow)*. *(From Bucholz RW, Heckman JD, editors: Rockwood and Green's fractures in adults, 5th ed, Philadelphia, 2001, Lippincott, Williams & Wilkins, p 1285.)*

In contrast to anterior dislocations, the complications of an unreduced posterior dislocation are numerous: thoracic outlet syndrome, vascular compromise inclusive of blunt subclavian arterial and venous injuries including thrombosis of these vessels, and erosion of the medial clavicle into any of the vital mediastinal structures that lie posterior to the sternoclavicular joint. Closed reduction for acute posterior sternoclavicular dislocation can usually be obtained, and is generally stable. Often, general anesthesia is necessary. However, when a posterior dislocation is irreducible or the reduction is unstable, an open reduction should be performed. Depending on the exact pathoanatomy, either open reduction with ligament repair or medial clavicle resection and ligament reconstruction may be performed.

Clavicle Fractures

The clavicle is one of the most commonly fractured bones, representing 4% of all fractures and over a third of all fractures in the shoulder region. Fractures in the medial third are quite rare; fractures of the middle third represent nearly 70%, and fractures in the lateral third account for 20% to 30% of all clavicle fractures. Despite a longstanding and widely held belief that virtually all clavicle shaft fractures do well without surgery, recent data, more carefully obtained, demonstrate that this is often not the case.

Initial studies on the natural history of clavicle fractures demonstrated union rates of greater than 99% with nonoperative management and nonunion rates of 5% to 10% or higher for clavicle fractures treated with surgery. Missing from these studies was information on the age of the patients, the severity of injury, and the nature of the fractures selected for surgery. More recent studies focusing on the natural history of clavicle fractures in adults have demonstrated nonunion rates of 4% to 6% for all fractures, with nonunion rates as high as 15% when the fractures are significantly displaced. Shortening of a fractured clavicle by greater than 2 cm has proved to be particularly problematic.

A recent published systematic review of 2144 previously reported clavicle fractures has confirmed a nonunion rate of 15% for displaced fractures and a relative reduction of 86% in the risk for nonunion when displaced fractures are treated operatively. Finally, a multicenter randomized comparative trial of nonoperative treatment versus plate fixation demonstrated faster, easier, and more complete recovery in the surgical group, with both doctors and patients rating the surgical results significantly better at all-time points, including the final result. Complications in the surgical group were primarily related to the hardware (plate) used.

Current teaching holds that surgical repair is very strongly indicated for shortening more than 20 mm, open injury or threatened skin, neurovascular compromise, scapulothoracic dissociation, and displaced pathologic fracture. Accepted relative indications are displacement more than 20 mm, floating shoulder, polytrauma, expected prolonged recumbency, a patient unable to tolerate immobilization, bilateral fractures, and ipsilateral upper extremity fracture. Complete displacement (no cortical contact between the main fragments on any radiograph view) is also a relative indication in an informed patient willing to accept the risk of surgery in order to obtain a faster and more complete recovery.

When patients with clavicle fractures are selected for nonoperative management, current recommendation is for sling immobilization without attempt at reduction of the fracture. When internal fixation is indicated, surgery may be performed with either a plate and screws or an intramedullary device (Fig. 3). Although both techniques have their proponents and detractors, no large study has demonstrated superiority of one technique over the other.

Fractures of the lateral, or distal, third of the clavicle are also fairly common, comprising approximately 20% to 30% of all clavicle fractures. In contrast to fractures of the midshaft, a propensity of distal clavicle fractures toward nonunion was noted early and nonunion rates in excess of 20% have been reported by Robinson. This had

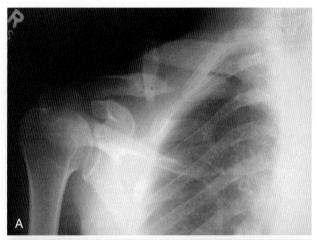

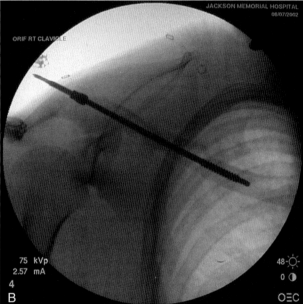

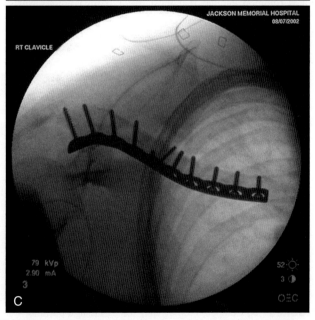

FIGURE 3 A comminuted displaced midshaft clavicle fracture (**A**) may be fixed with either an intramedullary device (**B**) or with a plate and screws (**C**).

led some authors to recommend early surgery although others have noted that many of these nonunions become asymptomatic with time, leading them to recommend nonoperative treatment for these fractures.

Although fractures of the lateral clavicle have not been as thoroughly studied as fractures of the midshaft, recent reports of surgery performed using newer techniques demonstrate excellent healing and function with a low rate of complications. One would expect that recommendations for the lateral clavicle might soon be similar to those for the midshaft—surgery will not be mandatory but will likely allow a faster and easier rehabilitation, with an "on average" better final result. When operative fixation is chosen, plate and screw fixation is probably the most familiar method, although numerous other methods, such as screw fixation alone, may be used.

Acromioclavicular Dislocation (Separated Shoulder)

The acromioclavicular (AC) joint is a strong, stable joint between the end of the clavicle and the acromion. In addition to the robust capsule that joins the acromion to the clavicle, there is a thick coracoclavicular (CC) ligament that suspends the scapula from the end of the clavicle. It has the distinction of being the only commonly dislocated joint that is routinely managed without reduction of the dislocation, and although it is predominantly injured in young adult males involved in collision sports such as ice hockey or rugby, AC separation can also occur in trauma patients who have sustained a direct downward blow to the lateral aspect of the shoulder. The dislocations are more often incomplete than complete, and the majority can be managed nonoperatively.

Classification of AC joint separation into three groups was originally proposed by Allman and subsequently modified by Rockwood to include six categories (Fig. 4). Grade I and II injuries (partial or complete disruption of the AC joint) are virtually always managed without surgery. There is no attempt at reducing the dislocation. Patients are given a sling for comfort and permitted to gradually resume use of the arm as their level of comfort allows. Grade IV to VI are uncommon and severe and are typically managed with surgery to restore the anatomy and either repair or reconstruct the CC ligament. Surgical techniques for this injury are numerous, with no clear consensus as to the optimal surgical technique. Management of grade III injuries (complete disruption of both the AC joint and the CC ligament) is controversial. The majority of American shoulder surgeons continue to manage these nonoperatively, although there are some advocates for routine surgical repair. The nonsurgical management is the same as for grade I and II injuries. There is some consensus that grade III separations in heavy laborers present future problems for return to work and ought to be treated surgically.

Scapular Fractures

Fractures of the scapula are relatively uncommon, accounting for just a few percent of all shoulder girdle injuries. These generally occur as the result of high-energy trauma, explaining the frequent association with other, often life-threatening, injuries that are of greater significance than the fracture itself. It is not uncommon for scapular fractures to be overlooked in polytrauma patients and often noticed incidentally on a chest radiograph or CT scan.

Associated injuries are quite common due to the high-energy mechanisms in which these fractures usually occur. In one study of 148 fractures in 116 scapulas, 96% had associated injuries, with upper thoracic rib fractures being the most common. Pulmonary injuries were also common, with an overall incidence of 37%, of which 29% were hemopneumothorax, and 8% pulmonary contusion. Head injuries were observed in 34%, ipsilateral clavicle fractures in 25%, and cervical spine injuries in 12%.

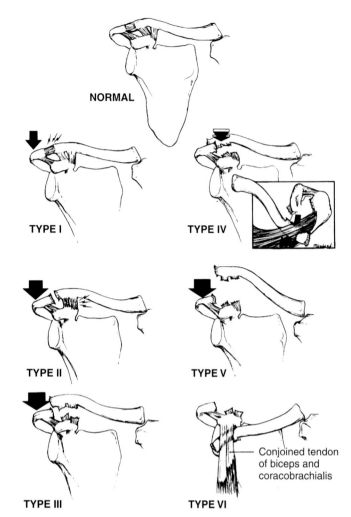

FIGURE 4 Classification showing the types of acromioclavicular (AC) separation: in grade I and II injuries the AC joint is either partially or completely disrupted. In grade III injuries the coracoclavicular ligament is completely disrupted as well. Types IV, V, and VI have extreme disruption of the joint, with the distal clavicle being displaced severely posteriorly, superiorly, or inferiorly. *(From Rockwood CA Jr, Matsen FA, Wirth MA, Lippitt SB, editors:* The shoulder, *3rd ed, Philadelphia, 2004, Saunders, Fig. 12–14.)*

Management of these fractures is usually nonsurgical because the thick, investing rotator cuff musculature provides both a rich blood supply that produces rapid healing and a layer of cushion that prevents most malunions from causing symptoms. When a high-energy mechanism is present, we recommend admission for a period of 24 hours to assess pulmonary and cardiac status. For fractures managed without surgery, a brief period of sling immobilization is initiated for comfort, followed by early range of motion. Most fractures are clinically united by 6 weeks and strengthening can begin at that time.

Clear operative indications include intra-articular glenoid fractures with 5 mm of step-off, coracoid fractures with intra-articular extension and more than 5 mm of step-off, and glenoid rim fractures with persistent or recurrent glenohumeral instability. Appropriate treatment of displaced fractures of the scapular spine and glenoid neck are more controversial, with some favoring surgery but others advocating for nonoperative management.

The injury pattern described as the *"floating shoulder"* deserves special mention here. This injury is perhaps better described as a "double disruption" of the superior shoulder suspensory complex.

This complex consists of a bone and soft tissue ring formed by the glenoid and its surrounding structures. This ring is suspended from the clavicle in the front and from the scapular body in the rear. Isolated disruption of one suspensory component is generally tolerated well; however, when both the front and back are disrupted, the potential for instability of the shoulder girdle increases. This is most commonly seen with ipsilateral clavicle and glenoid neck fractures.

The treatment of such injuries is somewhat controversial. Initial uncontrolled case series reported good results with fixation of both the glenoid and clavicle, and with fixation of the clavicle alone. However, subsequent studies comparing the results of nonoperative management to the data from previous operative studies demonstrated no clear benefit to operative management. Given these considerations, the general approach to treatment now is to evaluate the clavicle and scapula fractures independently and treat them according to the guidelines used for isolated fractures.

Scapulothoracic Dissociation

Scapulothoracic dissociation is an infrequent but devastating injury that is best thought of as an internal forequarter amputation. It is the result of a massive traction injury causing significant lateral displacement of the upper extremity between the scapula and its thoracic articulation. The impact required to cause this is so severe that many patients with this injury do not survive the initial associated thoracoabdominal injuries. According to Althausen et al, 88% have associated vascular compromise and 94% presented with severe neurologic injuries in conjunction with severe injuries to the brachial plexus and subclavian vessels. In this series 52% wound up with a flail extremity, 21% with early amputation, and 10% died.

Diagnosis is made clinically by the presence of massive swelling, weakness, pain, tenderness, and absent or diminished pulses. It is crucial not to attribute pulselessness to a more distal injury when a more proximal, life-threatening injury may be the underlying cause. Radiographically, an AP film of the chest may reveal lateral displacement of the scapula. An increased distance from the medial border of the scapula to the spinous processes when compared to the uninjured side should alert the physician to the possibility of a scapulothoracic dissociation. This may or may not be seen in conjunction with a sternoclavicular or AC dislocation or a distracted clavicle fracture.

Management is controversial but arterial injuries warrant immediate exploration. Brachial plexus exploration may be carried out locally at the same time. Although it is probably not necessary to explore the brachial plexus all the way up into the neck, the plexus is at times found to be in the field of the vascular exploration and completely avulsed from either the arm or the neck. The prognosis for recovery from a complete plexus avulsion is so bleak that many consider this to be an indication for an immediate above elbow amputation. When a complete plexus avulsion is not seen, vascular repair should proceed. Bony stabilization may be necessary to protect vascular repairs but the role of internal fixation is otherwise less clear. Because manipulation and stabilization of the bony injury could potentially disrupt a vascular repair the recommended operative sequence at our institutions is to: (1) control bleeding and shunt the vascular injury, (2) establish bony stability if needed, and then (3) perform definitive vascular repair.

Glenohumeral Dislocation

Because of its lack of bony constraint, the shoulder is the most commonly dislocated joint in the body. It is not a true ball-and-socket joint, but more like a golf ball resting on a tee. The static restraints to dislocation are composed of the osseous structures, the glenoid labrum, and the capsule and glenohumeral ligaments, and additional dynamic stability is provided by the rotator cuff musculature.

Anterior dislocations are by far the most common type. These are usually the result of an eccentric load applied to the arm while in an outstretched position as would be seen in a volleyball player while spiking the ball. Posterior dislocations may occur with a posteriorly directed force on an adducted, flexed arm or from overwhelming contraction of the internal rotators of the shoulder in patients having an electric shock or seizure.

An anteriorly dislocated shoulder will present with the arm at the side or in slight abduction and external rotation. Normal loss of the shoulder contour may be seen with a full appearance in the front and a prominent "sulcus" sign under the acromion in the back. Adduction and internal rotation are usually limited. In contrast, a patient with a posterior dislocation will hold the arm in an adducted, internally rotated position and have an anterior shoulder that appears flatter than normal with an extremely prominent coracoid and anterior acromion.

Evaluation should include a thorough neurologic examination and radiographic evaluation prior to any attempted reduction. Neurologic involvement is not infrequent, occurring in up to 50% of patients, with the axillary nerve being most commonly affected. Vascular status should likewise be documented, as vascular injuries can also occur. A standard radiographic trauma series as described earlier is extremely helpful in delineating any associated glenoid rim or proximal humeral fracture.

Reduction is most easily carried out with some form of sedation or injection of lidocaine into the joint. Gentle traction will reduce most dislocations. Irreducible dislocations and dislocations with accompanying humeral fractures are best managed in the operating room with general anesthesia. Postreduction films should confirm the glenohumeral reduction. If there is persistent displacement of either a proximal humeral or a significant glenoid fracture, surgery is required to reduce and fix the fracture. Otherwise, a period of sling immobilization for comfort followed by gradual mobilization of the shoulder is recommended. In the majority of cases patients will recover their range of motion without the need for a formal physical therapy program.

In younger patients the skeletal injury is typically an avulsion of the labrum and anteroinferior capsule (the Bankart lesion) off the glenoid rim. The best natural history studies have demonstrated additional dislocation in approximately 50% of young adults, with about half of those developing recurrent instability requiring surgical repair. In extremely young or active patients whose job or sport puts them at high risk of recurrent dislocation, one might consider a primary ligament repair after a first-time dislocation, but in general, the initial management of this injury is nonoperative, with surgery reserved for recurrent dislocators.

As patients age, ligament injury and recurrence become less common, and rotator cuff tears become more frequent. By the age of 40, rotator cuff tear becomes more common than ligamentous injury, and recurrence becomes infrequent. A careful physical examination for strength of the rotator cuff should follow all reductions, and weakness in the absence of proximal humerus fracture should prompt an MRI to rule out the possibility of a significant rotator cuff tear. Acute tearing of the rotator cuff following a dislocation is typically an indication for surgical repair.

Proximal Humerus Fractures

Proximal humerus fractures are common injuries, especially with our aging population. The majority of these injuries are minimally displaced or nondisplaced and can be treated nonoperatively. Factors to take into consideration in the treatment plan are age of the patient, hand dominance, bone quality, fracture type, and fracture displacement. Associated injuries in the multitrauma patient are also important in the decision-making process.

Assessment should consist of a thorough neurovascular examination along with a radiographic trauma series. The presence of an expanding axillary mass or an absent distal pulse is concerning for a vascular injury. Clinically evident nerve injuries occur in as many as one third of patients and are more common with increasing age. When EMG is used to detect them, the incidence of nerve injury is even higher, occurring in up to 82% of displaced proximal humeral fractures. If present, these injuries may take many months to recover, and functional recovery is at times incomplete.

These fractures are most commonly classified according to Neer. He used Codman's original description of the four "parts" of the proximal humerus—the articular segment, the greater and lesser tuberosities, and the shaft—and defined a part as displaced when it was shifted by 1 cm or angulated 45 degrees. Despite relatively poor interobserver reliability, this is by far the most frequently used classification system (Fig. 5). Subsequent work with Codman's original description has better defined the possible fracture patterns and implications for treatment. Fractures that isolate the articular segment, disrupt the "hinge" between the shaft and the articular segment, or leave the articular segment with less than 8 mm of bone at its inferior margin all potentially disrupt the blood supply to the humeral head. This has implications for treatment because disruption of the blood supply increases the likelihood of avascular necrosis of the head of the humerus.

Treatment varies from a period of immobilization in a sling followed by progressive mobilization of the shoulder in fractures managed nonoperatively to surgical repair or replacement in fractures with greater displacement. Fracture pattern and degree of displacement, age of the patient and ability to participate in rehabilitation, preinjury function of the limb, and the presence of concomitant injuries all have implications for choice of treatment. Surgical techniques and preferences between surgeons vary greatly, with plate and screw, intramedullary nail, suture, and percutaneous pin fixation all presenting viable options (Fig. 6). Humeral head replacement is classically used for severe fractures in the elderly. Although this generally results in a stable shoulder and good pain relief, functional outcome is unpredictable. Recently there has been a growing interest in reverse shoulder replacement for comminuted geriatric fractures because it does not rely on healing of the fractured tuberosities around the prosthesis in order for the shoulder to function.

Humeral Shaft Fractures

There is a bimodal distribution of diaphyseal humeral shaft fractures, the first mainly occurring in young adults injured in high-energy motor vehicle accidents, falls from height, or gunshots. The second peak is seen in elderly patients who sustain the fracture during a fall from a standing height.

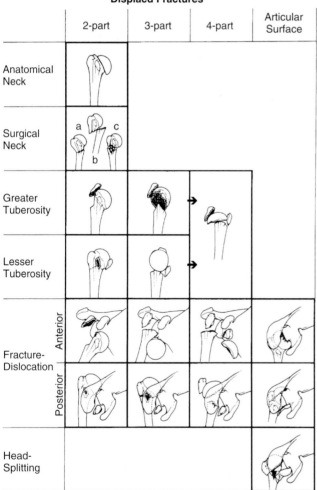

FIGURE 5 The Neer classification. The four "parts" of the proximal humerus—the articular segment, the greater tuberosity, the lesser tuberosity, and the shaft—are considered displaced if they are separated by more than 1 cm or angulated more than 45 degrees. Fracture lines that have not displaced are not considered to create "parts." *(After Neer CS: Displaced proximal humeral fractures. Part I. Classification and evaluation.* J Bone Joint Surg Am *52:1077–1089, 1970.)*

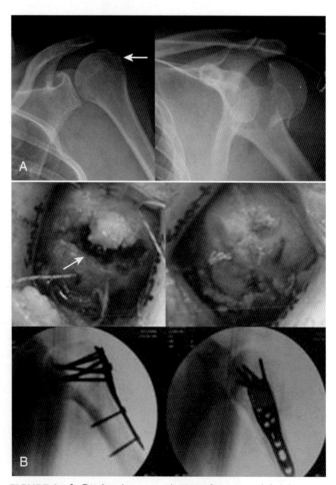

FIGURE 6 **A,** Displaced greater tuberosity fracture on left *(white arrow),* and displaced anatomic neck fracture on right. Both are considered "two-part fractures" according to the Neer classification. **B,** Intraoperative photographs of greater tuberosity fracture being repaired with suture and intraoperative fluoroscopy after open reduction and internal fixation of anatomic neck fracture.

Historically, treatment of these fractures has been successful with nonoperative management; initial splinting is followed by placement in a functional brace in the subacute phase. In one study of 922 patients whose fractures were selected for functional bracing, only 3% of fractures failed to heal and 98% of patients regained near-full motion of the shoulder and elbow. Even in severely displaced or comminuted fractures such as the one seen in Figure 7, functional bracing presents a treatment option that may minimize the risks associated with a major surgical procedure. However, recent investigations comparing plate fixation and management with a fracture brace have noted lower rates of nonunion, malunion, and surprisingly, radial nerve palsy in the operatively treated group. There was no significant difference in infection rate, time to radiographic union, or final range of motion between the nonoperative and operative groups.

Treatment of fractures with associated nerve injury remains controversial. The reported incidence of radial nerve palsy varies from 1.8% to 24% with shaft fractures. The nerve is most commonly contused, with a neuropraxia that recovers in the majority of cases. Transverse fractures of the middle third are more likely to have a neuropraxia than spiral fractures of the distal third. The more distal fractures do however have a higher incidence of laceration or entrapment of the radial nerve, as can be seen in Figure 8. Although exploration for acute nerve injury is not routinely recommended, one would certainly include exploration as part of the exposure for those fractures treated operatively, such as open fractures or those from high-energy gunshot wounds.

Standard indications for operative intervention include open fractures, fractures resulting from high-energy gunshot wounds, fractures

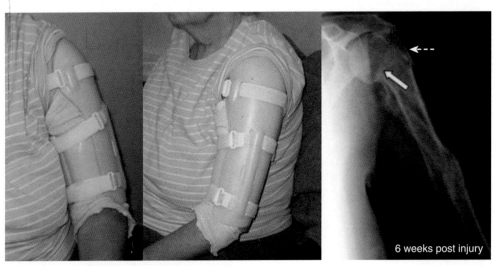

FIGURE 7   Clinical photographs of a humeral fracture brace. Radiograph on right shows complex fracture being treated in this brace at 6 weeks with acceptable alignment of all components. Greater tuberosity component *(dotted arrow)*, surgical neck *(solid arrow)*, and comminuted shaft with early callus formation. *(Courtesy of Robin M. Gehrmann, MD.)*

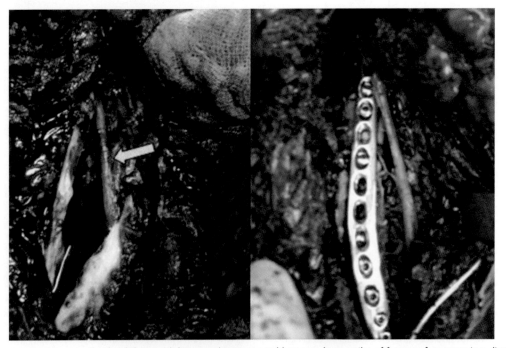

FIGURE 8   Intraoperative photograph of radial nerve *(white arrow)* incarcerated between bony spike of fracture fragments in a distal third humerus fracture *(left)*. After open reduction and internal fixation with radial nerve crossing plate proximally *(right)*. *(Courtesy of Robin M. Gehrmann, MD.)*

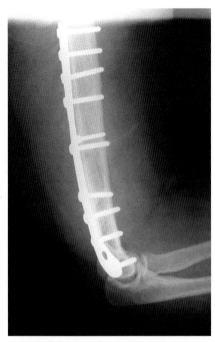

FIGURE 9   A similar fracture, internally fixed.

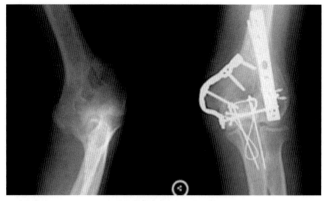

FIGURE 10   Preoperative anteroposterior (AP) radiograph of comminuted intra-articular distal humerus fracture *(left)*; postoperative AP film *(right)* with restoration of the articular surface and the medial and lateral columns. *(Courtesy of Robin M. Gehrmann, MD.)*

with vascular injury, patients with polytrauma, and patients whose injuries cannot be acceptably aligned in a splint or functional brace, which is a common problem in obese patients and in patients for whom prolonged recumbency is anticipated. Although intramedullary fixation has a small number of indications, plate and screw fixation is used for the vast majority of humeral shaft fractures treated with internal fixation (Fig. 9).

ELBOW

Distal Humerus Fractures

Distal humerus fractures are rare, accounting for a very small percentage of all adult fractures. Both operative and nonoperative treatments have historically reported poor outcomes due to pain, deformity, stiffness, nonunion, and ulnar neuropathy. The factors that appear to be most predictive of a good outcome are the ability to achieve an anatomic reduction of the joint surface and the ability to start early motion.

Nondisplaced or minimally displaced fractures can be treated nonoperatively with a brief period of immobilization. If they maintain acceptable position, then one may begin range of motion exercises in a few weeks' time. However, when there is a displaced intra-articular component, operative treatment is the only way one can restore articular congruity. With modern fracture treatment principles and fixation devices, an acceptable result can usually be obtained.

In adults, the goals of reconstruction are aimed at recreating the articular surface, reestablishing the medial and lateral columns of the humerus, and fixing the fracture stably enough to allow early motion (Fig. 10). An olecranon osteotomy is frequently necessary in order to provide adequate exposure of the articular surface. The ulnar nerve must always be identified and protected and is sometimes transposed to an anterior subcutaneous position after the fracture has been repaired. Complications of the fracture and surgical repair include joint contracture, ulnar neuropathy, heterotopic ossification, and prominent hardware. It is not uncommon for patients to undergo a delayed secondary operation to release a stiff elbow, remove heterotopic bone, or remove bothersome implants.

In the case of a badly comminuted joint surface in a low-demand elderly patient with poor bone quality, other options would include early range-of-motion exercises without fixation (so-called "bag of bones" treatment) or primary total elbow replacement. In current practice, the former is used only for the most infirm of patients, and elbow replacement has grown in popularity as a result of additional studies, which have demonstrated faster and easier recovery and improved functional results with arthroplasty. Although the choice of treatment for "fixable" geriatric fractures remains unclear, replacement is clearly becoming the treatment of choice for elderly patients in whom stable fixation cannot be obtained.

Elbow Dislocation

The elbow is the second most commonly dislocated joint (after the shoulder), accounting for 20% of all dislocations. Approximately half of the elbow's stability is due its highly congruent bony articulation, and half is due to the collateral ligaments. The anterior band of the medial collateral ligament is the primary stabilizer to valgus stress, and the lateral collateral ligament complex provides restraint to posterolateral rotatory instability.

Elbow dislocation usually occurs in adolescents and young adults, frequently from a fall onto an outstretched arm with the shoulder abducted and elbow extended. Patients present with pain and inability to move the elbow. Gross deformity may be apparent but can be underappreciated due to swelling. A thorough neurovascular examination with documentation is essential because a stretch injury of the ulnar or median nerve is not uncommon. The shoulder and wrist should be carefully evaluated to rule out associated injuries. Any forearm tenderness or instability of the distal radioulnar joint (DRUJ) should be recognized as potential signs of disruption of the interosseous membrane and DRUJ (known as an Essex-Lopresti injury).

Radiographs of the elbow are used to confirm the clinical diagnosis of dislocation. An elbow dislocation that does not involve a fracture is known as a simple dislocation and is classified according to the direction of the dislocation. Dislocation with associated fracture(s) of the radial head/neck or coronoid process (i.e., a complex dislocation) must be well defined with imaging studies because the fractures have implications for definitive treatment.

An acute elbow dislocation should initially be managed with prompt closed reduction with adequate analgesia and muscle relaxation. This can usually be achieved in the emergency room with intramuscular or intravenous medication(s). Several reduction techniques have been described but they all involve correcting the medial-lateral displacement, followed by longitudinal traction and flexion of the forearm. A "clunk" is often felt with reduction of the joint.

After reduction, stability is assessed by checking range of motion with valgus-varus stress. If there are no fractures, passive motion to within 30 degrees of full extension without instability suggests a stable reduction, and mobilization of the elbow can begin within a few days when the patient is more comfortable. If the elbow is unstable after reduction, then it should be immobilized in 90 degrees of flexion for approximately 1 to 2 weeks before beginning motion. Recently, some have suggested that early active flexion exercises may be helpful in establishing a stable joint.

Posterior elbow dislocation with associated fractures of the radial head and the coronoid process has been referred to as the "terrible triad of the elbow" because of the difficulties encountered in its management. Definitive treatment of these complex elbow dislocations usually involves surgery because they are highly unstable and are prone to numerous complications when inadequately treated. With operative treatment, the surgeon should attempt to restore elbow stability by: (1) reestablishing radiocapitellar contact by either repairing the radial head or replacing it with a prosthesis, (2) repairing the lateral collateral ligament, and (3) performing internal fixation of the coronoid fracture as needed. An example is shown in Figure 11.

The outcome of nonoperative management of a simple elbow dislocation is usually highly successful. Poor results can occur with prolonged immobilization (usually greater than 3 weeks) and inadequate rehabilitation. Other sequelae include heterotopic ossification and stiffness. Additionally, complex dislocations can also have recurrent instability, failure of fixation, and posttraumatic arthritis.

Radial Head Fractures

Radial head fractures are common injuries, accounting for one third of elbow fractures, and are frequently associated with elbow dislocations. The mechanism of injury is usually an axial load on a pronated forearm. Patients with radial head fractures often present with lateral elbow pain upon extension or forearm rotation. Most use the classification originally described by Mason. Type I fractures are nondisplaced, type II displaced, and type III comminuted. Subsequent modifications have included a type IV, which is a radial head fracture with an associated elbow dislocation.

Nondisplaced fractures are well managed with early mobilization. Operative indications for radial head fractures include displacement greater than 3 mm, a bony block to forearm rotation, an Essex-Lopresti lesion (i.e., associated disruption of the interosseous membrane), and an unstable elbow. Surgery for radial head fracture may entail excision, internal fixation, or prosthetic replacement. Isolated radial head fractures without elbow instability can be safely excised without compromising elbow stability or function, especially in the elderly patient. Ring et al have shown that internal fixation is best when the number of radial head fragments is three or fewer. Metallic prosthetic radial head replacement is performed when stable fixation of the head is not possible, typically in the setting of an Essex-Lopresti lesion or a Mason type III or IV fracture.

Coronoid Fractures

The coronoid process of the ulna serves both as a buttress that prevents posterior displacement of the forearm and as the attachment site for the anterior band of the medial collateral ligament. Therefore, it has an important role in providing stability to the elbow. Coronoid fractures are commonly associated with elbow dislocations. Originally, three types were identified and are best seen on a lateral elbow radiograph: type I, tip fracture; type II, less than 50%; and type III, greater than 50% of the coronoid height. More recently, an oblique or vertical fracture line about the anteromedial coronoid has also been recognized as a less common fracture that, if unrepaired, can cause persistent varus instability of the ulnohumeral joint and early posttraumatic arthritis (Fig. 12). This fragment is best seen on a CT scan. In general, type I coronoid fractures can be managed without fixation of the fragment itself. Because displaced type II and III fractures and anteromedial fractures can contribute to elbow instability, they should be treated with internal fixation as part of the overall surgical management of elbow dislocation.

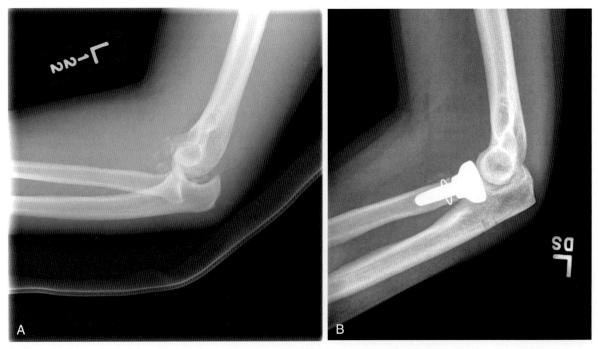

FIGURE 11 A, A 40-year-old man sustained a fracture dislocation of the elbow. Comminution of the radial head made it irreparable. **B,** Open reduction of the joint with replacement of the radial head and repair of the lateral ligament yielded a stable elbow.

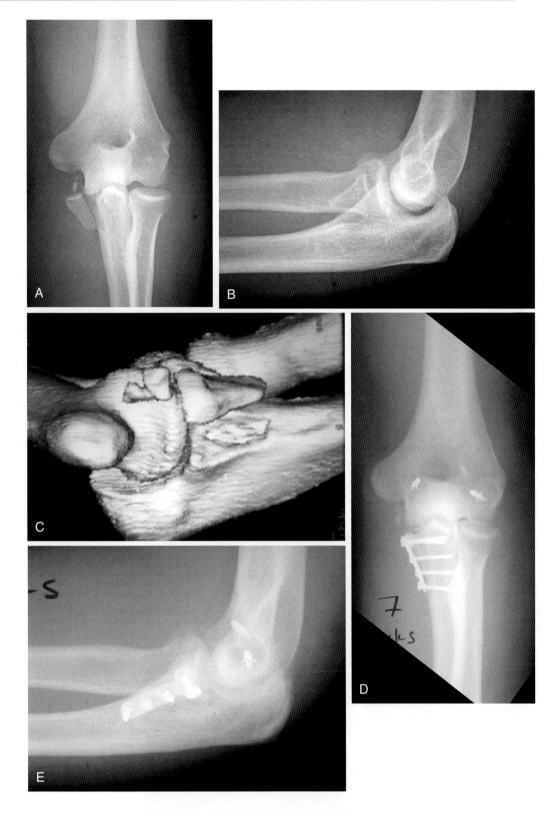

FIGURE 12   Anteroposterior lateral elbow radiographs (**A** and **B**) and a three-dimensional computed tomography scan (**C**) showing an anterior medial coronoid fracture. This patient had an elbow dislocation that was emergently reduced prior to these imaging studies. **D** and **E,** The patient subsequently underwent operative fixation of his coronoid fracture and repair of both the lateral and medial collateral ligaments with suture anchors. *(Courtesy of Virak Tan, MD.)*

Olecranon Fractures

The greater sigmoid notch of the ulna is formed by the olecranon and coronoid processes. The olecranon makes up the proximal half of the notch. Fractures involving this portion do not result in ulnohumeral instability. Olecranon fractures can result from direct force or from eccentric loading of the triceps. Minimally displaced fractures (less than 2 mm gap at 90 degrees of elbow flexion) are uncommon but can be treated with elbow splinting at 30 to 45 degrees of flexion. More commonly, the fractures are displaced and require operative fixation to restore the tricep mechanism and active elbow extension. Several options exist for fixing olecranon fractures, including tension band technique with supplemental Kirschner wires or screw(s), bicortical interfragmentary or intramedullary screw(s), and plating. Comminuted fractures are best managed with dorsal plate fixation. In cases of severe comminution, excision of the fragments and reattachment of the triceps to the remaining portion of the proximal ulna may be required.

Complications of olecranon fixation most commonly involve hardware prominence, which can be managed by removal after the fracture has healed. In addition, elbow stiffness, malunion, nonunion, and posttraumatic arthritis can also occur.

FOREARM

Fractures of the forearm commonly result from high-energy trauma and are often associated with systemic and other musculoskeletal injuries. Clinical evaluation should include careful examination of the entire patient and not just the injured extremity. It is essential to determine if there is an open wound, neurovascular deficit, and or impending forearm compartment syndrome. Radiographs should include AP and lateral views of the forearm, elbow, and wrist. Virtually all adult forearm fractures, except for the isolated nondisplaced or minimally displaced ulnar shaft fracture, require operative fixation. Although intramedullary nails and external fixation are occasionally used, the gold standard for fixation is compression plating (Fig. 13).

This permits early functional mobilization of the forearm and produces fracture union and good function in the vast majority of cases.

Monteggia Fracture

A Monteggia fracture is a fracture of the proximal ulna with dislocation of the radial head. It occurs in 1% to 2% of all forearm fractures. Bado described four types of injury patterns: type I, apex anterior ulnar fracture and anterior radial head dislocation; type II, apex posterior ulnar fracture and posterior radial head dislocation; type III, proximal ulnar metaphyseal fracture and lateral radial head dislocation; and type IV, proximal ulnar and radial shaft fractures with radial head dislocation (Fig. 14). The key to successful outcome of Monteggia fracture is anatomic reduction and fixation of the ulna fracture. Upon reduction of the ulna, there is typically concomitant stable relocation of the radial head. Irreducible radial head dislocation is usually

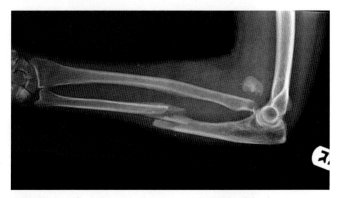

FIGURE 14 A single anteroposterior radiograph of the forearm showing a Monteggia type IV variant in which there are fractures of the midshaft of the ulna and radial neck and dislocation of the radial head. *(Courtesy of Virak Tan, MD.)*

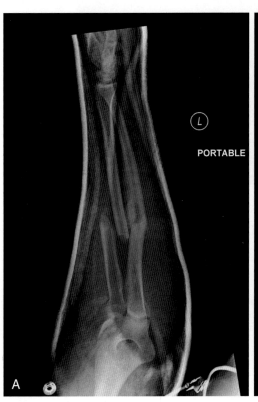
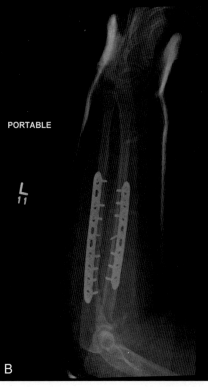

FIGURE 13 **A** and **B,** Both bone forearm fracture fixed with compression plating.

associated with soft tissue entrapment and requires open reduction of the radiocapitellar joint. In a type IV lesion, open reduction and internal fixation of both the ulna and radius is required.

Complications of Monteggia fractures often result from nonanatomic reduction or loss of fixation of the ulna fracture, leading to chronic malalignment or dislocation of the radial head. Poor outcome can also be due to heterotopic ossification or proximal radioulnar synostosis.

Radial and Ulnar Shaft Fractures

Fractures of both the radial and ulnar shafts ("both-bones" forearm fractures) are relatively common injuries in the adult trauma population. Most surgeons prefer compression plating of both bones using a separate incision for each. The anatomic bow of the radial shaft must be restored to prevent loss of forearm rotation.

Isolated radial shaft fractures are uncommon but can occur. If displaced, they are poorly controlled by casting and are therefore generally treated with internal fixation. A Galeazzi injury pattern in which a radial shaft fracture is accompanied by dislocation of the DRUJ is treated with anatomic reduction and plate fixation of the radius and either immobilization of the forearm in a position of DRUJ stability or by reducing and temporarily pinning the DRUJ.

Isolated ulnar shaft fractures are historically referred to as "night-stick fractures" because they occurred as a result of using the forearm to block a direct blow from a nightstick. In the modern era, motor vehicle accidents can also cause this injury. Fractures with less than 10 degrees angulation and 50% shaft displacement can be treated by nonoperative means. Plate fixation is indicated for displacement beyond those limits.

Galeazzi Fractures

A Galeazzi fracture is defined as a fracture of the distal radial shaft with subluxation or dislocation of the DRUJ. It is an uncommon injury with the incidence varying from 3% to 6% of all forearm fractures. The mechanism is a direct blow to the dorsoradial wrist or a fall onto an outstretched hand with forced pronation of the forearm. Radiographic signs suggesting a Galeazzi fracture include an ulnar styloid fracture, widened DRUJ on the AP view, dislocation of the distal ulna on the lateral view, and 5 mm or greater of radial shortening through the fracture site.

In adults, operative treatment is essential in all Galeazzi fractures because closed treatment has resulted in very high failure rates. After stable anatomic plate fixation of the radius, the DRUJ stability is assessed. If the joint is stable with forearm rotation, then immobilization is not necessary. However, if the DRUJ is reducible but unstable, then the arm must either be immobilized with the forearm rotated to the position of greatest DRUJ stability (typically supination) or the DRUJ must be pinned in a reduced position. Occasionally, open reduction of the DRUJ and repair of its soft tissue supports may also be required. Complication of this fracture include loss of forearm rotation due to malalignment of the radius and incongruity of the DRUJ leading to painful and limited forearm rotation.

For the chapter's Suggested Readings list, please visit the book at www.ExpertConsult.inkling.com.

LOWER EXTREMITY AND DEGLOVING INJURY

Peter G. Trafton, Herman P. Houin, and Donald D. Trunkey

Injuries of the lower extremity can be devastating (see Mangled Extremities, later in this chapter) and life threatening or minimal and quickly healed. Advanced Trauma Life Support (ATLS) assessments should be made on all patients. The history, if obtainable, should include the mechanism of injury, initial physical examination by emergency medical services, and any pertinent medical information. Control of exsanguinating hemorrhage and splint immobilization should take priority.

The physical examination should include localization of pain and assessment of pulses, sensation, color, motor function, and angulated or rotational deformities. The entrance and exit of foreign objects that have caused penetration injuries and potentially embedded foreign objects should be noted.

RADIOLOGIC EVALUATION

Thorough evaluation of lower extremity injuries should include anteroposterior and lateral radiographs of the injured area and the joint above and below. Penetrating injuries are best evaluated with entrance and exit site markers. Careful clinical evaluations can minimize needless overuse of angiography (and subsequently its complications and expense); however, if one or more pulses distal to a penetrating injury are absent, the patient needs angiography, computed tomographic arteriography (CTA), or immediate surgery. If pulses are present, ankle brachial indices (ABIs) should be obtained. If the dorsalis pedis and posterior tibialis ABIs are 1.0 or greater, the patient can be safely observed for other injuries and discharged, with follow-up ABIs taken at 1 week. If the dorsalis pedis or posterior tibialis ABI is less than 1.0 with clinical ischemia, emergency angiography, CTA, or surgery (if distal perfusion is clearly inadequate) should be done if duplex scanning is not available or wounds are extensive, such as shotgun injuries. If distal perfusion is clinically adequate with an ABI less than 1.0, duplex ultrasonography can be done electively. If it is negative or shows only a minor injury (small intimal defect or small pseudoaneurysm), the patient can be observed with follow-up ABIs obtained in 1 week. If duplex scanning reveals a major injury, such as a large intimal defect, large pseudoaneurysm, or intraluminal clot, angiography or exploration should be performed.

FRACTURES

It is now generally accepted that aggressive, appropriate early management of the trauma patient's musculoskeletal injuries contributes substantially to overall care by reducing morbidity, mortality, and costs. Rehabilitation and ultimate function are also improved. This section is not a "how-to" discussion, but rather provides recommendations for immediate and knowledgeable collaboration with an experienced orthopedic traumatologist. Specific details of management for musculoskeletal injuries are treated only briefly (and thus arbitrarily) here. Several acceptable alternative treatments exist for many fractures. Differences of opinion are thus unavoidable.

Skeletal injuries cannot be managed safely in isolation. The treating physician must always think beyond the broken bone and assess associated soft tissue trauma, the status of the entire injured limb, and the whole patient. Other injuries, age and anticipated activity level, preexisting musculoskeletal resources, and chances for meaningful participation in a rehabilitation program must also be considered. The choice of management for fractures and joint injuries may depend on whether an injury is isolated or is one of several problems in a patient with multiple injuries. Treatment is also affected by the resources available to the surgeon. In the absence of a well-equipped operating room (OR), effective radiographic monitoring, and an experienced surgical team, modern techniques of internal fixation are likely to fail.

EARLY CARE OF MUSCULOSKELETAL INJURIES

Extremity injuries may be obvious or occult. Initial care of obvious injuries includes control of bleeding with pressure dressings, splinting unstable injuries in an acceptable position, and urgent identification and treatment of arterial occlusion.

Once resuscitation is proceeding satisfactorily, a thorough and systematic search must be made for more occult injuries. All skin surfaces, from digits to trunk, must be inspected for deformity, swelling, ecchymosis, and laceration. Skin abrasions are significant. If they are present in the region of a musculoskeletal injury, any needed operation must be done promptly or delayed until the abrasion heals. Palpate each bone and joint for swelling, deformity, and tenderness. Manually stress each bone to confirm stability. Move each joint to demonstrate normal passive range of motion and absence of abnormal motion (instability). When emergency surgery is a part of the resuscitation or early care of a trauma patient, examination of the extremities should always be completed before terminating the anesthetic. Confirm the presence of peripheral pulses. Obtain radiographs of all abnormal areas.

When the patient is conscious and able to cooperate, active voluntary motion of each joint must be assessed to check motor nerve and myotendinous integrity. Check sensation in the isolated sensory area of each major peripheral nerve. For critically ill patients who are unable to cooperate initially, completion of this evaluation may take several days. Such follow-through is mandatory to avoid missing injuries. Resuscitation of patients with multiple injuries necessarily places diagnosis and treatment of musculoskeletal conditions at a relatively low priority. Many injuries are not initially appreciated. Repeated examinations during the early recovery period are frequently rewarded by the discovery of additional injuries in time for effective treatment.

OPEN FRACTURES

Identification and Classification

Open fractures require special attention to minimize risk of clostridial and pyogenic infections. Treatment is guided by classification of the severity of the injury, primarily according to the extent of soft tissue trauma, and level of contamination (Table 1). It is important to consider the entire soft tissue wound and not just the skin opening. In severe crush injuries, small lacerations may overlie extensively contused or necrotic soft tissue.

Identification of an open fracture is the first step of early management. Although they are usually obvious, open fractures occasionally are missed because of an incomplete examination. Posterior surfaces must be checked. Seemingly superficial wounds may communicate with underlying injuries to bones or joints. Neurovascular status, myotendinous function, and the possibility of multiple injuries must be checked. If completely satisfactory examination and treatment of a wound near a fracture cannot be done in the emergency department (ED) assume that the fracture is open and proceed to the OR where adequate anesthesia, assistance, hemostasis, and lighting usually confirm suspicions and facilitate treatment.

TABLE 1: Classification of Open Fractures

Type	Clinical Findings
Grade I	Small wounds caused by low-velocity trauma, with minimal contamination and soft tissue damage (e.g., skin laceration by bone end or a low-velocity gunshot wound).
Grade II	Wounds more extensive in length and width, but that have little or no avascular or devitalized soft tissue and minimal contamination.
Grade IIIA	Significant wounds caused by high-energy trauma, often with extensive lacerations and soft tissue flaps, but such that after final débridement, adequate local soft tissue coverage is maintained and delayed primary closure is feasible.
Grade IIIB	Major wounds with considerable devitalized soft tissue, contamination, or both. Bone is exposed in the wound, and extensive periosteal avulsion may be present. Coverage of the soft tissue defect usually requires a local or free microvascular muscle pedicle graft.
Grade IIIC	Open fracture with an associated arterial injury that requires repair.

Once an injured limb has been examined, control of bleeding is achieved with sterile compression dressings, and a splint is applied before transportation to the radiology department or the OR. If a patient arrives with a well-described open fracture already covered, the dressing should optimally be removed only in the OR. Radiographs of injured or suspect areas are essential for evaluating the trauma patient. Unfortunately, the quality of emergency studies varies greatly, and it is risky for the patient to languish, poorly monitored, in the radiology department. The responsible surgeon must be prepared at any moment to conclude that the radiographs already obtained are the best possible and that the patient should proceed to surgery. Chest, pelvis, and cervical spine radiographs have the highest priority. Those of the extremities are necessary for a complete evaluation. Without adequate radiographs, the orthopedic surgeon may not be able to diagnose the extent of the fracture and whether it is an intra-articular injury. Of course, such radiographs may be obtained in the OR once the patient has been stabilized.

Management

It is strongly recommended that each open fracture be cared for in a well-prepared OR, with adequate anesthesia, as soon as is safely possible.

Immediate Wound Care

The basic aspects of surgical wound care have changed little since their description by Desault in the late 18th century. Effective medical adjuncts are more recent. Tetanus prophylaxis is administered immediately. The use of an appropriate intravenous (IV) antibiotic promptly after diagnosis of an open fracture is required. The value of this adjunct to surgical treatment has been shown by several comparative studies. A good requirement is the use of 1 to 2 g IV cefazolin every 8 hours, beginning in the ED and continuing through the 48 hours after injury, regardless of whether the wound is left open. Depending on the source and extent of contamination, aminoglycosides for better gram-negative coverage or penicillin for anaerobic organisms should be added to the initial antibiotic regimen, especially for grade III open fractures. Alternative antibiotics are required for allergic patients.

The properly evaluated patient is brought to the OR as soon as the team and equipment are assembled. Adequate anesthesia is induced, and definitive care of the open fracture is begun simultaneously with or following higher-priority surgical treatment.

Care of the open fracture starts with a thorough reassessment of the injured limb, which takes place under anesthesia. Is salvage warranted or must primary amputation be considered? If amputation seems to be a possibility, an effort to discuss this with the patient and the family preoperatively in the ED is optimal. It is also optimal to have another surgeon agree and write a note in the patient's chart that amputation is the best treatment alternative.

A pneumatic tourniquet is applied, but inflated only if necessary to control bleeding or to assess tissue viability with postischemic hyperemia. In principle, further contamination of the wound of an open fracture should be avoided during cleansing of an injured limb. However, in practice it is hard to scrub the limb adequately while a sterile occlusive dressing is kept over the wound. Most detergents and soaps are injurious to tissue; therefore, the wound itself should be avoided during use of a scrub solution. The scrub is done with the limb lying on a sterile waterproof disposable drape, which is replaced twice during the 10-minute wash. Detergent suds are rinsed, and the skin is dried with sterile towels. At that point, the entire limb, including the wound, is disinfected with iodophor antiseptic solution, and new waterproof sterile drapes are applied.

Irrigation and Débridement

Irrigation and débridement are the next step. It is often necessary to enlarge the wound to permit adequate inspection and cleansing. This should be carefully planned to avoid devitalizing skin flaps or interrupting superficial veins that might be essential for blood return. If possible, incisions should avoid contused skin and preserve a healthy flap of tissue to cover the fracture site and any internal fixation device that may be implanted. With sufficient exposure, all foreign matter and any dead or questionable tissue are removed. Nerves, major vessels, and as much bone as possible are not discarded. Grossly contaminated bone surfaces are removed with a rongeur or curet. All joints that have been penetrated are opened and inspected for debris, including osteochondral fragments. It is useful to leave questionably viable bone, which can readily be assessed during the days after injury. Subcutaneous fat, fascia, and injured muscle are aggressively removed if dead or dirty, although it is important not to excessively undermine a viable skin flap. Contractility, consistency, and especially the presence of bleeding from small intrinsic vessels are more helpful than color as indicators of muscle viability.

A pulsatile irrigation system enhances cleansing of injured tissue, although it should be used gently to minimize additional soft tissue injury. Pulsatile lavage pumps may permit use of less than the 10 L or more of irrigant frequently recommended. Six liters of normal saline or Ringer's solution for the average grade II open fracture is recommended. Another adjunct, bacitracin solution (50,000 U in 1 L of normal saline, with 2 ampules of sodium bicarbonate to alkalinize) as a final antibiotic rinse, can be applied with a bulb syringe.

During débridement, decisions must be made about two other aspects of care for the injured limb: (1) fracture stabilization and (2) wound closure. Complications arising from either of these areas can considerably increase the patient's period of disability and can jeopardize the eventual result. Avoidance of failure is best achieved by use of techniques with which the surgeon is thoroughly familiar and for which the proper equipment is available. Adequate fracture stabilization is important, and external or internal fixation may reduce the risk for infection and facilitate overall management. Meticulous wound toilet and delayed primary closure are essential if internal fixation is used, and in all grade II and III open wounds.

Reduction and Fixation

Although articular surface fractures should be reduced anatomically, extra-articular fractures generally require only adequate restoration of angular and rotational alignment with preservation of length. How to stabilize an open fracture is becoming less controversial. Traction, plaster cast, external skeletal fixation, and the several forms of internal fixation are all useful, individually and in combination. Two problems must be solved anew for each fracture patient: (1) How much stability is necessary, or even possible? (2) What is the most beneficial and least hazardous way to obtain stability? Few direct comparative studies document the unequivocal superiority of one form of stabilization over another. We favor surgical fixation for all but the most minor open fractures, and prefer intramedullary nailing or external fixation to plate fixation in most cases because of the higher risk for infection and wound-healing problems associated with plate fixation of open fractures.

Patients with severe soft tissue wounds over fractures that can be stabilized better with internal than external fixation (e.g., ankle fracture, some radius shaft fractures, and proximal femur fractures) are also more easily managed this way, despite the risk for infection. Primary internal fixation of fractures adjacent to arterial anastomoses is not necessary to protect the vascular repair.

External skeletal fixation must be carefully coordinated with wound management and bone grafting. It offers a powerful and adaptable technique for stabilizing open fractures without additional exposure or devascularization of bone and without the encumbrance of plaster casts or traction. External fixation can be applied rapidly and with minimal additional bleeding. An external fixator can span unstable joints and complex fracture. This provides stable provisional surgical fixation that can later be replaced with definitive internal and external fixation when the patient can better tolerate prolonged anesthesia and blood loss associated with complex fracture fixation procedures. This application of external fixation typically permits mobilization of a patient who might not tolerate recumbency. External skeletal fixation is especially applicable to unstable open fracture of the pelvis. Such fractures are associated with a mortality rate that approached 35% without modern treatment emphasizing aggressive resuscitation, pelvic stabilization, wound débridement, open wound management, and usually a diverting colostomy.

Larger-diameter threaded pins placed in predrilled holes are preferable for diaphyseal fixation. Ring fixators, fixed to the bone with tensioned wires, although somewhat more cumbersome, provide better control of many metaphyseal fractures. By temporarily spanning the injured joint with a simple half-pin fixator, placement of more complicated external fixation devices can be deferred until the patient is more stable.

Skeletal traction may provide an appropriate provisional or definitive means to stabilize open fractures for the patient with an isolated injury. However, compared with internal and external fixation, the poorer outcomes and increased systemic complications associated with skeletal traction with enforced recumbency have resulted in its being used only rarely and temporarily in modern trauma centers.

Wound Coverage

Whether, when, and how to close an open fracture wound are as controversial as the question of stabilization. Skin closure over a contaminated wound is dangerous. The risk for infection is increased when hardware is implanted, tension on skin flaps is excessive, or dead space is created by the closure. Nonetheless, an important early goal of open fracture care is to convert the initially contaminated open wound to a clean closed one. Several techniques are advocated for this, ranging from leaving the wound open until it heals secondarily to primary closure with any of several plastic surgical procedures if simple suture is not possible.

For all but the most trivial wounds and especially when open fractures are internally fixed, it is best to avoid primary wound closure.

When wounds are left open, the use of antibiotic bead-pouch dressing technique developed by Henry and colleagues is still a good technique. Polymethylmethacrylate cement (one full batch) is mixed with 1.2 g of tobramycin powder. This is used to make beads of 5-mm diameter, which are molded onto twisted stainless steel wire, separated by 3 to 4 mm. Although this can be done by the surgical team in the OR, our pharmacy follows the procedures described by Henry and colleagues for prefabrication and gas sterilization of bead chains, which are made available to us in individual sterile peel-apart pouches. The beads are placed in the wound, and a large piece of Tegaderm or Opsite is used to cover and seal the opening and to keep the gentle traction of the wound flaps to prevent flap shrinkage.

Patients with more severe wounds should be returned to the OR in 1 to 2 days for a dressing change and further débridement as needed. As soon as all questionably viable tissues have been excised, the wound should be closed. Grades II and IIIA wounds can usually be sutured closed 5 to 7 days after injury but may require split-thickness skin grafts (STSGs). More extensive wounds often benefit from closure with muscle pedicle flaps using local tissue or free microvascular transfers. Carefully chosen fasciocutaneous flaps are occasionally helpful, but other tissue flaps are not as effective in severely injured limbs. STSGs can be used to cover healthy wound tissue at any time, although they are unsatisfactory over exposed blood vessels, tendons, and bare cortical bone. The multiple perforations produced by a meshing device minimize fluid accumulation under STSGs.

It is entirely possible to manage most severe open fractures without the use of elaborate plastic surgical procedures. Open fractures heal successfully despite exposure of bone and hardware for several months or more.

COMPARTMENT SYNDROMES

Various injuries can cause progressive elevation of tissue pressure within the confines of "compartments" formed by the normal fascial envelopes around groups of skeletal muscles. Once compartment pressure is elevated sufficiently to obstruct microvascular perfusion, muscle and nerve ischemia leads to necrosis of the involved tissue. The pressure eventually recedes to normal levels, leaving behind dead muscle and nerve, the causes of Volkmann's contracture.

The key to effective treatment is early diagnosis. This requires suspicion of compartment syndrome whenever an extremity sustains a crushing or severely contusing injury, with or without a fracture. Conscious patients with compartment syndrome develop pain and firm swelling of the entire involved compartment and soon lose function of the muscles and nerves that lie within it. Pulses and skin perfusion are often normal. Compartment syndromes may occur in open fractures, which do not necessarily provide an adequate surgical incisions made for débridement alone.

For a minimum of every 2 hours, patients with significant extremity injuries must be monitored for inordinate pain and for loss of sensation or motor function distal to the area of injury. Release of any constricting bandage or cast is the essential first step in treatment of a suspected compartment syndrome to permit examination and to avoid external compression of the involved compartment. This may reduce pressure sufficiently to restore tissue perfusion and prevent necrosis. If the patient is unconscious, or has an associated nerve injury that prevents clinical assessment, compartment pressures are measured with a commercially available tissue pressure measuring device (e.g., Stryker STIC or a slit-wick catheter made from polyethylene tubing with the terminal end slit about 1 mm longitudinally in several places). The device is filled with sterile saline solution and connected to a strain gauge, as used for monitoring intra-arterial pressure. The catheter is then introduced through a large-bore needle into the compartment in question. A satisfactory measurement system elicits a prompt response to manual pressure on the compartment, and pressure will fall to a reproducible level soon after such external compression is released. It is important to measure the

pressure in each compartment of the involved area. For the leg, this means anterior, lateral, deep posterior, and superficial posterior spaces. In the forearm, both flexor and extensor groups should be assessed at several sites. The pressure is typically highest close to the fracture.

If neuromuscular findings are normal, a patient with elevated compartment pressure may be monitored clinically or by repeated pressure measurements. If sensation of contractility is impaired or not accessible and compartmental pressure is within 30 to 40 mm Hg of mean arterial pressure, fasciotomy is required. All involved compartments must be released. For the leg, we use two incisions. One is lateral with identification and preservation of the superficial peroneal nerve, and is used for release of anterior and lateral compartments. The second is immediately posterior to the medial, tibial shaft for the deep and superficial posterior compartments. Skin incisions 8 to 10 cm long, with proximal and distal "blind" fasciotomies, may permit adequate decompression but are often insufficient in severely injured limbs. Such limbs are best treated with incisions that extend nearly the entire length of the compartment. The skin is left open for delayed closure by suture or STSG. If an associated fracture is present, fixing it at the time of fasciotomy simplifies wound management. Either external or internal skeletal fixation may be used, depending on the fracture configuration and the degree of additional soft tissue dissection required.

Forearm compartment syndromes may involve anterior (flexor) or posterior (extensor) muscles and may require releasing the intrinsic fascia of each involved muscle. An extensive surgical approach is required, such as McConnell's combined exposure of the median and ulnar nerves, as described by Henry in *Extensile Exposure*.

For any open wound of the lower extremity that is to be treated open, vacuum-assisted wound closure (VAWC) is becoming a routine technique in mitral management of these wounds. After the wound is cleansed and irrigated, polyurethane foam is cut to fit the wound, and a Silastic sheet is placed over the polyurethane. An incision is made in the middle of the Silastic sheet, an adaptor fitted over this incision, and continuous suction is begun at 100 to 125 mm Hg. The dressing can be changed on the ward or in the OR if closing the wound is also planned. This is possible when the edema decreases and distention of the circumferential diameter of the extremity lessens. This is usually associated with a diuresis of the patient. Using this technique, it is often possible to eventually close the wound primarily. If the defect is too large after multiple dressing changes, an STSG is indicated.

Quantitative biopsies comprise another technique that may help the surgeon in determining when a wound can be closed. These biopsies help differentiate wound colonization or contamination from bacterial invasion of the wound bed. With a VAWC, there is also a salutary effect in keeping the wound dry, and typically there is less invasive bacterial into the wound.

Compartment syndromes that are recognized after necrosis is far advanced are probably best left closed rather than treated with fasciotomy because of the significant risk for infection and the lack of benefit from decompressing dead tissue.

DEGLOVING INJURIES

Treatment of degloving injuries requires careful assessment of the extent of the devitalized tissue, the layers of tissue in the flap, and the direction of the avulsion (whether proximally or distally based) and a thorough understanding of the blood supply to the affected tissues.

Degloved skin that remains attached to a pedicle will try to live as a flap and obtain its nutrients from the pedicle rather than the underlying bed. Thorough understanding of the muscular and fascial perforators to the skin will help to predict which flaps can be preserved. Extensive avulsions of the skin with narrow or distal pedicles with or without superficial subcutaneous tissue and without damage to the deeper tissues are best addressed by completely dividing the pedicle, defatting the skin, and replacing the avulsed skin as a full-thickness skin graft.

If the wound is too contaminated or too swollen, the avulsed tissue should be cleansed with pulsatile lavage, left with little or no tension, and addressed at a second exploration. Intraoperative fluorescein examination is a reliable predictor of tissue survival. If arterial in-flow is adequate, the soft tissues can be débrided and closed; tension should be minimal during closure.

Diminished venous return is a common cause for the ultimate death of tissue in degloving injuries. Pharmacologic manipulation with an antithromboxane treatment, such as Dermaid aloe cream applied topically every 4 hours and 81 mg aspirin daily, coupled with the liberal use of leech therapy, has improved tissue survival with both delayed and immediate wound closures. Leeches are applied every 4 hours initially, and should remain on the wound until the cyanosis from venous congestion is relieved. Large flaps may require two leeches initially. Leeches can be stored on site with minimal tending or obtained within hours by calling a supplier (e.g., Leeches U.S.A., 1-800-645-3569). As venous recanalization occurs, the frequency of leech application can be reduced and leeches are usually unnecessary after 3 days.

MANGLED EXTREMITIES: DELAYED AMPUTATION

In a perfect world, it should be possible for a general or orthopedic surgeon to assess a patient with a mangled extremity and to make a perfect decision as to whether to do prompt amputation or to attempt reconstruction. Unfortunately, the literature does not help such surgeons in making these decisions, and most of the literature that addresses the mangled extremity focuses on the lower extremity. These fractures have been classified as 3C and are invariably open. Some have vascular injuries, and some do not. Some are insensate, and some are not.

Many scoring systems have been developed to predict those patients who should undergo immediate amputation and those who should have reconstruction. Our own bias is reflected by Bonanni et al, who state that predictive scoring is an exercise in futility. In their study, they could not show reliable sensitivity or specificity using the MESI (Mangled Extremity Syndrome Index), PSI (Predictive Salvage Index), MESS (Mangled Extremity Severity Score), or the LSI (Limb Salvage Index). Surgical judgment based on experience is still the gold standard.

In a recent study by Bosse et al, of 569 patients with severe leg injuries who underwent reconstruction or amputation, the sickness impact profile (SIP) showed no difference in outcomes between these two groups. Their study did show that there was a poorer score for the SIP if the patient was rehospitalized or had a major complication, lower educational level, nonwhite ethnicity/race, poverty, lack of private health insurance, poor social support network, low self-efficiency, smoking, and involvement in disability-compensation litigation. Interestingly, patients who underwent reconstruction were more likely to be rehospitalized than those who underwent amputation. Return to work in the two groups was similar. The fact that the groups are similar reflects good decisions made by the surgeons.

Few other areas in trauma care are as controversial as whether amputations for mangled extremities should be done early or delayed. The most common reasons for delayed amputation are loss of wound cover or infection in ununited fractures, an insensate limb, recurrent ulcerations, a dystrophic limb, sympathetic dystrophy, and phantom pain, to name a few. Some surgeons have argued that functional recovery is faster and less costly following amputation than with multiple procedures for salvage and reconstruction. In addition to the study by Bosse et al mentioned previously, Pozo et al studied 35 patients who had amputation following the failure of treatment for severe lower limb trauma. Seven of the amputations were performed for ischemia within 1 month of the injury; 13 were performed between 1 month and 1 year for infection, complicating loss of limb cover or ununited fractures; and 15 occurred later than 1 year after injury, mainly for infected nonunion. The latter group had an average of 12 operations and 50 months of treatments, including 8 months in hospital. Factors that contributed to salvage failure were vascular injuries, nerve damage, bone damage, muscle damage, skin cover, and sepsis. Overall, these authors concluded that if lower limb reconstruction is attempted, it should be assessed very early by two specialists, one in trauma surgery and the other in orthopedic or plastic surgery, as to whether failure is inevitable. Obviously, this requires experience, and persistent attempts at salvage can be extremely difficult.

Another study that might influence surgeons on whether to salvage comes from Case Western Reserve. Thirty-four patients were followed, of whom 16 had a successful limb salvage procedure, and 18 had an immediate below knee amputation (BKA). The patients who had a successful limb salvage procedure took significantly more time to achieve full weight bearing, were less willing or able to work, and had higher hospital charges than the patients who had been managed with an early BKA. Furthermore, patients who had limb salvage considered themselves severely disabled, and they had more problems than the amputation group with the performance of occupational and recreational activities. These quality-of-life evaluations, however, must be put into the perspective of Bosse and colleagues, mentioned previously.

In a final study for consideration, Roessler and colleagues reviewed 80 patients for a 4-year period and asked the question of when to amputate. They concluded that neurologic, bone, and tissue status influenced the decision regarding immediate amputation, but had little to do with delayed loss of limb or life. Somewhat surprisingly, they found that the circulation as determined by the presence or absence of a palpable or Doppler-detected pulse was critical. They concluded that in cases in which salvage is attempted, amputation should be performed at 24 hours if the patient's condition, including a markedly positive fluid balance, indicates systemic compromise. They also made the observation that in the absence of a distal pulse on presentation, the eventual amputation rate is high.

For the chapter's Suggested Readings list, please visit the book at www.ExpertConsult.inkling.com.

CERVICAL, THORACIC, AND LUMBAR FRACTURES

Nicholas Spoerke and Donald D. Trunkey

Injuries to the spinal column represent a major source of short- and long-term morbidity in trauma. There are over 10,000 injuries to the spinal column each year in the United States and approximately half of spinal column injuries (SCIs) result from motor vehicle collisions. Falls, penetrating trauma including gunshot wounds, and sports injuries make up the majority of the remainder. Just over half of all SCIs occur in the cervical spine with the rest occurring in the thoracic and lumbar spine.

Because of the energy involved and the blunt mechanism responsible for most injuries to the spinal column, most SCI patients are multiply injured. Almost 30% of SCI patients have extraspinal fractures, traumatic brain injury is common, and multiple fractures of the spinal column are frequently seen.

All patients with a mechanism capable of producing SCI should have proper immobilization of the entire spinal column during extraction, transport, and initial evaluation. This includes in-line cervical immobilization, usually achieved with a cervical collar or tape and a rigid backboard. As with other instances of suspected injury to the central nervous system (CNS), initial resuscitation efforts should attempt to avoid systemic hypotension and adhere strictly to Advanced Trauma Life Support (ATLS) protocols.

SPINAL CORD SYNDROMES

Neurologic deficit due to spinal cord trauma varies considerably based on location and severity of injury. Complete spinal cord injury is classified as absence of motor or sensory function for more than three segments below the level of injury. Incomplete injuries result in motor and sensory deficits correlating to the damaged portion of the cord. Three incomplete cord syndromes are commonly encountered in traumatic injury:

Anterior cord syndrome is frequently caused by vascular injury to the anterior portion of the spinal cord. The resulting neurologic deficit is characterized by motor and sensory deficits below the level of injury with preservation of proprioception and positional sense. This syndrome is associated with a poor prognosis, with only 10% of patients recovering functional motor control.

Central cord syndrome is characterized by weakness affecting the upper extremities to a greater extent than the lower extremities. It is commonly caused by a hyperextension mechanism in the setting of underlying cervical stenosis and carries a good overall prognosis with upward of 75% of patients showing recovery.

Brown-Séquard syndrome, which usually results from penetrating trauma and spinal cord hemitransection, classically presents with ipsilateral motor and contralateral sensory deficits. This syndrome carries the best overall prognosis.

STEROIDS IN SPINAL CORD INJURIES

Initial cellular neurologic damage is caused by the kinetic energy of the traumatic impact. Secondary damage is believed to occur through a number of biochemical and cellular pathways and represents an area of potential intervention to improve neurologic outcome. In an effort to prevent secondary damage to neurons and improve neurologic recovery, much research has been dedicated to the idea of neuroprotection. Avoidance of hypotension is an important initial step to prevent secondary CNS damage. Suppression of cellular neuron damage and lipid peroxidation has been extensively studied over the past 30 years, including the much debated National Acute Spinal Cord Injury Studies (NASCIS) trials. Although this debate is outside the scope of this chapter, there is still no overall consensus regarding the optimal timing, dose, or indications for the use of steroids in SCI. Current recommendations regarding the decision to administer methylprednisolone should be made early (ideally within 3 hours of injury and definitely within 8 hours of injury) and in conjunction with the managing spine surgeon. Methylprednisolone is also prescribed for nonpenetrating spinal cord injuries. It has been shown that an intravenous (IV) dose of 30 mg/kg followed by IV drip at 5.4 mg/kg/hour for 23 hours improves sensory and motor recovery if given within 8 hours of the injury.

CERVICAL SPINE INJURIES

Pertinent Anatomy of Cervical Spine

There are seven cervical vertebrae, which are generally divided into C1, C2, and the subaxial spine (C3–C7). The atlas (C1) is ring-shaped with an anterior and posterior arch and two lateral masses. C1 articulates with the occipital condyles and the odontoid and facets of C2 to form complex, highly specialized movements which allow rotation of the head. The axis (C2) is distinctive for the presence of the odontoid process (dens), which articulates with the anterior arch of C1 and is stabilized by the transverse ligament. The vertebrae of the subaxial spine (C3–C7) are more uniform with lateral masses protecting the course of the paired vertebral arteries (C6 to C1) and facet joints arranged at 45 degrees, which allow primarily for flexion and extension. The cervical spinal cord occupies relatively less space in the spinal canal than elsewhere in the spine, taking up only 33% of the spinal canal at C1.

Patterns and Management of Cervical Spine Injuries

Patients with suspected cervical spine injury should have their spines immobilized and maintained in anatomic alignment throughout their primary and secondary surveys. Focused neurologic examination should be performed as part of the secondary surveys with specific attention to motor and sensory function and pain or bony step-offs on palpation of the midline spine. When mechanism, tenderness on palpation, or neurologic deficit are present, or if the patient is obtunded and unexaminable (intubated and chemically paralyzed, for example), the radiographic workup should include dedicated spine computed tomography (CT). CT has, in fact, replaced plain radiographs and flexion/extension views as the imaging modality of choice for spine injuries. Magnetic resonance imaging, although more sensitive than CT for soft tissue injury, should not be used as the primary imaging study and is reserved for patients with physical findings not explained by CT or for more detailed evaluation of injures in conjunction with a spine surgeon. SCIs are best classified by the American Spinal Injury Association (ASIA) International Standards for Neurological and Functional Classification of Spinal Cord Injury (Fig. 1).

Occipital Condyle Fractures

Fracture to the occipital condyle is generally caused by a high-energy injury to an anatomically sensitive area and mortality rate in accidents involving occipital condyle fractures is relatively high. These fractures

A = **Complete.** No sensory or motor function is preserved in the sacral segments S4-S5.

B = **Incomplete.** Sensory but not motor function is preserved below the neurological level and includes the sacral segments S4-S5.

C = **Incomplete.** Motor function is preserved below the neurological level, and more than half of key muscles below the neurological level have a muscle grade less than 3.

D = **Incomplete.** Motor function is preserved below the neurological level, and at least half of key muscles below the neurological level have a muscle grade greater than or equal to 3.

E = **Normal.** Sensory and motor function is normal.

FIGURE I   American Spinal Injury Association impairment scale.

can be classified into three types, based on the Anderson and Montesano classification (Fig. 2):

Type I: impaction fractures due to axial loading (rare)
Type II: extension of basilar skull fracture into the condyle
Type III: avulsion fracture (common)

Type III fractures are generally caused by ligamentous avulsion of the condyle through distracting forces. Stable fractures of any type are best managed with a cervical collar. Type II or III injuries with fracture displacement require a halo vest. Unstable type III fractures require occiput to C2 fusion and are associated with a high incidence of occipitocervical dissociation.

Occipitocervical Dissociation (Atlantoaxial Dissociation)

Injuries causing occipitocervical dissociation are rare and frequently fatal. They usually consist of subluxations or dissociations with underlying devastating spinal cord injury or transection. They are typically unstable and require surgical fusion of occiput to C2 once alignment has been reestablished. The injury patterns are generally classified as type I (anterior displacement of the occiput on the atlas), type II (longitudinal facet distraction), and type III (posterior displacement of the occiput on the atlas).

Atlas Fracture

C1 fractures can involve the anterior or posterior arches, lateral masses, and transverse processes (Fig. 3) and rarely involve neurologic deficit. Burst fractures (also called Jefferson fracture) include bilateral fractures of both the anterior and posterior arches, usually as a result of axial loading. Lateral mass fractures should raise suspicion for vertebral artery injury and should prompt evaluation with cervical CT angiogram, especially if the vertebral foramen is involved. Treatment of stable fractures without transverse ligament disruption can be treated with a cervical collar. More unstable fractures with disruption of the transverse ligament with displacement may require gentle traction initially, followed by a halo vest.

Dens Fractures

Fractures to the dens (odontoid process) have been classified into three patterns (Fig. 4). Type I fractures generally result from apical ligament avulsion of the tip of the dens, are usually stable fractures, and generally require minimal treatment or a cervical collar. Type III fractures extend into the body of C2 and can likewise usually be treated by 6 to 8 weeks in a cervical collar. Type II injuries occur at the waist of the odontoid process and their treatment is more variable depending on the age of the patient, comorbid injuries, degree of fragment displacement, and overall stability. Minimally displaced stable fractures in young patients are best treated with a halo vest. Relative indications for surgical repair include fracture displacement greater than 6 mm, posterior angulation, fracture comminution, or patient age greater than 50.

Hangman's Fracture

Hangman's fracture is the broader name given for the types of injury to bilateral pars interarticularis (Fig. 5). They are classified by Levine and Edwards (Table 1). Type I injuries are treated by halo vest immobilization but type II and III injuries generally require surgery.

Subaxial Spine Fractures

Injuries to C3-C7 vertebrae are broadly classified as subaxial spine injures and consist of any combination of fractures, subluxations, and dislocations. Fractures of the spinous processes, laminae, and transverse processes are relatively common and are considered stable

FIGURE 2   Types of occipital condyle fractures. *(From Anderson PA, Mirza SK, Chapman JR: Injuries to the atlantooccipital articulation. In Clark CR, Dvorak J, Ducker TB, et al, editors: The cervical spine, 4th ed, Philadelphia, 2005, Lippincott-Raven, p 594.)*

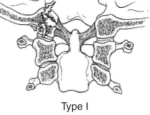
Type I

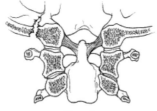
Type II

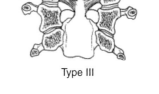
Type III

FIGURE 3   Types of C1 arch fractures. *(From Hasharoni A, Errico TJ: Fracture of the first cervical vertebra. In Clark CR, Dvorak J, Ducker TB, et al, editors: The cervical spine, 4th ed, Philadelphia, 2005, Lippincott-Raven, p 610.)*

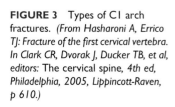
Posterior arch fracture

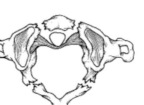
Burst fracture

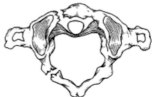
Lateral mass fracture

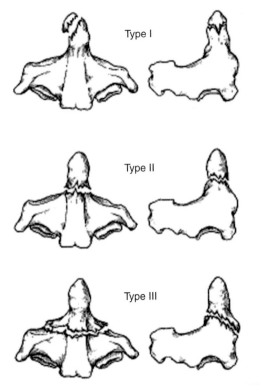

FIGURE 4   Types of odontoid fractures. *(From Anderson LD, D'Alonzo RT: Fractures of the odontoid process of the axis.* J Bone Joint Surg *56:1663–1674, 1974.)*

when isolated and when the facet joints are intact and there is no angular or translational displacement. More extensive fractures fall into three basic categories: (1) compression, (2) burst, and (3) teardrop.

Compression fractures result in wedging of the anterior portion of the vertebral body with an intact posterior body and spinal canal. When accompanied by minor angulation (<11 degrees), minimal height loss (<25%), and minimal translation (<2.5 mm) cervical collar immobilization is generally adequate. More unstable fractures include those with body height loss greater than 50% or those with posterior distraction and usually require surgical stabilization and fusion.

Burst fractures result from axial loading and characteristically involve disruption of the anterior and middle columns. Surgery is required if both the anterior and posterior longitudinal ligaments are injured or if reduction and alignment cannot be maintained. Halo vest is acceptable treatment if there is no neurologic deficit and alignment can be achieved.

Teardrop fractures can be anterior or posterior. Anterior teardrop fractures are usually avulsion injuries resulting from an extension mechanism, often occur at the C2–C3 junction, and are usually treated with a cervical collar. Posterior teardrop fractures usually occur from a flexion-compression mechanism, often involve all three columns of the spinal canal, and often involve neurologic compromise.

TABLE I: Classifications of Hangman's Fractures

Type	Clinical Findings
Type I	Fractures with <3 mm of displacement and no angulation due to axial compression and hyperextension
Type IA	Asymmetrical fracture line with minimal angulation or displacement due to hyperextension with lateral bending forces
Type II	Fractures with >3 mm of translation and angulation due to hyperextension and axial loading followed by rebound flexion
Type IIA	Fractures demonstrate angulation without translation due to a flexion-distraction injury
Type III	Fractures include C2-C3 facet dislocation due to hyperextension followed by flexion mechanism

From Levine AM, Edwards CC: The management of traumatic spondylolisthesis of the axis. *J Bone Joint Surg* 67:221–226, 1985.

Treatment of posterior teardrop fractures usually requires acute reduction and surgical fixation.

THORACIC AND LUMBAR SPINE INJURIES

Injuries to the thoracic spine are relatively infrequent due to the stabilizing support of the spine with the ribs and sternum. Fractures to the thoracic spine are often due to high-energy mechanisms and are therefore often accompanied by underlying injuries such as rib fractures, pulmonary contusions and pneumothoraces, and vascular injuries. When injures do occur, neurologic damage can be devastating owing to the high energy required to cause injury, the relatively small size of the neural canal, and the uniquely poor blood supply to the thoracic cord.

Pertinent Anatomy of the Thoracic and Lumbar Spine

Because of the bony attachments to the ribcage and overlapping lamina, the kyphotically curved thoracic spine is more rigid than the cervical or lumbar spine. This relative rigidity results in proportionally more fractures at the transition zones at T1 and T12 and the interface between these two areas is so susceptible to injury that it is the second most commonly injured area of the spinal column. The stability of these fractures generally depends on whether or not the spine can maintain anatomic relationships under physiologic loads. The determination of stability is often evaluated using Denis's three-column model of injury (Fig. 6). The anterior column consists of the anterior longitudinal ligament and anterior half of the vertebral bodies. The

FIGURE 5   Types of hangman's fractures. *(From Levine AM, Edwards CC: The management of traumatic spondylolisthesis of the axis.* J Bone Joint Surg *67:221–226, 1985.)*

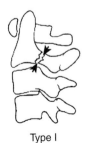
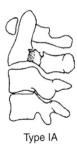
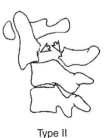
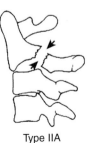
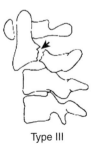

Type I   Type IA   Type II   Type IIA   Type III

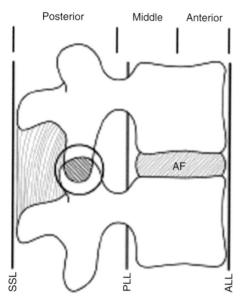

FIGURE 6   Spinal columns. AF, Annulus fibrosus; ALL, anterior longitudinal ligament; PLL, posterior longitudinal ligament; SSL, supraspinal ligament. *(Modified from McAfee PC, Yuan HA, Fredrickson BE, Lubicky JP: The value of computed tomography in thoracolumbar factures: an analysis of one hundred consecutive cases and a new classification.* J Bone Joint Surg 65:461–473, 1983.)

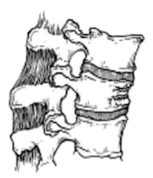

FIGURE 7   Compression fracture. *(From Holdsworth FW: Fractures, dislocations and fracture-dislocations of the spine.* J Bone Joint Surg Br 52:1534–1551, 1970.)

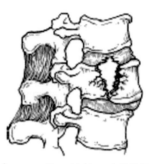

FIGURE 8   Burst fracture. *(From Holdsworth FW: Fractures, dislocations and fracture-dislocations of the spine.* J Bone Joint Surg Br 52:1534–1551, 1970.)

middle column consists of the posterior half of the vertebral body and the posterior longitudinal ligament. The posterior column is composed of the ligamentum flavum, supraspinal ligament, posterior bony arches, and the facet joints. By definition, unstable injuries involve disruption of two of the three columns or any fracture with a neurologic deficit. Additionally, percentage of vertebral height loss and degree of angulation are often used to estimate stability.

Thoracic and Lumbar Fractures

Fracture patterns are generally classified as compression, burst, and flexion-distraction.

Compression fractures are the most common subtype of thoracolumbar fractures. Morphologically, compression fractures consist of anterior vertebral body height loss without damage to the middle or posterior columns (Fig. 7). Though these fractures only involve one column, these fractures can still be unstable if greater than 50% of the vertebral height is lost or there is greater than 30 degrees of angulation. Stable fractures are treated in a brace but unstable fractures require surgical stabilization.

Burst fractures disrupt both the anterior and middle columns and have a higher risk of neurologic injury (Fig. 8). Unstable injuries present with greater than 50% height loss, greater than 25% angulation, or greater than 50% canal compromise and require surgical stabilization. Stable fractures with minimal height loss or angulation can generally be treated in an orthosis with close monitoring upon mobilization to ensure maintenance of alignment.

Flexion-distraction injuries have both bony and ligamentous components. These injuries are often the result of sudden deceleration in motor vehicle collisions with lap seat belts. The anterior column undergoes compression and the middle and posterior columns experience excessive tension (Fig. 9). Primary ligamentous injuries usually

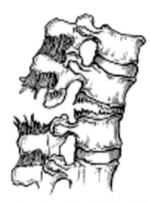

FIGURE 9   Flexion distraction. *(From Holdsworth FW: Fractures, dislocations and fracture-dislocations of the spine.* J Bone Joint Surg Br 52:1534–1551, 1970.)

require surgical reduction and fixation because of the poor propensity for healing. This injury pattern at the T12–L2 vertebrae should raise suspicion for concomitant injury to the duodenum, pancreas, or retroperitoneal vascular structures.

For the chapter's Suggested Readings list, please visit the book at www.ExpertConsult.inkling.com.

PELVIC FRACTURES

Christopher H. Perkins and Stephen M. Quinnan

Fractures of the pelvis are relatively uncommon injuries, composing only 2% of all fractures. However, 20% of polytrauma patients sustain pelvic fractures with a mortality rate approaching 15% to 20%. Common mechanisms of injury include motor vehicle accidents, motorcycle accidents, auto-versus-pedestrian accidents, and falls from height. A bimodal distribution exists with high-energy unstable fractures more common in young males and low-energy stable fractures more common in elderly females. Associated injuries occur in 12% to 62% of patients with pelvic fractures, with injuries to the bladder and urethra being most common (63%), followed by closed head injuries (35%), nerve injuries (24%), intestinal injuries (20%), and chest injuries (20%). Open pelvic fractures make up only 2% to 4% of pelvic fractures, but have a 25% to 50% mortality rate. The cause of death from pelvic fractures is often hemorrhagic shock from intrapelvic bleeding or associated abdominal injury. Because of the severity and prevalence of associated injuries, a coordinated multidisciplinary approach is necessary to manage these patients. A treatment algorithm that includes early involvement of orthopedic traumatologists and interventional radiologists has been developed and implemented at many Level I trauma centers to reduce fatality from these injuries.

ANATOMY

The pelvic ring comprises the sacrum and two innominate bones, which are joined anteriorly at the pubic symphysis and posteriorly at the sacroiliac joints. The innominate bones are formed by the fusion of the ischium, ilium, and pubis at the triradiate cartilage. Stability comes from the strength of the ligaments attached to the pelvic ring. Posteriorly, the interosseous, anterior, and posterior sacroiliac ligaments provide the majority of support with the iliolumbar, sacrotuberous, and sacrospinous ligaments also playing a role. Anteriorly, the pubic symphysis provides support and acts as a strut to prevent collapse. The pelvis functions to provide structural support during weight bearing and protects the organs and other structures housed within. The pelvis functions as a ring; therefore, injury to one part of the ring should raise suspicion of injury to another part of the ring. Biomechanical studies have shown that sectioning of the pubic symphysis allows for diastasis up to 2.5 cm. Further sectioning of the anterior sacroiliac ligaments allows for opening of the pelvis until bony abutment at the posterior superior iliac spine. However, the pelvis remains vertically stable until the posterior sacroiliac ligaments are sectioned.

There are also many major blood vessels within the pelvis that can be injured when a fracture occurs. The aorta divides into the common iliac arteries at the level of the L5 vertebra and further divides into the internal and external iliac arteries just anterior to the sacroiliac joints. The superior gluteal artery branches off the internal iliac and exits the pelvis through the sciatic notch and is the vessel most commonly injured with pelvic fractures. Other branches of the internal iliac within the pelvis that can be injured include the lateral sacral, iliolumbar, obturator, vesical, and inferior gluteal arteries. Multiple veins also run within the pelvis and are also subject to injury.

IMAGING

A plain radiograph should be obtained in patients with suspected pelvic fractures, along with chest and lateral cervical spine radiographs, which make up the trauma series that is a part of Advanced Trauma Life Support (ATLS) protocol. Most pelvic fractures can be diagnosed on this single anteroposterior radiograph, but inlet and outlet radiographs help further determine fracture morphologic characteristics. These radiographs are obtained with the patient supine with the beam angled 45 degrees cephalad for the inlet view and 45 degrees caudad for the outlet view. The inlet view shows anteroposterior and rotational displacement of the fracture and the outlet view shows vertical displacement and sacral fractures. If a binder has been placed and the initial radiographs do not show displacement, an additional anteroposterior radiograph may be necessary without the binder after the patient is adequately stabilized. Computed tomography (CT) with reconstructions is useful for delineating displacement and fracture patterns and is part of many blunt trauma protocols. A contrast trauma CT scan has a sensitivity of 60% to 84% and specificity of 95% for diagnosing arterial injuries associated with pelvic fractures. It is also important to diagnose concomitant intra-abdominal and chest injuries (Figs. 1 to 4).

CLASSIFICATION

Pelvic fractures are classified based on mechanism of injury or stability, depending upon the system used. The classification system developed by Young and Burgess is based primarily on mechanism and is the most widely used. Three mechanisms exist: anteroposterior compression (APC), lateral compression (LC), and vertical shear (VS). APC injuries involve injuries to the anterior ring with varying degrees of posterior injury with the involved hemipelvis externally rotating with increasing degree of injury. Lateral compression injuries involve pubic rami fractures with variable posterior injuries with the involved hemipelvis internally rotating with increasing degree of injury. VS injuries involve sacroiliac joint disruptions or sacral fractures associated with pubic rami or symphyseal injuries and result in vertical displacement of the involved hemipelvis. Because injuries can occur with multiple force vectors, the classification system allows for combined mechanism injuries (CMI).

The classification system developed by Tile is based on stability. The pelvis is divided into posterior and anterior arches relative to the acetabulum with fracture based on the stability of the posterior arch. Type A fractures are stable, type B fractures are rotationally unstable but vertically stable, and type C fractures are both rotationally and vertically unstable.

The classification system developed by the Orthopedic Trauma Association (OTA) is also based on stability. Type A fractures are stable pelvic fractures. Type B fractures are partially stable. Type C fractures are unstable injuries secondary to complete disruption of the posterior arch. Within this classification system are many subgroups and divisions, which are useful for research purposes but difficult for routine clinical use.

INITIAL ASSESSMENT

Prehospital management of pelvic fractures is guided by suspicion based on mechanism of injury. After extrication and airway assessment, emergency personnel can identify a pelvic fracture based on history if the patient is awake and alert and by brief clinical examination. Hemorrhage can be initially controlled by internally rotating both legs and binding the pelvis. Manual compression of the pelvis should be avoided in this setting as well as log rolling the patient more than 15 degrees. If the pelvis is bound in the prehospital setting, it should not be removed until appropriate evaluation in the emergency department.

Upon arrival to the emergency department, initial management follows ATLS protocol including primary and secondary surveys with

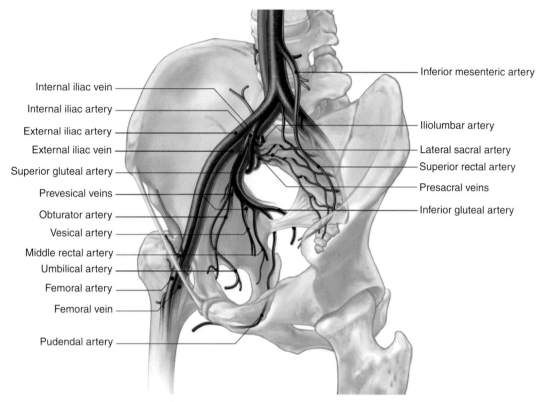

FIGURE 1   Vascular anatomy of the pelvis.   *(From Geeraerts T, Chhor V, Cheisson G, et al: Clinical review: initial management of blunt pelvic trauma patients with haemodynamic instability. Crit Care 11:204, 2007.)*

trauma series radiographs. Focused assessment with sonography in trauma (FAST) examination can be used to quickly identify intra-abdominal injuries. However, FAST examination is not reliable for detecting retroperitoneal hematoma; 25% of patients with pelvic fractures will have intra-abdominal injuries despite a negative FAST scan. Diagnostic peritoneal lavage (DPL) can also be used but should be performed via a supraumbilical incision to avoid false-positive findings due to pelvic fracture hematoma. CT scan is the best modality for assessing intra-abdominal and intrapelvic injuries along with retroperitoneal hematoma. Genitourinary injuries occur in 15% to 20% of pelvic fractures with greater anterior displacement associated with increased risk of injury. Retrograde cystourethrogram can be performed to diagnose genitourinary injuries.

Physical examination of the pelvis begins with questioning for pain in the pelvic region in awake and alert patients. Features suggestive of significant pelvic injury include deformity, ecchymosis or swelling over the pelvis and perineum, symphyseal gap, and leg-length discrepancy. Wounds over the pelvis or bleeding from the rectum or vagina may indicate an open fracture. Pelvic and rectal examinations are mandatory to rule out occult open fractures, and a high-riding prostate may be indicative of a urethral injury in males. Complete neurologic examination should also be performed when the patient's stability allows. Compression testing of the pelvis, or springing, is controversial because it has the potential for causing more soft tissue damage or dislodging clots. In addition, it is unreliable with a sensitivity of only 71% and specificity of only 59% for detecting pelvic instability. If pelvic compression testing is performed, it should be limited to a single attempt by an orthopedic traumatologist.

Prompt diagnosis of pelvic fractures is important because of the risk of significant hemorrhage and associated fatality. Tachycardia and peripheral vasoconstriction are early indicators of hemorrhage, with hypotension and low hematocrit being later findings. Initial fluid and blood resuscitation should follow accepted protocols,

and coagulopathy should be corrected if present. Base deficit and lactate levels are useful to monitor hemorrhage and resuscitation, and urine output is also a good indicator of resuscitation and systemic perfusion. Substantial hemorrhage in pelvic fractures comes from bleeding bone and arterial or venous injury within the internal iliac distribution, resulting in massive retroperitoneal hematoma. Risk of hemorrhage is greatest with APC III, VS, and Tile C pelvic fractures. Bleeding from the bone at the fracture site decreases when the fracture is reduced and stabilized. Arterial injury accounts for hemodynamic instability in 10% to 20% of patients with pelvic fractures. Identification of patients with pelvic fractures and persistent hemodynamic instability despite adequate resuscitation dictates further management with techniques to control bleeding and stabilize the pelvis. Modern resuscitation and techniques to control bleeding have reduced mortality rates from 40% to 80% down to 20% (Box 1; Fig. 5).

INITIAL TREATMENT

When a pelvic fracture with increased volume (APC type injury) is detected by physical examination and imaging, the simplest way to reduce and stabilize the fracture is by pelvic binding. This can be accomplished with a sheet or prefabricated binder. The binder is placed at the level of the greater trochanters and secured. The most common mistake is to place the binder over the iliac wings. It is imperative to assure the binder is located over the greater trochanters because when placed at the pelvic brim it will not reduce and control the pelvis. With this technique, bony bleeding is reduced by apposition of the fracture site, and reduced movement prevents disruption of a formed clot. It is also effective in reducing bleeding from venous origin, but does not reliably control bleeding from major arteries. Pelvic binding should not be performed on pelvic fractures with decreased volume (LC type injury) or transforaminal sacral fractures.

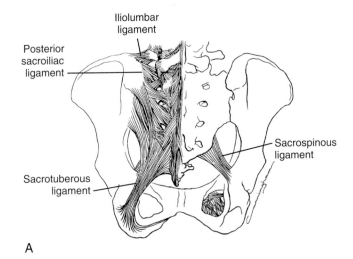

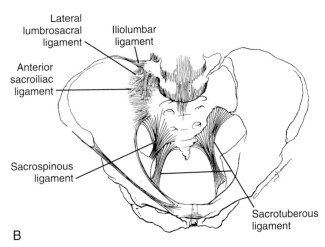

FIGURE 2 **A,** The bony pelvis and its major posterior ligaments. **B,** Anterior view. *(From Tile M, editor: Fractures of the pelvis and acetabulum, 3rd ed, Baltimore, 2003, Williams & Wilkins.)*

In addition, skin necrosis can occur if the binder is placed too tightly or if it remains in place for too long. Sometimes it is necessary to maintain the binder for an extended period of time because of continued profound instability, but it must be recognized that the longer a pelvic binder is used to maintain pelvic stability, the higher the risk of skin necrosis.

Another technique for reducing and stabilizing pelvic fractures is pneumatic antishock garments. They have the advantage of being able to control the amount of pressure being applied and are effective in reducing bleeding from a retroperitoneal hematoma. However, pneumatic antishock garments have the disadvantage of being bulky and can lead to ischemia and lower extremity compartment syndrome. They also make access to the abdomen and perineum difficult. For these reasons, pneumatic antishock garments are not as widely used as pelvic binders.

A C-clamp can also be used to reduce and stabilize pelvic fractures, but it is more popular in Europe than in the United States. It can be placed quickly outside the operating room and more directly reduces the posterior ring injury. The C-clamp is placed percutaneously in the same location as sacroiliac screw fixation, but is only temporary in comparison to external fixation. However, this technique also has a risk of potentially catastrophic complications when placed outside of the operating room, especially in comminuted sacral fractures.

Anterior external fixation is another technique used to reduce unstable pelvic fractures. This technique is effective in stabilizing the pelvic fracture and reducing hemorrhage. Pins can be placed in the anterior inferior iliac spine (AIIS) or in the iliac crest. External fixation is almost always placed in the operating room, but it is possible to place a fixator with iliac crest pins in the emergency room. Iliac crest pins can be placed more rapidly when needed and they can be safely placed without fluoroscopy, although when time permits, imaging is preferred. The AIIS pins require fluoroscopy for safe placement and are more time consuming; however, AIIS pins have greater pull-out strength, have increased rigidity, and provide a better axis for reduction. Placement of a pelvic fixator is usually performed in conjunction with other procedures such as laparotomy for concomitant injuries. The configuration of the external fixator frame chosen depends on a number of variables, but generally iliac crest pins are used for a "resuscitation frame" when the patient is in extremis. When the patient's physiology permits, a "definitive treatment frame" with AIIS pins is preferred. Anterior external fixation alone cannot fully control the posterior pelvis when vertical instability is present.

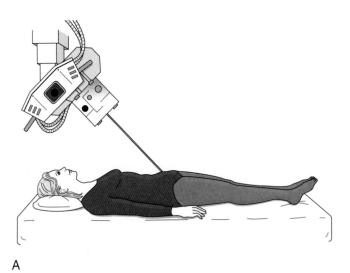

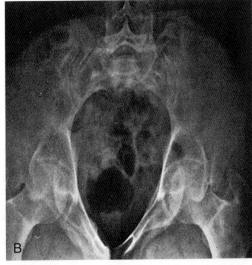

FIGURE 3   The inlet pelvic view. **A,** Patient positioning. **B,** Radiographic appearance. *(From Kellam JF, Browner BD: Fractures of the pelvic ring. In Browner BD, Jupiter JB, Levine AM, et al, editors: Skeletal trauma. Philadelphia, 1992, WB Saunders, pp 849–897.)*

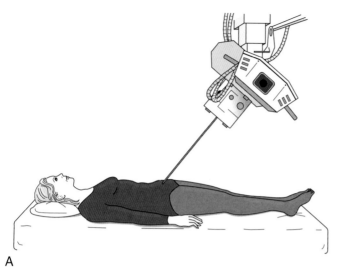
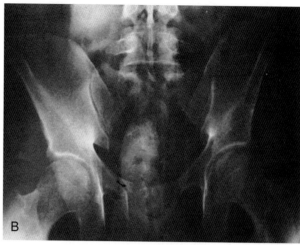

FIGURE 4   The outlet pelvic view. **A,** Patient positioning. **B,** Radiographic appearance.   *(From Kellam JF, Browner BD: Fractures of the pelvic ring. In Browner BD, Jupiter JB, Levine AM, et al, editors: Skeletal trauma. Philadelphia, 1992, WB Saunders, pp 849–897.)*

BOX 1 Classification of Pelvic Fractures

Tile Classification
Type A (stable)
  A1. Fractures of the pelvis not involving the ring; avulsion injuries
  A2. Stable, minimal displacement of the ring
Type B (rotationally unstable and vertically stable)
  B1. External rotation instability; open-book injury
  B2. LC injury; internal instability; ipsilateral only
  B3. LC injury; bilateral rotational instability (bucket-handle injury)
Type C (rotationally and vertically unstable)
  C1. Unilateral injury
  C2. Bilateral injury, one side rotationally unstable, with the contralateral side
  C3. Bilateral injury, both sides rotationally and vertically unstable, with an acetabular fracture

Young and Burgess System Classification
Lateral compression (LC): Transverse pubic rami fracture, ipsilateral or contralateral to posterior injury
  I. Sacral compression on side of impact
  II. Crescent (iliac wing) fracture on side of impact
  III. LC I or LC II injury on side of impact; contralateral open-book (APC) injury
Anteroposterior compression (APC): Symphyseal diastasis or longitudinal rami fractures
  I. Slight widening of pubic symphysis (less than 2.5 cm) or anterior sacroiliac (SI) joint; stretched but intact SI, sacrotuberous, and sacrospinous ligaments; intact posterior SI ligaments

  II. Symphyseal diastasis greater than 2.5; widened anterior SI joint; disrupted anterior SI, sacrotuberous, and sacrospinous ligaments; intact posterior SI ligaments
  III. Complete SI joint disruption with lateral displacement, disrupted anterior SI, sacrotuberous, and sacrospinous ligaments; disrupted posterior SI ligaments
Vertical shear (VS): Symphyseal diastasis or vertical displacement anteriorly and posteriorly, usually through the SI joint, occasionally through the iliac wing or sacrum
Combined mechanism injury (CMI): Combination of the injury patterns, LC/VS is most common

Orthopedic Trauma Association (OTA) Classification of Pelvic Ring Fractures
Type A: Lesion sparing (no displacement of posterior arch)
  1. Fracture of innominate bone, avulsion
  2. Fracture of innominate bone, direct blow
  3. Transverse fracture of sacrum and coccyx
Type B: Incomplete disruption of posterior arch, partially stable
  1. Unilateral, partial disruption of posterior arch, external rotation (open-book injury)
  2. Unilateral, partial disruption of posterior arch, internal rotation (LC injury)
  3. Bilateral, partial lesion of posterior arch
Type C: Complete disruption of posterior arch, unstable
  1. Unilateral, complete disruption of posterior arch
  2. Bilateral, ipsilateral complete, contralateral

From McCormack R, Strauss EJ, Alwattar BJ, Tejwani NC: Diagnosis and management of pelvic fractures. *Bull NYU Hosp Joint Dis* 68(4):281–291, 2010.

For vertically unstable injuries (VS type injuries), skeletal traction is also required to maintain reduction of the disrupted hemipelvis (Fig. 6).

Patients with pelvic fractures who remain hemodynamically unstable after resuscitation and stabilization of the pelvis are candidates for angiography. Hemorrhage from pelvic fractures is 90% venous and 10% arterial; however, arterial injuries are more common in cases of hemodynamic instability. During angiography, signs of macrovascular lesions are identified based on contrast extravasation, missing arteries, wall irregularities, and venous stagnation of contrast

agent. Embolization should be selective and sequential, addressing only the injured artery and leaving the remaining vessels intact to retain the blood supply to structures around the pelvis. Blind embolization with Gelfoam can occlude multiple small sources of bleeding. Proximal embolization should be avoided because of the potential for significant diffuse ischemia. Success rates with angiography have been reported to be 80% to 100% in the literature. However, for this technique to be effective, a skilled interventional radiologist must be available 24 hours a day 7 days a week. Complications from angiography occur 5% of the time and include puncture site hematoma, dissection,

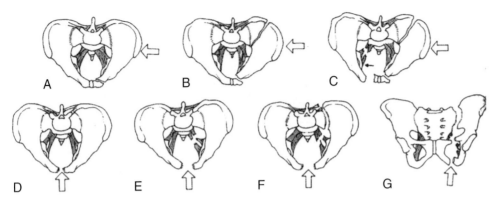

FIGURE 5 A graphic depiction of the Young and Burgess classification system. *(Reprinted with permission from Tornetta III P: Pelvis and acetabulum: trauma. In Beaty JH, editor:* Orthopaedic knowledge update, *ed 6, Rosemont, Ill., 1999, American Academy of Orthopaedic Surgeons, pp 427–439.)*

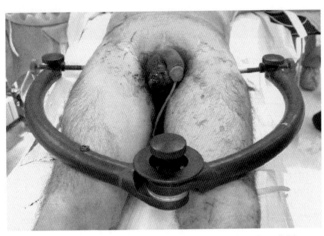

FIGURE 6 Pelvic C-clamp. *(From Mohanty K, Musso D, Powell JN, et al: Emergent management of pelvic ring injuries: an update.* Can J Surg *48:49–56, 2005.)*

thrombosis, downstream tissue necrosis, contrast agent sensitivity, and embolism dissemination in decreasing order. Second angiography can be performed in patients with persistent hemorrhage after initial angiography. Risk factors for recurrent bleeding include systolic pressure less than 90 mm Hg, base deficit greater than 10 mEq/L persisting for more than 6 hours, and absence of intra-abdominal hemorrhagic lesions.

Laparotomy for isolated pelvic fractures should be avoided secondary to the possibility of reexpansion of a retroperitoneal venous hematoma by decompression and the increased risk of deep infection

with later reconstruction. A 66% to 83% mortality rate has been reported in patients with unstable pelvic ring injuries and hemodynamic instability who underwent laparotomy for the purpose of vessel ligation. However, laparotomy is indicated for patients with common or external iliac arterial injuries. Placement of anterior external fixator before laparotomy for associated injuries is advised because the abdominal wall serves as a tension band for the anterior pelvis and disruption could cause increased widening of an open-book type fracture.

Pelvic packing has recently become a treatment option used in Europe and now in some centers in the United States. It is a damage control option used to restore hemostasis while waiting for arterial embolization to take place. It can also be used in patients necessitating immediate operative intervention for other causes and for residual hemodynamic instability after angiography. It is performed though a low midline or Pfannenstiel incision. Packing is pushed up against the peritoneum to increase the tamponade effect and then temporized with a vacuum dressing. It is most successful when combined with a pelvic reduction technique such as external fixation. The packing can be effective for arterial and venous lesions and has to be changed in 24 to 48 hours. This technique has not been evaluated in a large series of patients and the impact on infection with open reduction and internal fixation may also be of concern (Fig. 7).

DEFINITIVE TREATMENT

Up to the mid-1970s, pelvic fractures were generally managed nonoperatively using compression devices, plaster casts, and bed rest. Advances in surgical approaches, percutaneous techniques, and internal fixation have now led to the majority of significantly displaced pelvic fractures being treated operatively. Definitive reconstruction

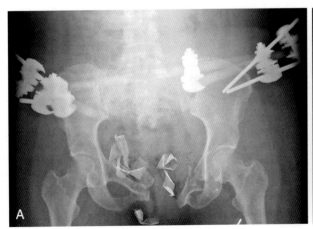
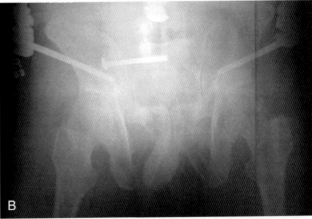

FIGURE 7 **A** and **B,** Pelvic external fixator. (*Left,* Iliac crest pins; *right,* anterior inferior iliac spine pins).

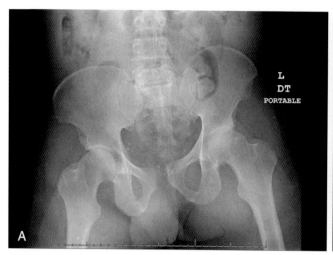
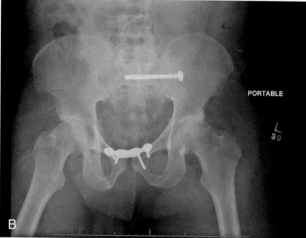

FIGURE 8 **A** and **B,** Definitive fixation of a pelvic ring injury.

is undertaken after adequate resuscitation and stabilization of the patient has been achieved. Stabilization of the pelvic ring facilitates patient care by allowing early mobilization, improved pulmonary toilet, and greater ease of nursing care. In addition, reconstruction of the anatomy leads to decreased long-term morbidity from malunion of the pelvic ring, which is very difficult to correct once it has occurred. Definitive fixation method depends upon the fracture type and displacement.

Reconstruction of the posterior ring is the most critical for long-term function and preventing leg-length discrepancy and sitting imbalance. Posterior ring injuries can be stabilized with percutaneous sacroiliac screws, plate and screw constructs, or lumbopelvic fixation. When adequate closed reduction can be obtained, percutaneous sacroiliac screws are preferred. If closed reduction is not possible or if the pattern cannot be stabilized with sacroiliac screws alone, then the other methods are employed. Fractures that only involve the iliac wing do not always require reconstruction, but when required, typically open reduction and internal fixation with plate and screws is used.

Anterior ring injuries can be treated with external fixation, plate and screw constructs, or internal screw and rod constructs. External fixation allows for percutaneous placement of hardware and the pins can be used to manipulate and reduce the pelvis. Pubic symphysis dislocations are more often managed with a plate and screw construct, which offers the advantage of no external hardware. More recently, anterior fixation with AIIS internal pedicle screws and a subcutaneous rod has been developed as a less invasive alternative. This technique has some advantages, but is most useful for injuries with pubic rami fractures that would make plating or screw fixation difficult and that do not require extensive reduction maneuvers. Postoperative weight bearing status is determined by the fracture pattern and stability of fixation.

Injuries to the urogenital system are very common in pelvic fractures. Their treatment often requires a multidisciplinary approach with urologists, gynecologists, and trauma surgeons. These injuries can lead to long-term complications such as stricture, incontinence, erectile dysfunction, dyspareunia, and difficulty with natural childbirth. Facilitating success in addressing these injuries is an important part of managing the musculoskeletal injuries of the pelvis (Fig. 8).

OUTCOMES

Very few quality studies exist in the literature regarding the outcomes of pelvic fractures. Union rates are 83% to 100% in nonoperatively treated fractures and 93% to 100% in operatively treated fractures. The quality of reduction is best and the malunion rate is lowest with fixation of posterior ring injuries. The incidence of long-term severe pain is related to the quality of reduction and presence of malunion. Infection rates are less than 5% in fractures treated with open reduction and internal fixation, but pin track infections occur in 20% of fractures treated definitively with external fixation. Loss of reduction and failure of fixation also occur in approximately 5% of patients. Residual gait abnormalities occur less often in patients treated with operative intervention and are also related to the quality of reduction. Approximately 66% to 75% of patients return to employment and SF-36 scores range from 64 to 75 in both mental and physical components, indicating that some residual disability may exist in patients with pelvic fractures. The most significant factor in this regard is the severity of the initial neurologic injury associated with the pelvic fracture. Overall, studies demonstrated that posttraumatic anatomic deformities and pelvic instability correlated with persistent pain and functional limitation.

SUMMARY

Pelvic fractures are common in polytrauma patients and represent a significant cause of morbidity and fatality. Initial assessment and interventions are aimed toward timely diagnosis, resuscitation, and control of hemorrhage. Understanding of the mechanism and fracture type helps predict stability and potential associated soft tissue injury. Stabilization of the fracture by multiple methods combined with angiography has reduced the mortality rate associated with these injuries. In addition, improvements in definitive fixation have improved the outcomes in this patient population. A coordinated multidisciplinary treatment algorithm is necessary to adequately manage patients with pelvic fractures.

For this chapter's Suggested Reading list, please visit the book at www.ExpertConsult.Inkling.com.

WRIST AND HAND FRACTURES: ORTHOPEDIC MANAGEMENT OF CURRENT THERAPY OF TRAUMA AND SURGICAL CRITICAL CARE

Patrick Owens

Please visit the book at www.ExpertConsult.inkling.com to read this chapter in full.

SCAPULOTHORACIC DISSOCIATION AND DEGLOVING INJURIES OF THE EXTREMITIES

Walter L. Biffl and Kyros Ipaktchi

Please visit the book at www.ExpertConsult.inkling.com to read this chapter in full.

EXTREMITY REPLANTATION: INDICATIONS AND TIMING

Haaris Mir, Morad Askari, and Zubin Jal Panthaki

Please visit the book at www.ExpertConsult.inkling.com to read this chapter in full.

Special Techniques for the Management of Complex Musculoskeletal Injuries: The Roles of Fasciocutaneous and Myocutaneous Flaps

Christopher Salgado, Ari Hoschander, and John Oeltjen

Please visit the book at www.ExpertConsult.inkling.com to read this chapter in full.

Special Issues and Situations in Trauma Management

Airway Management: What Every Surgeon Should Know about the Traumatic Airway (The Anesthesiologist's Perspective)

Shawn M. Cantie and Edgar J. Pierre

Acute airway trauma is a rare yet potentially lethal injury. The majority of blunt trauma to the airway is due to motor vehicle collisions, closely followed by sport-related and domestic violence–related trauma. Most penetrating injuries to the airway are secondary to gunshot or stab wounds. The primary goals of airway intervention are to relieve or prevent airway obstruction, to secure the unprotected airway from aspiration, to provide adequate gas exchange, and to maintain cervical spine stabilization. Gaining control of the traumatized airway is the ultimate test to the provider's adeptness and clinical acumen, as the provider must assume that the patient has a full stomach and an unstable cervical spine, two conditions that exacerbate the already difficult task. It requires knowledge of the hazards encountered secondary to the injury itself as well as those resulting from interventions by the anesthesiologist.

When a trauma patient arrives to the emergency room or resuscitation bay, the initial moments should be devoted to obtaining the most basic information about the overall condition: stable, unstable, moribund, or deceased. The primary survey of the Advanced Trauma Life Support protocol involves rapid evaluation and stabilization of the functions that are crucial to survival: airway patency, breathing, circulation with hemorrhage control, evaluation of disability with brief neurologic examination, and exposure of the entire patient by removal of all articles of clothing.

It is during these initial moments of the encounter that the physician must be attentive to any signs of airway trauma, as the most critical step in management of acute airway trauma is recognition of the condition. The physician should have a high index of suspicion in the setting of anterior cervical trauma. Symptoms such as hoarseness, dyspnea, dysphagia, dysphonia, and pain with phonation are frequently seen with laryngeal trauma, whereas crepitus, stridor, hemoptysis, anterior cervical edema, ecchymoses, and laceration are usually representative of laryngeal-tracheal injury. For patients with laryngeal-tracheal injury airway control is fundamental and should be accomplished as rapidly as possible.

The goal of manual in-line immobilization (MILI) is to apply sufficient force to the head and neck to limit the movement that might result from medical intervention, most notably airway management. MILI is typically provided by an assistant positioned either at the head of the bed or, alternatively, at the side of the stretcher facing the head of the bed. The patient is positioned supine with the head and the neck in neutral position. Assistants grasp both the mastoid processes with their fingertips and cradle the occiput (head-of bed assistant) or inferior neck and trapezii (side-of-bed assistant) in the palms of their hands. When MILI is in place, the anterior portion of the cervical collar can be removed to allow for greater mouth opening, facilitating airway interventions. During laryngoscopy, the assistant ideally applies forces that are equal in force and opposite in direction to those being generated by the intubating physician to keep the head and neck in the neutral position.

Avoiding traction forces during the application of MILI may be particularly important when there is a serious ligamentous injury resulting in gross spinal instability. Lennarson et al noted excess distraction at the site of a complete ligamentous injury when traction forces were applied for the purposes of spinal stabilization during direct laryngoscopy. Similarly, Kaufmann et al demonstrated that in-line traction applied for the purposes of radiographic evaluation resulted in spinal column lengthening and distraction at the site of injury in four patients with ligamentous disruptions. MILI may be effective in reducing overall spinal movements recorded during airway maneuvers but may have lesser restraining effects at the actual point of injury. This may be because spinal movement is restricted by the weight of the torso at the caudal end and the MILI forces at the cephalad end but is unrestricted by any force at its cervical midpoint. It is possible that application of traction forces during MILI would also reduce midcervical movement in some patients, but traction forces may also result in distraction at the site of injury. The use of such forces during application of MILI continues to be discouraged.

Control of the traumatized airway can be obtained by either routine intubation or by cricothyroidotomy. Although most anesthesiologists are extremely comfortable with intubation via direct or fiberoptic laryngoscopy, surgeons generally have more experience with the establishment of a surgical airway. At first glance, endotracheal intubation may seem to be the most helpful and efficient method of gaining airway control, but a cricothyroidotomy can be advantageous in certain situations. For injuries at or just below the level of the larynx, a tracheostomy provides space with which to examine the site of injury both at the site and from above with direct laryngoscopy. Endotracheal intubation might render further examination of the injury difficult and might aggravate an existing laryngeal injury. A surgical airway through a cricothyroidotomy should be established, recognizing the risk of laryngeal tracheal separation after cricothyroidotomy in patients with significant neck injuries.

Trauma to the face and upper airway poses particular difficulties. Failure to identify an injury to the face or neck can lead to acute or subacute airway obstruction secondary to swelling and hematomas. In patients with severe facial injuries, early oral intubation is recommended before swelling and edema compromise the airway.

Assuming no absolute contraindications to this position exist, these patients should be allowed and encouraged to remain seated until the trauma team is ready to manage their airway definitively. Facial and pharyngeal injuries also pose a particular danger as their appearance (i.e., cribriform plate injuries with cerebrospinal fluid leak) may serve to distract from other critical injuries that often occur in this setting such as cervical spine instability. Careful axial traction should be applied to stabilize the cervical spine during intubation.

Most facial injuries are obvious and can be recognized by hemorrhage, edema, erythema, fractures, and facial anatomic distortion. In a minority of cases, mainly isolated facial blunt trauma, edema and erythema may not appear in the very early stages. In this case crepitus upon palpation, hoarse voice, drooling, and refusal to maintain the supine posture should alert for facial injury and airway injury.

Because of the extreme urgency in these situations, assessment of the airway should be almost entirely clinical. Important findings to note include anxiety, stridor, ability or inability to phonate, adequacy of air movement through the mouth and nares, presence of tracheal deviation, the use of accessory muscles of respiration, and movement of the diaphragm.

Findings such as intraoral hemorrhage, pharyngeal erythema, mandibular injuries, and change in voice are all indications for early intubation. Bilateral mandibular fractures and pharyngeal hemorrhage may lead to upper airway obstruction, particularly in a supine patient. Therefore, a patient found in the sitting or prone position and refusing to lay supine because of airway compromise is best left in that position until the moment of anesthetic induction and intubation.

As facial and pharyngeal injuries pose difficult yet not impossible intubation situations, it is imperative that intubation be attempted in a controlled environment that is equipped to execute the difficult airway (DA) algorithm. An oropharyngeal or nasopharyngeal airway may be required to temporarily maintain airway patency until these conditions are met. Rapid sequence intubation with cervical in-line immobilization is the preferred method of intubating the trachea of the trauma patient.

However, prolonged struggle to intubate may be a misuse of the golden hour, compromising the patient's respiratory status and elevating intracranial pressure. Cricothyroidotomy is a useful alternative. Perhaps early cricothyroidotomy, rather than repeated multiple attempts to intubate, would result in less hypoxia and improved patient outcome. Emergency tracheostomy is not considered an appropriate method to establish emergency definitive airway as the procedure is lengthy and carries significant rate of complications. In a series of 71 patients with laryngeal-tracheal trauma, 39 (54.9%) required an emergency airway. Forty-eight percent of patients underwent initial orotracheal intubation, whereas tracheostomy and cricothyroidotomy were each performed in 4%. Patients with blunt laryngotracheal trauma required an emergency airway in 78.9% of cases, whereas those with penetrating injuries required 1 in 46 (2%). Intubation was successful in 14 of the 15 patients in the blunt trauma group and in 20 of the 24 patients in the penetrating trauma group.

The diagnosis of penetrating neck trauma is usually simple, as the injury is obvious. On the contrary, diagnosis of blunt neck trauma depends upon a high index of suspicion. Clinical examination remains the most reliable sign of laryngotracheal injury. The only hard diagnostic sign to laryngotracheal trauma is air escaping through the neck wound, which is often difficult to definitively identify. Equally as critical is the prompt identification of subcutaneous emphysema through the detection of crepitus to palpation over the anterior face, neck, and upper chest. Patients with neck injury may also have dyspnea, hemoptysis, hoarseness, stridor, and crepitus upon palpation. The symptoms associated with these injuries are secondary to the soft tissue swelling, including the sensation of choking, dyspnea, dysphagia, hoarseness, and stridor experienced by these patients. The quality of the victim's voice (i.e., hoarseness) is unpredictable. However, a hoarse patient suffers major airway injury until proved otherwise. A hoarse voice should be assumed to exist prior to the injury only if an awake and oriented patient can confirm this.

Trauma is a dynamic disease, especially in the acute phase. As the patient's condition can change very quickly, the frequent reassessment of the patient's state is essential. Frequent checks of the patient also help to identify the propagation of edema and hematoma that can lead to an insidious airway obstruction.

The most urgent priority in neck trauma is securing the airway. The end result should be a well-positioned orotracheal tube with an inflated, sealed cuff placed entirely distal to a laryngotracheal perforation. Nevertheless, intubation of the trachea might be extremely difficult, as pharyngeal or neck hematoma might obscure the vocal cords or distort the anatomy. Passing an endotracheal tube blindly is dangerous as it may follow or produce a false passage. In the instance of a partial transection, an endotracheal tube advanced with zeal may cause complete laryngotracheal separation.

In light of the possible hazards, the obvious conclusion is to avoid tracheal intubation on the scene or emergency department (ED), assuming a stable patient. The more common neck injuries such as stab wounds and low-velocity gunshot wounds do not mandate prehospital or ED intubation. In this case intubation should be performed in the operating room by the most experienced available anesthesiologist, equipped by appropriate instruments and availability of a surgical airway. On the contrary, high-velocity gunshot wounds and severe blunt neck injuries often mandate urgent airway control.

Traditionally, rapid sequence orotracheal intubation is necessary. Concomitant preparation for fiberoptic assurance of the proper tube position as well as continuing preparations for establishment of surgical airway via cricothyroidotomy is mandatory. The unstable patient with a slashed throat or large anterior neck lacerations can be intubated through the incision as a lifesaving act, which may be the only practical alternative for emergency medical services personnel if artificial airway establishment cannot be delayed until hospital arrival. In the past cricothyroidotomy or tracheostomy were the procedures of choice, even in the hospital.

Signs indicative of vascular injuries include hematoma, shock, and persistent bleeding. The hematoma may be limited without jeopardizing the airway. Bleeding and edema formation are more likely in patients treated with anticoagulants. In this case, a critical point might be reached in which the airway will be obstructed and the patient will deteriorate abruptly. It is reasonable to postpone tracheal intubation until the arrival at the hospital in these patients because of the inability to predict the clinical course. Nevertheless, close monitoring of the patient as well as the size of hematoma is crucial. Preventive intubation should be done if the hematoma enlarges or if the patient shows progressive signs of airway compromise. Low threshold for intubation is advocated if the transport time is long. In the prehospital, ED, and operating room settings a difficult intubation should be anticipated and the technique is to be planned accordingly.

Once the airway is secured, a meticulous diagnostic workup is to be started in order to verify the exact location of injury and to choose the appropriate surgical intervention. This workup will mostly include fiberoptic examination of the pharynx, larynx, trachea, and esophagus.

AMERICAN SOCIETY OF ANESTHESIOLOGISTS DIFFICULT AIRWAY ALGORITHM MODIFICATION FOR TRAUMA

The American Society of Anesthesiologists (ASA) Task Force on Difficult Airway Management presents guidelines for the management of the DA. The algorithm gives the physician a systematic approach to nonsurgical methods of ventilation before a surgical pathway is elected. The ASA algorithm is only generally applicable to the trauma patient. The time taken to obtain nonsurgical airway control may not be in the best interest of the trauma patient in whom hemorrhagic shock, risk of aspiration, and head trauma often exist. Indeed, in cases of severe trauma, the crisis approach to management often precludes continuing with nonsurgical methods of airway ventilation, and a surgical airway is sometimes elected at a point in time before that which would be the case in other patient populations. Ultimately, it is clinical judgment that guides the path taken in obtaining airway control in trauma patients.

Recently a trial to modify the DA algorithm to trauma was done. Maxillofacial and neck trauma falls into the category of suspected difficult intubation. The key points in the modified algorithm are as follows:

1. Stopping is seldom an option with trauma.
2. Surgical airway can be the first/best choice in certain conditions.
3. An awake endotracheal tube technique should be chosen in a DA patient provided the patient is cooperative, stable, and spontaneously ventilating.
4. If the patient is uncooperative/combative, general anesthesia (GA) may need to be administered—but if the airway is difficult, spontaneous ventilation (SV) should be continued (if possible).

The DA algorithm modification for trauma defines invasive airway access as surgical/percutaneous tracheostomy as well as cricothyroidotomy. It seems worth mentioning that many practitioners do not believe tracheostomy is a proper choice to gain emergency control of the airway surgically (Figs. 1 and 2).

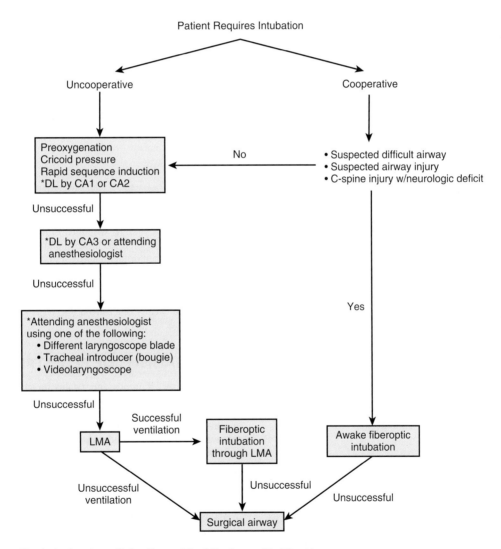

FIGURE 1 RTA airway algorithm. C-spine, Cervical spine; LMA, laryngeal mask airway.

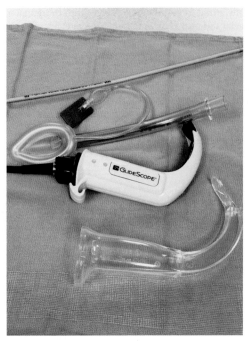

FIGURE 2   Three adjuncts to the difficult airway: the tracheal introducer, the laryngeal mask airway, and the GlideScope.

SUMMARY

Penetrating trauma to the airway is usually obvious but blunt trauma mandates a high index of suspicion to recognize its existence. A comprehensive understanding of the extent of the injury is mandatory in order to plan the best timing and method to secure the airway. If the airway is stable, it is advised that airway control will be carried out in the operating room, by the most experienced anesthesiologist available, with the availability of a surgical airway. It is better to maintain spontaneous ventilation in any case in which there is suspicion of a DA.

For the chapter's Suggested Readings list, please visit the book at www.ExpertConsult.inkling.com.

PEDIATRIC TRAUMA

David W. Tuggle and L.R. Tres Scherer

Pediatric trauma is the number one killer of children in the United States. It is also the number one cause of permanent disability in this population. It has often been said that children are not merely small adults, and this is never more accurate than in pediatric trauma. Although the principles of trauma care are the same for children as for adults, the differences in care required to optimally treat the injured child do require special knowledge, careful management, appropriate equipment, and attention to the unique physiology and psychology of the growing child or adolescent.

INCIDENCE OF PEDIATRIC TRAUMA

Although medical science has made vast strides in the surgical care of the neonate and child, unintentional injuries remain the leading cause of death in children under 19 years of age. From 2000 to 2009, the overall annual unintentional injury death rate decreased 29%, from 15.5 to 11.0 per 100,000 population, accounting for 9143 deaths in 2009. Child injury death rates varied substantially by state in 2009, ranging from less than 5 deaths per 100,000 children in Massachusetts and New Jersey to more than 23 deaths per 100,000 children in South Dakota, Montana, and Mississippi. For every childhood traumatic death, 25 pediatric patients are hospitalized, and 925 children are treated in an emergency department.

For children ages 1 to 4 years, drownings are the leading cause of death. Motor vehicle crashes are the second leading cause of injury-related death for children ages 1 to 4 years; nearly half of children age 4 and younger who died in motor vehicle crashes were riding unrestrained. Children under 5 years are among those most at risk for injuries from residential fires. For children ages 5 to 19 years, motor vehicle injuries are the leading cause of death. Drowning is the second leading cause of injury-related death among children 5 to 14 years. For children ages 15 to 19 years, suicide is the second leading cause of death. Nearly one third of bicyclists killed in traffic crashes are children ages 5 to 14 years.

MECHANISMS OF PEDIATRIC TRAUMA

The mechanism of injury and fatality in children has remained remarkably consistent. In children over 1 year and under 14 years of age, motor vehicle–related fatality remains the greatest killer of children, at 46.5% of all causes (2009). Drowning is the second cause, followed by suffocation under the age of 1 year. A detailed view of fatality statistics reveals the home as an area of continuing concern. Other areas of concern include falls and bicycle-related injuries; a growing area of death and disability now includes all-terrain vehicle (ATV) crashes (see CPSC 2009 report; Available at http://www.cpsc.gov//PageFiles/108615/atv2009.pdf).

Childhood injuries most commonly occur as energy is transferred abruptly either by rapid acceleration or deceleration or by a combination of both. The body of a child is very elastic, and energy can be transferred in a way that creates internal injuries without significant external signs. Because of the closer proximity of vital organs, children can have multiple injuries from a single exchange of energy, more so than older patients. Penetrating trauma is a much less common form of injury in small children, ranging from 1% to 10% in pediatric trauma centers. No matter the type of injury, the health care professional evaluating the injured child should keep in mind these significant differences during evaluation and management.

INITIAL ASSESSMENT, STABILIZATION, AND MANAGEMENT OF THE INJURED CHILD

Airway Management

Most children do not have preexisting pulmonary disease; therefore, an oxygen saturation of greater than 90% on room air is often proof of adequate pulmonary function. If oxygenation is difficult, then a lung injury, pneumothorax, or aspiration should be considered. Hypoventilation is common in the presence of a head injury or shock. If any of these conditions exist, assisted ventilation and subsequent advanced airway techniques are appropriate. Respiratory compromise requiring intubation commonly indicates a very severe injury. Although no criteria have been validated to determine what constitutes a "major resuscitation" in children, intubation and airway compromise have been shown to suggest a population that has a higher incidence of fatality compared with injured children who do not have airway issues. As with all patients, care should be taken to avoid cervical spine motion during intubation. It should be noted that nasotracheal intubation is generally not used in small children in the emergency setting.

Intubation also facilitates evaluation and resuscitation in many circumstances. The combative child should be evaluated for hypoxia in the acute setting, although an alert, uncooperative child may also indicate the presence of minimal injuries. The use of weight/length-based tape has become the standard for determining the weight, appropriate size for resuscitative equipment, and drug doses and drip concentrations during a resuscitation.

With the difficult airway, advanced airway techniques with laryngeal mask airway and bronchoscopy may be required. This advanced technique often requires the expertise of an anesthesiologist or intensivist. The use of gum elastic bougies to facilitate intubation is being promoted, but its use has been limited in children.

Postintubation management includes secondary confirmation of placement, gastric decompression, and performing a chest radiograph for pneumothorax and endotracheal tube positioning. End-tidal capnography or colorimetry should be used to confirm airway placement, but not positioning. Gastric decompression with a nasogastric or orogastric tube should be employed in every case because gastric distention will impair diaphragmatic excursion, with resulting respiratory compromise in the small child. If a pneumothorax is present, needle decompression can be employed, but this should be followed by immediate tube thoracostomy.

Vascular Access

The ideal initial sites for vascular access in children are the peripheral veins in the upper extremities, especially the antecubital fossa. If access cannot be achieved in these vessels, central venous access may be employed (Fig. 1). An advanced and skilled technique,

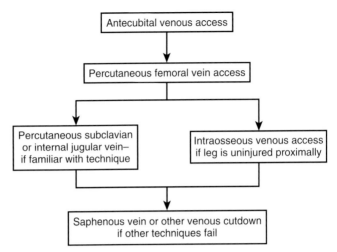

FIGURE I Algorithm for venous access in children.

percutaneous femoral venous catheterization, is the next best choice and the most commonly used route for emergency venous access in the child. This should be done without attempting a cut-down, preferably using the Seldinger technique. Surgeons familiar with subclavian catheterization in the child may use this route as the next choice. For surgeons comfortable with this technique in children, complications are rare. In the emergent situation, intraosseous access is the most acceptable in injured children. Contraindications include proximal fractures and sites of infection nearby. The anteromedial surface of the proximal tibia is used, 2 to 4 cm distal to the tibial tuberosity. For insertion in the proximal tibia, the needle is directed inferiorly at a 45-degree angle from the perpendicular. If the insertion site is the distal tibia, the needle should be angled 45 degrees superiorly. In both instances, the goal is to angle away from the region of the growth plate or joint. Specialized needles are readily available to use with this technique, including powered intraosseous insertion. Multiple entries into the medullary cavity should be avoided, as the leakage that occurs with multiple attempts may cause a compartment syndrome.

Circulatory Management

Age-specific hypotension is an indication for designating the necessity for major resuscitation in an injured child (Table 1). In an analysis of the National Pediatric Trauma Registry, 38% of recorded deaths occurred in children whose systolic blood pressure was less than 90 mm Hg. This group represented 2.4% of the study population. To determine if a child has "age-specific hypotension" requires knowledge of normal blood pressures in children. A child with an injury that produces significant blood loss may present with a normal blood pressure. The otherwise healthy child can readily compensate for blood loss by mounting a significant tachycardia coupled with

TABLE I: Normal Vital Signs and Weights for Various Age Groups in Pediatric Population

Age	Respiratory Rate (breaths/min)	Pulse (beats/min)	Systolic Blood Pressure (mm Hg)	Weight (kg)	Weight (lb)
Newborn	30–50	120–160	50–70	2–4	4–7
1–12 months	20–30	80–140	70–100	4–10	10–22
1–3 years	20–30	80–130	80–110	10–15	22–33
3–5 years	20–30	80–120	80–110	15–20	33–44
6–13 years	20–30	70–110	80–120	20–45	44–99
14 years and up	12–20	55–90	90–120	45 and up	99 and up

peripheral vasoconstriction. Therefore, a normal blood pressure in a child does not mean that circulating blood volume is at normal levels. A more accurate determination includes a blood pressure evaluation along with monitoring heart rate and assessing peripheral perfusion.

Clinical signs of poor perfusion in conjunction with altered mentation are classic findings in pediatric hypovolemic shock. If these signs are present, then an immediate bolus of 20 mL/kg of isotonic crystalloid is in order. If a second bolus of this amount is needed, and there is little improvement, blood transfusion should be started immediately (Fig. 2). Caution must be taken, as overresuscitation may be as problematic as underresuscitation, especially in the presence of a head injury. Enthusiastic administration of crystalloid solutions may exacerbate cerebral edema in certain circumstances. Overtreatment with crystalloid infusions may result in poor clot formation, worsening the compromised hemorrhagic state, and may have no impact on survival. Supranormal trauma resuscitation increases the likelihood of the abdominal compartment syndrome in adult trauma victims, and there are reports of the same problem in children. Typically, a bolus of 20 mL/kg of isotonic crystalloid in the presence of hypotension is the first treatment. If there is evidence of continuing instability, a second bolus of this amount may be given. If after two boluses of crystalloid the child does not have stable vital signs, blood transfusion should be started immediately. Type-specific packed red blood cells should be given, or O negative blood if necessary, in certain circumstances. Fresh frozen plasma and platelets should be considered early in the resuscitation period if large amounts of blood are needed for resuscitation. If there is a decreased level of consciousness without signs of hypovolemia, then modest fluid resuscitation is in order.

Hypothermia is an extremely common occurrence in injured children. Hypothermia in the injured child may occur at any time of the year, even during the extremes of summer. The response to hypothermia includes catecholamine release and shivering, with an increase in oxygen consumption and metabolic acidosis. Hypothermia as well as acidosis contribute to a posttraumatic coagulopathy. Prevention and treatment of hypothermia require attention to this serious complication during the initial evaluation of the injured child. A warm room, warmed fluids, heated air-warming blankets, or externally warmed blankets should be used during the initial resuscitation. An aggressive approach to rewarming should begin in the emergency department and should be continued in the radiology suite during evaluation. There is some evidence to suggest that early, carefully controlled hypothermia in the severely head-injured child who has no other injuries may be beneficial, but this treatment option is still experimental.

Diagnostic Assessment

The diagnostic assessment of the injured child begins with the initial evaluation and resuscitation phase of trauma management. The physical examination is a crucial first step, as it will direct all other forms of assessment. The initial physical examination also becomes the baseline for serial physical examinations by the trauma team performed later in the hospitalization. After the physical examination, other adjuncts may be employed.

Although the patient is undergoing resuscitation in the emergency department, the diagnosis of injuries begins with standard radiographs. The most frequently ordered imaging studies in the emergency department include plain radiographs of the chest, abdomen, pelvis, cervical spine, and extremities. Thoracic and lumbar spinal radiographs are commonly ordered when neurologic injuries are suspected, or when the physical examination reveals point tenderness over the spine. Detecting a pneumothorax, pneumoperitoneum, pelvic fracture, or long-bone fracture is an important component of the initial care of an injured child. Plain radiographs of the skull may document fractures, but they have little value in directing management of the head-injured child, except for penetrating injury and suspected child abuse.

Several studies by adult and pediatric trauma surgeons have attempted to determine the role of focused assessment with sonography in trauma (FAST) in the evaluation of the injured child. The most common FAST evaluation examines the heart, right and left upper quadrants, and the pelvis for fluid (Fig. 3). Some surgeons include an evaluation of the thorax for fluid in the pleural space and for pneumothorax.

Currently, non–radiologist-directed ultrasound evaluation in children should be coupled with the physical examination and should not be considered a conclusive diagnostic study. Although its sensitivity, specificity, and accuracy are high, it is used mostly as a screening tool to determine the need for more in-depth imaging studies or invasive

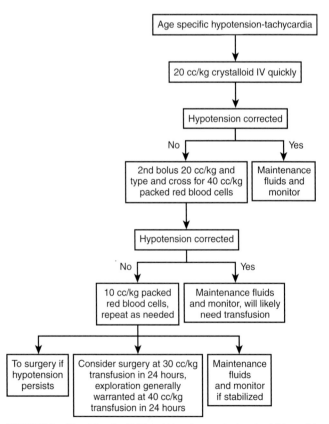

FIGURE 2 Algorithm for fluid and blood resuscitation in children. IV, Intravenous.

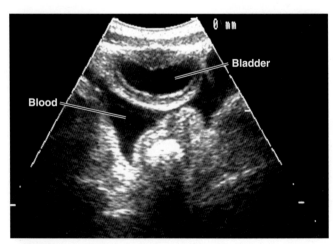

FIGURE 3 A positive focused assessment with sonography in trauma in a 4-year-old. Blood in the pelvis.

evaluation. The relative lack of subcutaneous tissue in most children makes this an easy study to perform on children, compared with adolescents and adults. Obvious benefits of the FAST evaluation include its portability, eliminating the need to transport the child to the radiology suite, and the child's decreased radiation exposure.

Computed tomography (CT) is the accepted diagnostic radiologic tool of choice for the vast majority of injured children suspected of having a potentially life-threatening injury. It is important to limit the amount of CT scanning of children whenever possible. It is commonly accepted that CT scanning for trauma is appropriate, yet multiple scans are frequently ordered and this practice leads to a potential risk of cancer caused by medical imaging.

Pan-scanning of the adult patient from head to pelvis is considered standard of care, but due to the risk of radiation and low yield of injuries, alternate algorithms to evaluate the neck and chest have been developed. Recently the Canadian Trauma Association has developed guidelines minimizing the amount of radiation required to clear the cervical spine. Almost all clinically significant thoracic injuries are identified by a plain chest radiograph. The majority of children with suspected intra-abdominal injuries, providing they are stable, should have a CT scan performed prior to instituting operative or nonoperative management, unless an absolute indication for surgery is present. Physiologically unstable children in the emergency department are evaluated by other modalities, such as diagnostic peritoneal lavage or ultrasound. Although CT scanning is the imaging modality of choice for evaluating a stable injured child, it is generally accepted that a high percentage of those scans will reveal no injuries. Abnormal abdominal CT scans are seen in only one fourth of patients (Fig. 4). A CT scan affects the decision to operate on children with a solid organ injury in a very small number of cases. Evidence, on a CT scan, of intra-abdominal injuries requiring operative correction may be subtle. Findings of free intraperitoneal or retroperitoneal air, extraluminal gastrointestinal contrast medium, bowel wall defects, and active hemorrhage are often obvious and have a high correlation with intestinal injury requiring operative intervention. There are, however, potentially life-threatening intestinal injuries that may be manifest only by focal bowel wall thickening or peritoneal fluid accumulation without solid organ injury. Other less specific findings associated with intestinal injuries include mesenteric stranding, fluid at the mesenteric root, focal hematomas, mesenteric pseudoaneurysm, and the hypoperfusion complex.

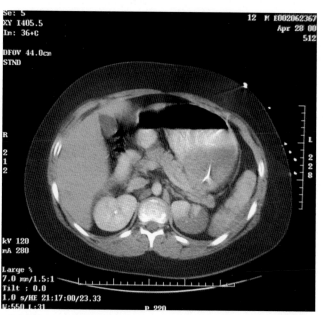

FIGURE 4 A positive computed tomography scan for a renal and spleen injury in an 8-year-old.

Other adjuncts to the management of the injured child may include interventional radiologic techniques, magnetic resonance imaging, and invasive and noninvasive vascular studies. The routine use of laboratory studies in the emergency department, in general, has not been shown to be of significant value in the pediatric trauma population. Some specific clinical laboratory testing, such as base deficit tests, urinalysis, and arterial blood gas tests, may be of limited benefit in selected circumstances. Most often, laboratory testing has lagged behind the clinical decision-making process occurring in the emergency department during evaluation and resuscitation. Point-of-care testing has not altered this concept. In the presence of a head injury, testing for a coagulopathy, thrombocytopenia, or hyperglycemia may be of benefit to establish a baseline for later determinations or to assist in assessing morbidity or mortality risks. During hospitalization, routine laboratory testing is appropriate as long as specific indications exist for monitoring, such as nonoperative management of a spleen or pancreatic injury, blood gases for patients receiving mechanical ventilation, and patients with head injuries.

MANAGEMENT OF SPECIFIC INJURIES

It should be noted that the scale used for every injured organ—namely, the American Association for the Surgery of Trauma's Organ Injury Scale—is the same for adults and children. The management of specific injuries in children is virtually identical to that used for adults, except when indicated.

Head and Central Nervous System Injury

Acute traumatic brain injury is the most common cause of death and disability in the pediatric population. In those who survive, minor injuries can be associated with reversible defects, but major injuries can result in severe disabilities. The mechanisms of head injury in children are related to age. Infants typically suffer more from falls, such as from a table or the arms of a caregiver. Intentional injury is a common cause of death in children under 2 years. Injury with intention, independent of severity, raises the mortality rate in brain-injured children. In older children, the usual cause of head injuries is from vehicle-related accidents or recreational activities. Although children have a better survival rate with head injury than adults do, this does not mean they have less morbidity with similar injuries. Children have a plasticity of the neuron related to the myelination and establishment of neuron interconnections. This allows a given focal injury to produce a less severe deficit as compared with a mature brain. But this same lack of maturity may also make the child more susceptible to a diffuse injury and subject to greater cognitive impairment.

During the initial evaluation and resuscitation of the brain-injured child, care should be taken to avoid secondary brain injury due to causes such as hypotension and hypoxia. Control of the cervical spine is also mandatory during this period. Clinical and radiologic evaluation of the cervical spine is important to rule out injury. The Glasgow Coma Scale (GCS) can be used for children over the age of 5, and some modification of the GCS is often used for children under 5. If a score of less than 9 is determined, that patient typically requires airway management, and intracranial pressure (ICP) measurement and treatment options should be considered. A score of less than 8 indicates the patient is comatose. Maintaining good oxygenation and perfusion is crucial during the entire resuscitation period, and this often mandates endotracheal intubation, taking care to protect the cervical spine, as injury may not be known.

Once the patient is initially evaluated and causes of secondary brain injury are managed, a head CT should be obtained. If there is evidence of brain swelling, monitoring of ICP is indicated. This is best done with a system that allows drainage of cerebrospinal fluid, such as a ventriculostomy. Avoiding hyperthermia is important, as this may cause secondary brain injury. Other management techniques include hyperosmolar therapy with mannitol or hypertonic saline solution. Sedation is used as needed to maintain a low ICP. Hyperventilation as prophylaxis should generally be avoided. High-dose barbiturate therapy to create a coma has been suggested to be of some benefit. Decompressive craniectomy is now considered an alternative for the surgical management of head-injured children in specific circumstances. It should be considered in head-injured children with cerebral edema and medically uncontrolled intracranial hypertension. It may be of some benefit in children with a potentially recoverable head injury. It is not likely to be useful in children who have suffered an extensive secondary brain injury, or those who have a GCS score of 3, with no improvement. Nutritional support, avoidance of steroid use, and treatment of postinjury seizures when indicated are also important aspects of the care of the head-injured patient.

Thoracic Injuries

Thoracic trauma is an important cause of morbidity and death in children. It accounts for 4% to 25% of pediatric trauma injuries, but these chest injuries are associated with a greater mortality rate when compared with other system injuries. Thoracic trauma can be anticipated in children who present with a low systolic blood pressure, an elevated respiratory rate, abnormalities on thoracic physical examination including abnormal chest auscultation, and femur fractures.

In general, the pediatric airway is more susceptible to mucus plugging and small amounts of airway edema. The chest wall is more compliant in children, with less muscle mass for soft tissue protection. This allows a greater transmission of energy to underlying organs when injury occurs. In children, the mediastinum is more mobile than in older patients, particularly in young children. Unilateral changes in thoracic pressure, such as with a tension pneumothorax, can lead to a shift of the mediastinum to the extent that venous return is markedly reduced. The pathophysiologic effect is similar to hypovolemic shock. This response is more pronounced in children than is typically in the case in an adult.

Rib fractures are relatively uncommon in young children and occur more frequently in adolescents. Even though rib fractures are uncommon, internal injuries of the organs lying underneath the ribs, such as liver or spleen injuries, and pulmonary contusion, are quite common. Flail chest is seen less commonly in children than in adults. One of the most common thoracic injuries in children is a pulmonary contusion. The flexible chest wall of the child allows contusion of the lung without rib fracture. The presence of a pulmonary contusion contributes to decreased pulmonary compliance, hypoxia, hypoventilation, and a ventilation/perfusion mismatch. A chest radiograph taken during the initial assessment may demonstrate a pulmonary contusion; however, a chest CT scan can show areas of pulmonary contusion not appreciated on the radiograph. Treatment includes appropriate fluid resuscitation, supplemental oxygen, pain management, and strategies to prevent atelectasis and pneumonia. Children with pulmonary contusions may have prolonged changes in respiratory function and radiographic abnormalities.

Pneumothorax and hemothorax are not uncommon injuries in children. A pneumothorax is typically treated with a chest tube appropriately sized for the patient. A hemothorax is also treated with a tube thoracostomy, typically with the largest tube that can be inserted. Intrathoracic blood loss of 15 mL/kg immediately or ongoing losses of 2 to 3 mL/kg/hour for 3 or more hours suggest the need for thoracic exploration to control bleeding in children. Cardiac injuries are extremely rare, as are tracheobronchial injuries and esophageal injuries. Injuries to the great vessels occur in older children (mean age of 12 years, and rare in children younger than 10 years) with rapid deceleration injuries. The mechanism of injury and an abnormal chest radiograph demonstrating a wide mediastinum, loss of the aortic knob or strip, deviation of the esophagus, or first rib fracture are signs of an injury. Helical CT of the chest with intravenous contrast is sensitive and provides an accurate negative prediction when normal.

Abdominal Injuries

Due to the relative thinness of the pediatric abdominal wall, a modest amount of force may cause a greater injury to one or more organs in the abdomen. Multiple organs may be injured from a single blow due to closer proximity. The assessment for abdominal injury begins with the physical examination. Inspection may reveal bruising, a lap belt mark, or abdominal distention. Tenderness on physical examination should prompt a higher level of suspicion and an evaluation with CT scanning. A nasogastric or orogastric tube should be placed to decompress the stomach.

During the course of routine nonoperative management of abdominal injuries, injuries requiring operative management may be overlooked for quite some time. It has been noted that a delay in diagnosis, although not uncommon, is not associated with increased fatality. However, an increase in septic complications has been seen when operative intervention occurred more than 24 hours after injury. Therefore, in-hospital observation with serial examinations should be employed in all children with abdominal examinations that are not perfectly normal. When abdominal injuries occur under suspicious circumstances, the diagnosis of child abuse should be entertained.

Blunt diaphragmatic rupture is an uncommon occurrence. The left diaphragm is involved more often than the right; however, bilateral injury can occur. The frequency of associated injuries, especially of liver and spleen, is very high. Blunt injury to the diaphragm may have several manifestations. An abnormal diaphragm contour, a high-riding diaphragm, or a questionable overlap of abdominal visceral shadows may indicate injury. Visceral herniation, the abnormal placement of a nasogastric tube into the hemithorax, or intestinal obstruction should be considered diagnostic. CT has been used to establish this diagnosis, but the CT scan may appear normal in some patients. Many diaphragmatic ruptures are not identified in the first few days after injury and may not be detected for a considerable period of time. Repair of an acute diaphragmatic rupture is often best accomplished with an abdominal approach. If a late diagnosis of a diaphragmatic injury is made, a thoracic approach to repair should be considered.

The child with a duodenal injury that requires surgery more often presents with abdominal distention, bilious vomiting, pneumoperitoneum, and peritonitis. A duodenal hematoma is usually treated nonoperatively with nasogastric decompression and total parenteral nutrition. This management is associated with a high rate of success, but may take as long as 3 weeks for the obstruction to resolve. A late diagnosis of duodenal perforation can occur with this injury and is usually associated with an increase in complications, but not fatality.

The small bowel, both jejunum and ileum, is the most common part of the intestinal tract to be injured in a child. The mechanism of injury to the small bowel is the result of its being trapped between the delivered force and the vertebral column. Adult-sized seat belts are often used to secure children in a car, and as a result the risk of small bowel injury rises. If a seat belt bruise is present, the risk of an intra-abdominal injury is much more likely, and therefore a higher index of suspicion should be employed. Children with small bowel injury due to blunt trauma invariably have an abnormal physical examination. Free fluid seen on an ultrasound or CT scan, coupled with a tender abdomen, and no solid organ injury, almost mandates an abdominal exploration for bowel injury. Even if no perforation is identified in surgery, care should be taken to evaluate for mesenteric rents, hematomas, and possibly retroperitoneal injuries. In this same setting, compression injury of the lumbar vertebrae (chance fracture) is also common; and when present, the patient usually requires a longer hospital stay due to pain management.

Injuries to the colon and rectum are not common in children. Accidental causes of colon and rectal injuries include motor vehicle collisions involving pelvic fractures and rectal wall penetration by bone shards. Nonaccidental injuries caused by child abuse, typically from blunt instrumentation, are also seen. If the mucosa is injured or the injury is superficial, observation is appropriate. Full-thickness injuries of the distal rectum can be managed with primary repair in many cases. Devastating colon injuries above the peritoneal reflection often need a temporary colostomy. Penetrating injuries often can be managed by primary repair, but in the face of complicating features may also need diversion at the time of repair.

The injured spleen in a child will almost always stop bleeding without any intervention. Nonoperative management is the standard of care, and the incidence of any potential operative intervention is very small. The rate of operative intervention is likely cut in half when a trained pediatric surgeon is managing the patient. Children who require surgery are those who have received or are likely to receive half their blood volume in transfusions within 24 hours of injury (40 mL/kg or remain unstable after 20 mL/kg). The physiologic response to splenic injury correlates with the grade of splenic injury. Most often children who need operative intervention will need splenectomy. If splenectomy must be performed, postsplenectomy immunization is appropriate. Many children are given penicillin on a daily basis if the splenectomy is performed before age 5 years of age. If immunosuppression is suspected, hepatitis B vaccine should also be administered.

When only the liver is injured, without major vascular or bile duct involvement, then observation will almost always succeed. This is especially true in patients with isolated solid organ injuries. However, it is possible that hepatic injuries may be associated with a slightly higher mortality rate than splenic injuries. The combination of hepatic and splenic injury is clearly associated with a higher mortality rate, which goes up as the severity of injury rises. The concept of operation when half of the blood volume has been transfused, as noted for splenic injury, is valid for liver injury as well. If a blush is seen on CT, angioembolization may be of benefit in the unstable child if immediately available prior to surgical exploration. Embolization is not indicated in the hemodynamically stable patient. Early operative intervention including damage-control laparotomy, coupled with angioembolization and early reoperation as a means to improve survival, has seen some success. The physiologic and hematologic effects of a massive transfusion in the child often make the operative management of liver injury very difficult.

Pediatric pancreatic injuries are uncommon and are most often due to blunt trauma. Bicycle-related injuries should be included in this category. The majority of pancreatic injuries in children may be treated successfully with nonoperative management, including gut rest, intravenous nutrition, and occasionally pancreatic antisecretory medication. Conservative management of children with a pancreatic transection may be more controversial. The beneficial effects of a spleen-sparing distal pancreatectomy, even in the face of a delayed diagnosis, have been noted. When the capabilities for pediatric endoscopic retrograde cholangiopancreatography (ERCP)

are available, ductal stenting may be of significant benefit. Other surgeons, as well as our group, have been able to employ laparoscopic distal pancreatectomy with splenic salvage for pancreatic transection when stenting could not be accomplished.

Blunt trauma is the most common mechanism of renal injury in children. Contusion is the most common injury seen. Renal injury can occur in the absence of hematuria. Nonoperative management of most pediatric renal injuries (grades I–III) can be accomplished safely. Nonoperative management for renal salvage appears to be successful in most cases, even with grade IV injuries, but operative renal salvage for grade V injuries appears to be uncommon. Ureteral stenting for urine leaks may be needed in patients with injuries of the collecting system. Rarely, nephrectomy for exsanguinating injury may be needed and would typically be initiated when 40 mL/kg of blood transfusion had been necessary and administered. Angioembolization may be considered in some cases; however, the majority of patients will not require emergency procedural intervention. Because most injured children now undergo abdominal CT scanning, CT cystography should be considered on every child to evaluate for bladder injury. The majority of bladder injuries can be treated successfully with urethral catheters, without the need for additional suprapubic drainage.

Vascular injuries in children are uncommon. Children can tolerate complete vascular occlusion to arms and legs to a greater degree than adults. Extremity vascular injuries are equally divided between blunt and penetrating mechanisms. Limb salvage is typically greater than 95%. Abdominal aortic injuries can occur due to seat belt injuries, bicycle injuries, and ATV-related injuries. Immediate direct vessel repair is an optimal management plan, due to related internal injuries. Endovascular stents have not been evaluated for long-term use in children and especially in the growing child.

Orthopedic injuries are the greatest cause of required operative intervention in injured children. These injuries are often of such magnitude that they distract the child from complaining of other, more serious injuries. Thus, orthopedic injuries are also a significant source of missed injury in the injured child. Missed injuries are the most important reason that a tertiary examination should be considered for all children admitted to the hospital. Cervical spine injuries are often misdiagnosed, and most of the missed injuries are due to normal variants.

ACKNOWLEDGMENT

Supported in part by the Paula Milburn Miller/Children's Medical Research Institute, Chair in Pediatric Surgery, Oklahoma City, Oklahoma.

For the chapter's Suggested Readings list, please visit the book at www.ExpertConsult.inkling.com.

TRAUMA IN PREGNANCY

Amy C. Sisley and William C. Chiu

The pregnant trauma patient presents significant challenges to the trauma surgeon. The physiologic changes in the mother during pregnancy represent both diagnostic and treatment dilemmas, and the need to treat two patients simultaneously may represent both clinical and emotional challenges for the trauma team.

EPIDEMIOLOGY

Trauma complicates 7% to 8% of pregnancies and is the leading non-obstetric cause of maternal death. The incidence of significant maternal and fetal injury increases with gestational age, with slightly over 50% of injuries occurring in the third trimester.

The most common mechanisms of injury for maternal trauma are motor vehicle collisions (MVCs) at 55% to 70%, followed by blunt trauma assault at 12% to 22% and falls at 9% to 22%.

Risk factors associated with adverse fetal outcome include Injury Severity Score (ISS) higher than 15, significant head injury as indicated by Glasgow Coma Scale score lower than 8, and Adjusted Injury

Score higher than 3 in the head, abdomen, thorax, or lower extremities. In addition, pelvic fractures, elevated maternal lactate level, and active uterine contractions are associated with increased risk of fetal demise.

Data from the American College of Surgeons National Trauma Data Bank has yielded the largest study of pregnant trauma patients to date ($n = 1195$). When compared to their nonpregnant counterparts, pregnant trauma patients were younger, more likely to be African American or Hispanic, and less likely to be wearing seat belts than their nonpregnant counterparts. These risk characteristics may be useful in designing prevention strategies in order to optimize efficacy.

MECHANISM OF INJURY

Blunt Trauma

Blunt trauma is the leading cause of both maternal and fetal death and is usually a consequence of MVCs, assaults, or falls. Although mortality rates are similar for pregnant versus nonpregnant blunt trauma patients, with equivalent ISSs, their patterns of injury are notably different. Pregnant patients injured in MVCs are more likely to sustain significant abdominal injuries and less likely to sustain head injuries than their nonpregnant counterparts. Splenic, hepatic, and retroperitoneal injuries occur more frequently in gravid trauma patients, partly because of the increased vascularity associated with pregnancy as well as to the displacement of the abdominal contents by the uterus. Up to 25% of pregnant blunt trauma patients sustain significant splenic or hepatic lacerations.

Direct injury to the fetus from blunt trauma is rare (<1%). The leading cause of fetal fatality after blunt trauma is maternal fatality followed by placental abruption. Because the uterus is elastic and the placenta is not, sheering forces can result in placental abruption, even in otherwise minor blunt abdominal trauma. The estimated incidence of abruption is 2% to 3% for minor trauma and up to 40% for severe blunt abdominal trauma. Uterine rupture occurs less commonly than placental abruption but increases in incidence with gestational age. Although uterine rupture is life threatening to both the mother and the fetus, its diagnosis is often difficult, given the variable and sometimes subtle clinical presentation. The clinician must maintain a high index of suspicion for both placental abruption and uterine rupture in any patient with blunt abdominal trauma, especially in late gestation.

Penetrating Trauma

Penetrating trauma is usually the result of either gunshot wounds (GSWs) or stabbing. This type of injury in pregnant patients is most often sustained at the hands of a spouse or intimate partner. Death rates for these injuries are actually decreased in pregnant patients compared with nonpregnant patients, owing to the protective effect for the mother of the gravid uterus. Unfortunately, the consequence to the fetus is a mortality rate of 71% for abdominal GSWs and 42% for abdominal stab wounds. It should also be noted that due to the upward displacement of intraabdominal content by the uterus in pregnancy, upper quadrant abdominal stab wounds carry a high risk for small bowel injury in pregnant patients.

Intimate Partner Violence

Intimate partner violence (IPV) is not uncommon in pregnancy. Between 7.4% and 21% of pregnant patients reported physical abuse at the hands of an intimate partner and fully two thirds reported an escalation of violence during pregnancy. Physically abused women have higher rates of miscarriage and low-birth-weight infants than nonabused women. Battering during pregnancy is not only associated with an increase in the frequency of abuse but also with a threefold increase in the risk of homicide compared with physically abused women who are not pregnant. Hence, intrapartum battering is a marker for a particularly violent and potentially lethal relationship.

PHYSIOLOGIC ALTERATIONS OF PREGNANCY

The extent of the anatomic and physiologic changes that occur during normal pregnancy is dependent on gestational age. During the first trimester, early changes are easily adapted to, so there is minimal functional alteration. By the third trimester, virtually every organ system has undergone change to compensate for the enlarged uterus and growing fetus. It is most important to remember that the presence of a fetus and the physical size of the abdomen are not the only aspects to consider when caring for the injured pregnant patient.

During the entire first trimester, the uterine size is small enough so that it remains relatively well protected by the bony pelvis. The earliest physiologic changes result from the presence of the placenta. Hormones released from the placenta include human chorionic gonadotropin (hCG), human placental lactogen (hPL), progesterone, estrogen, adrenocorticotropic hormone (ACTH), and thyroid-stimulating hormone (TSH). These hormones increase maternal insulin resistance and promote hyperglycemia. The subsequent increase in insulin and glucose levels translate into enhanced protein synthesis for the fetus. The reproductive hormones also inhibit gastrointestinal motility, which increases the potential for aspiration as early as 8 to 12 weeks of gestation.

Increased levels of estrogen and progesterone, as well as of renin and aldosterone, lead to increased sodium resorption and plasma volume expansion beginning at about 10 weeks of gestation. Although heart rate, mean arterial pressure, and central venous pressure are not yet altered, the cardiac output may start to increase by 1 to 1.5 L/minute (Table 1). Progesterone also promotes hypertrophy of the kidneys from 10 weeks of gestation and leads to impaired gallbladder contraction and bile stasis. Beginning at the end of the first trimester, there may be an increase in gallstone formation.

Second Trimester

During the second trimester, the uterus begins to rise out of the pelvis, and by 20 weeks, it may reach the umbilicus (Fig. 1). Blood pressure falls by about 5 to 15 mm Hg and reaches its lowest level of the pregnancy. In traumatic maternal hemorrhage, placental blood flow is preferentially reduced, and 30% of maternal blood volume may be lost prior to signs of shock. The "supine hypotensive syndrome" is caused by compression of the inferior vena cava by the gravid uterus,

TABLE 1: Cardiovascular Alterations during Pregnancy

Parameter	TRIMESTER		
	1st	2nd	3rd
Cardiac output	Increased	Increased	Increased
Stroke volume	Increased	Increased	Increased
Heart rate	Normal	Normal	Increased
MAP	Normal	Decreased	Normal
SVR	Normal	Decreased	Decreased

MAP, Mean arterial pressure; SVR, systemic vascular resistance.

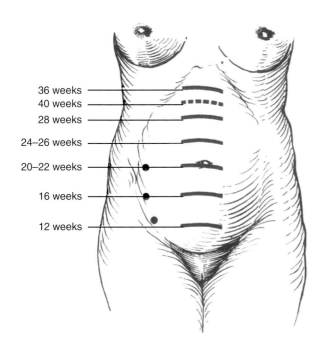

FIGURE 1 The height of the uterine fundus relative to the abdominal wall. *(Courtesy of David Gens, MD.)*

36 weeks
40 weeks
28 weeks
24–26 weeks
20–22 weeks
16 weeks
12 weeks

TABLE 2: Respiratory Alterations during Pregnancy

Parameter	Alteration
P_{CO_2}	Decreased
Minute ventilation	Increased
Tidal volume	Increased
Functional residual capacity	Decreased
2,3-DPG	Increased

2,3-DPG, 2,3-Diphosphoglycerate; P_{CO_2}, partial pressure of carbon dioxide.

The movement of gastrointestinal viscera cephalad is associated with a displacement of the gastroesophageal sphincter into the thorax. Placental release of gastrin augments the acid production of the stomach, making the risk for aspiration greatest at this time.

Uterine compression of the bladder and ureters results in a compensated hydronephrosis. The increase in blood volume and cardiac output is associated with increased renal blood flow of up to 80% and increased glomerular filtration rate of 50%. Blood urea nitrogen and serum creatinine are commonly reduced, but urine output volume does not significantly change.

DIAGNOSIS

Primary Survey

The initial evaluation of the pregnant trauma patient should include early consultation with the obstetrics service as well as neonatology if appropriate (>24 weeks of gestation). The general principles of evaluation of trauma patients are similar to those of the nonpregnant patient and include initial focus on assessing and stabilizing maternal vital signs. These include the standard Advanced Trauma Life Support (ATLS) primary survey, which is then followed by a rapid and brief assessment of the fetus for viability. Because pressure from the pregnant uterus on the inferior vena cava can result in a decrease in cardiac return, an effort should be made to displace the uterus laterally in pregnant patients. This may be accomplished by tilting the backboard to the side or by manually displacing the uterus to the left side.

Indications for intubation in the pregnant trauma patient are similar to those in the nonpregnant patient, although aspiration risk is higher during pregnancy. It should be kept in mind, however, that the fetus will not tolerate hypoxemia as well as the mother, so supplemental oxygen should always be applied and oxygen saturation monitored in all pregnant patients.

Accurate assessment of maternal volume status may be complicated by the physiologic changes of pregnancy. Because the fetus will be compromised by even minor maternal hypovolemia, aggressive volume replacement should be undertaken. Vasopressors and inotropes may actually reduce maternal blood flow to the fetus and should not be used as a substitute for volume resuscitation in alleviating maternal hypotension. Immediate jeopardy of the mother's life may occasionally necessitate the use of vasopressors or inotropes for circulatory support, but they should be used sparingly and discontinued as rapidly as possible.

Secondary Survey

The secondary survey is then performed in accordance with ATLS guidelines, with the caveat that examination of the perineum must include a formal examination of the vagina and cervix to evaluate

---

decreasing venous blood return and thereby decreasing preload and cardiac output. Turning the mother left side down increases cardiac output by about 30% after 20 weeks of gestation.

Third Trimester

By the seventh month, the pubic symphysis and sacroiliac joints widen. At approximately 36 weeks of gestation, the uterus reaches its maximal height near the costal margins. Intraperitoneal structures are displaced cephalad and laterally.

During the third trimester, blood pressure returns to more normal levels and heart rate increases up to 20 beats per minute relative to the nonpregnant state. This physiologic tachycardia must be considered when evaluating the pregnant trauma patient. Pulmonary capillary wedge pressure and left ventricular function remain normal, but systemic and pulmonary vascular resistances are decreased.

After 30 weeks of gestation, plasma volume has increased 40%, accompanied by a 15% increase in red blood cell mass. This discrepancy leads to the "physiologic anemia of pregnancy." Serum albumin declines by up to 30% because of this volume expansion. Benign physiologic pericardial effusion is more prevalent and may complicate the focused assessment with sonography for trauma (FAST). The decrease in colloid oncotic pressure may increase the risk for pulmonary edema. A hypercoagulable state is also induced because of an increase in nearly all coagulation factors, procoagulants and fibrinogen, and a reduction in fibrinolytic activity.

Anatomic changes in the thorax include the diaphragm rising about 4 cm and the chest diameter increasing by 2 cm. The most significant changes in respiratory function include an increase in minute ventilation by as much as 50%, mostly by an increase in tidal volume (Table 2). Functional residual capacity decreases largely due to elevation of the diaphragm. A state of compensated respiratory alkalosis results in a chronic reduced Pa_{CO_2} to approximately 30 mm Hg and reduced plasma bicarbonate level. Oxygen release to the fetus is also facilitated by increased levels of 2,3-diphosphoglycerate. These changes leave the pregnant patient with diminished oxygen reserve and buffering capacity.

for bleeding. The pelvic examination should be performed by an obstetrician if possible.

The physical examination of the abdomen is difficult in pregnancy because of displacement of abdominal contents from their normal position. Additionally, stretching of the abdominal wall by the uterus in late pregnancy may result in a relative insensitivity to peritoneal irritation, resulting in difficulty in detecting peritonitis on clinical examination alone. The FAST examination represents a rapid and noninvasive means of evaluating the patient for the presence of intra-abdominal fluid. The sensitivity of the FAST examination in pregnant patients, at 83%, is slightly lower than in the nonpregnant population; however, the specificity is similar at 96%. Although it does not replace formal fetal ultrasonography, the FAST examination may be used to get a rapid picture of the fetal status during the initial resuscitation by detecting the fetal heart rate. The FAST examination has also been reported to detect unsuspected pregnancies in some trauma patients, thus influencing subsequent management. The use of ultrasonography does not involve ionizing radiation and poses no known risk to the developing fetus.

Initial Evaluation of the Fetus

The initial evaluation of the fetus is part of the secondary survey and potentially includes ultrasonography, fetal monitoring, and obstetric consultation if not previously obtained. Formal pelvic ultrasonography can determine if the fetus is still viable and can calculate gestational age. It should be noted that ultrasonography is unreliable in predicting placental abruption.

Cardiotrophic monitoring is the mainstay of fetal assessment in the third trimester. The practice management guidelines of the Eastern Association for the Surgery of Trauma (EAST) include a recommendation that all pregnancies greater than 20 weeks of gestation should undergo fetal monitoring for a minimum of 6 hours. More prolonged monitoring has been recommended in cases of uterine contractions, abnormal fetal heart rate patterns, and severe maternal trauma. Fetal monitoring is used to evaluate both the state of the fetus and the presence and frequency of uterine contractions. It is the single most reliable tool available for the assessment of placental abruption. The use of fetal monitoring routinely, even in cases of apparently minor maternal trauma, must be emphasized. A recent multi-institutional study of 13 Level I and Level II trauma centers revealed that fetal monitoring was obtained on only 61% of trauma patients with third trimester pregnancies.

Exposure to Radiation from Diagnostic Radiographs

Invariably, the necessity of obtaining radiographs in the evaluation of the pregnant patient raises concern about radiation exposure and subsequent damage to the fetus. Because the most important predictor of fetal outcome is maternal outcome, the clinician caring for the injured pregnant patient should not hesitate to obtain diagnostic radiographs that are necessary for the evaluation of the mother. These diagnostic tests should be limited to those that will have impact on maternal outcome and for which there is no alternative test. Redundancy should be eliminated. Hence, if it is known that the patient will require computed tomography (CT) scans of the chest and abdomen, plain films of the chest and thoracolumbar spine need not be obtained. Radiation exposure is extremely low when the fetus is outside the CT field of view. CT scanning of the head, cervical spine, or extremities (excluding hip/pelvis) is considered safe during any trimester of pregnancy. The dose of ionizing radiation to the fetus can be further reduced by the use of lead shielding whenever possible.

Predicting teratogenicity as a consequence of fetal radiation exposure is difficult; however, no study has shown an increase above baseline for exposures of 10 rad (100 mGy). According to the recommendations on radiation exposure during pregnancy made by the

TABLE 3: Estimated Fetal Exposure from Radiographs

Procedure	Approximate Fetal Dose* (rad)
Plain Films	
Chest (two views)	0.00002–0.00007
Abdomen	0.1
Cervical spine	0.002
Pelvis	0.040
Thoracolumbar spine	0.370
CT Scans†	
Head CT	<0.05
Chest CT	<0.100
Abdominal CT	2.60

CT, Computed tomography.
*Dose varies depending on exact procedure used and on body habits.
†Estimate based on 10-mm slices.
Modified from Barraco RD, Chiu WC, Clancy, et al: Practice management guidelines for the diagnosis and management of injury in the pregnant patient: the EAST Practice Management Guidelines Work Group. *J Trauma* 69(1):211–214, 2010; Eastern Association for the Surgery of Trauma, World Wide Web site, http://www.east.org/tpg/pregnancy.pdf; and Wakeford R, Little MP: Risk coefficients for childhood cancer after intrauterine irradiation: a review. *Int J Rad Biol* 79(5):293–299, 2003.

American College of Obstetrics and Gynecology (ACOG), exposure of 5 rad (50 mGy) is not associated with any increase in risk of fetal loss or of birth defects. It should also be kept in mind that teratogenicity is a function of gestational age; the fetus is most vulnerable during the period of organogenesis (2–8 weeks after conception). Other than teratogenicity, the principal concern in exposing a fetus to radiation is that of increasing the risk of childhood cancers. The National Radiation Protection Board of Britain cites a 6% excess risk per 100 rad exposure.

Most of the common radiographic tests employed in the evaluation of trauma patients are associated with fetal radiation doses of 1/100 rad or less (Table 3). The exception to this is the abdominal CT, with a radiation dose of 2.60 rad for 10-mm slices. This is still only about half of the 5-rad dose cited by ACOG as safe. However, it should be kept in mind that the newer multiplanar scanners may have a higher radiation exposure. In addition, failure to account for variability in the body habitus of the patient as well as variability in the depth of the fetus from the maternal skin surface may result in significant errors in estimation of the fetal radiation dose. Consultation with the radiology department is strongly recommended in planning a diagnostic workup that will minimize the risk of radiation exposure.

SURGICAL MANAGEMENT

The majority of traumatic injuries to the pregnant patient are treated similarly to those in nonpregnant patients. In general, injuries requiring operative intervention would be the same in the pregnant patient and in the nonpregnant patient. The additional considerations necessary in pregnancy are that general anesthesia and abdominal surgery may precipitate premature labor. Direct injury to the uterus, maternal shock, or fetal distress may require emergency cesarean section.

Blunt Trauma

Uterine rupture occurs in only 0.6% of instances of blunt trauma during pregnancy. Direct fetal injury is also very rare and complicates less than 1% of cases. As it is in the nonpregnant patient, nonoperative management of abdominal solid organ injuries should be the treatment of choice in hemodynamically stable pregnant patients. The greatest difference in nonoperative management of abdominal injuries is that angiographic therapeutic adjuncts are not advisable because of the potential for large radiation exposure. In unstable patients, operative management may best limit maternal and fetal shock, and the indications for laparotomy are similar to those in nonpregnant patients. Hemodynamic instability in patients with blunt abdominal trauma and free intraperitoneal fluid found by ultrasonography are indications for urgent laparotomy (Fig. 2). At laparotomy, the uterus should be left intact unless there is direct uterine injury.

Pelvic fractures have several serious implications in the pregnant patient and may be associated with fetal demise in up to 25% of cases. Engorgement of pelvic and retroperitoneal vasculature renders any pelvic fracture at increased risk for significant hemorrhage. Fetal injury or death may result from direct placental injury or from maternal shock (Fig. 3). Pelvic angiography for embolization should be an adjunct used for life-threatening pelvic hemorrhage, as the radiation required for the procedure exceeds safe levels for the fetus.

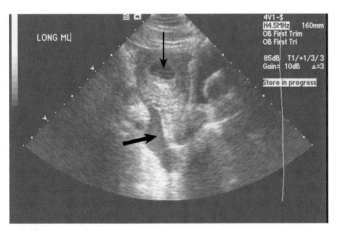

FIGURE 2   Ultrasound of a car crash victim showing an early intrauterine pregnancy (*small arrow*) and free fluid in the abdomen (*large arrow*).

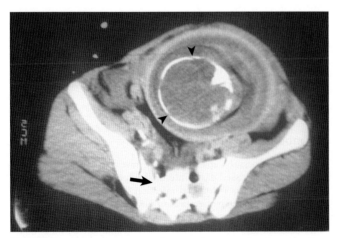

FIGURE 3   Computed tomography scan demonstrating fracture of the maternal pelvis (*long arrow*) with concomitant fracture of the fetal skull (*short arrows*).

Penetrating Trauma

As the uterus enlarges and rises out of the bony pelvis, the risk of injury from penetrating trauma increases. The muscular uterine wall is somewhat resilient to low-velocity stab wounds to the abdomen but is not an adequate barrier to GSWs. Patients who should have urgent laparotomy are those who are hemodynamically unstable, those with obvious transperitoneal penetration, and those with free intraperitoneal fluid found on ultrasonography. Although the diagnostic options available are similar to those of nonpregnant patients, the main concern would be the exposure of ionizing radiation. It may be prudent to use local wound exploration to evaluate superficial stab wounds whenever possible. Diagnostic peritoneal lavage (DPL) has relative contraindications in pregnancy, and there is the special consideration for the need of a supraumbilical location for access.

The use of CT scanning in penetrating torso trauma in the pregnant patient is an area that has not yet been well studied. In blunt trauma, the judicious use of abdominopelvic CT scanning to evaluate for abdominal injury is recommended. In penetrating trauma, the benefits and risks of the options must be considered. In penetrating torso trauma in nonpregnant patients, triple contrast abdominopelvic CT reliably excludes peritoneal penetration to prevent unnecessary laparotomy. The risks of CT scanning include the fetal exposure to ionizing radiation. The risks of general anesthesia and unnecessary laparotomy must be considered in balance. Without clear evidence and recommendations on the use of CT in penetrating torso trauma, careful individual decision making and judgment are required between immediate laparotomy and diagnostic CT scanning.

Cesarean Section

Although the importance of emergency cesarean section for fetal salvage is evident, the indications for perimortem cesarean section remain controversial (Table 4). Morris et al showed that emergency cesarean section for patients at greater than 25 weeks of gestation was associated with a 45% fetal survival rate and that 60% of infant deaths resulted from delay in recognition of fetal distress. In this multicenter study, infant survival was independent of maternal injury, and no fetus delivered without fetal heart tones survived.

Perimortem cesarean section refers to those cases of emergency cesarean section performed surrounding maternal death, whether fetal delivery is performed prior to or after actual maternal death, and should be considered in any moribund pregnant patient of at least 24 weeks gestational age if fetal heart tones are still present. When performed following maternal death, fetal neurologic outcome and survival are closely dependent upon the time interval between maternal death and fetal delivery. Fetal delivery must occur within 20 minutes of maternal death, but should ideally start within 4 minutes of maternal cardiac arrest. The anticipated fetal survival rate is up to 70% when delivery is performed within 5 minutes of maternal death.

TABLE 4: Indications for Emergency and Perimortem Cesarean Section

Fetal hypoxia or distress
Premature rupture of membranes
Uterine injury or rupture
Amniotic fluid embolism
Disseminated intravascular coagulation
Gravid uterus complicating management at laparotomy
Maternal refractory shock or cardiac arrest

MORBIDITY AND COMPLICATIONS MANAGEMENT

The pregnant trauma patient is at risk for complications specifically associated with the pregnancy and fetus. Changes in the anatomy and physiology of pregnancy may also place the pregnant patient at increased risk for some potential complications that are not directly related to the pregnancy.

Fetomaternal Hemorrhage

Fetomaternal hemorrhage occurs in up to 28% of pregnancies after trauma. The amount of Rh-positive fetal blood required to sensitize the Rh-negative mother is variable, but most patients are sensitized by as little as 0.01 mL of blood. The extent of fetomaternal hemorrhage and Rh alloimmunization is evaluated with the Kleihauer-Betke (KB) test. The test uses a stain that identifies fetal red blood cells with hemoglobin F in maternal blood. The ratio of fetal-to-maternal red blood cells can be assessed. Treatment with Rh immunoglobulin should be given early, along with obstetric consultation, but definitely within 72 hours of injury.

Premature Labor

Many cases of mild uterine contractions after trauma resolve spontaneously. Instances of true premature labor involve both preterm contractions and evidence of cervical dilation and may need to be treated with pharmacologic tocolytics. Several agents are available for tocolysis, including terbutaline and magnesium sulfate, and should only be administered with obstetric consultation. Traumatic injury, surgery, and general anesthesia may increase the risk of premature labor. Drost et al reported an 80% efficacy using tocolysis in a study of major trauma in pregnancy. Blunt abdominal trauma may cause premature rupture of membranes leading to premature labor.

Preeclampsia and Eclampsia

Systemic blood pressure is normally decreased beginning in the second trimester. Any hypertension in these patients may be a sign of preeclampsia. Control of pregnancy-induced hypertension is important to prevent uterine vasoconstriction and placental ischemia. The initial treatment includes fluid resuscitation to expand intravascular volume. These patients may also require vasodilator therapy or inotropic support to improve perfusion. Preeclampsia typically resolves following fetal delivery.

Pregnant trauma patients with altered sensorium, coma, or seizures may have eclampsia. Associated signs may include hypertension, oliguria, proteinuria, pulmonary edema, and disseminated intravascular coagulation (DIC). As in the treatment of preeclampsia, fluid resuscitation and hemodynamic support is necessary. Intravenous magnesium sulfate should be administered, and cesarean section should be considered in those patients at 28 weeks of gestation or greater.

Placental Abruption

In surviving pregnant trauma patients, placental abruption is the most common cause for fetal death and occurs in 30% to 70% of severely injured patients. The mechanisms for abruption in blunt trauma may be either from uteroplacental ischemia from maternal shock or from mechanical shearing as a result of deceleration forces. The uterus lacks autoregulation of perfusion and is very sensitive to changes in maternal blood pressure. Maternal hypovolemia or hypotension causes uterine vasoconstriction and hypoperfusion. Later in pregnancy, relatively minor blunt trauma may result in abruption.

In the setting of trauma, the signs of abruption may be as subtle as occult vaginal bleeding and abdominal pain, or may be severe enough to result in shock or DIC. The absence of vaginal bleeding does not exclude abruption. Uteroplacental separation of up to 25% may result in vaginal bleeding and premature labor. Separation of greater than 50% usually results in fetal demise. Delayed placental abruption has been reported up to 6 days after trauma.

Amniotic Fluid Embolization

Amniotic fluid embolism refers to the entrance of amniotic fluid into the maternal circulation. It more commonly presents during labor or the immediate postpartum period, and the risk of maternal mortality is up to 80%. Pregnant trauma patients suffering from premature labor may be at risk. The diagnosis is mostly made on clinical signs, and the manifestations include severe dyspnea, hypoxia, hypotension, altered sensorium or seizures, and possible cardiac arrest. Respiratory failure mimics that seen in the acute respiratory distress syndrome. Patients may develop thrombocytopenia or DIC. Following fetal delivery, the maternal treatment for this condition is largely supportive. These supportive measures include supplemental oxygen or mechanical ventilation, fluid resuscitation, inotropes, vasopressors, and blood product replacement.

Venous Thromboembolism

The hypercoagulable state associated with pregnancy is caused by an increase in coagulation factors and inhibition of fibrinolysis. The hypercoagulable state exacerbates conditions of prolonged immobilization in trauma patients with neurologic injury, pelvic or lower extremity fractures, and critical illness. Prophylaxis with subcutaneous low-molecular-weight heparin or low-dose unfractionated heparin, in combination with lower extremity intermittent pneumatic venous compression devices, is recommended. Heparin products do not cross the placental barrier and are considered safe during pregnancy. Although warfarin products are contraindicated during pregnancy, patients may be transitioned to warfarin post partum.

Acute deep vein thrombosis (DVT) should be treated with full anticoagulation doses of heparin. Although both unfractionated heparin and low-molecular-weight heparin are considered safe and effective during pregnancy, the ability to titrate continuous infusion heparin has advantages with acute traumatic injury and the potential need for unplanned delivery.

The method of radiologic diagnosis for pulmonary embolism (PE) remains controversial. Winer-Muram et al showed that the average fetal dose of ionizing radiation from a helical thoracic CT scan for PE is less than that with ventilation-perfusion lung scanning and was safe in all three trimesters. The use of inferior vena cava filters for PE prophylaxis and the safety of thrombolytic agents for severe cases of PE have not been well studied.

Intraabdominal Infection

Although unnecessary laparotomy may have a risk for maternal and fetal morbidity, missed gastrointestinal injury may result in greater complications. Intra-abdominal infection is particularly harmful to the fetus, and aggressive surgical or interventional therapy should be considered. Antibiotic therapy should be administered with infectious diseases and requires pharmacy consultation because many agents may have adverse effects on the fetus. Empiric antibiotic selection should consider both the likely etiologic organisms and the safety of the fetus.

Mortality

Reported fetal mortality rates due to trauma vary, but are as high as 61% for major trauma and 80% for maternal shock. Even minor trauma is associated with a 1% to 5% fetal mortality rate. The incidence of significant maternal and fetal injury increases with gestational age, with slightly over 50% of injuries occurring in the third trimester. The most common cause of fetal death is maternal death followed by placental abruption. The most common mechanism associated with fatality for both mother and fetus is the MVC. This mechanism alone accounts for 82% of fetal deaths. It should be noted that the fetal death rate is affected by maternal age, with peak fetal death rates in mothers aged 15 to 19. This may reflect the greater propensity for patients in that age group to participate in risk-taking behavior such as alcohol and substance abuse, with an increased incidence of both MVCs and interpersonal violence.

The single most important measure to be taken to reduce mortality rate among pregnant women is the promotion of seat belt use. The use of seat belts results in a significant decrease in maternal (and hence fetal) fatality. It has been shown that along with crash severity, the use of seat belts is the best predictor of maternal and fetal outcome. Three-point restraints should be used with the belt low on the pelvis, below the uterine fundus, with the shoulder belt placed between the breasts.

CONCLUSIONS

The evaluation and treatment of the pregnant trauma patient represent a significant challenge to the trauma team. Optimization of the outcome depends on an understanding of the physiologic changes that occur in pregnancy as well as a firm grasp of the strategies that are necessary to assess both the mother and the fetus. Care must be maternally directed at the outset because the best way to save the fetus is to save the mother. Fetal monitoring of third trimester pregnancies is essential in the early detection of both premature labor and fetal distress. Finally, a multidisciplinary approach, with early involvement of consultants from obstetrics, is an essential element of successful care.

For the chapter's Suggested Readings list, please visit the book at www.ExpertConsult.inkling.com.

TRAUMA IN OUR "ELDERS"

Daniel J. Grabo, Benjamin M. Braslow, and C. William Schwab

As the elderly population increases across America, it is important for surgeons and physicians to understand how age-related anatomic and physiologic changes in addition to chronic medical conditions can alter clinical presentation and management of older trauma patients. The United States is experiencing unprecedented growth in the number of older adults, which is commonly defined as age 65 and above. As the baby boomers continue to age and life expectancy continues to lengthen secondary to improved health care and preventive medicine, the population of older Americans will double during the next 25 years. By 2030 the number of adults over age 65 years is expected to increase by 70 million, and the number of "oldest old," those over 80 years, will increase to nearly 20 million persons. The younger cohorts of our "elders" will live longer, be more active, and enjoy better health.

As older Americans continue to age they will experience common age-related medical conditions, with 80% of our elders living with at least one chronic health problem and 50% living with two. Moreover, the consequences of age such as diminished postural stability, motor strength, coordination, vision, and hearing will predispose our elders to injury. Despite being injured less often than those under age 65, older Americans who are injured have higher case fatality rates. Trauma or unintentional injury is the fourth leading cause of death for Americans 55 to 64 years old and the ninth leading cause of death for Americans 65 years and older. Mechanisms of injury, such as falls and motor vehicle crashes (MVCs), are similar in frequency in younger and older Americans; however, injury patterns, effects, and outcomes differ significantly in these two groups. With decreasing activity, the "oldest old" experience age-related changes that limit their functional status and ability. Falls, especially from ground level, account for a significant number of emergency department visits and hospital admissions. Trauma in the elderly when compared to younger adults results in sicker patients, despite low Injury Severity Scores (ISS), increased hospital length of stay, and increased mortality rate.

As the number of older Americans increases, those providing emergency care for them need to appreciate that the common injuries sustained frequently result in significant morbidity. Understanding the age-related physiologic changes, the common mechanisms of injury, and the organ specific injuries that are sustained will more than likely result in better emergency care and improved outcomes for this unique group of injured patients. Moreover, the integration of geriatric medicine consult service with the trauma team may also serve to assess for fall risk, delirium/dementia, and polypharmacy. In addition, the presence of geriatric consultation may aid the trauma team with the often difficult ethical and end-of-life issues that can be associated with severely injured elders.

PHYSIOLOGIC CHANGES

Older individuals are known to have a diminished ability to handle the stress of surgery, trauma, and infection. This change is the result of normal age-related anatomic and physiologic changes that affect each organ system. The presence of chronic disease and certain medications (i.e., anticoagulants and cardiovascular drugs) can have deleterious effects on the older trauma patient.

The central nervous system (CNS) in the older adult is affected by cortical atrophy and pathologic changes such as amyloid deposition and arteriosclerotic cerebrovascular disease. Clinically, this is manifested by blunted sensation (visual, auditory, tactile, and pain perception) and altered cognition. These changes in addition to alterations in cerebellar function, gait, and balance increase the risk of injury, especially falls. Injury and polypharmacy can make the injured older adult more susceptible to anxiety, agitation, and delirium.

Cardiovascular disease is one of the most common chronic medical conditions and is present in up to 80% of octogenarians. A progressive loss of cardiac myocytes with compensatory hypertrophy leads to reduced compensatory capacity and myocardial dysfunction. Fibrosis of cardiac autonomic tissue often results in conduction abnormalities in the form of arrhythmias and varying degree of heart block. Arteriosclerotic vascular disease predisposes to impaired blood flow to organs and tissues. Older adults often take medications that affect the cardiovascular system such as beta blockers, calcium channel blockers, antihypertensive agents, and diuretics. As a result of age-related changes to the cardiovascular system and common medications, the older adult is often unable to improve cardiac contractility and heart rate in response to exogenous stress and endogenous catecholamines. They are often preload dependent and thus do poorly in hypovolemia.

Decreases in chest wall compliance, respiratory muscle strength, and lung elasticity results in a decline in respiratory function with increased age. Alveolar collapse can diminish surface area available for gas exchange, causing decreases in arterial oxygenation. In the setting of injury, respiratory insufficiency and failure can result from age-related changes in pulmonary compliance, an inability to mount an effective cough, and impaired gas exchange. Adequate treatment of injury-related torso pain (specifically chest wall pain) is of vital importance or poor inspiratory effort, atelectasis, and pneumonia may develop. Epidural anesthesia/analgesia has become an adjunct to commonly used opioids, often in the form of patient-controlled analgesia, and nonsteroidal anti-inflammatory drugs (NSAIDs).

With increasing age, anatomic and physiologic changes occur in the kidney. Effective renal cortex mass decreases and can result in a functional cortical loss of as much as 25%. In addition, there is a decrease in glomerular filtration rate (GFR) and impaired renal tubule reabsorption and secretion. The elderly patient often has problems with solute clearance and fluid balance. Due to a decrease in lean body mass and creatinine production, serum creatinine levels can remain within normal range despite significantly decreased renal function. Calculation of creatinine clearance should be based on age and body mass.

With advanced age, there is a decrease in muscle mass, strength, and responsiveness. Bone density is also greatly decreased. The frequency and severity of bony fractures increases with age-related osteoporosis. The prevalence of osteoarthritis is high and is associated with compromised mobility and pain. The vertebral column becomes stiffened and shortened, resulting in altered pulmonary mechanics. Spinal canal stenosis and vertebral osteophytes can be the result of osteoarthritis and predisposes to clinically significant spinal cord injury with only minimal mechanisms of injury. These anatomic changes in the elderly bones, joints, and spinal column also affect their ability to avoid injury. Increased activity has been shown to increase muscle mass and strength and as such slow the aging process.

Increasing age is thought to inhibit the older adult from mounting an appropriate inflammatory response to infection and injury. The neutrophil is the first-line defense against infection and also exhibits age-related decline in function, such as decreased phagocytic ability. Changes in the autonomic nervous system (sympathetic and parasympathetic) can have deleterious effects on homeostasis and temperature control. Markers of stress, for example, tumor necrosis factor and interleukin 6, in the elderly have been shown to be markedly elevated in response to even minor trauma, surgery, and infection. The systemic inflammatory response syndrome (SIRS) may result from this disproportionate increase in cytokines that are released in the elderly trauma patient.

Older adults exhibit increased sensitivity to benzodiazepines, anesthetics, opioids, and other CNS active drugs. Cardiovascular active medications, such as beta blockers, can blunt reflexive and catecholamine-induced tachycardia. Common medications, such as antibiotics, diuretics, and vasoactive medications, can have deleterious side effects on renal function. Computed tomography (CT) is commonly used in the evaluation of trauma patients. Despite the common fear, the use of intravenous (IV) contrast media in elderly trauma patients has not been shown to increase disproportionately the risk of acute kidney injury.

Antiplatelet agents, NSAIDs, and anticoagulants (warfarin) are common medications used in the management of chronic health conditions. Aspirin and clopidogrel irreversibly inhibit platelet activity, and platelet transfusion is the treatment of choice for platelet-associated coagulopathy. Desmopressin or DDAVP is an alternative to platelet transfusion in treating platelet-associated coagulopathy in the uremic patient. In an evaluation of the National Trauma Data Bank (NTDB), Cotton et al reported that warfarin use is increasing, especially in patients age 65 and older. Moreover, not only is warfarin

use common in injured patients, its use is a powerful marker of mortality rate. Plasma transfusion, containing coagulation factors, has traditionally been used to reverse warfarin-induced coagulopathy. Limited cardiopulmonary reserve is often present in elderly patients, and as such, the large volumes of plasma (10 to 15 mL/kg; 4 to 6 units; 800 to 1200 mL) that are commonly used to reverse a high international normalized ratio (INR) in younger patients can result in pulmonary edema in the older population. Vitamin K (5 to 10 mg, IV) can be used as an adjunct to plasma transfusion. Also, vitamin K–dependent coagulation factor containing prothrombin complex concentrates that are derived from human plasma has been shown to be effective in the elderly in decreasing time to reversal of INR as well as doing so with a limited volume. Recombinant factor VIIa (rFVIIa), which enhances thrombin generation and results in a stable hemostatic plug, has been used to treat moderate coagulopathy in traumatic brain injury and has been shown to be both safe and effective in the elderly cohort.

MECHANISM OF INJURY

The major type of geriatric injury is blunt trauma, with falls being the most common mechanism of injury followed by motor vehicle traffic injury. The NTDB reports 148,382 falls in persons age 55 and older who presented to designated trauma centers. Elderly women tend to fall more frequently than men, but case fatality rates for men, age 55 or older, are significantly higher for falls than their female counterparts. Older adults tend to fall from the standing or sitting position, known as ground level falls (GLFs), but younger adults are more likely to fall from height. Although the mechanism of a GLF is considered minor, undertriaging the elderly is a potential risk for morbidity and fatality as the severity of injury might be more than expected from this low-energy mechanism. Age older than 55 was found to be an independent risk factor of fatality in patients who presented after a GLF. Up to 6% of falls in the elderly result in clinically significant fractures, with 1% to 2% of these being hip fractures. Age-related changes, such as gait disturbances, declines in proprioception, and peripheral neuropathy, may contribute to the prevalence of falls. The frequent use of medications, such as beta blockers and sedatives, may cause orthostatic hypotension or alter proprioception and cognition and are risk factors for falls. Chronic medical conditions may contribute to syncopal events and weakness. Fall intervention programs include environmental modifications and modification of medications and have been shown to reduce fall incidence by 19% when implemented at elderly residence facilities. Moreover, physical strength and conditioning programs are successful at improving bone density and overall fitness, also reducing fall potential.

According to the National Highway Traffic and Safety Administration (NHTSA) in 2009, 187,000 people over the age of 65 were injured in motor vehicle traffic crashes and 5288 died. The elderly accounted for 16% of all traffic fatalities and 8% of motor vehicle traffic injuries. There were 32 million licensed older drivers in 2008, and this number is expected to increase as the population continues to age. Elderly drivers are more likely to have vehicular accidents during daylight hours, on weekdays, and in good weather. The same age-related changes and chronic medical conditions that compromise the mobility of older Americans will have adverse effects on their driving skills as well, such as declining reaction time and impaired vision. Alcohol intoxication, however, seems to play less of a role in older age group related motor vehicle traffic crashes than in younger cohorts. Discussion continues on the evaluation of elderly drivers as to their cognitive and physical abilities, but currently no federal or state mandates for driving restrictions are in effect.

Elderly pedestrians are at increased risk for being struck by moving vehicles. Declines in vision, hearing, and walking speed, as well as cognition and judgment, seem to be predisposing factors. Pedestrian being struck is the third most common mechanism of injury and accounts for greater than 20% of automobile versus pedestrian fatalities. Age plays a critical role in the distribution of injuries as well as severity. Time allotted for traversing crosswalks may be insufficient for the slowed walking speed of many elderly persons. Nearly one third of all pedestrian fatalities in people age 65 and older occurred within a crosswalk. Identification of dangerous intersections and appropriate safety measures, such as crossing guards, may help to decrease pedestrian fatalities in the older age groups.

Although attacks on the elderly primarily involve blunt instruments, penetrating injuries account for over 50% of assault-related fatalities in the elderly. Although the elderly make up a small portion of the number of assault victims in this country, they are four times more likely to die than younger assault victims. Mortality rate from penetrating trauma remains steady in younger cohorts (approximately 10%) and increases after age 55 (14%–26%). In elderly gunshot wound (GSW) patients, low admission Glasgow Coma Scale score, ISS 16 and above, and hypotension are more predictive of fatality than increased age alone. Decreased strength and mobility are the major factors that impair the elderly in self-defense. Impairments in cognition and judgment may affect situational awareness and decision making, leading to worse outcomes in assaults upon the elderly.

Declines in physical strength and mobility as well as impaired judgment and cognition have led to increases in domestic abuse as a source of nonaccidental trauma in the elderly. Female gender and age greater than 80 are more often associated with elderly abuse. Injuries are often afflicted in the home or apartment by someone who knows or provides care for the victims. Neglect often precedes violence, and financial difficulties and altered family dynamics are often reasons for mistreatment. Physical injury that is inconsistent with the described mechanism and chronic signs of poor general hygiene should be investigated with a high degree of suspicion in order to identify the possibility of worse impending violence.

For the elderly, the suicide rate is 14 per 100,000 people per year in the United States, and the number is even higher in urban areas. The presence of chronic medical conditions, depression, and pain are common reasons for the frequency of suicide attempts in this population. Nearly 40% of gunshot injuries in the elderly are found to be self-inflicted.

The elderly seem to be particularly vulnerable to thermal injury due to decreased cutaneous sensation and reaction times. At a regional burn center in Marseille, France, 16% of all burn admissions were age 65 and older, and the mortality rate in this elder population reached 30%. Scalding, typically from bath water, appears to be the most common form of burn injury in the elderly. Mortality rates are higher than for age-matched younger patients. Burns exceeding 50% of total body surface area are uniformly fatal, and inhalation injuries are poorly tolerated. The massive volume of resuscitation needed in the management of burn patients can have deleterious effects on the elderly patient with limited cardiovascular reserve.

As the population ages, the activity level of our elders will increase. The elderly will be affected by the drawbacks of physical overloading, mostly due to the limited ability of the older adult to tolerate physical stress. Exertional injuries are common as a result of diminished reserve. Acute injuries most often will affect the musculoskeletal system and will be the result of sports activities. Some of these injuries will result in long-term inactivity and require prolonged rehabilitation. Treatment of these injuries should be aggressive and similar to that used in younger cohorts in order to prevent prolonged immobility and the possibility of permanent disability.

OUTCOMES

Elderly trauma patients fare worse than their age-matched cohorts in both the immediate postinjury phase as well as the long term. Trauma in the elderly and the subsequent management of injury often result in complications, such as congestive heart failure (CHF), respiratory insufficiency, acute kidney injury, and infection. There is an increased risk of reinjury or death in elderly trauma patients for as long as 5 years from the time of hospitalization for the initial injury. The presence and number of chronic medical conditions increase the risk of trauma-related fatality. As ISS rises above 15, however, the association of chronic medical conditions with fatality ceases to be significant. Moreover, ISS above 25 is independently associated with increased fatality in the elderly. Perdue et al found that when controlling for injury severity, comorbid conditions, and complications, the elderly were five times more likely to die after trauma when compared to younger cohorts.

The survival of severely injured patients can be significantly improved by the early presence of a trauma team, under the direction of an experienced trauma surgeon. Presenting physiology, mechanism of injury, and anatomic location are classically used to identify injured patients who would benefit from the high level of care provided at a mature trauma center. The mortality rate of elderly trauma patients when taken as a whole is in the range of 15% to 30%, as compared to less than 10% in younger cohorts. Evaluation of the geriatric trauma patient can be difficult as the physiologic response to trauma and injury may be blunted. Age-related declines in physiologic reserve, the presence of one or more comorbid conditions, and medications used to treat chronic health conditions may interfere with the normal physiologic response to injury. For example, tachycardia in response to hypovolemia may be blunted in the older adult who receives beta blockers. Moreover, a perceived normal blood pressure may be present in the elderly trauma patient with hypertension despite severe hemorrhage. More than 60% of elderly patients with severe injuries (ISS >15) and 25% with critical injuries (ISS >25) do not meet the hypotension (SBP <90 mm Hg) criteria for trauma team activation. Cardiovascular collapse, respiratory deterioration, and many complications can be prevented by early resuscitative efforts and continuous reassessment by the trauma team followed by admission to the intensive care unit (ICU) when appropriate. The expertise of the trauma team and ICU staff can limit unnecessary diagnostic testing, provide a rapid and comprehensive list of injuries and physiologic derangements, expedite therapeutic interventions, and accurately provide monitoring. The early identification of shock and limitation of hypoperfusion and hypoxia can prevent multiorgan failure as well as improve survival.

The "oldest old," age 80 and older, are twice as likely to die during the initial postinjury phase. They are also more likely to require discharge to an extended care facility if they survive their hospitalization. Trauma patients age 80 or older have a significantly greater mortality rate (46%) compared to younger elder patients (ages 65 to 79) with similar ISS. Of course, withdrawal of medical support in the "oldest old," whether at the time of disclosure of end-of-life wishes by family or the recognition of the futility of further care, likely serves to increase the mortality rate.

MANAGEMENT OF SPECIFIC ORGAN INJURIES

The initial evaluation and management of elderly trauma patients follows the age-independent protocols of the American College of Surgeons (ACS) Committee on Trauma Advanced Trauma Life Support (ATLS). Special attention, however, should be given early to preexisting medical conditions, chronic medications (i.e., beta blockers and anticoagulants), and the potential for blunted physiologic response. In addition, although the trauma team is performing initial diagnostic procedures and resuscitation, attempts should be made to contact family members or caregivers for medical information and advanced directives as the potential for early deterioration is very real. Traditional vital signs have been shown to be inadequate predictors of shock in the elderly non-neurologically injured blunt trauma patient. Early and comprehensive diagnostic testing via CT, ultrasound, and cardiac monitoring is imperative! Although pain control is essential, dosing of narcotics and other sedatives must be done with extreme caution secondary to altered pharmacokinetics and often paradoxical results.

TABLE I: An Age-Related Approach to Trauma Care in Our "Elders"

Age	Considerations
55 through 69 years	Assume some mild decrease in physiologic reserve. Suspect the presence of some common disease of middle age (diabetes, hypertension). Suspect use of prescription or over-the-counter medication. Assume TBI with history of LOC or cognitive abnormalities and obtain head CT. Proceed with standard diagnostic and management schemes.
70 through 80 years	Accept the presence of age-related and acquired physiologic alterations. Accept the presence of medications to control acquired diseases. Determine competency for medical history; involve relatives and personal physician. Monitor patient and control physiologic parameters to optimize cardiac performance. Brain imaging is mandatory for any alterations in cognition. Proceed with standard diagnostic and management schemes. Prepare for early, aggressive operative management. Be aware of poor outcomes, especially with severe injury to the CNS. Check for advanced directives.
80 years or older	Proceed as previously mentioned. Assume a poor outcome with moderately severe injury, especially in the CNS or any injury causing physiologic disturbance. After aggressive initial resuscitation and diagnostic maneuvers, discuss appropriateness of care with patient and family members. Attempt to be humane; recognize the legal and ethical controversies involved. Consider early ethics consultation and social services.

Modified from Schwab CW, Kauder DR: Trauma in the geriatric patient. *Arch Surg* 127(6):701–706, 1992. Copyright 1992 American Medical Association. All rights reserved.
CNS, Central nervous system; CT, computed tomography; LOC, loss of consciousness; TBI, traumatic brain injury.

Table 1, An Age-Related Approach to Trauma Care in Our "Elders," reviews many of the axioms of care for this patient population.

Head trauma in the elderly continues to carry the highest mortality rate (12%; 19% in head Abbreviated Injury Scale [AIS] 3 and higher). Assessment of the elderly trauma patient for brain injury is difficult because physical examination might be misleading if there is underlying dementia. In addition, the presence of opioids and sedatives might be problematic when attempting mental status examination. A high index of suspicion and early CT scanning of the brain are critical to appropriate triage of traumatic brain injury. Decreased brain tissue mass results in loss of intracranial volume and increased vascular shearing injuries, which can be associated with frequent intracranial hemorrhage. In addition, there is more intracranial space that needs to fill before elevated intracranial pressure (ICP) results in

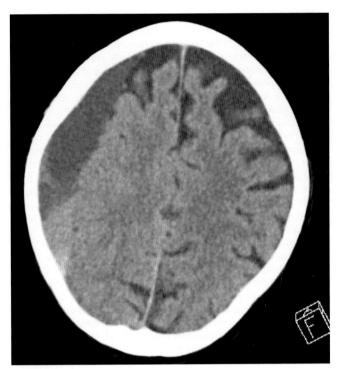

FIGURE I This is a representative noncontrast head computed tomography scan, axial view, of a patient with known chronic right frontoparietal subdural hemorrhage who presented after a fall and was found to have a Glasgow Coma Scale score of 14. Notice the chronic subdural hemorrhage with new layering of acute subdural hemorrhage in the dependent parietal region. In addition, there is evidence of cerebral volume loss, which is not uncommon in the elderly population and can allow for accumulation of intracranial hemorrhage with minimal increase in intracranial pressure or mass effect.

midline shift or herniation, as can be seen in Figure 1. Although elderly patients with traumatic brain injury are known to have worse functional outcomes, resources of care should not be refused to the "oldest old." Elderly trauma patients age 80 and above do not show worse outcomes with respect to traumatic brain injury when compared to younger cohorts.

Preexisting neurologic disease, both central and peripheral, can make the evaluation of spinal cord injury in geriatric trauma patients problematic. Degenerative joint disease can manifest in the cervical spine as canal stenosis and osteophyte formation. Cervical injuries predominate in the elderly with odontoid fractures being the most common. Management of elderly patients with odontoid fractures by halo vest (HV) is associated with increased mortality rate and major complications, such as pneumonia, when compared with operative fixation or nonoperative management via rigid cervical collar. Forward falls can result in cervical hyperextension, acute compression of the spinal cord, and injury to the central portion of the spinal cord. This injury pattern often results in central cord syndrome, which carries poor prognosis in the elderly with approximately 50% mortality rate, which is usually linked to respiratory failure that arises from complications of cervical immobilization devices. Diagnostic imaging, such as CT and magnetic resonance imaging (MRI), should be obtained early when spinal cord injury is suspected.

Torso trauma is the second leading cause of death in elderly trauma patients after traumatic brain injury. Blunt chest injury is commonly encountered and can account for significant morbidity and even fatality. Treatment of the complications of pneumothorax, hemothorax, and pulmonary contusions is similar to that in younger patients. In patients age 65 and older, mortality rate increases 19% and risk of pneumonia increases 27% for each rib fracture present.

In older trauma patients with rib fractures, admission to a trauma center, preexisting CHF, intubation, increasing age, and increasing ISS were the strongest predictors of fatality. In addition, the presence of rib fractures can be indicative of solid abdominal organ injury such as liver and spleen injury. The presence of flail chest, which is defined as rib fractures in three or more consecutive ribs in two or more places, is associated with significant increase in fatality. Managing pain from rib fractures, however, is imperative as respiratory insufficiency can rapidly ensue, especially in the elderly patient who seems comfortable. The judicious use of opioids, NSAIDs, and epidural analgesia/anesthesia are all important methods of pain control. Rib fixation has improved outcomes in the elderly.

Traumatic aortic injury (TAI) results from rapid deceleration associated with falls and MVCs and is often lethal. Those with a mechanism of injury that includes acute deceleration and a widened mediastinum on chest radiograph should be suspected of having TAI. A normal chest radiograph does not exclude TAI and as such a high index of suspicion for aortic injury is required. CT of the chest and aorta is the modality of choice for the diagnosis of TAI. Although management of TAI is similar to that in younger patients, endovascular repair (EVAR) has reduced stability of the endograft in the elderly. There are increasing problems being noted in the young with type 2 endoleaks. Medical management for stable patients includes beta blocker therapy as well as vasodilators to reduce wall stress on the injured aorta. Surgical repair is reserved for the unstable patient or after the initial resuscitation phase. Delay is often undertaken in order to plan for endovascular procedures, which have largely replaced traditional open surgical techniques. Endovascular therapy is of particular benefit in the elderly trauma patient with comorbid conditions that might make the morbidity of traditional open surgery prohibitive, but vascular calcifications and tortuosity can complicate this technique.

The evolution in management of blunt abdominal solid organ injury has tended toward a nonoperative approach with liberal use of interventional radiology procedure in diagnosis and arterioembolization therapy. This management plan is only employed in the hemodynamically stable patient without signs of peritonitis. A reliable examination is paramount if this treatment paradigm is to be followed. In the elderly patient, who for a host of reasons is unable to participate with a physical examination, early laparotomy for suspected solid organ injury with hemoperitoneum and hemodynamic instability is still recommended. In an evaluation of Pennsylvania Trauma Systems Foundation (PTSF) database, the majority of elderly trauma patients (age 55 and older) with blunt splenic trauma were managed nonoperatively. Increasing age was associated with a higher failure rate of nonoperative management. ISS and splenic injury grade were also predictive of failure. Mortality rate was high regardless of treatment choice, and failure of nonoperative management was associated with increased hospital and length of ICU stay.

Because of anatomic changes associated with increasing age, such as osteoporosis, falls, from even minimal height, are likely to result in pelvic fractures, suggesting that even small amounts of energy can result in significant injury in the elderly. In an analysis by Dechert et al, the elderly who died from pelvic trauma were observed to have had lower rates of interventional angiography or operative intervention. Of note, the elderly with pelvic fractures exhibited less hypotension than younger cohorts. Morbidity and fatality are the result of not only the initial injury but also the subsequent prolonged immobilization that follows. In addition, pelvic fractures are associated with increased hospital length of stay as well as increased resource use.

Damage control surgical principles and resuscitative strategies have led to improved outcomes in patients with severe, life-threatening injuries. Damage control laparotomy (DCL) has been shown to be effective in severely injured elderly trauma patients. Elderly trauma patients undergoing DCL are reported to have a higher mortality rate (42.9% age 55 to 80 vs. 12.5% age 16 to 54) and earlier time to death (9.8 days vs. 26 days) when compared to the younger cohort. Most outcomes, such as prolonged hospital stay in survivors, length of ICU stay, and ventilator days, in elderly trauma patients undergoing DCL were not significantly different from the younger cohort. The mechanism of injury, though, is very different, with only 14% of the elderly being injured by penetrating mechanisms as compared to 60% in the younger cohort. DCL has been shown to be beneficial in both emergent general and trauma surgery in octogenarians. Despite an overall complication rate of 62% and in-hospital mortality rate of 37%, long-term survival in this population can be increased for those surviving to hospital discharge.

CONCLUSIONS

As the population continues to age, our emergency departments and trauma teams will face an increase in the number of elderly patients presenting with injury. These elderly trauma patients will exhibit altered physiology, profound injury severity even for low-velocity mechanisms, and unique injury patterns due to the presence of chronic health conditions, medications, and a blunted response to injury. As such, an appreciation of the physiologic changes that are inherent in the elderly patient as well as the unique results of injury mechanics will serve to improve the care provided the geriatric trauma patient and, ideally, will improve outcomes. A high index of suspicion for occult shock and injuries is mandatory, as is early and comprehensive diagnostic imaging, especially for suspected brain injury. In addition, in the face of limited physiologic reserve, early operative management including damage control procedures is often indicated in the elderly trauma patient who might not tolerate failure of nonoperative management strategies. The addition of geriatric medicine consultation is often beneficial in assessing trauma patients for age-related conditions and end-of-life issues.

For the chapter's Suggested Readings list, please visit the book at www.ExpertConsult.inkling.com.

BURNS

John T. Schulz III, Kimberly A. Davis, and Richard L. Gamelli

The frequency of burn injury and its subsequent multisystem effects make the treatment of burn patients a commonly encountered management challenge for the trauma/critical care surgeon. The emergency surgery components of initial burn care include fluid resuscitation and ventilatory support, as well as preservation and restoration of remote organ function. Following appropriate resuscitation, burn patient management is focused on wound care and provision of the necessary metabolic support. The involvement of the emergency/trauma surgeon in burn wound management is dependent on the extent and depth of the wound and the rapid identification of those patients who are best cared for at a burn center.

INCIDENCE

The precise number of burns that occur in the United States each year is unknown because only 21 of 50 states mandate the reporting of burn injury. An estimated total number of burns has been obtained

TABLE 1: Burn Center Referral Criteria

Partial-thickness burns involving more than 10% of the total body surface area

Full-thickness burns in any age group

Burns involving face, hands, feet, genitalia, perineum, or major joints

Significant electrical burns, including lightning injury

Chemical burns

Inhalation injury

Burns in patients with preexisting medical conditions that can complicate management, prolong recovery, or affect survival

Lesser burns in association with concomitant trauma sufficient to influence outcome*

Any size burn in a child in a hospital without qualified personnel or the equipment needed for the care of children

Any size burn in a patient who will require special social or psychiatric intervention or long-term rehabilitation

*If the mechanical trauma poses the greater immediate risk, the patient may be stabilized and receive initial care at a trauma center before transfer to a burn center.
Modified from American Burn Association: Stabilization, transfer and transport. In *Advanced life burn support course instructors manual.* Chicago, American Burn Association, 2001, Chap. 8, pp 73–78.

by extrapolation of those data. At present, 1.25 million is regarded as a realistic estimate of the annual incidence of burns in the United States, 80% of which involve less than 20% of the total body surface. Approximately 150 to 170 patients per million population are estimated to require admission to a hospital for burn care each year. In the population of burn patients requiring hospital care, there is a smaller subset of approximately 20,000 burn patients who, as defined by the American Burn Association (Table 1), are best cared for in a burn center each year. This subset consists of 42 patients per million population with major burns, and 40 patients per million population having lesser burns but a complicating cofactor.

MECHANISM OF INJURY

Certain populations are at high risk for specific types of injuries that require treatment by the trauma/critical care surgeon. Scald burns are the most frequent form of burn injury overall, causing 58% of burn injuries and over 100,000 emergency department visits annually. Sixty-five percent of children age 4 and under who require hospitalization for burn care have scald burns, the majority of which are due to contact with hot foods and liquids. The occurrence of accidental tap water scalds can be minimized by adjusting the temperature settings on hot water heaters or by installing special faucet valves that prevent delivery of water at unsafe temperatures. Scald burns resulting from child abuse are often accompanied by an inconsistent or changing history and are remarkable on physical examination for being sharply demarcated. These injuries typically involve the feet, posterior legs, and buttocks (and sometimes the hands) and are most often caused by immersion in scalding water by an abusive caretaker. Children suspected of experiencing abuse should undergo a radiologic skeletal survey. It is important that the trauma/critical care surgeon identify and report child abuse, because when abuse is

undetected and the child is returned to the abusive environment, repeated abuse is associated with a high risk of fatality.

Fire and flame sources cause 34% of burn injuries and are the most common causes of burns in adults. One fifth to one quarter of all serious burns are related to employment. Kitchen workers are at relatively high risk for scald injury, and roofers and paving workers are at greatest risk for burns due to hot tar. Workers involved in plating processes and the manufacture of fertilizer are at greatest risk for injury due to strong acids, and those involved with soap manufacturing and the use of oven cleaners are at greatest risk of injury due to strong alkalis.

Electric current causes approximately 1000 deaths per year. Young children have the highest incidence of electrical injury caused by household current as a consequence of inserting objects into an electrical receptacle or biting or sucking on electrical cords and sockets. Adults at greatest risk of high-voltage electrical injury are the employees of utility companies, electricians, construction workers (particularly those manning cranes), farm workers moving irrigation pipes, oil field workers, truck drivers, and individuals installing antennae. Lightning strikes result in an average of 107 deaths annually. The vast majority (92%) of lightning-associated deaths occur during the summer months among people engaged in outdoor activities such as golfing or fishing.

Abuse is a special form of burn injury, affecting the extremes of age. Child abuse is typically inflicted by parents but also perpetrated by siblings and child care personnel. The most common form of thermal injury abuse in children is caused by intentional application of a lighted cigarette. Burning the dorsum of a hand by application of a hot clothing iron is another common form of child abuse. Scald burns, as previously discussed, are also common. In recent years, elder abuse by caretakers or family members has become more common, and it too should be reported and the victim protected.

PATHOPHYSIOLOGY

Local Effects

The cutaneous injury caused by a burn is related to the temperature and heat capacity of the energy source, the duration of the exposure, and the tissue surface involved. At temperatures less than 45° C, tissue damage is unlikely to occur even with an extended period of exposure. In the adult, exposure for 30 seconds when the temperature is 54° C will cause a burn injury, but an identical burn will occur with only a 10-second exposure in a child. When the temperature is elevated to 60° C, a common setting for home water heaters, tissue destruction can occur in less than 5 seconds in children. It is not surprising, therefore, that significant injury can occur when patients come in contact with boiling liquids or open flames. Both intentional and unintentional scald injuries frequently lead to litigation: consequently, providers should be familiar with the correlation between water temperature and time to burn injury summarized in Table 2.

Burn injury causes three zones of damage. Centrally located is the zone of coagulation or necrosis. In a full-thickness burn, the zone of coagulation involves all layers of the skin, extending down through the dermis and into the subcutaneous tissue. In partial-thickness injuries, this zone extends down only into the dermis, and there are surviving epithelial elements that may ultimately be capable of resurfacing the wound. Surrounding the zone of coagulation is an area of nonlethal cell injury, the zone of stasis. In this area, blood flow is altered but is restored with time as resuscitation proceeds. If patients are inadequately resuscitated, thrombosis can occur and the zone of stasis can be converted to a zone of coagulation. The most peripheral zone is an area of minimally damaged tissue, the zone of hyperemia, which abuts undamaged tissue. The zone of hyperemia is best seen in patients with superficial partial-thickness injuries as occur with severe sun exposure.

TABLE 2: Water Temperature and Exposure Time Necessary for Dermal Injury

TEMPERATURE		
Fahrenheit (°)	Celsius (°)	Time
120	48.9	>5 min
125	51.7	1.5–2 min
130	54.4	30 sec
135	57.2	10 sec
140	60	<5 sec
145	62.8	<3 sec
150	65.6	1.5 sec
155	68.3	1 sec

Along with the changes in wound blood supply, there is significant formation of edema in the burn-injured tissues. Factors elaborated in the damaged tissues and released as local mediators include histamine, serotonin, bradykinin, prostaglandins, leukotrienes, interleukin 1, interleukin 6, interleukin 10, tumor necrosis factor alpha, and interleukin 17, all of which cause alterations in local tissue homeostasis and increases in vascular permeability. Complement is also activated, which can further modify transcapillary fluid flux. The net effect of these various changes is significant movement of fluid into the extravascular fluid compartment. Maximum accumulation of both water and protein in the burn wound occurs at 24 hours after injury and can persist beyond the first week after burn. Additionally, patients who have greater than a 20% to 25% body surface burn have similar fluid movement in undamaged tissue beds. This fluid accumulation is due to systemic changes in transcapillary fluid flux, but may be exacerbated by overaggressive fluid resuscitation.

Systemic Response

The physiologic response to a major burn injury results in some of the most profound changes that a patient is capable of enduring. The magnitude of the response is proportional to the burn size, reaching a maximum at about a 50% body surface area burn. The duration of the changes is related to the persistence of the burn wound and therefore resolves with wound closure. The organ-specific response follows the pattern that occurs with other forms of trauma, with an initial level of hypofunction, the "ebb phase," followed by a hyperdynamic "flow" phase.

Changes in the cardiovascular response are critical and directly impact the initial care and management of the burn patient. Immediately following burn injury, there is a transient period of decreased cardiac performance and elevated peripheral vascular resistance, which can be exacerbated by inadequate volume replacement. Systemic hypoperfusion can result in further increases in systemic vascular resistances and reprioritization of regional blood flow. Failure to adequately resuscitate a burn patient worsens myocardial performance. Conversely, adequate resuscitation restores normal cardiac performance values within 24 hours of injury, and by the second 24 hours, those values further increase to supranormal levels, resulting in a hyperdynamic state, which will revert back to more normal levels with wound closure.

Pulmonary changes following burn injury are the consequences of direct parenchymal damage that occurs with inhalation injury. In patients without inhalation injury, pulmonary changes following

burn injury are reflective of the generalized hyperdynamic state of the patient. Lung ventilation increases in proportion to the total body surface area of the burn, with increases in both respiratory rate and tidal volume. Worsening of the burned patient's respiratory status in the absence of smoke inhalation injury indicates a supervening process, including sepsis, pneumonia, occult pneumothorax, pulmonary embolism, congestive heart failure, or an acute intra-abdominal process. In patients without these events, pulmonary gas exchange is relatively preserved, and there is little change in pulmonary mechanics.

The renal response to burn injuries is largely dependent on the cardiovascular response. Initially there is a reduction in renal blood flow, which is restored with resuscitation. If a patient is underresuscitated, renal hypoperfusion will persist, with early onset renal dysfunction secondary to renal ischemia. This can be exacerbated if the patient exhibits myoglobinuria or hemoglobinuria (from, for instance, thermal myonecrosis, extremity compartment syndrome, or accompanying soft tissue trauma), either of which is capable of causing direct tubular damage.

Burn injury is capable of affecting both gastrointestinal motility and mucosal integrity, usually as a result of underresuscitation leading to intestinal hypoperfusion. Conversely, patients who are massively resuscitated will have significant edema of the retroperitoneum, bowel mesentery, and bowel wall contributing to a paralytic ileus. With near-immediate initiation of enteral feedings, gastrointestinal motility can be preserved, mucosal integrity protected, and effective nutrient delivery achieved. Delay in the initiation of enteral feeding is associated with the onset of ileus, which can also occur when the burn resuscitation has been complicated.

From a neuroendocrine standpoint, burn injury results in an elevated hormonal and neurotransmitter response similar in magnitude to that of the "fight or flight" response. The duration of the neurohumoral response is prolonged and is exacerbated by surgical stress. The increases in glucocorticoids and catecholamines are necessary to support the stress response of the injured patient. When there is an insufficient stress hormone response, an otherwise survivable insult can become fatal. Many of the multisystem changes occurring after burn can be related in part to the alterations in catecholamine secretion, particularly the changes in resting metabolic expenditures, substrate use, and cardiac performance. As wound closure is accomplished, the increased neurohumoral response abates and anabolic hormones become predominant.

Burn injury affects the hematopoietic system, resulting in the loss of balance in both leukocyte and erythrocyte production and function. Burns of greater than 20% of total body surface area are associated with both alterations in red blood cell production and increases in red blood cell destruction at the level of the cutaneous circulation, resulting in anemia. Such anemia can be further compounded by frequent phlebotomy, surgical blood loss, hemodilution due to resuscitation, and transient alterations in erythrocyte membrane integrity. Longer-term changes appear to be related to hyporesponsiveness of the erythroid progenitor cells in the bone marrow to erythropoietin. During the early stages of resuscitation, reductions in platelet number, depressed fibrinogen levels, and alterations in coagulation factors return to normal or near normal values with appropriate resuscitation. Changes in white blood cell number occur early, with an increase in neutrophils due to demargination and accelerated bone marrow release. With uncomplicated burn injury, bone marrow myelopoiesis is preserved.

In addition to the changes occurring in the bone marrow, there are significant further depressions in the immune response. Burn injury causes a global impairment in host defense. Alterations of the humoral immune response include reductions in IgG and IgM secretion, decreased fibronectin levels, and increases in complement activation. Cellular changes include alterations in T-cell responsiveness and cell populations, leading to alterations in antigen presentation and impairment of delayed-type hypersensitivity reactions. Leukocyte function is adversely affected. Granulocytes have been noted to have impaired chemotaxis, decreased phagocytic activity, decreased antibody-dependent cell cytotoxicity, and a relative impairment in their capacity to respond to a second challenge. The clinical significance of these observations is that the burn patient is at significant risk for postburn infectious complications.

GRADING OF BURN WOUND DEPTH

The injuries that will be apparent on examination are the consequences of the level of tissue destruction. Wounds that are superficial, dry, and hyperemic; blanch easily; and do not blister represent first-degree burns. The injury is only to the epidermis, and the basal layer of the epidermis does not separate form the dermis. Unlike first-degree burns, second-degree, or partial-thickness, burns involve some injury to the dermis. Superficial partial-thickness burns (minimal destruction of the dermis) are associated with hyperemia, blistering, increased sensation, and exquisite pain upon palpation or air contact of the exposed dermal surface. The wounds are hyperemic and warm and readily blanch. With a deeper partial-thickness burn (deeper extent of dermal necrosis), the wound presents with intact or ruptured blisters or may be covered by a thin layer of necrotic dermis termed "eschar." The key physical finding is preservation of sensation in the burned tissue, although it is reduced (Table 3). With proper care, superficial and even deeper partial-thickness injuries are capable of spontaneous healing without grafting; but very deep partial-thickness burns leave too little intact dermis and epidermal appendages to stabilize epithelialization and are functionally equivalent to full-thickness burns The risk of infection in deep partial-thickness wounds is significant, and if an infection develops it can lead to a greater depth of skin loss (wound conversion). A full-thickness wound (third degree) occurs when the injury penetrates all layers of the skin or extends into the subcutaneous or deeper tissues (fourth degree). These wounds will appear pale or waxy; be anesthetic, dry, and inelastic; and contain thrombosed vessels. Occasionally in the elderly, in children, and in young women, the initial appearance of a wound may be more that of a brick red coloration due to extravasation of heme from ruptured erythrocytes in the dermis. Such wounds will have significant edema and are inelastic and insensate. Full-thickness wounds are infection-prone wounds, as they no longer provide any viable barrier to invading organisms and if left untreated become rapidly colonized and a portal for invasive burn wound sepsis.

RESUSCITATION PRIORITIES

Fluid Administration

Immediately following burn injury, the changes induced in the cardiovascular system must receive therapeutic priority. In all patients with burns of more than 20% of the total body surface area and those with lesser burns in whom physiologic indices indicate a need for fluid infusion, a large-caliber intravenous cannula should be placed in an appropriately sized peripheral vein, preferably underlying unburned skin. Central venous access is indicated if there are no peripheral veins available or if the patient is going to be intubated and will require multiple infusions. Lactated Ringer's solution should be infused at an initial rate of 1 L/hour in the adult and 20 mL/kg/hour for children who weigh 50 kg or less. That infusion rate is adjusted following estimation of the fluid needed for the first 24 hours following the burn.

Resuscitation fluid needs are proportional to the extent of the burn (combined extent of partial- and full-thickness burns expressed as a percentage of total body surface area) and are related to body size (most readily expressed as body weight) and age (the surface area per unit of body mass is greater in children than in adults). The patient should be weighed on admission and the extent of partial- and full-thickness burns estimated according to standard nomograms (Fig. 1). The fluid needs for the first 24 hours can be estimated on the basis of the Advanced Burn Life Support and Advanced Trauma Life Support consensus formula (Table 4). Although a detailed comparison of various resuscitation formulas is beyond the scope of this chapter, a summary of all previously described burn resuscitation formulas is listed in Table 5.

Because of the greater surface area per unit of body mass in children, the volume of fluid required for the first 24 hours is relatively greater than that for an adult. In all patients the systemic capillary leak is greatest in the first 8 hours, and consequently, one half of the estimated volume should be administered in the first 8 hours after the burn. If the initiation of fluid therapy is delayed, the initial half of the volume estimated for the first 24 hours should be administered in the hours remaining before the eighth postburn hour (i.e., time starts with the injury, NOT with the time of arrival in the emergency department). The remaining half of the fluid is administered over the subsequent 16 hours.

TABLE 3: Clinical Characteristics of Burn Injuries

Feature	PARTIAL-THICKNESS BURNS		FULL-THICKNESS BURNS
	First Degree	**Second Degree**	**Third Degree**
Cause	Sun or minor flash	Higher intensity or longer exposure to flash Relatively brief exposure to hot liquids, flames	Higher intensity or longer exposure to flash Longer exposure to flames or "hot" liquids Contact with steam or hot metal High-voltage electricity Chemicals
Color	Bright red	Mottled red	Pearly white Translucent and parchment-like Charred
Surface	Dry No bullae	Moist Bullae present	Dry, leathery, and stiff Remnants of burned skin present Liquefaction of tissue
Sensation	Hyperesthetic	Pain to pinprick inversely proportional to depth of injury	Surface insensate Deep pressure sense retained
Healing	3–6 days	Time proportional to depth of burns, 10–35 days	Requires grafting

From Pruitt BA Jr, Gamelli RL: Burns. In Britt LD, Trunkey DD, Organ CH, Feliciano DV, editors: *Acute care surgery.* New York, Springer, 2007, p 128.

BURN ESTIMATE AND DIAGRAM
AGE vs AREA

Area	Birth 1 yr	1–4 yr	5–9 yr	10–14 yr	15 yr	Adult	2°	3°	Total	Donor Areas
Head	19	17	13	11	9	7				
Neck	2	2	2	2	2	2				
Ant Trunk	13	13	13	13	13	13				
Post Trunk	13	13	13	13	13	13				
R. Buttock	2 ½	2 ½	2 ½	2 ½	2 ½	2 ½				
L. Buttock	2 ½	2 ½	2 ½	2 ½	2 ½	2 ½				
Genitalia	1	1	1	1	1	1				
R. U. Arm	4	4	4	4	4	4				
L. U. Arm	4	4	4	4	4	4				
R. L. Arm	3	3	3	3	3	3				
L. L. Arm	3	3	3	3	3	3				
R. Hand	2 ½	2 ½	2 ½	2 ½	2 ½	2 ½				
L. Hand	2 ½	2 ½	2 ½	2 ½	2 ½	2 ½				
R. Thigh	5 ½	6 ½	8	8 ½	9	9 ½				
L. Thigh	5 ½	6 ½	8	8 ½	9	9 ½				
R. Leg	5	5	5 ½	6	6 ½	7				
L. Leg	5	5	5 ½	6	6 ½	7				
R. Foot	3 ½	3 ½	3 ½	3 ½	3 ½	3 ½				
L. Foot	3 ½	3 ½	3 ½	3 ½	3 ½	3 ½				
						TOTAL				

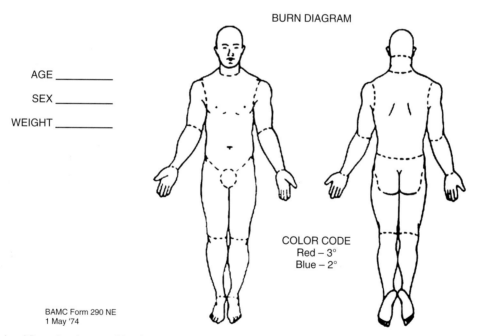

BURN DIAGRAM

AGE _____

SEX _____

WEIGHT _____

COLOR CODE
Red – 3°
Blue – 2°

BAMC Form 290 NE
1 May '74

FIGURE 1 The Lund-Browder chart used for documenting extent of burn. Figure outlines are filled in with a blue pencil and a red pencil to indicate distribution of partial-thickness and full-thickness burns, respectively. Note the columns indicating how the percentage of total body surface area represented by body part surface changes with time. *(From Martin RR, Becker WK, Cioffi WG, Pruitt BP Jr: Thermal injuries. In Wilson RF, Walt AJ, editors: Mangement of trauma: pitfalls and practice, 2nd ed. Baltimore, Williams & Wilkins, 1996, p 765.)*

The limited glycogen stores in a child may be rapidly exhausted by the marked stress hormone response to burn injury. Serum glucose levels in the burned child should be monitored, and 5% dextrose in lactated Ringer's solution administered if serum glucose decreases to hypoglycemic levels. In the case of small children with small burns, the resuscitation fluid volume as estimated on the basis of burn size may not meet normal daily metabolic requirements. In such patients, maintenance fluids should be added to the resuscitation regimen: all children weighing less than 30 kg (66 lb) should get maintenance fluid with 5% dextrose in water (D_5W) in addition to resuscitation volume.

The infusion rate is adjusted according to the individual patient's response to the injury and the resuscitation regimen. The progressive

TABLE 4: Fluid Required for the First 24 Hours After Burn

Adults: 2–4 mL LR/%TBSAB/kg BW
Children: 3–4 mL LR/%TBSAB/kg BW + maintenance in children weighing < 30 kg

BW, Body weight; LR, lactated Ringer's solution; TBSAB, total body surface area burned.

edema formation in burned and even unburned limbs commonly make measurements of pulse rate, pulse quality, and even blood pressure difficult and unreliable as indices of resuscitation adequacy. Therefore, hourly urine output should be used as a measure of the adequacy of resuscitation. The fluid infusion rate is adjusted to obtain 30 mL of urine per hour in the adult and 1 mg/kg of body weight per hour in children weighing less than 30 kg. The administration of fluid is increased or decreased only if the hourly urinary output is one third or more below, or 25% or more above, the target level for 2 successive hours. Capillary refill in unburned skin is an excellent surrogate for visceral perfusion and should be maintained and checked hourly along with urine output. If in either adults or children the resuscitation volume infused in the first 12 hours will result in administration of 6 mL or more per percent of body surface area burned per kilogram of body weight in the first 24 hours, human albumin diluted to a physiologic concentration in normal saline should be infused and the volume of crystalloid solution reduced by a comparable amount.

Failure to respond appropriately to fluid resuscitation even after the addition of colloid should prompt a careful reconsideration of the injury history: Is it possible that there is a missed occult traumatic injury with associated hemorrhage? Clearly, fluid resuscitation will not effectively address ongoing hemorrhage and any patient presenting with a severe burn and history of mechanical trauma needs a thorough trauma assessment. In addition, for those patients arriving with no obtainable history, the safest initial stance is that patients have a traumatic mechanism until proved otherwise.

Additionally, some patients with no other occult injuries do not respond well to fluid resuscitation. When a patient has received 1.5 times the calculated resuscitation volume with the albumin modification (or 250 mL/kg) and shows no sign of being able to tolerate lowering the infusion rates, one should consider the addition of vasopressors. Severe inflammation is sometimes accompanied by a relative deficiency of endogenous vasopressin. Provision of vasopressin for these patients can rapidly rectify their response to fluid resuscitation. In addition, some patients will require norepinephrine. Negotiating the difficult resuscitation with appropriate fluids and vasoactive infusions is challenging and should be guided by the most experienced provider available.

Restoration of functional capillary integrity occurs at or near 24 hours after burn injury. Consequently, the volume of fluid needed for the second 24 hours after burn is less, and colloid-containing fluids can be infused to reduce further volume and salt loading. Human albumin diluted to physiologic concentration in normal saline is the colloid-containing solution of choice, infused in a dosage of 0.3 mL per percent of burn per kilogram of body weight for patients with 30% to 50% burns, 0.4 mL per percent of burn per kilogram of body weight for patients with 50% to 70% burns, and 0.5 mL per percent of burn per kilogram of body weight for patients whose burns exceed 70% of the total body surface area. Water containing 5% dextrose is also given in the amount necessary to maintain an adequate urinary output. The colloid-containing fluids for children are estimated according to the same formula, but half normal saline is infused to maintain urinary output and avoid inducing physiologically significant hyponatremia by infusion of large volumes of

TABLE 5: Burn Resuscitation Formulas, Current and Past

Crystalloid formulas: Usually use lactated Ringer's solution, although newer isotonic fluids may be used.	Parkland (Baxter) formula: 4 mL/kg/% TBSA burn, give half in the first 8 hours and half in the next 16 hours. Adjust rate based on urine output. For second 24 hours, give 20% to 60% of calculated plasma volume as colloid. (The recommendation for the second 24 hours is usually not followed.) Modified Brooke formula: 2 mL/kg/% TBSA burn, give half in the first 8 hours and half in the next 16 hours. Adjust rate based on urine output. For the second 24 hours, give 0.33 to 0.5 mL/kg/% TBSA burn as colloid plus D$_5$W (dextrose 5% in water) to maintain urine output.
Hypertonic formulas: No colloid.	Monafo: 250 mEq/L Na$^+$ + 150 mEq lactate + 100 mEq Cl$^-$. Adjust rate based on urine output. For second 24 hours, give one third of isotonic salt orally. Warden: lactated Ringer's solution + 50 mEq NaHCO$_3$ (180 mEq of Na$^+$) per liter for first 8 hours (based on the Parkland formula). Switch to lactated Ringer's when pH normalizes or at 8 hours. Adjust rate based on urine output.
Colloid formulas	Burn budget formula of F.D. Moore: lactated Ringer's 1000–4000 mL + 0.5 normal saline 1200 mL + 7.5% of body weight colloid + 1500–5000 mL D$_5$W. For second 24 hours, use same formula except for colloid 2.5% of weight. Evans formula: normal saline at 1 mL/kg/% TBSA burn + colloid at 1 mL/kg/% TBSA burn. For second 24 hours, give half of first 24 hour requirements + D$_5$W 2000 mL. Brooke formula (original): lactated Ringer's at 1.5 mL/kg/% TBSA burn + colloid at 0.5 mL/kg/% TBSA burn. Switch to D$_5$W 2000 mL for second 24 hours. Slater formula: lactated Ringer's 2000 mL + fresh frozen plasma at 75 mL/kg/24 hours. Adjust rate based on urine output. Haifa formula: plasma at 1.5 mL/kg/% TBSA burn + lactated Ringer's at 1 mL/kg/% TBSA burn. Adjust rate based on urine output. Demling formula: Dextran 40 in normal saline at 2 mL/kg/hr for 8 hours. Fresh frozen plasma at 0.5 mL/kg/hr starting at 8 hours. Lactated Ringer's should be given to maintain urine output.

TBSA, Total body surface area.
From Greenhalgh DG: Burn resuscitation. *J Burn Care Res* 28(4):555–565, 2007.

electrolyte-free fluid into the relatively small intravascular and interstitial volume of the child. Fluid infusion "weaning" should also be initiated during this period, to further minimize volume loading. In a patient who is assessed to be adequately resuscitated, the volume of fluid infused per hour should be arbitrarily decreased by 25% to 50%. If urinary output falls below target level, the prior infusion rate should be resumed. If urinary output remains adequate, the reduced infusion rate should be maintained over the next 3 hours, at which time another similar fractional reduction of fluid infusion rate should be made. This decremental process will establish the minimum infusion rate that maintains resuscitation adequacy in the second postburn day.

Fluid management the first 48 hours after burn should permit excretion of the retained fraction of the water and salt loads infused to achieve resuscitation, prevent dehydration and electrolyte abnormalities, and allow the patient to return to preburn weight by postburn days 8 to 10. Infusion of the large volumes of lactated Ringer's solution required for resuscitation commonly produces a weight gain of 20% or more and a reduction of serum sodium concentration to approximate that of lactated Ringer's solution—that is, 130 mEq/L. Correction of that relative hyponatremia is facilitated by the prodigious evaporative water loss from the surface of the burn wound, which is the major component of the markedly increased insensible water loss that is present following resuscitation. Inadequate replacement of insensible water loss makes hypernatremia the most commonly encountered electrolyte disturbance in the extensively burned patient following resuscitation. Such hypernatremia should be managed by provision of sufficient electrolyte-free water to allow excretion of the increased total body sodium mass and replace insensible water loss to the extent needed to prevent hypovolemia.

Electrolyte abnormalities are frequently encountered in the immediate postburn period. Hyperkalemia is frequently encountered and is typically a laboratory sign of hemolysis but may also be a sign of muscle destruction by high-voltage electrical injury or a particularly deep thermal burn. Hyperkalemia may also occur in association with acidosis in patients who are grossly underresuscitated. In the case of patients with high-voltage electrical injury and severe hyperkalemia, emergent dialysis and excision/amputation of nonviable tissue/extremities may be necessary to stabilize the serum potassium and salvage the patient. Hypophosphatemia is also extremely common after burn resuscitation and is due to either prolonged administration of parenteral nutrition or failure to supply sufficient phosphate to meet the needs of tissue anabolism following wound closure. Hypophosphatemia can be prevented and treated by appropriate dietary phosphate supplementation.

Ventilatory Support

The most critical factor in the initial assessment of a burn patient is the patency of the airway and the ability of the patient to maintain and protect the airway. Standard criteria should be used to determine the need for mechanical stabilization of the airway, also keeping in mind the systemic response to a major burn and the local response to an airway injury, which may combine to cause progressive airway swelling and edema that will impair airflow. Circumferential torso burns will further impair the ability of the patient to respire. Allowing airway compromise to proceed to a critical state before intubating the patient and stabilizing the airway is not appropriate care. The safest approach when there is concern about the airway, particularly in a patient needing transport for definitive care, is to perform early intubation.

Patients suffering both inhalation injuries and thermal burns have a significantly increased incidence of complications and probability of death. Although an inhalation injury alone carries a mortality rate of 5% to 8%, a combination of a thermal injury plus inhalation injury can easily result in a mortality rate 20% above that predicted on the basis of age and burn size. Injuries to the airway are due to the direct damage by the inhaled products of combustion that cause inflammation and edema. Damage to the oropharynx and upper airway is related to the heat content of the inhaled material. Conversely, the heat exchange capability of the pharynx is sufficient that injury below the glottis is principally related to the particulate material contained within the smoke and the chemical composition of inhaled materials. Moist heat, which occurs with steam, has 4000 times the heat-carrying capacity of dry smoke and is capable of causing more extensive thermal damage of the tracheobronchial tree.

Presenting signs and symptoms of an inhalation injury are stridor, hypoxia, and respiratory distress. The probability that a patient has suffered an inhalation injury is highly correlated with being burned in an enclosed space, having burns of the head and neck, and having elevated carbon monoxide levels. The extent and severity of the inhalation injury are directly related to the duration of exposure and the types of toxins contained within the smoke, and all these factors exacerbate the ensuing host inflammatory response. Activation of the inflammatory cascade results in the recruitment of neutrophils and macrophages, which propagate the injury. Altered surfactant release causes obstruction and collapse of distal airway segments. As part of the response to injury, there is a marked and near-immediate increase in bronchial artery blood flow, which is associated with marked alterations in vascular permeability within the lung. The net effect is that extensive destruction and inflammation reduce pulmonary compliance and impair gas exchange, resulting in altered pulmonary blood flow patterns and ventilation-perfusion mismatches.

Part of the initial management of the patient with inhalation injury should include a thorough evaluation of the airway, including bronchoscopy. The clinical findings of an inhalation injury on bronchoscopy include airway edema, inflammation, increased bronchial secretions, presence of carbonaceous material that can diffusely carpet the airway, mucosal ulcerations, endoluminal obliteration due to sloughing mucosa, mucus plugging, and cast formation. Signs of gastric aspiration may also be evident. Repeat bronchoscopy can be performed for removal of debris and casts as well as surveillance for infection.

Carbon monoxide and cyanide gases are present in smoke and when inhaled are rapidly absorbed and cause systemic toxicity as well as impaired oxygen use and delivery. Carbon monoxide is an odorless, nonirritating gas that rapidly diffuses into the bloodstream and has a 240-fold greater affinity for hemoglobin than dose oxygen, thus easily displacing oxygen. The diagnosis of carbon monoxide poisoning is made in a burn patient on the basis of circumstances of injury, physical findings, and the measurement of blood carboxyhemoglobin level. It is important to note that pulse oximetry values do not differentiate between carboxyhemoglobin and oxyhemoglobin. Patients with significant carbon monoxide intoxication can have normal oxygen saturations but will not have satisfactory blood oxygen content. Signs and symptoms of carbon monoxide poisoning are typically mild to absent when carbon monoxide–hemoglobin (carboxyhemoglobin) levels are 10% or less. When carboxyhemoglobin levels are between 10% and 30%, symptoms are present and often manifested by headache and dizziness. Severe poisoning is seen in patients with carboxyhemoglobin levels of greater than 50%, which may be associated with syncope, seizures, and coma. The primary treatment modality for carbon monoxide intoxication is the administration of increased levels of inspired oxygen.

Cyanide poisoning, which can occur in combination with carbon monoxide intoxication, disrupts normal cellular use of oxygen by binding to cytochrome oxidase, the terminal electron acceptor in the mitochondrial electron transport system. Oxidative phosphorylation comes to a halt, resulting in cellular lactic acid production, severe ischemia at the cellular level, and generation of toxic free radical reactive oxygen species. Blood concentrations of cyanide greater than 0.5 mg/L are toxic. Treatment of cyanide poisoning includes the administration of oxygen as well as decontaminating agents such as amyl and sodium nitrates. These compounds induce the formation of methemoglobin, which can act as a scavenger of cyanide. Hydroxycobalamin is the antidote of choice.

The goal of mechanical ventilation following inhalation injury is to minimize further damage to the airway and lung parenchyma while providing adequate gas exchange. This is best achieved through careful control of airway pressures, thereby limiting ventilation-induced barotrauma. Lung damage following burn injury is not homogeneous but patchy in distribution and requires that the level of positive end-expiratory pressure (PEEP) used to maximize airway recruitment be limited to avoid ventilator-induced lung injury. In severe lung injury, mechanical ventilation can lead to increases in alveolar sheer forces and changes in pulmonary blood flow. High inflation pressures exacerbate these problems, promoting injury to the functional areas of the lung. This development, in association with reductions in elasticity and alterations in lung compliance, results in further lung injury and ventilation-perfusion abnormalities.

For patients who have signs of inhalation injury on bronchoscopy, it is beneficial to initiate aggressive management of retained secretions with the use of bronchodilators and mucolytic agents. Meticulous control of airway pressure should be practiced, with the early performance of torso escharotomies and prompt treatment of abdominal compartment syndrome. Mean airway pressures should be maintained at less than 32 to 34 cm H_2O and chemical paralysis liberally used, with a low threshold for conversion to pressure-controlled ventilation with titration of tidal volumes to lessen further the risk of ventilator-induced barotrauma. This may require the acceptance of smaller than usual tidal volumes and permissive hypercapnia, which is acceptable as long as arterial blood pH is above 7.26 and the patient is hemodynamically stable. Airway pressure release ventilation (APRV), a relatively new mode of ventilation in which the lungs are maintained at a constant inflation pressure (P_{high}) with regular release of pressure for expiration (P_{low}) is also useful in the patient with a large pulmonary shunt fraction.

Initial Wound Care

Initial wound care is focused on preventing further injury. Burning clothing should be removed, contact disrupted with metal objects that may retain heat, and only molten materials adherent to the skin surface should be cooled. Attempted cooling of burn wounds should not be done, as local vasoconstriction can impair wound blood flow and extend the depth of the injury, as well as exacerbate systemic hypothermia. Patients being prepared for transport or admitted for definitive care should be placed in sterile or clean, dry dressings and kept warm. Items of clothing or jewelry should be removed prior to the onset of burn wound edema to prevent further compromise of the circulation. In cases of chemical injury, the removal of contaminated clothing with copious water lavage of liquid chemicals and removal by brushing of powdered materials at the scene can limit the extent of the resultant burn injury. No attempt should be made at chemical neutralization, as such treatment would result in an exothermic reaction and cause additional tissue damage. The care provider must exercise extreme caution when working with victims of chemical injury to prevent self-contamination and personal injury.

After admission to the hospital and as soon as resuscitative measures have been instituted, the burn wounds should be cleansed with warm fluids and a detergent disinfectant, such as chlorhexidine gluconate, which has an excellent antimicrobial spectrum. During cleansing, hypothermia must be avoided. Materials that are densely adherent to the wound, such as wax, tar, plastic, and metal, should be gently removed or allowed to separate during the course of subsequent dressing changes. Sloughing skin, devitalized tissue, and ruptured blisters should be gently trimmed from the wound. Careful wound cleansing should be done at each dressing change, with serial débridement of devitalized tissue performed as necessary. The wound should be monitored for signs of infection and change in depth from the initial assessment.

The damaged skin surface can serve as the portal for microbial invasion if it becomes progressively colonized. As microbial numbers increase within the wound to levels of 100,000 organisms per gram of tissue, an invasive wound infection and ultimately systemic sepsis may occur. Topically applied antimicrobial agents, which penetrate the burn eschar, are capable of achieving sufficient levels to control microbial proliferation within the wound. Systemic antibiotics are not indicated, as they do not adequately penetrate eschar. Topical antimicrobial agents are used in the prophylactic treatment of the burn wound and as a part of the management of burn wound infections. Topical agents do not heal the wound but prevent local burn wound infection from destroying viable tissue in wounds capable of spontaneous healing.

Silver sulfadiazine, the most widely used agent, is available as a 1% suspension in a water-soluble micronized cream base. The cream is easily applied and causes little or no pain on application. The cream can be directly applied to the wound as a continuous layer and covered over with a dressing. At each dressing change, the cream should be totally removed and not allowed to form a caseous layer (termed "pseudoeschar") that will obscure the wound bed. The most common toxic side effect of silver sulfadiazine is a transient leukopenia which, when it does occur in up to 15% of treated patients, resolves spontaneously without discontinuation of the drug. Silver sulfadiazine is active against a wide range of microbes, including *Staphylococcus aureus*, *Escherichia coli*, *Klebsiella* spp., many but not all *Pseudomonas aeruginosa*, *Proteus* spp., and *Candida albicans*.

Mafenide acetate was one of the first effective topical agents introduced for the management of the burn wound. It was initially available as Sulfamylon burn cream, which is highly effective against gram-positive and gram-negative organisms but provides little antifungal activity. Mafenide acetate readily diffuses into the eschar and is the agent of choice for significant burns of the ears because it is also capable of penetrating cartilage. Drawbacks with the use of mafenide acetate include pain on application to partial-thickness burns, and limited activity against methicillin-resistant *S. aureus*. Mafenide acetate also inhibits carbonic anhydrase and may cause a self-limiting hyperchloremic acidosis. Mafenide acetate has more recently become available as a 5% aqueous solution and is an excellent agent to use on freshly grafted wounds and is not associated with the problems found with the cream formulation.

Silver nitrate as a 0.5% solution is effective against gram-positive and gram-negative organisms but does not penetrate the eschar. Silver nitrate solution leaches sodium, potassium, chloride, and calcium from the wound, in association with transeschar water absorption, which can result in mineral deficits, alkalosis, and water loading. Those side effects can be minimized by giving sodium and other mineral supplements and modifying fluid therapy. These problems and the labor required to use silver nitrate effectively limit its routine use, and most see silver sulfadiazine as a highly acceptable alternative.

Silver-impregnated dressings have recently become available for clinical use. When the fabric base is in contact with wound fluids, the silver is released continuously and serves as the antimicrobial agent deposited onto the wound. The treatment interval with such a composite may extend up to several days depending on the fabrication design, with dressing changes needed only once or twice per week. The effectiveness of this membrane in treating extensive full-thickness burns is unconfirmed, and at present it is used to treat partial-thickness burns.

In superficial partial-thickness burns, the use of bacitracin ointment represents a satisfactory alternative, particularly in patients with a known sulfa allergy. It may be used open, especially with superficial facial burns, or as a component of a closed dressing. Worldwide, bacitracin is one of the most commonly used topical agents, but it should not be used on large surface areas because when absorbed it has significant nephrotoxicity. Other topical agents include antibiotic combinations such as triple antibiotic ointment (neomycin, bacitracin zinc, and polymyxin B) and Polysporin (bacitracin zinc and polymyxin B). In the case of methicillin-resistant staphylococci, mupirocin is a useful agent.

The application of topical antimicrobial agents to the burns of patients who will be transferred to a burn center may preclude the use of biologic membrane dressings that must adhere to the wound surface to be effective. Additionally, as soon as a patient is admitted to a burn center, any previously placed dressing must be removed to permit the burn team to make a precise assessment of the extent of the burn and the depth of injury. Unless there will be an extended period of time before the patient is transferred to a burn center, the preferred initial management entails placing the patient in a dry dressing, particularly one with a nonadherent lining, and keeping the patient warm.

Burn Wound Excision and Grafting

Excision of the burned tissue and grafting are required for wounds that are full thickness in depth; this treatment is also now considered the optimal management of wounds with a mixed depth of injury. Wounds that are capable of spontaneous closure within 2 to 3 weeks after injury can be managed expectantly, provided the cosmetic and functional outcomes will be acceptable. Wounds needing excision and closure should undergo excision as soon as possible, as this reduces the period of disability and the overall cost of the injury. In patients with a large burn wound, the timing and extent of the surgery are based on the patient's relative physiologic stability and his or her capacity to undergo a major operative procedure. Early burn wound excision and closure in patients with large wounds shortens the length of hospitalization, reduces cost, may attenuate the hyperinflammatory response, and favorably impacts overall burn mortality rate.

Wounds that are small or linear in shape can be managed by excision of the burn and primary wound closure. This is useful in burns of the upper inner arm in the elderly, localized burns of a pendulous breast, abdominal burns, buttock injuries, and thigh burns. This approach works quite well when these wounds are excised early, before significant microbial colonization of the wound occurs, and should be employed whenever feasible.

In selected cases, the injury may be such that amputation of the burned part is most appropriate. In the patient with significant multisystem trauma, the expeditious removal of the burn injury might be the best option for the patient's overall survival. A mangled extremity, which has also suffered a severe burn that is deemed nonsalvageable, should undergo early amputation. It is not necessary to extend the amputation to a level that allows closure with unburned tissue. If viable muscle is available to close the amputation site, the wound bed can be resurfaced with an autogenous skin graft. A grafted amputation site can, with a modern prosthesis, function as a durable stump. In a patient who is paraplegic and suffers an extensive, deep lower extremity burn injury, amputation can be a viable alternative to excision and grafting. A similar option may need to be considered for the patient in whom significant preexisting peripheral vascular disease makes the likelihood of a healed and functional extremity very low.

Excision and grafting will be required for wounds not amenable to primary closure. The extent of the procedure that a patient can undergo is related to the patient's age and physiologic status. Implicit in this approach is the use of experienced operating teams, an anesthesiologist who thoroughly understands the unique problems of the patient with a major body surface area burn, and an operating room fully equipped to treat such a patient, as well as ready availability of blood products and the capacity to care for the patient postoperatively. A patient having this extent of surgery in essence undergoes a doubling of the surface area of "injury"—the now excised and grafted wound along with the partial-thickness wound produced by the donor site. In patients with wounds of a larger size (>30% total body surface area) or those who cannot tolerate a single procedure to achieve closure, staged excision of burned tissue is performed and the resulting wounds are closed with available cutaneous autografts or a biologic dressing.

The technique of burn wound excision is based on the depth of the wound and anatomic site to be excised. The most common method of excision is tangential. Excision of deep partial-thickness wounds to the level of a uniformly viable bed of deep dermis by tangential technique and immediate coverage with cutaneous autograft results in rapid wound closure with a typically excellent result. Optimally, the desired wound bed is achieved in one pass of the Weck blade as evidenced by diffuse bleeding. A frequent error is attempting this technique in wounds of an inappropriate depth and assuming that punctuate bleeding indicates a viable bed. Such wounds will heal with a poor take, as the bed contains marginally viable tissue incapable of supporting the cutaneous autograft (the bleeding, although sometimes profuse in this type of wound, is arteriolar, not capillary: perfusion is inadequate to support a graft). During the performance of this procedure, the amount of blood loss can be minimized with the use of a tourniquet on extremity burns or subeschar clysis containing epinephrine. An alternative to tangential excision is fascial excision, which involves excision of the burn wound to fascia or deep subcutaneous tissue. Viability of the fascia should be carefully assessed, and if the viability is questionable, the excision should be carried down to the underlying muscle prior to grafting. Alternatively, beds of questionable viability may be allografted as should beds of relatively poorly perfused subcutaneous fat in adults. The subsequent fate of the allograft determines whether or not a deeper excision need be performed.

The blood loss occurring with burn wound excision is related to the time of excision after burn, the area to be excised, the presence of infection, and the type of excision. Donor sites can also represent a significant portion of the blood loss. The quantity of blood loss has been estimated to range from 0.45 to 1.25 mL/cm² of burn area excised. Adjunctive measures that can be used to control blood loss include elevation of limbs undergoing excision, applications of topical thrombin or vasoconstrictive agents in solutions to the excised wound and donor site, clysis of skin graft harvest sites or the eschar prior to removal, and application of tourniquets. Spray application of fibrin sealant can also reduce bleeding from the excised wound after release of the tourniquet. Blood loss will be compounded if the patient becomes coagulopathic, hypothermic, or acidotic during the procedure, a triad that can be avoided by partnership with an experienced anesthesiologist. Some judgment must be used in timing, extent, and nature of surgery on the severely burned patient, remembering that autograft harvest increases the patient's wound burden and the metabolic demand on the patient.

Grafting of the burn wound is usually done at the time of excision. However, in some instances it is advisable to stage the skin grafting procedure. The surgeon must be aware of the patient's status throughout the surgical procedure and, if necessary, truncate the procedure. It may be best to perform only the excision, and stage the timing of the grafting. Additionally, if the viability of the wound bed is suspect, only excision should be performed. The wound can be dressed with a 5% Sulfamylon solution dressing or covered with a skin substitute and subsequently reevaluated. Staging wound closure is also appropriate in the patient who is severely malnourished.

Several skin substitutes exist. The two most commonly used naturally occurring biologic dressings are human cutaneous allograft and porcine cutaneous xenograft. Allograft skin, which becomes vascularized, can provide wound coverage for 3 to 4 weeks before rejection of the alloepidermis. Xenograft tissue, which does not vascularize, is available as reconstituted sheets of meshed porcine dermis or as fresh or prepared split-thickness skin. Xenograft skin, essentially an inert biologic dressing, can be used to cover partial-thickness injuries or donor sites, which reepithelialize beneath the xenograft. Additionally, various synthetic membranes have been developed that provide wound protection and possess vapor and bacterial barrier properties. An example is Biobrane (Dow-Hickham, Sugarland, Tex.), which can be used interchangeably with porcine xenograft. Integra (Integra Life-Science Corporation, Plainsboro, N.J.), on the other hand, is a tissue regeneration matrix consisting of a dermal analog of crosslinked collagen and glycosaminoglycan and a Silastic epidermal analog. It can be placed over freshly excised full-thickness wounds, providing wound fibroblasts with the information necessary to create a neodermis of native protein mimicking the architecture of the dermal analog. Once the dermal analog is fully vascularized (at least 2 weeks in an acutely burned patient), the Silastic epidermal analog is removed and the vascularized "neodermis" is covered with a thin split-thickness cutaneous autograft. A permanent skin substitute for burn care victims continues to represent the Holy Grail. Presently, cultured epithelial autografts are commercially available but are limited in their use because of suboptimal graft take, fragility of the skin surface, and high cost (dermis or a dermal equivalent is necessary to stabilize epidermis). Use of any biologic dressing requires that the excised wound and the dressing that has been applied be meticulously examined on at least a daily basis. Submembrane suppuration or the development of infection necessitates removal of the dressing, cleansing of the wound with a surgical detergent disinfectant solution, and even reexcision of the wound if residual nonviable or infected tissue is present.

The proper management of the patient's burn wounds is critical to achieve the optimal cosmetic and functional outcome and the timely return of the patient to full activity. In patients with major burns, the wound must be properly cared for and closure achieved expeditiously to lessen the level of physiologic disruption that accompanies a major burn. Failure to do so can result in invasive wound infection, chronic inflammation, erosion of lean body mass, progressive functional deficits, and even death.

Specialized Injuries: Electrical Burns

The principal mechanism by which electricity damages tissue is by conversion to thermal energy. Currents of 1000 volts and above are classified as high voltage. Upon contact with such currents, the body acts as a volume conductor. The electric current may induce cardiac and respiratory arrest, necessitating cardiopulmonary resuscitation at any time after injury. Arrhythmias may also occur, necessitating electrocardiogram monitoring for at least 24 hours after the last recorded episode of arrhythmia.

Two characteristics of high-voltage electrical injury increase the incidence of acute renal failure in patients. First, there is often extensive unapparent subcutaneous tissue injury in a limb underlying unburned skin. The limited cutaneous injury may lead to gross underestimation of resuscitation fluid needs. Second, the mass of muscle injured by the electric current may cause rhabdomyolysis, resulting in direct damage to the renal tubules. Resuscitation fluids should be based on the extent of burn visible plus the estimated daily needs of the patient, adjusted according to the patient's response. If the urine contains hemochromogens (dark red pigments), fluid should be administered to obtain output of 75 to 100 mL of urine per hour, with sodium bicarbonate added to the fluids to alkalinize the urine. If the hemochromogens do not clear promptly, or the patient remains oliguric, 25 g of mannitol should be given as a bolus and 12.5 g of mannitol added to each liter of lactated Ringer's solution until the pigment clears. The addition of mannitol, an osmotic diuretic, makes measurements of urine output unreliable as a monitor of the adequacy of resuscitation, and central venous monitoring is indicated.

When the body functions as a volume conductor, current density is inversely proportional to the cross-sectional area of the body part involved. Consequently, severe tissue destruction may occur in a limb with a relatively small cross-sectional area, whereas relatively little tissue damage may occur as current flows through the trunk. With high voltage (greater than 1000 V) and high current, the tissue with the highest resistance heats the most, such that soft tissues next to bone in the extremities are usually the most injured. Damage to the muscle in a limb is often associated with marked increase in the pressure within the compartment containing the damaged muscle, which, if unrelieved, may cause further tissue necrosis. A limb compartment, which is hard to palpation, should alert one to the need for immediate surgical exploration. Operative intervention and extensive fasciotomy are mandated by extensive deep tissue necrosis, compartment syndrome, or persistent or progressively severe hyperkalemia. The extent of destruction may necessitate amputation at the time of exploration, particularly if the nonviable muscle is the source of persistent hyperkalemia. Following débridement or amputation, the wound should be dressed open. The patient is returned to the operating room in 24 to 36 hours for reinspection and further débridement of nonviable tissue if necessary. When all tissue in the wound is viable, it may be closed definitively.

Tissue damage can also be caused by low-voltage or house current. Burns of the oral commissure occur in young children who bite electrical cords or suck on the end of a live extension cord or an electrical outlet. The lesion may have the characteristics of full-thickness tissue damage, but early surgical débridement may only accentuate the defect and should be avoided. These injuries will usually heal with minimal cosmetic sequelae, which can be addressed electively if needed. For the worst injuries, significant experience is required to perform a cosmetically acceptable reconstruction.

Specialized Injuries: Chemical Injuries

A variety of chemical agents can cause tissue injury as a consequence of an exothermic chemical reaction, protein coagulation, desiccation, and delipidation. The severity of a chemical injury is related to the concentration and amount of chemical agent and the duration with which it is in contact with tissue. Consequently, initial wound care to remove or dilute the offending agent takes priority in the management of patients with chemical injuries, brushing away dry material and instituting immediate, copious water lavage. For patients in whom extensive surface injury has occurred, the irrigation fluid should be warmed to prevent the induction of hypothermia.

The appearance of skin damaged by chemical agents can be misleading. In the case of patients injured by strong acids, the involved skin surface may have a silky texture and a light yellow-brown appearance, which may be mistaken for a sunburn rather than the full-thickness injury that it is. Skin injured by delipidation caused by petroleum distillates may be dry, show little if any inflammation, and appear to be undamaged and yet found to be a full-thickness injury on histologic examination.

Specialized Injuries: Cold Injuries

Injuries occurring secondary to environmental exposure can result in local injuries, frostbite, or systemic hypothermia. The pathophysiology of frostbite is crystal formation due to freezing of both extracellular and intracellular fluids. Patients presenting with frostbite will have coldness of the injured body part, with loss of sensation and proprioception. On initial examination, the limb may well appear pale, cyanotic, or have a yellow-white discoloration. During rapid rewarming at 40° to 42° C in water for 15 to 30 minutes, hyperemia will occur followed by pain, paresthesias, and sensory deficits. Greater than 1 week may pass before a true determination of the depth and extent of the injury can be obtained. The injured extremity should be elevated in an attempt to control edema and padded to avoid pressure-induced ischemia as a secondary insult. Frostbite wounds are tetanus-prone wounds, and therefore, tetanus toxoid should be administered based on the patient's immunization status.

MORBIDITY AND COMPLICATIONS MANAGEMENT

Early Complications

As resuscitation proceeds and edema forms beneath the inelastic eschar of encircling full-thickness burns of a limb, blood flow to

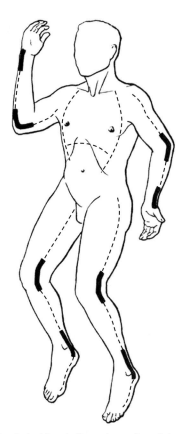

FIGURE 2 The dashed lines indicate the preferred sites of escharotomy incisions for the limbs (midlateral and midmedial lines), thorax (anterior axillary lines and costal margin), and neck (lateral aspect). The thickened areas of the lines on the limbs emphasize the importance of carrying the incisions across involved joints. *(From Martin RR, Becker WK, Cioffi WG, Pruitt BP Jr: Thermal injuries. In Wilson RF, Walt AJ, editors: Management of trauma: pitfalls and practice, 2nd ed. Baltimore, Williams & Wilkins, 1996, p 765.)*

underlying and distal unburned tissue may be compromised. Cyanosis of distal unburned skin and progressive paresthesias, particularly unrelenting deep tissue pain, which are the most reliable clinical signs of impaired circulation, may become evident only after relatively long periods of relative or absolute ischemia. In limbs threatened by circumferential deep burns, escharotomy can be performed at bedside without anesthesia because the full-thickness eschar is insensate. The escharotomy can be performed using a scalpel or an electrocautery device. Care should be taken not to injure large, patent, subcutaneous veins. On an extremity, the escharotomy incision, which is carried only through the eschar and the immediately subjacent superficial fascia, is placed in the midlateral (midradial for the upper extremity) line and must extend from the upper to the lower limit of the burn wound (Fig. 2). The circulatory status of the limb should then be reassessed. If that escharotomy has not restored distal flow, another escharotomy should be placed in the midmedial (midulnar for the upper extremity) line of the involved limb. A fasciotomy may be needed when there has been a delay in restoring the patient's limb circulation and in particular if the patient is receiving a massive fluid load.

Edema formation beneath encircling full-thickness truncal burns can restrict the respiratory excursion of the chest wall. If the limitation of chest wall motion is associated with hypoxia and elevated peak inspiratory pressure, chest escharotomy is indicated to restore chest wall motion and improve ventilation. These escharotomy incisions are placed in the anterior axillary line bilaterally and must be

connected by transverse escharotomies to fully release the chest eschar. If the entire anterior trunk is involved, transverse escharotomies should be performed at the level of the anterior posterior iliac spine (ASIS) and sternal notch (see Fig. 2).

The timely administration of adequate fluid as detailed previously has essentially eliminated acute renal failure after burn injury. Far more common today are the complications of excessive resuscitation—that is, compartment syndromes and pulmonary compromise. Compartment syndromes can be produced in the calvarium, muscle compartments beneath the investing fascia, and the abdominal cavity.

Excessive fluid administration may also cause formation of enough ascitic fluid and edema of the abdominal contents resulting in intraabdominal hypertension. The abdominal compartment syndrome represents progression of intraabdominal hypertension to the point of organ dysfunction, including decreased cardiac output with resultant hypotension, increased peak airway pressures, oliguria, and worsening metabolic acidosis due to hypoperfusion. Bladder pressure measurements serve as an indirect measurement of intraabdominal pressures. Elevation of the bladder pressure above 25 mm Hg should prompt therapeutic intervention, beginning with adequate sedation, reduction of fluid infusion rate, diuresis, and paracentesis. If organ failure becomes evident, decompressive laparotomy is indicated.

Compartment syndromes may also occur in the muscle compartments underlying the investing fascia of the limbs of burn patients, even in limbs that are unburned. To assess compartment pressure, the turgor of the muscle compartments should be assessed on a scheduled basis by simple palpation. A stony hard compartment is an ominous finding that should prompt direct measurement of intracompartmental pressure. A muscle compartment pressure of 25 mm Hg or more necessitates performing a fasciotomy of the involved compartment in the operating room using general anesthesia.

Metabolic and Nutritional Support

Burn injury alters the distribution and use of nutrients as well as the metabolic rate, and the severely burned patient will lose significant muscle mass during his or her illness. All of these postburn metabolic changes must be considered in planning nutritional support of the hypermetabolic burn patient in order to minimize loss of lean body mass, accelerate convalescence, and restore physical abilities. Bedside indirect calorimetry is the most accurate means of determining metabolic rate and nutritional requirements, but bedside metabolic care may not always be available. A rule of thumb estimate for nutritional needs of patients whose burns exceed 30% of the body surface area is 2000 to 2200 kcal and 12 to 18 g of nitrogen per square meter of body surface per day (up to 2.5 g protein/kg/day).

At the time of admission, patients should have a nasogastric or nasoduodenal tube placed. It is preferable to start enteral feedings as soon as possible after the patient is admitted. When feedings are initiated early, the desired rate of administration can typically be reached within 24 to 48 hours after admission. If the patient is intolerant to gastric feedings, the administration of metoclopramide will often resolve the problem. If a patient fails to respond to metoclopramide, an attempt should be made to pass a feeding tube distal to the ligament of Treitz. In patients who become intolerant of enteral feedings, or who develop gastrointestinal complications that prevent enteral feeding, total parenteral nutrition will be required.

Burn injury induces insulin resistance, which may lead to hyperglycemia. The maintenance of blood glucose values below 120 mg/dL with aggressive insulin infusion has been demonstrated to have a favorable impact on the outcome of critically ill patients. Potassium and phosphorus must also be given to meet the patient's needs, which often exceed initial estimates, particularly when large loads of glucose are being given with exogenous insulin. Over the course of the patient's care, as the open wound area decreases and the hypermetabolic state slowly resolves, the nutrient load should be adjusted so that balance is maintained between metabolic needs and substrate delivery, preventing overfeeding. Anabolic steroids have been shown to increase net protein retention in burned patients and oxandrolone is routinely used in critically ill burned patients for this purpose. Recombinant human growth hormone promotes anabolism in children, but its use in critically ill adults is associated with increased mortality rate.

TRANSPORTATION AND TRANSFER

Many important advances have been made in the care and management of burn-injured victims. One of the more significant advances has been the recognition of the benefits of a team approach in the care of critically injured burn patients. The American College of Surgeons and the American Burn Association have developed optimal standards for providing burn care and a burn center verification program that identifies those units that have undergone peer review of their performance and outcomes. Patients with burns and associated injuries and conditions listed in Table 1 should be referred to a burn center.

Once the decision has been made to transfer a patient to a burn center, there should be physician-to-physician communication regarding the patient's status and need for transfer. It is critical that the patient be properly stabilized in preparation for the transfer. During transport, the need to perform lifesaving interventions such as endotracheal intubation or reestablishing vascular access may be very difficult to accomplish in the relatively unstable and limited space of a moving ambulance or a helicopter in flight. That difficulty makes it important to institute hemodynamic and pulmonary resuscitation and to achieve "stability" prior to undertaking transfer by either aeromedical or ground transport. A secure large-bore intravenous cannula must be in place to permit continuous fluid resuscitation. Patients should be placed on 100% oxygen. If there is any question about airway adequacy, an endotracheal tube should be placed and mechanical ventilation instituted. The hourly urinary output should also be monitored, with fluid infusion adjusted as necessary. All patients should be placed NPO (nothing by mouth), and those with a greater than 20% body surface area burn require placement of a nasogastric tube. The burn wound should be covered with a clean or sterile dry sheet. The application of topical antimicrobial agents is contraindicated prior to transfer because they will have to be removed on admission to the burn center. Maintenance of the patient's body temperature is vital. The patient should be covered with a heat-reflective space blanket to minimize heat loss. Burn wounds, as tetanus-prone wounds, mandate immunization in accordance with the recommendations of the American College of Surgeons.

TABLE 6: Changes in Burn Patient Mortality Rate at U.S. Army Burn Center, 1945–1991

Age Group	PERCENTAGE OF BODY SURFACE BURN CAUSING 50% MORTALITY RATE (LA$_{50}$)	
	1945–1957	1987–1991
Children (0–14)	51	72*
Young adults (15–40)	43	82†
		73‡
Older adults	23	46§

From Pruitt BA Jr, Gamelli RL: Burns. In Britt LD, Trunkey DD, Organ CH, Feliciano DV, editors: *Acute care surgery.* New York, Springer, 2006, p 155.
*5 years.
†21 years.
‡40 years.
§60 years.

MORTALITY

Early postburn renal failure as a consequence of delayed or inadequate resuscitation has been eliminated, and inhalation injury as a comorbid factor has been tamed. Invasive burn wound sepsis has been controlled and early excision with prompt skin grafting and general improvements in critical care have reduced the incidence of infection, eliminated many previously life-threatening complications, and accelerated the convalescence of burn patients. Mortality rate for various ages and burn sizes is reported in Table 6. Not only has survival improved, but the elimination of many life-threatening complications and advances in wound care have improved the quality of life of even those patients who have survived extensive, severe thermal injuries. Challenges, however, remain. Although we are capable of restoring to the burned patient an envelope that is a reasonably effective barrier to microbes, heat loss, and water loss, we remain quite poor at restoring a normal social interface to the patient. Burned patients with visible scars remain "other" every time they walk into a room. The challenge for this century is to restore an aesthetically "normal" envelope to the patient along with saving his or her life.

For the chapter's Suggested Readings list, please visit the book at www.ExpertConsult.inkling.com.

SOFT TISSUE INFECTIONS

Sharon Henry

The skin is the largest organ of the body. It is flexible yet tough and acts as a structural barrier to invasion by microbes. Skin and soft tissue infections vary from trivial to life threatening. These infections may involve the epidermis, dermis, subcutaneous tissue, deep fascia, and muscle. They are the result of diverse causes and the host may be either healthy or compromised. In order to assure effective treatment, a prompt diagnosis should be made. The severity of the patient's illness must be assessed, the probable pathogen determined, specific antibiotic choices made, and prompt surgical therapy undertaken when appropriate. A myriad of microbes are capable of producing soft tissue infection and to confound issues there is considerable overlapping of clinical presentation.

Severe soft tissue infections have been described throughout the medical literature since ancient times. Celsius in the first century described the classic signs of inflammation: rubor, dolor, calor, and tumor. Necrotizing fasciitis was described in the fifth century BC by Hippocrates, though Wilson coined the term in 1952.

Much of our knowledge regarding the treatment of soft tissue infection has been based on the experience gained during military conflicts. For instance, hospital gangrene was described first by Joseph Jones, a Confederate surgeon during the Civil War. The treatment of battlefield infections has influenced civilian practice.

INCIDENCE

Soft tissue infections occur frequently and account for approximately 48.3 in 1000 outpatient visits. Infections of the skin and soft tissue are among the most common infections treated in hospitals. Estimated acute care hospital admissions for skin and soft tissue infection have risen from 675,000 in 2000 to 869,800 in 2004. This represents an increase of 29%. The increased admission is mainly for the treatment of cellulitis and abscess and seems to involve children, young adults, African Americans, and communities served by high safety net status hospitals disproportionately. In hospitalized patients, somewhere between 4.3% and 10.5% of septic episodes are caused by soft tissue infections. The incidence of serious soft tissue infection is thankfully far less common. The exact incidence, however, is not known. A 1994 WHO report estimates 500 to 1500 cases of necrotizing fasciitis annually. Though uncommon, it is not rare. The Centers for Disease Control and Prevention monitors group A streptococcal (GAS) infections and estimates 10 to 20 cases per 100,000 population. In Ontario, Canada, a population study estimated an incidence of 0.6 per 100,000.

MECHANISM OF INJURY

The skin is the largest organ in the body and is designed to protect by maintaining a mechanical barrier to microbes. It additionally maintains temperature homeostasis; excretes fluids and electrolytes, lipids, and acids; is a sense organ; produces vitamin D; and allows for non-verbal communication. Figure 1 depicts the anatomy of the skin.

The skin is colonized with a microbacterial flora. Common organisms include staphylococcal species, corynebacteria, propionibacteria, and yeast. The number of organisms per surface area varies extending from a few hundred in drier areas to several thousand in moist areas like the axilla and groin. Primary soft tissue infections occur most commonly following the disruption of the protective skin barrier. The indigenous microbes may prevent the growth of pathogenic species. Infection of the skin and soft tissue occurs frequently following damage to the skin. This can occur through injury, surgery, bites (insect, spider, animal or human), burns, medical injections, or parenteral drug use. Secondary infections occur when a skin lesion such as dermatitis exists. Chronic ulcers (diabetic, venous, or vascular) or

dermatologic skin lesions like psoriasis also become secondarily infected. Direct spread from nearby structures can result in soft tissue infections as with gastrointestinal or genitourinary perforations. Minor tissue trauma can be the portal of entry of bacteria. This may be as innocuous as skin cracks resulting from tinea pedis, xerosis, skin abrasion following vigorous scratching, or irritation at a hair follicle or sweat gland. Frequently no etiologic lesion can be identified. Less commonly, secondary infection of the soft tissue results from hematogenous spread. This is most frequently seen in the immunosuppressed patient. Injection drug users with endocarditis are at risk for the development of skin and soft tissue infections through this mechanism as well.

Most skin and soft tissue infections are caused by *Staphylococcus aureus* and beta-hemolytic streptococcus groups A, C, and G. Group B beta-hemolytic streptococcus is seen most commonly in patients with diabetes mellitus. Gram-negative and anaerobic organisms are more likely to be found in infections following surgical procedures involving the abdominal wall or in infections that occur around the anus. Infections that are caused by both gram-negative and gram-positive organisms are more likely to occur in tissues where there is compromise to perfusion. This is seen most commonly in the patient with diabetes mellitus and arterial or venous insufficiency. The bacterial flora of patients previously treated with antimicrobials will change the likely causative organisms. Therefore, chronic infections are frequently polymicrobial. In addition, the use of antibiotics results in the emergence of resistant strains of microorganisms. Methicillin-resistant *S. aureus* (MRSA) has reached endemic proportions. MRSA was identified in 1960 and was initially a problem confined to the hospitalized patient population. In the late 1990s community-associated MRSA (CA-MRSA) appeared in patients without discernible risk factors. A 2007 study noted the incidence of MRSA isolates in patients with soft tissue infections averaged 35.9% and in 2004, the last year of the study period, that increased to 47.4%. Table 1 lists the most commonly isolated bacterial pathogens from cultures of skin and soft tissue infections.

Many bacteria produce endotoxins and exotoxins that facilitate their movement along fascial planes and ultimately through fascial planes. These toxins produce tissue injury, ischemia, and liquefaction necrosis. In severe cases they can cause rapid progression of the infection by as much as 1 inch per hour. *Clostridium*, *Staphylococcus*, and *Streptococcus* are best known for this (Table 2). Most importantly,

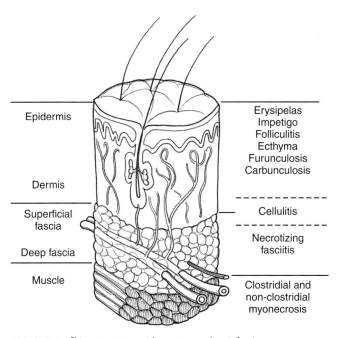

FIGURE 1 Skin structures with corresponding infection.

Epidermis

Dermis

Superficial fascia

Deep fascia

Muscle

Erysipelas
Impetigo
Folliculitis
Ecthyma
Furunculosis
Carbunculosis

Cellulitis

Necrotizing fasciitis

Clostridial and non-clostridial myonecrosis

TABLE 1: Ten Most Common Bacterial Isolates for Skin and Soft Tissue Infections

Rank	Organism
1	*Staphylococcus aureus*
2	*Pseudomonas aeruginosa*
3	*Enterococcus* species
4	*Escherichia coli*
5	*Enterobacter* species
6	*Klebsiella* species
7	Beta-hemolytic streptococcus
8	*Proteus mirabilis*
9	Coagulase-negative staphylococcus
10	*Serratia* species

TABLE 2: Bacterial Toxins and Effects

Organism	Toxic Substance	Effects
Clostridia	Alpha toxin	Tissue necrosis Cardiovascular collapse
Streptococci and Staphylococci	M-1 and M-3 proteins Exotoxins A, B, and C Streptolysin O Superantigen	Increased ability to adhere and escape phagocytosis Damage endothelium, cause loss of microvascular integrity and tissue edema and impair blood flow at the capillary Stimulate CD4 cells and macrophages to produce TNF-α, IL-1, and IL-6 Stimulate T cells to produce excessive cytokine Emesis

IL, Interleukin; TNF, tumor necrosis factor.

TABLE 3: Risk Factors and Associated Pathogens

Risk Factor	Pathogen
Human bite	*Eikenella corrodens*
Cat bite	*Pasteurella multocida*
Dog bite	*Capnocytophaga canimorsus*
Rat bite	*Streptobacillus moniliformis* *Spirillum minus*
Animal hides	*Bacillus anthracis* *Francisella tularensis*
Medical leeches	*Aeromonas hydrophila* *Aeromonas sobria* *Serratia marcescens* *Vibrio fluvialis*
Water exposure	
Salt water	*Vibrio* species
Freshwater	*A. hydrophila*
Hot tub	*Pseudomonas aeruginosa*
Fish tank	*Mycobacterium marinum*
Salon foot spa	*Mycobacterium fortuitum*
Reptile contact	*Salmonella* species
Injection drug use	*Clostridium botulinum*, anaerobes, *E. corrodens*
Travel	*Leishmania* (leishmaniasis) *Ancylostoma braziliense* (cutaneous larva migrans) Fly larvae causing myiasis *Cordylobia anthropophaga* *Dermatobia hominis*
Cirrhosis	*Campylobacter fetus*, *Klebsiella pneumoniae*, *Escherichia coli*, *C. canimorsus*, other gram-negative bacilli, *Vibrio vulnificus*
Neutropenia	*P. aeruginosa*

these toxins stimulate macrophages to produce inflammatory cytokines TNF-α (tumor necrosis factor), interleukin 1, and interleukin 6. Systemically these cytokines produce the systemic inflammatory response that may lead to sepsis, organ failure, and death. Locally, neutrophil degranulation and superoxide release produce injury to endothelium. Superantigens produced by the bacteria cause massive T-cell stimulation, amplifying the inflammatory response. They also activate the complement system as well as the coagulation cascade. This effect causes thrombosis of small vessels and further tissue ischemia and injury.

Though common things occur commonly, other less usual pathogens can be responsible for skin and soft tissue infection. These organisms are often associated with particular risk factors, including human or animal bites or contact with water (Table 3).

Several classification schemes have been suggested to simplify the discussion of soft tissue infection as well as to guide the treatment. For the purpose of clinical study of antimicrobials the Food and Drug Administration uses a simple uncomplicated as well as a complicated stratification system (Table 4).

Simple Uncomplicated Infections

Superficial infections are limited anatomically to the epidermis and the dermis. These infections can occur spontaneously or secondary to minor trauma. Impetigo usually presents with vesicles that leak, producing a thick yellow crust. These lesions are typically located on the face, neck, and extremities. *S. aureus* and *Streptococcus pyogenes* are the most common causative agents. Bullous impetigo, like impetigo, is most commonly caused by *S. aureus*. It is characterized by small vesicles that coalesce to form large bullae. The peak incidence is in childhood at ages 2 to 5, though it does occur in older children and adults. Generally skin colonization is thought to precede the development of this infection by an average of 10 days. It occurs most commonly on exposed areas such as the face or extremities. The lesions may be multiple but are well localized. Ecthyma is a deeper ulcerated form of impetigo. Systemic symptoms are unusual.

Folliculitis develops as a superficial inflammation of the hair follicle. The lesions appear as pustules or papules, commonly on the extremities, scalp, or beard and are anatomically located in the epidermis. Whirlpool folliculitis is associated with immersion in inadequately chlorinated pools, whirlpools, or hot tubs. Diffuse pustules

are seen. *Pseudomonas aeruginosa* is the classic causative agent. Swimmer's itch is a folliculitis that develops after freshwater exposure. Moist heat application will usually promote drainage at this stage.

Furuncles, deeper inflammatory nodules, can develop from folliculitis, when the suppuration extends through the dermis and into the subcutaneous tissue. *S. aureus* is often the causative agent. Carbuncles are coalescing furuncles formed by connecting sinuses. The nape of the neck is the most common anatomic location. *S. aureus* is frequently cultured. Furuncles and carbuncles require incision and drainage. Systemic antibiotics are necessary when there is surrounding cellulitis or associated fever. When recurrent infection with resistant *S. aureus* occurs, patients are advised to be meticulous in their personal hygiene. Areas that may harbor the organism should be thoroughly cleansed, and decontamination through use of antimicrobial soaps and thorough laundering of towels and bed sheets may be necessary. Nasal decontamination with mupirocin ointment twice daily for 5 to 10 days may be useful in cases of recurrent infection.

Erysipelas is a term frequently used interchangeably with cellulitis. It is distinguished by a clear line of demarcation between normal and involved skin and it is usually raised above the skin level. It is usually

TABLE 4: Classification of Skin, Skin Structure, and Soft Tissue Infections

Uncomplicated Skin and Soft Tissue Infection		Complicated Skin and Soft Tissue Infection	
Superficial	Impetigo Ecthyma	Secondary infection of diseased skin Acute wound infections	Traumatic Bite related Postoperative
Deeper	Cellulitis/erysipelas	Chronic wound infections	Diabetic foot infections Venous stasis ulcers Pressure sores
Hair follicle associated	Folliculitis, furunculosis	Perianal cellulitis/abscess	
Abscess	Carbuncle, other cutaneous abscess	Necrotizing fasciitis	Type I Type II Type III
		Myonecrosis	Clostridial Nonclostridal

caused by group A hemolytic streptococcus but groups C or G may also cause it. It is less commonly caused by *S. aureus*. It is most common in children or the elderly and affects the lower extremities most frequently. Historically, the face was the most common site, but currently the extremities are more often affected.

Cellulitis is an inflammation of the subcutaneous tissue and is therefore deeper than erysipelas. There is erythema, pain, and edema of varying severity. Lymphangitis and regional lymph node swelling may be present. The skin may have a peau d'orange appearance as a result of the edema surrounding the hair follicles, which remain attached to the dermis producing a dimpled appearance. Vesicles and bullae of the skin may occur. Petechiae and ecchymoses may be seen on the inflamed skin. A portal of entry for the bacteria is usually present. It may be as mundane as a crack in the skin from dryness or tinea pedis. Systemic symptoms may manifest and include fever, chills, malaise, and (infrequently) organ failure. Streptococcus (groups A, B, C, and G) as well as staphylococcus are frequent culprits. Areas of compromised venous or lymphatic drainage are prone to this infection, and recurrence is common. Pelvic radiation or having had lymphadenectomy, mastectomy, or venectomy makes the development of cellulitis more likely. Other infectious organisms may be responsible in special circumstances (see Table 3).

Complicated Infections

Necrotizing Soft Tissue Infection

Deeper infections are more frequently life and limb threatening. The literature concerning the potentially life-threatening infections is confusing. Multiple terms are used to describe the same disease, depending on the clinical setting in which it arises. The treatment is the same regardless of the term used to describe it. It therefore seems that anatomic classification is more logical and more easily remembered.

In the medical literature, deep structure infection has masqueraded under a variety of pseudonyms. The term "necrotizing soft tissue infection" (NSTI) is used here. Table 5 lists a variety of terms that may appear in the medical literature to describe this infective process.

All the terms describe an infection involving the subcutaneous fat and fascia, with variable skin involvement. In severe cases the muscle may also be involved. There is often vast tissue destruction that, if not fatal, is mutilating. The ability of an organism to cause infection is dependent on the virility of the organism and the resistance of the

TABLE 5: Terms Used to Describe Necrotizing Soft Tissue Infection

Meleney's synergistic gangrene	Hospital gangrene
Streptococcal gangrene	Fournier's gangrene
Gas gangrene	Acute dermal gangrene
Suppurativa fasciitis	Necrotizing erysipelas
Phagedena	Phagedena gangrenosum
"Flesh-eating disease"	Necrotizing fasciitis
Clostridial cellulitis	

host. In about 80% of cases the infection has spread from a discernible lesion. Table 6 contains a list of potential sites. The remaining 20% will not have an identifiable origin. This disease is unique in that it affects both the compromised and the uncompromised host. Multiple reviews identify multiple risk factors associated with increased susceptibility; however, exceptionally virulent bacteria such as GAS are able to affect otherwise uncompromised hosts. These bacteria produce exotoxins that result in the release of cytokines, leading to a robust systemic response. At the cellular level, the toxins and enzymes (hyaluronidases and lipases) facilitate the spread of bacteria along fascial planes and through the subcutaneous tissue. Necrosis of the superficial fascia and fat often produce a thin, watery, foul-smelling fluid (dishwater pus). The skin necrosis that may accompany this infection results when thrombosis of the skin's nutrient vessels occurs. Microscopic findings are usually severe subcutaneous fat necrosis, severe inflammation of the dermis and subcutaneous fat, vasculitis, endarteritis, and local hemorrhage (Fig. 2). The fascia may be edematous and suppurative, and thrombosis of vessels may be seen. Myonecrosis may also be seen in advanced cases.

Pyomyositis

Pyomyositis occurs when there is pus within muscle groups. Its clinical presentation is usually of severe pain often initially thought to be secondary to muscular strain. Diagnosis is often delayed as treatment with rest and nonsteroidal anti-inflammatory medications are prescribed. The pain symptoms worsen and muscle spasm is noted

TABLE 6: Potential Sites and Causes of Necrotizing Soft Tissue Infection

Site	Etiology
Perineum	Anal abscess
	Bartholin's abscess
	Genitourinary infection
	Postgenitourinary tract surgery or catheterization
	Postanal procedure
	Bulky neoplasm
Extremity	Diabetic foot ulcer
	Venous stasis ulcer
	Arterial insufficiency ulcer
	Injection drug use
	Traumatic wound or fracture
	Animal or human bite
	Decubitus ulcer
Trunk	Surgical site infection
	Extension from intra-abdominal source
	Decubitus ulcer
	Strangulated hernia
Head and neck	Dental abscess
	Pharyngeal/tonsillar abscess
	Surgical site infection

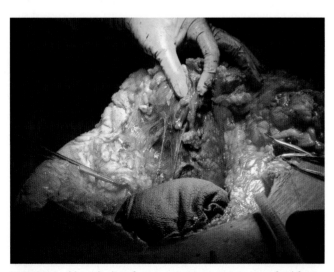

FIGURE 2 Note the liquefaction necrosis present in superficial fascia and fat in this patient with necrotizing soft tissue infection following cesarean section.

and, if not suppressed, fever develops. Early in the course, abnormalities may not be palpable as the infection is deep. As the infection enlarges and myonecrosis ensues, woody firmness or even bulging of an abscess may be appreciated. The organism isolated is usually *S. aureus*.

Surgical Site Infections

Surgical site infections are a common adverse event affecting the hospitalized patient. Superficial infections involve only the subcutaneous space and develop within 30 days of an operative procedure. There is at least one of the following present:

Purulent drainage
Positive fluid or tissue culture from the wound
Local signs and symptoms of pain, swelling, tenderness, and erythema
Diagnosis of infection made by attending surgeon or physician

Deep surgical site infections are defined as involving the fascia or muscle and develop within 30 days of the operative procedure.

DIAGNOSIS

Clinical Presentation

Signs and symptoms of NSTI can be quite nonspecific (Table 7). Pain, erythema, and swelling of the affected area are most frequently present. This same constellation of symptoms may be seen in pathologic processes that have a much more benign course and respond effectively to antibiotic therapy alone. "Hard signs" of necrotizing infection include tense erythema, bullae, skin discoloration, and crepitus, pain out of proportion to examination, or anesthesia of the affected area (Fig. 3). Unfortunately, these hard signs are present in a minority of patients. In addition, once these signs are recognized the infective process is well established.

Signs of systemic toxicity may also be present and include pyrexia, tachycardia, hypotension, and organ dysfunction. The progression of symptoms may be rapid over the course of hours to days or more indolent over the course of days to weeks. The rate of progression of symptoms may be ameliorated by partial treatment. Several clinical features suggest the diagnosis of necrotizing fasciitis and are listed in Table 8.

Laboratory data are equally nonspecific. Leukocytosis, hyponatremia, and elevated creatine phosphokinase (CPK) have been evaluated in clinical studies and may be markers of the disease. Wall et al matched 21 patients with necrotizing fasciitis with control subjects with non-necrotizing infections and attempted to identify parameters that would distinguish the groups. White blood cell (WBC) count 15.4×10^9/L, serum sodium (Na) less than 135 mmol/L, or both, were the best factors to distinguish necrotizing fasciitis from non-necrotizing infection. The sensitivity was 90%, and the specificity was 76%. In this study, 40% of the patients with necrotizing fasciitis lacked "hard signs." Wong and colleagues developed the Laboratory Risk Indicator for Necrotizing Fasciitis (LRINEC) score. The score was developed retrospectively based on WBC count, hemoglobin (Hb), serum Na, C-reactive protein, creatinine, and glucose in patients with necrotizing fasciitis and patients with other severe soft tissue infections. A score of greater than 6 had a positive predictive value of 92% and a negative predictive value of 96%. In a cohort of prospectively evaluated patients, the model was found to have a positive predictive value of 40% and a negative predictive value of 95%. CPK elevation was found by one group to distinguish patients with GAS necrotizing fasciitis from non–GAS necrotizing fasciitis. CPK elevations were higher than 600 IU/L in the GAS group. Serum lactate and base deficit should be measured in physiologically abnormal patients to guide their resuscitation.

TABLE 7: Frequency of Clinical Signs of Necrotizing Soft Tissue Infection

Author	Erythema (%)	Crepitans (%)	Edema (%)	Year Published	No. Patients in Study
Callahan	77	3	20	1998	30
McHenry	72	12	75	1995	65
Brook	89	39	77	1995	83
Elliot	66	45	75	1996	197
Tang	50		58	2001	24
Theis	54			2002	13
Wong	100	13	92	2003	89

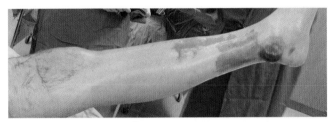

FIGURE 3 Note the hemorrhagic bullae around the ankle.

TABLE 8: Clinical Features of Necrotizing Soft Tissue Infection

1. Severe constant pain

2. Bullae resulting from perforator vessel occlusion

3. Skin necrosis or ecchymosis prior to skin necrosis

4. Gas in the tissues by palpation or radiography

5. Edema or induration beyond the margin of erythema

6. Cutaneous anesthesia

7. Systemic toxicity fever, leukocytosis, delirium, acute kidney disease

8. Rapid spread despite antibiotic therapy

Diagnostic Imaging

Imaging may be useful in cases in which the diagnosis is in doubt or in defining the extent of disease. The hallmark of NSTI, air in subcutaneous tissues, can be seen with a variety of imaging techniques. Plain radiographs will demonstrate subcutaneous air in only 16% of patients. Plain films may also demonstrate foreign bodies. This is especially important when treating intravenous drug users. Ultrasonography, computed tomography (CT) scan, and magnetic resonance imaging (MRI) are more sensitive than plain radiography in demonstrating air in the tissues. These modalities may additionally identify fluid collections in the subcutaneous tissues or within the muscle. They may be very helpful in cases without significant skin changes in planning incisions and evaluating the extent of the infection. MRI has the advantage of not requiring the administration of intravenous contrast material, which may be toxic to the kidneys. This is especially helpful in patients who already have compromised renal

TABLE 9: Computed Tomography Scoring for Necrotizing Soft Tissue Infection

Finding	Points
Fascial air	5
Muscle/fascial edema	4
Fluid tracking in subcutaneous space	3
Lymphadenopathy	2
Subcutaneous edema	1

function. However, systemically compromised patients are often logistically poor candidates for MRI scanning. In most cases, diagnostic imaging is only confirmatory, as patients with nonspecific findings on evaluation, such as edema, may still harbor the disease. Failure to improve with appropriate antibiotics, development of systemic toxicity, or profound elevation of the WBC count should markedly raise the index of suspicion. Recently a CT scoring system has been advocated to differentiate patients with necrotizing and non-NSTIs. It is based on a retrospective analysis of patients discharged with a diagnosis of necrotizing fasciitis, abscess, or cellulitis. The CT scan images of the study patients were reviewed and a scoring system developed based on the findings (Table 9). Patients with a score of 6 or greater were found to have NSTI with a sensitivity of 86.2% and specificity 91.5%, a negative predictive value of 85%, and a positive predictive value of 63.3%.

Enron and his colleagues devised a classification system based on the severity of the local and systemic signs of infection. They also included the presence of comorbid conditions. They intended this to be a useful guide to the need for admission and appropriate therapy (Table 10). NSTIs are often classified by the bacteria that cause the infection. Type I is a polymicrobial infection and is the most common variety. Typically this infection is seen in patients with comorbid conditions. Gram-negative enteric bacteria are seen in combination with gram-positive organisms and anaerobes. As many as 15 different organisms have been cultured from such patients with an average of 5. Type II is GAS either alone or in combination with *S. aureus*. This type takes a more virulent course and occurs in younger, healthier patients. Clostridial infections classically produce air in the soft tissues, although the polymicrobial type I infections may also produce air as well. *Vibrio vulnificus* and *Aeromonas hydrophilia* should be suspected when the patient has been exposed to shellfish or freshwater and are considered to be type III by some.

Others suggest classifying the disease by its clinical course. Fulminant disease presents in patients with acute onset and rapid

TABLE 10: Eron's Classification of Soft Tissue Infections

Class	Patient Criteria	Probable Treatment	Location
1	Afebrile and healthy, other than cellulitis	Drainage if needed and oral antibiotic	Outpatient treatment
2	Febrile and ill appearing, but no unstable comorbid conditions	Drainage if needed and oral or intravenous (IV) antibiotics	Short inpatient observation with outpatient treatment
3	Toxic appearing or at least one unstable comorbid condition or a limb-threatening infection	IV antibiotics	Inpatient treatment
4	Sepsis syndrome or life-threatening infection	IV antibiotics	Inpatient intensive care unit treatment Surgical consultation

Eron LJ: Infections of skin and soft tissue: outcomes of a classification scheme. *Clin Infect Dis* 31:287, 2000.

TABLE 11: Clinical Settings of Necrotizing Soft Tissue Infections

Type	Progression	Prior/Partial Antibiotic Use	Systemic Symptoms	Organ Failure	Persistent Local Symptoms
I, II, III	Hyperacute	−	✓	✓	−/✓
I, II, III	Acute	−	✓	✓	−/✓
I, II	Subacute	✓	−	−	✓

progression over the course of hours with shock. Acute disease presents with large surface area involvement and over the course of days. Subacute disease presents for weeks and is usually localized (Table 11). Differentiating this process from cellulitis or simple abscess can be a challenge. Clinically, failure to improve with appropriate antibiotics or worsening systemic toxicity portends this diagnosis.

Lastly, Wong and his colleagues (2003) observed the progression of disease in a group of patients with NSTI. They performed a retrospective review of patients who were diagnosed with necrotizing faciitis and had a delay in surgery of more than 96 hours. They describe a progression of clinical findings over time from stage I to III (Table 12).

TABLE 12: Clinical Findings of Necrotizing Soft Tissue Infections, Stages I to III

Stage I: Early Stage

Tenderness to palpation (extending beyond the apparent area of skin involvement)

Erythema

Swelling

Calor (warm skin)

Stage II: Intermediate

Blister or bullae formation (serous fluid)

Stage III: Late

Crepitus

Skin anesthesia

Skin necrosis with dusky discoloration

SURGICAL MANAGEMENT

The management of the patient with soft tissue infection begins with an assessment of the general physiologic state. Stable patients without comorbid conditions, the uncomplicated patient, may require no more than topical or oral antimicrobial agents or incision and drainage. On the other hand, patients with evidence of organ failure or hemodynamic abnormality require immediate resuscitation with adherence to the sepsis guidelines listed in Table 13.

TABLE 13: Surviving Sepsis Guidelines Abridged

Stage	Goal	Intervention
Initial resuscitation ≤6 hr	CVP 8–12 mm Hg MAP ≥ 65 mm Hg Urine output ≥ 5 mL/kg/hr MVo_2 ≥ 65%	Fluid resuscitation Transfuse PRBCs if Hct <30% or Dobutamine infusion
Diagnosis	Prior to administering antibiotics if it won't delay	Obtain two or more blood cultures Culture other sites if indicated
Antibiotic therapy	Within the first hour of recognizing severe sepsis/septic shock	Broad-spectrum bacterial/fungal therapy, ensure good penetration to source Consider two drugs with *Pseudomonas* Consider combination in neutropenia
Source control	≤6 hours	Drain abscess, débride tissue

CVP, Central venous pressure; Hct, hematocrit; MAP, mean arterial pressure; MVo_2, myocardial oxygen consumption; PRBC, packed red blood cell.

Necrotizing fasciitis is a surgical emergency. The mainstay of treatment is surgical débridement. These procedures can be quite disfiguring, requiring the removal of large amounts of skin, subcutaneous fat, fascia, and possibly muscle or bone. Explorations on the extremities are usually begun by making generous vertical incisions. When involvement is diffuse, fasciotomy incisions on the extremities are often a useful starting place. The dissection must extend down to the level of the deep fascia. The muscle should also be inspected to confirm its viability (Fig. 4). Formal fasciotomies may be necessary in cases with very intense edema in order to prevent myonecrosis (Figs. 5 and 6).

The integrity of the tissue plane between the subcutaneous fat or superficial fascia and the deep fascia is tested with either a finger or clamp (Fig. 7). Lack of resistance to this probing is the hallmark of the diagnosis in early cases. "Dishwater pus" may be encountered as this plane is opened. In more advanced cases, frankly necrotic or purulent material is encountered. Cultures and stat Gram stain for aerobic and anaerobic cultures should be obtained. If the patient is immunosuppressed, cultures for *Mycobacterium* and fungus should also be sent. It is imperative to widely open all affected tissue planes and débride all obviously devitalized tissue (Fig. 8).

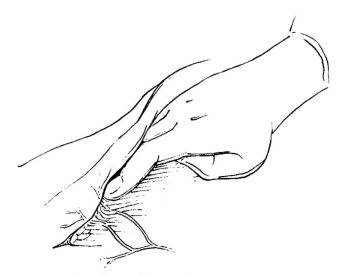

FIGURE 7   Loss of tissue plane integrity.

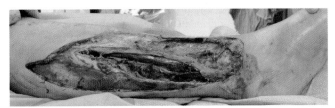

FIGURE 4   Postdébridement appearance of patient in Figure 3; necrosis and purulence extended through the deep fascia and involved the soleus and gastrocnemius muscles.

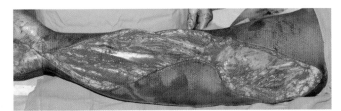

FIGURE 5   Decompression with upper extremity dorsal fasciotomy.

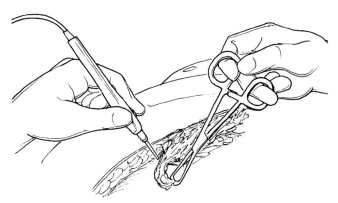

FIGURE 8   Thorough débridement.

When the presentation is more focal, incisions can be placed over the area of maximal skin abnormality and the incision extended as abnormalities of the deeper tissue are encountered (Figs. 9 and 10). A colostomy may be helpful in cases with extensive perianal involvement to prevent ongoing stool contamination. Surgical feeding tube placement should be considered in critically ill patients or in patients with large surface area wounds that are likely to remain open for some time.

Plans should be made at the end of the case for return to the operating room for reevaluation of the wounds within 48 hours. Adequate evaluation of these deep and often painful wounds is not possible at the bedside. A variety of wound dressings can be applied. Negative pressure wound therapy (NPWT) is optimally suited for this purpose. It allows removal of exudate, which may further decrease bacterial counts. It prevents maceration of the surrounding tissue and keeps the patient and the bed linens dry. It is often helpful to be able to quantify the fluid losses that are occurring. Replacement of these losses may be necessary. The skin surrounding the wound can be evaluated for advancing cellulitis or edema. The character of the fluid can also be assessed.

It is imperative if this type of wound care is to be used that hemostasis is meticulous and coagulopathy corrected. Parameters must be given to the nursing staff regarding volume and character of the fluid loss that is acceptable. When this type of dressing is not available or prudent, the wounds may be packed with Kerlix (Kendall Kerlix AMD) or gauze impregnated with antimicrobial material. Although some of these materials may be cytotoxic, the antimicrobial properties may outweigh the negative effect of the cytotoxicity on normal tissues. Once the infection is controlled, noncytotoxic products should be used. Silver ion–based products are a good choice.

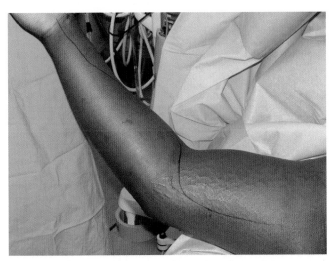

FIGURE 6   Patient with severe swelling and erythema of the upper arm and forearm.

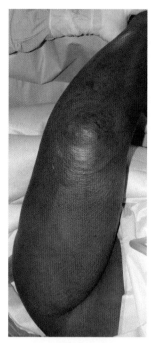

FIGURE 9 Preoperative appearance of patient in Figure 10. Note the area of discoloration and blistering at the elbow with tense edema and erythema.

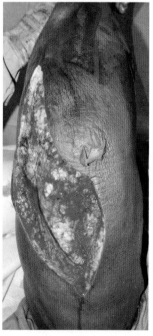

FIGURE 10 Postoperative photo of patient in Figure 9, which is the predébridement appearance of this wound. This demonstrates the necrosis of the superficial fascia and fat found extending from the elbow.

PHARMACOLOGIC THERAPY

Initial treatment of the patient in shock should be aimed at resuscitation. Fluids and blood products are given as needed to replace deficits. Coagulation abnormalities should be corrected. It must be stressed that resuscitation is begun, but all abnormalities will not and need not be fully corrected before proceeding to surgery. Resuscitation must continue throughout the preoperative, operative, and postoperative phases. Many abnormalities will not fully correct until there is adequate source control. Pressors and steroids may be

necessary in severe cases. When GAS is involved, intravenous immunoglobulin (IVIG) may also be given. Broad-spectrum antibiotic therapy is initiated to cover the most likely causative organisms (Table 14). Extended spectrum penicillins are a good first-line choice. Clindamycin should be added in cases that may involve GAS. Methicillin resistance is emerging in the community, and this must be considered in choosing antibiotics. Vancomycin or daptomycin should be considered when resistance is suspected or in cases in which the patient is severely compromised. Patients with penicillin allergies can be treated with fluoroquinolones in combination with gram-negative and anaerobic therapy or carbapenems.

HYPERBARIC OXYGEN

Hyperbaric oxygen (HBO) is an adjunct to resuscitation, surgical débridement, and broad-spectrum antibiotics. A variety of salutary affects have been attributed to HBO therapy (Table 15). There are no prospective randomized studies to scientifically validate the efficacy of HBO therapy; however, a number of retrospective studies seem to support its use in severe necrotizing infections. Several studies demonstrated decreased mortality rate in patients treated with HBO compared with historical control groupss. Other studies demonstrated improved preservation of tissue as evidenced by a decrease in the number of débridements to achieve control of the infection. Some studies, however, have questioned the efficacy of HBO. These studies showed no statistically significant difference in mortality rate between patients treated with HBO and those who received only surgical débridement. HBO therapy is not uniformly available throughout the country, so it is not an option for every patient who presents with this problem. When available, given the relatively high mortality and morbidity rates, use of this modality as an adjunct makes sense.

MORTALITY, MORBIDITY, AND COMPLICATIONS MANAGEMENT

The morbidity following the treatment of severe NSTIs can be severe. Most of the morbidity results from the tissue destruction brought about by the infection. The extent of morbidity depends on the area involved and the extent of the necessary débridement. During débridement, iatrogenic injury to nerves and blood supply can compound dysfunction. This is most common in the management of extremity infections. Tissues may be distorted by the inflammation and necrosis or scarred by prior surgery, making the identification of vital structures a challenge. It is vitally important to be familiar with the anatomy of the area. Patients may be left with significant deficits in function solely related to the magnitude of the surgical débridement. Amputation rates from 17% to 33% have been documented in patients with extremity severe soft tissue infections. Large wounds are frequently associated with significant pain. Acute and chronic pain management may be necessary in these patients.

Patients with abdominal sites of infection, who require débridement of their abdominal wall, are subject to the development of enterocutaneous fistulas. Management of the output of the fistula and providing for adequate nutrition are the treatment goals in the early management of this problem.

Mortality rates as high as 76% have been recorded, although contemporary studies report overall mortality rates in the range of 8% to 25%. Multiple factors affect mortality rate. Clinical presentation and speed to surgery appear to be the two most important determinants. Patients who suffer delays in obtaining surgical treatment had higher mortality rates. Patients who present with organ failure or increased serum lactate also have higher mortality rates. Comorbid conditions such as diabetes mellitus, renal failure, and advanced age and the need for large surface area débridements have also been noted to increase mortality rate. Anaya recently evaluated a large dataset of patients with severe soft tissue infections and identified several predictive factors including WBC count, hematocrit (Hct), creatinine, temperature, and heart rate. They developed a score that stratifies fatality (Table 16). Finally, a recent

TABLE 14: Antibiotics for Serious Soft Tissue Infections

Antibiotic	Organisms Treated	Comment
Penicillin β-lactam antibiotic inhibits bacterial cell wall X linking	Streptococcus *Clostridium* Peptostreptococcus	High incidence of *Staphylococcus aureus* resistance
Clindamycin lincosamide antibiotic inhibits bacterial protein synthesis	*Bacteroides fragilis* *Fusobacterium* Peptostreptococcus MRSA but induces resistance	May be used with GAS to inhibit toxin production. Is bacteriostatic
Metronidazole nitroimidazole antibiotic deactivates bacterial enzymes	Anerobes (above) and *Prevotella*	
Vancomycin glycopeptides antibiotic bacterial cell wall synthesis inhibitor	MRSA MSSA	For penicillin-allergic patients Redman syndrome, thrombophlebitis occur Drug levels must be monitored Has been parenteral drug of choice for treatment of infections caused by MRSA
Daptomycin lipopeptide antibiotic disrupts cell membrane function	MRSA Gram–positive organisms	Bactericidal may cause myopathy, not useful in treating pneumonias
Linezolid oxazolidinone antibiotic disrupts bacterial protein synthesis	MRSA VRE	Long-term use associated with bone marrow suppression and thrombocytopenia, lactic acidosis, and peripheral neuropathy
Quinupristin/dalfopristin streptogramin antibiotic inhibits protein synthesis	MRSA VRE	Each drug alone is bacteriostatic but combined are bactericidal Myalgias, nausea, and vomiting
Piperacillin-tazobactam extended spectrum penicillin	Gram-negative organisms including *Pseudomonas* Gram-positive organisms	
Cefotaxime third-generation cephalosporin	Gram-negative organisms Gram-positive organisms No enterococcal activity	
Ciprofloxacin fluoroquinolone DNA gyrase inhibitor	Gram-positive organisms Gram-negative organisms	Many drug interactions
Impinem, meropenem, ertapenem carbapenem β-lactamase resistant	Aerobes including *Pseudomonas* Anerobes Does not cover MRSA	Wide-spectrum efficacy, and inhibition of endotoxin release from aerobic organisms

GAS, Group A streptococci; MSSA, methicillin-sensitive *Staphylococcus aureus*; MRSA, methicillin-resistant *Staphylococcus aureus*; VRE, vancomycin-resistant enteroccoci.

TABLE 15: Beneficial Effects of Hyperbaric Oxygen

Inhibits growth of anaerobic organisms

Reduces the production of clostridial toxin

Improves leukocyte bacterial killing

Bactericidal and bacteriostatic effects on a variety of organisms

Enhances efficacy of certain antibiotics

Modulates cytokine levels

Decreases tissue edema

Increases collagen formation

TABLE 16: Clinical Score Predictive of Death for Patients with Necrotizing Soft Tissue Infection

Variable (on Admission)	Number of Points
Heart rate >110 beats/min	1
Temperature <36° C	1
Serum creatinine >1.5 mg/dL	1
Age >50 years	3
White blood cell count >40,000/μL	3
Hematocrit >50%	3

Group Category	Number of Points	Mortality Risk (%)
1	0–2	6
2	3–5	24
3	≥6	88

COMPLICATED SOFT TISSUE INFECTION MANAGEMENT ALGORITHIM

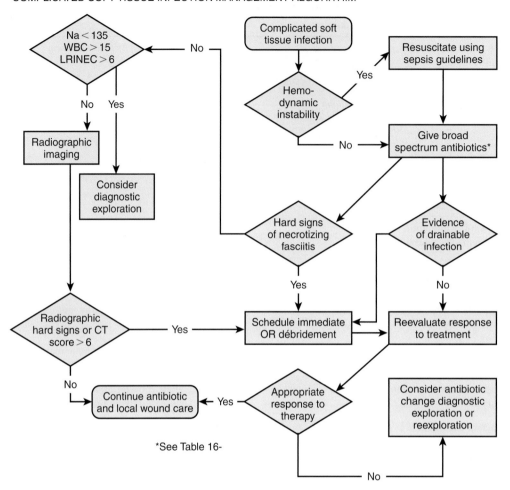

FIGURE 11   Complicated soft tissue infection management algorithm. CT, Computed tomography; LRINEC, Laboratory Risk Indicator for Necrotizing Fasciitis; Na, sodium; OR, operating room; WBC, white blood cell.

NSQIP dataset study demonstrated patients with discharge diagnosis of necrotizing fasciitis have a mortality rate of only 12% but that their length of hospital stay was nine times that of the average hospitalized patient.

CONCLUSIONS

NSTI can occur under a variety of clinical conditions. It should be considered in postsurgical, posttraumatic wounds as well as in wounds from insect or animal bites. Differentiation from superficial infection is mandatory to assure appropriate surgical therapy is performed.

Patients who fail to respond to appropriate medical therapy or who present with evidence of shock or organ dysfunction often harbor deeper infections. Patients with leukocytosis, hyponatremia, hyperglycemia, elevated creatinine, C-reactive protein, or CPK on laboratory evaluation should elicit an aggressive evaluation. This may include radiographic workup or surgical exploration. Progression of physical findings, including worsening edema, blistering, and crepitans or skin necrosis, mandates surgical exploration. Figure 11 represents a rational treatment algorithm. Delays in treatment result in increased mortality and morbidity rates.

For the chapter's Suggested Readings list, please visit the book at www.ExpertConsult.inkling.com.

COMMON ERRORS IN TRAUMA CARE

R. Stephen Smith, Allan S. Philp, and Stepheny D. Berry

Errors in management occur frequently in medicine. A recent Institute of Medicine report estimated that 44,000 to 98,000 deaths each year were caused by medical errors. This represents more deaths in the United States each year than are caused by breast cancer or AIDS (acquired immunodeficiency syndrome). Most of these errors occur in low-intensity, nonemergent scenarios. Obviously, trauma care is a much more difficult setting to perform in an errorless fashion. Care of injured patients must occur in an emergent fashion. Decisions must be made rapidly, based on limited information. In many instances, interventions must be initiated before a complete clinical and radiographic evaluation is performed. Frequently, the history of the mechanism of injury is obscure, or injured patients involved in socially unacceptable or criminal activities may mislead the trauma team. Moreover, injured patients are frequently unresponsive, have a decreased level of consciousness, or are uncooperative due to intoxication. Seriously injured patients frequently present with multiple injuries that require the involvement of multiple providers.

Routinely, numerous surgeons, surgical subspecialists, emergency medicine physicians, and residents must accurately communicate and coordinate care for an optimal outcome. Residents as members of the trauma team add complexity to communication, organization, and supervision.

The list of potential causes for errors in trauma care is infinite. Because of these many difficulties, the surgeon who cares for trauma patients must pay particular attention to factors that cause errors in management and should make every effort to prevent these errors. In this chapter, a number of common errors in the management of injured patients are discussed. This discussion includes missed diaphragmatic injury, failure to recognize extremity compartment syndrome, failure to prevent or treat abdominal compartment syndrome, delayed damage-control laparotomy, missed hollow viscus injuries, failure to perform a tertiary survey, futile emergency department (ED) thoracotomy, and the dogma of mandatory colostomy.

MISSED DIAPHRAGMATIC INJURY

Traumatic diaphragm injuries have been described since the 16th century and surgical repair of both penetrating and blunt injuries to the diaphragm were cited in the literature in the 1880s and 1900s, respectively. Incidence of diaphragmatic injuries varies based on mechanism of injury, with blunt trauma having a reported incidence of 0.5% to 8% and penetrating trauma having 3.4% to 40% incidence. Only 1% to 2% of patients have bilateral diaphragmatic injury. Bilateral injury is associated with higher mortality rate. Associated solid and hollow organ injuries are common with both blunt and penetrating diaphragmatic injuries. Up to 66% of injuries may be missed during the initial diagnostic workup, resulting in herniation of solid and hollow viscera, incarceration, and strangulation. Mortality rates as high as 36% are reported in the literature when diagnosis is delayed.

Intraabdominal pressure (IAP) can be significantly increased in persons involved in motor vehicle collisions, particularly if they are restrained. It is this significant pressure gradient that has been suggested as the pathophysiologic mechanism that causes the majority of blunt diaphragmatic ruptures. In addition, the negative intrathoracic

pressure generated during inspiration contributes to herniation of intraabdominal organs into the thoracic cavity. There is a strong association between thoracic aortic transection and diaphragmatic rupture in deceleration injuries with up to 10% of patients with aortic injuries also having a diaphragmatic injury. Other associated injuries include liver and splenic lacerations, long-bone fractures, and traumatic brain injury. Penetrating thoracoabdominal injuries also often result in diaphragmatic injuries. Because these injuries are typically much smaller than blunt ruptures, the diagnosis may be unrecognized even if appropriate diagnostic modalities are used.

Physical examination is unreliable for diaphragm injuries in most patients. The signs and symptoms are often nonspecific and include pleuritic chest pain, abdominal and epigastric tenderness, auscultation of bowel sounds in the chest, and hemodynamic instability. Respiratory distress may be present with large injuries causing tension viscerothorax. Diagnostic modalities routinely used for trauma including chest radiograph, focused assessment with sonography in trauma (FAST), and computed tomography (CT) imaging have had varying degrees of success in diagnosing diaphragmatic injuries in the acutely injured patient. Up to 50% of initial chest radiographs in patients with confirmed diaphragmatic injuries are reported as normal. Case reports and small series have suggested that abnormal movement of the diaphragm on FAST supports the diagnosis; however, this technique is not widely accepted. CT technology has improved with sensitivity and specificity as high as 82% and 99.7%, respectively; however, these results have not been duplicated.

Despite technological advances, operative evaluation (laparotomy, laparoscopy, thoracotomy, or video-assisted thoracoscopy) of the diaphragm remains the diagnostic tool with the highest sensitivity, specificity, and accuracy. Nontherapeutic operations are not without risk; therefore, a high index of suspicion combined with the available diagnostic technologies should be used to evaluate these patients. Patients with equivocal imaging studies and a high index of suspicion warrant further scrutiny. Diaphragm injuries identified by any diagnostic modality should be repaired to avoid the risk of strangulation and perforation. Most injuries may be repaired primarily with permanent sutures. Some large defects may require prosthetic reinforcement. However, there are numerous reports of successful thoracoscopic and laparoscopic repairs of diaphragmatic injuries. The surgical approach should reflect the surgeon's expertise and experience in treating such injuries, the patient's clinical condition, and the presence of associated injuries.

FAILURE TO RECOGNIZE EXTREMITY COMPARTMENT SYNDROME

Development of a compartment syndrome occurs commonly in patients with injuries to the upper and lower extremities. Compartment syndrome may also occur in any muscular compartment encased by fascia. This includes the hand, shoulder, arm, buttocks, thigh, and foot. A commonly held misconception is that patients with open fractures are protected from the development of compartment syndrome. Approximately 10% of patients with open fractures develop a limb-threatening compartment syndrome. Compartment syndrome is diagnosed on history and physical findings as well as a few adjunctive evaluations. Physical findings suggestive of compartment syndrome include a tense extremity with increased pain. Paresthesia indicates advanced ischemia involving nerves. It is an error to assume that a compartment syndrome is not present if a distal pulse is palpable. In fact, pulselessness is a late sign of compartment syndrome and may only occur after irreversible nerve and muscular injury have taken place.

Compartment syndrome develops in injured extremities secondary to a number of factors. Hemorrhage and muscle edema within a compartment may occur secondary to fracture. As pressure within the compartment increases and compartment pressure exceeds perfusion pressures, muscle and nerve ischemia will occur. Additionally, venous outflow obstruction results when compartment pressures rise. Compartment syndrome is a well-recognized complication of electrical burns. Ischemia with reperfusion is also a well-known cause of compartment syndrome. Iatrogenic causes of compartment syndrome include misplaced intravenous (IV) catheters into a muscle compartment followed by infusion of fluids into the compartment. Prolonged use of military antishock trousers (MAST) has also been associated with the development of compartment syndrome.

The diagnosis of compartment syndrome is based on clinical assessment and invasive evaluation of compartment pressure. Measurement of compartment pressure is easily accomplished using a number of techniques. If pressures within a muscular compartment are greater than 30 mm Hg, then compartment syndrome must be considered. A more elegant approach to determining compartment syndrome is measurement of the compartment perfusion pressure. The compartment perfusion pressure is calculated by subtracting the compartment pressure from the mean arterial blood pressure. If the compartment perfusion pressure is less than 40 mm Hg, then compartment syndrome must be considered.

Definitive therapy for compartment syndrome exists in the form of fasciotomy. Techniques of fasciotomy for both the upper and lower extremities are well known and involve decompression of all compartments of the involved extremity.

ABDOMINAL COMPARTMENT SYNDROME

The abdominal compartment syndrome (ACS) is defined as the pathophysiology and organ dysfunction that occurs as a result of intraabdominal hypertension (IAH). The renal, cardiovascular, and pulmonary systems are most affected. Treatment of the syndrome is early decompression. However, even when treated appropriately, mortality rate approaches 50%.

Appreciation of the adverse affects of IAH began in the 19th century. Marey and Burt demonstrated the affects of IAH on respiratory function. In 1890, Heinricius observed increased fatality in cats and guinea pigs when IAP increased from 27 to 46 cm H_2O.

Emerson showed the relationship between IAH and adverse cardiovascular affects in 1911. In 1913, Wendt demonstrated the relationship between IAH and renal dysfunction. Later in the century, pediatric surgeons became aware of the adverse physiologic affects of IAH and developed techniques to allow expansion of the abdominal contents. In 1984, Kron described a technique to measure IAP and first used the phrase "abdominal compartment syndrome."

The cardiovascular effects of IAH are consistent and well defined. Cardiac output is reduced as a result of decreased venous return secondary to increased intrathoracic pressure. This phenomenon occurs at IAP greater than 20 mm Hg, although venous return has been shown to be impaired at pressures as low as 15 mm Hg. Elevated intrathoracic pressure also contributes to a reduction in ventricular compliance, which reduces cardiac contractility. The diminished cardiac output seen with IAH has been shown to be exacerbated by hypovolemia and inhalational anesthetics.

The respiratory effects of IAH are mechanical. As the diaphragm is displaced cephalad, increased airway pressures are required to maintain adequate ventilation. Ultimately, this leads to ventilation/perfusion mismatch with resultant hypoxia and hypercarbia.

The mechanism of renal failure with ACS is multifactorial. Inadequate renal perfusion secondary to poor cardiac output, decreased perfusion, obstruction of renal venous outflow, and compression of the kidney all contribute to the renal failure associated with increasing IAP. Numerous studies have demonstrated that the oliguria and anuria seen with ACS are reversible with abdominal decompression.

Very little evidence exists on the effects of ACS on other organ systems. However, decreased blood flow in all abdominal organs occurs when IAP is more than 40 mm Hg. Hepatic artery, portal vein, and microcirculatory perfusion decrease when IAP surpasses 20 mm Hg. Intracranial hypertension and decreased cerebral perfusion pressure consistently improve with abdominal decompression when IAH is present.

Many causes exist for the development of ACS. Massive fluid resuscitation with crystalloid solutions plays a prominent and potentially preventable role in the development of this syndrome. Any condition associated with intraabdominal hemorrhage places the patient at risk for ACS. Such conditions include abdominal trauma, ruptured abdominal aortic aneurysm, retroperitoneal hemorrhage, elective abdominal operations, complications of pregnancy, and hepatic transplantation. In addition to blood, other intraperitoneal fluid collections may contribute to the development of ACS. Edema of the bowel and retroperitoneum, abdominal packing, ileus, ascites, massive volume resuscitation for shock, and inadvisable closure of abdominal fascia all increase the risk of IAH and ACS.

The diagnosis of ACS is based on clinical parameters and the measurement of IAP. Findings of oliguria (<0.5 mL/kg/hour), hypoxia (oxygen delivery <600 mL/minute/m^2) with increasing airway pressures (peak >45 cm H_2O), systemic vascular resistance (SVR) greater than 1000, and a distended abdomen, are all suggestive of ACS. Two methods of IAP measurement are clinically useful: (1) intragastric and (2) intravesicular. The latter is the most widely employed. First described by Kron et al, the technique involves clamping the bladder catheter, followed by the injection of 50 to 100 mL of sterile saline into the bladder. The catheter is then connected to a pressure manometer.

Based on the adverse physiologic changes at different IAP levels, most experienced surgeons suggest that the abdomen be decompressed with IAP above 25 mm Hg and that all patients be decompressed above 35 mm Hg. Early decompression, which may be performed in the intensive care unit (ICU), can reverse the pathophysiology of ACS. To avoid hypotension upon decompression, it is important to ensure that adequate intravascular volume resuscitation has been accomplished. Complications of abdominal decompression include hyperkalemia, respiratory alkalosis, hemorrhage, and reperfusion injury. The final step in decompressive laparotomy is to provide temporary abdominal closure that prevents recurrent IAH. Additional concerns include infection, fluid loss, evisceration, enterocutaneous fistula formation, and exposure of the abdominal viscera. Many methods of closure are available, including absorbable mesh, plastic IV (Bogota) bags, and vacuum-assisted closure. The large ventral hernia that results from temporary closure frequently requires delayed repair with nonabsorbable mesh. The mortality rate of ACS, despite decompression, still approaches 50%. Left untreated, it is routinely fatal. Early clinical suspicion in patients at risk, combined with aggressive measurement of IAP, can lead to lifesaving decompression.

THE MYTH OF MANDATORY COLOSTOMY

Interpersonal violence remains prevalent in North America. The colon is the second most commonly injured organ in penetrating abdominal trauma, and concomitant injuries and complications from such wounds are common (Table 1). When these patients present, the surgeon must decide whether to primarily repair the colon, resect and perform an anastomosis, or create a colostomy. There is continuing debate as to the optimal treatment for penetrating colon injuries. During World War I, many patients underwent primary repair. Colostomy was reserved for extensive injuries or left colon injuries. Regardless of the approach, a high mortality rate existed. These dismal survival statistics, however, occurred in an era of delayed treatment, inadequate volume resuscitation, lack of blood transfusions or antibiotics, and the

TABLE I: American Association for the Surgery of Trauma (AAST) Colon Injury Scale

Grade I	Hematoma or contusion without devascularization
Grade I	Laceration: partial thickness without perforation
Grade II	Laceration <50% of circumference
Grade III	Laceration >50% of circumference
Grade IV	Transection of colon
Grade V	Transection of colon with segmental tissue loss

absence of supportive critical care. The dogma of mandatory colostomy began after the U.S. Army Surgeon General W. H. Ogilvie published a letter in 1943 that mandated the performance of colostomy for colon injuries:

> The treatment of colon injuries is based on the known insecurity of suture and the dangers of leakage. Simple closure of a wound of the colon, however small, is unwarranted; men have survived such an operation, but others have died who would still be alive had they fallen into the hands of a surgeon with less optimism and more sense. Injured segments must either be exteriorized, or functionally excluded by a proximal colostomy.

This declaration was based on scant evidence but was issued in response to a mortality rate greater than 50%. From Ogilvie's own data, 50% of patients primarily repaired died, and 59% of patients treated with colostomy died. As military surgeons returned home, they perpetuated the dogma of treating all colonic injuries with colostomy. Notably, as early as 1951, Woodhall and Ochsner reported decreased mortality rate with primary repair compared to colostomy in civilian practice (8.3% vs. 35%). In recent decades, surgeons have become more comfortable with primary repair of colon injuries that previously would have been diverted. Many surgeons are comfortable with repair or resection with anastomosis of right colon injuries, but treatment of left colon injuries are increasingly treated without colostomy as well. In previous decades, surgeons were forced to justify primary repair of a colon injury, but more recent data have changed this position. Stone and Fabian published a landmark prospective series in 1979 suggesting that many injuries could be managed without colostomy in stable patients, and in 1991, Chappuis et al reported a prospective, randomized study of primary repair versus diversion in penetrating colon injuries. Patients were randomized irrespective of injury, contamination, transfusions, or shock. There was no difference in morbidity between the groups (17.9% vs. 21.4%) and length of hospitalization was 6 days longer in the colostomy group.

A 1996 prospective, randomized study by Gonzalez evaluated patients with penetrating colon injuries and was randomized to either primary repair with or without resection versus mandatory colostomy. Randomization occurred regardless of concomitant injuries or other risk factors. Septic complications were lower in the primary repair group (20% vs. 25%), although this did not reach statistical significance. In severely injured patients with a PATI (penetrating abdominal trauma index) score higher than 25, there was a lower complication rate in the primary repair group as compared with the diversion group. Although these differences were not statistically significant, this experience demonstrated that primary repair was at least equal to mandatory colostomy and might be superior.

Several authors (Cornwell et al) have cautioned against colonic repair or anastomosis in the setting of highly destructive injuries, larger transfusion requirement (>6 units packed red blood cells [PRBCs]), or a longer time out from injury with contamination

(>6 hours). The Eastern Association for the Surgery of Trauma (EAST) practice guidelines from 1998 also urged caution in patients with shock, peritonitis, or significant comorbid conditions and injuries.

Several randomized trials appear to support repair or anastomosis in these populations. Gonzalez et al reported their 6-year experience with 181 patients with penetrating colon injury. These patients were again randomized to primary repair or colostomy, regardless of other injuries, heavy fecal contamination, or hypotension. Septic complications were lower in the primary repair group (18% vs. 21%, $P = .05$). In hemodynamically unstable patients, the complication rate was also lower in the primary repair group (26% vs. 50%). Complications declined over time in both groups, which can likely be explained by improvement in the overall care of trauma victims.

Similarly, Sasaki et al's prospective randomized study of 71 patients with penetrating colon injuries had no exclusionary criteria used in the randomization. Sixty percent of patients were treated with primary repair or resection and anastomosis. There was no significant difference in the grade of injury. There was a 19% complication rate (colon and noncolon related) in the primary repair group as compared with a 36% complication rate in the diversion group. In patients with a PATI greater than 25, the complication rate was 33% in primarily repaired patients and 93% in diverted patients. The PATI score has been used as an argument for mandatory colostomy in the past, but in this and other studies, the complication rate is higher in patients with higher PATI scores regardless of the choice of treatment. The authors also reported a 7% complication rate at the time of colostomy reversal. Berne et al performed a retrospective review of 40 patients who underwent colostomy reversal after trauma. They found a morbidity rate of 55% in patients initially treated with colostomy for colon injury.

A note of caution was introduced by Ott et al with a review of 174 patients that showed a sixfold increase in leak rates in anastomoses performed in the setting of an open abdomen after damage control celiotomy, suggesting that scenarios still exist in which either delayed reconstruction when abdominal closure is possible or diversion may have a role.

The decision to perform a diverting colostomy may seem theoretically sound, but contemporary trauma care must be based on evidence and not intuition. In addition to not clearly showing a short-term benefit in most instances, diverting colostomy condemns patients to a subsequent operation for reanastomosis and exposes them to stoma-specific complications, including hernia, ostomy stenosis or retraction, necrosis and skin breakdown at the ostomy site, and the lifestyle limitations attached to ostomy management. Based on current evidence, mandatory colostomy for penetrating colon injury should be abandoned. Consideration of colostomy for any colon injury, regardless of the coexisting injuries or comorbid conditions, must be justified based on patient physiology in the operating room and the realization that repair or anastomosis presents an equivalently safe or even superior option in many instances.

DELAYED DAMAGE-CONTROL LAPAROTOMY

"Damage control," a term originating from the U.S. Navy definition of a ship's ability to absorb damage and maintain mission capability, is now a phrase that describes a surgical strategy used in many body regions. It describes a modified operative sequence in which the immediate repair of all injuries is abandoned in favor of a staged approach. This is done in recognition of the physiologic insult suffered by the critically injured patient, and the continued deterioration during the operation, which may render that insult irreversible. The concept of abbreviated laparotomy dates to 1908, when Pringle described the principles of compression and hepatic packing for control of portal venous hemorrhage. This practice fell out of favor after World War II, but reports emerged in the 1960s and 1970s that suggested improved outcomes with this technique. In 1983, Stone et al introduced the modern concept of the abbreviated laparotomy with subsequent resuscitation and interval completion laparotomy after physiologic restoration. In 1993, Rotondo and associates popularized the term "damage control," and it has rapidly become a standard in the treatment of critically injured patients with deteriorating physiologic parameters in many areas of trauma and emergency surgery.

Three stages of damage-control laparotomy were originally described—control of hemorrhage and contamination, ongoing resuscitation, and subsequent definitive repair of injuries. The first step is the truncated laparotomy in the face of life-threatening physiologic circumstances. It involves the control of hemorrhage with intra-abdominal packing and control of enteric contamination with rapid sutures, stapling, or resection. Lengthy vascular repairs are not pursued, but temporary shunting is used liberally. No attempt at definitive reconstruction of bowel continuity is required. Overpacking can lead to increased IAP and a secondary ACS. Underpacking may fail to stop hemorrhage. Packing should provide pressure in vectors that recreate the disrupted tissue planes, but it must be remembered that it is difficult to obtain hemostasis of arterial injuries with packing alone. If rapid repair, ligation, or stenting cannot be accomplished, then other methods, such as angiographic embolization, should be employed. Biliary tract and pancreatic injuries can be managed with external tube drainage in nearly all acute settings. Once the abbreviated laparotomy is completed, the abdomen is closed by temporary methods. Many techniques for temporary closure have been described, including penetrating towel clamp closure, running skin sutures without fascial closure, use of an IV bag attached to the skin (Bogota bag), and vacuum closure devices. Whichever method is used, the goals are identical: prevent evisceration, protect the bowel, and minimize the risk of IAH and ACS. For this reason, either commercial or modified vacuum dressings have largely become the dressings of choice in these instances.

The second phase of damage control involves ongoing resuscitation in the ICU with the reversal of the lethal triad: (1) hypothermia, (2) acidosis, and (3) coagulopathy. Each of these devastating physiologic complications has a compounding effect on the others. Hypothermia, defined as a core temperature less than 35° C, is exacerbated by prolonged exposure, inadequate perfusion, and inadequate warming in the ED or operating room. Hypothermia exists in as many as half of injured patients following trauma laparotomy and increases the requirement for fluid resuscitation, vasopressors, inotropes, and transfusions. It is independently associated with increased morbidity, organ dysfunction, coagulopathy, and mortality rate. In the ICU, the ambient temperature, airway circuit, IV fluids, and blood products should all be warmed. Warm blankets and a forced-air heater should be used aggressively. Acidosis results from inadequate oxygen delivery secondary to hemorrhage, which results in anaerobic metabolism and the release of lactic acid. Acidosis worsens coagulopathy, depresses myocardial contractility, diminishes inotropic response to catecholamines, and predisposes to dysrhythmias. Correction of acidosis is directed at improvement of oxygen delivery and optimizing cardiac output. Failure to correct elevated lactic acid levels or base deficit within 48 hours is associated with rates of mortality approaching 100% in some series. Coagulopathy is worsened by the combined effects of hypothermia, acidosis, and dilution of clotting factors by massive crystalloid resuscitation. Correction of coagulopathy is achieved by the reversal of hypothermia and acidosis, as well as the aggressive replacement of clotting factors with fresh frozen plasma, cryoprecipitate, and platelets. Several other pharmacologic adjuncts exist that may assist in the correction of coagulopathy (tranexamic acid, recombinant factor VIIa, prothrombin complex concentrate), but the precise application and survival benefit of these measures continue to be investigated.

The third phase of damage control refers to definitive operative repair of injuries after reversal of physiologic impairments. The timing of definitive repair is based on normalization of physiology and not temporal parameters. It may be necessary to perform more than one subsequent laparotomy to repair all injuries.

The decision to employ damage control techniques is ultimately that of the surgeon. This should be made early if the benefits of the technique are to be fully realized because once physiologic reserve is exhausted, even the highest quality care will prove ineffective. Indications for the damage control approach include the inability to achieve hemostasis, inaccessible source of hemorrhage, multiple severe injuries, poor response to resuscitation, and as dictated by the direct measurement of physiologic parameters of temperature, pH, and the vital signs. Complications of damage control include wound infection, abscess formation, enterocutaneous fistula formation, dehiscence, bile leak, pancreatic pseudocyst formation, intestinal necrosis, ACS, multisystem organ failure, acute respiratory distress syndrome (ARDS), and death.

Damage control represents a surgical approach that can be lifesaving in a select population of critically injured patients. Success is dependent on early application, patient selection, rapid operative control of hemorrhage and contamination, aggressive resuscitation, and the reversal of the lethal triad of hypothermia, acidosis, and coagulopathy.

MISSED HOLLOW VISCUS INJURY

With the increasing use of nonoperative management of solid organ injuries in blunt trauma, the incidence of missed hollow viscus injury and its timely diagnosis must be considered. Hollow viscus injury affects about 1% of all trauma patients and 15% of patients with blunt abdominal trauma. Motor vehicle collisions are the most common mechanism of injury, with small bowel being the organ most commonly involved. Even as diagnostic imaging has progressed, it is still inferior to laparotomy in establishing the diagnosis of hollow viscus injury and so the diagnostic quandary remains. Some of these injuries are evident on close examination of initial CT scans, but others do not become apparent for hours or days. Although the FAST examination has proved useful to diagnose hemoperitoneum, it is not capable of reliably identifying hollow viscus injury. Physical examination, diagnostic peritoneal lavage (DPL), and laboratory tests are similarly unreliable.

In 1999, Fang et al examined patients with a delayed diagnosis of small bowel injury. Their retrospective review of 111 blunt trauma victims with small bowel injury showed no difference in mortality rate if the injury was treated within 24 hours. But patients with a delay in diagnosis of greater than 4 hours had an increased incidence of wound infection, abscess formation, enterocutaneous fistula, wound dehiscence, and sepsis. Those whose injury was repaired after 24 hours averaged a 20-day increase in hospital stay. Fakhry et al found an increase in mortality and morbidity rates with diagnostic delays in small bowel injuries. Mortality rate was 2% when the injury was treated within 8 hours, 9.1% when treated between 8 and 16 hours, 16.7% when treated between 16 and 24 hours, and 30.8% when delayed more than 24 hours. The large multicenter EAST trial showed an increase from 5% to 16% in mortality rate if operative intervention was delayed past 24 hours.

CT technology has advanced substantially over the past 2 decades, but its ability to identify solid organ injuries remains far superior to that for hollow viscus injury. Killeen et al examined 150 CT scans of blunt trauma victims and compared these to operative findings. Helical CT scan showed a sensitivity of 94% for bowel injuries and 96% for mesenteric injuries. The number of solid organ injuries influences the diagnosis of hollow viscus injuries. With a single solid organ injury, a hollow viscus injury was found in 7.3% of patients. The incidence doubled (15.4%) with two solid organ injuries and was 34.4% with three solid organ injuries. Malhotra et al found that the following findings on CT were predictive of hollow viscus injury: unexplained intraperitoneal fluid, pneumoperitoneum, bowel wall thickening, mesenteric fat streaking, mesenteric hematoma, extravasation of luminal contrast agent, and extravasation of vascular contrast agent.

Missed injuries are not isolated to blunt mechanism of injury. Sung et al found, in a retrospective review of 607 patients with penetrating trauma, a missed injury rate of 2% at the initial operation. Forty-two percent of patients with missed injuries developed sepsis, 17% developed renal failure, and mortality rate was significantly higher at 17% versus 6.4%.

What remains unclear is the optimal strategy for evaluating patients at risk for hollow viscus injury, as no consensus regarding a specific pathway exists. Malhotra et al have proposed CT imaging with DPL or operative intervention for one or more significant radiographic findings. Mitsuhide suggests a combination of initial physical examination, CT imaging, and diagnostic laparoscopy may decrease both delays in diagnosis and nontherapeutic laparotomy. Regardless of the specific algorithm employed, it is clear that early and attentive management is mandatory to avoid the well-demonstrated complications of delays in diagnosis and definitive care.

FAILURE TO PERFORM TERTIARY SURVEY

Missed injuries, or the more politically popular "delay in diagnosis," plague all trauma centers. The Advanced Trauma Life Support (ATLS) course has become the gold standard for initial recognition and treatment of life-threatening injuries in the initial evaluation period through the use of a primary and secondary survey. However, it is clear from published reports that although this system effectively identifies immediate threats to life, it is less effective in identifying injuries completely. Although there is no consensus on the specific criteria to define a missed injury, it typically refers to any injury not appreciated in the initial evaluation. The reported rates of missed injuries vary from 2% to 50%. The majority of these may not be clinically significant, but some are potentially fatal. Buduhan reported that 15% of their missed injuries were clinically significant, with a 2% preventable mortality rate in that subset. Even less severe injuries can cause prolonged disability, expense, pain, and deterioration in the relationship between the trauma team and the patient and family. Factors that contribute to the prevalence of missed injuries include the attention focused on more urgent treatment priorities, altered patient sensorium, poorly appreciated physical findings, and radiologic studies that are not appropriately performed, are misinterpreted, or are not reviewed. Missed injuries are more common in patients involved in motor vehicle crashes, those with higher Injury Severity Scores (ISSs), and those with a greater number of injuries. One other factor reported to increase the frequency of missed injuries is inexperience of the treating physician.

A number of reports recommend the use of a tertiary survey as a mechanism to address this issue. The tertiary survey is a thorough reexamination of the trauma patient within the first 24 hours of admission and after many contributing factors to limited examination have resolved. This examination includes symptom review, physical examination, and review or ordering of appropriate radiologic or laboratory studies. Because factors of hemodynamic instability and altered sensorium may still exist after 24 hours of treatment, it is important to complete the tertiary survey again when a patient is stabilized and neurologically competent as the delay in diagnosis has been described as long as weeks after injury. Many surgeons have suggested formal radiology rounds as a standard part of the tertiary survey because over 25% of missed injuries can be correctly identified on the original radiograph studies. Enderson et al reported identifying additional injuries in 9% of blunt trauma patients with the routine use of a tertiary survey. Janjua et al detected 56% of early missed injuries and 90% of clinically significant missed injuries with the performance of a tertiary survey within 24 hours of admission. Biffl et al were able to reduce the incidence of missed injuries from 2.4% to 1.5% after implementation of a standardized tertiary survey policy, and Soundappan et al reported similar results in a pediatric population. More recently, Lawson et al reported a decrease in delayed diagnosis rate in the head/neck/trunk to less than 0.4% using routine CT imaging of those regions triggered by trauma activation criteria. This practice has yet to be established as a standard, however, given the expense and concern for radiation exposure.

Missed injuries occur with disappointing frequency and with the potential for significant morbidity and fatality. The tertiary survey is a comprehensive patient evaluation that occurs after the initial resuscitation period and should include a thorough physical examination combined with targeted radiographic imaging (plain film, ultrasound, or CT based on examination findings). The demonstrated success in decreasing delays in diagnosis of potentially life-threatening injuries indicates that a tertiary survey should become a standard and necessary feature of the care of every trauma patient.

FUTILE RESUSCITATIVE THORACOTOMY

One of the most dramatic procedures in trauma care is the ED thoracotomy. This procedure is performed in a hectic environment, but when carried out in the properly selected patient, it can be lifesaving. Unfortunately, this technique is frequently performed in poorly selected patients without valid indications, with predictably dismal results. There is little doubt that a patient with cardiac tamponade secondary to a small stab wound to the right ventricle who loses vital signs in the trauma bay may be salvaged. But in many instances, indications for resuscitative thoracotomy are less clear. Futile thoracotomy performed for patients with lethal injuries is distressingly common.

Rhee et al retrospectively reviewed a 25-year multicenter experience with resuscitative thoracotomy. Blunt trauma victims undergoing ED thoracotomy had a survival rate of 1.4%. Survival rate of blunt trauma victims ranged from 0% to 12.5% for various trauma centers. If the 12.5% rate of survival from one center is excluded, most survival rates are less than 2%. Many blunt trauma "survivors" of ED thoracotomy were not neurologically intact. In 2004, Powell et al evaluated their experience with ED thoracotomy for victims of penetrating and blunt trauma who required prehospital cardiopulmonary resuscitation (CPR). They documented four blunt trauma survivors, all of whom had severe neurologic deficits. Even in blunt trauma patients with cardiac tamponade, the outcome after ED thoracotomy is routinely fatal. In a retrospective review of ED thoracotomy patients, Grove et al reported four blunt trauma victims with cardiac tamponade who survived ED thoracotomy and were admitted to the ICU; all died within 9 days. Clearly, blunt trauma victims without signs of life in the field or upon arrival in the trauma bay should be declared dead. The blunt trauma patient who loses vital signs shortly after arrival in the ED will have a dismal outcome with any therapy, and we believe that thoracotomy should not be performed.

Some victims of penetrating trauma clearly benefit from ED thoracotomy. Proper selection of potentially salvageable patients is key. Powell et al found that the duration of CPR was critical. All survivors of ED thoracotomy had CPR for 15 minutes or less. Any penetrating trauma patient with prolonged CPR (>15 minutes) and no signs of life on arrival to the trauma bay should be pronounced dead.

Few patients will survive if the duration of prehospital CPR is greater than 5 minutes. ED thoracotomy is a potentially lifesaving procedure, but there are few survivors. Use of this intervention should be limited to patients with penetrating mechanisms of injury. Those with noncardiac injuries have a poor prognosis. The FAST examination may help to delineate treatable intrathoracic injury and decrease the number of futile ED thoracotomies in the future.

SUMMARY

The circumstances involved in the evaluation and treatment of injured patients makes errors likely. It is inevitable that delays in diagnosis and intervention will occur in multiply injured patients. Excessive use of diagnostic modalities does not eliminate variations in care. However, it is incumbent upon all those who care for trauma patients to recognize common errors so that the frequency of these may be minimized. A high index of suspicion for injuries that are difficult to diagnose must be maintained if optimal care is to be delivered. Futile efforts to salvage lethally injured patients are costly and time-consuming and should be minimized.

For the chapter's Suggested Readings list, please visit the book at www.ExpertConsult.inkling.com.

COMBAT TRAUMA CARE: LESSONS LEARNED FROM A DECADE OF WAR

Colonel Matthew J. Martin and Colonel (retired) Brian Eastridge

OVERVIEW OF MODERN FORWARD TRAUMA CARE

The modern battlefield is a highly complex and deadly arena that continues to drive innovation and advancements in both civilian and military trauma care. Prior to World War I, the vast majority of battlefield morbidity and fatality was due to infectious and other medical diseases. Simultaneous advances in medicine and weaponry subsequently resulted in trauma becoming the predominant focus of battlefield medicine. The historical practice of deploying civilian health care personnel who were activated only during times of war has given way to the development of a full-time dedicated military medical service that maintains constant readiness to provide comprehensive battlefield trauma care. The terrorist attacks of September 11, 2001 resulted in the first large-scale and prolonged forward deployment of military medical assets since the Vietnam War. Although a full description of the breadth and depth of trauma experience gained from these conflicts is not possible here, the purpose of this chapter is to highlight some of the major lessons learned (and relearned) over the past decade of sustained combat medical operations.

Although the exact configuration and manpower requirements vary widely between specific types of units and between military services (Army, Navy, Air Force, etc.), they all follow some basic principles of organization and capabilities. This allows for both the flexibility and stability required to function in a variety of combat environments and circumstances. Battlefield medicine always starts at the point of injury, with immediate care provided by fellow soldiers ("buddy aid") and combat medics or corpsman. Formal medical care is then organized in a series of levels, from Level 1 through Level 5 as outlined in Table 1. Surgical care is first available at Level 2 facilities, and focuses on damage control and stabilization. Of note, an important lesson learned is that the more severely injured patient should be transported immediately to the most appropriate facility, which often means bypassing Level 1 or even Level 2 and going directly to a Level 3 facility.

TABLE 1: Echelons of Care System for Management of Military Combat Trauma During Operation Enduring Freedom and Operation Iraqi Freedom

Echelon	Example	Surgical Capability	Other Capabilities	Comments
Level 1	Battalion Aid Station, Shock Trauma Platoon	None	"Aid bag," limited supplies, maybe ultrasound	Medics and PA or primary care MD; no hold capability
Level 2	Army/Air Force: Forward Surgical Team (FST) Navy: Forward Resuscitative Surgical System (FRSS)	Yes, general and orthopedics; sustained OR capability for 24–48 hours	Damage control surgery, basic lab, basic radiograph and ultrasound, oxygen, limited blood product supply	Focus on damage control and immediate MEDEVAC to Level 3; Team may move to follow operational unit or split to cover two areas
Level 3	Army: Combat Support Hospital Air Force: Theater Hospital Navy: Hospital Ship	Yes, general and orthopedic surgery, surgical and medical subspecialties	Multiple specialists, advanced lab and blood product support, advanced radiology and CT, physical therapy	Damage control surgery and definitive management; stabilization and evacuation portal to Level 4
Level 4	Regional Medical Center (Landstuhl, Germany)	Extensive, excellent subspecialty support	Major medical center capabilities	More definitive surgical intervention; burns may bypass directly to Brooke Burn Center
Level 5	CONUS National Medical Centers (Walter Reed, Bethesda, Balboa, Brooke)	Full tertiary care	Full rehabilitation and specialty intervention	Performs most delayed and reconstructive care

From Martin M, Beekley A, editors: Front line surgery, New York, 2010, Springer Publishing.
CONUS, Continental U.S. Naval hospitals; CT, computed tomography; MEDEVAC, medical evacuation; OR, operating room; PA, physician assistant.

BATTLEFIELD INJURIES

An understanding of the predominant injury mechanisms, patterns, and anatomic wound distributions is critical to adequately deploying and maximizing battlefield medical assets. These may be unique to each combat theater, and may even vary significantly by the phase of operations. This was seen in current combat operations in Iraq and Afghanistan, with a marked difference in wounding mechanisms and lethality between the initial invasion phase and the subsequent insurgency and stabilization phases. Unlike civilian trauma, battlefield injuries are characterized by a predominance of penetrating and often high-velocity mechanisms, severe multisystem trauma, and mangled and amputated extremities. The majority of these injury types require some type of operative intervention. One of the defining factors of the current combat operations has been the widespread use of the enemy weapon of choice, the improvised explosive device, or IED (Fig. 1). These devices can be assembled around almost any explosive source and vary widely in size, triggering mechanisms, and resultant blast force (Fig. 2). In contrast to previous conflicts, only a small portion of traumatic wounds in the current conflicts are from firearms (25%), and the majority (60%) have been from explosive mechanisms. The resultant combination of explosive injury with associated blast, blunt force trauma, and penetrating fragment wounds often creates a severe and complex battle injury that has no true civilian counterpart.

As a result of the detailed and thorough collection of wounding data, therapy, and outcomes with the Joint Theater Trauma Registry (JTTR), the anatomic distribution and severity of combat injuries can be analyzed and used to drive real-time changes in prevention and treatment. Modern developments such as advanced body armor, explosive-resistant vehicles, and changes in operational tactics have been partially based on this data. Figure 3 shows the composite distribution of anatomic sites of battlefield injuries seen during the current combat operations, and Table 2 shows the various anatomic wound distributions compared to previous conflicts. The exact distribution and severity will also be greatly dependent on individual factors, such as the presence of body armor, vehicular or dismounted injury, and the wounding mechanism.

Battlefield deaths are a particular point of interest and have been analyzed in great detail over the past decade of combat operations. Two excellent analyses of autopsy and clinical data from Operation Iraqi Freedom/Operation Enduring Freedom (OIF/OEF) have described the predominant mechanisms (blast and gunshot) and injury sites (head and trunk) resulting in death on the battlefield. Of interest, up to 28% of deaths were deemed to be potentially survivable with the majority of those (80%) being due to hemorrhage.

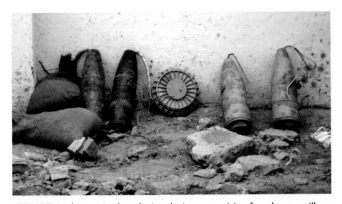

FIGURE 1 Improvised explosive device comprising four large artillery shells and an antitank mine wired together (or "daisy-chained") with detonating cord. *(Courtesy of U.S. Department of Defense.)*

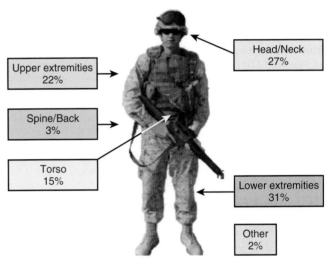

FIGURE 3 Distribution of combat injuries in Iraq and Afghanistan. *(Data from the Joint Theater Trauma Registry (JTTR) 2001–2009.)*

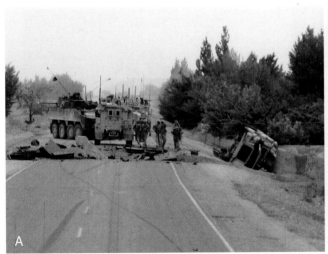
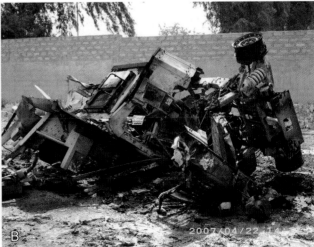

FIGURE 2 **A,** Blast crater and overturned vehicle from an improvised explosive device (IED) placed on a main roadway. **B,** Military vehicle destroyed by an IED. *(Courtesy of U.S. Department of Defense.)*

TABLE 2: Distribution of Combat Wounds by Body Region in Operation Iraqi Freedom and Operation Enduring Freedom Compared to Prior Conflicts

	Body Surface Area (%)	WWII	Korea	Vietnam	OIF/OEF
Head/neck	12	21%	21%	16%	30%
Thorax	16	14%	10%	13%	6%
Abdomen	11	8%	8%	9%	9%
Extremities	61	58%	60%	61%	55%

Modified from Owens BD, Kragh JF Jr, Wenke JC, et al: Combat wounds in Operation Iraqi Freedom and Operation Enduring Freedom. *J Trauma* 64(2):295–299, 2008.
OEF, Operation Enduring Freedom; OIF, Operation Iraqi Freedom; WWII, World War Two.

Another analysis of these data has demonstrated that the case fatality rate (CFR) for Iraq/Afghanistan was approximately half of that seen in prior conflicts (10.5% vs. 20.2%), possibly attributed to improved protective equipment, evacuation capability, and prehospital care. However, there has been a concurrent increase in those who died of wounds (DOW) after reaching a medical facility, from 3% in WWII and Vietnam to as high as 6% to 8% for Afghanistan. This concerning statistic likely reflects the ability to get more severely injured patients quickly evacuated to a medical facility, and highlights the need for forward medical facilities and personnel prepared to deal with these high acuity injuries. A detailed analysis of in-hospital deaths from a Combat Support Hospital in Iraq highlights the need for rapid definitive intervention, with the majority of deaths occurring within the first hour of arrival (78%) and attributable to hemorrhage (62%).

PREHOSPITAL AND EN ROUTE CARE

The sharp decline in killed in action and CFRs during current combat operations is multifactorial, and has been attributed to both improvements in personal protective equipment and vehicles as well as improved medical care. Initial improvements to enhance survivability from IED blasts included modifications to currently available military vehicles, followed by the deployment of new vehicles (mine-resistant

ambush protected, or MRAP) specifically designed to withstand larger explosive forces (Fig. 4). Although definitive data is lacking, there appears to be a significant (up to 90%) reduction in IED-related fatalities among passengers in MRAP-type vehicles. Arguably, an equally important factor in improving battlefield survival in OIF/OEF has been the massive investment in equipping and training military first responders and medical evacuation (MEDEVAC) personnel. The Tactical Combat Casualty Care (TCCC) course is the military adaptation of the widely used civilian prehospital trauma courses, and provides realistic and up-to-date training and information aimed at maximizing survival on the battlefield. Unlike most civilian settings, combat medics have to deliver initial care in a hostile environment and often while receiving direct or indirect fire from enemy forces. The TCCC course outlines principles and priorities for three phases of prehospital care: (1) care under fire, (2) tactical field care, and (3) tactical evacuation care as shown in Table 3. In distinction from the commonly taught ABCs (airway, breathing, circulation) for civilian trauma, combat medics are trained to prioritize hemorrhage control (C) first, and then move on to airway and breathing issues.

Analysis of battlefield deaths and preventable deaths has resulted in rapid training and fielding initiatives to better equip military first responders. One of the most important interventions during the early phases of these conflicts was the widespread deployment of manually operated extremity tourniquets, and currently each soldier carries his or her own tourniquet so that it is readily available and can be applied if needed (Fig. 5). More recently, devices designed to control "junctional" bleeding (axilla and groin) have been developed and deployed. Early results with these junctional tourniquets have shown great promise, particularly for groin wounds or high above-knee amputations. In addition to the standard gauze field dressing, medics were equipped for the first time with advanced hemostatic dressing products, including the HemCon bandage (HemCon Medical Technologies, Portland, Ore.) and the granular agent QuikClot (Z-Medica, Wallingford, Conn.). Subsequently, a next-generation kaolin-coated gauze roll (Combat Gauze, Z-Medica) has been widely deployed and is the current TCCC recommended hemostatic dressing. In 2014 two additional chitosan-based dressings were also approved for use in addition to Combat Gauze. Current research is focused on developing the next generation of hemostatic dressings that contain active clotting factors and advanced biomaterials that may be more efficacious even in patients with major acidosis and coagulopathy. Other equipment items and changes include longer large-bore needle thoracostomy catheters (3.25 inches), intraosseous access devices, and self-contained hypothermia prevention and management kits (HPMK). Prehospital fluid resuscitation has also undergone

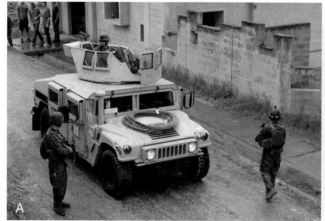 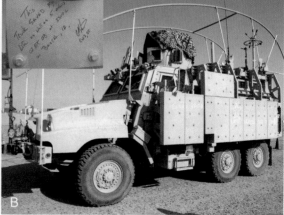

FIGURE 4 Improvement in military vehicles to enhance survival from explosive blasts: **A,** Enhancement ("up-armoring") of current vehicles such as the high mobility multipurpose wheeled vehicle (HMMWV or "Humvee"). **B,** The deployment of newly designed mine-resistant ambush protected (MRAP) vehicles. The inset shows an inscription written on the side panel of an MRAP that was struck by an improvised explosive device with no passenger injuries. *(Courtesy of U.S. Department of Defense.)*

TABLE 3: Three Phases of Prehospital Combat Trauma Care and Associated Priorities

Care under fire	Return fire and take cover, direct casualty to return fire if able
	Move casualty to cover, direct self-aid if casualty is awake and responsive
	Extricate from burning vehicles or buildings
	Stop life-threatening external hemorrhage with pressure or tourniquet
Tactical field care	Disarm casualty if mental status altered
	Open airway with maneuvers, cricothyroidotomy if necessary
	Decompress tension pneumothorax with 3.25-inch catheter, dress any open chest wounds
	Hemorrhage control with tourniquet, combat gauze as needed
	Administer 500 mL of Hextend if in shock, otherwise hold fluids
	Analgesia, antibiotics, topical dressings
Tactical evacuation care	Assess airway and breathing as previously mentioned
	Chest tube if needle thoracentesis inadequate or prolonged transport anticipated
	Assess hemorrhage control, expose and time/date all tourniquets
	If persistent shock, administer 500 mL Hextend followed by blood products if available
	Prevent hypothermia by removing wet clothing, apply hypothermia prevention equipment
	Start burn resuscitation per clinical practice guideline if needed
	Prepare casualty for medical evacuation, complete prehospital documentation

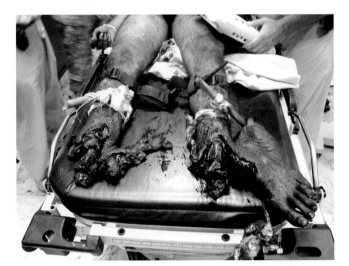

FIGURE 5 Combat application tourniquets applied to the bilateral legs after an improvised explosive device blast.

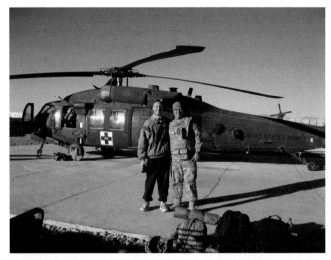

FIGURE 6 Blackhawk helicopters are used for the majority of medical evacuation and patient transport missions in Iraq and Afghanistan. (Chapter authors Matthew Martin and Brian Eastridge are in the foreground at Forward Operating Base Ghazni, Afghanistan.)

significant changes based on current combat experience, with a focus on low-volume initial resuscitation, avoidance of large volumes of crystalloid, and earlier use of blood products for evidence of shock. If a rapid assessment for shock (mental status and radial pulse) is normal, then no fluids are given. If abnormal, then the current TCCC fluid of choice is a 500-mL bolus of Hextend (6% hetastarch).

Although the military uses a wide variety of vehicular platforms for front-line evacuation of wounded patients, the vast majority of MEDEVAC missions in Iraq and Afghanistan are performed by rotary wing aircraft, typically using the Blackhawk helicopter (Fig. 6). Although the exact staffing and training of the MEDEVAC crew members vary widely between military services, there is a common focus on rapid evaluation of the patient, continuing prehospital care and resuscitation, and evacuation to a Level 2 or 3 facility as quickly as possible. Frequent challenges encountered during these missions include danger from enemy fire, heat and noise, a dirty/dusty environment, operating in low light or blackout conditions (particularly during night operations), multiple simultaneous casualties, and the difficulty of performing in-flight advanced care or procedures. Current initiatives are examining ways to mitigate some of these limitations, and include pilot projects assessing the impact of deploying advanced skill providers (critical care nurses, physicians, surgeons) and resuscitation supplies (blood products, rapid infusers) with MEDEVAC crews to provide oversight and additional advanced "golden hour" care capabilities.

TRIAGE AND IMMEDIATE CARE

The importance of rapid, accurate, and organized triage in combat situations cannot be overemphasized, particularly during mass casualty (MASCAL) scenarios. A hallmark of forward combat care is severely constrained resources and personnel that must be used wisely in order to maximize patient outcomes and the unit's ability to continue to provide care. The senior triage officer should be one of the more experienced trauma providers in the unit, and is typically best staffed by a surgeon or emergency medicine physician. An often overlooked principle is that the first step in triage is assessing the current capabilities and supply situation of the facility, which will significantly impact triage decisions. Triage is a dynamic process of sorting, categorizing, and continually reevaluating the available resources balanced against the patient needs and likelihood of survival with intervention. Those with a low likelihood of survival or with injuries that will require more resources than can be safely allocated should be categorized as expectant, with the remainder triaged to receive either immediate or delayed care.

TABLE 4: Combat Mass Casualty Policies

Triage "expectant" casualties to a separate area and provide comfort care as needed

Hemorrhage control first, then airway and breathing

Do not remove any tourniquets until other life-threatening injuries have been ruled out

The only urgent radiograph is usually a chest radiograph—no extremity radiographs until all chest radiographs are done

Most lab tests are unnecessary, but a blood type and crossmatch are critical to obtain on arrival

Prioritize emergent CT scans (usually head) and defer all nonemergent scans

Unstable patients almost always belong in the OR, and require minimal workup

No ED thoracotomies during a MASCAL; move on to someone with vital signs

Be prepared to retriage patients who were mistriaged or have clinical deterioration

Conduct an after action review meeting with all involved personnel after every MASCAL

CT, Computed tomography; ED, emergency department; MASCAL, mass casualty; OR, operating room.

The process of triage does not stop at the door, and should continue throughout the entire period of acute care in a MASCAL setting. Obtaining radiologic and laboratory studies will typically be a rate-limiting factor that can be overcome by establishing simple protocols and ground rules (Table 4). Development of an in-depth MASCAL plan coupled with realistic rehearsal drills is the best way to minimize and control the inevitable chaos associated with these events. Hemorrhage remains the most common cause of early deaths at forward medical facilities, so immediate care priorities start with control of recognized ongoing bleeding and rapidly identifying sources of occult bleeding, coupled with a resuscitation strategy aimed at restoration of the hemostatic system as well as organ perfusion (see next section).

One of the most common causes of preventable fatality and morbidity among combat casualties is a delay to operative intervention, frequently as a result of applying standard civilian blunt trauma practices to this unique patient population. Approximately two thirds of preventable battlefield deaths from hemorrhage are due to proximal (groin, axilla) or internal bleeding that can only be managed by immediate operative intervention. Common sources of delay include system-level factors (transport times, operating room [OR] availability and staffing, administrative processes) that may not be modifiable, but more often are related to provider-level factors that represent a target for process and quality improvement. These include failure to recognize occult hemorrhage or shock, performing unnecessary and time-consuming tests or procedures, prolonged diagnostic and imaging workups, and prolonged preoperative resuscitations to "stabilize" the patient prior to operative intervention. Most of these interventions are unnecessary or nonemergent and can be safely deferred, and the remainder (such as intubation, central line placement, transfusion) can be done in the OR in tandem with surgical intervention. The fact that 80% of in-hospital combat deaths occur within 1 hour of arrival at a medical facility highlights the critical importance of early and effective prioritization and delivery of immediate care.

DAMAGE CONTROL RESUSCITATION AND MASSIVE TRANSFUSION

Standard initial trauma resuscitation strategies for the bleeding patient have historically relied on the early administration of large volumes of crystalloid solutions, followed by infusion of cold stored packed red blood cell (PRBC) products. Increasing recognition of the adverse effects of this strategy such as volume overload, immune dysfunction, metabolic disturbances, and induced or worsened coagulopathy have prompted a search for superior alternatives. One of the most widely lauded and discussed advances in combat trauma care over the past decade has been a radical change in resuscitation strategy, now known as damage control resuscitation (DCR). The core principle of this strategy is to replace blood loss with a balanced resuscitation of red blood cells, plasma, platelets, and clotting factors. This is achieved by either the use of fresh whole blood or with component therapy including PRBCs, fresh frozen or thawed plasma, and platelets. The optimal ratio of administration of each type of product remains a matter of ongoing study and debate, with the current practice being to aim for a 1:1:1 ratio starting with the initial administration and continuing through the early resuscitation period. Although this concept has not yet been validated with Level 1 evidence, multiple series have suggested a significant benefit in achieving hemostasis and overall survival with DCR. The DCR resuscitative paradigm has been associated with a decrease in massive transfusion mortality rate from 40% to less than 20% after battlefield injury. More important than the exact ratio of products is adhering to the basic principles of early and aggressive balanced hemostatic resuscitation coupled with avoidance of large-volume crystalloid infusion and allowing relative hypotension until definitive hemorrhage control has been achieved.

The only way to routinely and reliably provide adequate DCR is through development of a comprehensive and facility-specific protocol for massive transfusion. Adhering to a 1:1:1 ratio is made easier by automatically providing blood products for initial resuscitation in transfusion packs rather than individual components. As an example, the Combat Support Hospital in Baghdad protocol provided initial packs containing 4 units PRBCs and 4 units of fresh frozen plasma (FFP), followed by "massive packs" containing 6 units of each and an apheresis platelet pack. In addition, there is growing recognition of the adverse effects associated with prolonged storage of blood products ("storage lesion") and that minimizing the time from collection and storage to administration may have clinical benefit. Thus, the current combat guidelines recommend using the least aged blood products for massive transfusions, also known as "last-in/first-out," or LIFO. However, the availability of component blood products will vary widely depending on the size and location of the forward facility and the robustness of the resupply chain. This can severely limit the ability to administer a balanced resuscitation, particularly in more austere locations or during the earlier phases of combat operations. These limitations can be countered by developing a "walking blood bank"; a pool of local whole blood donors who have been prescreened and can be activated as needed. The use of fresh whole blood in our combat experience has been safe and effective, has allowed the extension of DCR to even far-forward and austere locations, and has demonstrated outcomes equivalent to or better than standard component therapy.

Triggers for initiating DCR and massive transfusion have been widely debated, and there are no simple rules or algorithms that can adequately replace experience and clinical judgment. Multiple factors have been identified that predict the need for massive transfusion in combat, including hypotension, altered mental status, elevated base deficit, abnormal prothrombin time, low hemoglobin, and injury pattern recognition, such as multiple mangled/amputated extremities. If more than one of the factors mentioned is present, then massive transfusion should be initiated in most situations. One simple rule that we have found extremely useful in avoiding under resuscitation or delayed resuscitation after explosive-type injuries is to immediately administer 4 units each of PRBCs and FFP for each mangled or amputated extremity. Administration of recombinant activated factor VII (Novoseven, Novo Nordisk) was widely used as a massive transfusion adjunct during the first several years of combat operations, but was subsequently abandoned based on lack of efficacy data and safety concerns about the prothrombotic potential. There is currently great interest in the use of an antifibrinolytic agent, tranexamic acid (TXA), which has demonstrated a mortality rate benefit in the civilian trauma setting. Two published analyses of the outcomes with the use of TXA among combat casualties (Military Application of Tranexamic Acid in Trauma Emergency Resuscitation Study 1 and 2) have demonstrated a significant mortality rate benefit among all patients, and a larger benefit among patients requiring greater amounts of blood products. The use of TXA has now been included in the Joint Theater Trauma System (JTTS) Clinical Practice Guidelines (CPG) for DCR (dose 1 g intravenous [IV] bolus followed by 1 g IV infusion over 8 hours), and ongoing research will help clarify questions about the optimal indications, timing, and dosing of this product. Another exciting subject of ongoing research is the use of lyophilized, or "freeze-dried," plasma that would be immediately available for administration after simple reconstitution in fluid. This could overcome the current problems of storage and time delay for thawing with standard FFP.

COMBAT SURGERY

A full discussion of the broad spectrum of combat trauma surgical principles and techniques is beyond the scope of this chapter, but there are now several excellent books available that cover this in detail (see Suggested Readings). Although most of the surgical techniques used in combat trauma are identical to civilian practice, the principles of how and when they are applied are unique. As emphasized earlier, the majority of combat trauma patients will require some type of operative intervention and undergo multicavity and multisystem operative intervention much more frequently than civilian trauma. All efforts should be made to minimize unnecessary delays to the OR in severely injured patients, and in some cases the patient is best served by a "direct to OR" triage that bypasses the typical emergency department (ED) evaluation entirely.

Subspecialty consultation or patient transfers are often not available options, so the combat surgeon must become proficient in the initial operative management of traumatic injuries from head to toe. This includes procedures such as emergency craniotomy, complex facial reconstruction, cardiac or pulmonary repair, and fracture/amputation management that is infrequently or never performed by general trauma surgeons outside of combat. Predeployment training initiatives have been developed by all of the military services to provide general trauma refresher training and hands-on exposure to specialty techniques such as basic craniotomy/craniectomy, external fixation of fractures, vascular repair, etc. In addition, military surgeons have made extensive use of technologic advancements such as videoteleconferencing and Internet-based instruction to enhance their capabilities and provide remote "virtual" subspecialty consultation to even far-forward facilities.

The nature and type of surgical procedures performed will be largely dictated by the location and capabilities of the facility. As described in Table 1, a forward Level 2 facility will principally perform abbreviated damage control procedures for life and limb preservation with rapid evacuation to a more robust hospital. In contrast, a Level 3 facility has full staffing and holding capability, and can provide both initial emergent surgery as well as the more complex definitive or reconstructive procedures. In either location, the same basic principles apply when dealing with acute trauma surgery. A damage control approach should be the default, and should preferably be initiated BEFORE the development of worsening acidosis, hypothermia, and coagulopathy. The goals of initial operation should be at a minimum to (1) control hemorrhage, (2) control any ongoing aerodigestive spillage, and (3) provide initial cleaning and débridement of contaminated or devitalized tissue. This is followed by rapid temporary closure or dressing application with a plan for subsequent definitive operation(s). In addition to helping achieve physiologic stabilization, this approach serves to minimize valuable OR time when there are often more casualties waiting, and conserves scarce resources (equipment and personnel).

The goal of minimizing operative time is frequently in conflict with the multisystem nature and severity of combat injuries. In the civilian setting, these patients are typically managed by several different teams of surgeons operating in series with prolonged operative times. In the combat setting these procedures are performed in parallel as resources permit, with multiple teams of surgeons working simultaneously on different areas of the body (Fig. 7). All involved or injured areas are prepped and draped into the same operative field, allowing for simultaneous intervention and for observation of all injured areas to avoid occult intraoperative bleeding under the drapes. In this manner, a patient could undergo a damage control laparotomy, mangled extremity débridement and fixation, and repair of facial injuries in under 60 minutes by three teams working simultaneously. One of

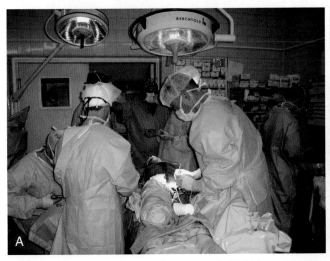
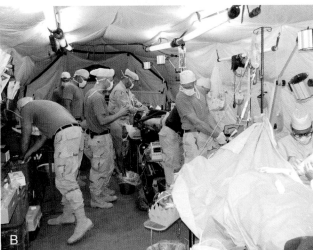

FIGURE 7 Team approach to combat trauma. **A,** Multiple surgical teams operating simultaneously on the trunk, arms, and legs of an injured child at a Combat Support Hospital. **B,** Operating tables arranged head to head at a Forward Surgical Team allowing a single anesthesia provider to monitor both cases simultaneously.

the most important basic principles in combat damage control is to leave wounds open (trunk and extremity) and avoid primary closure at the initial surgery. This allows for easy reoperation and inspection at the next level of care, repeat débridements of often massively contaminated wounds, and avoidance of infection or compartment syndromes (particularly during prolonged transport periods).

An additional unique factor in combat-related injuries, particularly with explosive or blast injuries, is the degree of tissue injury and nature of contamination that is in the wound on initial presentation. Massive amounts of soft tissue loss, damage, or subsequent necrosis result in large and deep cavities that can be difficult to cover or subsequently close. In addition, there is a remarkable amount of gross wound contamination from a variety of sources that is frequently driven deeply into the wound bed and adjacent tissue planes by the blast. This typically includes dirt, debris, fabric, and bullet or metallic fragments from both the explosive device and the clothing or uniform and equipment. Larger metallic objects such as ball bearings or nuts and bolts are frequently seen as either components of the explosive device (such as a "suicide vest") or in passengers of vehicles struck by an IED. Bone fragments may be found in the absence of any identifiable fracture, and represent tissue fragments from the suicide bomber or nearby victims ("bioshrapnel") that are blown into the wound (Fig. 8A). Finally, all battlefield health care providers must also be cognizant of the potential for unexploded ordnance to be present in extremity or truncal wounds (Figs. 8B and 8C). These pose a grave risk to not only the patient, but to the health care providers and

other nearby patients. Once identified, these patients should be segregated, necessary treating personnel should don full protective gear, and removal under controlled conditions should be expedited with assistance of expert explosive ordnance technicians. Operative removal should include avoidance of metallic contact with the device and any use of cautery and ultrasound devices.

Like civilian trauma, combat damage control typically involves multiple staged procedures performed over set time intervals. A drastic difference is that in the modern combat setting these procedures are performed by multiple different providers at facilities spread out over three continents, often within 48 to 72 hours of the initial injury. This has mandated a massive and successful effort at close coordination between military services, medical facilities, providers, and the aeromedical transportation assets. As a result, these disparate elements now function as a unified system providing continuous high-level surgical and critical care from the point of injury on the battlefield to the recovery and rehabilitation phase in the United States.

POSTOPERATIVE CARE AND EVACUATION

The importance of planning for the disposition and subsequent care issues when dealing with combat casualties cannot be overemphasized. With the limited bed space and resources available, any delays or breakdown in patient movement out of the facility can hinder the

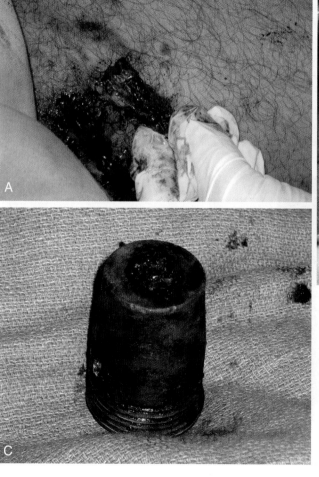

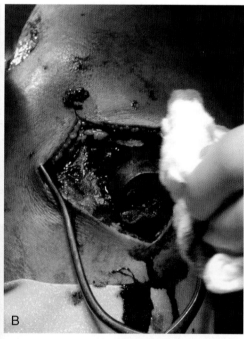

FIGURE 8 Combat wounds may be contaminated with a variety of objects. **A,** Fragments of bone ("bioshrapnel") from the body of a suicide bomber that were blown into the leg wound of a nearby victim. **B,** Metallic object identified in a wound cavity that was recognized as an unexploded rocket-propelled grenade and **C,** after removal by a U.S. Army surgeon.

ability to care for incoming patients. Consideration must be given to the reality that these facilities will not just be caring for U.S. military personnel, but will also be treating coalition forces, local national forces, contractors, and civilian casualties, each with their own evacuation or disposition chain. A typical patient mix at most facilities is at least 50% of patients being local national forces or civilians, and their disposition will require close coordination with local host nation facilities and transportation assets. The creation of specific positions for bilingual local nationals with some medical training to coordinate disposition has greatly streamlined this process.

Postoperative care priorities will typically focus on continued resuscitation, stabilization, and preparation for transfer. As in civilian centers, the military has recognized the importance of having dedicated medical and surgical intensivists to augment combat hospitals. This is particularly critical during times of higher operational tempo when the surgical personnel will be busy in the ED and OR, and not able to devote full attention to postoperative intensive care unit (ICU) care. However, the care remains a team effort with coordination between both the primary surgeon and the ICU team in a cooperative model. Most Level 2 facilities have very limited postoperative holding capacity (1–2 beds) and ICU-level equipment. Level 3 facilities typically have more robust ICU capabilities, including ICU nurses and intensivists, modern ventilators, infusion pumps, pressors, etc. Some advanced ICU therapies such as hemodialysis and salvage modes of ventilation (high-frequency ventilation, extracorporeal membrane oxygenation [ECMO]) are not routinely available in-theater, and thus any indication for these therapies should prompt immediate arrangements for transfer.

Preparing the severely injured combat patient for evacuation to the next level of care is often a difficult balancing act, considering the need for evacuation to a higher level of care versus the potential for deterioration or other problems during transport. Frequently patients are evacuated within several hours of major damage control surgery and with ongoing resuscitation. This has necessitated the development of standard protocols to prepare the patient for transfer, including preflight order sets and checklists. In addition, specialized training courses for in-flight personnel including medics, nurses, and physicians have been developed to augment their abilities to provide a continuous and high level of care during both rotary wing and fixed wing transport. Immediately prior to transfer the patient should have a thorough review of vital signs, laboratory results, and close inspection of all surgical sites and dressings. If a prolonged transport period is anticipated, then protocols have been initiated to perform a final washout or dressing change immediately prior to evacuation. All dressings are marked with the time and date of the last change or washout, and a full copy of the available medical records should accompany the patient. This is now also augmented with increasingly robust Internet-based electronic medical record systems that have greatly enhanced the flow of information and coordination of patient care. However, sometimes the most effective medical records in far-forward care are as low tech as a handwritten note with a color marker (Fig. 9).

One of the most important initiatives in the creation of a system that delivers seamless high-level trauma care across large distances has been the development of the U.S. Air Force Critical Care Air Transport Team (CCATT) program. The CCATT consists of a physician-led team of specialists trained in both critical care and aeromedical care who are able to operate on a wide variety of fixed wing platforms. They have the equipment and training to provide advanced ventilator support, monitoring, and infusion therapies including blood products and pressors. In special circumstances they can be further augmented to deliver advanced ICU therapeutics such as hemodialysis, high-frequency ventilation, and even ECMO during transportation from Level 3 facilities in a combat zone to a Level 4 or 5 facility for definitive care. In the current conflicts this has primarily involved transporting patients from the Air Force Theater Hospitals in Iraq (Balad) and Afghanistan (Bagram) to Landstuhl Regional Medical Center in Germany, and then on to the United States.

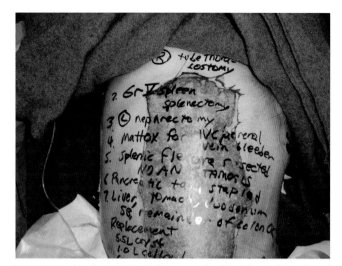

FIGURE 9 Handwritten operative report on the abdominal dressing of a patient who underwent damage control laparotomy at a Forward Surgical Team (Level 2) and then transferred to a Combat Support Hospital (Level 3) in Iraq.

COORDINATION AND QUALITY IMPROVEMENT INITIATIVES

Administrative oversight and review functions that are critical to a complete and mature civilian trauma system have often been a low priority in the austere and hectic setting of a forward combat medical unit. One of the hallmarks of the current conflicts has been the implementation of system-wide process and quality improvement initiatives like those found at civilian Level 1 trauma centers. The establishment of the JTTS has allowed for robust data collection, centralization of trauma care coordination, and global implementation of quality improvement initiatives. The JTTS director position is filled by senior trauma surgeons on a rotating basis, and has responsibility for theater-wide oversight of trauma operations.

Trauma coordinator nurses under the leadership of the JTTS director have been emplaced at all forward Level 3 facilities. They perform prospective data collection and entry into the JTTR (currently contains over 25,000 U.S. military patients) and oversee a number of quality improvement processes at individual facilities. There are currently 48 completed combat-specific JTTS CPGs covering a wide variety of clinical topics to assist deployed providers (http://www.usaisr.amedd.army.mil/clinical_practice_guidelines.html). Unit level educational and mortality and morbidity conferences have been installed, frequently with CME (continuing medical education) credits awarded for attendance. One of the most important aspects of unifying care across the entire system has been fostering communication and real-time feedback via a weekly video teleconference (VTC) run by the JTTS staff. This VTC includes participants from each level of care, from point of injury to stateside Level 5 and rehabilitation facilities. Each patient is reviewed, the patient's care at each level is presented by someone who was directly involved, the current status is updated for all interested parties, and active discussion of positive and negative aspects of the trauma care is fostered.

The recognized importance of both data collection and then productive use of the data for both research and quality improvement projects has resulted in the creation of a well-staffed Deployment Combat Casualty Research Team (DCCRT). This team consists of a physician-scientist director, a nursing research expert, scientific advisors, and administrative support staff who are deployed to the theater of operations and support all aspects of deployment-related research. This includes facilitating protocol development and approval, assisting with data collection, statistical and data analysis consultation, human subject research protection review, and assistance with preparation of abstracts

Top Ten Combat Trauma Lessons

1. Patients die in the ER, and

2. Patients die in the CT scanner;

3. Therefore, a hypotensive trauma patient belongs in the operating room ASAP.

4. Most blown up or shot patients need blood products, not crystalloid.

5. For mangled extremities and amputations, one code red (4 PRBC + 4 FFP) per extremity.

6. Patients in extremis will code during rapid sequence intubation; be prepared and intubate these patients in the OR (not in the ER) whenever possible.

7. This hospital can go from empty to full in a matter of hours; don't be lulled by the slow periods.

8. The name of the game here is not continuity of care, it is throughput. If the ICU or wards are full, you are mission incapable.

9. MASCALs live or die by proper triage and prioritization – starting at the door and including which x-rays to get, labs, and disposition.

10. No personal projects!!! They clog the system, waste resources, and anger others. See #8 above.

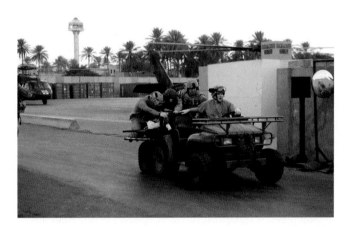

Reprinted from "The Volume of Experience (January 2008 edition)", a document written and continuously updated by U.S. Army trauma surgeons working at the Ibn Sina Hospital, Baghdad, Iraq.

FIGURE 10 List of top 10 combat trauma lessons. ASAP, As soon as possible; CT, computed tomography; ER, emergency room; FFP, fresh frozen plasma; IC, intensive care unit; MASCAL, mass casualty; OR, operating room; PRBC, packed red blood cell. *(From "The Volume of Experience" [January 2008 edition], a document written and continuously updated by U.S. Army trauma surgeons working at the Ibn Sina Hospital, Baghdad, Iraq.)*

or manuscripts for presentation. In addition to contributing to scientific knowledge, this initiative has fostered numerous real-time data-driven changes and improvements in combat care that have doubtless had an immense impact on fatality, morbidity, and the quality of combat care.

CONCLUSIONS

A detailed overview of all aspects of the modern military combat medical system would be beyond the scope of a single book chapter, so we have attempted to provide a summary of some of the key points and developments over the past decade of combat operations (Fig. 10). The unique wounding mechanisms and issues associated with operating in a variety of austere environments require the development of a specialized skillset and knowledge base that is separate but complementary to standard civilian trauma practices. One of the few positive aspects of war is the associated advances in trauma care, and we must continue to maximize and use these lessons that have come at such a high human cost.

For the chapter's Suggested Readings list, please visit the book at www.ExpertConsult.inkling.com.

CARDIAC HEMODYNAMICS: THE PULMONARY ARTERY CATHETER AND THE MEANING OF ITS READINGS

D. Dante Yeh, Mitchell J. Cohen, and Robert C. Mackersie

The pulmonary artery catheter (PAC) is a physical object creating a conundrum. Since its introduction in the 1970s, the PAC has been simultaneously hailed for its ability to provide physiologic data not easily obtainable by other means and condemned as a useless and potentially harmful invasive monitor. Very little hard data support continued use of the PAC, and some data support avoiding its use altogether. Despite considerable controversy over the clinical use and safety of the PAC, the PAC provides an important means of invasive intensive care unit (ICU) monitoring. This chapter reviews the history of right-sided heart catheterization; examines the basis of insertion, data collection, interpretation, and troubleshooting; and explores the clinical evidence for and against the use of PA catheterization and determination of resuscitation in critically ill surgical patients.

HISTORY OF CONTROVERSY

The PAC was introduced in the late 1960s, approved for clinical use in 1970, and was quickly incorporated into the armamentarium of the critical care physician. By 1999, 1.5 million catheters were sold, and presumably used, each year in the United States. The PAC is classified by the Food and Drug Administration (FDA) as a class II device and requires general and specific controls to reasonably assure safety and effectiveness. Even as considerable controversy and political debate over its use continues, the catheter has never been considered a lifesaving device and, as a result, is exempt from licensing and required evaluation.

Since its development, the PAC has enjoyed growing use and acceptance as a monitoring device. Indeed, its popularity has followed closely the advent of critical care as a specialty, and thus is considered by many a primary tool of the critical care physician. After years of use, and with little data supporting its benefits, concerns about the overall use and safety of the PAC appeared in several papers beginning in the late 1980s. Gore and colleagues examined 3000 patients with acute myocardial infarction (MI) and the relationship of outcome to PA catheterization. This study of over 3000 patients with acute MI reported a higher mortality rate in patients with hypotension who received a PAC (42% vs. 32%). Higher mortality rate was also reported in the subgroup of patients with congestive heart failure (CHF) who received a PAC (44% vs. 25%). In addition, patients who received a PAC had longer hospital stays. Several observational and retrospective studies quickly followed with similar results. Many in the critical care community discounted these trials, believing that PAC placement was more common in patients with more severe illness, with attributable mortality rates. A 1990 Canadian trial was the first to attempt to prospectively study the use of PAC in critically ill patients. In what was to become a recurring theme, however, the study failed because of a 35% exclusion rate, with many clinicians refusing to randomize their patients. A lack of clinical consensus regarding PAC use followed, and the PAC enjoyed continued widespread use until the debate was reignited in 1996. Connors et al studied PAC use in 5735 critically ill ICU patients, carefully matching illness severity and other confounding variables between the PAC and control groups. Ultimately, this study found that patients treated with PAC had increased 30-day mortality rate, mean cost, and ICU stay. Subset analysis was unable to identify any group of patients who actually benefited from PAC.

As a result of these and similar data, and in the same issue of the *Journal of the American Medical Association*, Bone and Dalen called for a National Heart, Lung, and Blood Institute (NHLBI) randomized prospective clinical trial to test the efficacy and safety of the PAC. They went on to spark considerable controversy by suggesting that the FDA issue a moratorium on the use of the PAC until such time that the safety and use be measured in an appropriate clinical trial. In response to this call for a moratorium, both NHLBI and Society of Critical Care Medicine (SCCM) consensus conferences were convened in 1997. The Pulmonary Artery Catheter Consensus Conference Consensus Statement was published later that same year. This statement did not support a moratorium on PACs, citing adequate level IV evidence to support the possibility of benefit of PAC in patient groups including MI and trauma patients, but conceded that appropriate clinical trials were needed to measure its use and safety. The NHLBI conference came to similar conclusions. Many trials followed, all with limited numbers of patients or low randomization rates, increasing the likelihood of a type II error and selection bias. Additionally, protocols and therapies backed by quality evidence were rarely used.

In 2003, a Canadian group published the first prospective randomized study with sufficient patient enrollment to have statistical power and authority. In this study, 1994 patients were randomized to surgery without a PAC versus with a PAC. The authors found there were no differences in hospital survival and in 6- and 12-month survival. There was, however, an increase in the number of pulmonary embolism (PE) events, with eight reported in the catheter group versus none in the observation group. The authors concluded that no benefit from PA catheterization could be found in elderly high-risk surgical patients. Although this study was important in that it was the first to randomize a significant cohort of patients, the randomization rate, 52%, remained low. Furthermore, it included a disproportionate number of older critically ill patients, excluding younger trauma or septic patients. Other trials have followed that also showed mixed results. More recently Shah et al performed a meta-analysis of 13 randomized clinical trials between 1985 and 2005. This study totaling 5051 patients was performed using a random effects model to estimate the odds ratio for death, hospital days, and pressors and found no difference between patients with and without a PAC.

A 2006 Cochrane Collaboration meta-analysis of all randomized controlled trials in adults comparing management with and without a PAC was published. Importantly, of the 12 trials identified, only one reported any systematic differences in the care provided to the patients other than the presence of a PAC. However, the authors described possible sources of bias for each of the studies: allocation bias, performance bias, attrition bias, and detection bias. The majority of patients in the surgical trials underwent routine major surgery and most of the trials were small and single center; only one study was adequately powered. The authors ultimately concluded there was no evidence of benefit or harm from a PAC.

In the same year, the Fluid and Catheter Treatment Trial (FACTT) was published in which the ARDSnet trialists randomized 1000 patients with acute lung injury/acute respiratory distress syndrome (ALI/ARDS) to management using the PAC or the less invasive alternative, the central venous catheter. Additionally, patients were randomized to receive a conservative versus a liberal fluid management strategy. Trauma patients composed less than 10% of all patients. One of the strengths of this trial was the detailed, explicit management protocol, ensuring standardization of treatment across 36 centers. Additionally, all study personnel underwent extensive training in measurement and interpretation of PAC-derived data. Pressure tracings also underwent centralized review. Similar to other studies, this trial was characterized by a low enrollment rate: 91% of screened patients were excluded. In this study, the PAC-guided therapy did not improve survival and was associated with twice as many catheter-related complications (predominantly arrhythmias). Serious complications were rare and there were no deaths related to insertion.

No randomized prospective trial to date, however, has been able to demonstrate an overall benefit to PA catheterization in critically injured patients. In data limited to trauma patients, there is some recent evidence to show a benefit for PAC use in the injured. A retrospective database study of over 53,000 patients drawn from the National Trauma Data Bank showed a reduction in mortality rate in older patients and patients with higher injury severity scores. Overall, PAC use was shown to be beneficial in patients with severe shock with a base deficit of 11 or more, injury severity scores higher than 25, and age over 61. This large nonrandomized cohort database study is the first and only study to show a clear benefit from PAC use in the severely injured patient.

One bias confounding PAC use and study are disparate factors that affect which patients are treated with the PAC. In 2000, Rapoport et al reported a comprehensive look at the characteristics of PAC use. This group retrospectively examined 10,217 patients in 34 ICUs in the United States and showed that full-time ICU staffing was associated with a decreased likelihood of PAC use. Catheter use was associated with white race/ethnicity and private insurance. Patients admitted to a surgical ICU were two times more likely to have a PAC. This study is revealing in that it is indicative of the lack of an established protocol and the presence of an established bias in PAC placement.

Another factor confounding many PAC studies is the absence of quality control measures to ensure accurate interpretation of PAC-derived data. A survey of critical care practitioners revealed that 47% of physicians were unable to correctly determine the pulmonary artery occlusion pressure (PAOP) from a pressure trace with a clearly identified end-expiration. Even more concerning, 61% did not

Rates among all medical patients

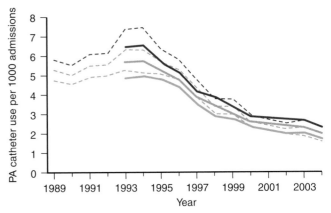

FIGURE 1   Rates among all medical patients. PA, Pulmonary artery. *(From Wiener RS: Trends in the use of the pulmonary artery catheter in the United States, 1993-2004. JAMA 298:423–429, 2007.)*

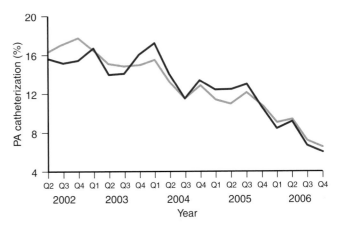

FIGURE 2   Pulmonary artery (PA) catheterization percentages. *(From Koo KK, Sun JC, Zhou Q, et al: Pulmonary artery catheters: evolving rates and reasons for use. Crit Care Med 39:1615–1618, 2011.)*

recognize an unambiguous indication that the introducer had been placed in a systemic artery. Another study reported that "experienced physicians' accuracy in predicting confirmed-valid PAOP tracings using waveform analysis was no better than a coin toss." Similarly, a survey of critical care nurses revealed that only 57.7% could correctly read a PAOP tracing on a clear pressure trace. Considering the mounting concerns regarding inaccurate measurement, incorrect interpretation of data, absence of protocols to guide action based on PAC-derived data, and scant evidence of patients benefiting from those actions, it is not surprising that enthusiasm for PAC use has waned. PAC use decreased by 65% from 1993 to 2004 and decreased more than 50% by 2006 (Figs. 1 and 2). This declining experience has further skewed the risk/benefit ratio as the current and future generations of ICU physicians will be more prone to error in insertion, interpretation, and appropriate application of PAC-related data.

PULMONARY ARTERY CATHETER USE AND INSERTION: WHAT IT IS AND HOW IT WORKS

PACs are commonly 100 cm long with an exterior French diameter of 7.5. Available with or without a heparin or antibiotic coating, they commonly contain latex rubber, an important consideration in latex-allergic patients. The 7.5 F diameter is further separated into three lumens. At the far distal end of the catheter is the PA port, which is used to transduce PA pressure and draw mixed venous blood. Just proximal to this port is a 1.5-mL balloon, which facilitates both the "floating" of the catheter and is also used to distally occlude the PA to measure PAOP. Another side infusion port, used for instillation of fluid, vasoactive agents, and medications, is located 15 cm proximal to the end of the catheter. Proximal to the side infusion port is the right atrium (RA)/central venous pressure (CVP) port, which is designed to be positioned at the vena cava/RA junction. This RA/CVP port is transduced to measure the CVP. Like the proximal infusion port, it can also be used as an infusion port for medication and fluids.

Along with ports that allow for pressure transduction and fluid infusion, the PAC also incorporates a thermal coil and proximal and distal thermistors for the measurement of cardiac output. Cardiac output is calculated by measurement of the change in temperature of blood between a proximal thermistor and a more distally placed thermistor. Traditionally, a cooled fluid bolus was injected proximally and the temperature of this bolus (now slightly warmed by blood flow) was measured by the thermistor at the tip of the catheter. Using formulas discussed later in this chapter, the cardiac output could be calculated. Most modern catheters now use a proximally placed thermal coil incorporated into the catheter which gently warms blood proximally and extrapolates from the temperature difference proximally and distally to give a continuous calculation of cardiac output. (A more detailed discussion of cardiac output monitoring appears later in the chapter.)

Insertion Tips and Guidelines

Insertion of the catheter is done through the gasketed introducer port of a Cordis catheter. Full sterile technique is paramount in order to reduce infection rates. We commonly place the introducer catheter and the PAC sequentially with one sterile prep and setup, which prevents contamination at the introducer gasket as well as the necessity of reprepping of a previously placed introducer. At times, however, this cannot be avoided, or a PAC will be placed through a previously located introducer line. In this instance, the introducer catheter and surrounding skin should be prepped widely with chlorhexidine preparation. In all cases, wide sterile prep with chlorhexidine and full sterile precautions including gown, hat, mask, and sterile gloves are essential. Any break in sterile technique has been shown in many studies to significantly increase the infection rate, and implementation of the preceding precautions has been reported to reduce the infection rate to near zero. Another tip is to prep widely. We cannot stress this seemingly trivial point too strongly. Opening, preparing, and inserting a PAC results in an often-unwieldy octopus of catheter, tubing, and transducers that have to cross through a sterile to unsterile transition zone. Wide prep of all or most of the bed with a sterile half-sheet facilitates easy handling and reduced risk of contamination. Once an introducer catheter is in place, the PAC is removed from the packaging and the proximal end is passed to a nurse or assistant who will connect and flush the catheter ports. At this time, the transducer is connected, zeroed, and tested. The balloon is also tested. Placement of the catheter sheath allows future adjustments without additional sterile prep.

Constant verbal communication between the floater and the assistant is essential. Once the tip of the catheter is passed through the introducer and into the blood vessel, it must be advanced only when the balloon is inflated (up), and conversely it must never be withdrawn unless the balloon is deflated (down). The slang term "floating" a swan refers to the fact that the catheter advances by floating along with the blood flow. Direct advancement can cause vascular injury or perforation. A constant communicative banter—"balloon up?" "balloon up"; "balloon down?" "balloon down"—can prevent injuries such as arterial, cardiac, and PA rupture.

Initially the catheter is inserted to the 10- to 15-cm mark, allowing the balloon to pass through the introducer. Once the catheter tip is safely past the introducer, the balloon is inflated and the catheter slowly advanced by feeding slack catheter and allowing the catheter to be pulled downstream by the blood flow. A combination of clinical experience, length of catheter inserted, and careful attention to the monitored transducer tracing allow successful placement. As the catheter tip enters the vessel, the initial pressure reading will be the CVP, which first transduced at less than 15 to 25 cm depending on patient size and insertion site. With another 5 to 10 cm of advancement, the catheter passes into the right atrium and the transducer will register a distinct right arterial waveform. Another few centimeters of advancement passes the catheter tip through the tricuspid valve (around 30 cm) and the easily recognizable spike of right ventricle (RV) pressure will register on the monitor. Slow careful advancement of another 5 to 10 cm will pass the catheter into the PA (tracing), and will soon wedge the catheter to produce a flattening of the waveform and characteristic wedge tracing.

Often several attempts to ensure proper wedging are required. When an RV waveform is not evident after 35 to 45 cm or no wedge tracing occurs after the catheter has advanced 10 to 15 cm past the RV tracing, the balloon should be deflated, and the catheter pulled back to the RA or RV. Once a distinct tracing identifies the catheter location, another careful attempt at reinsertion and wedging can begin. When the catheter is inserted and wedged, the pulmonary capillary wedge pressure (PCWP) is noted and the balloon deflated. The catheter is locked into place and the sterile covering advanced to cover the full length of the catheter. Placement of the catheter is confirmed by a chest radiograph.

Serious complications can occur during central venous access, the PA catheterization process, balloon inflation, and subsequent care. Complications during central venous access (including arterial puncture and pneumothorax) are common to all access procedures and are not unique to PAC insertion. The most common complication, arrhythmia, is often temporary and minor and generally occurs during balloon flotation through the right ventricle. Other more serious complications such as cardiac perforation, pulmonary artery rupture, pericardial tamponade, sustained right bundle branch block, and catheter knotting are extremely rare (less than1%) in experienced hands with modern, softer catheters. Thromboembolic events and catheter infection have become increasingly uncommon with the introduction of heparin-bonded catheters and prompt removal of the PAC once it is no longer indicated.

INTERPRETATION: WHAT DOES IT MEASURE AND WHAT DOES IT MEAN?

Initial Warnings and Potential Measurement Problems

Although the PAC provides a lot of otherwise unobtainable data, only diligent attention and educated interpretation make PA catheterization worth the risk, time, and cost. Without proper placement, all obtained data are erroneous and will lead to false interpretation and incorrect (and possibly harmful) intervention. Careful attention to the PAC waveform helps confirm catheter placement. Entry into the pulmonary artery is evidenced by a decrease in mean pressure and characteristic waveform. Upon entering the PA, a triphasic waveform is seen, which reflects atrial and ventricular contraction. From the PA, careful advancement of the catheter will "wedge" the catheter.

From the PAOP and CVP, we begin the pressure-volume measures. Once wedged or occluded, the inflated balloon prevents forward blood flow from the right ventricle or proximal pulmonary artery and allows only back-pressure to be transduced at the catheter tip. This transduced "wedge" pressure reflects a contiguous fluid column from the PA through the pulmonary vasculature to the left atrium (LA). The unobstructed column continues through the mitral valve into the (when open) left ventricle (LV), and hence,

$$PA < LA < LV < LVEDP$$

where LVEDP is left ventricle end-diastolic pressure. It is crucial to note that this relationship holds true only when there is a contiguous fluid column between the PA and LV. Improper interpretation of PAOP commonly occurs when this contiguous fluid column is interrupted or affected. Examples of interrupted fluid column include mitral valve disease (stenosis or insufficiency) and pulmonary venous obstruction. Also affecting the relationship between PAOP and left ventricle end-diastolic volume (LVEDV) is the ability to extrapolate volume from pressure measurements. Because PCWP is ultimately used as a measure of ventricular filling (volume), this necessitates the ability to predictably extrapolate volume from pressure, which is only possible with normal compliance. Indeed, LVEDP is analogous to LVEDV only in a normally compliant heart and thorax. Many factors influence the ability to use PCWP as an accurate measure of left-side heart–filling pressures. As described previously, the analogous relationship between LVEDP and LVEDV is accurate only insofar as the ventricle is normally compliant. In cases when left-side heart compliance is reduced, such as ventricular hypertrophy or ischemic myocardial damage, the PCWP will be elevated for a corresponding left ventricular pressure/volume and cannot be considered an accurate measure. Although trend analysis can be used to monitor fluid resuscitation in these patients, injured or septic patients often manifest rapidly changing cardiac compliance, making interpretation difficult and suspect. Indeed, multiple animal models have shown a rapid flux of cardiac edema resulting from injury, resuscitation, and inflammation, all of which can rapidly change ventricular compliance and render the PAC an unreliable measure of cardiac filling.

Along with proper wedging in the pulmonary artery and a normally compliant heart, the pulmonary catheter must be placed in the proper lung zone. In order for PCWP to reflect a vascular rather than alveolar pressure, the catheter must be placed in West zone 3 of the lung. Here $P_A > PV > PA$, so the measured pulmonary venous (PV) pressure reflects vascular pressure instead of pulmonary alveolar (P_A) pressure. If the catheter is in zone 1, $PA > P_A > PV$, or $2 P_A > PA > PV$, the catheter will reflect alveolar pressure rather than the PA pressure.

Constantly changing thoracic pressures from ventilation (spontaneous or mechanical) are reflected in the PAC tracing. In a positive pressure–ventilated patient, the PCWP should be measured at end-expiration when the pleural pressures are closest to zero. This is reversed if the patient is spontaneously breathing. In a spontaneously breathing patient the pressure normalizes somewhere between expansion and inhalation and by convention, the pressure is measured at end-inspiration. Direct monitoring and examination of the tracing rather than reliance on automatically collected single number display is always better. In an extreme situation, brief paralysis might be necessary to get a useful pulmonary artery wedge pressure (PAWP) tracing in an agitated or ventilatory dyssynchronous patient.

Positive end-expiratory pressure (PEEP) also affects the PAC tracing, and interpretation of the PCWP in a patient affected by intrinsic or intrinsic PEEP is the subject of much conjecture and misinformation. PEEP (both intrinsic and extrinsic) causes transmural thoracic pressure, which positively affects PAWP measurements. To correctly determine the PAWP, the PEEP can be temporally disconnected (for a few seconds or breath cycles). Alternatively, the effect of intrinsic or extrinsic PEEP can be estimated by adding 2 to 3 cm H_2O to each 5 cm H_2O of PEEP higher than 10.

Cardiac output (CO) is measured by thermodilution. Traditionally, a cooled saline bolus was injected proximally, and the temperature of the bolus was measured by a thermistor at the catheter tip. CO is calculated by determining the area under the curve and plotting the integral. An average of three to five injections were used to minimize variability. Newer catheters measure CO continuously by integrating

a thermal coil, which gently heats the proximal blood, measures the temperature drop at the catheter tip and uses a similar method to calculate CO. In either method, intracardiac shunt and tricuspid regurgitation will lead to unpredictable error in CO measurement. At least one set of authors suggest that greater reliability can be had by calculating CO through plotting of the Fick curve and extrapolating CO.

Pressure, Volume, and Work Measures

Although modern PAC monitoring units or ICU nurses provide continuous data readouts of hemodynamic parameters, it remains essential to have a grounded understanding of the physiologic principles and calculations involved in PAC monitoring. Actual measured parameters begin with CVP. CVP is directly transduced from the proximal or CVP port of the catheter. Without obstruction between the right atrium and the vena cava, CVP is analogous to right atrial pressure (RAP), which is again analogous to right ventricle end-diastolic pressure (RVEDP) and right ventricle end-diastolic volume (RVEDV). Hence,

$$CVP \sim RAP < RVEDP < RVEDV$$

CVP is a directly measured extrapolation of RVEDV or cardiac preload. Just as CVP is a measure of right-side heart filling, PCWP measures left-sided pressure and volume. As described previously, when the catheter is "wedged" in the pulmonary artery, there is a continuous fluid column between the PA and LV. Hence,

$$PCWP < LAP < LVEDP < LVEDV$$

CO is also measured directly through the previously mentioned thermodilution. CO is converted to a more normalized cardiac index (CI) by dividing CO by body surface area (BSA). BSA is derived from height and weight nomograms but can also be easily calculated with the Mosteller formula as follows (where W is weight in kg and H is height in cm):

$$BSA = \sqrt{W \times H} / 60$$

Once CO is known, stroke volume (SV) can be calculated as follows:

$$SV = CO / HR$$

where HR is heart rate.

Right-sided ejection fraction (RVEF) is then calculated as follows:

$$RVEF = SV / RVEDV$$

Calculation of RVEDV requires a continuous thermistor, which is capable of dividing CI into systolic and diastolic components. Knowing RVEF allows RVEDV to be calculated:

$$RVEDV = SV / RVEF$$

Right-sided heart work estimates the work of the right side of the heart as it pumps blood through the lungs back to the LV. The right ventricle stroke work index (RVSWI) is estimated as follows:

$$RVSWI = (PAP - CVP) \times SVI \times 0.0136$$

where PAP is pulmonary artery pressure, and SVI is stroke volume index.

The left side of the heart volume and work are calculated similarly to the right. The left ventricular work is the work of the blood circulating through the systemic circulation. This is estimated by

$$LVSWI = (MAP - PCWP) \times SVI \times 0.0136$$

where LVSWI is left ventricle stroke work index, and MAP is mean arterial pressure.

Among the most useful calculated measures provided by the PAC is the pulmonary vascular resistance (PVR) and systemic vascular resistance (SVR). Each estimates the resistance across the pulmonary or systemic circulation and is an extrapolation of vascular tone. SVR is the drop in pressure across the systemic circulation times the flow and is calculated as

$$SVR = (MAP - RAP) \times 80/CI,$$

in which RAP is right atrial pressure.

PVR is the drop in pressure across the pulmonary circulation multiplied by right-sided flow:

$$PVR = (PAP - PCWP) \times 80/CI$$

Goal-Directed Therapy Using Pulmonary Artery Catheter

There is little disagreement regarding the large amount of data provided by a properly placed and interpreted PAC. Whether the data provided result in better patient outcome is the source of considerable debate. Much clinical research has been done in an attempt to determine which PAC-derived physiologic parameters should be measured and which are predictive of outcome. Shoemaker and his group provided the initial work toward defining and grouping patient physiologic response to trauma. As early as 1973, Shoemaker and colleagues showed in several studies that PAWP measured reduced CO. They further showed that decreased oxygen delivery along with increased peripheral vascular resistance characterized nonsurvivors after trauma. Based on these and other similar study results, many groups targeted resuscitation of severely injured trauma patients to achieve physiologic values retrospectively associated with survival. Ten years after his initial studies, Shoemaker and colleagues showed an overall survival benefit in patients who achieved normal physiologic values. Finally, this group showed there was less oxygen debt as measured by oxygen consumption (Vo_2) in surviving patients. Interestingly, there was no difference in oxygen consumption between the groups. In similar research, Bishop et al examined physiologic parameters in 90 trauma patients and found that patients who achieved higher levels of CI, oxygen delivery (Do_2), and Vo_2 within the first 24 hours after admission had a lower incidence of ARDS and reduced overall mortality rate. Based on these and similar findings, several groups then randomized patients to supernormal resuscitation versus traditional resuscitation with the intent of proving that invasive monitoring of aggressive resuscitation would allow achievement of supranormal physiology and better outcome. These studies showed mixed results. Bishop's group randomized patients to be supranormally resuscitated to a CI of more than 4.5, Do_2 index greater than 670, and a Vo_2 index greater than 166, versus traditional resuscitation as defined by achievement of normal urine output and CVP. The supranormally resuscitated group showed significantly lower mortality rate and decreased organ failure. Interestingly, optimal parameters were reached in 70% of the study group and 29% of the control group. Similarly, Fleming et al randomized trauma patients with blood loss of more than 2000 mL to supernormal CI, Do_2, and Vo_2, and found that attainment of these goals resulted in statistically significant decreases in organ failure, ICU stay, and ventilator days, and a trend toward decreased mortality rate.

Other studies, however, pointed out that attainment of resuscitation was more important than the means by which it was achieved and many more recent studies have been unable to show similar benefit to monitoring or goal-directed resuscitation. Velmahos et al randomized severely injured patients to supranormal resuscitation versus traditional hemodynamic monitoring. Although there was no difference in mortality rate, organ failure, sepsis, ICU days, or hospital stay between the two groups, they found that 70% of the supranormal group and 40% of the traditional group achieved supranormal physiologic parameters, and that attainment of these optimal values was associated with better outcome independent of treatment protocol. There were no outcome differences between the two groups. What was perhaps most interesting in this study, however, was the finding that nonresponders (those who failed to reach the set goals despite volume and inotropic manipulation) fared significantly worse than the control group. This suggests the likelihood that aggressive resuscitation toward supranormal physiology will be harmful in those whose physiology cannot attain it, and is in fact exhausted by such attempts. Other groups have reported similar results, which indicate that the ability to achieve normal parameters is associated with the mortality rate benefit, and is ultimately more important than whatever treatment was designed to achieve them. Taken together, these results cast doubt regarding the usefulness of interventional monitoring and resuscitation. To date, a study that randomizes "intervention responders" (those whose physiology is below goal, but respond to interventions) to "continue treatment" and "stop treatment" groups has never been performed. The ultimate efficacy of $Vo_2/Do_2/CO$-based interventions, therefore, has never really been tested.

Many believe that aggressive resuscitation should be instituted in all patients without any need for invasive monitoring. Others argue for limited supraphysiologic resuscitation. Some data point to poorer outcome from PAC use. Indeed, deleterious consequences of aggressive resuscitation and the PAC have been reported. Hayes et al reported that increasing oxygen delivery with inotropic augmentation with dobutamine was associated with increased mortality rate. Others have reported similar increased mortality rate in supranormally resuscitated patients. At least one group has purported to show that the PAC is itself a predictor of morbidity independent of protocol-driven resuscitation. Rhodes et al performed a prospective randomized trial of 200 patients in which no protocol-driven resuscitation was instituted. In this study, patients were randomized to PAC versus no PAC when patients were resuscitated based upon the clinical judgment of the ICU staff. Data were obtained prospectively and examined retrospectively, and revealed that the PAC group received significantly more fluid in the first 24 hours and exhibited increased morbidity. Evidence for the deleterious effects of PAC protocol-driven resuscitation was seen in a study by Hayes et al that showed an increased mortality rate in PAC-treated patients (54% vs. 34%). In this study there was a rigorous goal-directed attempt to achieve supranormal physiologic parameters. To achieve these goals, aggressive fluid resuscitation and inotropic support were used.

These measures were not benign, however, as one consequence of overzealous fluid administration is the development of intra-abdominal hypertension (IAH) and the abdominal compartment syndrome (ACS). In its full-blown clinical manifestation, ACS adversely affects every major organ system and early descriptions reported near universal mortality rates. This may have contributed to the negative outcomes reported when PAC use was followed by more aggressive fluid resuscitation. With increased awareness, ACS and IAH are now being recognized at earlier stages. Preventive measures have resulted in decreasing incidence of ACS and improved outcomes.

In an attempt to make sense of the huge amount of data regarding PACs and end points of resuscitation, Kern and Shoemaker performed a meta-analysis on 21 randomized clinical trials and found that early hemodynamic optimization achieved significant mortality rate reduction only if optimized parameters were achieved prior to the onset of sepsis or organ dysfunction. Heyland and associates analyzed seven studies and found no significant reductions in mortality rate achieved with optimization. Lastly, an analysis by Poeze et al showed that physiologic optimization resulted in decreased mortality rate. In this analysis the entire benefit was from patients who were hemodynamically optimized perioperatively. Patients with established sepsis or organ failure prior to treatment were unlikely to benefit from "optimization." In trauma patients undergoing emergency surgery, all optimization occurs afterward, and optimization, therefore, is of questionable benefit.

Others have questioned the accuracy of the actual PAC measurements. Epstein et al studied the accuracy of Vo_2 measurements by the calculated reverse Fick method versus direct measurement by indirect calorimetry in an attempt to determine the accuracy of PAC determined oxygen consumption measures. Their study showed a bias of 41 mL/minute/m^2, indicative of an undermeasurement of V_{O_2} by PAC measures. Finally, Luchette and colleagues studied the accuracy of continuous CO measurements and found there was higher signal-to-noise ratio and degraded accuracy when patient temperature was above 38.5° C, resulting in further questioning of the accuracy and usefulness of PAC measurements in severely injured or septic patients.

Mixed Venous Saturation: Monitoring Tissue Metabolism

Although the results of supranormal resuscitation are mixed, many believe that the best use of a PAC is as a measure of tissue perfusion. PAC sampling of mixed venous saturation should serve as an adjunctive measure of tissue-level perfusion. Even if supranormal resuscitation remains controversial with mixed data, surely $S\bar{V}_{O_2}$ should provide useful data. Unfortunately, this measure of tissue perfusion, although seemingly useful as a measure of tissue oxygenation and subsequent outcome, has also not ultimately been shown useful as the targeted end point of resuscitation. Gattinoni and associates published a randomized prospective trial involving 762 patients across 56 ICUs who were randomized to either traditional resuscitation or targeting of CI more than 4.5 or $S\bar{V}_{O_2}$ greater than 70%. There was no difference in mortality rate or organ dysfunction among the three groups. Like the studies discussed earlier, subgroup analysis showed that patients who achieved hemodynamic targets had similar mortality rates independent of the group to which they were randomized.

Right Ventricle End-Diastolic Pressure as Measure of Cardiac Index and Cardiac Function

As predicted by the Starling curve, end-diastolic volume is the best predictor of preload. Unfortunately, PAC pressure measurements as discussed previously are confounded in the setting of changing intrinsic ventricular compliance and extrinsic PEEP. RVEDV monitoring provides the first actual measurement of preload. Rather than being a pressure surrogate for volume, RVEDV uses a PAC with a fast thermistor to give a directly measured volume. In an attempt to find an alternative to PAOP as a measure of cardiac function, Cheatham et al showed that CI correlated better with RVEDVI than PAOP. The same group then studied 64 patients with respiratory failure and high PEEP requirements, and suggested that RVEDVI was a better measure of CI than PAOP at all levels of PEEP. CI was inversely correlated with PCWP at PEEP levels over 15. Taken together, these findings caused this group to conclude that RVEDVI should be used in lieu of PAOP as a measure of cardiac function.

Despite initial reservations that mathematical coupling was responsible for the close correlation between RVEDV and CI, several groups have shown that the directly measured volumes are superior to extrapolations from pressure (CVP and PAWP) measures. Chang and colleagues showed that splanchnic malperfusion was better predicted by RVEDV than PCWP, which was in turn associated with multiple-organ dysfunction syndrome (MODS) and mortality rate. Other correlations among RVEDV, tissue perfusion, and outcome have been similarly reported by several groups. Lastly, Kincaid et al presented data to show that optimal RVEDV could be calculated for each individual patient. Taken together, these data support the use of RVEDV as a superior measure of cardiac function and goal-directed resuscitation.

Evidence of proper application of accurately obtained and interpreted PAC data is also lacking. In a simulation survey of critical care practitioners using a real life low-complexity case scenario, greater than 15% of respondents would have administered a treatment considered by experts to be potentially harmful. There were no differences according to country of origin or specialty. According to the observed responses, the authors state that inappropriate application of PAC data may cause a 30% decrease in the potential beneficial effects of PAC on mortality rate in prospective randomized studies.

ALTERNATIVES TO THE PULMONARY ARTERY CATHETER

Since the turn of the new century, attention has been increasingly turned toward developing and validating less invasive technologies aimed at providing the clinician with useful hemodynamic parameters to assist in critical decision making. These include esophageal Doppler, transthoracic echocardiography, and pulse contour analysis.

Esophageal Doppler technology allows evaluation of the descending thoracic aorta: blood flow velocity or corrected flow time (FTc) and aortic diameter. Recently, a goal-directed randomized trial demonstrated superior outcomes using a treatment algorithm using esophageal Doppler-derived data in the resuscitation of trauma patients. The disadvantages of this technique include the requirement for specialized operator training and interpretation and the difficulty of maintaining correct positioning for prolonged periods.

As an alternative to the "static" measures of intravascular volume such as CVP, PAOP, and RVEDI, "dynamic" measures of intravascular volume include stroke volume variation (SVV), systolic pressure variation (SPV), and pulse pressure variation (PPV). SVV is calculated from the product of the velocity time integral and the outflow track area, both obtained from the esophageal Doppler. Alternatively, it can be calculated from a pulse contour analysis. PPV may be measured directly from an arterial pressure tracing; neither SVV nor PPV requires pulmonary artery cannulation. Both measures rely on heart-lung interactions during mechanical ventilation, whereby positive-pressure ventilation displaces blood in the pulmonary circulation into the LA and LV, resulting in an early inspiratory augmentation of LV preload and increased in stroke volume and systolic blood pressure (termed Δup). Simultaneously, the RV preload is decreased (via decreased venous return) and RV afterload increased (via increased transpulmonary pressure). The decreased RV ejection fraction results in a decreased LV preload two to three heartbeats later, resulting in a late inspiratory decrease in LV stroke volume (termed Δdown). In hypovolemic patients, Δdown is the predominant component of PPV but in patients in CHF, Δup is dominant. These effects are more pronounced on the steep, ascending portion of the Frank-Starling curve and therefore can be used to predict fluid responsiveness. Although early studies used tidal volumes ranging between 8 and 12 mL/kg, it has been demonstrated that PPV remains with high specificity even at low tidal volumes and high PEEP settings. A recent systematic review concluded these "dynamic" measures are more accurate than traditional "static" measures in predicting fluid responsiveness. Although this is attractive, it is important to remember that PPV and SVV provide no information about ventricular function. Additionally, these "dynamic" measures are only accurate in patients on fully controlled mechanical ventilation without cardiac arrhythmias. The lure of and blind acceptance of new technologies must not be repeated.

SUMMARY

Since its inception, the PAC has been a data tool of the critical care physician. As can be seen from a careful review of the literature, little prospective, conclusive data exist to support its continued use. At the same time, however, there is recent literature and clinical support for early goal-driven resuscitation of critically ill patients. The optimal resuscitation goals for trauma patients, however, remain to be determined. Trauma patients are often hyperprotocolized based on their mechanism and injuries. The PAC is also subject to extreme difficulties in proper measurement and interpretation of collected data, and it is impossible to know the precise accuracy of collected data and how well they were interpreted in the many PAC and resuscitation trials. In the midst of controversy, however, it is important to remember that the PAC is not a drug or intervention, and its use therefore cannot be directly assessed. The PAC has been subject to intense scrutiny and one might point out that the use of other diagnostic and monitoring devices such as electrocardiograms, chest radiographs, arterial lines, and pulse oximeters is widely accepted, yet a survival benefit has not been definitely confirmed by level I evidence. The potential effectiveness of the PAC depends on a number of other factors, many of which are not measured or assessed in clinical studies. These include proper indications and risk assessment, proper placement and risk reduction measures, knowledgeable use and interpretation, and the contextual relevance and use of the data obtained from the PAC.

Because of these confounders and the powerful data that can be procured from measurement, we advocate continued selected and diligent use of the PAC as a tool for proper resuscitation in the critically injured and ill patient. Although the proper resuscitative parameters and goals may not be absolutely known, and may change from minute to minute in our patients, more frequent and better data collection properly filtered through clinical judgment should only benefit patient care. To be used correctly, however, perfect attention to proper and safe placement and use must be assumed. From there,

continued data collection and monitoring corroborated with patient state is also essential. It is not enough to intermittently examine a few select physiologic variables. Indeed, at any given moment a patient's physiology and subsequent predicted outcome are the sum of a huge number of measured and unmeasured variables and the interactions between these patterns of variables. As technology becomes sufficiently advanced to allow for pattern recognition of more than a few variables, the use of each measure should increase and be revealed. To discount the important measures derived from the PAC based on studies that failed to find use of these independent measures is probably shortsighted, and ignores the use of these otherwise unobtainable data. Indeed, the continued use of the PAC despite multiple studies reflects the clinician's belief that the PAC data combined with other monitoring and clinical acumen will be beneficial on a patient-to-patient basis, which might not be measured in a large trial. That said, use of the PAC requires continual attention, monitoring, and intervention, and we believe that much of the confusion and negative data regarding PA catheterization results from a once-a-day glance at the Swan numbers (usually without regard to their accuracy) without careful perusal of the ongoing flux of the patient's state. Discounting the PAC is foolish. It is a tool that can only be made useful and better through physician education and diligence.

For the chapter's Suggested Readings list, please visit the book at www.ExpertConsult.inkling.com.

OXYGEN TRANSPORT

Patricio Polanco, Juan Carlos Puyana, Mitchell Fink, and Andrew B. Peitzman

The primary role of the cardiorespiratory system is to meet the steady state demands of the body by delivering adequate amounts of oxygen (O_2) to meet metabolic requirements, to sustain aerobic respiration in the tissues, and to remove excess carbon dioxide (CO_2). Adequate tissue oxygenation is determined by the balance between the oxygen delivered into the tissues/organs and the oxygen required to sustain aerobic metabolism.

Unicellular organisms evolved to efficiently harness large amounts of energy from organic molecules (especially glucose) through the use of oxygen as an electron acceptor. In this process, CO_2 is generated and chemical energy is transferred to high-energy molecules of adenosine triphosphate (ATP). Oxygen cannot be stored in our cells; therefore, the generation of energy through aerobic (oxygen-consuming) processes is completely dependent on its supply. Without oxygen, death rapidly ensues.

In unicellular organisms, the oxygen consumed and the CO_2 produced easily diffuses across the cell membrane. This cannot occur in multicellular organisms such as humans. Instead, complex mechanisms of oxygen delivery and CO_2 removal needed to evolve to maintain aerobic metabolism. We are therefore totally reliant on the coordinated function of respiratory, cardiovascular, and hematologic systems to maintain energy production.

At a molecular-cellular level, *shock* is defined as the pathologic state that occurs when oxygen supply becomes the rate-limiting step in the generation of energy; a condition of hypoperfusion at a cellular level when oxygen delivery (Do_2) to the cells is below the tissue oxygen consumption (Vo_2) needs. Oxygen delivery is a product of blood flow (cardiac output) and arterial oxygen content. The degree of

failure in the supply and use of oxygen during shock can be measured, and in fact using these variables, we can monitor the effectiveness of therapy. This chapter explains how we can quantify the delivery and consumption of oxygen.

ENERGY GENERATION IN THE CELL

The process of glucose breakdown to CO_2, water, and energy is the metabolic backbone of the energy production of the cell, although other molecules such as amino acids and fatty acids can also enter at different steps of this process.

Glycolysis (the first step in the process of glucose metabolism) requires the breakdown of glucose to two molecules of pyruvate. This first step occurs universally in the cytoplasm of all mammalian cells, yielding two molecules of ATP. This constitutes only 5.2% of the total potential energy that can be released from glucose. In the absence of oxygen, pyruvate is metabolized by lactic dehydrogenase to lactate. Under anaerobic conditions, such as that seen in intense physical activity or during shock, lactate rapidly accumulates in the circulation. Lactate uptake with regeneration of glucose occurs in the liver. Lactate concentrations in blood of less than 2 mmol/L are considered normal. Increased lactate production, poor lactate clearance, and accumulation in plasma reflect increased anaerobic metabolism and a state of shock. The degree of increase in plasma lactate is a reliable prognostic sign. Lactate levels can also be used as an end point of therapy in trauma resuscitation so that successful treatment of shock should be followed by normalization of lactate in plasma. Inability or delay in clearance of lactate is associated with increased mortality rate from injury.

In the presence of oxygen, pyruvate is oxidized to and ultimately metabolized to CO_2 and water. This aerobic phase of glucose metabolism is called respiration, and occurs entirely in the mitochondria. The generation of energy from pyruvate involves three stages. The first stage generates acetyl-coenzyme A (acetyl CoA), an irreversible process. In the second stage, acetyl-CoA is metabolized in an eight-step process (the citric acid cycle) through enzymatic oxidation generating CO_2, and energy that is conserved in nicotinamide adenine dinucleotide (NADH) and flavin adenine dinucleotide ($FADH_2$). In the final stage (the electron transfer chain), NADH and $FADH_2$ are oxidized through an electron-carrying process that uses oxygen as the final electron acceptor.

In the aerobic portion of glucose metabolism, 36 molecules of ATP are generated. Thus, cellular respiration yields 18 times more energy than anaerobic glycolysis. Most of the cells in our body are dependent on cellular respiration for the generation of energy and ultimate survival. Organic molecules that generate pyruvate are not limited to glucose because other molecules, such as certain amino acids and fatty acids, can be used. Therefore, oxygen, not pyruvate, becomes the rate-limiting step in the generation of energy in our patients.

Pathologic states that involve abnormal mitochondrial use of oxygen are observed in various clinical processes. For example, cyanide poisoning of the electron transfer chain results in a rapid development of a severe energy deficit, accumulation of lactate, and death. More commonly, states of septic shock are thought to cause "mitochondrial disease" that renders these organelles incapable of efficiently using oxygen for the generation of energy.

MICROCIRCULATION AND OXYGEN DELIVERY

The diffusion of oxygen into the cell is limited by the distance between the cell itself and the source of oxygen, and is limited to only 100 to 200 μm. A highly complex capillary network (microcirculation) exists to distribute the oxygen to cells and tissues. The surface area in the microcirculation far exceeds the circulating blood volume. Thus, a hypovolemic state would occur if all capillary beds were open at any given time. To avoid this, blood flow is selectively distributed to various vascular beds as needed to meet oxygen demands.

A breakdown in the regulation of oxygen distribution (dysoxia) across the microcirculation occurs in septic shock; thus, septic shock is a form of distributive shock. Excessive amounts of nitric oxide, a potent vasodilator, are thought to be a central aspect of sepsis dysoxia. In addition, the resultant tissue edema increases the distance between the cells and the capillaries, which also contributes to poor oxygen diffusion. Maldistribution of capillary flow is also a major component of sepsis. Thus, sepsis is characterized by poor oxygen extraction.

Hemoglobin, the Ultimate Oxygen Carrier

Oxygen is carried in the blood in two forms: dissolved and bound to hemoglobin (Hb). Approximately 98% of O_2 is carried by Hb and 2% is carried in the dissolved state. Hb serves as a unique oxygen carrier capturing oxygen in the alveoli, distributing it through the microcirculation, and ultimately discharging it in the pericellular environment. Adult human Hb consists of two α and two β polypeptide chains, each bound to a heme group capable of binding one molecule of O_2. Each gram of Hb binds 1.34 mL of O_2. Because Hb concentration is easily measured, the content of O_2 carried per 100 mL of blood can be calculated as follows:

$$1.34 (mL/g) \times Hb \, (g/dL) \times O_2 \text{ saturation } (Sao_2, \text{ fraction of } 1)$$
$$= Hb \text{ oxygen content}/100 \, mL$$

Example:

$$1.34 \times 15 \times 0.98 = 19.7 \, mL/100 \, mL$$

The degree of oxygen saturation in Hb through spectrophotometric absorption of light (pulse oximeter) is a widely used tool in intensive care. The saturation of Hb is highly nonlinear, roughly following an S curve (Fig. 1). This determines that Hb can easily upload or download O_2 under physiologic conditions. It also determines that

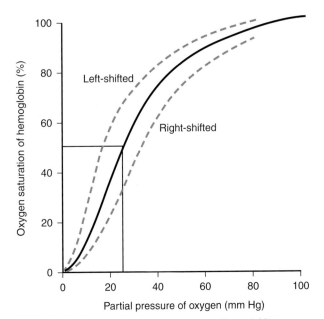

FIGURE 1 Oxyhemoglobin dissociation curve. The solid line represents the oxyhemoglobin dissociation curve for normal adult hemoglobin. The right- or left-shifted curves represent increase or decrease capacity of hemoglobin to delivery of oxygen at a define partial pressure of oxygen.

minor drops in Sao_2 at saturations of less than 90% reflect higher degrees in the change of the partial pressures of O_2 (Po_2) than drops at a lower Sao_2. Roughly, a 90% Sao_2 reflects a Po_2 of 60 mm Hg. Pathologic alterations of the Hb-oxygen saturation curve are observed with alterations in pH, temperature, and the concentration of 2,3-diphosphoglycerate (2,3-DPG).

A small percentage of O_2 is also carried by the plasma and is a function of the Po_2. This concentration is approximately

$$0.003 \, mL/100 \, mL \, (\text{of plasma})/(Po_2) \, mm \, Hg$$

Thus, we can calculate the total amount of O_2 contained in a given amount of blood *arterial oxygen content* (Cao_2) as follows:

$$(1.34 \, [Hb] \times Sao_2) + 0.003 \, (Po_2) = Cao_2$$

Based on this formula, we could assume that increasing levels of serum Hb through blood transfusion will increase Cao_2 and therefore oxygen delivery. This is theoretically true; however, attempts to achieve normal levels of serum Hb in critically ill patients are not uniformly beneficial. The Transfusion Requirements in Critical Care trial by Hebert et al showed increased mortality rate in patients who were treated with a liberal transfusion strategy (transfused when Hb falls below 10 g/dL) versus those with a restrictive transfusion therapy (Hb maintained at 7 to 9 g/dL). However, oxygen consumption and delivery were not measured in this study. In addition, it has been shown that red blood cell transfusion in septic patients may increase oxygen delivery but generally does not increase oxygen consumption.

Considerable interest and efforts have been invested in the development of hemoglobin-based oxygen carriers (HBOCs). The potential benefits of HBOCs include universal compatibility, useful vascular half-life, absence of infectious agents, and better storage life than banked red blood cells. Although promising effects of these products on oxygen transport and microcirculation have been identified, further investigation is needed. A recent meta-analysis reported that the administration of HBOCs in surgical, stroke, and trauma patients was associated with a significant risk of myocardial infarction and death.

Heart as Oxygen Delivery Pump

How much oxygen is ultimately delivered (Do_2) to the cells is determined by the amount of blood pumped by the heart (cardiac output), making cardiac performance an essential aspect in analyzing oxygen-dependent cellular energy production. Cardiac output (Q) is calculated at the bedside through several methods. Although the use of the Swan-Ganz catheter has been questioned, it is still the most practical tool to determine Do_2:

$$Q \times Cao_2 = Do_2 \, (mL/minute/m^2)$$

Cardiac output is determined by preload (intravascular volume), contractility, afterload (vascular resistance), and heart rate. Inappropriate cardiac performance rapidly leads to shock. Thus, inadequate contractility observed after myocardial infarction leads to inadequate oxygen delivery, a state known as cardiogenic shock. Cardiogenic shock occurs in 7% of patients after myocardial infarction and is the most common cause of early death in these patients. Other complications of a myocardial infarction that can cause cardiogenic shock include papillary muscle rupture with acute mitral insufficiency and ventricular wall rupture with pericardial tamponade.

PUTTING IT ALL TOGETHER: MEASURING CELLULAR OXYGEN CONSUMPTION AND EXTRACTION IN PATIENTS

We can easily quantify the amount of oxygen consumed in whole organisms using the functions developed previously. The amount of oxygen taken up by the cells (Vo_2) is a function of measuring Q and the difference in arterial (Cao_2) and venous (Cvo_2) oxygen content. Cvo_2 is calculated using the same variables as in arterial content with the exception that venous oxygen saturation (Svo_2) is measured in the central circulation (right atrium or ventricle):

$$Q(Cao_2 - Cvo_2) = Vo_2$$

Not all oxygen delivered to the periphery is consumed or extracted in the periphery. In fact, only approximately 25% of the oxygen delivered is normally extracted, although there are significant variations by organ. Oxygen extraction ratio (O_2ER) is calculated as a percentage of the oxygen consumed divided by the oxygen delivered:

$$(Vo_2/Do_2) = O_2ER$$

The amount of oxygen extracted by the tissues can be increased significantly under physiologic conditions to satisfy cellular needs. This provides an important buffer that allows the maintenance of adequate oxygen consumption during times of increased demand. In addition, oxygen extraction allows tissues to maintain adequate oxygen consumption when delivery is decreased.

Several authors have described the use of oxygen delivery and Svo_2 as a valid end point of resuscitation in what has been defined as early goal-directed therapy (EGDT). Despite its widespread use, the validity of Svo_2 as a tool for monitoring resuscitation remains controversial. Shoemaker reported that mortality rate was decreased when high-risk surgical patients were treated to supranormal values for cardiac index (greater than or equal to 4.5 L/minute/m²) and oxygen delivery (greater than or equal to 600 mL/minute/m²). Gattinoni et al and Hayes et al found no improvement in outcome using cardiac index, oxygen delivery, and Svo_2 compared with traditional treatments of resuscitation. In contrast, Rivers et al showed that EGDT in septic shock patients using a constant measurement of central venous oxygen saturation using a central line instead of a pulmonary artery catheter (defined as $Scvo_2$) was associated with lower mortality rate (30.5%) when compared to patients receiving standard therapy (46.5%). The role of invasive hemodynamic monitoring such as pulmonary artery catheters to obtain cardiac index, Svo_2, and calculate Do_2 for shock resuscitation is still controversial. It has been described that the sole measurement of these parameters is a futile effort if it is not coupled with a treatment protocol that by itself improves outcomes.

Relationship of Oxygen Consumption and Oxygen Delivery during Pathologic States

During physiologic states, oxygen delivery exceeds oxygen consumption; it is therefore said that oxygen consumption is independent of the delivery (Fig. 2). In experimental models, a gradual decrease in oxygen delivery is associated with an increase in O_2ER and maintenance of normal aerobic metabolism. A critical point in Do_2 is reached (cDo_2) when oxygen consumption becomes dependent on oxygen delivery and aerobic energy generation fails. As a result, lactate accumulates in the blood. Not surprisingly, variables that measure the state of oxygen delivery and consumption are good predictors of clinical outcome.

Serum levels of lactate and base deficit have been described as indirect indicators of tissue perfusion and cellular oxygen use. Several authors have determined a strong correlation of serum lactate or base deficit with outcome in hemorrhagic shock. Broder and Weil in 1964, and later Vincent et al and Dunham et al, confirmed the previous findings, both in clinical studies and animal models.

Determining the cDo_2 in a given patient would give clinicians the advantage of confirming the presence of shock. However, cDo_2 is not easily determined using conventional technology. The cDo_2 varies from patient to patient, and differs according to pathologic state. In addition, Vo_2 and Do_2 share several variables including Hb and cardiac performance. Varying one or more of these shared variables will alter both Vo_2 and Do_2, a phenomenon known as "mathematical coupling."

Despite these limitations, measuring oxygen transport and consumption remains an essential tool for clinicians treating shock states. Careful measurements of oxygen variables allow the "fine-tuning" of resuscitation—optimizing oxygen transport and cardiac performance and minimizing physiologic costs. An array of variables is routinely manipulated by the clinician, including increasing oxygen saturation, increasing Hb concentrations, optimizing preload and myocardial contractility, altering afterload, and decreasing cellular oxygen

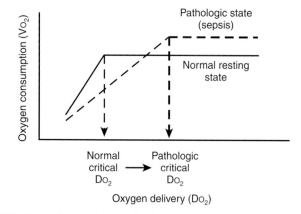

OXYGEN DELIVERY AND CONSUMPTION

FIGURE 2 Oxygen delivery (Do_2) and consumption (Vo_2). Solid line represents the normal state in which Vo_2 stays constant over a decrease of Do_2 until it falls below a critical Do_2 ($cDco_2$). The dashed line represents a pathologic state (sepsis) with an increase of Vo_2 and cDo_2 due to impaired oxygen use.

consumption. How these variables are changed in a given patient depends in great part on the type of shock present.

Characteristic Oxygen Transport Variables in States of Shock

Hemorrhagic Shock

Hemorrhagic shock is characterized by the loss of blood (loss of Hb), thereby decreasing oxygen-carrying capacity, and by loss of intravascular volume to negatively affect preload. Thus, in hemorrhagic shock, there is a decrease in Do_2 due to decreased Hb and cardiac output, associated with an increase in O_2ER. Hemorrhagic shock is best treated by early control of the site of bleeding and restoration of intravascular volume and Hb levels. Early source control and rapid payback of *oxygen debt* are critical to optimize outcomes. Whole fresh blood, although not normally available, should ideally be used in cases of severe hemorrhagic shock. Provision of adequate volumes restores cardiac output and Hb levels.

Cardiogenic Shock

Cardiogenic shock is characterized by decreased myocardial contractility most often as a result of myocardial infarction. Other less common causes of cardiogenic shock include acute myocarditis, sustained dysrhythmia, acute valvular catastrophe, and decompensation of end-stage cardiomyopathy from multiple causes. Cardiogenic shock is characterized by hypotension and a reduced cardiac output and cardiac index (less than 2.2 L/minute/m^2) in the presence of elevated pulmonary capillary occlusion pressure (greater than 15 mm Hg) and increased O_2ER.

Septic Shock

With adequate volume resuscitation, septic shock generally results in a hyperdynamic state characterized by high cardiac output, increased oxygen delivery, and decreased afterload or systemic vascular resistance. Sepsis results in increased microvascular stopped-flow. The maldistribution of capillary blood flow in septic shock results in a mismatch of oxygen delivery and oxygen demand. Oxygen consumption is increased, but impaired oxygen extraction ability in the peripheral tissues results in lactic acidosis. Mitochondrial dysfunction and decreased ATP production can lead to organ failure and death in sepsis. The basic pathogenesis of this organ dysfunction is still unclear; both tissue hypoxia and mitochondrial dysfunction resulting in impaired oxygen use seem to be contributory. O_2ER is decreased, and therefore characteristically elevated Svo_2 is observed.

Neurogenic Shock

Neurogenic shock is observed after traumatic high spinal cord injuries and is associated with a normal cardiac output, an absence of reactive tachycardia, and decreased afterload. Neurogenic shock is a distributive type of shock attributed to the disruption of the autonomic pathways within the spinal cord. Hypotension occurs due to decreased systemic vascular resistance resulting in pooling of blood within the extremities lacking sympathetic tone.

CONCLUSIONS

Use of oxygen in mammalian cells is necessary for the production of adequate amounts of energy. Oxygen must be transported to the pericellular environment, as it only diffuses through small distances in tissues. A complex network of capillaries is designed so that adequate delivery of oxygen transported by Hb can occur. Hb is the main oxygen carrier and increasing its concentration may increase oxygen delivery but does not increase oxygen consumption; therefore, liberal strategies of transfusions are not recommended. Different disease processes, cardiorespiratory disorders, and types of shock present with distinct profiles of oxygen transport variables. Systemic assessment of oxygen delivery and consumption can be readily performed to provide important prognostic information that also allows optimization of therapeutic approaches to the treatment of various forms of shock.

For the chapter's Suggested Readings list, please visit the book at www.ExpertConsult.inkling.com.

PHARMACOLOGIC SUPPORT OF CARDIAC FAILURE

John W. Mah and Orlando C. Kirton

Cardiovascular disease affects more than 82 million people, according to statistics from the American Heart Association in 2008, with congestive heart failure affecting approximately 5.7 million of these adult Americans. Although survival from heart failure has improved, the risk of death remains high with a 5-year survival rate of approximately 50% after diagnosis. Admission for acute decompensated heart failure (ADHF) often results from exacerbation of preexisting disease or following any number of events, including acute myocardial infarction, valvular disease, and arrhythmias. Additionally, patients today are older and sicker and may be undergoing cardiac and noncardiac surgery as well as developing other causes of acute heart failure such as from sepsis or pulmonary embolus. Patients with ADHF are often triaged to the medical intensive care unit (ICU); however, these patients are also presenting for urgent exploratory and elective surgery. Whether presenting with acute or chronic heart disease, this sicker population represents an increasingly difficult challenge for the surgical intensivist. Diagnosing and treating the initiating cause are imperative; the mainstay of therapy is optimal pharmacologic hemodynamic management.

PATHOPHYSIOLOGY

The pathophysiologic mechanisms leading to ADHF, as well as the goals of pharmacologic treatment, must be identified in order to successfully treat patients with ADHF. Understanding the complex nature of each specific disease process and its physiologic response is crucial for improving function and outcome. Cardiac failure is usually a result of derangement in any number of physiologic factors, including preload, afterload, contractility, heart rate, and heart rhythm.

Increased preload is common in ADHF and is usually secondary to volume overload but can also occur with myocardial ischemia and valvular dysfunction. The body's natural compensatory response is to increase filling pressures to improve myocardial contractility by increasing wall stress on the ventricle (moving up on the Frank-Starling curve). Heart failure generally causes a decrease in renal blood flow and subsequently activates the renin-angiotensin-aldosterone axis (RAAA). The end results of these compensatory mechanisms are vasoconstriction by angiotensin II with increased renal blood flow; release of aldosterone, which increases sodium absorption in exchange for potassium; and promotion of ventricular hypertrophy, fibrosis, and remodeling that ultimately leads to increased ventricular stiffness.

Increased cardiac afterload is common in the perioperative setting and is due to multiple causes such as preexisting hypertension, catecholamine surge, postoperative hypertension, and release of cytokines and inflammatory mediators. Moreover, pulmonary artery hypertension is increased owing to similar causes, but can be exacerbated as well by relative hypoxic vasoconstriction and acidosis. In the failing heart, the sympathetic nervous system (SNS) is stimulated as the body acts to increase systemic vascular resistance (SVR) to maintain normal perfusion to vital organs. The failing heart is further strained as it attempts to increase cardiac output against higher outflow pressures. The increased sympathetic tone also stimulates the release of renin, further activating the RAAA and its inherent problems in heart failure. Subsequently, there is an increase in myocardial oxygen demand, worsening sodium and water retention, and a heightened potential to exacerbate lethal cardiac arrhythmias. Furthermore, higher plasma levels of circulating catecholamine have been correlated with worse prognosis.

Myocardial contractility is largely affected by stimulation of the SNS. Adrenergic agents increase intracellular cyclic adenosine monophosphate (cAMP), which in turn, increases calcium influx and strengthens the contraction. However, with chronically increased sympathetic tone, the failing heart becomes less responsive to circulating catecholamines, seemingly protecting the myocytes from the excessive catecholamines and their resulting inotropic and chronotropic drive. This dampened response is due to decreased sensitivity and downregulation of the β-receptors from the chronically elevated catecholamine levels that persist in congestive heart failure. Contractility becomes impaired and is less responsive to physiologic needs as well as to pharmacologic agents that act at the β-adrenergic receptors. In addition, the failing heart responds inadequately to volume overload. The Frank-Starling mechanism is blunted, and significant increases in preload are poorly tolerated, further exacerbating congestive symptoms.

Right ventricle (RV) failure is becoming increasingly recognized as a significant cause of morbidity and fatality in the ICU. The RV is thin-walled and compliant relative to the left ventricle (LV) and is designed to function in a low-pressure, low-resistance environment. Contraction occurs in three stages: (1) papillary muscle contraction, (2) RV movement toward the interventricular septum, and (3) LV contraction with twisting of the RV. There is minimal time spent in isovolumic contraction and relaxation, resulting in almost continuous flow to the lungs. The RV is perfused primarily from the right coronary artery (RCA), with perfusion occurring in systole and diastole as long as the low-pressure system remains intact. The RV is vulnerable to elevation in pulmonary vascular resistance, which will increase the time spent in isovolumic contraction and relaxation, decreasing overall forward blood flow. Both ventricles are dependent on movement of the interventricular septum, which can shift toward either the RV or LV, both of which can impair adequate filling and increase end-diastolic pressures.

Following cardiac surgery, ventricular function is transiently impaired even in patients with normal preoperative ventricular function. This is due to several factors, including aortic cross-clamping, inadequate myocardial protection, hypothermia and cardioplegia, and reperfusion injury, as well as excessive levels of inotropes in the perioperative setting. There is a biphasic pattern, with initial recovery following weaning from cardiopulmonary bypass (CPB), a nadir at about 3 to 6 hours, and then full recovery at 8 to 24 hours.

This pattern can obviously be delayed by poor preoperative ventricular function. Pharmacologic support is frequently necessary until adequate function returns.

TREATMENT

The general pharmacologic goals of supporting the acutely decompensated heart are to ameliorate afterload, optimize preload and myocardial performance while modulating myocardial oxygen consumption, and minimize further activation of the neurohormonal cascade. Additional support is often needed to maintain an adequate mean arterial blood pressure to ensure sufficient coronary blood flow.

Diuretics

Diuretics are the mainstay and building block in treating patients with ADHF, as volume overload is a common occurrence. However, there are no randomized clinical trials demonstrating the efficacy of diuretics on survival in ADHF. Nonetheless, diuretics remain an effective therapy for the volume-overloaded patient; they act by decreasing preload and intravascular volume and relieving the symptoms of dyspnea and pulmonary congestion. Also, hypervolemia is common in the surgical patient who has preexisting congestive heart failure due to volume resuscitation from trauma, sepsis, major surgery, or perioperative fluid management. Loop diuretics such as furosemide are commonly used; more potent alternatives such as bumetanide or torasemide are useful in the diuretic-resistant patient. Intravenous bolus or continuous infusions can be used. Although "gentle" diuresis in many smaller studies using continuous infusions have been shown to be less toxic and even more efficacious, more recent evidence suggests that there is no difference between bolus dosing and continuous infusion in regard to global symptoms and renal function. Volume status should be addressed clinically or with invasive monitoring if needed, as overdiuresis or diuresis of the normovolumic patient can cause hypotension or hypoperfusion of end organs. Diuretics may be detrimental in the face of an acute myocardial infarction or other organ dysfunction, as well as in the early postoperative setting in the presence of capillary leak and third space fluid sequestration. Other concerns include the use of high-dose diuretics, which can activate the RAAA and the SNS, and which have their own adverse long-term effects.

Vasodilators

Nitroglycerin (NTG) can be an effective agent for the rapid treatment of cardiogenic pulmonary edema and ADHF and provides rapid relief of symptoms. The primary effect of NTG is venodilation, with vasodilation occurring at higher dosing more than 30 μg/minute). NTG has minimal effects on cardiac and skeletal muscle and causes smooth muscle relaxation mainly in the venous system, allowing for increased venous capacitance. It effectively and rapidly reduces ventricular filling pressures (preload), relieves unwanted ventricular wall stress, and more importantly, reduces myocardial oxygen demand. In addition, NTG can improve coronary blood flow by reducing coronary artery resistance and prolonging diastole. The half-life of NTG is short, allowing for rapid escalation and discontinuation of the drug, but tachyphylaxis occurs and often requires persistently increasing dosage. Other unwanted side effects include headache and abdominal pain related to the powerful vasodilation. Volume status must be determined, and diuretics can be helpful in negating the increasing resistance to nitrates.

Nitroprusside induces a more balanced dilation of arterial and venous systems independent of dosing. Venous tone is reduced, producing benefits of decreased preload. In addition, nitroprusside causes a dramatic reduction in afterload, allowing for improvement in cardiac output, stroke volume, and reduced LV filling pressures and ventricular wall stress and ultimately decreased myocardial oxygen demand. It can be especially useful in ADHF for rapid afterload reduction in conditions such as acute mitral or acute aortic regurgitation. Nitroprusside also causes coronary vasodilation and can improve myocardial perfusion if ventricular diastolic pressure reduction exceeds aortic diastolic pressure reduction. Patients with coronary artery disease, however, have the potential to develop a "coronary steal," redirecting blood flow away from ischemic to nonischemic myocardium. Specific cautions include precipitous drops in blood pressure and cyanide and thiocyanate toxicity.

Nesiritide is a recombinant form of a human brain type natriuretic peptide (hBNP) that binds to vascular and endothelial receptors to increase the intracellular levels of cyclic guanosine monophosphate (cGMP). This results in smooth muscle relaxation with predominant vasodilation and some venodilation. Although considered a "natriuretic," diuresis has not been shown to be a major effect. It may, however, potentiate the effects of other diuretics. Nesiritide has been used in controlling the symptoms of congestive heart failure and lowering pulmonary capillary wedge pressures (PCWP). Symptomatic hypotension can occur, and subsequently its use is limited in the setting of volume depletion, hypotension, or malperfusion. Furthermore, investigators have brought to light nesiritide's increased incidence of renal failure and overall increased short-term risk of death in a pooled analysis of randomized controlled trials (RCTs) and suggest that its use be limited to failure of traditional therapy with combination of diuresis and NTG. In fact, a recent large randomized controlled study of 7141 patients admitted for acute heart failure suggested that nesiritide appears to be better than placebo in controlling symptoms and resulted in no change in mortality rate or readmission to the hospital.

Inotropes and Vasopressors

The ideal inotropic agent would increase contractility without increasing heart rate, afterload, preload, or myocardial consumption. The receptor-based agonists exert their effects through α_1, α_2, β_1, β_2, or dopaminergic receptor agonism, and the phosphodiesterase (PDE) III inhibitors increase intracellular cAMP concentrations to enhance the contractile force in cardiac muscle (Table 1). Vasopressors, although having some intrinsic inotropic activity, are most useful in treating hypotension and maintaining an appropriate mean arterial blood pressure to ensure adequate coronary flow.

Inotropic Agents

Dobutamine is a synthetic catecholamine with predominant β_1- and weak β_2-agonist effects as well as weak α_1-agonist activity; its main effect is enhanced contractility and heart rate, augmenting cardiac output and stroke volume (Table 2). Systemic vasodilation occurs secondary to dobutamine's β_2-agonist activity, affecting peripheral circulation as well as the pulmonary circulation. Although dobutamine increases myocardial oxygen consumption, this effect is balanced with improvement in myocardial oxygen supply by coronary vascular

TABLE 2: Hemodynamic Actions and Infusion Rates

Agent	CO	Inotropy	HR	SVR	Infusion Rate
Dobutamine	↑↑	↑↑	↑↑	↑↓	2–40 µg/kg/min
Epinephrine	↑↑	↑↑	↑	↑	1–4 µg/min
	↑	↑↑	↑↑	↑↑	4–7 µg/min
	↑↓	↑↑	↑↑	↑↑↑	>7 µg/min
Milrinone	↑↑	↑↑↑	↑↓	↑↓	50 µg/kg bolus, then 0.375–0.75 µg/kg/min
Norepinephrine	↑↓	↑	↓	↑↑↑	0.01–0.1 µg/kg/min
Dopamine	↑↓			↑↓	0.5–2 µg/kg/min
	↑			↑↓	2–5 µg/kg/min
	↑↓	↑↑	↑↑↑	↑↑	5–10 µg/kg/min
Phenylephrine	↓		↓	↑↑	20–400 µg/min

CO, Cardiac output; HR, heart rate; SVR, systemic vascular resistance.

dilation. However, this beneficial effect occurs only if the deleterious increase in heart rate can be avoided. Dobutamine is contraindicated in idiopathic hypertrophic subaortic stenosis due to an increasing pressure gradient between the LV and aorta. Dobutamine should be used with caution in patients with atrial fibrillation or flutter because of its proarrhythmic pharmacologic effect. Its use may also be limited in the patient already taking doses of long-term beta blockers or those with preexisting chronic heart failure, because of the need for higher levels of medication to achieve effect. In these circumstances, combination therapy with PDE inhibitors has been shown to be useful.

Epinephrine acts predominantly at the α_1-, β_1-, and β_2-receptors, and its cardiac effects are most beneficial when used at lower doses (up to 0.02 µg/kg/minute) when the β effects predominate. Contractility is improved along with peripheral vasodilatation and increase in heart rate. The end result in the normovolumic patient is increased cardiac output and systolic pressure with decreased diastolic pressure, SVR, and pulmonary vascular resistance (PVR). In fact, following cardiac bypass, epinephrine produces equal increases in stroke volume as dobutamine or dopamine, with less significant tachycardia at lower dosing. At higher dosing, arrhythmias become more frequent and α-receptor activity significantly increases, which tends to encourage alternative inotropic support.

TABLE 1: Catecholamine Activity at Adrenergic Receptor Sites

Catecholamine	Dopamine	β_1-Receptor	β_2-Receptor	α-Receptor
Dopamine	+++	++	+	+++
Dobutamine	0	+++	++	+
Norepinephrine	0	+++	0	++
Epinephrine	0	+++	++	+++

0, No activity; +, minimal activity; ++, moderate activity; +++, predominant activity.

PDE inhibitors are a unique class of drugs that inhibit the PDE III isoenzyme found in myocardial and vascular smooth muscle cells, leading to increased levels of cAMP. This higher level of intracellular cAMP results in increased myocardial contractility and myocardial and vascular smooth muscle relaxation. Systemic vasodilation is also enhanced, with significant reduction in both peripheral vascular resistance (PVR) and SVR. Mean arterial blood pressure can decrease, but there is usually minimal effect on myocardial oxygen consumption and heart rate. This unique mechanism of action improves contractility in these situations when desensitization secondary to downregulation of β-receptors has occurred. PDE inhibitors may in fact work synergistically with the β-agonists, thereby decreasing the necessary concentrations of these agents and reducing their harmful side effects. The addition of even small doses of PDE inhibitor can have a large impact on cardiac index without augmenting systolic blood pressure. PDE inhibitors have been found to be beneficial for RV failure due to its inotropic ability and pulmonary vasodilatory properties (decreased RV afterload). The PDE inhibitors have a longer half-life than most inotropes but have a fairly quick onset of action. Milrinone has essentially replaced amrinone because of its improved safety profile and potency. It is 20 times as potent as amrinone and reaches peak concentration in 2 minutes, with a half-life of approximately 2 to 4 hours. The half-life is significantly longer than the adrenergic agents, and the risk of systemic hypotension must be taken under consideration prior to its use. It causes significantly more vasodilation compared with dobutamine at similar increases in cardiac output. Also, the half-life is further prolonged by its decreased elimination in patients with congestive heart failure or renal insufficiency. Other cautions of its use include ventricular and supraventricular arrhythmias, hypotension, headache, and rare occurrences of thrombocytopenia.

Vasopressors

Dopamine is a naturally occurring agent and stimulates different receptors based on serum concentration. At least part of its effect is due to release of norepinephrine from nerve terminals in myocardial cells. Dopamine is usually the drug of choice for acute heart failure with associated hypotension, also deemed cardiogenic shock. At lower doses (up to 3 μg/kg/minute), it is mainly a dopaminergic agonist. As the rate increases to 5 to 10 μg/kg/minute, it acts at the β_1-receptor. It is in this range that cardiac contractility is stimulated, with minimal increase in heart rate, blood pressure, and SVR. Higher doses result in increasing α_1-receptor stimulation. Because dopamine has no β_2-adrenergic effects, the overwhelming result is strong systemic as well as coronary vasoconstriction. At higher dosing, dopamine usually becomes limited by its profound tachycardia, arrhythmias, and coronary vasoconstriction. Hence, in cardiac failure dopamine is best used at low to moderate dosing.

Norepinephrine is of little value in the treatment of acute heart failure and remains in use only after other drugs have failed. Its predominant activity is at the α-receptor, with only mild β_1-agonist activity. Any β-receptor activity is usually countered by the strong vasoconstriction and increase in afterload, further offsetting the myocardial oxygen supply and demand ratio. It is, however, one of the first-line agents useful in septic shock or other causes of marked vasodilatory shock. Its use in cardiac failure is supportive to keep arterial blood pressure adequate for coronary artery perfusion, such as in cardiogenic shock.

Arginine vasopressin (AVP) is an endogenous hormone released from the posterior pituitary gland usually in response to changes in volume as well as blood pressure and osmolality. Its role is limited in treatment of acute heart failure but it has recently been found to be useful in refractory septic shock. In early septic shock, AVP levels are high, followed by a relative depletion in circulating AVP and a relative vasoplegic state by 36 hours. Replacement of low-dose AVP to physiologic levels has been shown to restore normal vascular tone while providing paradoxical vasodilation and increased blood

flow to other organs. AVP binds to motor (V_1) and renal (V_2) receptors, allowing some potential for renal protection, and may have pulmonary vasodilatory or rather minimal pulmonary vasoconstricting effects. Regardless, administration of low-dose AVP (0.01 to 0.04 U/minute) can potentially restore a catecholamine-resistant state while reducing the high dosage of additional first-line vasopressors and their added harmful effects.

Other Agents

Thyroid hormone has been used in transplant organ donors to improve cardiac function. Sick euthyroid syndrome is being frequently diagnosed, and other nonthyroidal illnesses are relatively common in the critically ill patient. Replacement of thyroid hormone has been suggested to improve cardiac performance and enhance recovery of ventricular function after an ischemic event. In the cardiac patient, triiodothyronine (T_3) hormone levels have been shown to be significantly decreased following CPB, unrelated to dilution or heparin administration. These levels then return to normal after 12 to 24 hours. Although there is some evidence that administration of T_3 improves cardiac function, studies are conflicting for using T_3 in the perioperative setting to wean patients from CPB. Although no adverse effects have been reported with the use of thyroid hormone in the T_3-deficient patient, its use has not been clearly supported and remains relatively controversial.

Methylene blue is mentioned for its potential use in refractory shock but obviously lacks strong evidence-based studies. It is mentioned for its unique and untapped potential as a mechanism of action in sepsis or other systemic inflammatory response syndrome (SIRS) resulting in shock. The SIRS state results in increased production of nitric oxide (NO) and subsequently smooth muscle cGMP leading to hypotension, decreased response to catecholamines, and myocardial depression. Methylene blue inhibits the production of NO and cGMP, increasing arterial blood pressure, improving myocardial function, and maintaining oxygen transport, and has been shown in a few small studies to be effective in refractory septic shock, reducing the requirement of adrenergic agents. There have been some reports of worsening hypoxia in those patients with acute lung injury who have been administered methylene blue, due to apparent pulmonary vasoconstriction. This result appears to be lessened by lower dosing and continuous infusions.

SPECIAL CIRCUMSTANCES

Heart Failure in Septic Shock

Multiple factors contribute to the hypotensive state and relative cardiac failure associated with septic shock. Although sepsis usually results in a high-output cardiac state, there is, nevertheless, a reduction in the contractile performance that is often unable to meet the metabolic demands of the tissues. RV and LV contractility is directly impaired. Preload is reduced owing to a marked drop in the SVR and a loss of fluid from capillary leakage and thus poor venous return. Endogenous vasopressin, although initially enhanced, is thought to be quickly exhausted from prolonged intense stimulation of neurohypophyseal stores. Although dopamine, epinephrine, norepinephrine, phenylephrine, and vasopressin have all been shown to increase blood pressure in septic shock, dopamine and norepinephrine are the recommended first-line agents for maintenance of normal blood pressure along with adequate fluid resuscitation. Of note, dopamine compared with norepinephrine when used in septic shock has resulted in a significantly higher rate of arrhythmias. Although commonly used as a second-line agent, the addition of low-dose vasopressin has not been shown to reduce mortality rate and to be no more effective than norepinephrine alone. Marked depression of myocardial contractility can occur, requiring inotropic support. Dobutamine has been shown to be effective in maintaining a normal range of cardiac output and subsequently increasing Svo$_2$. In general, acceptable end points of resuscitation include establishing a mean arterial blood pressure to at least 65 mm Hg, central venous pressure (CVP) between 8 and 12 mm Hg (12 to 15 mm Hg if requiring mechanical ventilation), and Scvo$_2$ equal to or greater than 70%.

Right Ventricular Failure

Acute RV failure had been a fairly neglected entity in the ICU until recent times. The incidence has been reported to be similar to that of LV failure and can occur in a variety of clinical settings, including heart or lung transplant, acute respiratory distress syndrome (ARDS), presence of an LV assist device (LVAD), RV infarction, positive-pressure mechanical ventilation, or significant pulmonary embolism. Any impairment of RV preload, afterload, or LV function can result in damage to the RV. The RV is very sensitive to increased afterload. If pulmonary vascular resistance is persistently elevated, it may allow progression to RV dilation, tricuspid regurgitation, increased myocardial consumption, and worsening RV output, and initiate a degenerating cycle of RV failure. Additionally, RCA perfusion of the RV, which normally continues throughout systole and diastole, degenerates into only diastolic perfusion in the presence of significant pulmonary hypertension. Increased RV end-diastolic volume can also have ill effects on LV function if it is significant enough to cause interventricular septal deviation impairing LV filling. RV insufficiency during the initial few days following LVAD insertion occurs because of this leftward septal shift as the LV is unloaded.

Maintaining higher filling pressures can restore normal hemodynamics if RV contractility, PVR, and interventricular septal function are normal. However, volume loading may be counterproductive if mean pulmonary artery pressures are already greater than 30 mm Hg. Dobutamine and PDE inhibitors such as milrinone increase RV contractility while allowing pulmonary (and systemic) vasodilation and help establish improved filling of the LV by increasing right-to-left blood flow. Epinephrine and isoproterenol are also effective agents in improving RV contractility. Vasopressors are indicated to increase arterial blood pressure and improve coronary perfusion. Norepinephrine has been recommended over other α-adrenergic agents to enhance RCA perfusion in hypotensive patients. Inhaled NO has been shown to be effective in reducing PVR, improving oxygenation, and subsequently improving RV function due to its selective pulmonary vasodilation and improved ventilation-perfusion (V/Q) matching. Its inhaled route avoids significant effects on systemic blood pressure. However, outcome studies are lacking, and effects on mortality rate have not been well studied. Other provocative selective pulmonary vasodilators, such as inhaled prostacyclin with or without inhaled PDEs, have been used with anecdotal success. They boast similar pulmonary selectivity and avoidance of systemic hypotension and are much cheaper than inhaled NO, but these strategies are very labor intensive. Regardless of the pharmacologic treatment, the diagnosis must be determined and underlying cause must be corrected to reestablish intrinsic RV function. Pulmonary artery monitoring and echocardiography can be very helpful in establishing the correct diagnosis and may aid in augmenting treatment.

Blunt Cardiac Injury

Blunt cardiac injury (BCI) infrequently requires the use of inotropic support, except in the patient with preexisting heart disease. When it does occur, BCI results either from energy transfer from the direct blow to the chest, a deceleration-type injury, or a compression injury between the spine and sternum. There are no standard treatment guidelines, and care must be supportive based on injury pattern and the clinical picture. One must then familiarize oneself with all the potential causes of cardiac failure and treat accordingly. Blunt cardiac injury is a general term and encompasses all types of injury. The term "myocardial commotion" is used in the literature and occurs when no identifiable lesion exists on histologic examination or imaging study. This is most commonly a low-impact event, such as in contact sports. Nevertheless, cardiac arrest may occur from timed impact 15 to 30 ms before the peak of the T wave initiating ventricular fibrillation or impact during the QRS complex, causing complete heart block. Contusion implies a myocardial lesion and most commonly will involve the RV and septum due to its proximity anteriorly. RV dysfunction can also occur, as it is sensitive to increases in RV afterload that can result from ARDS, high levels of positive-end expiratory pressure (PEEP), or severe chest trauma and pulmonary contusions. Invasive monitoring and echocardiography can help guide treatment in the hypotensive patient, the elderly, and patients with preexisting heart disease. There are also reports of perioperative concerns including increased risk of systemic hypotension, arrhythmias, and cardiac arrest, which have been shown to persist at least up to 1 month following injury. Treatment is largely supportive, ensuring adequate preload and inotropic support. RV contusion again is common, and dysfunction must first be suspected. Treatment of increased RV afterload must be addressed, including correction of acidosis, hypoxia, and pulmonary hypertension, and avoidance of conventional mechanical ventilation and high PEEP.

■ SUMMARY

ADHF is a common occurrence in the surgical ICU, with urgent surgical problems becoming progressively more complicated by preexisting heart failure or cardiac compromise. These patients bring additional challenges to the surgical intensivist. Although the pathophysiology of ADHF remains the same, treatment of the surgical patient becomes increasingly complex due to the additional, simultaneously occurring perioperative pathophysiology. Recognition and optimal pharmacologic support can improve patient outcome in ADHF and allow opportunity for recovery from the initial insult.

For the chapter's Suggested Readings list, please visit the book at www.ExpertConsult.inkling.com.

DIAGNOSIS AND MANAGEMENT OF CARDIAC DYSRHYTHMIAS

Kareem R. AbdelFattah and Joseph P. Minei

The care of the patient with multiple comorbid conditions unrelated to their surgical disease has become commonplace for today's surgeon. A common knowledge of most major medical issues, and the potential consequences thereof, is required for any surgeon caring for inpatients after complex surgery. Given that the majority of patients undergoing major surgery will be placed in settings allowing for continuous monitoring techniques, the rapid identification and treatment of dysrhythmias has become common practice in the Surgical Intensive Care Unit (SICU). Cardiac dysrhythmias in the postoperative setting can have several causes, with some of the most common causes including hypoxia, cardiac ischemia, catecholamine excess, routine medications, and electrolyte abnormalities.

Cardiac dysrhythmias can be diagnosed with a focused physical examination, a standard 12-lead electrocardiogram (ECG), and from the response to specific maneuvers or drug therapy. The acute management of most dysrhythmias is dependent upon the stability of the patient, an accurate classification of the dysrhythmia, and an understanding of the mechanisms causing the dysrhythmia. Management may range from simple pharmacologic intervention to cardioversion in the acutely unstable patient, and may occasionally require percutaneous or transvenous pacing, pathway ablation, or implantation of pacemakers or defibrillators.

INCIDENCE AND RISK FACTORS

The incidence of cardiac dysrhythmias in the postoperative setting ranges from 9% in noncardiac surgical patients without a significant history of cardiac disease to over 40% in cardiac surgery patients. In one study that took place in a standard intensive care unit (ICU) admitting cardiac, noncardiac, and medical critical care patients, an average of 20% of admitted patients experienced dysrhythmias during their stay. The most commonly encountered dysrhythmia, other than sinus tachycardia, is atrial fibrillation (AF), which in cardiac surgery patients, may be seen in nearly half of that patient population. Up to 15% of patients with inferior wall myocardial infarction (MI) will present with atrioventricular (AV) nodal conduction disturbances or complete heart block. Patients who have preexisting cardiac or pulmonary disease have an increased risk of dysrhythmia, which is compounded in the face of noncardiac surgery, trauma, or critical illness. Vasopressor requirement is associated with an increased risk of dysrhythmia, caused by the proarrhythmic properties of catecholamines on cardiac tissue. Only 10% of the dysrhythmias encountered are bradyarrhythmias. Dysrhythmias are distributed equally between atrial and ventricular origins, with AF and ventricular tachycardia (VT) being most common, respectively. Patients who have dysrhythmias have been shown to have longer ICU stays and have shown lower survival rates overall in several studies, indicating that a dysrhythmia may be a marker of more severe critical illness.

Risk factors for the development of cardiac dysrhythmias have been examined in a number of retrospective studies. In patients undergoing cardiac surgery, risk factors have included advanced age, the type of surgery performed (e.g., valve replacements combined with

coronary artery bypass grafting [CABG] have higher rates of dysrhythmia than CABG alone), the need for pacemaker placement, any inotropic support during surgery, increasing New York Heart Association classification Table 1, and complicated weaning from cardiopulmonary bypass. Other risk factors include obesity, positive fluid balance during surgery, and the metabolic syndrome. Finally, some groups have pointed toward genetic predispositions for certain patient populations to develop postoperative dysrhythmias.

BRADYARRHYTHMIAS

Although not as commonly encountered as tachyarrhythmias, bradyarrhythmias can represent potentially life-threatening illness. They can be classified according to the node from which they originate, that is, the AV or sinoatrial (SA) nodes. Bradyarrhythmias may be caused by either extrinsic factors or intrinsic disease in the conduction system of the heart. Extrinsic causes include medications, myocardial ischemia, metabolic abnormalities, increased vagal tone, and acute respiratory failure. Further classification of bradyarrhythmias depends on the reversibility of the rhythm, whether the patient is symptomatic due to the rhythm, and the likelihood that the particular rhythm will progress or recur. Management options may be as simple as withholding a causative agent or as complicated as placing a permanent pacing device.

Sinus Node

The normal heartbeat arises from the SA node, which serves as the pacemaker of the heart under normal conditions. Bradycardia arising from SA nodal dysfunction originates from either failure of impulse generation or failure of the conduction of that impulse. The older term "sick sinus syndrome" was used to describe a range of conditions that reflect these dysfunctions. Currently, bradyarrhythmias arising from the SA node are described as one of the following: inappropriate sinus bradycardia, sinus pause or arrest, sinus exit block, and bradycardia-tachycardia syndrome.

Sinus bradycardia is defined as a heart rate below 60 beats per minute (bpm). This alone does not signify SA nodal dysfunction, as heart rates below 40 bpm can be asymptomatic and considered normal in well-trained athletes. Sinus bradycardia is considered pathologic, then, when patients are symptomatic (e.g., syncope) or when there is a failure to appropriately increase the heart rate during activity. Sinus pause or arrest occurs when the SA node transiently fails to exhibit automaticity and does not fire. Sinus exit block similarly results in a pause but the SA node does not fire. The impulse is either delayed or fails to propagate beyond the SA node, resulting in failure of atrial depolarization. Bradycardia-tachycardia syndrome refers to sinus node dysfunction with both bradycardia and tachycardia. Typically, bradycardia episodes follow the termination of tachycardia events, and can be associated with clinical symptoms of presyncope or syncope. Management can be challenging, as pharmacotherapy to treat fast rhythms often predisposes patients to slow ones, and vice versa. Commonly, insertion of a pacemaker for the symptomatic bradycardia, in conjunction with pharmacologic treatment for the tachycardia, is required.

Treatment for SA node dysfunction depends on the clinical status of the patient and the presumed cause. If the bradycardia is transient and not associated with hemodynamic compromise, no therapy is necessary. Investigation into the cause of bradycardia should include correction of metabolic and electrolyte abnormalities, minimizing maneuvers which could increase vagal tone, and the cessation or reduction in dosage of potentially offending medications, such as beta blockers, calcium channel antagonists, and lithium. If the bradycardia is sustained, or severe enough to lead to hemodynamic instability,

TABLE 1: Baseline Characteristics by NYHA Class*

Characteristic	NYHA class I (n = 10 592)	NYHA class II (n = 3242)	NYHA class III (n = 869)	P
Male sex	8702 (82)	2517 (78)	651 (75)	<.001
Age, mean ± SD, years	60 ± 7	61 ± 7	60 ± 7	<.001
Current smoking	1092 (10)	353 (11)	109 (13)	.04
Hypertension	3336 (32)	1185 (37)	318 (37)	<.001
Diabetes mellitus	1860 (18)	718 (22)	216 (25)	<.001
Past myocardial infarction	7749 (73)	2222 (69)	605(70)	<.001
Angina pectoris	5285 (50)	2913 (90)	799 (92)	<.001
Peripheral vascular disease	326 (3)	168 (5)	65 (8)	<.001
Body mass index, mean ± SD, kg/m²	26.6 ± 3.4	26.9 ± 3.7	27.3 ± 3.9	<.001
Glucose, mean ± SD, mg/dL	112 ± 44	118 ± 49	123 ± 56	<.001
Total cholesterol, mean ± SD, mg/dL	224 ± 39	225 ± 41	225 ± 43	.24
HDL cholesterol, mean ± SD, mg/dL	37.9 ± 10	37.7 ± 10.6	37.1 ± 10.2	.07
Triglycerides, mean ± SD, mg/dL	155 ± 86	164 ± 100	167 ± 94	<.001
LDL cholesterol, mean ± SD, mg/dL	156 ± 34	155 ± 35	156 ± 38	.92
Percent HDL out of total cholesterol, mean ± SD	17.3 ± 5.0	17.1 ± 5.1	16.9 ± 5.0	.03
Antihypetensive medications	8024 (76)	2782 (86)	768 (88)	<.001
Antidiabetic medications	1082 (10)	451 (14)	140 (16)	<.001
Antiplatelets	6497 (61)	1706 (53)	458 (53)	<.001

From Koren-Morag N, Goldbourt U, Tanne D: Poor functional status based on the New York Heart Association classification exposes the coronary patient to an elevated risk of ischemic stroke. *Am Heart J* 155(3):515–520, 2008, pp 515-520.

HDL, High-density lipoprotein; LDL, low-density lipoprotein; NYHA, New York Heart Association; SD, standard deviation.

*Data are presented as number (percent in parentheses) unless otherwise indicated.

therapy with antimuscarinic agents such as atropine or beta-agonists such as isoproterenol should be considered. Percutaneous or transvenous pacing may be necessary in some patients in the acute setting and can bridge those patients until a permanent pacemaker is placed. Patients who are hemodynamically stable but symptomatic from sinus node dysfunction almost invariably require permanent pacing.

Atrioventricular Node

Disturbances in conduction through the AV node or His-Purkinje system are classified as AV blocks. These blocks may be temporary or permanent, depending on the cause of the delayed conduction. In adults, the most common causes are drug toxicity, coronary artery disease, and degenerative disease of the conduction system. Many other conditions, such as electrolyte disturbances, myocarditis, sarcoidosis, scleroderma, and hypervagal responses, can cause AV block. The PR interval is a measure of the conduction time through the AV node and bundle of His. When the PR interval is prolonged (more than 210 ms), a patient has first-degree AV block. Second-degree AV block occurs with intermittent failure of the conduction of the impulse to the ventricles. In Mobitz type I, second-degree AV block (Wenckebach block), there is progressive prolongation of the PR interval until failure of conduction to the ventricle occurs (Fig. 1). The PR interval then shortens following the dropped beat. This failure

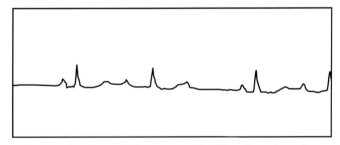

FIGURE 1   Rhythm strip shows progressive PR prolongation and a subsequent "dropped" QRS complex, followed by shortening of the PR interval which is diagnostic of Mobitz type I, second-degree atrioventricular block.

in conduction originates from the AV node itself and the QRS complex remains narrow. In Mobitz type II, second-degree AV block, there is intermittent failure of conduction reaching the ventricles that is not associated with progressive prolongation of the PR interval. There is not a shortened PR interval following the dropped beat. This failure in conduction is considered "infranodal" and originates from the His-Purkinje system. The QRS complex may be prolonged, and this type of AV block is more concerning. There is a significant likelihood of progression to complete heart block associated with

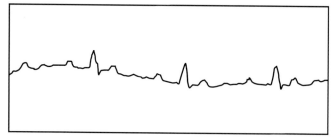

FIGURE 2   Rhythm strip shows atrial P waves and ventricular QRS complexes occurring at different rates and with no relationship between them, which is characteristic of third-degree atrioventricular block.

inadequate ventricular response with this rhythm. Third-degree or complete heart block results from failure of all impulses through the AV node and His-Purkinje system, resulting in AV disassociation. The ventricles rely on their innate automaticity, which produces a typical wide QRS escape rhythm between 40 and 50 bpm. The atrial rate is commonly faster, producing multiple P waves with no relationship to the ventricular QRS complexes (Fig. 2).

Management of AV block depends on the hemodynamic stability of the patient, the transient nature of the dysrhythmia, and where the focus originates from within the conduction system. Acute pharmacotherapy relies upon atropine and isoproterenol. Isoproterenol use should be avoided in patients with ischemic heart disease because of the associated increase in myocardial oxygen demand. There is no long-term pharmacotherapy for AV block, and removal of any of the common offending agents, such as digitalis or beta blockers, should first be attempted. Temporary pacing is used for those with ongoing instability, and permanent pacing is typically required for Mobitz type II second-degree AV block and third-degree AV block. It should be noted that the 2010 guidelines from the American Heart Association now recommend chronotropic pharmacotherapy as an alternative to pacing, as it has been shown to be as effective as external pacing when atropine is ineffective.

TACHYARRHYTHMIAS

Tachyarrhythmias are classified according to their anatomic origin in relation to the AV node, and as such, the first step in the management of any tachyarrhythmia depends on determining whether the arrhythmia originates above the SA node (supraventricular tachyarrhythmias, or SVT), or below the SA node (ventricular tachyarrhythmia, or VT). These can also be thought of as producing a narrow QRS complex (SVTs) versus a wide QRS complex (VTs) on ECG. Narrow complex tachyarrhythmias include sinus tachycardia, AV nodal reentrant tachycardia (AVNRT, sometimes called paroxysmal SVT), AV reentry from an accessory pathway (Wolff-Parkinson-White syndrome, also called AVRT, atrioventricular reentrant tachycardia), AF, and atrial flutter. In contrast, VTs originate from below the AV node and include ventricular tachyarrythmia and ventricular fibrillation (VF). Important determinants of the malignant potential of tachyarrhythmias are the duration, the hemodynamic consequences, and the presence of significant structural heart disease. The acute management depends on a basic understanding of the mechanism, the choices for pharmacologic intervention (Table 2), and the indications for urgent cardioversion for each situation. Interventional techniques, such as aberrant pathway ablation and implantation of pacemakers and defibrillators, have drastically improved long-term outcome once patients have left the ICU setting, and have added significantly to our armamentarium in treating these dysrhythmias.

The mechanisms by which tachyarrhythmias arise are categorized into (1) abnormal automaticity, (2) triggered activity, or (3) reentry. Abnormal automaticity occurs when cells outside the normal conduction system generate spontaneous impulse formation. Triggered activity occurs during an "afterdepolarization," which causes the membrane potential to reach threshold early and generate abnormal impulse formation. Reentry, the most common mechanism, occurs when an impulse can travel down two pathways separated by an area of unexcitable tissue. One of the pathways contains a unidirectional block, with slowed conduction, so that recovery and further excitation can subsequently occur. This defines an area of cardiac tissue that can self-propagate and thus becomes the focus for the generation of the tachyarrhythmia (Fig. 3).

TABLE 2: Classification of Common Tachyarrhythmia Drug Therapies

Class	Examples	Mechanism of Action	Prolong QT Interval
Class I IA IB IC	Quinidine, procainamide, disopyramide Lidocaine, mexiletine Flecainide, propafenone	Sodium channel blockade Varying effects on prolongation of action potential, and dissociation from the sodium channel	Yes
Class II	Metoprolol, esmolol	Blocks β-adrenergic receptor Sympatholytic	No
Class III	Amiodarone, bretylium, sotalol, ibutilide	Blocks the delayed rectifier potassium current Significant prolongation of action potential	Yes
Class IV	Verapamil, diltiazem	Calcium channel blockade Slows primarily AV node conduction	No
Other	Adenosine Digoxin	Activation of an inward rectifier K^+ current and inhibition of calcium current Extremely short acting, primarily on AV node Blocks sodium-potassium ATPase and increases intracellular calcium Slow onset of action and toxicity can be common	No

Modified from Brunton L, editor: *Goodman & Gilman's the pharmacological basis of therapeutics,* 11th ed, New York, 2005, McGraw-Hill.
ATPase, Adenosine triphosphatase; AV, atrioventricular.

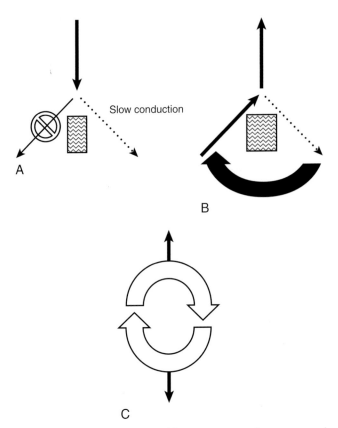

FIGURE 3 **A,** Conditions required for reentry; two pathways separated by unexcitable tissue, unidirectional block, and slowed conduction. **B,** Initiating factors allow retrograde conduction up the prior blocked pathway. **C,** A reentrant circuit is formed.

TABLE 3: Responses to Increased Vagal Tone

Arrhythmia	Response to Increased Vagal Tone
Sinus tachycardia	Temporary slowing, with resumption of tachycardia
AVNRT	Abrupt termination or a transient slowing
Atrial fibrillation or atrial flutter	Increased AV block with slowed ventricular response rate
Multifocal atrial tachycardia	Increased AV block with slowed ventricular response rate
Ventricular tachycardia	No response

Modified from Tarditi DJ, Hollenberg SM: Cardiac arrhythmias in the intensive care unit. *Semin Respir Crit Care Med* 27(3):221–229, 2006.
AV, Atrioventricular; AVNRT, atrioventricular nodal reentry tachycardia.

In attempting to classify a tachyarrhythmia seen on 12-lead ECG, maneuvers that increase vagal tone can assist in the diagnosis. Through carotid massage or administration of adenosine, AV nodal conduction time can be slowed and refractoriness increased. This can demonstrate to the clinician the presence of P waves on ECG, or can interrupt reentry pathways. The response to such maneuvers can often suggest the type of tachyarrhythmia that the clinician is dealing with (Table 3).

Sinus Tachycardia

Sinus tachycardia should not be considered a true dysrhythmia, but instead a physiologic reflex related to an increased demand for oxygen, and as such, it is an important sign for which the cause must be sought. Fever, hypovolemia, and anemia all appropriately increase heart rate to at least maintain or increase cardiac output. Blunting this reflex with pharmacotherapy without knowledge of the cause can be dangerous. Less common causes include thyrotoxicosis, pheochromocytomas, or side effects of sympathomimetic drugs, which also cause sinus tachycardia without regard for reflex mechanisms. The primary goal for management of sinus tachycardia is to find and appropriately treat the confounding condition. Sinus tachycardia will resolve with resolution of this inciting process.

Paroxysmal Supraventricular Tachycardia

The term "paroxysmal supraventricular tachycardia" actually describes a diverse group of tachyarrhythmias commonly known as the SVT, the most common being AVNRT. AVNRT is more common in women than men, and can present at any age. The underlying pathologic condition consists of a dual conduction pathway, each with different rates of conduction. As described previously, this allows for the possibility of reentry and the potential for a self-propagating tachyarrhythmia focus. In AVNRT, the two pathways reside in or around the AV node itself. Antegrade conduction typically occurs through the slower pathway, and the retrograde conduction occurs through the faster pathway. Rates of 140 to 220 bpm are typical, and P waves are not seen on ECG because retrograde atrial activation and antegrade ventricular activation occur simultaneously. The QRS complex is typically narrow because the antegrade conduction to the ventricles uses the normal AV node and His-Purkinje system.

A similar system is present in AVRT. In comparison, AVRT also has two conduction pathways, but the additional pathway is remote from the AV node and resides in the AV groove, where it is commonly referred to as an "accessory pathway." Antegrade conduction occurs through the AV node and His-Purkinje system, and retrograde conduction occurs via the accessory pathway. The QRS complex for AVRT is also narrow, and because the accessory pathway only conducts retrograde, it is not seen on ECG and is considered "concealed." The antegrade conduction through the AV node combined with retrograde conduction through the accessory pathway is sometimes termed "orthodromic" tachycardia. In contrast, electrical conduction can progress in the opposite configuration (that is, antegrade impulse through the accessory pathway and retrograde impulse through the AV node) and is termed "antidromic" tachycardia. This form of reentry tachycardia is distinguished by its wide-complex QRS on ECG, and is much less common than the orthodromic form.

Acute management depends on the stability of the patients with paroxysmal SVT. Urgent direct-current cardioversion is indicated when myocardial ischemia, acute heart failure, or hypotension result. In hemodynamically stable patients, pharmacologic intervention with the intent to slow or break AV nodal conduction is the mainstay of treatment. Intravenous adenosine is the first-line drug of choice because of its potent yet short-lived depressant effects on AV nodal conduction. Adenosine will successfully terminate greater than 90% of tachyarrhythmias due to AVNRT and AVRT (see Table 3). Calcium channel blockers or beta blockers (verapamil/diltiazem or metoprolol) are also useful, particularly when adenosine is not successful, although they should be used with caution because of their possible hypotensive and bradycardic effects.

Wolff-Parkinson-White Syndrome

Wolff-Parkinson-White syndrome occurs when an accessory pathway (the bundle of Kent) allows both antegrade and retrograde

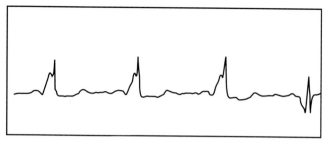

FIGURE 4 Lead II in this electrocardiogram shows a prominent delta wave consistent with the diagnosis of Wolfe-Parkinson-White syndrome.

conduction, and commonly a delta wave or preexcitation can be seen in the early QRS complex (Fig. 4). This syndrome occurs in 0.1% to 0.3% of the population, usually presenting in early adulthood, and the initial presentation can be VF. Management in these patients where conduction occurs antegrade through the accessory pathway varies from narrow complex AVRT as described previously. Adenosine will only be effective if the antegrade conduction occurs through the AV node. Otherwise it can precipitate AF, which can result in degeneration to VF when an antegrade accessory pathway exists in these patients. This degeneration occurs secondary to the 1:1 ratio of conduction of atrial impulses to the ventricles. This situation in patients diagnosed with Wolff-Parkinson-White syndrome occurs in 0.1% of patients per year as a part of the natural history of the condition. Calcium channel blockers and digoxin are contraindicated, because they will slow conduction in the AV node and enhance conduction through the accessory pathway. Class I and class III antiarrhythmics, which include flecainide, procainamide, and ibutilide, are able to depress the conduction across the accessory pathway, decrease the ventricular rate, and likely terminate the wide QRS tachyarrhythmia. Direct-current cardioversion is used with hemodynamic instability or if antiarrhythmic therapy fails. Ultimately, the treatment of choice for these patients will require ablation of the accessory pathway.

Multifocal Atrial Tachycardia

Multifocal atrial tachycardia is thought to be due to abnormal automaticity and is commonly associated with chronic respiratory disease, congestive heart failure, and pulmonary embolus. It has an irregular rate and rhythm that is characterized by the presence of three or more morphologically different P waves on ECG, and rates of 110 to 140 bpm (Fig. 5). It can easily be confused with AF if P waves are not prominent on a rhythm strip. First-line therapy consists of treating the underlying condition, correction of hypercarbia or hypoxia, and electrolyte repletion. Calcium channel blockers typically can provide rate control but beta blockers should be used with caution in those with obstructive pulmonary disease. Amiodarone can be helpful in patients refractory to first-line therapies.

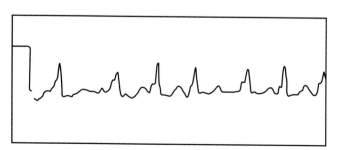

FIGURE 5 Rhythm strip shows an irregular tachycardia with greater than three morphologically different P waves, characteristic of multifocal atrial tachycardia.

Atrial Flutter

Atrial flutter is due to a reentrant circuit from within atrial tissue and is associated with atrial enlargement. It is commonly grouped with AF because of similar associated causes and similar treatment regimens. Atrial rates of 250 to 350 bpm are typical. The AV node refractory period allows only a proportion of these atrial beats to pass to the ventricle, typically in a 2:1 ratio. When a ventricular pulse rate is measured to be 150 bpm, atrial flutter should be considered. By increasing AV nodal refractoriness with adenosine or beta blockade, the atrial "flutter waves," characterized by a sawtooth appearance, can usually be seen on ECG, and most commonly in the inferior leads (Fig. 6). Adenosine may be useful for diagnosis, but as with AF, it rarely converts the rhythm back to sinus. Beta blockers and calcium channel blockers allow ventricular rate control for long-term management, but more commonly antiarrhythmic drug therapy or electrical cardioversion is required if the rhythm remains persistent. In patients who present with hemodynamic instability, direct-current synchronized (DC-synchronized) cardioversion with 50 J is used, with very high success rates. Pharmacotherapies such as ibutilide, sotalol, and procainamide have been used but with much lower rates of conversion in the acute setting.

Atrial Fibrillation

AF is the most common SVT identified in the ICU (VT is the most common) and can portend a number of negative sequelae. AF and atrial flutter account for greater than 60% of the SVTs in noncardiac surgical patients and can affect up to 40% of patients following cardiac surgery. AF is commonly associated with left atrial distention, whether from acute fluid shifts or chronic dilatation secondary to structural heart disease. Other associations that must be ruled out include electrolyte imbalances, myocardial ischemia, pericarditis, diabetes, hyperthyroidism, hypoxia/hypercarbia, pulmonary embolus, and pneumonia. Risk factors identified in the general population include chronic hypertension, valvular disease, and left ventricular hypertrophy. It is an "irregularly irregular" rhythm with an absence of P waves on ECG (Fig. 7). It is thought to arise from multiple

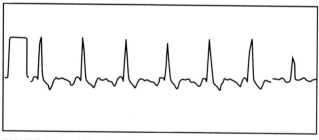

FIGURE 6 Lead II in this electrocardiogram shows the characteristic "sawtooth" flutter wave of atrial flutter with 2:1 conduction. The rate is approximately 150 beats per minute.

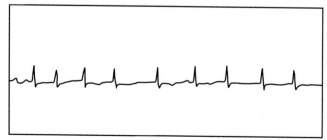

FIGURE 7 Rhythm strip shows an irregular, normal complex tachycardia without P waves, consistent with atrial fibrillation.

shifting reentrant circuits that bombard the AV node with a multitude of impulses, from which only a proportion initiate ventricular contraction, 110 to 190 bpm. Patients without structural heart disease tolerate the loss of the atrial component of ventricular filling well. However, in patients with known structural heart disease, hypotension, acute congestive failure, and myocardial ischemia can be precipitated by AF. Another concerning consequence is the possibility of mural thrombus formation, and the associated embolic risk, from within the noncontracting left atrium. Thrombus can occur in up to 10% of patients with new-onset AF lasting longer than 3 days.

The overall goals of treatment include ventricular rate control, resumption and maintenance of sinus rhythm, and prevention of embolic events. Acutely, if the patient is hemodynamically unstable, in acute heart failure, or the rhythm is precipitating myocardial ischemia, direct-current cardioversion should be performed. This is successful in restoring sinus rhythm in up to 90% of patients with recent-onset AF, but carries up to a 7% risk of stroke if not anticoagulated. The 2010 Advanced Cardiovascular Life Support (ACLS) guidelines recommend a biphasic energy dose for conversion of 120 to 200 J. In the hemodynamically stable patient, ventricular rate control should be the main priority. Calcium channel blockers, beta blockers, amiodarone, and digoxin are all shown to be of benefit owing to enhancement of the AV nodal refractory period. Beta blockers have been shown to provide more effective rate control than calcium channel blockers at rest and during exercise. Secondary hypotension can be a common side effect, which may require concomitant fluid administration and calcium infusion. Digoxin is not associated with hypotension, but requires approximately 30 minutes for its effects to take place when given intravenously, thus limiting its usefulness in many ICU settings.

A variety of treatment methods may be used to terminate AF and restore sinus rhythm. Common options include the use of antiarrhythmic drugs, alone or in conjunction with electrical cardioversion, but these must be tailored to each individual case. Therapy with class III antiarrhythmic drugs such as amiodarone, ibutilide, and propafenone have been shown to terminate AF, alone or in conjunction with electrical cardioversion, in 30% to 80% of cases if initiated within 7 days of onset. The use of antiarrhythmic therapy must keep in mind the side-effect profile of this class of drugs, including the risk of drug-induced torsades de pointes, VT, and other serious dysrhythmias. Controversy exists concerning what emphasis should be placed on pharmacologic or electrical cardioversion of AF back into sinus rhythm. The results from the Atrial Fibrillation Follow-up Investigation of Rhythm Management (AFFIRM) study, a multicenter trial examining elderly high-risk patients, showed no difference in the long-term outcome in those patients treated with ventricular rate control versus rhythm control. Despite these controversies, up to one third of patients with new-onset AF spontaneously convert to sinus rhythm without antiarrhythmic therapy in the perioperative period. In those in whom AF continues unabated, options include pharmacologic or electrical cardioversion, versus ventricular rate control alone. Currently, level I evidence supports the use of beta blockers as first-line therapy in the postsurgical patient for rate control and conversion to sinus rhythm. In patients who are hemodynamically unstable or have a known ejection fraction (EF) of less than 40%, amiodarone may be considered first-line therapy.

The risk of atrial thrombus and emboli become more concerning over time in AF, and anticoagulation therapy should be considered if return to sinus rhythm has not occurred after 48 hours. The American College of Chest Physicians recommends that in these patients, anticoagulation should be continued for 3 weeks before cardioversion and 4 weeks afterward, unless emergent cardioversion is warranted. In some situations, the use of a transesophageal echocardiogram (TEE) to identify the presence or absence of a thrombus may be used to allow for immediate cardioversion along with concurrent heparinization. The potential benefits of anticoagulation must be weighed against the risk of postoperative bleeding. The embolic risk is increased when transition occurs from AF to sinus rhythm and vice versa. If TEE is positive for atrial thrombus, anticoagulation should be continued for 4 to 6 weeks, and resolution of thrombus should be proved prior to elective cardioversion.

Ventricular Tachyarrhythmias

Appropriate management of newly diagnosed VTs depends on accurate rhythm classification and patient risk factor stratification so that appropriate therapy can be provided in a timely fashion. Serious VTs occur in less than 2% of patients following cardiac surgery, and in noncardiac surgery they are most commonly associated with postoperative myocardial ischemia and significant structural heart disease. The position of intravascular hardware should always be evaluated because dislodgement can be associated with mechanically induced dysrhythmias. Metabolic, acid-base, and oxygenation disturbances in the context of myocardial ischemia and exogenous or endogenous catecholamine excess have all been implicated in promoting triggered activity, abnormal automaticity, and reentry phenomenon in ventricular tissue. The presence of significant structural heart disease is the most important predictor of future malignant VTs and sudden cardiac death. A typical ECG will show a wide QRS complex tachycardia, which can originate from a supraventricular source or, more commonly, is due to VT. If differentiation is not feasible, a wide complex tachycardia should be treated as probable VT. Attention to the QT interval is imperative because treatment without regard for QT interval prolongation can have drastic consequences. The majority, if not all, of antiarrhythmic drugs are "proarrhythmic" themselves. Torsades de pointes (see later) accounts for the majority of these drug-induced VTs, and thus, it is most advantageous to use single antiarrhythmic drug therapy and avoid the proarrhythmia effects of combination therapy. VF is an inherently unstable rhythm, and a detailed discussion on ACLS is not the focus of this chapter. More pertinent is an understanding of the rhythms with the propensity to degenerate into VF and the ability to intervene in an appropriate fashion to prevent this from happening.

VT is classified into monomorphic and polymorphic subtypes. Monomorphic VT is thought to originate from a single ventricular focus and has a wide QRS pattern, each with similar morphologic appearance (Fig. 8). Polymorphic VT, in contrast, is characterized by an irregular, undulating appearance, with significant variation in QRS morphologic appearance. Differentiation is important because polymorphic VT commonly degenerates to VF. Further classification is determined by the persistence of the rhythm. Compared with sustained VT, nonsustained VT typically lasts less than 30 seconds and spontaneously terminates. In a study following patients aged 60 to 85 years of age over a course of 10 years, nonsustained VT did not predict coronary events, although if it occurred within 1 week of an MI, the risk of sudden cardiac death was doubled.

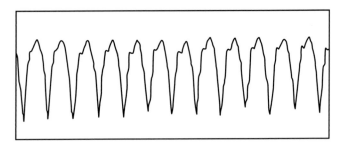

FIGURE 8 Rhythm strip shows a classic wide QRS tachycardia with similar QRS morphologic appearance characteristic of sustained monomorphic ventricular tachycardia.

Premature Ventricular Contractions

Premature ventricular contractions (PVCs) are common in postoperative critical care patients. They can be unifocal or may present as couplets or as bigeminy. They are associated with many electrolyte imbalances and metabolic abnormalities, such as hypokalemia, hypomagnesemia, alkalosis, hypoxia, and catecholamine excess. Correction of these abnormalities, along with the use of beta blockers, commonly eliminates the majority of PVCs. In asymptomatic patients without structural heart disease, further treatment or suppression of PVCs is rarely required, and there are no associated short- or long-term consequences. In patients with coronary artery disease, history of MI, or impaired left ventricular function (EF <40%), PVCs may be a sign of more malignant dysrhythmias to come. Correction of any reversible precipitating factors, including myocardial ischemia, should first be performed, followed with attempts to reduce vasopressor or inotropic support. In symptomatic patients who do not generate sufficient stroke volumes in the face of multiple PVCs, temporary suppression with antiarrhythmic drug therapy may be of benefit in critically ill patients.

Monomorphic Ventricular Tachycardia

Nonsustained monomorphic VT can be considered as a prolonged version of PVCs. The rhythm is associated with similar electrolyte and metabolic abnormalities that promote or initiate triggered activity, abnormal automaticity, or reentry mechanisms. Beta blockade, and reversal of any of the preceding precipitating factors, will reduce the frequency and duration of this rhythm. The use of antiarrhythmic drug therapy or electric cardioversion is required only for those patients who manifest symptoms or hemodynamic compromise. The long-term prognosis associated with nonsustained monomorphic VT again depends on the presence of structural heart disease. There is an overall increased risk of sudden cardiac death in those with coronary artery disease and left ventricular dysfunction (EF <40%). Due to this association, patients with structural heart disease should be referred for electrophysiologic (EP) testing. Patients found to have an inducible rhythm at the time of EP testing benefit from placement of an implantable cardioverter-defibrillator (ICD). In patients without structural heart disease, nonsustained monomorphic VT carries no added long-term risk.

The most common mechanism causing sustained monomorphic VT is reentry. This rhythm is most commonly due to a healed scar from a prior MI, which allows a reentry circuit to occur. This typically portends a poor prognosis, with in-hospital mortality rates exceeding 40% following surgery, with recurrence in more than 30% of patients who initially survive. Up to 20% of patients discharged from the hospital will succumb to cardiac death within 24 months. Because the substrate (e.g., the scar) for sustained monomorphic VT persists, in those who survive their acute illness, EP testing and subsequent ICD placement is similarly recommended.

The acute management for monomorphic VT is dependent on the hemodynamic status of the patient. Direct-current synchronized cardioversion (monophasic or biphasic waveform cardioversion starting at 100 J) is the mainstay of treatment for those symptomatic or unstable. Electric cardioversion is highly effective and is also recommended for hemodynamically stable VT in conjunction with adequate short-term anesthesia. In those patients who are stable, or when electric cardioversion is not appropriate or available, either intravenous procainamide, sotalol, or amiodarone is the current antiarrhythmic drug recommendation. Amiodarone is the drug of choice for those patients with impaired cardiac function. The American Heart Association's 2010 update to ACLS has also recommended that adenosine can be considered for assistance in evaluation and treatment of undifferentiated, regular, wide-complex monomorphic tachyarrhythmias. Antitachycardia pacing is also an option in those with transvenous or an internal pacemaker already in place, although the potential for tachycardia acceleration exists and a defibrillator should be at the bedside if attempted.

Polymorphic Ventricular Tachycardia

Polymorphic VT should be considered an ischemic rhythm with a significant predisposition to degenerate into VF. The distinction between nonsustained and sustained is less pertinent, because short bursts of this rhythm commonly evolve into sustained polymorphic VT. This rhythm is invariably symptomatic and requires prompt direct-current cardioversion. The most important step once the patient's condition is more stable is the determination of the QT interval by ECG analysis. In patients without QT prolongation, the most likely cause is acute cardiac ischemia and associated severe left ventricular dysfunction. Correction of any associated electrolyte and metabolic abnormalities and minimization of exogenous catecholamine support and beta blockade should be initiated. In those patients with severe coronary vascular disease, revascularization will be required, and the use of an intra-aortic balloon pump may be needed to bridge the patient until revascularization can be performed. Antiarrhythmic drug therapy with intravenous amiodarone, procainamide, or sotalol can promote maintenance of sinus rhythm, but emphasis should be placed on treating the underlying cardiac ischemia. Prognosis depends on the hemodynamic status of the patient rather than the presence of ongoing VT. In those who acutely recover, ICD placement has been shown to improve long-term outcome.

Polymorphic VT in the setting of a prolonged QT interval (QT >460 ms) is commonly referred to as the syndrome of *torsades de pointes* or "twisting of the points." The ECG shows a wide QRS tachycardia that appears to twist around the ECG baseline. This syndrome requires a different management algorithm because the mechanism is attributed to triggered activity secondary to early after depolarization rather than reentry. Acquired QT prolongation can result from many electrolyte abnormalities and a myriad of medications (Table 4). Common causes seen in an ICU setting include hypokalemia, hypomagnesemia, specific antibiotics and psychoactive drugs, and most importantly, class I and III antiarrhythmics. The first priority in the management of torsades de pointes is identification and removal of offending agents along with correction of any electrolyte abnormalities. Direct-current cardioversion is used for the hemodynamically unstable, and it is important that any medication that could further prolong the QT interval not be given. Intravenous magnesium should be given to all patients with suspected torsades. Because the length of the QT interval is proportional to the RR interval (time between each beat), patients can benefit from overdrive pacing with isoproterenol or transvenous pacing. Isoproterenol should be used with caution in patients with coronary vascular disease. Antiarrhythmic drugs that do not prolong the QT interval can be used and include lidocaine and phenytoin. Long-term management depends on avoiding the use of drugs that prolong the QT interval. The overall prognosis is generally good, and no long-term therapy is typically recommended.

TABLE 4: Common Intensive Care Unit Drugs That Can Promote Torsades de Pointes

Drug Class	Examples
Antiarrhythmics	Procainamide, quinidine, amiodarone, sotalol, ibutilide
Antimicrobial	Erythromycin, trimethoprim-sulfamethoxazole
Psychoactive	Haloperidol, lithium, chloral hydrate, tricyclic antidepressants
Miscellaneous	Tacrolimus, vasopressin

Modified from Parrillo J, Dellinger R, editors: *Critical care medicine: principles of diagnosis and management in the adult,* 2nd ed, St. Louis, 2001, Mosby.

CONCLUSION

The diagnosis and management of cardiac dysrhythmias depend on accurate rhythm classification, knowledge of the underlying mechanisms, and a thorough understanding of appropriate treatment regimens. Measures aimed at prevention of electrolyte and metabolic disturbances that promote these dysrhythmias must not be understated. The use of antiarrhythmic drugs must be limited to those who are symptomatic or hemodynamically unstable so as to limit their potential for inducing a proarrhythmic state. Direct-current cardioversion should be used without hesitation in appropriate patients with instability and in those with a propensity to degenerate into VF. Particular emphasis should be placed on diagnosis of the more uncommon dysrhythmias, including Wolfe-Parkinson-White syndrome and torsades de pointes, because following standard treatment algorithms can lead to disastrous consequences. Consultation with a cardiology team is essential in regard to long-term management, patient risk stratification, and the plethora of interventional procedures that can improve both acute and long-term outcomes in patients with dysrhythmias. Physical examination, ECG interpretation, and experience are the required tools necessary to manage dysrhythmias appropriately. In just about every ICU setting, these tools can be sharpened and fine-tuned so that, ultimately, patients receive the maximum benefit.

For the chapter's Suggested Readings list, please visit the book at www.ExpertConsult.inkling.com.

FUNDAMENTALS OF MECHANICAL VENTILATION

Soumitra R. Eachempati, Jerry A. Rubano, Jared M. Huston, Philip S. Barie, and Marc J. Shapiro

KEY POINTS

- New technology now provides several modes by which a patient may be ventilated, with the goals of improved gas exchange, better patient comfort, and rapid liberation from the ventilator.
- Noninvasive ventilation (NIV) may avoid intubation or reintubation for awake, cooperative patients with marginal oxygenation or ventilation.
- Basic modes of assisted ventilation include assist-control ventilation (ACV), intermittent mandatory ventilation (IMV), and pressure support ventilation (PSV).
- Ventilation of patients with acute lung injury (ALI) and acute respiratory distress syndrome (ARDS) using a low tidal volume (6 mL/kg) decreases morbidity and mortality from mechanical ventilation (MV).
- Sedation should be used judiciously and withdrawn transiently each day during a "sedation holiday" to assess readiness for liberation from MV.
- Adherence to a "ventilator bundle" (e.g., prophylaxis of stress-related gastric mucosal hemorrhage and venous thromboembolic disease, head-of-bed up 30 degrees at all times unless contraindicated medically, daily sedation holiday, oral care with topical chlorhexidine solution) decreases the length of MV and the incidence of ventilator-associated pneumonia (VAP).

MV is often required to manage trauma or critical illness, whether for airway protection, administration of general anesthesia, or management of acute respiratory failure (ARF) (Table 1). New technology now provides several modes by which a patient may be ventilated, with the goals of improved gas exchange, better patient comfort, and rapid liberation from the ventilator. Moreover, noninvasive positive-pressure ventilation permits some cases of ARF to be managed without insertion of an artificial endotracheal airway and some patients who are extubated with marginal reserves to avoid reintubation. Nearly all ventilators can be set to allow full support of the patient on the one hand, and periods of exercise on the other. Thus, the choice of ventilator settings for the majority of patients is a matter of physician preference (Table 2). Controlled ventilation with suppression of spontaneous breathing leads rapidly to respiratory muscle atrophy, and therefore, modes of assisted ventilation are preferred wherein machine-delivered breaths are triggered by the patient's own inspiratory efforts. Basic modes of assisted ventilation include ACV, *synchronized intermittent mandatory ventilation* (SIMV), and PSV.

Most patients are started on MV for management of ARF, during which the work necessary to initiate a breath increased by a factor of 4 to 6. The most common reason to initiate MV is to decrease the work of breathing by the patient. Additional potential benefits of MV include improved gas exchange, enhanced coordination between support and the patients' own efforts, resting of respiratory muscles, prevention of deconditioning, and prevention of iatrogenic lung injury while promoting healing. However, unless settings are chosen carefully to synchronize with the patients' own central respiratory drive, MV can cause an increase in work. Regardless of the mode chosen, all MV is a modification of the manner in which positive pressure is applied to the airway and the interplay of the mechanical support and the patients' own efforts.

TABLE 1: General Indications for Mechanical Ventilation

Airway maintenance or protection
Airway obstruction
General inhalational anesthesia
Hemodynamic instability
Hypoxemia
Metabolic acidosis
Pulmonary toilet (excessive secretions)

NONINVASIVE VENTILATION

Ventilatory support delivered without establishing an endotracheal airway is NIV. NIV was administered previously with intermittent negative pressure, but the current technique uses positive-pressure ventilation delivered through a nasal or face mask, and usage is expanding in the management of acute and chronic respiratory failure and possibly for some patients with heart failure.

TABLE 2: A Glossary of Basic Terminology of Mechanical Ventilation

Control: regulation of gas flow:

Volume-controlled—Airway pressure is variable (volume limited, volume targeted)
Pressure-controlled—Volume delivered is variable (pressure limited, pressure targeted)
Dual-controlled—Seldom used in practice (volume targeted [guaranteed], pressure limited)

Cycling: ventilator switching:

Time-cycled—Example: pressure-controlled ventilation
Flow-cycled—Example: pressure support ventilation
Volume-cycled—Example: volume-controlled ventilation

Triggering: causes the ventilator to cycle to inhalation:

Time-triggered—The ventilator cycles at a set frequency as determined by the controlled rate.
Pressure-triggered—The ventilator senses the patient's inspiratory effort from a decrease of airway pressure.
Flow-triggered—A constant flow of gas is delivered throughout the respiratory cycle (flow-by). Altered flow caused by patient inhalation is detected by the ventilator, which delivers a breath. Less work is done by the patient than with pressure-triggering.

Breaths: cause the ventilator to cycle from inhalation to exhalation:

Mandatory (controlled)—Determined by the respiratory rate
Assisted—Examples: assist control, synchronized intermittent mandatory ventilation, pressure support
Spontaneous—No additional assistance, as in continuous positive airway pressure (CPAP)

Flow pattern: constant, decelerating, or sinusoidal:

Sinusoidal—Examples: spontaneous breathing and CPAP
Constant—Flow continues at a constant rate until the set tidal volume is delivered; seldom used in practice
Decelerating—Inhalation slows from a high initial flow rate as alveolar pressure increases; example: pressure-targeted ventilation, often used in volume-targeted ventilation, as it causes lower peak airway pressures than constant flow

Mode (breath pattern):

Controlled medical ventilation—Controlled ventilation, without allowances for spontaneous breathing, typical of anesthesia ventilators
Assist-control—Assisted breaths simulate controlled breaths
Intermittent mandatory ventilation—Admixes controlled and spontaneous breaths, which may also be synchronized to prevent "stacking"
Pressure support—The patient controls all aspects of the breath except the pressure limit

---

Putative benefits of NIV are numerous, owing to avoidance of the complications of endotracheal intubation. NIV preserves swallowing, feeding, speech, cough, and physiologic air warming and humidification by the naso-oropharynx. Nonintubated patients communicate more effectively, require less sedation, and are more comfortable. In addition, patients are often able to continue with standard oral nutrition. NIV eliminates complications such as trauma with tube insertion, mucosal ulceration, aspiration, infection (e.g., pneumonia, sinusitis), and dysphagia after extubation.

In a randomized, prospective trial following pulmonary resection of 48 patients with acute hypoxemic respiratory insufficiency, Auriant et al compared standard invasive MV with nasal mask NIV. The need for postoperative reintubation and the mortality rate were clearly reduced in patients receiving NIV as a part of respiratory support. Similarly, Squadrone et al randomized 209 patients with respiratory failure in the postanesthesia care unit after major abdominal surgery to oxygen alone, or with continuous positive airway pressure (CPAP) by mask. Patients who received oxygen plus CPAP had a significantly lower intubation rate, and also lower rates of pneumonia, infection, and sepsis.

Contraindications to Noninvasive Ventilation

Crucial to successful NIV is an awake, cooperative patient who is breathing spontaneously. Airway, electrocardiographic, or hemodynamic instability argues against the use of NIV. An additional requirement is an intact cough reflex and ability to clear secretions, the absence of which is a common reason for failure of NIV. Relative contraindications include the inability to fit and seal the mask adequately, inability to cough with prompting, or inability to remove the mask in the event of emesis. A hypothetical contraindication is recent gastrointestinal surgery with aerophagia and gut distention. If pressures used to ventilate the patient are kept below 30 mm Hg, the closing pressure of the lower esophageal sphincter should not be exceeded, and aerophagia should be avoided. Morbid obesity is also a relative contraindication secondary to increased ventilatory pressure requirements arising from body habitus and the weight of the chest wall and abdominal viscera while the patient is supine.

Complications of Noninvasive Ventilation

The most common complication of NIV is focal skin necrosis, which is most common over the bridge of the nose but may also occur over the zygoma. The incidence is 7% to 10% among patients receiving full-face mask NIV. Other complications (incidence, 1% to 2% each) include gastric distention, aspiration, and pneumothorax. Conceptual concerns with gastric distention are subsequent vomiting, aspiration, and pneumonia. Conjunctivitis may develop secondary to air leaks near the eyes in about 2% of patients.

The most serious complication is failure to recognize when NIV is not providing a patient with adequate ventilation, oxygenation, or airway patency. Delayed placement of an artificial airway, or failure of placement thereof, may cause continued deterioration or the death of a patient.

PRESSURE SUPPORT VENTILATION

Pressure support is a method of assisting spontaneous breathing in a ventilated patient, either partially or fully. The patient controls all parts of the breath except the pressure limit. The patient triggers the ventilator, which delivers a flow of gas in response up to a preset pressure limit (for example, 10 cm H_2O) depending on the desired minute ventilation ($\dot{V}E$). Gas flow cycles off when a certain percentage of peak inspiratory flow (usually 25%) has been reached. Tidal volumes (V_T) may vary, just as they do spontaneously.

Positive end-expiratory pressure (PEEP, also called CPAP) is added to restore *functional residual capacity* (FRC) to normal for the patient. When lung volumes are low, the work of breathing during early inhalation is reduced. Noncompliant lungs require higher intrapleural pressures to inflate to a normal V_T, even with CPAP. Addition of pressure support assists the patient to move up the pressure-volume curve (larger changes in volume for a given applied pressure; i.e., increased lung compliance). The term *pressure support ventilation* describes the combination of pressure support and PEEP (or CPAP). Although useful in the patient breathing spontaneously, pressure support may be used to assist spontaneous breaths in SIMV. Weaning may be facilitated using this combination, as the backup (SIMV) rate is weaned initially, and then the pressure support.

HELIOX

Helium has lower density than air or nitrogen. Substituting helium for nitrogen reduces the density of the gas in direct proportion to the amount of helium admixed. Breathing *heliox* (the concentration in clinical use ranges from 80:20 to 60:40 ratio of helium to oxygen) results in more laminar flow, reduced airway resistance, and reduced work of breathing. Heliox may be useful in clinical situations when resistance to airflow is high, including asthma, acute exacerbations of chronic bronchitis or chronic obstructive pulmonary disease (COPD), other causes of bronchospasm, and upper airway obstruction with stridor. Breathing heliox is well tolerated, without appreciable adverse effects. Disadvantages include high cost and limited use when a high *fraction of inspired oxygen* (FIO_2) is required. Ventilators must also be recalibrated when heliox is delivered by ventilator rather than nebulizer (the usual route), to ensure that the flow of gas is measured correctly.

MODES OF MECHANICAL VENTILATION

Assist-Control Ventilation

The ACV mode is the most commonly used mode in medical/surgical critical care units. Set parameters in ACV mode are inspiratory flow rate, frequency (*f*), and V_T. The ventilator delivers a set number of equal breaths per minute each of a given V_T. Tidal volume and flow determine inspiratory (I) and expiratory (E) time and the I:E ratio. Plateau or alveolar pressure is related to V_T and respiratory system compliance. The patient has the ability to trigger extra breaths by exerting an inspiratory effort exceeding a preset trigger level. Typically, each patient will display a preferred rate for a given V_T and will trigger all breaths when *f* is set a few breaths/minute below the patient's rate. In this mode, the control rate serves as adequate

support should the patient stop initiating breaths. When high inspiratory effort continues during a ventilator-delivered breath, the patient may trigger a second superimposed breath. Patient effort can be increased, if desired, by increasing triggering threshold or lowering V_T.

Synchronized Intermittent Mandatory Ventilation

In a passive patient, SIMV cannot be distinguished from ACV. Ventilation is determined by *f* and V_T. However, if the patient is not truly passive, respiratory work may be performed during mandatory breaths. In addition, the patient may trigger additional breaths by spontaneous effort. If the triggering effort comes in a brief, defined interval before the next mandatory breath, the ventilator will deliver the mandatory breath ahead of schedule to synchronize with patient inspiratory effort. If a breath is initiated outside the synchronization window, V_T, flow, and I:E ratio are determined by patient effort and respiratory system mechanics, not by ventilator settings. These spontaneous breaths tend to be of low V_T and are variable from breath to breath. The SIMV mode is often used to augment patient work of breathing gradually by lowering the mandatory breath frequency or V_T, compelling the patient to breathe more rapidly in order to maintain adequate $\dot{V}E$. Some ventilators allow combinations of modes. A useful combination is SIMV plus PSV as a means to add "sigh" breaths and decrease atelectasis. Because SIMV plus PSV guarantees some backup $\dot{V}E$ that PSV alone does not, this combination may be particularly useful for patients at high risk for deteriorating central respiratory drive, and it is also popular as an adjunct to weaning from the ventilator.

Positive End-Expiratory Pressure

Although it is a ubiquitous form of ventilatory support, PEEP can be confusing because the positive pressure is actually applied throughout the respiratory cycle and is more correctly termed CPAP. Using PEEP accomplishes three goals: (1) prevention of alveolar derecruitment by restoring FRC, which is decreased in ALI and atelectasis, to the physiologic range; (2) protection against injury during phasic opening and closing of atelectatic units; and (3) assisting cardiac performance during heart failure, by increasing mean intrathoracic pressure.

The FRC is the lung's physiologic reserve; loss of chest wall or lung compliance (the rate of change of volume in response to pressure) causes reduced FRC. The FRC is the volume of gas that remains in the lungs at the end of a normal tidal breath ($\sim$2.5 L); gas exchange does occur. At FRC, the tendency for the lungs to collapse is balanced by the tendency for the chest wall to move outward. Slight negative intrapleural pressure relative to atmospheric pressure assists in maintaining equilibrium, which is lost when pneumothorax is present.

The FRC is determined by the compliance of the lung and chest wall. Anything that constrains chest wall expansion reduces its compliance; likewise, anything that reduces lung volume reduces lung compliance. The FRC is composed of two volumes, the expiratory reserve volume (ERV) and the residual volume (RV). Below FRC, exhalation is active; lung tissue must be compressed to express gas. The RV ($\sim$−1 L in adults) is the point at which no more gas can be expressed from the lungs regardless of the pressure applied, because alveolar pressure exceeds atmospheric pressure and the gradient along the airway is reversed. Being filled with gas and coated with surfactant, alveoli are difficult to compress, but airways are compressible. When intrathoracic pressure exceeds pressure in the small airways, "dynamic airway collapse" occurs and gas is trapped in alveoli. Airway collapse increases the work of breathing and leads to *ventilation-perfusion ($\dot{V}/\dot{Q}$) mismatch*. Collapsed airways are difficult to reinflate, leading to a huge increase in the work of breathing and oxygen consumption.

The concept behind PEEP is to increase FRC; in essence, to allow alveoli to deflate only to the point just above where inflation remains easy (called the lower inflection point of the pressure-volume curve). The patient requires sufficient PEEP to prevent alveolar derecruitment, but not so much PEEP to create alveolar overdistention, *dead space ventilation* ($\dot{V}_{DS}$) from collapse of the alveolar microcirculation, or hypotension due to reduced right ventricular preload, right ventricular output, and ultimately cardiac output.

Auto-PEEP is caused by gas trapped in alveoli at end-expiration. This gas is not in equilibrium with the atmosphere and is at positive pressure, increasing the work of breathing. In patients with obstructive airways disease, increased bronchial tone leads to resistance to both inhalation and exhalation. Shortening of E (e.g., small airways disease, mucus plugging, pressure-controlled ventilation with inverted I:E ratio) results in gas trapping at end-expiration, hyperinflation, and increased intrathoracic pressure, which abolishes the airway pressure gradient. Auto-PEEP can be ameliorated by lengthening E, shortening I, or decreasing the respiratory rate.

The ideal level of PEEP is controversial (Table 3). It may be that which prevents derecruitment of the majority of alveoli, while causing minimal overdistention; alternatively, application of PEEP is a recruitment maneuver, arguing for higher pressures to be applied to overcome alveolar collapse. Applying PEEP to put the majority of lung units on the favorable part of the pressure-volume curve will maximize gas exchange and minimize overdistention, but it is easier said than done because the lower inflection point is sometimes indistinct. Undoubtedly, the combination of PEEP and low V_T prevents *volutrauma*, but the exact amount of PEEP that should be applied is controversial. The reason for this is hysteresis—the tendency of the lungs, due to surfactant, to be inflated at higher volumes in exhalation than in inhalation.

Ventilator "Bundle"

Care of the patient who requires MV is more than just a matter of providing ventilation and oxygenation. Such patients are often critically ill and at risk of numerous complications, not all of which are related directly to ARF or MV. Therefore, it is important for the clinician to bear in mind the total patient. The patient may be at

TABLE 3: Protocol Summary for Institution of Mechanical Ventilation for ALI/ARDS

Initial Ventilator Settings

Use a volume-controlled mode initially to ensure that V_T is delivered.

Initial V_T 8 mL/kg; reduce by 1 mL/kg/2 h until 6 mL/kg is reached. Minimum V_T 4 mL/kg.

Set ventilator rate at 12–20 breaths/min. Maximum ventilator rate 35 breaths/min.

Adjust ventilator subsequently based on goals of arterial pH (7.25–7.45; ventilator rate) and end-inspiratory plateau pressure (P_{plat}) (<30 cm H_2O; V_T).

Measure arterial pH upon admission to the ICU, each morning, and 15 min after each change in respiratory rate or V_T.

Alkalemia is managed by decreasing ventilator rate by at least 2 breaths/min.

Mild acidemia (pH 7.15–7.25) is managed by increasing ventilator rate until pH >7.25 or $Paco_2 < 25$ mm Hg up to 35 breaths/min. If ventilator rate = 35 breaths/min or $Paco_2 < 25$ mm Hg, give sodium bicarbonate.

Severe acidemia (pH <7.15) is managed by increasing the ventilator rate up to 35 breaths/min. If ventilator rate = 35 and pH <7.15, and sodium bicarbonate has been given, increase V_T in increments of 1 mL/kg until pH >7.15. It may be necessary to exceed the target P_{plat} under these conditions.

Keep $P_{plat} < 30$ cm H_2O. Measure P_{plat} at least every 8 h, and 5 min after each change in PEEP or V_T, and more frequently when changes in lung compliance are likely. Accurate measurement of P_{plat} requires a patient who is not moving or coughing.

If P_{plat} cannot be measured because of an air leak, peak inspiratory pressure may be substituted.

Target ranges for Pao_2 are 55–80 mm Hg, or $Sao_2 > 88\%$. The combination of PEEP and Fio_2 is discretionary, but Fio_2:PEEP should generally be ≤ 5 if $Fio_2 > 0.45$.

When increasing PEEP above 10 cm H_2O, increase by 2–5-cm increments up to a maximum of 35 cm H_2O, until target ranges for Pao_2 are reached. Reduce PEEP to the previous level of PEEP if the change does not increase $Pao_2 > 5$ mm Hg or if decreased oxygen delivery results from a decrease of cardiac output.

Assess arterial oxygenation by blood gas determination or oximetry at least every 4 h.

If arterial oxygenation is below the target range, increase Fio_2 incrementally (up to 1.0) then PEEP (up to 35 cm H_2O within 30 min). Reassess every 15 min after each adjustment until target ranges for Pao_2 are regained. Brief periods of $Sao_2 < 88\%$ (<5 min) may be tolerated. $Fio_2 = 1.0$ may be used transiently (<10 min) for arterial desaturation or during suctioning or bronchoscopy.

Modified from Nathens AB, Johnson JL, Mine JP, et al; Inflammation and the Host Response to Injury Investigators: inflammation and the host response to injury, a large-scale collaborative project: patient-oriented research core—standard operating procedures for clinical care. I. Guidelines for mechanical ventilation of the trauma patient. *J Trauma* 59:764–769, 2005.
ALI, Acute lung injury; ARDS, acute respiratory distress syndrome; ICU, intensive care unit; PEEP, positive end-expiratory pressure.

prolonged bed rest, and at risk for deconditioning, venous thromboembolic complications, and the development of pressure ulcers. Neurologic compromise from disease or sedative/analgesic drugs may impair the sensorium sufficiently that the patient cannot protect his or her airway, increasing the risk of pulmonary aspiration of gastric contents. Oversedation may be one component aspect of prolonged MV, which is a definite risk factor for development of VAP. Prolonged MV (longer than 48 hours) is itself a marker of critical illness, specifically the development of stress-related gastric mucosal hemorrhage, a rare but serious (~50% mortality rate) harbinger of adverse outcomes of critical illness.

Using the principles of evidence-based medicine, several "best practices" have been combined into a *ventilator bundle* to optimize the outcomes of MV. The bundle, originally four maneuvers, now consists of five: (1) keeping the head of the patient's bed up at least 30 degrees from level *at all times* unless contraindicated medically; (2) prophylaxis against venous thromboembolic disease; (3) prophylaxis against stress-related gastric mucosal hemorrhage; (4) a daily "sedation holiday" to assess for readiness to liberate from MV through assessment of a trial of spontaneous breathing; and most recently, (5) the addition of oral care with topical chlorhexidine mouthwash. Careful adoption and adherence to all facets of the bundle decrease the risk of VAP, along with other maneuvers such as adherence to the principles of infection control.

Routine Settings

Ventilator settings are based on the patient's ideal body mass and medical condition. The risk of oxygen toxicity from prolonged exposure to FIO_2 greater than 60% is minimized by using the lowest FIO_2 that can oxygenate arterial blood satisfactorily (e.g., arterial oxygen tension (PaO_2) of 60 mm Hg or an oxygen saturation (SaO_2) of 88% (see Table 3).

The normal lung (e.g., during general anesthesia) may be ventilated safely with VT 8 to 10 mL/kg for prolonged periods. Historically, critically ill patients with *ALI/ARDS* have been ventilated with VT 10 to 15 mL/kg of ideal body mass, which is now considered inappropriate because overdistention can produce endothelial, epithelial, and basement membrane injuries associated with increased microvascular permeability and iatrogenic (ventilator-induced) lung injury (VILI). Direct monitoring of alveolar volume is not feasible. A reasonable substitute is to estimate peak alveolar pressure as obtained from the plateau pressure (P_{plat}) measured in a relaxed patient by occluding the ventilator circuit briefly at end-inspiration. In patients with pulmonary dysfunction, many clinicians reduce the VT delivered to 4 to 6 mL/kg or less in order to achieve a P_{plat} no higher than 35 cm H_2O. The incidence of VILI increases markedly when P_{plat} is high. Low VT ventilation may lead to an increase in $PaCO_2$. Acceptance of elevated CO_2 tension in exchange for controlled alveolar pressure is termed *permissive hypercapnia*. It is important to focus on pH rather than $PaCO_2$ if this approach is employed. If the pH falls below 7.25, increase $\dot{V}E$ or administer $NaHCO_3$.

The *f* that is set depends on the mode. With ACV, the backup rate should be about 4 breaths/minute less than the patient's spontaneous rate to ensure that the ventilator will continue to supply adequate $\dot{V}E$ should the patient have a sudden decrease in spontaneous breathing. With SIMV, the rate is typically high at first and then decreased gradually in accordance with the patient's tolerance.

An inspiratory flow rate of 60 L/minute is used with most patients during ACV and SIMV. In patients with COPD, better gas exchange may be achieved at a flow rate of 100 L/minute, probably because the resulting increase in E allows for more complete emptying of trapped gas. If the flow rate is insufficient to meet the patient's requirements, the patient will strain against his or her own pulmonary impedance and that of the ventilator, with a consequent increase in the work of breathing.

In the ACV, SIMV, and pressure control modes (discussed in the chapter Advanced Techniques in Mechanical Ventilation), the patient must lower airway pressure below a preset threshold (usually minus 1-2 cm H_2O) in order to trigger the ventilator to deliver a tidal breath. In most situations, this is straightforward: the more negative the sensitivity, the greater the effort demanded of the patient. When auto-PEEP is present, the patient must lower alveolar pressure by the amount of auto-PEEP in order to have any impact on airway opening pressure, then further by the trigger amount to initiate a breath, increasing dramatically the work of breathing. Flow triggering systems have been used to reduce the work of triggering the ventilator. In contrast to the usual approach in which the patient must open a demand valve in order to receive assistance, continuous flow systems maintain a high continuous flow, then augment flow further when the patient initiates a breath. These systems reduce the work of breathing slightly below that present using conventional demand valves but do not solve the triggering problem when breath stacking occurs.

Sedation

Most patients who require MV will require sedation, but only a minority (~10%) will also require neuromuscular blockade. A panoply of agents are available for both (Table 4), so the choice of agent can be individualized for the patient, but caution must be exercised so that patients receive only what they need and are not oversedated. Titration of sedation such that patients are comfortable is facilitated by ordering sedation to be titrated to a sedation score of 3 to 4 points on the Ramsay or Riker scale (Table 5). Intermittent doses of sedatives are preferred to continuous infusions, also to attempt to minimize the amount of sedation. Neuromuscular blockade should be avoided whenever possible.

Prolonged or excessive sedation increases the duration of MV and increases the likelihood of tracheostomy. Protocolized weaning of sedative medications, and daily sedation "holidays" to permit spontaneous breathing trials (see later) shorten the duration of MV and decrease the risk of VAP and other complications.

MONITORING

Blood Gases

Blood gas analyzers report a wide range of results, but the only parameters measured directly are the partial pressures of oxygen (PO_2) and carbon dioxide (PCO_2), and blood pH. The arterial blood hemoglobin saturation (SaO_2) is calculated from the PO_2 using the oxyhemoglobin dissociation curve, assuming a normal P_{50} (the PO_2 at which SaO_2 is 50%, normally 26.6 mm Hg), and that hemoglobin is normal structurally. Some blood gas analyzers incorporate a co-oximeter that measures the various forms of hemoglobin directly, including oxyhemoglobin, total hemoglobin, carboxyhemoglobin, and methemoglobin. The actual HCO_3^-, standard HCO_3^-, and base excess are calculated from the pH and PCO_2.

A freshly drawn, heparinized, bubble-free arterial blood sample is required. Heparin is acidic; if present to excess, the measured PCO_2 and calculated HCO_3^- are reduced spuriously. Delayed analysis allows continued metabolism by erythrocytes, reducing pH and PO_2 and increasing PCO_2; keeping the specimen iced preserves accuracy for up to 1 hour. Air bubbles cause a decrease in PCO_2 and an increase in PO_2.

The solubility of all gases in blood, including CO_2 and O_2, increases with a decrease in temperature. Thus, hypothermia causes the PO_2 and PCO_2 to decrease and pH to increase. As analysis of a sample taken from a hypothermic patient occurs at 37° C, the PO_2 and PCO_2 results are artificially high, but the error is usually too small to be meaningful clinically.

TABLE 4: Selected Formulary for Analgesia, Anesthesia, and Sedation in the ICU

Agent	Initial IV Adult Dose	Comments
Induction Agents		
Etomidate	0.3 mg/kg or more	Maintains CO and BP. Reduces ICP but maintains CPP. Short $T_{1/2}$; use infusion for maintenance. Possible adrenal suppression.
Ketamine	1–2 mg/kg	Rapid onset, short duration agent for induction of anesthesia. Can be given by maintenance continuous infusion, and at lower dose for sedation without anesthesia. Transiently increases BP and HR. Raises ICP and intraocular pressure. Usually does not depress breathing. Generally safe in pregnancy and for neonates and children. Concurrent narcotics or barbiturates may prolong recovery. Can cause anxiety, disorientation, dysphoria, and hallucinations, which may be reduced by a short-acting benzodiazepine during emergence. Atropine pretreatment is recommended to decrease secretions but may increase incidence of dysphoria. Hepatic metabolism.
Propofol	1.5–2.5 mg/kg	Provides no analgesia. Potent amnestic effect. Causes apnea and loss of gag reflex. Can cause marked low BP. Infuse at 0.05–0.3 mg/kg/min for prolonged sedation. Minimal accumulation (hepatic insufficiency) facilitates rapid elimination. Account for 1 kcal/mL (lipid infusion) in nutrition prescription. Use of same vial >12 h associated with bacteremia. Safety for children still debated.
Intravenous Analgesics		
Midazolam	0.5–4 mg	Short $T_{1/2}$, but accumulates during infusion owing to active metabolites. Only benzodiazepine with potent amnestic effect. Can cause low BP and loss of airway. Primary use is short-term sedation for ICU procedures. Renal elimination.
Lorazepam	1–4 mg	Effective anxiolytic. Preferred agent for continuous infusion of benzodiazepine (starting dose 1 mg/h). Can cause low BP, especially with hypovolemia and paradoxical agitation. Hepatic elimination.
Morphine	2–10 mg	Analgesic and sedative effects. Can cause low BP, CO, and apnea. Tolerance and withdrawal possible after long-term use. Can be given as IV infusion or by PCA for analgesia or to facilitate prolonged mechanical ventilation or withdrawal of care. Hepatic elimination.
Hydromorphone	0.5–2.0 mg	Hydrated ketone of morphine with similar use and risk profiles. Approximately eightfold more potent than morphine. Hepatic elimination.
Fentanyl	50–100 μg	Approximately 50-fold potency compared with morphine, but less likely to cause low BP in appropriate dosage (less histamine release). Versatile for ICU use given IV or by epidural infusion or PCA. Less potent than local anesthetics for epidural analgesia or abrogation of surgical stress response. Can cause truncal rigidity and apnea with inability to ventilate by hand (use neuromuscular blockade to facilitate intubation in that setting). Hepatic elimination.
Neuromuscular Blocking Agents		
Succinylcholine	0.75–1.5 mg/kg	Only depolarizing NMBA (occupies ACh receptor). Rapid onset, effect dissipates within 10 min of single dose. Causes hyperkalemia. Can precipitate malignant hyperthermia. Increases ICP and intraocular pressure. Contraindicated in TBI, spinal cord injury, neuromuscular disease, and burns. Metabolized by plasma cholinesterase, absence of enzyme (relatively common) causes prolonged paralysis.
Atracurium and cisatracurium	0.2–0.5 mg/kg	Short-acting nondepolarizing NMBAs (competitive inhibitors of ACh). Relatively slow in onset. These drugs are similar, except atracurium causes histamine release and can cause high HR, low BP. Cisatracurium is now used preferentially. Short-acting, requires IV infusion for prolonged effect. Effect potentiated by hypokalemia. Many drug interactions. Metabolized by Hoffman elimination/ester hydrolysis; thus used for patients with renal/hepatic insufficiency.
Pancuronium	0.05–0.1 mg	Rapid onset, prolonged effect. Causes increased BP and HR. Used for induction of neuromuscular blockade, but should be converted to a drug such as continuous-infusion cisatracurium for maintenance. Renal/hepatic elimination, accumulates in organ dysfunction.

Continued

TABLE 4: Selected Formulary for Analgesia, Anesthesia, and Sedation in the ICU—Cont'd

Agent	Initial IV Adult Dose	Comments
Vecuronium	0.08–0.10 mg/kg	Nondepolarizing NMBA with rapid onset and short duration of action. Less potential for histamine release. Can cause malignant hyperthermia. Metabolized by the liver.
Miscellaneous Agents		
Dexmedetomidine	1 µg/kg load, then 0.2–0.7 µg/kg/h	Central selective α_2-receptor agonist used for short-term (<24 h) sedation. Sympatholysis lowers HR and BP. Can achieve light sedation, does not depress respirations. No anamnestic effect. Useful for drug/alcohol withdrawal and sedation when liberation from mechanical ventilation is imminent. Expensive.
Haloperidol	2–5 mg	Used commonly for anxiolysis (often over lorazepam), especially when respiratory depression is undesirable. IV administration, not FDA-approved, is commonplace. Antidopaminergic properties contraindicate use in Parkinson disease. Causes extrapyramidal effects. Hepatic elimination.
Ketorolac	15–30 mg q6h	Parenteral NSAID used in lieu of opioids or for opioid-sparing effect in combination. Irreversible platelet dysfunction; can cause incisional or GI hemorrhage and acute renal failure. Use strictly limited to less than 5 days in postoperative period.
Reversal Agents		
Flumazenil	0.1–0.2 mg	Benzodiazepine antagonist. Rapid onset and short duration. Adverse effect of benzodiazepine can persist after drug wears off. Repeated doses of up to 0.8 mg can be used. Abrupt antagonism of chronic benzodiazepine use can precipitate seizures.
Naloxone	Up to 0.4 mg	Opioid antagonist. Rapid onset and short duration. Often diluted 0.4 mg/10 mL and titrated 0.04–0.08 mg at a time to reverse undesirable side effects but preserve analgesia. Repeated doses of up to 0.4 mg or continuous IV infusion can be used. Abrupt opioid antagonism can precipitate hypertension; increased HR, pulmonary edema, or myocardial infarction.
Edrophonium with atropine	0.5–1.0 mg/kg, 0.1 mg q5–15 min up to 4 doses	Anticholinesterase inhibitor with antidysrhythmic properties. Rapid onset, short duration, therefore used usually in concert with atropine, which counteracts the increased secretions, decreased HR, and bronchospasm. Not effective for reversal of neuromuscular blockade caused by depolarizing agents. Renal and hepatic elimination (edrophonium). Atropine may cause fever.
Neostigmine with glycopyrrolate	0.5–2. 0 mg, 0.1–0.2 mg	Neostigmine causes salivation and severe low HR. May cause laryngospasm or bronchospasm. Renal metabolism. Not effective for reversal of neuromuscular blockade caused by depolarizing agents. Because of profound low HR, given in same syringe with glycopyrrolate (or sometimes atropine). Glycopyrrolate counteracts low HR and unopposed causes increased HR. May cause fever. Glycopyrrolate is contraindicated in GI ileus/obstruction and in neonates.

ACh, Acetylcholine; BP, blood pressure; CO, cardiac output; CPP, cerebral perfusion pressure; FDA, U.S. Food and Drug Administration; GI, gastrointestinal; HR, heart rate; ICP, intracranial pressure; ICU, intensive care unit; IV, intravenous; NMBA, neuromuscular blocking agent; NSAID, nonsteroidal anti-inflammatory drug; PCA, patient-controlled analgesia; $T_{1/2}$, elimination half-life; TBI, traumatic brain injury; Vo_2, oxygen consumption.

Pulse Oximetry

Pulse oximetry calculates Sao_2 by estimating the difference in intensity of signal between oxygenated and deoxygenated blood from the red (660 nm) and near-infrared (940 nm) regions of the light spectrum. To function accurately, pulse oximetry must detect pulsatile blood flow, but all things being equal, pulse oximetry data can be obtained from a detector on the finger, the earlobe, or even the forehead. Pulse oximetry is generally accurate ($\pm2\%$) over the range of Sao_2 70% to 100%, but less accurate below 70%.

Several aspects of the technology and patient physiology limit the accuracy of pulse oximetry. If the device cannot detect pulsatile flow, the waveform will be damped and unable to provide an accurate estimation. Consequently, patients with hypothermia, hypotension,

hypovolemia, or peripheral arterial disease, or who are treated with vasoconstrictor medications (e.g., norepinephrine), may have inaccurate pulse oximetry readings. Additionally, an elevated carboxyhemoglobin concentration will lead to falsely elevated Sao_2 because reflected light is absorbed at the same wavelength as oxygenated hemoglobin. Other situations contributing to inaccurate pulse oximetry include the presence of ambient light and motion artifact.

Capnography

Capnography measures changes in the concentration of CO_2 in expired gas during the ventilatory cycle. This technique is most reliable in ventilated patients and employs either mass spectroscopy or

TABLE 5: Sedation Scales in Common Use

Scale	Value	Clinical Correlate
Ramsey Sedation Scale		
Awake scores 1–3	1	Anxious, agitated, or restless
	2	Cooperative, oriented, tranquil
	3	Responsive to commands
Asleep scores 4–6	4	Brisk response to stimulus*
	5	Sluggish response to stimulus
	6	No response to stimulus
Riker Sedation-Agitation Scale		
Dangerous agitation	7	Pulling at catheters, striking staff
Very agitated	6	Does not calm to voice, requires restraint
Agitated	5	Anxious, responds to verbal cues
Calm and cooperative	4	Calm, awakens easily, follows commands
Sedated	3	Awakens to stimulus
Very sedated	2	Arouses to stimulus, does not follow commands
Unarousable	1	Minimal or no response to noxious stimulus

Modified from Ramsay M, Savege T, Simpson B, et al: Controlled sedation with alphaxalon-alphadolone. *BMJ* 2:656–659, 1974; and Riker RR, Picard JT, Fraser GL: Prospective evaluation of the Sedation-Agitation Scale for adult critically ill patients. *Crit Care Med* 27:1325–1329, 1999.
*Stimulus is light glabellar tap or loud auditory stimulus.

infrared light absorption to detect the presence of CO_2. The gas may be collected by sidestream or mainstream sampling; the former is most common and has the advantage of a lightweight analyzer. However, sidestream sampling is susceptible to accumulation of water vapor in the sampling line. In the intensive care unit (ICU), when respiratory gases are humidified, mainstream sampling may be preferable.

The peak CO_2 concentration occurs at end-exhalation and is regarded as the patient's "end-tidal CO_2" ($ETCO_2$), at which time $ETCO_2$ is in close approximation to the alveolar gas concentration. Capnography is useful in the assessment of successful tracheostomy or endotracheal tube placement, to monitor weaning from MV, and as a monitor of resuscitation. The ability to detect hypercarbia during ventilator weaning can diminish the need for serial blood gas measurements. In conjunction with pulse oximetry, many patients can be weaned successfully from MV, without reliance upon arterial blood gases or invasive hemodynamic monitoring.

Other information is acquired from capnography as well. Prognostically, an $ETCO_2$ to $PaCO_2$ gradient of 13 mm Hg or more after resuscitation has been associated with increased mortality rate in trauma patients. A sudden decrease or even disappearance of $ETCO_2$ can be correlated with potentially serious disease or events, such as a low cardiac output state, disconnection from the ventilator, or pulmonary thromboembolism. A gradual increase of $ETCO_2$ can be seen with hypoventilation; the converse is also true. Another cause of gradually decreasing $ETCO_2$ is hypovolemia.

INVASIVE HEMODYNAMIC MONITORING

Arterial Catheterization

Measurement of arterial blood pressure is one of the simplest, most reproducible methods of evaluating hemodynamics. Automated non-invasive blood pressure cuff devices are accurate (margin of error, $\pm 2\%$), but take measurements only periodically. If fluctuations require more frequent monitoring, continuous monitoring is available via an indwelling arterial catheter. Indications for invasive arterial monitoring include prolonged operations or prolonged MV (longer than 24 hours), unstable hemodynamics, substantial blood loss, a need for frequent blood sampling, or a need for precise blood pressure control (e.g., neurosurgical patients, patients on cardiopulmonary bypass). Although there is morbidity from insertion and from indwelling catheters, there is also morbidity from repetitive arterial punctures; the risk/benefit analysis is a matter of clinical judgment for "less unstable" patients.

Arterial catheters may be placed in any of several locations. The catheter should be a special-purpose thin-walled catheter to maintain fidelity of the waveform and to avoid obstructing the vessel lumen; a standard intravenous cannula should not be used. The radial artery at the wrist is the most commonly used site; although the ulnar artery is usually of larger diameter, it is relatively inaccessible percutaneously. Careful confirmation of a patent collateral circulation to the hand is mandatory before cannulation of an artery at the wrist, to minimize potential tissue loss from arterial occlusion or embolization. In neonates, the umbilical artery may be catheterized; intestinal ischemia is a rare complication. The axillary artery is relatively spared by atheromas, supported by good collateral vessels at the shoulder, and easy to cannulate percutaneously, making it a suitable choice. The superficial femoral artery may also be used, but is not a location of choice because the burden of plaque (and therefore the risk of distal embolization) is higher, as is the infection rate. The superficial temporal artery is difficult to cannulate because of small caliber and tortuosity. The dorsalis pedis artery is accessible, but should be avoided in patients with peripheral vascular disease. The brachial artery should be strictly avoided, because the collateral circulation around the elbow is poor and the risk of ischemia of the hand or forearm is high. Severe peripheral vasoconstriction due to vasopressor therapy may necessitate a longer catheter at a more central location (e.g., axillary, femoral) in order to place the catheter tip into an artery in the torso that would be less affected. Nosocomial infection of arterial catheters is unusual provided basic tenets of infection control are honored and femoral artery catheterization is avoided. Other complications from arterial catheterization include bleeding, hematoma, and pseudoaneurysm.

Central Venous Pressure Monitoring

The central venous pressure (CVP) is an interplay of the circulating blood volume, venous tone, and right ventricular function. The CVP measures the filling pressure of the right ventricle, providing an estimate of intravascular volume status. Central venous access can be obtained via the basilic, femoral, external jugular, internal jugular, or subclavian vein. In the ICU, the internal jugular, subclavian, and femoral veins are used, in decreasing frequency. The internal jugular site is most popular because of ease of accessibility, a high technical success rate of cannulation, and a low rate of complications. However, it is difficult to keep an adherent dressing in place, and the infection rate is higher than for subclavian catheters. Subclavian insertion is technically demanding, and has the highest rate of pneumothorax (1.5% to 3%), but the lowest rates of infection. The femoral vein site is least preferred, despite the relative ease of catheter placement. It is accessible during cardiopulmonary resuscitation or emergency intubation, so procedures can occur concurrently. However, the site is particularly prone to infection, and the risks of arterial puncture (9% to 15%) and venous thromboembolic complications are higher than for jugular or subclavian venipuncture. Overall complications are comparable for internal jugular and subclavian vein cannulation (6% to 12%) and higher for femoral vein cannulation (13% to 19%). The incidence of carotid puncture during internal jugular cannulation (6% to 9%) is higher than that for puncture of the subclavian artery during subclavian vein catheterization (3% to 5%).

PULMONARY ARTERY CATHETERIZATION

A *pulmonary artery catheter* (PAC) is a balloon-tipped, flow-directed catheter that is usually inserted percutaneously via a central vein and transits the right side of the heart into the PA. Data from PACs are used mainly to determine cardiac output (Q) and preload, which is most commonly estimated in the clinical setting by the *PA occlusion pressure* (PAOP), or "wedge" pressure. PA diastolic pressure corresponds well to the PAOP. Diastolic pressure can exceed the PAOP when pulmonary vascular resistance is high (e.g., pulmonary fibrosis, pulmonary hypertension).

Normally, PAOP approximates left atrial pressure, which in turn approximates left ventricular end-diastolic pressure (LVEDP), itself a reflection of left ventricular end-diastolic volume (LVEDV). The LVEDV represents preload, which is the actual target parameter. Factors that may cause PAOP to reflect LVEDV inaccurately include mitral stenosis, high levels of PEEP (greater than 10 cm H_2O), and changes in left ventricular compliance (e.g., due to myocardial infarction, pericardial effusion, or increased afterload). Inaccurate readings may result from balloon overinflation, improper catheter position, alveolar pressure exceeding pulmonary venous pressure (as with ventilation with PEEP), or severe pulmonary hypertension (which may make PAOP measurement hazardous). Elevated PAOP occurs in left-sided heart failure. Decreased PAOP occurs with hypovolemia or decreased preload.

A desirable feature of PA catheterization is the ability to measure mixed venous oxygen saturation ($S\bar{V}O_2$); although controversial, sampling from the superior vena cava via a central venous catheter may provide data of comparable use. True mixed venous blood is blood from both the superior and inferior vena cavas admixed in the right atrium, which may be sampled for blood gas analysis from the distal port of the PAC. Some catheters have embedded fiberoptic sensors that measure $S\bar{V}O_2$ directly. Causes of low $S\bar{V}O_2$ include anemia, pulmonary disease, carboxyhemoglobinemia, low Q, and increased tissue oxygen demand. The SaO_2:($SaO_2 - S\bar{V}O_2$) ratio determines the adequacy of O_2 delivery (DO_2). Ideally the $P\bar{V}O_2$ should be 35 to 40 mm Hg, with a $S\bar{V}O_2$ of about 70%. Values of $P\bar{V}O_2$ lower than 30 mm Hg are critically low.

CLINICAL USE OF THE PULMONARY ARTERY CATHETER

Many indications have been championed for the PAC, but no studies have demonstrated unequivocally that PAC use decreases morbidity or mortality rates. PACs may still be useful in cardiomyopathy, shock of various causes, suspected pulmonary hypertension, or an unpredicted or poor response to conventional fluid therapy. Critically ill patients receiving inotropic agents despite resuscitation with large volumes of fluid may also benefit from monitoring by PAC. However, a recent ARDSnet trial demonstrated no differences in outcome when ALI/ARDS was managed by PAC versus CVP monitoring.

Transesophageal echocardiography is a less invasive alternative for assessment of Q that is available increasingly in ICUs. Bioreactance

and bioimpedance are noninvasive technologies that measure cardiac output and other hemodynamic variables such as stroke volume and cardiac index. Bioimpedance and bioreactance are noninvasive measurements; the latter is now available via a commercial device. Bioimpedance detects electrical changes occurring with altering fluid volumes in the thorax. Volumes change as the left ventricle contracts and blood flows into the thoracic aorta. This causes a corresponding change in resistance within the thorax because the fluid volume in the aorta increases. This change in impedance can be measured as a change in voltage passing between electrodes placed on a patient's chest. In essence, bioimpedance measures the amplitude of the voltage change across the thorax. By contrast, bioreactance tracks the phase of electrical currents traversing the chest; the higher the stroke volume, the more marked these phase shifts become.

The technological advancement is similar in concept to that of an amplitude modulation (AM) versus frequency modulation (FM) radio. Because FM radio detects and analyzes radio signals based on their frequency rather than amplitude difference in the waveform, greater fidelity is achieved with respect to noise cancellation. In monitoring, high signal/noise ratio provides greater accuracy and precision with unstable hemodynamics, motion, and variations on electrode location and with thoracic fluid shifts.

LIBERATION FROM MECHANICAL VENTILATION

Objective measures and proactive tactics are available to hasten the moment when patients on MV can be liberated from the ventilator. The stakes are high, because each day of MV via artificial airway (e.g., endotracheal or tracheostomy tube) increases the need for sedation, which may postpone "liberation day." Moreover, each day of MV increases the risk of VAP, which may prolong further the need for MV.

Some patients do not wean readily from the ventilator, which may be due to disease- or therapy-related reasons. Most clinical cases of failed liberation from the ventilator are multifactorial, but respiratory muscle fatigue is a common factor, in that the load on the respiratory system exceeds the capacity to breathe (Table 6). The increased load may take the form of a demand for increased $\dot{V}E$, or increased work of breathing. Increased $\dot{V}E$ may result from increased CO_2 production, increased VD ventilation, or increased ventilatory drive. Increased CO_2 production may be caused by a catabolic state, or excess carbohydrate administered during nutritional support. Increased VD (ventilation of unperfused or underperfused lung) may be caused by decreased Q, pulmonary embolism, pulmonary hypertension, severe ALI, or iatrogenically from positive-pressure ventilation. Increased

TABLE 6: Load on the Respiratory System

Demand for increased minute ventilation	Increased carbon dioxide production Increased dead space ventilation Increased ventilatory drive
Increased work of breathing	Airway obstruction Decreased respiratory system compliance
Decreased respiratory system capacity	Impaired central drive to breathe Integrity of phrenic nerve transmission Impaired respiratory muscle force generation

ventilatory drive may occur from muscle fatigue or failure, stimulation of pulmonary J receptors (usually by lung inflammation or parenchymal hemorrhage), or lesions of the central nervous system. Psychological stress is also an important factor that may manifest itself as tachypnea, hypoxemia, agitation, or delirium. Stress may be caused by inadequate analgesia or sedation or by untreated delirium. Acute alcohol or drug withdrawal is a major factor in some patients.

Increased work of breathing results from either increased airflow resistance or decreased thoracic compliance. Airway obstruction can result from reversible small airways disease (e.g., bronchospasm), tracheal stenosis, tracheomalacia, glottic edema or dysfunction, mucus plugging, or muscle weakness or fatigue. Muscle dysfunction may be caused by nutritional or metabolic causes (including hypocalcemia, hypokalemia, or hypophosphatemia). The *critical illness polyneuropathy* syndrome has poorly understood pathophysiology, but is associated with sepsis and *multiple organ dysfunction syndrome* and is often diagnosed when sought specifically by electromyography. Other potential causes of muscular failure or weakness include hypoxemia, hypercarbia, and possibly anemia.

Patients who "fight" the ventilator technically have the syndrome of *patient-ventilator dyssynchrony*. The cause can usually be found and must be sought; to sedate the patient more deeply (or administer neuromuscular blockade) before correctable causes are identified and remedied is incorrect and may be catastrophic if an unstable airway is the cause. A systematic approach to evaluation is advocated; recognizing that the patient and the ventilator are supposed to be working in concert facilitates an understanding that the problem may be the patient or the ventilator. The cause may be found anywhere on the continuum from the alveolus to the power outlet or the source of respiratory gases and must be sought systematically (Table 7). The first step is always to ensure that the patient has a patent airway that is positioned properly.

Liberation from MV can be easy in patients requiring short-term support. However, as many as 25% of patients will experience respiratory distress such that ventilation has to be reinstituted; patients recovering from ARF, necrotizing VAP, or major torso trauma can be especially challenging. Patients who cannot be weaned have a characteristic response to trials of spontaneous breathing. There is an almost-immediate increase in respiratory rate and decrease in V_T. As the trial of spontaneous breathing continues over 30 to 60 minutes, work of breathing increases substantially by fourfold to sevenfold. Increased oxygen demand is met by increased oxygen extraction, which eventually caused decreased Do_2 and arterial hypoxemia. Pulmonary compliance decreases, and gas trapping from lengthened I:E ratio doubles measures auto-PEEP. The rapid, shallow breathing pattern causes CO_2 retention because of increased dead space ventilation despite increased $\dot{V}_E$. There is considerable cardiovascular stress also, with pulmonary and systemic hypertension and increased afterload on both ventricles, likely from the extreme changes in intrathoracic pressure generated by the struggling patient.

Timing is important; if weaning is delayed unnecessarily, the patient remains at risk for a host of ventilator-associated complications. If weaning is performed prematurely, failure may lead to cardiopulmonary decompensation and further prolonged MV. In general, discontinuation of MV is not attempted in the setting of cardiopulmonary instability or Pao_2 lower than 60 mm Hg with a Fio_2 of 0.60 or higher. However, satisfactory oxygenation does not predict successful weaning reliably; rather, a more important determinant is the ability of respiratory muscles to perform increased respiratory work. Decisions based solely on clinical judgment are frequently erroneous. Parameters gathered traditionally, including maximal negative inspiratory pressure, vital capacity, and $\dot{V}_E$, have limited predictive accuracy. Measurement of f/V_T during 1 minute of spontaneous breathing (the Rapid Shallow Breathing Index, or Tobin Index) is a more accurate predictor (95% probability of success) if f/V_T is lower than 80 after a 30-minute trial of spontaneous breathing. Calculation of f/V_T during PSV is considerably less accurate.

TABLE 7: Therapies to Reverse Ventilatory Failure

Improve Muscular Function

Treat sepsis—avoid aminoglycosides

Nutritional support without overfeeding (follow indirect calorimetry)

Replete electrolytes to normal

Assure periods of rest—do not exhaust the patient

Limit neuromuscular blockade

Avoid oversedation

Identify/correct hypothyroidism

Reduce Respiratory Load

Airway resistance

Ensure airway patency/adequate caliber

Compliance (elastance)

Treat pneumonia

Treat pulmonary edema

Identify/reduce intrinsic PEEP (auto-PEEP)

Drain large pleural effusions

Evacuate pneumothorax

Treat ileus (promotility agents)

Decompress abdominal distention/treat abdominal compartment syndrome

Position patient 30 degrees head-up

Minute ventilation

Treat sepsis

Antipyresis (T > 40° C)

Avoid overfeeding

Correct metabolic acidosis

Identify/reduce intrinsic PEEP (auto-PEEP)

Bronchodilators

Maintain least possible PEEP

Resuscitate shock/correct hypovolemia

Identify and treat pulmonary embolism

PEEP, Positive end-expiratory pressure.

The process of weaning begins by determining patient readiness (Table 8). Patients should be screened carefully for hemodynamic stability, cooperative mental status, respiratory muscle strength, consistent and adequate wakefulness, ability to manage secretions, nutritional repletion, normalization of acid–base and electrolyte status, and an artificial airway of adequate size. Particular attention should be given to acceptance of hypercapnia if present chronically (e.g., COPD) and avoidance of new metabolic alkalosis. Finally,

TABLE 8: Cornell Protocol for Liberation from Mechanical Ventilation

Screening (performed at least once daily, usually in early AM, by respiratory therapist, nurse, or physician, according to local protocol)

Resolution of the underlying disease process
No vasopressors or sedative infusions (except propofol or dexmedetomidine)
No neuromuscular blocking agents
Intermittent doses of sedatives are permissible
No active myocardial ischemia or cardiac rhythm disturbances
$\dot{V}_E$ <15 L/min
$Pao_2:Fio_2$ > 120 on Fio_2 < 0.55
$Paco_2$ < 50 mm Hg
Physiologic pH (7.30–7.50)
PEEP <8 cm H_2O
Pressure support <8 cm H_2O
Adequate cough/clearance of secretions
↓

YES/NO ➜Return to Screening
↓

Proceed with spontaneous breathing trial—turn off enteral feedings and monitor serum glucose concentration closely, especially if on continuous infusion of insulin

Spontaneous breathing trial
Calculate RSBI; target <105
↓

YES/NO ➜ Return to Screening—treat to reduce respiratory load
↓

Continue spontaneous breathing trial

CPAP with flow-by trigger, no change in CPAP or Fio_2 over course of 1-hour trial
Failure criteria:
RR >35 breaths/min for 5 min
Sao_2 <90% for 30 sec or more
HR >140 beats/min, or sustained Δ >20% in either direction
BP_{syst} >180 mm Hg or <90 mm Hg
Increased anxiety, agitation, or diaphoresis
↓

PASS/FAIL ➜ Return to Screening
↓

Does not require suctioning more than 4 h/day
Present evidence of ability to protect airway (cough, gag reflex)
No evidence of upper airway obstruction in previous 48 h
No history of reintubation for excessive tracheal secretions in previous 48 h
↓

T-piece trial (optional)
↓

EXTUBATE

BP, Blood pressure; CPAP, continuous positive airway pressure; HR, heart rate; RR respiratory rate; RSBI, rapid shallow breathing index.

normality of electrolytes affecting muscle function (e.g., calcium, phosphate, and potassium) must be assured. If the aforementioned conditions are addressed, weaning may be attempted.

There are four methods of weaning. Simplest is to perform spontaneous breathing trials each day with a T-piece circuit providing oxygen-enriched gas. Initially brief (5 to 10 minutes), the trials can be increased in frequency and duration until the patient can breathe spontaneously for several hours. An alternative is to perform a single daily T-piece trial of up to 2 hours in duration; if successful, the patient is extubated; if not, the next attempt is made the following day. Much more common (and popular) are SIMV and PSV, which in fact are often combined. Ventilatory assistance is decreased gradually by decreasing f or the amount of pressure. When combined, f is set to zero before the level of pressure is decreased. Pressure support of 5 to 8 cm H_2O is used widely to compensate for the resistance inherent in the ventilator circuit, and patients who can breathe comfortably at that level should be able to be extubated, although the minimal level of assistance in these modes has never been well defined. Randomized, controlled trials indicate that the process of weaning takes up to three times as long when IMV is used rather than trials of spontaneous breathing. Approximately 10% to 20% of patients require reintubation, defining a subgroup of patients with mortality rate that is sixfold higher, which may be a marker of more severe underlying illness. Use of NIV following extubation may improve the likelihood of successful extubation.

SPECIAL AIRWAY CONSIDERATIONS

Unplanned Extubation

Unplanned extubation (usually by the patient) is a morbid event that occurs in approximately 10% of patients receiving MV. Risk factors include chronic respiratory failure, poor fixation of the airway device, orotracheal intubation (which is decidedly uncomfortable), and inadequate sedation. The associated complications include reintubation (required in one half of cases), pneumonia, vocal cord trauma, and rarely loss of the airway with attendant cardiovascular and neurologic complications. Reintubation is more likely in the setting of accidental intubation, decreased mentation, occurrence outside a process of active weaning, and $Pao_2:Fio_2$ ratio lower than 200. The risk of unplanned extubation can be reduced by adequate, appropriate sedation, vigilance during position of the patient and bedside procedures, durable fixation of the airway device, and daily screening and assessment of patient readiness for liberation from the ventilator.

Reintubation

Approximately 20% of patients will require reintubation, which can occur even if protocols are followed and the patient meets all criteria for extubation. The rate varies widely among units; a rate that is "too low" may imply that patients are not being weaned aggressively enough, whereas a rate that is "too high" may reflect a high proportion of patients with neurologic impairment, who are at highest risk. Interestingly, weaning protocols, which are designed to liberate patients from MV sooner, are associated paradoxically with lower rates of reintubation. Reintubation may be a marker of severity of illness, but it is associated with substantially increased risks of pneumonia and death. The cause may either be airway compromise or failure of lung/chest wall mechanics (weaning failure).

Tracheostomy

It is challenging to identify patients who will not be able to be removed from the ventilator. Possible reasons include airway obstruction, anxiety or agitation (requiring heavy doses of sedatives), aspiration syndromes, alkalosis, bronchospasm/wheezing, COPD, critical illness polyneuropathy or other forms of neuromuscular disease, electrolyte abnormalities, heart disease, hypothyroidism, morbid obesity, nutrition (overfeeding or underfeeding), opioids, oversedation, pleural effusion (if large), pulmonary edema, and sepsis.

The timing of tracheostomy remains controversial. There is no consensus definition of when a tracheostomy is "early" (fewer than 10 days?) or "late" (more than 21 days?), although trends are toward earlier performance, with decreased sedation requirements and putative decreased risk of VAP, greater patient comfort,

and facilitated weaning subsequently. The shorter tube decreases airway resistance and work of breathing, and facilitates pulmonary toilet by suctioning. Percutaneous tracheostomy has decreased the morbidity of tracheostomy substantially. However, modern high-volume, low-pressure cuffs on endotracheal tubes permit translaryngeal intubation for several weeks with relative safety. Patients who are unstable hemodynamically, coagulopathic, or on high levels of PEEP may benefit from having tracheostomy postponed until they are more stable.

For the chapter's Suggested Readings list, please visit the book at www.ExpertConsult.inkling.com.

ADVANCED TECHNIQUES IN MECHANICAL VENTILATION

Jared M. Huston, Marc J. Shapiro, Soumitra R. Eachempati, and Philip S. Barie

KEY POINTS

■ Mechanical ventilation (MV) must support gas exchange and promote patient comfort while minimizing lung injury due to elevated airway pressures.

■ Protective, low tidal volume ventilation reduces morbidity and mortality rates in patients following acute lung injury (ALI) and acute respiratory distress syndrome (ARDS).

■ Pressure-controlled ventilation (PCV) determines inhaled tidal volumes via a preset inspiratory pressure and intrinsic respiratory mechanics.

■ Airway pressure release ventilation (APRV) allows for spontaneous and nonspontaneous ventilation, and may reduce patient-ventilator asynchrony and overall work of breathing.

■ Permissive hypercapnia allows CO_2 concentrations to increase in conjunction with reduced tidal volumes, in order to decrease airway pressures and prevent barotrauma.

■ Proportional assist ventilation varies gas flow in response to patient demand as a form of synchronized partial ventilatory assistance (closed-loop model).

■ Neurally adjusted ventilator assist delivers support in proportion to respiratory drive, which is measured via electrical activity of the diaphragm (EAdi).

■ Administration of nitric oxide (NO) or surfactant has theoretical advantages for improving oxygen exchange, but is used sparingly outside the neonatal population.

■ Additional methods of ventilatory support that may benefit select patient populations include extracorporeal membrane oxygenation (ECMO), high-frequency oscillatory ventilation (HFOV), positive end-expiratory pressure (PEEP), and prone positioning.

Modern positive-pressure MV emerged more than 50 years ago. The primary goal is to assist patients who cannot maintain adequate exchange of oxygen and carbon dioxide between the alveolar air spaces and capillaries. Clinical experience has taught that assisting gas exchange is but one important function of MV. Avoiding lung injury from high positive airway pressures, referred to as *ventilator-induced lung injury* (VILI), is another essential task. As a result, methods for noninvasive ventilation, such as *bilevel positive*

airway pressure (BiPAP), have emerged as useful alternatives to endotracheal intubation.

The science of ventilator management is advancing rapidly. Clinicians can now support critically ill patients who otherwise would have died owing to human and machine limitations. This chapter focuses on innovations in ventilatory support and introduces some newer technologies that may provide benefits to patients with *acute respiratory failure* (ARF) secondary to ALI and ARDS.

IMPAIRED OXYGENATION FOLLOWING ACUTE LUNG INJURY

Patients with ALI (PaO_2:$FIO_2 < 300$) or the more severe ARDS (PaO_2:$FIO_2 < 200$) are difficult to oxygenate because of reactive airways, lung edema, and inflammation. This condition is characterized pathologically by increased permeability of the alveolar-capillary barrier, and accelerated influx of neutrophils. Lung edema and inflammation in ALI and ARDS is heterogeneous, and matching of ventilation and perfusion ($\dot{V}/\dot{Q}$) varies throughout different lung regions. It is recognized that MV can increase lung inflammation, exacerbate tissue injury, and increase risks of morbidity and mortality.

Ventilator-Induced Lung Injury

VILI results from excessive mechanical stresses causing alveolar overdistention, usually from high tidal volumes (V_T) and airway pressures. Alveolar overdistention induces a local pulmonary and systemic proinflammatory cytokine response. Limiting alveolar overdistention and phasic alveolar recruitment and derecruitment of lung tissue (*atelectrauma*) can reduce inflammation. Experimental and clinical data suggest that the proinflammatory response driving VILI is attenuated by protective, low V_T ventilation tactics. New modes of MV are designed specifically to minimize iatrogenic injury, and this approach is now a fundamental tenet of modern critical care (Table 1).

Alveolar overdistention secondary to elevated airway pressures or high V_T is referred to as *barotrauma* or *volutrauma*. As such, peak and plateau airway pressures and V_T are critical parameters to monitor during MV. The Acute Respiratory Distress Syndrome Network (ARDSnet) trial is a landmark study that highlighted the lethal consequences of high V_T and airway pressures in patients requiring MV. In this randomized, multicenter trial, patients with ALI received either traditional ventilation with initial V_T of 12 mL/kg and plateau pressures of 50 cm H_2O or less, or lower V_T of 6 mL/kg and plateau pressures of 30 cm H_2O or less. The trial was stopped early because of a statistically significant survival advantage in the lower V_T group.

In addition to demonstrating improved outcomes following ALI/ARDS with lower V_T, the ARDSnet trial found that ventilating

TABLE 1: Modes of Ventilation

Ventilatory Mode/Strategy	Advantages	Disadvantages
Volume-controlled ventilation	Predetermined respiratory rate and tidal volume	Barotrauma
Low tidal volume ventilation	Lower airway pressures, decreased mortality rate	Hypoventilation, hypoxemia
Pressure-controlled ventilation	Predetermined airway pressures	Hypoventilation, hypoxemia
Inverse-ratio ventilation	Increases alveolar recruitment	Auto-PEEP, barotrauma
Airway pressure release ventilation	Predetermined airway pressure, allows for spontaneous breathing	Hypoventilation
Permissive hypercapnia	Allows for lower tidal volumes and airway pressures	Increased ICP, arrhythmias
Proportional assist ventilation	Decreases patient-ventilator asynchrony, adapts to respiratory mechanics	No predetermined tidal volume, requires measurable inspiratory drive
Adaptive support ventilation	Predetermined minute ventilation	Higher tidal volumes
Neurally adjusted ventilatory assist	Decreases patient-ventilator asynchrony	Requires invasive monitor to measure electrical activity of diaphragm
Mandatory minute ventilation	Predetermined minute ventilation, allows spontaneous breathing	Atelectasis, variable airway pressures
Extracorporeal membrane oxygenation	Avoids mechanical lung stress	Requires cardiopulmonary bypass
High-frequency oscillatory ventilation	Allows for lower tidal volumes	Higher mean airway pressures, requires heavy sedation
Prone positioning	Decreases $\dot{V}/\dot{Q}$ mismatch	Pressure sores, increased sedation

ICP, Intracranial pressure; PEEP, positive end-expiratory pressure.

patients with a lower V_T results in less circulatory, coagulation, and renal failure. The lower V_T group also had greater reductions in plasma interleukin 6 concentration. Taken together, these findings suggest a reduced systemic inflammatory response to VILI.

ALTERNATIVES TO CONVENTIONAL MECHANICAL VENTILATION

Pressure-Controlled Ventilation

Most conventional MV is volume-cycled, in which the desired V_T is determined by a setting on the ventilator. Airway pressures depend on the volume of gas delivered and the patient's underlying respiratory mechanics. PCV is a unique modality in that inspiratory pressure is set beforehand, and the V_T delivered to the patient is dependent on airway resistance and lung compliance. Inspiratory airway pressure increases early in the respiratory cycle and is maintained throughout the delivery phase. The inspiratory flow decreases exponentially during lung inflation in order to keep the airway pressure at the preselected value. This flow pattern can improve gas exchange, and it is believed to be the major benefit of PCV. PCV is a nonspontaneous modality, and requires no active patient participation. The primary disadvantage of PCV is that V_T depends on airway pressures and mechanical properties of the lungs. For example, with a constant peak airway pressure, inflation volume will decrease as airway resistance increases or lung compliance decreases. Inflation volumes can vary substantially during PCV. In patients with ARDS and damaged, noncompliant lungs, PCV can result in hypoventilation and hypoxemia.

A recent randomized controlled trial compared targeted low airway pressures (plateau pressure <30 cm H_2O) with an ARDSnet (low V_T)

control ventilation strategy in 20 patients with ARDS. There were no significant differences in duration of ventilation, duration of intensive care unit (ICU) stay, or duration of hospital stay between groups. The treatment group had significantly lower systemic proinflammatory cytokine concentrations, which could result in less organ damage. Additional larger studies are needed to evaluate differences in mortality rate.

Open Lung Ventilation

The concept of "open lung" ventilation refers to preventing repetitive opening and closing of alveoli, which may maximize gas exchange and prevent atelectrauma and associated proinflammatory cytokine production. Atelectasis occurs most often during exhalation when gas exits the lungs. Delivering high gas pressures during exhalation via PEEP is one method of preventing alveolar collapse. Recent studies examined the effects of "open lung" ventilation and recruitment strategies combined with PCV and low V_T on outcomes in patients with ALI and ARDS. Villar et al conducted a multicenter, randomized controlled trial comparing high PEEP and low V_T ventilation with conventional V_T (9 to 11 mL/kg) ventilation, and observed significant reductions in ICU and hospital mortality rate and ventilator-free days in the high PEEP/low V_T group. It is unclear whether the survival benefits resulted from low V_T, high PEEP, or both. To address this question, Meade et al conducted a multicenter, randomized study comparing low V_T ventilation with a combined approach of low V_T, high PEEP, and recruitment maneuvers in patients with ALI and ARDS. The authors did not observe any differences in all-cause hospital mortality rate, but found that the experimental group had lower rates of refractory hypoxemia and death with refractory hypoxemia. The additive benefits of an "open lung" approach to low V_T ventilation require further evaluation.

Inverse-Ratio Ventilation

Inverse-ratio ventilation (IRV) is a combination of PCV (hence, PC-IRV), when the ratio of inspiratory time (I) and expiratory time (E) is adjusted. It is often the first modality attempted after conventional MV fails (Fig. 1). A normal I:E ratio is 1:4. Decreasing the inspiratory flow rate will increase I and I:E to 2:1 or even 4:1. Increasing I can improve alveolar recruitment by preventing alveolar collapse. Studies of PC-IRV in ARDS demonstrate improvements in oxygenation. The early use of PC-IRV can facilitate tapering of high *fractions of inspired oxygen* (FIO_2) and decreasing high PEEP and *peak inspiratory pressures* (PIPs). A potential drawback to PC-IRV is stacking of breaths (auto-PEEP), with resulting alveolar hyperinflation, high airway pressures, and barotrauma. Increased transthoracic pressures from auto-PEEP can reduce cardiac output (Q) via decreased central venous return. To date, there are no studies comparing mortality rate differences between conventional and IRV.

Airway Pressure Release Ventilation

APRV is a pressure-limited, time-cycled, "open lung" ventilatory strategy. APRV is similar to *continuous positive airway pressure* (CPAP), with the addition of regular, brief, intermittent reductions of airway pressure to facilitate exhalation. APRV is feasible in patients breathing spontaneously and apneic patients requiring full ventilatory support. APRV can decrease peak airway pressures, lower intrathoracic pressures, reduce interference with venous return and cardiac output, and improve $\dot{V}/\dot{Q}$ matching. APRV in patients breathing spontaneously can reduce sedation requirements and help avoid neuromuscular blockade. Patient-ventilator asynchrony is potentially reduced as well. Facilitated exhalation during APRV may benefit patients with bronchospasm or small-airways disease. APRV is also useful as a weaning mode. Disadvantages of APRV include those of PCV, increased effects of airway and circuit resistance on ventilation, decreased transpulmonary pressure, and potential interference with spontaneous ventilation.

The terminology of APRV differs from other ventilation modes. Programmable variables include high pressure (P_{high}), low pressure (P_{low}), time high (T_{high}), and time low (T_{low}). The P_{high} term refers to the baseline airway pressure, alternatively called CPAP, inflation pressure, or P1 pressure. P_{low} describes the airway pressure following pressure release (alternatively called PEEP, release pressure, or P2 pressure). T_{high} refers to the duration of P_{high} (T1), whereas T_{low} refers to the duration of P_{low} (T2). Mean airway pressure can be calculated from the equation:

$$\frac{(P1 \times T1) + (P2 \times T2)}{T2 + T1}$$

There are no standardized initial settings for transitioning patients to APRV. Pressure settings are derived from conventional MV values.

FIGURE 1 Hierarchical ventilator management in a patient with acute respiratory distress syndrome (ARDS). ECMO, Extracorporeal membrane oxygenation; PBW, predicted body weight; PCV, pressure-controlled ventilation; PEEP, positive end-expiratory pressure; VT, tidal volume. *(Modified from Haas CF, Bauser KA: Advanced ventilator modes and techniques.* Crit Care Nurs Q 35:27–38, 2012.)

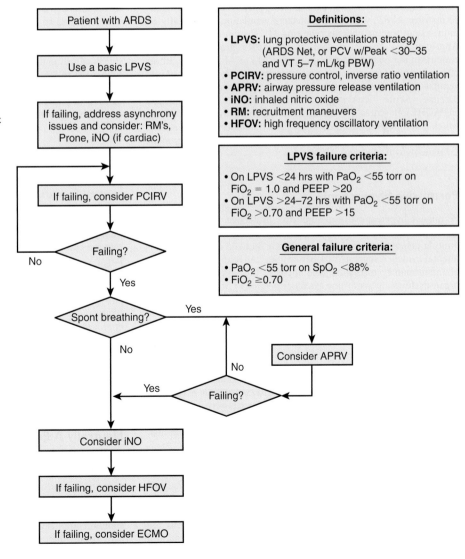

For example, the plateau airway pressure (P_{plat}) from conventional ventilation (if not higher than 35 cm H_2O) is converted to P_{high}, aiming for a $\dot{V}_E$ of 2 to 3 L/minute (lower than with conventional ventilation). P_{low} is set initially at 0 cm H_2O. T_{high} is a minimum of 4 seconds, and T_{low} is set at 0.8 second (0.5 to 1.0 second). A higher P_{high} (40 to 45 cm H_2O) is required occasionally for patients with low compliance (e.g., morbid obesity, abdominal distention). As lung mechanics improve, T_{high} is lengthened progressively to 12 to 15 seconds, usually in 1- to 2-second increments. Longer T_{high} prevents cyclic opening and closing of small airways that is responsible for VILI. T_{low} is optimized when expiratory flow decreases to 25% to 50% of peak expiratory flow. Spontaneous breathing is permitted throughout the ventilator cycle.

Clinical improvement is often delayed after transitioning to APRV. Studies suggest that maximum improvement may not occur until 8 to 16 hours after initiating APRV. Discontinuation of APRV is guided by general principles of weaning. In APRV, changes are made in P_{high} and T_{high}. P_{high} is decreased in increments of 2 to 3 cm H_2O down to approximately 15 cm H_2O, and T_{high} is lengthened progressively to 12 to 15 seconds, usually in 1- to 2-second increments. Minute ventilation is monitored for signs of hypoventilation. The goal is to transition to pure CPAP of 6 to 12 cm H_2O, at which point the patient may be evaluated as a candidate for extubation.

Currently, there are no randomized controlled trials comparing APRV with protective, low V_T ventilation in patients with ALI and ARDS. Retrospective studies suggest that APRV can improve oxygenation while reducing peak airway pressures in patients with ALI and ARDS. Maxwell et al conducted a prospective, randomized study comparing APRV with lung protective ventilation in critically ill, multisystem trauma patients requiring MV for more than 72 hours. Approximately 45% of patients in the APRV group and 34% of patients in the lung protective group had ALI or ARDS. The authors observed a trend for increased ventilator days, ICU length of stay, and ventilator-associated pneumonia in the APRV group. Of note, the baseline Acute Physiology and Chronic Health Evaluation (APACHE) II scores are significantly higher in the APRV group, which could have contributed to the poor outcomes. Further studies are required before APRV is considered a standard ventilatory tactic for patients with ALI and ARDS.

Permissive Hypercapnia

Permissive hypercapnia is an adjunctive protective ventilatory strategy for ARF. Permissive hypercapnia aims to avoid barotrauma by limiting airway pressure to approximately 30 to 35 cm H_2O. Experimental evidence suggests that barotrauma can stimulate the release of inflammatory mediators, and increase the severity of multiple organ dysfunction syndrome. As described for PCV, limiting airway pressure in noncompliant lungs can result in hypoventilation and hypercapnia. This strategy is employed purposely during permissive hypercapnia, thus permitting Pa_{CO_2} to increase considerably above normal concentrations. Hickling et al evaluated the adjunctive benefits of permissive hypercapnia with low V_T synchronized intermittent mandatory ventilation (SIMV), reporting that limiting PIPs to 30 to 40 cm H_2O but allowing Pa_{CO_2} to increase results in decreased expected mortality rates in patients with ARDS. Amato et al reported similar results in the first controlled study of permissive hypercapnia in patients with ARDS. Mortality rates with protective ventilation and permissive hypercapnia were lower at 28 days, but differences in hospital survival were not significant.

Despite the few studies demonstrating a benefit of permissive hypercapnia in ARDS, many concerns remain over the physiologic consequences of hypercapnia on the nervous, cardiovascular, and renal systems. The physiologic limits of permissive hypercapnia (e.g., Pa_{CO_2} up to 80 mm Hg, arterial pH down to 7.20) are not widely achieved. Safe levels of Pa_{CO_2} and respiratory acidosis are unknown. There is also concern for alveolar derecruitment and possible worsening of $\dot{V}/\dot{Q}$ mismatching. Permissive hypercapnia is contraindicated with elevated intracranial pressure, cerebral edema, depressed cardiac function, arrhythmias, increased pulmonary vascular resistance, and biochemical disturbances related to systemic acidosis.

Proportional Assist Ventilation

Proportional assist ventilation (PAV) is a form of synchronized partial ventilatory support that augments the flow of gas in response to patient-generated effort. The ventilator augments the patient's inspiratory effort without using a preselected target volume or pressure. PAV is a newer ventilator mode referred to as *closed-loop* ventilation, whereby intrinsic respiratory drive is used to determine the level of mechanical support. The patient initiates and determines the depth and frequency of the breaths independent of the ventilator. In theory, closed-loop ventilation allows the patient to achieve a pattern of ventilation and breathing that is adequate and comfortable, while avoiding patient-ventilator asynchrony. Advantages of PAV may include reduced peak airway pressures, less hyperventilation and alveolar overdistention, preservation and enhancement of respiratory drive, and improved efficiency of negative-pressure ventilation.

Effective use of PAV requires an understanding of the patient's ventilatory mechanics. This entails measuring the patient's airway resistance, compliance, and intrinsic PEEP (auto-PEEP), in order to determine the ventilatory load and assistance required. Younes et al proposed an innovative method for the noninvasive determination of passive elasticity during PAV. Once the patient's elastance and resistance are determined, the PAV parameters are set followed by PEEP, adjusting the peak pressure limit to 30 cm H_2O, adjusting volume assist to 8% of elastance, and then observing the patient's ventilation, breathing pattern, and peak airway pressure. The efficacy of PAV in patients with ALI and ARDS is unclear, and clinical use of this modality remains limited.

Adaptive Support Ventilation

Adaptive support ventilation (ASV) is a novel mode of ventilation that purportedly provides lung-protective levels of V_T and respiratory rate. A target $\dot{V}_E$ is set, and the ventilator determines an optimal V_T and rate combination that result in the least work of breathing. Theoretically, if lung compliance is reduced, a smaller V_T and faster rate are chosen, whereas in patients with obstructive lung disease, a larger V_T and slower rate are chosen to minimize air trapping. A ventilator mode that automatically adjusts inspired volume on the basis of the patient's actual respiratory mechanics may help to minimize iatrogenic lung injury, particularly in settings in which constant vigilance and frequent manual adjustments are impractical. Dongelmans et al reported data on 346 patients after cardiothoracic surgery who were placed on ASV ($n = 262$) or pressure control ventilation with pressure support (PCV/PS) ($n = 84$) targeted to a V_T of approximately 6 mL/kg. Mean V_T for ASV was 8.3 mL/kg versus 7.3 mL/kg for PCV/PS. Of note, V_T in ASV was more than 8 mL/kg in 55% of patients and more than 10 mL/kg in 12% of patients.

Neutrally Adjusted Ventilator Assist

Neutrally adjusted ventilator assist (NAVA) is another form of "closed-loop" ventilation when the duration and level of ventilator support is determined from measures of intrinsic respiratory effort. A primary goal of partial assist modes is to synchronize the beginning and end of ventilatory assist with the beginning and end of spontaneous inspiration. NAVA functions by measuring electrical activity of the diaphragm (EAdi) via an esophageal electrode positioned at the level of the diaphragm. The EAdi waveform is processed and then used to control MV. In theory, using the EAdi to guide ventilation may help synchronize patient efforts and ventilator support.

Clinical studies of NAVA are limited. Spahija et al conducted a prospective, comparative, crossover study of 14 (12 with chronic obstructive pulmonary disease) nonsedated ICU patients receiving MV to compare NAVA with standard PSV. The authors observed significantly reduced delays in ventilator triggering and cycling in the NAVA group. Arterial blood gases were similar between groups. Terzi et al conducted a prospective, interventional study on 11 consecutive medical ICU patients with ARDS attributable to pulmonary disease. In these spontaneously breathing patients, the authors observed that NAVA decreased patient-ventilator asynchrony compared with PSV.

Mandatory Minute Ventilation

Mandatory minute ventilation (MMV) is a ventilator mode in which the minimum level of $\dot{V}E$ required by the patient is provided. If the patient's pressure-supported, spontaneous ventilation fails to meet the predetermined $\dot{V}E$, the ventilator makes up the difference. If spontaneous breathing exceeds the target $\dot{V}E$, no support is provided. MMV is also a closed-loop ventilation mode because the ventilator varies its parameters in response to the patient's ventilatory requirements. MMV is believed to be best suited for patients with severe neuromuscular disease, with drug overdose, or under heavy sedation. A disadvantage of MMV is that alveolar ventilation may not be matched equally with exhaled $\dot{V}E$, thus diminishing closing volumes and leading to atelectasis. MMV and other closed-loop ventilator modes require additional evaluation and testing before they can be incorporated widely into clinical practice.

High-Frequency Oscillatory Ventilation

HFOV is a ventilatory tactic that has seen success in neonates and children. This modality limits alveolar distention with small V_T (often smaller than anatomic dead space) and a high-frequency respiratory rate (2.5 to 30 Hz). HFOV achieves many of the goals of protective lung ventilation strategies, including alveolar derecruitment and overdistention. In adults, HFOV is used to support complex thoracic surgical procedures (e.g., one-lung or split-lung ventilation), or to facilitate fiberoptic bronchoscopy or healing of a bronchopleural fistula. Limited studies suggest that HFOV improves oxygenation more rapidly compared with higher V_T conventional MV, but these effects are short-lived, and 30-day mortality rates are unchanged. A recent meta-analysis of eight randomized controlled trials including both adults and children with ARDS showed significantly reduced mortality rate with HFOV, and a significantly lower incidence of treatment failure (refractory hypoxemia, hypercapnia, hypotension, or barotrauma). Additional, ongoing large multicenter trials should help determine the effectiveness of HFOV, particularly in comparison to newer protective, low V_T strategies.

▓ PHARMACOTHERAPY

Surfactant Administration

ALI is characterized by pulmonary and endothelial inflammation causing pulmonary edema, hypoxemia from $\dot{V}/\dot{Q}$ mismatching, pulmonary hypertension and fibrosis, and destruction and impaired synthesis of surfactant, all resulting in worsening atelectasis and poor pulmonary compliance. Intratracheal administration of surfactant is a potential means of improving lung mechanics and gas exchange. Whereas surfactant administration has clinical use for neonatal

respiratory disress syndrome, trials of adult patients do not demonstrate a survival benefit for any of several variations of natural or synthetic surfactant. Of note, a recent pooled analysis of five multicenter studies of patients with ARDS treated with recombinant surfactant protein-C (rSP-C) demonstrated reduced mortality rate on post hoc analysis in the subgroup of patients with ARDS secondary to pneumonia or aspiration. The overall patient population did not benefit from surfactant administration, but this group of patients also sustained trauma or sepsis. Additional clinical trials consisting of more homogenous patient populations are necessary before surfactant administration is considered a standard therapy.

Inhaled Nitric Oxide

NO is a selective pulmonary vasodilator that acts on the alveolar endothelium to produce regional vasodilation in well-ventilated lung units where it is distributed. Inhaled nitric oxide (iNO) at a dose of 40 ppm can improve $\dot{V}/\dot{Q}$ mismatching, hypoxemia, and pulmonary hypertension in patients with ALI and ARDS. By contrast, administration of systemic vasodilators can cause pulmonary vasodilation in poorly ventilated lung regions, interfere with hypoxic vasoconstriction, and lead to hypoxemia and worsened $\dot{V}/\dot{Q}$ mismatch. Nitric oxide is also a bronchodilator and has anti-inflammatory properties that may benefit lung transplant patients. iNO eventually diffuses into the bloodstream, where it is metabolized rapidly and excreted via the urine, thus minimizing any systemic effects. A recent meta-analysis of 14 randomized controlled trials showed no statistically significant benefit of iNO on overall mortality rate, duration of ventilation, ventilator-free days, or hospital or ICU length of stay. There is a statistically significant improvement in oxygenation within the first 24 hours of treatment. There is also a significantly increased risk of renal impairment with iNO. Currently, iNO is not recommended for patients with ALI and ARDS.

▓ UNCONVENTIONAL METHODS OF VENTILATION

Extracorporeal Membrane Oxygenation

ECMO permits oxygenation of blood and removal of CO_2 via an extracorporeal circuit. ECMO requires institution of intermediate-term cardiopulmonary bypass for the treatment of potentially reversible cardiac or pulmonary failure. ECMO can provide sufficient gas exchange to allow reduced positive-pressure ventilation. The theoretical benefits of ECMO for ARF is that severely inflamed and damaged lungs can rest and heal rather than endure the mechanical stresses of high-level ventilator support necessary to achieve adequate gas exchange. Reports of successful use of ECMO for adult trauma patients date back to the early 1970s. The National Institutes of Health (NIH) sponsored a randomized, multi-institutional trial of ECMO in 1979, but that study failed to demonstrate a significant survival benefit. In 2006, Cordell-Smith et al reported in a retrospective study that a high proportion of adult trauma patients treated with ECMO for severe lung injury survived. In 2010, Arit et al reported on the use of ECMO in severe trauma patients with resistant cardiopulmonary failure and coexisting hemorrhagic shock. These retrospective findings compare favorably to conventional ventilation outcomes but still lack the power of randomized controlled trials. Interestingly, a recent meta-analysis of eight randomized controlled trials including both adults and children with ARDS showed significantly reduced mortality rate with HFOV, and a significantly lower incidence of treatment failure (refractory hypoxemia, hypercapnia, hypotension, or barotrauma).

ECMO is currently an option for support of adult patients with ARDS when other treatment options have failed. This recommendation is paradoxical because ECMO is most effective when instituted early. Indeed, mortality rates from ARF increase the longer a patient receives MV before initiation of ECMO. Technical advances in ECMO have resulted in greater biocompatibility and a lower rate of procedure-related complications. These improvements are leading to a reevaluation of the role for ECMO in patients with ARDS.

Prone Positioning

Prone positioning is accomplished using specialized rotary beds and equipment that allows the patient to be transitioned periodically (e.g., every 12 hours) from supine to prone. Ventilated lung segments tend to be in nondependent portions of lung, whereas perfused lung segments (and higher pulmonary vascular pressures and lung edema) reside in dependent lung regions. Positive-pressure ventilation can exacerbate this mismatch further. Prone positioning can improve oxygenation by decreasing $\dot{V}/\dot{Q}$ mismatch. Prone positioning reverses the dependent lung regions. Newly dependent, well-ventilated lung segments then receive perfusion until the effects of gravity and positive airway pressures restore the prior $\dot{V}/\dot{Q}$ inequalities over a period of several hours. Prone positioning can also facilitate drainage of secretions from the lungs and airways. A large, multicenter, randomized controlled trial by Gattinoni et al showed a significant improvement in 10-day mortality rate with prone positioning, but this benefit did not persist beyond ICU discharge. A recent meta-analysis of seven randomized controlled trials including ALI and ARDS patients showed no significant reduction in ICU mortality rate. When the four more recent studies including only ARDS patients were reevaluated, however, a significant ICU survival advantage for prone positioning was noted in retrospect. Prone positioning is not associated with increased major airway complications (e.g., tube dislodgement), a fear of many clinicians while the patient is prone. Complications of prone positioning can include pressure sores, need for increased sedation, facial edema, and difficulty maintaining airway patency or restoring it when the patient is inverted. Further studies are needed to evaluate the efficacy of prone positioning in patients with respiratory failure.

THE FUTURE

MV remains a vital component of modern critical care. Current practices encourage minimizing the risks of barotrauma and atelectrauma by instituting protective, low V_T strategies. Advances in microprocessor technology have led to the development of new, sophisticated ventilatory modalities. The precise role for these newer modes is unclear because rigorous scientific evaluation is lacking. Future studies are needed to help clinicians apply this rapidly developing technology to our critically ill patients.

For the chapter's Suggested Readings list, please visit the book at www.ExpertConsult.inkling.com.

MANAGEMENT OF RENAL FAILURE: RENAL REPLACEMENT THERAPY AND DIALYSIS

Joseph M. Gutmann, Christopher McFarren, Lewis M. Flint, and Rodney Durham

Acute renal failure (ARF) is a common and devastating problem that contributes to morbidity and fatality in critically ill patients. ARF prolongs hospital stays and increases mortality rate. Although effective renal replacement therapy (RRT) is available, it is not ideal and the best therapy is prevention.

The kidneys are the primary regulators of volume and composition of the internal fluid environment and their excretion. Renal failure leads to regulatory function impairment, causing retention of nitrogenous waste products and disturbance in fluid, electrolyte, and acid-base balance. Renal injury in intensive care unit (ICU) patients is a progressive process, usually starting with a prerenal insult—which progresses to severe renal injury. Other systemic issues can worsen the renal injury.

ARF in critically ill patients is a growing clinical problem. Options for RRT in these patients use convective and diffusive clearance, which may be intermittent (as in classic hemodialysis) or continuous. RRT needs to be tailored to the needs of each patient. Current and future research studies are essential in improving outcomes.

INCIDENCE

ARF is defined as an abrupt and sustained decline in the glomerular filtration rate (GFR), which leads to accumulation of nitrogenous waste products and uremic toxins. In critically ill patients, more than 90% of the episodes of ARF are due to acute tubular necrosis (ATN) and are the result of ischemic or nephrotoxic cause (or a combination of both). ARF affects nearly 5% of all hospitalized patients and as many as 15% of critically ill patients. Like many other medical conditions, there is no gold standard of diagnosis, no specific histopathologic confirmation, and no uniform clinical picture.

The mortality rate of an isolated episode of ARF is approximately 10% to 15%. When it occurs in association with multiple organ dysfunction, as in the ICU setting, mortality rates are much greater and vary in published series between 40% and 90%.

In some cases, preexisting conditions may worsen. New major complications, such as sepsis and respiratory failure, may also develop after the onset of renal failure. Although ARF that requires RRT carries a high mortality rate, there is emerging evidence to suggest that milder forms of ARF that do not require supportive therapy with RRT have better patient outcomes.

Many aspects of surgical diseases and their care have the potential to impair renal function, either by toxic effects on the renal parenchyma or by reducing renal perfusion (or a combination of the two). The prevention of ARF in critical patients consists of minimizing toxicity and ensuring adequate blood flow. Avoidance of renal failure is preferred to any treatment. Therefore, renal function should be monitored closely so that adverse circumstances can be limited.

Given the impact of ARF on mortality rate, it is important to prevent ARF or hasten the resolution of even the mildest forms of ARF. The goals of a preventive strategy for the syndrome of ARF are to preserve renal function, to prevent death, to prevent complications of ARF (volume overload, acid-base disturbances, and electrolyte abnormalities), and to prevent the need for chronic dialysis (with minimum adverse effects).

This chapter explores preventive strategies, the major challenges ARF presents, and key issues to be considered. Can the patient be managed conservatively or will RRT be needed? If RRT is required, which form of RRT is most appropriate?

MECHANISM OF INJURY/ETIOLOGY

Diagnosis

Renal failure is measured routinely and easily in the ICU: the excretion of water-soluble waste products of nitrogen metabolism, urea, and creatinine and the production of urine. To understand renal failure, we need to reflect on some important aspects of renal physiology.

Water and Fluid Homeostasis

Because body water is the primary determinant of the osmolality of the extracellular fluid (ECF), disorders of body water homeostasis can be divided into hypo- and hyperosmolar disorders depending on whether there is an excess or deficiency of body water relative to body solute. The end result of any change in circulating blood volume is a change in sodium excretion by the kidneys. This is brought about by the activation of the sympathetic nervous system, the renin-angiotensin-aldosterone axis, and release/suppression of natriuretic peptides.

Assessment of Renal Function

Serum concentrations of blood urea nitrogen (BUN) and creatinine are the most commonly used markers of renal function. Urea is the end product of protein and amino acid catabolism. Under normal conditions, 80% to 90% of total nitrogen excretion is by the kidneys. Creatinine is formed in muscle by the nonenzymatic degradation of creatine and phosphocreatine, and is excreted primarily by glomerular filtration. A small percentage of creatinine is actively secreted into the glomerular filtrate and tubular reabsorption of creatinine is negligible.

Circulating concentrations of BUN and creatinine are determined not only by how efficiently they are excreted by the kidneys but by their rate of production. Urea formation depends on the amount of protein and amino acids catabolized. It is increased with high-protein diets, reabsorption of hematomas, and digestion of blood in the gastrointestinal (GI) tract. It is reduced in starvation. These factors may change the value of the BUN, even though renal function is adequate. Creatinine production reflects muscle mass. It is constant over the short term, and steadily diminishes if muscle mass is lost. Muscle mass diminishes with age, together with intrinsic renal function. Therefore, serum creatinine stays relatively constant over time.

Creatinine Clearance

Determination of the creatinine clearance (Ccr) provides a measure of renal function. Creatinine secretion and reabsorption in the kidneys is negligible. Clearance is defined as the volume of plasma or serum cleared by the kidneys over a period of time. It is calculated as:

$$Ccr (mL/minute) = (Ucr \times V)/Pcr$$

where Ucr is urine creatinine, Pcr is serum creatinine, and V is volume.

The clearance reflects the net effect of GFR, which is the amount of fluid filtered from the plasma in a given time by the kidneys. The most commonly used method for estimating Ccr is the Cockcroft-Gault formula:

TABLE 1: Adequate Urine Output

Age	Urine Output (mL/kg/min)
Infant (<10 kg)	2.0
Toddler (10–20 kg)	1.5
Child (20–50 kg)	1.0
Adult (>50 kg)	0.5

$$Ccr_{men} = GFR(mL/minute) = (140 - age) \times (ideal\ body\ weight\ [kg]/72 \times serum\ creatinine[mg/dL])$$

$$Ccr_{women} = Ccr_{men} \times 0.85$$

Normal GFR is 125 ± 15 mL/minute/1.73 m^2 body surface area (BSA).

Sodium has the highest serum concentration of all cations in the ECF. Any transport of sodium necessarily involves the transport of water. Renal sodium clearance is an important mechanism for the regulation of ECF volume and tonicity. Aldosterone promotes tubular reabsorption of sodium, and it is elaborated in response to changes in hydrostatic pressure within the glomerular arterioles. If renal blood flow or pressure is reduced, tubular sodium reabsorption is increased—thus preserving ECF volume. The ratio of sodium clearance to Ccr is known as the fractional excretion of sodium (FENa):

$$FENa = ([Una \times Pcr/Ucr \times Pna]) \times 100$$

Here, Una and Ucr are the urinary concentrations of sodium and creatinine, and Pna and Pcr are the serum levels of sodium and creatinine, respectively. If the FENa is very low (less than or equal to 1%), it may indicate inadequate renal arteriolar pressure—suggesting that factors other than intrinsic renal dysfunction are responsible for clinically inadequate renal function.

Urine Production and Output

The end result of renal function is the production of urine. Quantitative measurements of urine are important for assessing renal function. Urine output is highly sensitive to renal blood flow, making it a key indicator of renal function and total body vascular perfusion (Table 1).

MANAGEMENT OF PATIENTS

Conservative Management

Despite many advances in medical technology, the mortality and morbidity rates attributed to ARF in the ICU remain high. Primary strategies to prevent ARF still include adequate hydration, maintenance of mean arterial pressure (preferably MAP greater than 60 mm Hg), and minimization of exposure to potentially nephrotoxic agents. Although hydration was shown to be beneficial, the type of fluid to be used in a hydration regimen remains controversial.

Considering its low cost, low toxicity, and consistent benefit, NAC (N-acetylcysteine) administration with intravenous (IV) hydration should be considered to decrease the prevalence of nephropathy in high-risk patients. Note that the routine use of NAC is controversial and is not well studied.

Nonpharmacologic Strategies for Acute Renal Failure Prevention

Nonpharmacologic strategies to prevent ARF include ensuring adequate hydration (limiting dehydration), maintenance of adequate mean arterial pressures, and minimizing exposure to nephrotoxic agents. Four particular strategies are worth reviewing: (1) fluids, (2) aminoglycoside dosing, (3) lipid-soluble preparations of amphotericin, and (4) nonionic contrast agents.

Fluids

Adequate hydration is the cornerstone of renal failure prevention. One randomized controlled trial ($n = 1620$) compared hydration using 0.9% saline infusion with 0.45% saline in dextrose for prevention of radiocontrast-induced nephropathy in patients who underwent coronary angiography. Hydration with 0.9% saline infusion significantly reduced contrast nephropathy compared with 0.45% saline in dextrose hydration (0.7% vs. 2%, respectively; $P = .04$). This effect was greater in women, diabetics, and patients who received a large volume (greater than 250 mL) of a contrast agent. A recent single-center randomized controlled trial compared the efficacy of sodium bicarbonate with 0.9% saline hydration in preventing contrast nephropathy. In this study, 119 patients who had stable serum creatinine of at least 1.1 mg/dL were randomized to 154 mEq/L infusion of sodium chloride ($n = 59$) or sodium bicarbonate ($n = 60$) before and after contrast (iopamidol) administration. One of 59 patients (1.7%) in the group that received bicarbonate developed contrast nephropathy (defined as an increase of greater than or equal to 25% in serum creatinine from baseline within 48 hours) compared with 8 of 60 patients (13.3%) in the group that received saline ($P = .02$).

Nephrotoxin Exposure

Minimizing exposure to potentially nephrotoxic agents is an important strategy to prevent ARF in the ICU setting. Aminoglycosides, other antibiotics, amphotericin, and radiocontrast agents are the nephrotoxins encountered most commonly in the ICU. A systematic review in patients who had neutropenic fever and received aminoglycosides, however, found no significant differences in efficacy or nephrotoxicity between once daily and three times daily dosing.

The use of lipid formulations of amphotericin B seems to cause less nephrotoxicity compared with standard formulations, but direct comparisons of long-term safety are lacking. With regard to contrast media, one systematic review (31 randomized controlled trials, 5146 patients) compared low osmolality contrast media with standard contrast media. The study showed that low osmolality contrast media did not influence the development of ARF or the need for dialysis.

Pharmacologic Strategies for Acute Renal Failure Prevention

Loop Diuretics

Multiple small clinical trials studied the efficacy of loop diuretics in preventing ARF and have provided conflicting results. They have been underpowered, nonrandomized, or methodologically flawed. One systematic review that compared fluids with diuretics in people who were at risk for ARF from various causes did not show any benefit from diuretics with regard to prevalence of ARF, need for dialysis, or mortality.

N-Acetylcysteine

Systematic reviews found that NAC plus hydration reduced the incidence of contrast nephropathy more than hydration alone in people who had baseline renal impairment and underwent radiocontrast studies. A recent study, however, suggested that NAC could decrease

serum creatinine independently without any effect on GFR (as evaluated by other surrogate outcomes, such as serum cystatin C levels). Hence, the current implications of reduction in serum creatinine after contrast agent administration with the use of NAC remain unclear and need to be explored further.

INDICATIONS FOR RENAL REPLACEMENT THERAPY IN ACUTE RENAL FAILURE

As in chronic kidney disease, overt disturbances of ECF volume and body fluid composition remain the objective indications for initiation of RRT in patients with ARF (Table 2). These include volume overload, hyperkalemia, severe metabolic acidosis, uremia, and azotemia.

Volume Overload

Volume overload is generally recognized as an indication for RRT in ARF. All modalities of RRT are effective at diminishing intravascular volume. Subjective criteria for initiation of therapy include impairment of cardiopulmonary function by pulmonary vascular congestion or compromise of cutaneous integrity and wound healing by peripheral edema.

Mehta and colleagues performed a retrospective analysis of data from 522 critically ill patients who had ARF. Fifty-nine percent of these patients had been treated with diuretics. After adjustment for relevant covariates and the propensity for diuretic use, they observed a significant increase in the risk of death or nonrecovery of renal function (odds ratio 1.77, 95% confidence interval 1.14 to 2.76). On the basis of this, they concluded that diuretic therapy was potentially deleterious in patients who had ARF. They noted, however, that the increased risk was borne largely by patients who were unresponsive to diuretics. This suggested that this increased risk might reflect selection for a more severe degree of renal injury.

Hyperkalemia

The treatment of hyperkalemia with evidence of myocardial toxicity was one of the early indications for hemodialysis in ARF. Hyperkalemia is a well-recognized complication of ARF, which, if not treated, may be rapidly fatal. Most medical therapies for hyperkalemia (e.g., IV calcium to directly antagonize the effects of hyperkalemia on the myocardial cell membrane, and IV insulin/dextrose and IV or inhaled β-adrenergic agonists to shift potassium into the intracellular compartment) are primarily temporizing measures. Three modalities are available to decrease the total body potassium burden: (1) diuretic therapy, (2) enteric potassium-binding resins, and (3) dialysis.

In patients who have severe renal failure, diuretic therapy is generally ineffective in promoting kaliuresis due to lack of diuretic response. Although sodium polystyrene sulfonate can enhance fecal potassium losses, its use is limited in patients with recent intraabdominal or GI surgery, ileus, or bowel ischemia. Dialysis provides the most

TABLE 2: Indications for Renal Replacement Therapy

Volume overload
Hyperkalemia
Metabolic acidosis
Uremia
Azotemia

rapid means of decreasing the serum potassium concentration. However, because of variability in study design and evolution of dialysis techniques it is difficult to determine the expected potassium removal during a single dialysis treatment.

Even greater clearances of potassium may be achieved by using more permeable synthetic hemodialysis membranes and greater blood flow rates. However, the rate of potassium removal is ultimately limited by the rapid decrease in the concentration gradient between plasma and dialysate. As with volume status, a specific threshold level of serum potassium cannot be established as an indication for initiation of RRT. Myocardial toxicity from hyperkalemia is uncommon when the serum potassium concentration is less than 6.5 mmol/L. Therefore, decisions regarding the initiation of treatment for control of hyperkalemia must take into consideration the absolute level and rate of increase of serum potassium, the patient's overall condition, and the likely efficacy of medical therapy.

Metabolic Acidosis

The role of alkali therapy in the treatment of metabolic acidosis, particularly lactic acidosis, is controversial. The use of RRT as an alternative to alkali replacement in metabolic acidosis can avoid some of the deleterious effects ascribed to aggressive alkali replacement, specifically volume overload and hypernatremia. Although progressive metabolic acidosis is a generally accepted indication for RRT, clinical trials to establish a threshold blood pH or serum bicarbonate concentration or to demonstrate improved patient outcomes have not been performed.

Other Electrolyte Disturbances

RRT may be used for the treatment of a variety of other electrolyte disturbances that can occur in the setting of ARF. These include severe hyponatremia and hypernatremia, hyperphosphatemia, hypocalcemia and hypercalcemia, and hypermagnesemia. In the treatment of hyponatremia, caution must be used to ensure that rapid correction does not predispose to the development of the osmotic demyelination syndrome. A rapid decrease of serum phosphate and uric acid levels and control of acidemia using RRT are necessary in patients who have the tumor lysis syndrome to support recovery of renal function.

Uremia

The development of overt uremic signs or symptoms represents an obvious indication for initiation of RRT in ARF. Early manifestations of uremia, such as anorexia, nausea and vomiting, and pruritus, are nonspecific and may be difficult to differentiate from other comorbid conditions in patients who have critical illness. Mental status changes, which may represent uremic encephalopathy, also may be difficult to differentiate from other causes of delirium in the critically ill patient. Uremic pericarditis is usually a late complication, but requires urgent initiation of renal support given the high risk of intrapericardial hemorrhage and tamponade. As was emphasized more than 4 decades ago by Teschan et al, optimally RRT should be initiated before the onset of overt uremic manifestations.

Azotemia

In many patients, the sole indication for initiation of RRT in ARF is the presence of progressive azotemia in the absence of uremia or other indications for renal support. There is no consensus, however, on the degree of azotemia that warrants initiation of therapy. In a multicenter trial that evaluated the dosing strategies for RRT in critically ill patients who had ARF, we observed substantial variation in practice regarding the degree of azotemia deemed appropriate for initiation of treatment between practitioners within individual institutions and

between institutions (unpublished data). There are many experts in nephrology who feel that RRT should be initiated in critically ill patients with a BUN higher than 60 mg/dL.

TIMING OF INITIATION OF RENAL REPLACEMENT THERAPY

Beginning with the studies by Paul Teschan and colleagues, in the years following the Korean War numerous studies have attempted to define the criteria for timing of initiation of RRT in ARF. These studies attempted to determine the balance between three major competing risks: the inherent risk that results from delay in therapy; the potential risk of harm as a result of RRT, including complications of therapy and the potential that dialysis may prolong the course of ARF; and the risk that early initiation of therapy will result in patients undergoing treatment who, if managed conservatively, might recover renal function without requiring RRT.

In their landmark report, Teschan et al described a prospective uncontrolled series of 15 patients who had oliguric ARF who were treated with "prophylactic" hemodialysis defined as the initiation of dialysis before the BUN reached 100 mg/dL. Patients received daily dialysis (average duration 6 hours) using twin-coil cellulosic dialyzers at a blood flow of 75 to 250 mL/minute to maintain a predialysis BUN of less than 75 mg/dL. Caloric and protein intake were unrestricted. All-cause mortality rate was 33%. Mortality rate due to hemorrhage or sepsis was 20%. Although no control group was studied, the investigators reported that the results contrasted dramatically with their own past experience in patients in whom dialysis was not initiated until "conventional" indications were present.

Modalities for Renal Replacement Therapy in Acute Renal Failure

ARF is a common complication in critically ill patients and is associated with a mortality rate greater than 50%. As many as 70% of these patients require RRT, making it an important component of the management of ARF in the ICU. Ideally, RRT controls volume, corrects acid-base abnormalities, improves uremia through toxin clearance, promotes renal recovery, and improves survival without causing complications (such as bleeding from anticoagulation and hypotension). The available RRT options include intermittent hemodialysis (IHD), continuous RRT (CRRT), and sustained low-efficiency dialysis (SLED). Currently, there is insufficient evidence to establish which modality of RRT is best for ARF in the critically ill patient. There is a general consensus that patients receiving CRRT using lower blood flow rates and lower fluid removal rates have less cardiovascular instability/morbidity. Clearly, there is no significant difference in mortality rates with any of the available modalities. Understanding the advantages and limitations of the various dialysis modalities is essential for appropriate RRT selection in the ICU setting.

Principles of Renal Replacement Therapy

All forms of RRT rely on the principle of allowing water and solute transport through a semipermeable membrane and then discarding the waste products. Ultrafiltration is the process by which water is transported across a semipermeable membrane. Diffusion and convection are the two processes by which solutes are transported across the membrane. The available RRT modalities use ultrafiltration for fluid removal and diffusion, convection, or a combination of diffusion and convection to achieve solute clearance.

Ultrafiltration achieves volume removal by using a pressure gradient to drive water through a semipermeable membrane. This pressure gradient is known as the transmembrane pressure gradient and is the difference between plasma oncotic pressure and hydrostatic pressure. Determinants of the ultrafiltration rate include the membrane surface area, water permeability of the membrane, and transmembrane pressure gradient.

Diffusion occurs by movement of solutes from an area of higher solute concentration to an area of lower solute concentration across a semipermeable membrane. The concentration gradient is maximized and maintained throughout the length of the membrane by running the dialysate (an electrolyte solution usually containing sodium, bicarbonate, chloride, magnesium, and calcium) countercurrent to the blood flow. Solutes with a higher concentration in the blood, such as potassium and urea, move down their concentration gradient across the membrane to the dialysate compartment. Conversely, solutes with a higher concentration in the dialysate (such as bicarbonate) diffuse into the blood. Solute concentrations that are nearly equivalent in the blood and dialysate, such as sodium and chloride, move very little across the membrane. Because smaller solutes (such as urea and creatinine) diffuse more rapidly than larger solutes, lower-molecular-weight molecules (less than 500 daltons) are cleared more efficiently than heavier molecules. The rate of solute diffusion depends on blood flow rate, dialysate flow rate, duration of dialysis, concentration gradient across the membrane, and membrane surface area and pore size.

Convection occurs when the transmembrane pressure gradient drives water across a semipermeable membrane (as in ultrafiltration) but then "drags" with the water both small-molecular-weight (BUN, creatinine, potassium) and large-molecular-weight (inulin, β_2-microglobulin, tumor necrosis factor, vitamin B_{12}) solutes. Membrane pore diameter limits the size of the large solutes that can pass through. Increasing the transmembrane pressure difference allows more fluid and solutes to be "pulled" through the membrane. Because the efficiency of solute removal depends mainly on the ultrafiltration rate, typically at least 1 L of water needs to be pulled through the membrane each hour. The process of increasing the ultrafiltration rate to provide convective clearance of solutes is known as hemofiltration. Ultrafiltration rate is determined by the transmembrane pressure, water permeability of the membrane, and membrane surface area and pore size.

CLASSIFICATION OF RENAL REPLACEMENT THERAPIES

RRT for ARF can be classified as intermittent or continuous, based on the duration of the treatment. The duration of each intermittent therapy is less than 24 hours, whereas the duration of continuous therapy is at least 24 hours. The intermittent therapies include IHD and SLED. The continuous therapies include peritoneal dialysis and CRRT. Peritoneal dialysis is rarely used in the acute setting because it provides inefficient solute clearance in critically ill catabolic patients, increases the risk of peritonitis, compromises respiratory function by impeding diaphragmatic excursion, and is contraindicated in patients with recent abdominal surgery or abdominal sepsis.

Intermittent Hemodialysis

Traditionally, nephrologists have managed ARF with IHD—empirically delivered three to six times a week, 3 to 4 hours per session, with a blood flow rate of 200 to 350 mL/minute and a dialysate flow rate of 500 to 800 mL/minute. In IHD, solute clearance occurs mainly by diffusion—whereas volume is removed by ultrafiltration. The degree of solute clearance, also known as the "dialysis dose," is largely dependent on the rate of blood flow. Increasing the blood flow increases solute clearance. Decisions regarding dialysis duration and frequency are based on patient metabolic control, volume status, and presence of any hemodynamic instability.

Advantages of IHD include rapid solute and volume removal, which results in rapid correction of electrolyte disturbances, such as hyperkalemia, and rapid removal of drugs or other substances in fatal intoxications within a matter of hours. IHD also has a decreased need for anticoagulation compared with other types of RRT because of the higher blood flow rates and shorter duration of therapy.

The main disadvantage of IHD is the risk of systemic hypotension caused by rapid electrolyte shifts and fluid removal. Hypotension occurs in approximately 20% to 30% of hemodialysis treatments. Sodium modeling, cooling the dialysate, increasing the dialysate calcium concentration, IV albumin, and intermittent ultrafiltration may be used to improve hemodynamic stability during IHD. Despite this, approximately 10% of ARF patients cannot be treated with IHD because of hemodynamic instability. Systemic hypotension can limit the efficacy of IHD and result in poor solute clearance, insufficient acid-base correction, and persistent volume overload, because the rate of ultrafiltration necessary to maintain fluid balance is seldom achieved within the 4-hour dialysis session.

Rapid solute removal from the intravascular space can cause cerebral edema and increased intracranial pressure. ARF patients with head trauma or hepatic encephalopathy are at a significant risk of brain edema and even herniation. Finally, there is a lack of consensus as to how to assess solute clearance (dialysis dose) and what constitutes an adequate dose in ARF because the kinetics of urea in the end-stage renal disease patient cannot be extrapolated to patients with ARF.

Although the results of some studies suggested an advantage of daily HD over conventional IHD, it is unclear whether the increased dialysis dose improved outcome by improving uremic control or by reducing the volume of fluid removed during each dialysis session and resulting in less hemodynamic instability.

Continuous Renal Replacement Therapy

Although the worldwide standard for RRT is IHD, CRRT has emerged as a viable modality for management of hemodynamically unstable patients with ARF. Continuous therapies have evolved from systems that relied on arterial access and blood pressure to maintain blood flow through the extracorporeal circuit to pump-driven systems that use double-lumen venous catheters. The continuous arteriovenous hemofiltration (CAVH) circuit is now rarely used in CRRT because of poor solute removal and complications from arterial cannulation. Unlike IHD, CRRT is a continuous treatment occurring 24 hours a day—with a blood flow of 100 to 200 mL/minute and a dialysate flow of 17 to 40 mL/minute if a diffusive CRRT modality is used. The different CRRT modalities can use diffusion, convection, or a combination of both for solute clearance.

All types of CRRT use membranes that are highly permeable to water and low-molecular-weight solutes. CRRT modalities are classified by access type and method of solute clearance. Venovenous circuits are now the standard, and the various venovenous modalities of CRRT differ by their mechanism of solute removal. The four main types of CRRT in order of increasing complexity are slow continuous ultrafiltration, continuous venovenous hemofiltration (CVVH), continuous venovenous hemodialysis (CVVHD), and continuous venovenous hemodiafiltration (CVVHDF).

In slow continuous ultrafiltration, low-volume ultrafiltration at a rate of 100 to 300 mL/hour is performed to maintain fluid balance only and does not result in significant convective clearance of solutes. No fluids are administered either as dialysate or replacement fluids, and the purpose of treatment is for volume overload with or without renal failure. Indications include volume overload in patients with congestive heart failure refractory to diuretics.

In CVVH, solute clearance occurs by convection. Solutes are carried along with the bulk flow of fluid in a hydraulic-induced ultrafiltrate of blood. No dialysate is used. Clearances are similar for all solutes that have a molecular weight in the range at which the membrane is readily permeable. The rate at which ultrafiltration occurs is the major determinant of convective clearance. The ultrafiltration rate is determined by the transmembrane pressure, water permeability, pore size, surface area, and membrane thickness. Typically, hourly ultrafiltration rates of 1 to 2 L/hour are used to provide adequate solute removal. These high ultrafiltration rates rapidly cause volume contraction, hypotension, and loss of electrolytes. IV "replacement fluid" is provided to replace the excess volume being removed and to replenish desired solutes. Replacement fluid can be administered prefilter or postfilter.

In CVVHD, a dialysate solution runs countercurrent to the flow of blood at a rate of 1 to 2.5 L/hour. Solute removal occurs by diffusion. Unlike IHD, the dialysate flow rate is slower than the blood flow rate, allowing small solutes to equilibrate completely between the blood and dialysate. As a result, the dialysate flow rate approximates urea and Ccr. Ultrafiltration is used for volume control but can allow for some convective clearance at high rates. CVVHDF combines the convective solute removal of CVVH and the diffusive solute removal of CVVHD. As in CVVH, the high ultrafiltration rates used to provide convective clearance require the administration of IV replacement fluids.

Replacement fluids can be administered prefilter or postfilter. Postfilter replacement fluid results in hemoconcentration of the filter and increased risk of clotting, especially when the filtration fraction is greater than 30%. The filtration fraction is the ratio of ultrafiltration rate to plasma water flow rate and is dependent on the blood flow rate and hematocrit. Prefilter replacement fluid dilutes the blood before the filter, resulting in reduced filter clotting. Dilution of solutes before the filter reduces solute clearance by up to 15% by lowering the diffusion driving force and convective concentration.

Advantages and Disadvantages

The advantages of CRRT include hemodynamic tolerance caused by slower ultrafiltration rates. The gradual continuous volume removal makes control of volume status easier and allows administration of medications and nutrition with less concern for volume overload. Because it is a continuous modality, there is less fluctuation of solute concentrations over time and better control of azotemia, electrolytes, and acid-base status. The improved hemodynamic stability may be associated with fewer episodes of reduced renal blood flow, less renal ischemia, and more rapid renal recovery. Mehta et al examined this issue in a prospective study in which 166 ICU patients with ARF were randomized to IHD or to CRRT. CRRT patients who survived were significantly more likely to show renal recovery than those treated with IHD. Because CRRT does not cause rapid solute shifts, it does not raise intracranial pressure like IHD.

The cumulative solute removal with CRRT is greater than that achievable with IHD. Ronco et al provided convincing evidence that increasing solute clearance with CRRT can improve outcome in critically ill patients with ARF. In a prospective randomized controlled trial, 425 critically ill patients with ARF were assigned to CVVH using ultrafiltration rates of 20 mL/kg/hour (group 1), 35 mL/kg/hour (group 2), or 45 mL/kg/hour (group 3). The ultrafiltration rate of 20 mL/kg/hour was based on the average rate used in clinical practice as reported in the literature at the time of the study. The blood flow rates ranged from 120 to 240 mL/minute and the replacement fluid was administered postfilter. The primary study outcome was survival at 15 days after discontinuation of CVVH. Secondary outcomes were recovery of renal function and CRRT-related complications. Patient survival after discontinuing CVVH was 41%, 57%, and 58% in groups 1, 2, and 3, respectively. Survival in group 1 was significantly lower than in group 2 ($P =.0007$) and group 3 ($P =.001$), demonstrating a survival advantage for patients treated with CVVH at an ultrafiltration rate of at least 35 mL/kg/hour. It is unclear, however, whether the reduction in mortality was solely caused by small-molecule (urea) clearance or by both small-molecule clearance and increased midsize-molecule clearance.

Intermittent Hemodialysis Versus Continuous Renal Replacement Therapy: Outcomes

There are few prospective studies comparing IHD with CRRT with respect to outcomes, such as fatality or recovery of renal function.

Mehta et al randomized 166 patients to CRRT (CVVH or CVVHDF) or IHD. Univariate intention-to-treat analysis revealed a higher mortality rate among patients receiving CRRT. Patients randomized to CRRT had higher Acute Physiology and Chronic Health Evaluation (APACHE) III scores and had a higher prevalence of liver failure, confounding the results. Multivariate analysis revealed no impact of RRT modality on all-cause mortality rate or recovery of renal function. Instead, severity of illness scores (such as APACHE III scores and number of failed organs) were more important prognostic factors. The authors concluded that insufficient data existed to draw strong conclusions, mainly because of the lack of randomized controlled trials and the influence of biases and confounding variables.

Sustained Low-Efficiency Dialysis or Extended Daily Dialysis

SLED and extended daily dialysis are slower dialytic modalities run for prolonged periods using conventional hemodialysis machines with modification of blood and dialysate flow rates. Typically, SLED and extended daily dialysis use low blood-pump speeds of 200 mL/minute and low dialysate flow rates of 300 mL/minute for 6 to 12 hours daily. SLED and extended daily dialysis combine the advantages of CRRT and IHD. They allow for improved hemodynamic stability through gradual solute and fluid removal, as in CRRT. At the same time, they are able to provide high solute clearances (as seen in IHD) and eliminate the need for expensive CRRT machines, costly customized solutions, and trained staff.

Because SLED and extended daily dialysis can be done intermittently based on the needs of the patient, they also avoid the interruption of therapy for various diagnostic and therapeutic procedures that may be required in such patients. Kumar et al described their prospective experience of 25 patients treated with extended daily dialysis and 17 patients treated with CVVH at University of California Davis Medical Center. No significant differences in mean arterial pressure or inotrope requirements were observed between the two groups. Mortality rate was higher in the extended daily dialysis group (84% vs. 65%). The APACHE II scores were higher, however, in the extended daily dialysis group at the onset of treatment. The authors argued that extended daily dialysis was more cost effective by removing the need for constant monitoring of dialysis equipment and reducing nursing workload.

■ SUMMARY

ARF in critically ill patients is a significant clinical problem. Options for RRT in these patients use convective and diffusive clearance. The renal replacement modality may be intermittent, as in classic hemodialysis, or continuous. RRT needs to be tailored to the needs of each patient. Future research studies are needed to determine criteria for RRT.

Given the impact of ARF on mortality, it is important to prevent or hasten the resolution of even the mildest forms of ARF. The main goal is a preventive strategy for the syndrome of ARF to preserve renal function, prevent death, prevent complications of ARF (volume overload, acid-base disturbances, and electrolyte abnormalities), and prevent the need for chronic dialysis, with minimum adverse effects.

In this chapter, we discussed preventive strategies, and offered several options for treatment of ARF. Advances in RRT in the last few years have resulted in multiple RRT modalities available for treating ARF in the ICU. CRRT is gaining greater acceptance with the use of venovenous access and its advantages in hemodynamically unstable patients. There is little scientific data as to the best modality of RRT. There are few randomized controlled trials. Most existing studies are retrospective and poorly controlled. Many confounders exist, such as severity of illness and cause of renal failure, which are probably the most important factors affecting outcome in ICU patients with ARF. Some recent studies also suggest that higher doses of dialysis confer a survival advantage.

The choice of dialytic modality to be used should be tailored to the needs of the individual patient. IHD is best for patients requiring rapid metabolic control (e.g., in hyperkalemia), whereas volume overload is best managed with CRRT. Patients who are hemodynamically unstable or who have increased intracranial pressure are best treated with CRRT. Patients in whom anticoagulation is contraindicated

might be better managed with IHD unless CRRT with citrate is used. CRRT is limited by its greater cost, demands on nursing time, and the constraint it places on a patient's mobility. Theoretically, the choice of RRT might also depend on the underlying disease and cause of ARF. The choice of modality should be based on the clinical status of the patient and the resources available in a given institution.

For the chapter's Suggested Readings list, please visit the book at www.ExpertConsult.inkling.com.

MANAGEMENT OF COAGULATION DISORDERS IN THE SURGICAL INTENSIVE CARE UNIT

Christopher P. Michetti and Samir M. Fakhry

Surgeons commonly encounter coagulation disorders in the course of caring for patients, especially those with serious injury and those undergoing or recovering from surgery. Whereas bleeding is a condition well known to humankind since the beginnings of time, understanding the pathophysiology of bleeding and coagulation and developing effective therapies for them have come relatively recently and continue to undergo change as more is learned about the complex mechanism of blood coagulation and fibrinolysis. The ability to treat hemorrhage effectively had to await the discovery of blood types A, B, and O by Karl Landsteiner in 1900 and the AB blood type by Alfred Decastello and Adriano Sturli in 1902.

It would be nearly 40 years before the first blood bank was established in the United States in 1937. The development of reliable techniques of cross-matching, anticoagulation, and storage of blood was followed by the introduction of plastic bags for storage and devices for plasmapheresis, making component therapy possible. The discovery of blood coagulation pathways and the development of reliable tests of coagulation made it possible to provide treatment for a variety of coagulation disorders, including those encountered as a result of the newfound ability to keep humans alive by the infusion of blood and the surgical control of bleeding.

The ability to replace blood loss is critically important in modern surgical practice and in trauma care. Equally important is the ability to provide therapy to patients who need individual blood components. Effective use of the precious resource that blood and its products represents is increasingly important as problems of supply continue to exist even while demand increases. The purpose of this chapter is to familiarize the practicing surgeon with the types of coagulation disorders encountered in critically ill or injured patients, reliable ways of diagnosing these disorders, and effective therapeutic strategies for treating them.

INCIDENCE AND MECHANISM OF DISEASE

Congenital Bleeding Disorders

Von Willebrand Disease

Von Willebrand disease (vWD) is the most common inherited bleeding disorder, occurring in 1/100 to 1/1000 live births via autosomal

inheritance. The disease consists of deficiency or dysfunction of von Willebrand factor (vWF), which promotes platelet adhesion to damaged endothelium and stabilizes factor VIII. There are three types of vWD. Knowing the specific type is important to direct therapy. In type 1, a deficiency of vWF exists. In type 3, vWF is absent. The main subtypes of type 2, 2a, and 2b, both consist of a qualitative functional defect in vWF.

Diagnosis of vWD is supported by prolonged partial thromboplastin time (PTT), and in types 1 and 3 reduced levels of vWF antigen. Factor VIII activity may be reduced, and bleeding time or other platelet functional assays may be abnormal. The ristocetin cofactor assay is a test that measures the ability of vWF to induce platelet aggregation.

DDAVP (1-deamino-8-D-arginine vasopressin) may be used to stimulate production of vWF and increase factor VIII levels in type 1 and type 2a disease. It is ineffective in type 3, however, and contraindicated in type 2b because of the risk of thrombocytopenia and increased bleeding. Concentrates of factor VIII vWF are virus inactivated and are used commonly in types 2 and 3, but also in type 1 that is unresponsive to DDAVP. Cryoprecipitate contains vWF and factor VIII and may be used in all types of vWD. However, it is pooled and not virus inactivated. It is only recommended as a third-line therapy. Antifibrinolytic amino acids, such as aminocaproic acid and tranexamic acid, are used as adjuvant therapy in all types of vWD along with the previously cited treatments.

Hemophilia A

Hemophilia A is a congenital bleeding disorder that results from factor VIII deficiency. It is phenotypically expressed in males because of its X-linked inheritance pattern, whereas females maintain a carrier state. Bleeding tendency is inversely related to factor VIII levels. As with most factor deficiencies, clinical coagulopathy is usually not evident until factor levels fall below 30% of normal (mild hemophilia). Spontaneous bleeding may occur at levels less than 5% (moderate hemophilia), and those with levels less than 1% (severe hemophilia) are especially at risk. Coagulation studies will show a prolonged PTT, normal prothrombin time (PT), and low factor VIII levels.

Patients with clinically significant bleeding or those undergoing surgery should receive factor VIII concentrates, preferably recombinant products. DDAVP increases endogenous factor VIII levels and may be used in mild cases. Up to 20% of individuals may develop IgG antibodies ("inhibitors") to factor VIII after factor infusion, rendering future treatments ineffective. In such cases, recombinant activated factor VIIa (rFVII) may be used to induce hemostasis. This is discussed in more detail later in this chapter. Cryoprecipitate contains factor VIII in lower concentrations than in factor VIII concentrates, but its use is tempered by risks of viral transmission. Viral transmission from pooled factor concentrates is now extremely rare, and virtually eliminated with use of recombinant factors.

Hemophilia B

Hemophilia B (Christmas disease) is an X-linked disorder of factor IX deficiency. It is clinically similar to hemophilia A, and coagulation tests also show prolonged PTT with normal PT and low factor IX levels. Recombinant factor IX concentrates are available, as well as pooled donated concentrates. Development of inhibitors is less common (1%) than in hemophilia A, and treatment of severe bleeding may also include rFVIIa. Therapy in such cases should be given in conjunction with a hematologist.

Acquired Bleeding Disorders

Coagulopathy of Hemorrhagic Shock

Hemorrhagic shock causes a complex coagulopathy whose cause is multifactorial, and is frequently misinterpreted as disseminated intravascular coagulation (DIC) or a simple dilutional coagulopathy, which may misdirect treatment. In hemorrhagic shock, blood loss and tissue hypoperfusion result in acidosis from anaerobic metabolism— leading to the generation of lactate. Decreased ATP (adenosine triphosphate) production from tissue ischemia contributes to hypothermia and inability to maintain core temperature, resulting in coagulopathy, which exacerbates bleeding and perpetuates the "bloody vicious cycle." Resuscitation with room-temperature fluids worsens hypothermia. In massive resuscitation from hemorrhagic shock, variable degrees of dilution of coagulation factors occur.

Recent investigations suggest that hemorrhagic shock induces a complex set of processes that contribute to coagulopathy, including an early postinjury coagulopathy. Cellular ischemia resulting from shock and exposed tissue factor promotes this early coagulopathy, and it appears independent of factor levels and thus not responsive to component transfusion. Hypothermia and acidosis are the two major contributors to the coagulopathy of hemorrhagic shock and are discussed in more detail in material following. In the operating room and postoperatively in the intensive care unit (ICU), multiple treatments are obviously conducted simultaneously. However, the priorities in general are to stop the bleeding, resuscitate with crystalloid and blood products to reverse ischemia and acidosis, and prevent and treat hypothermia. Because of the overwhelming influence of hypothermia and acidosis, coagulopathy is primarily that of ineffective clotting. This is in contrast to DIC, which implies an overactivated coagulation system with unregulated microvascular thrombosis.

Dilution of clotting factors can result from massive hemorrhage and the fluid resuscitation that is used to treat it. Clotting factor concentrations as low as 30% of normal are sufficient for hemostasis, as are fibrinogen levels greater than 75 mg/dL. Even replacement of an entire blood volume leaves one with about a third of the normal coagulation factor concentration. This is probably the minimum volume of transfusion that can lead to a true dilutional coagulopathy. Although dilution of factors may result in abnormalities in laboratory measures of coagulation such as PT and PTT, these alterations do not necessarily affect hemostasis in vivo. Furthermore, platelet count cannot reliably be predicted based on volume of blood loss. Newer hemorrhagic shock resuscitation techniques attenuate dilutional coagulopathy through use of a higher ratio of clotting factors to red cells transfused. Recent reports suggest that an association exists between higher ratios of plasma to red cell transfusion volumes and improved survival. There remains uncertainty as to whether this is a causal relationship or one that reflects a "survival bias" or other undetected effect. Current guidelines from national groups, including the AABB, leave significant room for variability and many centers have adopted high plasma to red cell transfusion ratios as their standard approach for severe bleeding pending further evidence from controlled trials. For further informations, see the chapter on shock resuscitation.

Hypothermia

Hypothermia is often seen in the critical care setting in association with the systemic inflammatory response syndrome (SIRS), sepsis, and shock, in which decreased oxygen consumption prevents maintenance of core body temperature. It routinely accompanies major surgery for hemorrhagic shock, in which it exacerbates the coagulopathy and should prompt a "damage control" strategy. In addition, heat loss from hemorrhage is compounded by the administration of room-temperature fluids and blood products. In trauma patients, temperatures less than 32° C have been associated with 100% mortality rate.

Hypothermia slows the rate of reaction of the proteolytic enzymes of coagulation, resulting in impaired hemostasis. Both coagulation enzyme activity and platelet function are impaired at temperatures below 34° C in trauma patients. Platelet dysfunction is multifactorial, and is caused by defective adhesion and aggregation and decreased thromboxane production.

Prompt and efficient rewarming is essential in the hypothermic coagulopathic surgical patient. Although controlled hypothermia has proved beneficial in other conditions, such as cardiac arrest, no clear benefit has been proved in trauma or general surgery. The priority of therapy is to treat the underlying cause, whether by stopping any ongoing surgical bleeding, evacuating an undrained abscess, treating infection, or débriding necrotic tissue. External rewarming methods, although slow and inefficient, help to prevent further heat loss. Ambient room temperature should be raised, and warm air blankets and fluid pads applied to the patient (including the head). Core rewarming is far more efficacious than external techniques. At the very least, all infused fluids and blood products should be run through a fluid warmer, and warm humidified air given via the mechanical ventilator. When available, the more aggressive rapid technique of continuous arteriovenous rewarming may be used. A randomized prospective study suggests improved early survival and reduced fluid resuscitation requirements with this method when compared with slower methods.

Acidosis

Metabolic acidosis has long been recognized as a consequence of, and contributor to, coagulopathy. However, the specific pathways whereby acidosis impairs coagulation have yet to be clearly defined. Animal data suggest that hypothermia induces a delayed onset of thrombin formation, whereas acidosis decreases the overall thrombin generation rate. The association of severe acidosis (pH <7.1) with hypotension and hypothermia in severely injured patients virtually guarantees life-threatening coagulopathy. Therapy is again directed at the cause of acidosis and not merely the correction of the pH. While simultaneously addressing the inciting events, lactic acidosis is treated with fluid resuscitation to optimize tissue perfusion. It can be guided by following the trend in base deficit or lactate level. Sodium bicarbonate administration is ineffective and potentially harmful in lactic acidosis, and is not recommended.

Thrombocytopenia

Thrombocytopenia is generally defined as a platelet count lower than 100,000/mm³. Counts of 50,000/mm³ to 100,000/mm³ increase risk of bleeding with surgery or major trauma, and spontaneous bleeding is a risk below 10,000/mm³ to 20,000/mm³. Thrombocytopenia in the ICU setting has a lengthy differential diagnosis, but its cause can be broadly divided into three categories: decreased production of platelets, consumption or sequestration of platelets, and dilution. Malignancies or chemotherapy may affect platelet production, and massive transfusion and fluid resuscitation can lead to dilution of the total platelet count. In critically ill surgical patients, sepsis can cause a consumptive coagulopathy that in its most severe form manifests as DIC. Platelet consumption also occurs through immune mechanisms (antibodies to platelet glycoproteins), most notably in response to certain drugs. The list of such drugs includes heparin, H_2 antagonists, sulfa, rifampin, quinidine, hypoglycemics, and gold salts.

Heparin-induced thrombocytopenia is a rare but highly morbid condition associated with a greatly increased risk of thrombosis. Dilutional thrombocytopenia may occur with massive transfusion because stored blood contains negligible levels of platelets. However, the decrease in platelet count is not proportional to the volume of blood transfusion. Thus, simple dilution is unlikely to be the sole determinant of the low platelet count. Release of platelets from the spleen and bone marrow may partly account for this variability. As with coagulation factors, dilutional thrombocytopenia alone does not account for microvascular bleeding. Treatment and transfusion guidelines are discussed later in this chapter.

Disseminated Intravascular Coagulation

DIC is a syndrome involving diffuse systemic hypercoagulation and fibrinolysis that occurs in response to specific clinical conditions. Disorders associated with DIC in the surgical ICU include sepsis, trauma, severe pancreatitis, malignancies, fulminant liver failure, and transfusion reactions—among others. The syndrome involves excessive fibrin deposition in the microvasculature, with platelet aggregation and microvascular thrombosis. The pathophysiology of DIC is linked to the inflammatory cascade and tissue factor (TF) pathway, and is reviewed in more detail elsewhere. The condition ranges in severity from a subclinical low-grade acceleration of thrombosis and fibrinolysis to overt pathologic bleeding. Fulminant DIC is associated with multiple-organ dysfunction and death.

Diagnosis of DIC is made with a few laboratory tests in the proper clinical setting, after other causes of coagulopathy have been excluded. Scoring systems and algorithms have been proposed to aid the diagnosis. However, treatment is mainly supportive and targets the underlying cause, clinical end points, and associated laboratory abnormalities. Given the nonspecific nature of DIC, setting a defined threshold for making the diagnosis in the clinical setting is unnecessary—whereas set criteria are still needed for therapeutic trials and research. In addition, the label of DIC is often applied to patients receiving massive transfusion and resuscitation when their coagulopathy stems from other more common and reversible causes. It has also been observed that trauma patients with DIC have a thrombotic and fibrinolytic profile distinct from the usual hemostatic response to trauma.

DIC may be suspected in the setting of a generalized coagulopathy and clinical microvascular bleeding associated with an underlying process such as those described previously. The laboratory profile includes a low platelet count, prolonged PT and PTT, and elevated fibrin split products (FSPs). D-dimer levels are increased in up to 94% of patients diagnosed with DIC, and the D-dimer assay is the most sensitive test for this condition. Fibrinogen levels may be maintained except in severe forms of DIC.

Therapy for DIC centers on treatment of the underlying disease process to remove the proinflammatory stimulus of the syndrome. Clinical hemostasis is the goal. Platelet counts and the PT/PTT are used to guide response to therapy, but are not end points themselves. FFP and platelet transfusion are indicated in patients with active bleeding and those with significant laboratory derangements undergoing surgery or procedures. Cryoprecipitate may be considered to replace fibrinogen if fibrinogen levels fall below 100 mg/dL and are not corrected with FFP infusion.

Many other therapeutic agents have been investigated, but to date no specific treatment has proved successful in improving outcome in patients with DIC. Anticoagulation has been used to attempt to control the hypercoagulation in DIC, and although improvement in certain laboratory parameters has been reported, no survival benefit has been demonstrated with low-molecular-weight heparin (LMWH), thrombin inhibitors, or antifibrinolytics.

Severe Sepsis

Research in recent years continues to elucidate the complex interrelationship of the inflammatory process and the coagulation mechanism. The initial manifestation of this relationship leads to a hypercoagulable state. Inflammation in sepsis induces TF expression on circulating monocytes, tissue macrophages, and the endothelial surface—and fibrinolysis is inhibited. As fibrinolysis is impaired, fibrin deposition in the microvasculature proceeds unchecked. In addition, most patients with severe sepsis have low levels of the natural anticoagulants protein C and antithrombin III. Diffuse thrombosis leads to tissue ischemia and the multiple-organ dysfunction syndrome (MODS).

Coagulopathy in sepsis is multifactorial. Sepsis-induced thrombocytopenia occurs through immune mechanisms, platelet sequestration on activated endothelium, and consumption in DIC. Extensive

thrombin generation consumes clotting factors, and fibrinogen is often reduced (although levels may be normal due to its generation as an acute-phase reactant). Pathologic bleeding may be due to lack of circulating clotting factors and platelets that have been consumed, but this development is relatively uncommon. Although DIC is estimated to occur in 15% to 30% of patients with severe sepsis, the incidence of serious bleeding episodes in a recent study of septic patients was only 5%.

Transfusion of FFP or platelets in septic patients is indicated for active bleeding, or those at high risk for bleeding. As mentioned previously, transfused factors and platelets usually have only a transient impact because they are depleted by the ongoing consumption in the microvasculature. However, in the face of active bleeding aggressive therapy is warranted while every effort is made to treat or remove the source of the sepsis.

Traumatic Brain Injury

Traumatic brain injury (TBI) is associated with changes in the coagulation system, thought to result from release of the brain's abundant concentration of TF (thromboplastin). Exposed TF incites hypercoagulation, followed by fibrinolysis—similar to the changes seen in trauma patients without TBI. Although laboratory tests may confirm coagulation and fibrinolysis in many patients, the manifestations of this process have a spectrum of severity ranging from clinically undetectable to occasional pathologic bleeding from consumptive coagulopathy. Coagulopathy is associated with increased mortality rate in blunt and penetrating TBI, but the mechanism is not clear.

The importance of the hemostatic changes may lie in promotion of secondary brain injury through cerebral microvascular thrombosis, which may exacerbate cerebral ischemia. Currently, it is not known whether therapy should target hemostasis to prevent further bleeding in the injured brain or block part of the coagulation pathway to prevent microthrombosis and ischemia. Until the pathophysiology is better understood, treatment should be directed only toward clinical end points and maintenance of platelets and clotting factors as necessary for hemostasis (as outlined elsewhere in this chapter).

Vitamin K Deficiency

Vitamin K is a necessary cofactor in the enzymatic reactions of coagulation factors II, VII, IX, and X; protein C; and protein S—known as the vitamin K–dependent factors. When vitamin K is deficient, calcium binding is impaired—resulting in inactive factors. These factors make up the extrinsic portion of the traditional coagulation cascade, and their function can be measured with the international normalized ratio (INR) or PT assays. Vitamin K deficiency may be due to inadequate dietary intake, malabsorption of adequate intake, destruction of vitamin K–producing enteric bacteria by antibiotics, insufficient supplementation during parenteral nutrition, renal insufficiency, and hepatic dysfunction. Vitamin K may be given orally or parenterally to correct coagulopathy from deficiency or to reverse the effects of warfarin, and is discussed in more detail in material following.

Anticoagulant Drugs

The list of drugs that affect hemostasis is extensive and expanding rapidly. Drugs that affect platelet function and fibrinolysis have no specific antidote, but some of the thrombin inhibitors and glycoprotein (GP) IIb/IIIa blockers have short half-lives and are able to be removed by hemodialysis. Serious bleeding associated with aspirin and other antiplatelet agents may be partially ameliorated with platelet transfusion, but a functional platelet count or platelet function test may be warranted to assess the level of thrombocytopathy prior to transfusion. Heparin and warfarin are undoubtedly the most common drugs associated with bleeding complications in the surgical ICU. More recently, a group of novel oral anticoagulants (NOAC) have been approved for various indications, including nonvalvular atrial fibrillation. NOACs include direct thrombin inhibitors and factor Xa inhibitors, and at this time they have no antidote that provides effective reversal of their effect. Reversal and management of these agents is discussed later in this chapter.

Cirrhosis and End-Stage Liver Disease

Severe liver disease is associated with abnormal coagulation from multiple hemostatic defects. The diseased liver's ability to synthesize coagulation factors is impaired and fibrinogen levels are low in end-stage liver disease (ESLD) and decompensated cirrhosis but may be normalized by its acute-phase reaction to inflammation. Thrombocytopenia may be due to decreased production of thrombopoietin in the liver, and platelets may be destroyed or sequestered. Platelet function may be altered as well, by an excess of circulating inhibitors of platelet aggregation such as nitrous oxide. Systemic fibrinolysis occurs, in part by reduced clearance in the liver of profibrinolytic enzymes. Patients with ESLD may appear to have a baseline low-grade DIC (e.g., elevated FSPs) and are at higher risk of declining into overt DIC. The frequency and severity of DIC generally advance with the stage of the liver disease.

Cirrhotic patients who require surgery pose a significant challenge to the surgeon. Morbidity and mortality rates are increased in such patients, especially for emergent operations (for which mortality rate may reach 50%). In one study, patients undergoing trauma laparotomy with intraoperatively diagnosed cirrhosis had 45% mortality rate compared to 24% in injury severity–matched control subjects. Postoperative ICU stay was significantly longer as well. Patients with ESLD undergoing surgery may have an enhanced fibrinolytic response as a result of release of tissue plasminogen activator (tPA) and other factors, hindering stable clot formation. Compounding the risk of bleeding from coagulopathy in ESLD is the presence of large intra-abdominal and abdominal wall varices, which can make even the laparotomy incision itself a daunting task. Given all of these obstacles, the decision to undertake any invasive procedure on a patient with cirrhosis or ESLD must be made with the utmost discretion.

The goal of treatment of coagulopathy in ESLD should be clinical hemostasis, and not complete normalization of laboratory values (which is often not possible). Mild aberrations in laboratory assays are frequent and may not result in a bleeding diathesis. FFP is used for factor and fibrinogen replacement, but cryoprecipitate may be necessary if fibrinogen levels are lower than 100 mg/dL. Owing to the short half-life of some clotting factors, large volumes of FFP may be needed to maintain the hemostatic state. Continuous FFP infusion is sometimes warranted and can be titrated to clinical end points. In cases of life-threatening bleeding or the need for emergency surgery, rFVIIa may be used to correct the INR acutely. However, its short half-life may necessitate repeated dosing after a few hours to maintain hemostasis. Transfusion guidelines for thrombocytopenia are the same as described elsewhere in this chapter. However, patients with splenomegaly may sequester transfused platelets and the rise in platelet count may be less than expected. The presence of microvascular bleeding with a normal platelet count may indicate platelet dysfunction, and a platelet function test may be considered. However, transfusion in these cases may result in brief or no improvement in hemostasis unless the underlying cause of the thrombocytopathy has been corrected. Administration of DDAVP may be considered, but its efficacy is unproved in this setting.

Despite an underlying coagulopathy, risk for thrombosis remains. Cirrhotic patients should not be presumed protected by an "auto-anticoagulation." In fact, hepatic and portal vein thromboses are common in these patients, especially in advanced disease. The INR may be misleading, in that an elevated INR in ESLD does not necessarily correlate with the same level of anticoagulation as if that value were achieved with warfarin therapy. Deficient factor VII synthesis may produce a measurable abnormality in laboratory tests owing to its short half-life, but clinical clotting abnormalities may not be apparent. Maintenance of normal fibrinogen levels is usually sufficient to aid in coagulation, except in late stages.

Renal Failure

Renal failure and uremia impair primary hemostasis through platelet dysfunction, specifically decreased platelet adhesion to the subendothelium and platelet aggregation. However, the exact mechanisms are not known. Uremic toxins such as urea, creatinine, phenolic acids, and guanidinosuccinic acid contribute to the platelet dysfunction. Hemodialysis may be the most effective therapy for the platelet dysfunction due to uremia. However, hemodialysis is typically not used solely to correct coagulopathy. DDAVP may be used if active bleeding is present, given intravenously in a dose of 0.3 μg/kg. DDAVP can reduce bleeding associated with procedures in renal failure patients. Cryoprecipitate and conjugated estrogens are additional second-line treatment options. Despite their platelet dysfunction, chronic renal failure patients on dialysis may also be prone to thrombotic complications due to defective fibrinolysis.

Liver Injury

Liver injury may be indirectly associated with coagulopathy. Severe hepatic trauma may lead to hemorrhagic shock and all of its attendant causes of coagulopathy, as described previously. The liver has considerable compensatory function even with extensive direct damage, and thus a small percentage of normal parenchyma is sufficient to produce adequate amounts of coagulation factors and to clear profibrinolytic substances from the circulation. Given that normal hepatic function is maintained with resection of up to 75% of a normal liver, it is unlikely that parenchymal damage alone will result in a clotting abnormality.

DIAGNOSIS

Clinical Evaluation

Bleeding in a critically ill patient should be evaluated in a systematic fashion to detect the cause and direct the treatment of the bleeding (Fig. 1). In the surgical ICU, the first critical decision in a bleeding patient is to differentiate surgical bleeding from nonsurgical coagulopathic microvascular bleeding. This may be one of the most difficult decisions a surgeon can face. A nontherapeutic operation on a coagulopathic patient may exacerbate the vicious cycle, but leaving a surgically correctable source of bleeding untouched can prove fatal.

The evaluation begins with a detailed history, especially review of operative notes if the patient has had surgery or invasive procedures. Physical examination may reveal blood in operative wounds, tubes, or drains that indicate a source of bleeding requiring reoperation. Conversely, oozing of blood from multiple sites or seemingly minor wounds (e.g., intravenous catheter sites) may indicate coagulopathy. All recently administered medications should be reviewed for drugs that may affect hemostasis, in addition to reviewing the patient's medical history.

Postoperative bleeding may be considered in the broad categories of loss of surgical hemostasis versus coagulation disorders. Loss of surgical hemostasis is bleeding at the operative site, which may be due to technical problems such as slipped ligature or inadequate hemostasis from the procedure. During an operation, vasoconstriction may prevent visible bleeding—but with warming and resuscitation bleeding resumes. Loss of surgical hemostasis usually requires definitive control through reoperation. Postoperative surgical bleeding may be associated with signs and symptoms ranging from hypovolemia to hemorrhagic shock. The physician should intervene based on early signs of shock (tachycardia, restlessness, anxiety, pallor, oliguria), and not wait until shock is glaringly obvious. Anxiety or agitation in a postoperative surgical patient should prompt first an assessment of perfusion and oxygenation, before analgesics or sedatives are given. Hypotension is a late sign of hemorrhage, indicating severe volume deficit.

Coagulation disorders may be grouped into those affecting primary hemostasis (formation of initial platelet plug) or secondary hemostasis (clotting factors and the coagulation cascade). These

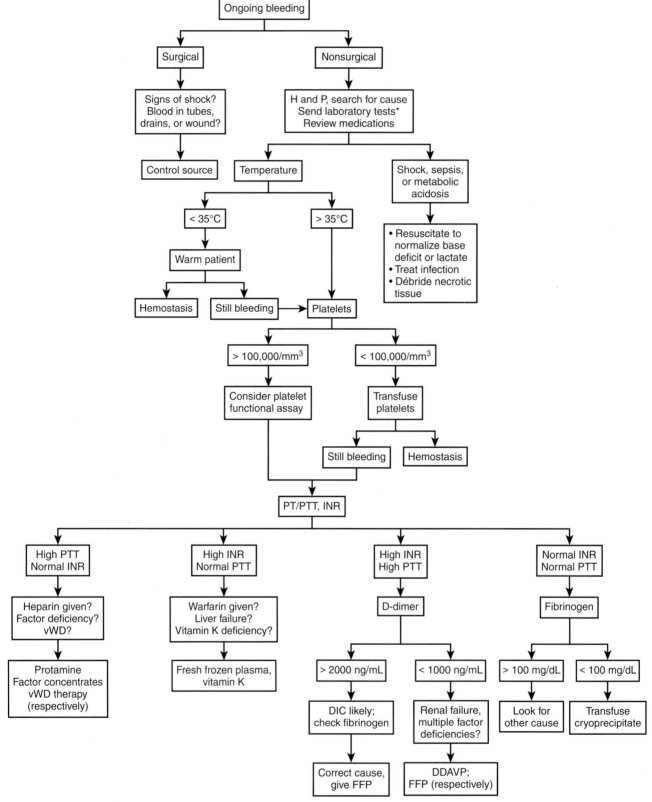

FIGURE I Approach to patients with bleeding. DDAVP, 1-Deamino-8-D-arginine vasopressin; DIC, disseminated intravascular coagulation; FFP, fresh frozen plasma; H, history; INR, international normalized ratio; P, physical; PT, prothrombin time; PTT, partial thromboplastin time; vWD, von Willebrand disease. *INR, PT/PTT, platelet count, arterial blood gas for base deficit or lactate; consider platelet function assay and thromboelastogram.

groups may be subdivided into qualitative defects (e.g., dysfunctional platelets, factor inhibition by heparin) or quantitative defects (e.g., thrombocytopenia, factor deficiencies). Furthermore, these conditions may be congenital or acquired. The algorithm presented in Figure 1 represents one example of a systematic approach that can help guide therapy in most surgical patients, even if the exact cause of the coagulopathy is not evident. It is intended to aid rapid assessment and initiation of treatment in the ICU, rather than as a definitive guide to diagnosis of specific bleeding disorders.

A few basic laboratory tests are helpful in guiding diagnosis and treatment of coagulopathy. It is worthwhile first to reiterate that the primary goal of therapy is clinical hemostasis, and not complete normalization of every clotting parameter. Platelet count, PT, INR, and PTT are the minimum basic laboratory tests needed to help differentiate problems with primary or secondary hemostasis. A baseline hematocrit level should be checked, keeping in mind that acute hemorrhage will not be reflected by a change in hematocrit until dilution of the intravascular space occurs from fluid shifts and intravenous fluid administration. Thromboelastography (TEG) is a global test of coagulation that may help define the cause of a coagulopathy. FSPs, D-dimer, and fibrinogen levels are rarely necessary in the setting of hemorrhagic shock-induced coagulopathy but may help confirm a clinical diagnosis of DIC. Each test is discussed in more detail in the following section.

Laboratory Tests of Coagulation

Prothrombin time: This test is done by adding a thromboplastin-containing TF, phospholipid, and calcium to citrated plasma and measuring the time in seconds until a fibrin clot is formed compared to a control time. The PT measures the activity of the extrinsic pathway (factor VII) and the common pathway (fibrinogen, factors II, IX, and X). It is used to monitor warfarin therapy, and is affected by depletion of the vitamin K–dependent factors (factors II, VII, IX, and X, and proteins C and S).

International normalized ratio: The INR is used to adjust for individual laboratory variation in the PT, using the formula INR = (log patient PT/log control PT) raised to the power of c, where c is the international sensitivity index (ISI). The thromboplastin used in individual laboratories is thus calibrated against a reference thromboplastin. The INR was developed to monitor the degree of warfarin anticoagulation.

Partial thromboplastin time: The PTT is calculated by adding a partial thromboplastin (mixture of phospholipids), an activating substance, and calcium chloride to citrated plasma. It measures the activity of the intrinsic pathway (high-molecular-weight [HMW] kininogen, prekallikrein, and factors VIII, IX, XI, and XII) and the common pathway (fibrinogen, factors II, IX, and X). Only factor VII activity is not measured by the PTT.

Bleeding time: The bleeding time is a test of platelet function and primary hemostasis. However, owing to variation in the performance of the test it is relatively insensitive and nonspecific in identifying platelet function abnormalities and may not predict surgical bleeding.

Platelet function tests: Several tests of platelet function are available through the laboratory or as point-of-care tests. Our hospital has abandoned the bleeding time in favor of the PFA-100 (Platelet Function Analyzer, Dade-Behring). The PFA-100 measures platelet function by the time it takes whole blood to occlude an aperture in a filter as it flows under high shear conditions. It is a global test of primary hemostasis that may detect platelet dysfunction due to certain disorders or medications, and congenital diseases such as vWD, but its role has not yet been completely defined. Other tests measure the percentage of platelets working normally to determine the functional platelet count, and are used often during cardiac surgery. Several point-of-care tests are available to assess platelet inhibition by drugs such as aspirin or GPIIb/IIIa inhibitors. Platelet aggregation tests use several agonists in different concentrations to induce aggregation in platelet-rich plasma, and will reveal quantitative or qualitative defects. It is a gold standard test but takes hours to perform, making it less useful in acute coagulopathy management.

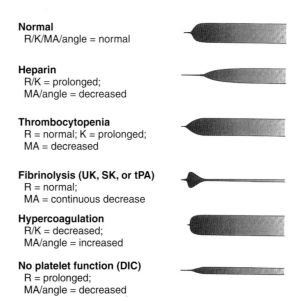

Normal
R/K/MA/angle = normal

Heparin
R/K = prolonged;
MA/angle = decreased

Thrombocytopenia
R = normal; K = prolonged;
MA = decreased

Fibrinolysis (UK, SK, or tPA)
R = normal;
MA = continuous decrease

Hypercoagulation
R/K = decreased;
MA/angle = increased

No platelet function (DIC)
R = prolonged;
MA/angle = decreased

FIGURE 2   Thromboelastogram. DIC, Disseminated intravascular coagulation; K, kinetics; MA, maximum amplitude; R, reaction time; SK, streptokinase; tPA, tissue plasminogen activator; UK, urokinase. *(Modified from Kaufmann CR, Dwyer KM, Crews JD, et al: Usefulness of thromboelastography in assessment of trauma patient coagulation. J Trauma 42:716, 1997.)*

Thromboelastography: TEG is reported as a graph of clot formation in a sample of whole blood (Fig. 2). The TEG tracing is drawn based on several factors, including rate of clot formation, fibrin cross-linking, and platelet-fibrin interaction. By measuring various parameters of the tracing, TEG provides an assessment of platelet function, coagulation enzyme activity, and the overall degree of coagulability. It can identify conditions such as primary fibrinolysis, consumptive coagulopathy, anticoagulant therapy, and the effect of hypothermia. TEG is used frequently during cardiopulmonary bypass, during liver transplantation, and in intensive care settings due to its rapid availability and ability to assess the components of coagulation in an integrated fashion. TEG and updated technologies such as ROTEM have proven useful in guiding resuscitation and component therapy for coagulopathy in patients requiring massive transfusion and may provide opportunities to optimize efficient and effective resuscitation and component therapy.

Thrombin time: The thrombin time (TT) is determined by adding thrombin to citrated plasma ± calcium. The TT measures the time for conversion of fibrinogen to fibrin, which is induced by thrombin. It is prolonged when fibrinogen is deficient (<100 mg/dL) or abnormal, in the presence of circulating anticoagulants (including FSPs and heparin), and during excessive fibrinolysis. Its high sensitivity to exogenous anticoagulants such as heparin limit its usefulness in hospitalized patients, but it can be used to detect low levels of circulating heparin that do not cause changes in the PTT.

Fibrinogen: Fibrinogen is a large protein that is cleaved by thrombin to produce fibrin monomers, which crosslink to form a fibrin clot in the presence of factor XIII. Fibrinogen levels may fall with the excess clotting seen in consumptive coagulopathy or with overanticoagulation by thrombolytic agents. It is also an acute-phase reactant, increasing in response to physiologic stress.

Fibrin split products: FSPs are fragments of the fibrin molecule that result from breakdown of fibrin by plasmin. The test is nonspecific, but elevated levels may indicate fibrinolysis and support a clinical picture of consumptive coagulopathy. The D-dimer is a specific form of FSP that is most closely associated with DIC.

Factor assays: Specific coagulation factor levels can be used to help diagnose certain diseases or deficiencies (for example, factor VIII for hemophilia A and factor IX for hemophilia B). Other assays may detect deficiencies in factors V, VII, X, XI, and XII (Hageman factor), prekallikrein, and HMW kininogen, all of which are very rare. Factor assays are used infrequently in the ICU setting.

MANAGEMENT

Blood Product Transfusion

Fresh Frozen Plasma

FFP is prepared by extracting the noncellular portion of blood and freezing it within hours of donation. One 250- to 300-mL unit of FFP contains all clotting factors and about 400 mg of fibrinogen, and will increase clotting factor levels by about 3%. The PT and PTT should be used during FFP therapy to gauge the efficacy of transfusion.

Indications for FFP administration in the surgical ICU are relatively few. These include coagulopathy with clinical bleeding, accompanied by measured or suspected factor deficiency as indicated by a PT or PTT more than 1.5 times normal, and emergent correction of a prolonged PT due to acquired coagulopathy from warfarin, liver disease, or DIC. FFP should not be used for volume replacement, for nutrition, to promote wound healing, or to treat hypoalbuminemia. Empirically during massive transfusion, or as part of a preset formula based on number of red blood cell transfusions. Avoiding unnecessary transfusion is important to reduce risks of transfusion reaction, bacterial infection, and transfusion-related acute lung injury (TRALI), as well as for cost control. The dose of FFP should be aimed at a minimum of 30% of normal plasma factor concentration and clinical hemostasis. Practically, 10 to 15 mL/kg of FFP are sufficient for this purpose, although lower volumes are usually adequate (5 to 8 mL/kg) to reverse warfarin.

Platelets

Treatment of thrombocytopenia or platelet dysfunction centers on the underlying cause and the patient's clinical condition. In the absence of active bleeding or imminent surgery, platelet counts above 10,000/mm^3 do not require treatment—whereas counts below 10,000/mm^3 warrant platelet transfusion to prevent spontaneous bleeding. Patients with microvascular bleeding and thrombocytopenia may benefit from platelet transfusion after excluding hypothermia because the transfused platelets will not function properly at low temperatures. Evidence-based guidelines are lacking for surgical patients with platelet counts between 50,000/mm^3 and 100,000/mm^3, and therapy should take into account the patient's condition, risk of significant bleeding, and plans for surgery or high-risk invasive procedures (e.g., ventriculostomy). In general, platelet transfusion to reach a threshold of 100,000/mm^3 may be necessary before surgery of the brain, spine, and eye, and to 50,000/mm^3 for other major operations.

In general, platelet transfusion is not indicated at these levels in the absence of microvascular bleeding. Patients with consumptive coagulopathy rarely benefit from platelet transfusion because the same process consumes newly transfused platelets. However, microvascular bleeding in the presence of sepsis or DIC usually warrants treatment. If surgery or invasive procedures are necessary in the presence of a consumptive process and low platelet count, platelet transfusion should be given just before or during the procedure to maximize the number of circulating platelets available for hemostasis.

Different platelet concentrates are available. The traditional "six-pack" from random donor concentrates contains platelets from multiple individuals and equals 6 units of platelet concentrates. One unit of single-donor platelets, also called apheresis platelets, contains roughly the same volume of platelets as 6 random donor units but has the advantage of originating from one person and thereby exposing the recipient to only one set of antigens. One can expect a rise in platelet count by about 30,000/mm^3 for each unit of single-donor platelets and

for each 6 units of random donor. Repeated platelet transfusion may lead to alloantibody formation in some patients, making them refractory to further platelet transfusions. Human leukocyte antigen (HLA)-matched or crossmatched platelets may be required in such cases. The use of single-donor platelet transfusions has been adopted by many institutions to minimize antibody formation and preserve the response to a platelet transfusion for as long as possible.

Cryoprecipitate

Cryoprecipitate is prepared by thawing FFP to 1° C to 6° C and then removing and refreezing the insoluble precipitate that forms. Each bag of cryoprecipitate has a volume of approximately 15 mL and contains 150 to 250 mg fibrinogen per bag, along with 80 to 100 factor VIII units and other components such as vWF and fibronectin. It is usually given as a pooled product containing 8 to 10 bags, resulting in transfusion of 1200 to 2500 mg of fibrinogen. Although it is not virus inactivated, it is thoroughly screened for virus—resulting in extremely low risk of transmission. Cryoprecipitate is used for treatment of hemophilia A, vWD, hypofibrinogenemia, in DIC when serum fibrinogen levels fall below 100 mg/dL, and when the previously cited factors need to be replaced in a low volume of fluid. Cryoprecipitate has less of a role in treating the coagulopathy of hemorrhagic shock, where factor replacement (when needed) is accomplished with FFP because volume is not an issue and fibrinogen replacement is rarely necessary.

Reversal of Warfarin

The prevalence of preinjury warfarin use among trauma patients increases with age. The effect of this drug on morbidity and mortality rates in trauma is variable, but potentially significant. Emergent reversal of warfarin anticoagulation is occasionally required in patients with TBI or serious injury associated with hemorrhage, and slower reversal is often used for patients with increased risk of bleeding due to trauma or perioperative status. Before initiating therapy, several factors should be considered—including urgency of warfarin reversal, expected length of time until reanticoagulation, and cardiac function of the patient (i.e., tolerance of volume loading).

Reversal of warfarin is guided by the INR and is best managed by standardized evidence-based guidelines. Vitamin K takes 8 to 12 hours to take effect, and is the first-line choice for nonemergent treatment of a high INR. However, it has a long half-life and high or repeated doses should be avoided if reanticoagulation with warfarin is anticipated in the next several days. Oral vitamin K is preferred for nonemergent reversal of warfarin, whereas the subcutaneous route is not recommended because of inefficient absorption. Patients receiving intravenous vitamin K should have continuous cardiac monitoring due to the risk of anaphylaxis. FFP is the standard therapy for patients with a high INR and significant bleeding or need for invasive procedures.

Many elderly patients on warfarin have concomitant heart disease, and caution must be used to avoid precipitating congestive heart failure with overly aggressive fluid loading. In our experience, an INR greater than 2 is rarely normalized with only 1 or 2 units of FFP. In addition, patient factors vary considerably—resulting in an unpredictable and nonlinear dose-response relationship. rFVIIa may be used when immediate reversal of anticoagulation is required in emergent situations such as severe TBI or life-threatening bleeding. However, data on its proper use in these conditions is limited. rFVIIa's half-life is only a fraction of that of warfarin, and thus it must be used in conjunction with FFP and vitamin K to maintain normal coagulation. Four-factor prothrombin complex concentrate (PCC-4) was made available in the U.S. in 2014. This product contains Factors II, VII, IX, and X, and provides rapid and often complete reversal of warfarin, in a very low volume of fluid (about 150mL). PCC-4 administration is a viable reversal strategy in the context of life-threatening bleeding or the need for emergent surgery. Consideration for use in these conditions is advocated in the updated 2015 guidelines from the American Society of Anesthesiologists. Table 1

TABLE 1: Management Options for Patients with Warfarin Anticoagulation and Bleeding Risk

Clinical Context	Treatment Options
INR <5, no significant bleeding	Hold warfarin
INR >5, no significant bleeding	Vitamin K 1–5 mg orally
INR >1.5, bleeding or high risk of bleeding, nonemergent	FFP in 2- to 4-unit doses, recheck INR after each dose until bleeding stopped or INR <1.5 Consider vitamin K 5 mg orally
INR >1.5, life-threatening bleeding or emergent surgery or invasive procedure required	FFP in 4-unit doses, recheck INR after each dose, *and* vitamin K 10 mg slow IV infusion PCC-4 (dosing based on Factor IX units/kg weight): INR 2- <4: 25 units/kg INR 4–6: 35 units/kg INR >6: 50 units/kg Consider factor VIIa (repeat in 2–3 hours if still bleeding)

FFP, Fresh frozen plasma; INR, international normalized ratio; IV, intravenous; PCC-4, four-factor prothrombin complex concentrate.

lists management schemes for patients on warfarin with an elevated INR and risk of bleeding.

Reversal of Heparin

Unfractionated heparin (UFH) and LMWH are used commonly in the surgical ICU for venous thromboembolism prophylaxis or treatment of other conditions. Although risk of major bleeding events with prophylactic doses is low, full anticoagulation is associated with higher risk. When nonsurgical bleeding occurs in patients anticoagulated with heparin, reversal of the drug's effects may be necessary. The half-life of UFH is about 1 hour, and thus most treatment doses are reversed by holding the infusion for 6 hours. When immediate reversal is desired, protamine may be used. Protamine binds heparin and neutralizes its effects. The dose is 1 mg of protamine for each 100 units of heparin given. The half-life of heparin must be taken into account when calculating the protamine dose, such that the dose of heparin must be halved for each hour since its injection. If a continuous infusion has been used, the cumulative dose must be estimated. Protamine administration carries risks of hypotension, which may be avoided by slow injection over 10 minutes, and a 1% risk of anaphylaxis in patients who have had previous exposure to protamine or NPH insulin.

The half-life of LMWH varies with the particular agent used, but in general ranges from 2 to 5 hours. LMWH is only partially neutralized by protamine, which reverses most of the anti-factor IIa (thrombin) activity but only some of the anti-factor Xa activity. The reversal is based on the level of anti-Xa activity, in a dose of 1 mg protamine per 100 anti-Xa units.

Reversal of Novel Oral Anticoagulants

In recent years a newer generation of oral anticoagulants has been FDA-approved for use in the management of atrial fibrillation and venous thromboembolism. While these agents share the advantage of having no need for laboratory tests for routine therapeutic monitoring, they also share the significant drawback of lacking an effective antidote.

The first of these, dabigatran, is a direct thrombin inhibitor. A normal thromboplastin time rules out significant anticoagulation from dabigatran, but only the ecarin clotting time correlates with its degree of effect. Standard tests such as PT/PTT and INR are not reliable for monitoring its effect. Rivaroxaban and apixaban are factor Xa inhibitors, whose effect can be identified by the PT. While patients on these drugs with a normal PT likely do not require reversal, a normal PT does not guarantee complete drug elimination.

Due to the lack of specific reversal agents, management of bleeding can be challenging in patients taking these medications. Currently, data on the efficacy of various reversal techniques is very limited, and available agents are only partially effective in normalizing coagulation. This is an evolving area, and it is advisable for practitioners to establish a multidisciplinary approach to this problem that works for their facility. One such approach is provided here. For dabigatran and rivaroxaban, activated charcoal may be used if the drug was ingested within 2 hours, and within 6 hours for apixaban. Hemodialysis is the most effective method to eliminate dabigatran and induce coagulation, but is labor and resource intensive. For serious or life-threatening bleeding, one may use either FEIBA (factor VIII inhibitor bypassing activity) or rFVIIa. FEIBA contains factors II, IX, and X (mostly nonactivated) and factor VIIa. For attempted reversal of rivaroxaban and apixaban one may use 4-factor PCC (described for warfarin reversal previously). For all agents time and supportive care, as well as judicious surgical and minimally invasive interventions, are reasonable adjuncts.

In nonurgent situations or for elective surgery, the direct thrombin inhibitor or Factor Xa inhibitor may be discontinued for a time, and eliminated through normal metabolism. The half life of these drugs depends on the specific agent, and for dabigatran and rivaroxaban, on the creatinine clearance (CrCl). When estimated CrCl is >50ml/min, elective surgery should be delayed for 24 hours after stopping dabigatran or rivaroxaban, and for 48 hours after stopping apixaban. In operations where the risk or consequences of bleeding are significant (e.g., cardiac, neurological, major abdominal, or orthopedic surgery), one should delay surgery for 2 days for dabigatran and rivaroxaban, and for 2 to 3 days for apixaban. These suggested observation periods need to be extended for the drugs whose half-life is prolonged in the context of a lower CrCl. In these situations, consultation with a pharmacist is beneficial.

Recombinant Activated Factor VIIa

Recombinant activated factor VIIa is a synthetic form of coagulation factor VII, intended to promote hemostasis. It is a Food and Drug Administration (FDA)-approved drug for bleeding in hemophilia patients with inhibitors, but has also been used in a variety of other conditions. The primary mechanism of action has been debated. When bound to exposed TF in the subendothelium, rFVIIa can activate factors X and IX—which then promote thrombin formation. This mechanism would explain its localized activity at sites of injury. Other data suggest that high-dose rFVIIa acts independently of TF by activating factor Xa on the platelet surface.

Recombinant activated factor VIIa has proved efficacious in reducing blood loss and improving survival in multiple animal studies of its use for the coagulopathy of hemorrhagic shock, and in reducing blood loss and operative time in humans undergoing radical prostate surgery. In blunt trauma patients, rFVIIa reduces the need for blood transfusion and for massive transfusion. A similar significant benefit was not seen in patients with penetrating trauma, however. The CONTROL trial randomized massively bleeding, predominantly blunt trauma patients, defined as the transfusion of 4 to 8 units of red blood cells within the first 12 hours after injury, to receive either three doses of rFVIIa or placebo. The doses of rFVIIa were 200 mcg/kg initially, followed by 100 mcg/kg at 1 and 3 hours. The study was terminated early for futility due to overall low mortality in both arms.

The rFVIIa group required less red blood cell transfusion than the placebo group, but no mortality advantage was seen. Initial concerns about an increased risk of thrombosis with rFVIIa have not been borne out. Studies have revealed no evidence of systemic thrombi or increased risk of thrombotic complications in animals or humans.

The optimal dose of rFVIIa for surgical patients has not yet been determined. Doses ranging from 20 to 200 µg/kg have been used successfully in clinical trials. Owing to the drug's short half-life, certain conditions such as severe coagulopathy may require a second or third dose within a few hours of the first to maintain hemostasis while other contributing factors are aggressively treated. Given the lack of survival benefit in randomized studies, routine use of rFVIIa in traumatic hemorrhagic shock is not recommended.

CONCLUSIONS

Coagulopathy is commonly encountered in critically ill or injured patients. When bleeding is encountered, the first priorities should be control of bleeding and resuscitation with crystalloids and blood. Congenital disorders should be considered. Patients should also be evaluated for acquired coagulopathies, including those resulting from medications. Coagulopathy frequently accompanies massive bleeding and resuscitation, and its cause in this setting is multifactorial. Although dilution is frequently invoked as the primary pathophysiologic process, hypothermia, acidosis, and shock generally play more important roles. Newer resuscitation strategies that employ increased ratios of plasma and platelets to red blood cells have been more effective in aiding hemostasis.

The use of blood components should be guided by objective evidence of coagulation abnormalities (including clinical findings and laboratory data) rather than resorting to formula-based replacement. Selective use of components (especially platelet transfusion) will yield safer and more effective therapy. Such an approach should lead to more effective management of coagulopathy and more judicious use of blood component therapy. Continued advances in the field present novel opportunities to affect coagulation, but the fundamental principles still apply in the patient with hemorrhage: control bleeding rapidly, expeditiously resuscitate from shock, manage temperature carefully, and monitor the patient for clinical and laboratory evidence of coagulation abnormalities.

For the chapter's Suggested Readings list, please visit the book at www.ExpertConsult.inkling.com.

Management of Endocrine Disorders in the Surgical Intensive Care Unit

Anthony Falvo and Mathilda Horst

KEY SURGICAL POINTS

1. The head-injured patient with high-volume diuresis should be suspected of having diabetes insipidus (DI).
2. A careful workup of hypernatremia should occur because cerebral salt wasting and syndrome of inappropriate secretion of antidiuretic hormone (SIADH) have completely different treatments.
3. SIADH causes volume expansion but cerebral salt wasting causes volume depletion.
4. Include thyroid storm in the differential diagnosis for fever workup.
5. Do not delay treatment for thyroid storm while waiting for laboratory results.
6. Many common intensive care unit (ICU) medications can affect thyroid hormone and antidiuretic hormone (ADH).
7. Suspect adrenal insufficiency when hypotension is unresponsive to vasopressors and fluids.
8. Patients with proven adrenal insufficiency have better outcomes when treated with corticosteroids.
9. Often patients have preexisting signs and symptoms of endocrine abnormalities.
10. Tight glycemic control improves outcomes.

The endocrine system as a part of the neuroendocrine axis (hypothalamic-pituitary-adrenal axis) influences the response to stress and critical illness. Endocrine abnormalities within this axis change and modify the physiologic response to trauma and stress. Critically ill patients with a known diagnosis of an endocrine problem are treated with replacement therapy; however, an unrecognized endocrine abnormality often creates management difficulties and increases morbidity. Endocrine problems occur at all levels of the neuroendocrine axis from primary or secondary disease, medications, or end-organ failure.

The neuroendocrine axis is responsible for the stress response and is controlled by the hypothalamus, pituitary, and autonomic nervous system (Fig. 1). This axis is activated by baroreceptor response to intravascular volume, sympathetic response from tissue injury, and inflammatory mediators released from tissue trauma. The hormones released in response to injury act through binding to cell surface receptors or intracellular receptors and produce a complex series of responses and feedback loops that maintain cellular processes. This chapter addresses abnormalities in the endocrine system that affect the course of critically ill patients.

BRAIN PROBLEMS: ABNORMALITIES IN HYPOTHALAMIC/PITUITARY RESPONSE

Injuries that affect the brain can interrupt the hypothalamus or pituitary production of hormone. Head injury, brain surgery, mass lesions or infiltrative diseases, vascular or hypoxic injuries, and cerebral infections cause failure of the releasing of pituitary hormones, resulting in single or combined abnormalities. Cerebral edema or increased intracranial pressure is thought to restrict the blood flow to the hypothalamic-pituitary area. Frequently encountered abnormalities are DI, SIADH, and cerebral salt wasting. These syndromes cause abnormalities of sodium and water balance. Evaluation of volume status, urine and serum sodium, and osmolality are required to determine which syndrome is present in order to provide appropriate treatment (Table 1).

Diabetes Insipidus

Central DI is caused by lack of vasopressin (antidiuretic hormone, ADH) which causes water diuresis of more than 3 L/day, dehydration, and hypernatremia. The urine is dilute with urine osmolality of less than 300 mOsm/kg and urine specific gravity less than 1.005. Urine osmolality greater than 800 mOsm/kg excludes DI.

FIGURE I Neuroendocrine axis. E, Epinephrine; NE, norepinephrine.

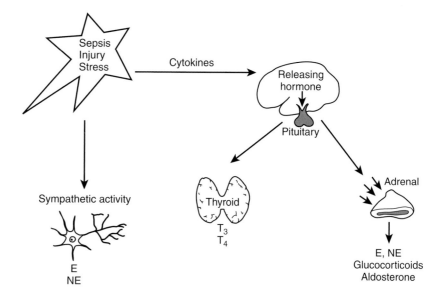

Hypothalamus: releasing hormones
• Corticotropin-releasing hormone: stimulates the release of adrenocorticotropic hormone (ACTH)
• Thyrotropin-releasing hormone (TRH): stimulates the release of thyroid-stimulating hormone (TSH)
• Antidiuretic hormone (ADH)/vasopressin: increased production in the hypothalamus and release from the posterior pituitary

Pituitary: stimulating hormones
• ACTH: stimulates the adrenal gland
• TSH: stimulates the thyroid gland
• ADH/vasopressin: multiple organs affected including the vascular system and the kidney

TABLE 1: Comparison of Central Causes of Sodium and Water Abnormalities

Feature	Diabetes Insipidus	Cerebral Salt Wasting	SIADH
Serum sodium	↑	↓	↓
Serum osmolality (mOsm/kg)	>290	<280	<280
Urine osmolality (mOsm/kg)	<300	>100	>100
Urinary sodium (mEq/L)	Variable	>20	>20
Volume depletion	Yes	Yes	No
Treatment	DDAVP, water replacement	Normal saline	Fluid restriction

DDAVP, 1-Deamino-8-D-arginine vasopressin; SIADH, syndrome of inappropriate secretion of antidiuretic hormone.

The diagnosis is usually made when dilute urine output exceeds 200 mL/hour for 2 consecutive hours. A dramatic rise in serum sodium occurs in the ICU patient population unless fluids are aggressively replaced. In the neurosurgery patient population the incidence of

TABLE 2: Formula for Calculating Water Deficit

$$\text{Water deficit} = 0.6^* \times (\text{Wt kg}) \times ([\text{Na}/140] - 1)$$

*0.5 for females.

DI is 3.7% with a mortality rate of 70%. DI commonly occurs in association with severe brain injury and herniation. The treatment is fluid rehydration and vasopressin replacement, intravenous (IV) DDAVP (1-deamino-8-D-arginine vasopressin) 2 to 4 μg/day or intranasally 10 to 60 μg/day. Frequent monitoring of electrolytes and central venous pressure (CVP) is necessary. The water deficit is calculated and slowly replaced. Caution is used when severe hypernatremia is present with half the water deficit replaced in 24 hours to avoid demyelination (Table 2).

SIADH and Cerebral Salt Wasting

The SIADH and cerebral salt wasting are linked together through a common cause—traumatic brain injury—and common result—hypotonic hyponatremia. Cerebral salt wasting is most often associated with subarachnoid hemorrhage but SIADH is also associated with brain injury, tumors, and medications (Table 3). The cause of SIADH is excessive release of ADH that leads to water retention and an increase in extracellular fluid volume. Volume expansion increases renal sodium excretion, producing hyponatremia. Cerebral salt wasting is thought to involve disruption of the neural input to the kidney or central secretion of a natriuretic factor. Sodium is wasted by the kidneys, causing extracellular volume depletion and stimulation of ADH secretion. Hyponatremia develops with extracellular volume depletion.

In both syndromes the diagnosis begins with serum sodium less than 135 mmol/L. Serum osmolality is less than 280 mOsm/kg and the urine osmolality is greater than 100 mOsm/kg in both diseases. The differentiating factor is the effective blood volume (CVP), which is normal in SIADH and low in cerebral salt wasting. Low effective blood volume normally causes orthostatic blood pressure, tachycardia, low CVP, low urine sodium, chloride, and fractional excretion of sodium with high blood urea nitrogen (BUN). Both disease states have low uric acid level. With correction of the salt deficit, uric acid levels normalize in SIADH and not in cerebral salt wasting. The treatment of SIADH is fluid restriction (800 to 1000 mL/day) and occasional hypertonic saline. Demecloycline, phenytoin, and lithium are used for treatment of chronic SIADH. The treatment for cerebral salt wasting is normal saline fluid replacement to expand the extracellular fluid compartment (see Table 1).

ABNORMALITIES IN THYROID RESPONSE

Untreated or unrecognized thyroid problems (excess or deficit) create life-threatening illness in critically ill patients. Thyroid hormones are responsible for the metabolic rate in all tissues. Critical illness may alter the production of thyroid hormone through thyroid-stimulating hormone (TSH) regulation, peripheral metabolism, or alteration in binding proteins. Cytokines as well as commonly used ICU medications (see Table 3) affect thyroid hormone function.

TABLE 3: Medications That Interfere with Thyroid Hormone and Antidiuretic Hormone

Drugs Causing Syndrome of Inappropriate Secretion of Antidiuretic Hormone

ADH analogs: vasopressin, oxytocin, desmopressin

Stimulating ADH release: opiates, opioids, barbiturates, nicotine, thiazides, isoproterenol, cyclic antidepressants, MAO inhibitors, haloperidol, risperidone, acetylcholine

Enhancing renal sensitivity: NSAIDs, acetaminophen

Stimulating ADH release and enhancing renal sensitivity: chlorpropamide, tolbutamide, cyclophosphamide, chlorambucil

Phosphodiesterase inhibition: theophylline

Other: amiodarone, ACE inhibitors, loop diuretics, thiazide diuretics, general anesthesia

Drugs That Influence Thyroid Function

Influence conversion: glucocorticoids, beta blockers, contrast agents, amiodarone, propylthiouracil

Increase TSH: cimetadine, dopamine antagonists, haloperidol, iodide, lithium, contrast agents, metoclopramide

Decrease TSH: adrenergic agonists, dopamine, steroids, opiates, phenytoin, phentolamine

Increase binding: estrogens, methadone, fluorouracil (5-FU), heroin, tamoxifen

Decrease binding: steroids, androgens, heparin, salicylates, seizure medications, furosemide

ACE, Angiotensin-converting enzyme; ADH, antidiuretic hormone; MAO, monoamine oxidase; NSAID, nonsteroidal anti-inflammatory drug; TSH, thyroid-stimulating hormone.

Nonthyroidal illness has been described in critically ill patients. Symptoms from thyroid function abnormalities are a continuum from hyperthyroidism to thyroid storm and hypothyroidism to myxedema coma.

Thyroid Excess

Hyperthyroidism with a 3% incidence in outpatients is caused by Graves disease, goiter, and adenoma. Treatment with amiodarone increases the incidence to 9%. Thyroid storm (severe hyperthyroidism) was first recognized after thyroidectomy in unprepared patients and now encompasses 1% to 2% of all admissions for thyrotoxicosis with a mortality rate of 20% to 30%. It is precipitated by physiologic stress related to specific events such as surgery, trauma, childbirth, severe illness, overdose of thyroid medication, or iodine in medications or contrast agent. The classic symptoms include fever, cardiovascular abnormalities, and mental status changes. The tachycardia is out of proportion to the fever. Fever is the hallmark of this disease with temperatures up to 106° F. A state of high-output cardiac failure can develop with bounding pulses, rales and hepatomegaly, and thyroidal bruit. Atrial fibrillation and congestive heart failure are common in elderly patients with hyperthyroidism and can occur without fever (thyrocardiac crisis). The mental status changes include a broad spectrum from anxiety to coma. There can be nonspecific gastrointestinal (GI) complaints and clinical findings of Graves disease.

This syndrome is recognized by clinical signs and symptoms. Laboratory testing turnaround time is long and treatment should be started based on clinical suspicion. TSH is not detectable and both triiodothyronine (T_3) and thyroxine (T_4) are elevated, with T_3 higher than T_4. There is an associated elevation of white blood cells (WBCs), calcium, blood glucose, and liver function tests. The treatment is directed toward decreasing the production of thyroid hormone and preventing its release, blocking the peripheral action, providing supportive care, and treating the cause (Table 4).

Thyroid Deficit

Hypothyroidism occurs in patients over age 50 years, in 8% of women and 2% of men in this age group. Previous surgery, radiation, and autoimmune disease are the most common causes. Myxedema coma

TABLE 4: Treatment of Thyroid Storm

Inhibit hormone synthesis: propylthiouracil 1000 mg loading dose then 300 mg orally every 6 hours

Blunt end organ effects: propranolol 1 to 10 mg IV push then 20 to 120 mg orally every 6 hours OR esmolol 250 µg/kg loading dose IV over 1 minute, then 50 µg/kg/minute infusion

Stop hormone release: sodium iodide 500 mg orally or IV every 8 hours.

Block peripheral conversion: propranolol or hydrocortisone 50 to 100 mg IV every 8 hours

Volume replacement

Treatment of precipitating event

Supportive treatment:

ICU monitoring

Treat CHF

Treat hyperthermia with cooling blanket or acetaminophen

CHF, Congestive heart failure; ICU, intensive care unit; IV, intravenously.

is severe hypothyroidism. Myxedema coma is rare but has a mortality rate of more than 60%. It is precipitated by physiologic stress of trauma, surgery, burns, infections, cardiovascular events, or cold temperatures, or failing to take thyroid medication. Medications can decrease hormone production and function (see Table 3). The cardinal findings relate to reduced metabolic rate and oxygen consumption and include hypothermia, bradycardia, hypotension, hypoventilation, and mental status changes. The mental status changes range from lethargy to coma and are associated with decreased deep tendon reflexes. Low cardiac output with both right- and left-sided failure and decreased myocardial contractility occur. There is slowing of the GI system with constipation or ileus. Skin, nail, and hair changes associated with hypothyroidism are present. The name myxedema comes from the infiltration of mucopolysaccaride of the skin. This is a clinical diagnosis with elevated TSH, very low T_4 and sodium, low blood glucose, elevated creatine phosphokinase (CPK), low Pao_2, and elevated $Paco_2$. There are characteristic electrocardiogram (ECG) changes (Table 5).

The treatment of myxedema coma includes supportive care in an ICU setting and replacement of thyroid hormone. ICU care includes ECG monitoring and possibly cardiac pacing, arterial blood gas monitoring with possible intubation, warming with blankets and external warmers, IV fluid containing glucose, temperature monitoring, and neurologic checks. IV T_4 is given 300 to 500 µg on day 1 and then 50 to 100 µg every day until oral replacement is started. Adrenal insufficiency should be tested for with the rapid cosyntropin (ACTH) test and treated with 100 mg of IV hydrocortisone every 8 hours.

Sick Euthyroid Syndrome

Sick euthyroid or nonthyroidal illness is a common finding in the ICU patient population. It is not completely clear if this syndrome represents a pathologic process or a means of adapting to critical illness. There are three patterns of abnormal thyroid function that represent a progression of disease severity: (1) decreased T_3, (2) decreased T_4 and decreased T_3, and (3) decreased T_3, T_4, and TSH (Table 6). Patients with decreased T_3 alone usually have mild to moderate illness. This pattern is the most common pattern of the sick euthyroid syndrome. The peripheral conversion of T_4 to T_3 is decreased. Mainly this pattern is the effect of medications (see Table 3). Serum T_4 levels

are increased early in acute illness related to decreased conversion or increased binding levels. These elevated T_4 levels then return to normal levels with progressing illness. This pattern is seen with elderly patients and patients with psychiatric problems. The most severe pattern has decreased T_3, T_4, and TSH. The free T_4 may be low, normal, or elevated. In addition to conversion problems, the binding proteins are low, as is TSH. The decline in T_4 correlates with prognosis. Mortality rate increases as the T_4 level drops below 4 µg/dL and is 80% at T_4 levels of 2 µg/dL.

The diagnosis requires trending thyroid function tests. These tests may serve as markers of the severity of disease rather than treatable thyroid disease. The treatment of sick euthyroid syndrome is unclear. Both thyroid replacement and no treatment are advocated. Animal studies show improvement with thyroid replacement, but human studies have not shown similar results, so currently treatment is not advised.

ABNORMALITIES OF ADRENAL FUNCTION

The adrenal glands are an important part of the neuroendocrine axis. The adrenals produce glucocorticoids, catecholamines, mineralocorticoids, and sex hormones. Clinical problems arise with either excess production or insufficient production. Cortisol is required for normal function of all cells, and deficiency states in critical illness are associated with increased morbidity and mortality rates. Catecholamines are produced in the adrenal medulla and require cortisol for synthesis. Sex hormones are not required for recovery from critical illness and there is some compensation for loss of mineralocorticoid activity. The two abnormalities discussed here are pheochrocytoma and adrenal insufficiency (AI).

Pheochromocytoma

Pheochromocytomas produce excess catecholamines, and these tumors follow the rule of 10s: 10% are malignant, 10% are extra-adrenal, 10% are incidental findings on radiographic studies, and 10% are multiple. Less than 0.2% of patients with hypertension have pheochromocytoma as their diagnosis. The diagnosis is usually not made in the ICU, but patients require ICU management for hypertensive crisis or perioperative care. The patients usually have the classic triad of headache, sweating, and tachycardia or palpitations. Weekly paroxysms of hypertension occur in at least 50% of patients and are due to rapid release of catecholamines from an inciting event. Other symptoms include blurred vision, orthostatic hypotension, weight loss, polyuria, and polydipsia.

Clinical suspicion leads to urinary and plasma evaluation for catecholamines and metabolites. These tests confirm the diagnosis 95% of the time. If these tests are inconclusive, a clonidine suppression test is performed with 0.3 mg of clonidine given orally 12 hours after antihypertensive drugs have been stopped. No beta blockers, diuretics, or tricyclic antidepressants can be used. Alpha blockers will not affect the test. Patients without a pheochromocytoma have a fall of the plasma catecholamines to less than 500 pg/mL. The tumor is then localized with computed tomography (CT) or magnetic resonance imaging (MRI). The CT scan has a risk of exacerbating the hypertension with its contrast agent. Failure to detect the tumor with these studies leads to MIBG (metaiodobenzylguanidine) scan, octreoscan, total body MRI, or selected venous sampling.

Acute hypertensive crisis requires treatment with sodium nitroprusside or phentolamine. Phentolamine is given as an IV bolus of 2.5 to 5 mg and then repeated every 5 minutes until the blood pressure is controlled. Nitroprusside is dosed at 0.5 to 10 µg/kg/minute.

Preparation for surgery requires alpha blockade, which is initiated with phenoxybenzamine 10 mg orally daily and increased every few days until symptoms and blood pressure are under control. Beta

TABLE 5: Electrocardiogram Findings in Hypothyroidism

Sinus bradycardia
Low-voltage QRS complex
Flat or inverted T waves
Prolonged intervals of PR, QRS, QT
Heart block

TABLE 6: Abnormalities in Thyroid Response

Hormone	Myxedema Coma	Thyroid Storm	SICK EUTHYROID		
			Mild	Moderate	Severe
TSH	↑	↓	↔	↔	↓
T_3	↓	↑	↓	↓	↓
T_4	↓	↑	↔	↓	↓

TSH, Thyroid-stimulating hormone.

blockade can then be initiated to control the tachycardia, but only after alpha blockade has been performed. Surgery will generally proceed in 10 to 14 days. Postoperatively patients require monitoring and fluid resuscitation. The alpha blockade is continued.

Adrenal Insufficiency

Controversy exists over the incidence, diagnosis, and treatment of adrenal insufficiency in ICU patients. The incidence is less than 0.01% in the general population but up to 28% in seriously ill patients. Reported mortality rate is as high as 25%, but this mortality rate may be reduced with early recognition to rates ranging from 6% to 11%. Cortisol is needed in the critically ill patient for appropriate response to acute inflammation and vasomotor stability. Cortisol has metabolic, catabolic, anti-inflammatory, and vasoactive properties. The most common cause of adrenal insufficiency remains adrenal suppression from the administration of steroids. This effect lasts up to a year after the discontinuation of steroids. In the ICU adrenal gland destruction can occur from infection, bleeding, or system inflammation, but decreased cortisol concentration during critical illness without anatomic disruption is the more common cause. This secondary adrenal insufficiency is usually related to sepsis.

In critically ill patients the usual signs and symptoms of adrenal insufficiency are not usually apparent. These critically ill patients often have hemodynamic instability despite fluid resuscitation and vasopressor use. This picture is a tipoff to adrenal insufficiency and should lead to evaluation of cortisol level and treatment. The most common abnormalities in ICU patients with adrenal insufficiency are listed in Table 7. Several signs and symptoms exist if the patient had preexisting adrenal insufficiency and include fatigue, weight loss, nausea, abdominal pain, arthralgias, syncope, hyperpigmentation of the skin, vitiligo, anorexia, and decreased libido.

The diagnosis and treatment of adrenal insufficiency in critical illness have evolved over time. Some might say that it has become even more confusing. Clinical suspicion leads to a random total cortisol level. If the total cortisol is less than 10 µg/dL adrenal insufficiency is present. Alternatively or concomitantly a stimulation test can be performed with 250 µg of IV synthetic adrenocorticotropic hormone (ACTH). Cortisol levels are drawn at 0, 30 minutes, and 60 minutes after the ACTH dose. If the cortisol level changes 9 µg/dL or more, then adrenal insufficiency is unlikely. If the cortisol changes less than 9 µg/dL, then adrenal insufficiency is likely and treatment is needed.

Laboratory diagnosis is not always required to begin treatment for adrenal insufficiency, however. Patients in septic shock requiring vasopressor support after adequate fluid resuscitation, patients not responding to vasopressor support in septic shock, and patients with early or progressive acute respiratory distress syndrome (ARDS) after 48 hours of treatment may be started on glucocorticoid therapy without laboratory diagnosis. If the previous criteria are met or if the laboratory tests confirm adrenal insufficiency, then treatment is started. IV hydrocortisone 200 to 300 mg/day is administered. IV administration of hydrocortisone 50 mg every 6 hours or 100 mg every 8 hours is the most common method, but a continuous infusion has been described. Fludrocortisone is not needed. Treatment is continued for at least 7 days ± a taper. If ARDS is present, the therapy should continue for 14 days with a taper. If the clinical condition worsens during the taper or after therapy is finished, the steroids are restarted at the original dose.

With the preceding being said, we would be remiss to not mention the CORTICUS (Corticosteroid Therapy of Septic Shock) study from the *New England Journal of Medicine*, published in January 2008. This was a multicenter, randomized, double-blind, placebo-controlled trial. They used 50 mg IV hydrocortisone versus placebo every 6 hours for 5 days and then a 6-day taper with the primary outcome of death among those who did not respond to a corticotropin test. They concluded that hydrocortisone did not improve survival in septic shock but did reverse shock earlier in those patients.

PROBLEMS WITH HYPERGLYCEMIA

Hyperglycemia occurs in most critically ill patients. Diabetes and undiagnosed diabetes may contribute to hyperglycemia; however, in critically ill patients increased sympathetic activity and the activation of the cytokine cascade are the major causes of elevated blood glucose. Medications (total parenteral nutrition, beta blockers, cyclosporine, catecholamines, and glucocorticoids) promote hyperglycemia. Electrolyte imbalance (hypokalemia) decreases insulin release and contributes to hyperglycemia. The stress-induced increased sympathetic activity leads to increased glycogenolysis, increased hepatic gluconeogenesis, and peripheral insulin resistance, which cause an increase in the serum glucose levels. Cytokines produced by the inflammatory process promote insulin resistance and activate the hypothalamic-pituitary-adrenal axis. All or many of these factors comes into play in the critically ill patient and produce an imbalance between glucose production and uptake, resulting in hyperglycemia.

Regardless of the mechanism of hyperglycemia, organ system dysfunction occurs in the cardiovascular, cerebrovascular, neuromuscular, and immunologic systems. Hyperglycemia in the cardiovascular population has been widely studied. An increased risk of in-hospital fatality has been found in patients with myocardial infarction and hyperglycemia. Insulin deficiency/resistance is associated with increased free fatty acids, which the heart uses as a fuel source. These free fatty acids are toxic to the ischemic myocardial cells and lead to arrhythmias. Hyperglycemia also causes an osmotic diuresis leading to volume depletion and increased oxygen consumption from increased contractility.

Hyperglycemic patients with ischemic stroke and head injury have worse outcomes than patients who are euglycemic. With elevated blood glucose levels, there is an increased risk of in-hospital fatality after ischemic stroke in nondiabetic patients. Persistent hyperglycemia is an independent predictor of infarct expansion and is associated with worse functional outcome in patients with ischemic stroke. There may be an association with tissue plasminogen activator and hemorrhagic transformation in hyperglycemic patients with ischemic stroke. In patients with head injury, both the Glasgow Coma Scale score and fatality appear related to blood glucose levels, with an inverse relationship to the Glasgow Coma Scale score and survival.

Increased brain glucose levels contribute to the acidosis from the glycolysis induced by anerobic metabolism of the ischemic brain

TABLE 7: Abnormalities in the Intensive Care Unit Patient Suspicious for Adrenal Insufficiency

Hypotension unresponsive to vasopressors and fluids

Abdominal pain

Nausea/vomiting

Recent steroid use

Tachycardia

Fever

Hypoglycemia

Hyponatremia

Hyperkalemia

Eosinophilia

tissue. The lactic acidosis promotes the formation and accumulation of free radicals, which impede mitochondrial activity. This effect is most important at the edge of the infarct where neurons, which may survive, are recruited into the infarct. Many animal models have shown infarct size increasing with hyperglycemia. Both disruption of the blood–brain barrier and hemorrhagic infarct conversion are suggested mechanisms for deterioration of brain function.

Polyneuropathy of critical illness appears to be related to blood glucose levels. Van den Berghe et al screened for polyneuropathy in critically ill patients and found that patients with control of hyperglycemia were less likely to have critical-illness neuropathy and in those patients who developed neuropathy, there was more rapid resolution. There was a positive linear correlation between blood glucose levels and risk of polyneuropathy. The mechanism of polyneuropathy and its association with hyperglycemia has yet to be defined.

Postoperative wound infections, pneumonias, urinary tract infections, and bacteremias are increased in patients with hyperglycemia. The immunologic system is impaired by hyperglycemia through action on the WBCs. Polymorphonuclear cells have impaired chemotaxis, phagocytosis, and oxidative burst pathways. Macrophages have impaired phagocytosis and deceased complement fixation. Collagen deposition is impaired, granulocyte adherence is irregular, and there is decreased bactericidal activity.

Evidence is accumulating that control of blood glucose improves outcomes from critical illness. Two large patient population studies showed that control of blood glucose to less than 200 mg/dL in cardiothoracic surgery patients reduced the incidence of deep wound infections. Improved survival after myocardial infarction occurs with glycemic control. Evidence is lacking for improved neurologic outcomes with glycemic control. Van den Berghe et al (Fig. 2) concluded that intensive insulin control (blood glucose 80 to 110 mg/dL) improved the morbidity and mortality rates of surgical ICU patients when compared to conventional insulin control (blood glucose 180 to 200 mg/dL). The NICE-SUGAR study investigators further clarified

the target range for blood glucose control as less than 180 mg/dL. In their comparison with intensive insulin control showed lower ICU and 90-day mortality rates and significantly less hypoglycemia, with similar length of hospital and ICU stay and similar rates of organ system failure, times of ventilation, and renal replacement therapy.

Hyperglycemia should be rapidly controlled with IV insulin to a blood glucose less than 180 mg/dL (Table 8). Rapid control can be achieved easily with continuous insulin infusion. Patients with renal failure, liver failure/resection, and renal transplantation are susceptible to hypoglycemia.

OTHER ENDOCRINE CONTRIBUTIONS: PROCALCITONIN

Procalcitonin is a prohormone of the hormone calcitonin. It is produced by the thyroid and the neurodendocrine cells of the lungs and intestine. Although calcitonin affects calcium balance, procalcitonin has been identified as a marker for possible bacterial infection. It has come to light in recent literature as a guide to antibiotic length of therapy coupling with other clinical and laboratory indicators of infection.

Several clinical uses of procalcitonin have been proposed. First, serial measurements may be used to determine when the levels drop enough to indicate that antibiotic therapy should be discontinued. Second, as a guide to empiric antibiotic treatment, procalcitonin can help determine if an infection actually exists and thus may guide the length of the therapy. Third, the level of procalcitonin has been suggested to correlate with mortality rate of the critically septic patient. Fourth, it may help determine if the infection therapy has been successful. Levels should fall after infection control, be it surgical or chemical therapy.

There are several limitations to using procalcitonin levels for detection of infection. Procalcitonin has been found to be increased with cirrhosis, ischemic bowel, cadiogenic shock, hemorrhagic shock, severe burns, and major trauma. This may relate to translocation of bacteria but has not been proved. Procalcitonin level has not been shown to increase with viral infection.

Normal circulating levels of procalcitonin in a noninfected individual are about 0.033 ± 0.003 ng/mL. Levels that indicate a patient is not infected or infection has cleared are less than 0.1 ng/mL. Levels of 0.25 to 0.5 ng/mL suggest bacterial infection that needs to be treated. Levels less than 0.25 ng/mL suggest that severe infection is unlikely but that there may be local infection. Levels of procalcitonin rise after about 2 hours and peak at about 24 hours. C-reactive protein has a slow rise and peaks at 48 hours in comparison.

A multicenter randomized controlled trial in France was published in 2010 looking at procalcitonin to reduce length of antibiotics use. The study was the PRORATA trial (Open label PROcalcitonin to Reduce Antibiotic Treatments in Acutely ill patients). Two groups were studied. The procalcitonin group used the procalcitonin level to determine whether antibiotics should be started and when they should be stopped. Antibiotics were encouraged to be started when levels were higher than 0.5 µg/L. Antibiotics were encouraged to be discontinued when the procalcitonin level was lower than 80% of the peak concentration or an absolute concentration of less than 0.5 µg/L. The procalcitonin group was compared to the control group. The number of days without antibiotics was found to be statistically different with the procalcitonin group, which had 2.7 fewer days of antibiotics.

A meta-analysis was conducted in 2010 and published in *Critical Care Medicine*. The authors found seven randomized controlled trials investigating procalcitonin-guided algorithms for antibiotic therapy in the ICU. A total of 1010 patients were in the seven studies. The authors concluded that procalcitonin-guided therapy in the ICU may decrease antibiotic exposure without compromising clinical outcomes. The body's endocrine system via procalcitonin shows promise in helping us manage our critically ill patients.

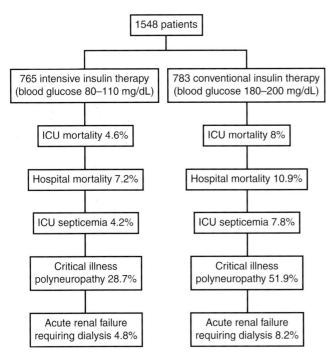

FIGURE 2 Outcome of tight glycemic control. ICU, Intensive care unit. *(Data from Van Den Berghe G, Wouters P, Weekers F, et al: Intensive insulin therapy in critically ill patients. N Engl J Med 345:1359–1367, 2001.)*

TABLE 8: Tight Glycemic Control Protocol for the Surgical Intensive Care Unit of Henry Ford Hospital, Detroit, Michigan

STARTING INSULIN INFUSION		
Glucose	181–219 mg/dL	>220 mg/dL
Starting insulin dose	Give 2 units regular insulin IVP and start 2 units/hr. If renal failure (creatinine > 2 mg/dL), liver failure, liver transplant, or kidney transplant start at 1 unit/hr.	Give 4 units regular insulin IVP and start 4 units/hr. If renal failure (creatinine >2 mg/dL), liver failure, liver transplant, or kidney transplant start at 2 units/hr.

MAINTENANCE INSULIN DRIP		
Glucose Level	**Insulin Rate 1–3 units/hr**	**Insulin Rate >3 units/hr**
<41 mg/dL	Verify result, D/C infusion. Give 1 amp dextrose 50% IVP, notify physician. Check glucose hourly until glucose greater than 80 mg/dL, then every 2 hr. When two in a row every 2-hr glucose checks are greater than 139 mg/dL restart drip at 0.5 unit/hr and use the insulin-sensitive nomogram. Notify physician when glucose greater than 80 mg/dL.	Verify result, D/C infusion. Give 1 amp dextrose 50% IVP, notify physician. Check glucose hourly until glucose greater than 80 mg/dL, then every 2 hr. When two in a row every 2-hr glucose checks are greater than 139 mg/dL restart drip but reduce rate by 50% and use insulin-sensitive nomogram. Notify physician when glucose greater than 80 mg/dL.
41–60 mg/dL	D/C infusion. Give ½ amp dextrose 50% IVP, notify physician. Check glucose hourly until glucose greater than 80 mg/dL, then every 2 hr. When two in a row every 2-hr glucose checks are greater than 139 mg/dL restart drip at 0.5 unit/hr and use the insulin-sensitive nomogram. Notify physician when glucose greater than 80 mg/dL.	D/C infusion. Give ½ amp dextrose 50% IVP, notify physician. Check glucose hourly until glucose greater than 80 mg/dL, then every 2 hr. When two in a row every 2-hr glucose checks are greater than 139 mg/dL restart drip but reduce rate by 50% and use insulin-sensitive nomogram. Notify physician when glucose greater than 80 mg/dL.
	Current Insulin Rate 1–3 units/hr	**Current Insulin Rate >3 units/hr**
61–139 mg/dL	D/C infusion: Recheck glucose *every hour* for glucose 61–80 mg/dL or every 2 hr for glucose 81–139 mg/dL. When glucose greater than 139 mg/dL restart drip at 1 unit/hr.	D/C infusion. Recheck glucose *every hour* for glucose 61–80 mg/dL or every 2 hr for glucose 81–139 mg/dL. When glucose greater than 139 mg/dL restart insulin infusion, but decrease dose rate 50%.

If insulin drip turned off for glucose less than 140 mg/dL (but greater than 60 mg/dL) check every hour until greater than 80 mg/dL, then every 2 hr. If three in a row every 2-hr checks are less than 140 mg/dL restart protocol from beginning. Change glucose check to every 4 hr and start insulin drip for first glucose greater than 180 mg/dL.

	Current Insulin Rate 1–3 units/hr	**Current Insulin Rate >3 units/hr**
140–180 mg/dL	No change unless: If previous glucose levels higher by 40 mg/dL reduce drip by 1 unit/hr. (If current dose 1 unit/hr, do not change.)	No change unless: If previous glucose higher by 40 mg/dL then reduce per below: Infusion Rate · Decrease Dose by 4–7 units/hr · 1 unit/hr 8–12 units/hr · 2 units/hr 13–17 units/hr · 3 units/hr 18–22 units/hr · 4 units/hr >22 units/hr · 5 units/hr

Glucose	Insulin Dosage All Others	Insulin Dosage for: Renal Failure (Creatinine >2), Liver Failure, Liver or Kidney Transplant, or Glucose <61 mg/dL
181–216 mg/dL	Give 2 units regular insulin IVP and increase drip rate by 1 unit/hr. If previous glucose higher by 30 mg/dL maintain same infusion dose/rate.	Give 2 units regular insulin IVP and increase drip rate by 0.5 unit/hr. If previous glucose higher by 30 mg/dL maintain same infusion dose/rate.
217–252 mg/dL	Give 4 units regular insulin IVP and increase drip rate by 1 unit/hr. If previous glucose higher by 30 mg/dL maintain same infusion dose/rate.	Give 4 units regular insulin IVP and increase drip rate by 0.5 unit/hr. If previous glucose higher by 30 mg/dL maintain same infusion dose/rate.
253–400 mg/dL	Give 6 units regular insulin IVP and increase drip rate by 2 unit/hr. Recheck glucose in 1 hr. If previous glucose higher by 50 mg/dL maintain same infusion dose/rate.	Give 6 units regular insulin IVP and increase drip rate by 1 unit/hr. If previous glucose higher by 50 mg/dL maintain same infusion dose/rate.
>400 mg/dL	"Out of critical range" message is displayed on glucometer; verify result. Call MD for new order.	"Out of critical range" message is displayed on glucometer; verify result. Call MD for new order.

D/C, Discontinue; IVP, intravenous push.

SUMMARY

Although the neuroendocrine axis is important for maintaining homeostasis, abnormalities in hormone production occur frequently in the critically ill. Clinical suspicion is required to diagnose the abnormalities. Early aggressive treatment appears to improve morbidity and mortality risks related to these disorders.

For the chapter's Suggested Readings list, please visit the book at www.ExpertConsult.inkling.com.

TRANSFUSION: MANAGEMENT OF BLOOD AND BLOOD PRODUCTS IN TRAUMA

Lena M. Napolitano

Approximately 15% of all blood transfusions in the United States are used in the care of patients who have sustained traumatic injury. Blood transfusion in trauma is lifesaving for those patients in hemorrhagic shock who are unresponsive to crystalloid fluid resuscitation. Importantly, concomitant attempts at prompt cessation of hemorrhage are also necessary. Trauma patients in hemorrhagic shock manifest an acute coagulopathy of trauma (ACOT), and early administration of blood and blood products (plasma, platelets, cryoprecipitate, fibrinogen concentrate [FC]) in ratios close to whole blood composition (hemostatic resuscitation, damage control resuscitation), with attempts to correct the ACOT, is associated with improved outcomes in prospective and retrospective cohort studies. Randomized trials are underway to confirm these preliminary results of noncontrolled clinical studies.

Blood transfusion in trauma has also been identified as an independent predictor of multiple-organ failure (MOF), systemic inflammatory response syndrome (SIRS), increased postinjury infection, and increased mortality rate in multiple studies. The cumulative risks of blood transfusion have been related to the number of units of packed red blood cells (PRBCs) transfused, increased storage time of transfused blood, and possibly donor leukocytes. Lack of efficacy of RBC transfusion in critically ill patients who are hemodynamically stable has also been documented. Therefore, once hemorrhage control has been established in acute trauma we should attempt to minimize the use of blood transfusion for the treatment of asymptomatic anemia in trauma patients.

A number of potential mechanisms that may mediate adverse effects associated with blood transfusion in trauma have been proposed, including increased systemic inflammatory response, immunomodulation, microcirculatory dysfunction due to altered RBC deformability, increased nitric oxide binding by free hemoglobin and vasoconstriction, and others. These data have led some to conclude that blood transfusion in the injured patient should be minimized whenever possible.

INCIDENCE: WHO NEEDS BLOOD TRANSFUSION IN TRAUMA?

The majority of potentially preventable early trauma deaths still result from uncontrolled hemorrhage including noncompressible torso hemorrhage. Trauma patients in hemorrhagic shock have an absolute indication for PRBC transfusion if they are unresponsive to isotonic crystalloid fluid resuscitation, have ongoing significant hemorrhage, and manifest physiologic signs of persistent shock (hypotension, tachycardia, oliguria, lactic acidosis, abnormal base deficit [BD])—indicating that oxygen consumption is dependent on hemoglobin concentration (critical oxygen delivery). In these patients, the prompt transfusion of PRBCs and blood products in conjunction with prompt hemorrhage control is lifesaving.

Patients with hemorrhagic shock, identified by a metabolic acidosis and increasing BD, have been documented to require increased blood and plasma transfusion (Table 1). A single-institution study documented that 8% (479 of 5645) of acute trauma patients received PRBCs, using 5219 units. The majority (62%) of transfusions were administered in the first 24 hours of care. Only 3% of patients ($n = 147$) received more than 10 units of PRBCs, and these patients also received plasma and platelet transfusions to treat actual or anticipated dilutional coagulopathy. Mortality rates in trauma patients who require blood transfusion is high, ranging from 27% to 39%.

MASSIVE TRANSFUSION

Massive blood transfusion is most commonly defined as complete replacement of a patient's blood volume within a 24-hour period or more than 10 units of PRBCs in 24 hours. Newer definitions include an ongoing blood loss of more than 150 mL/minute, or the replacement of 50% of the circulating blood volume in 3 hours or less. These newer definitions have the benefit of allowing early recognition of major blood loss and of the need for effective intervention to prevent hemorrhagic shock and other complications of massive hemorrhage and transfusion.

Massive transfusion (MT) therapy for the treatment of hemorrhagic shock requires a coordinated and detailed approach with the fundamental components listed in Table 2. In the absence of a predefined MT protocol, access to the appropriate blood products (and adequate volume of these products) may be significantly delayed. Without prompt replacement of these blood products, the resultant coagulopathy may worsen and bleeding will continue. In fact, the implementation

TABLE 1: Blood Transfusion Requirements in Trauma Patients and Admission Base Deficit

Admission Base Excess	Interpretation	Units PRBCs in First 24 Hours	Total Units PRBCs	Total Units FFP
≥ −2	Normal	0–1	1–2	0–1
−3 to −5	Mild base deficit	1–2	2–3	0–1
−6 to −9	Moderate base deficit	3–4	5–6	1–2
≤ −10	Severe base deficit	8–9	9–10	3–4

Modified from Davis JW, Parks SN, Kaups KL, et al: Admission base deficit predicts transfusion requirements and risk of complications. *J Trauma* 41:769–774, 1996.

FFP, Fresh frozen plasma; PRBCs, packed red blood cells.

TABLE 2: Management of Massive Transfusion for Hemorrhagic Shock

Provide adequate ventilation and oxygenation

Expedite control of the source of hemorrhage

Restore the circulating volume
Minimize or discontinue crystalloid fluid resuscitation
Hypotensive resuscitation, systolic blood pressure 80–100 mm Hg

Start blood component therapy: RBCs, FFP, Plts, Cryo
Initiate massive transfusion protocol
Anticipate and treat coagulopathy, thrombocytopenia

Maintain or restore normothermia

Evaluate the therapeutic response
Test for coagulopathy, thrombocytopenia, and DIC
Consider TEG or ROTEM

Know and implement specific local procedures for dealing with the logistic demands of massive transfusion

Cryo, Cryoprecipitate; DIC, disseminated intravascular coagulation; FFP, fresh frozen plasma; Plts, platelets; RBCs, red blood cells; ROTEM, thromboelastometry; TEG, thromboelastography.

of an organized "Massive Transfusion Policy" to address exsanguinating hemorrhage in the trauma population has proved to be of benefit in patient outcomes and in reducing blood product use. Studies have demonstrated an increase in survival rate (16% to 45%) in patients with exsanguinating hemorrhage following the implementation of such an MT protocol. Guidelines for the treatment of acute massive blood loss are listed in Table 3. The Joint Theater Trauma System Clinical Practice Guidelines for damage control resuscitation in military combat casualty care are an excellent resource as an evidence-based guideline and provide a template for MT protocol (Table 4). Our University of Michigan Trauma Massive Transfusion protocol is provided as a template for a civilian MT protocol (Fig. 1).

Data from a large prospective multicenter cohort study evaluating outcomes in blunt injured adults with hemorrhagic shock was used to examine resuscitation strategies over time (2004–2009) and determined that the percentage of patients who required MT overall significantly decreased over time. Over the study period for the MT group ($n = 526$), initial BD and admission international normalized ratio (INR) were unchanged, but Injury Severity Score (ISS) was significantly higher. No significant differences were found over time for 6-hour, 12-hour, and 24-hour FFP:PRBC and Plt:PRBC (platelet: PRBC) transfusion ratios in MT patients. Sub-MT patients ($n = 344$) had significantly higher 6-hour FFP:PRBC ratios and significantly higher 6-hour, 12-hour, and 24-hour Plt:PRBC ratios in the recent time period. The 6-hour/24-hour percent total for FFP and platelet transfusion was significantly greater in the recent time period (FFP: 54% vs.70%, $P = .004$; and Plt 46% vs. 61%, $P = .048$). This study documented that in a severely injured cohort requiring MT, FFP: PRBC and Plt:PRBC ratios have not changed over time, whereas

TABLE 3: Acute Massive Blood Loss: Template for Guidelines

Goal	Procedure	Comments
Arrest bleeding	Prompt cessation of hemorrhage Surgical intervention Interventional radiology Angiographic embolization	All attempts at early hemorrhage cessation should be initiated, and may include multiple modalities
Restore circulating volume Resuscitate to a level that restores or maintains vital organ perfusion, but restoration of normal blood pressure should not be attempted until definitive measures have been taken to control hemorrhage	Insert large-bore peripheral venous lines Give adequate volumes of warmed crystalloid, colloid, blood Aim to maintain adequate mean arterial pressure and urine output (0.5 mL/kg/hour)	Use 14 gauge or larger Blood loss often underestimated Refer to Advanced Trauma Life Support guidelines Keep patients warm
Request laboratory testing	PT, PTT, INR, CBC, blood bank sample for type and crossmatch, DIC screen Ensure correct sample identity Repeat testing after each one third blood volume replacement, every 4 hours Repeat testing after component infusion	Take initial samples on admission Misidentification is the most common transfusion risk Give FFP and platelets before coagulation tests available if clinical evidence of coagulopathy/bleeding
Request red blood cells	Severity of hemorrhage determines choice Immediate need: use group O Rh D–negative blood Need in 15–60 min: uncrossmatched ABO group-specific will be provided when blood group known Need in 60 min or longer: fully crossmatched blood When time permits, use blood warmer or rapid infusion device Employ blood salvage if available and appropriate (i.e., minimal contamination)	Emergency use of Rh D-positive blood is acceptable if patient is male or postmenopausal female Laboratory will complete crossmatch after issue Further crossmatch not required after replacement of one blood volume (8–10 units PRBCs) Blood warmer indicated if large volumes are transfused rapidly to prevent hypothermia Salvage contraindicated if wound heavily contaminated

TABLE 3: Acute Massive Blood Loss: Template for Guidelines—Cont'd

Goal	Procedure	Comments
Request platelets 10 mL/kg body weight for neonate/child One adult therapeutic dose	May have delayed delivery time Anticipate platelet count $<50 \times 10^9$/L after $2 \times$ blood volume replacement Repeat platelet count 10 minutes and 1 hour after platelet transfusion to assess efficacy	Target platelet count: $>100 \times 10^9$/L for multiple/CNS trauma or if platelet function abnormal; $>50 \times 10^9$/L for other situations May need to use platelets before lab results available (take sample before platelets transfused)
Request FFP 15 mL/kg body weight or 4 units (1 L) for an adult	Anticipate coagulation factor deficiency after blood loss of $1.5 \times$ blood volume Aim for PT and PTT $<1.5 \times$ control Allow for 30 minutes thaw time (if prethawed FFP not available in hospital)	PT and PTT $>1.5 \times$ control correlates with increased surgical bleeding May need to use FFP before lab results available (take sample before FFP transfused)
Request cryoprecipitate	To replace fibrinogen and factor VIII Aim for fibrinogen >1 g/L Allow for delivery and 30 min thaw time	Fibrinogen <0.8 g/L strongly associated with microvascular bleeding Fibrinogen deficiency develops early when plasma-poor PRBCs transfused for hemorrhage
Suspect DIC	Treat underlying cause if possible	Shock, hypothermia, acidosis leading to risk of DIC Mortality rate from DIC is high

Modified from Stainsby D, Maclennan S, Hamilton PJ: Management of massive blood loss: a template guideline. *Br J Anaesth* 85:487–491, 2000; and McClelland DBL: Clinical use of blood products. In McClelland DBL, editor: *The handbook of transfusion medicine*, 3rd ed, London, 2001, The Stationery Office, p 79. CBC, Complete blood (cell) count; CNS, central nervous system; DIC, disseminated intravascular coagulation; FFP, fresh frozen plasma; INR, international normalized ratio; PRBCs, packed red blood cells; PT, prothrombin time; PTT, partial thromboplastin time.

TABLE 4: Joint Theater Trauma System Clinical Practice Guidelines for Damage Control Resuscitation

Example of a Massive Transfusion Procedure at a USCENTCOM Level III Facility

Considerations for use with massive transfusion (MT): A flexible procedure for use in the emergency department (ED), operating room (OR) and intensive care unit (ICU) which can be initiated or ceased by the site-specific provider as dictated by the patient's needs when in that specific venue. It consists of batches as defined below, which vary in composition, but are directed toward approximating a 1:1:1:1 ratio of PRBC, FFP, platelets and cryoprecipitate (cryo). **Note:** 1 unit of apheresis platelets is approximately the equivalent of 6 units random donor platelets, therefore 1 unit apheresis platelets should be given for every 6 units of PRBC to approximate 1:1:1 resuscitation.

Initiate MT procedure if patient has received 4 units PRBC/4 units FFP emergency release blood products.

Pack One: 4 units PRBC, 4 units FFP, 1 unit apheresis platelets, 1 10-unit bag cryo. **Strongly consider the *early* use of TXA:** Infuse 1 g of tranexamic acid in 100 mL of 0.9% NS over 10 minutes intravenously in a separate IV line from any containing blood and blood products. (More rapid injection has been reported to cause hypotension.). **Hextend should be avoided as a carrier fluid.** Infuse a second 1-g dose intravenously over 8 hours infused with 0.9% NS carrier.

Pack Two: 4 units PRBC and 4 units FFP

Pack Three: 4 units PRBC, 4 units FFP, 1 unit apheresis platelets, 1 10-unit bag of cryo and +/− rFVIIa (obtained from pharmacy)

Pack Four: 4 units PRBC and 4 units FFP

Pack Five: 4 units PRBC, 4 units FFP, 1 unit apheresis platelets, and 1 10-unit bag of cryo.

A reassessment of the progress of the resuscitation, hemostasis and the need to continue the MT procedure should be conducted between the providers taking care of the patient at that time.

From Joint Theater Trauma System Clinical Practice Guidelines, Approved 2/1/13. Available at http://www.usaisr.amedd.army.mil/assets/cpgs/Damage%20Control%20Resuscitation%20-%201%20Feb%202013.pdf. Accessed December 2014.
FFP, Fresh frozen plasma; IV, intravenous; NS, normal saline; PRBC, packed red blood cell.

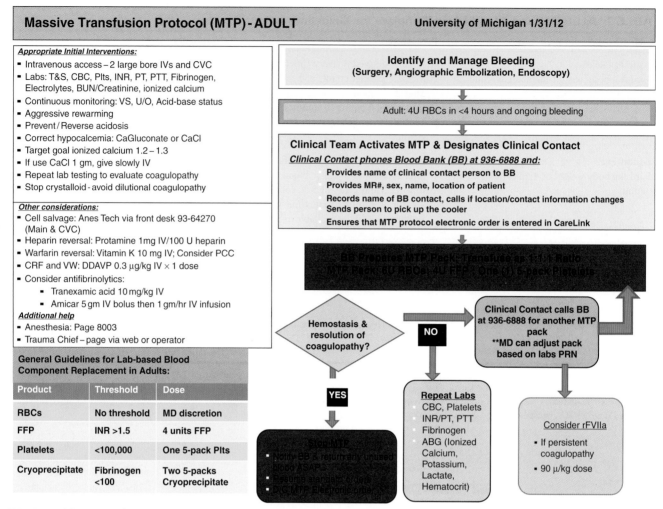

FIGURE I   Massive transfusion protocol. ABG, Arterial blood gases; ASAP, as soon as possible; BUN, blood urea nitrogen; CBC, complete blood count; CRF, chronic renal failure; CVC, central venous catheter; FFP, fresh frozen plasma; INR, international normalized ratio; IV, intravenous; PCC, prothrombin complex concentrate; Plts, platelets; PRN, as needed; PT, prothrombin time; PTT, partial thromboplastin time; RBCs, red blood cells; T&S, type and screen; U/O, urine output; VS, vital signs; VW, von Willebrand disease. *(Courtesy of the University of Michigan.)*

the rate of MT overall has significantly decreased. During the recent time period (after December 2007), significantly higher transfusion ratios and a greater percent of 6-hour/24-hour FFP and platelet transfusion were found in the sub-MT group, those patients just below the PRBC transfusion threshold definition of MT. These data suggest early, more aggressive attainment of high blood product transfusions ratios may reduce the requirement for MT and may shift overall blood requirements below those that currently define MT. Further prospective evidence is required to verify these findings.

Identification of Trauma Patients Who Will Require Massive Transfusion

Time to initiation of hemostatic/damage control resuscitation is thought to be associated with improved outcomes in MT patients. The identification of early predictors of MT in trauma would prevent undertriage of trauma patients likely to require MT. A recent study validated triggers using the Prospective Observational Multicenter Major Trauma Transfusion (PROMMTT) study. This study prospectively examined the predictive ability of individual triggers to expeditiously identify trauma patients who are likely to receive MT using individual triggers adapted from the Individual Transfusion Trigger study (Cincinnati ITT study, CITT) and the Assessment of Blood

Consumption (ABC) score, both of which have shown promise for predictive use of MT and ease of use in the civilian population. The CITT triggers were adapted from previously published military triggers and included systolic blood pressure (SBP) less than 90 mm Hg, hemoglobin (Hb) level less than 11 g/dL, temperature less than 35.5° C, INR greater than 1.5, and BD of 6 or greater. The ABC score includes SBP less than 90 mm Hg, heart rate (HR) 120 beats per minute (bpm) or greater, positive result for focused assessment with sonography in trauma (FAST), and penetrating mechanism of injury. From the CITT and ABC studies, eight unique triggers were identified for study inclusion. In 297 patients who received MT, all triggers except penetrating injury mechanism and heart rate were valid individual predictors of MT, with INR as the most predictive (adjusted odds ratio [OR], 2.5; 95% confidence interval [CI], 1.7 to 3.7) (Table 5).

BLOOD TRANSFUSION COMPONENTS

Red Blood Cells

For severe hemorrhagic shock, uncrossmatched type O blood should be transfused due to immediate availability. Advanced trauma life support (ATLS) encourages a transition to RBC products immediately after

TABLE 5: Likelihood of Massive Transfusion and Mean RBC Transfusion Volume for Individual Transfusion Triggers in Trauma*

Trigger	Data Available n = pts	Data Available % pts	MEAN UNITS RBCs TRANSFUSED			LIKELIHOOD OF MT (OR, 95% CI)			% MT IF TRIGGER EXCEEDED (PPV)		
			Trigger, Yes	Trigger, No	P-value	MT 24 h	MT 24 h+	MT 6 h+	MT 24 h	MT24h+	MT6h+
INR >1.5	1081	87%	13.5 ± 1.0	6.6 ±0.3	P<.0001	3.4 (2.5–4.7)	4.0 (2.9–5.5)	5.8 (4.0–8.2)	43%	49%	40%
SBP <90 mm Hg	1213	97%	11.2 ±0.7	6.5 ±0.3	P<.0001	2.6 (1.9–3.4)	2.5 (1.9–3.3)	2.4 (1.7–3.3)	36%	37%	25%
Hb <11 g/dL	1198	96%	10.3 ±0.6	6.8 ±0.3	P<.0001	2.4 (1.9–3.2)	2.6 (2.0–3.4)	3.5 (2.6–4.8)	34%	37%	28%
BD ≥6	960	77%	10.5 ±0.6	5.5 ±0.3	P<.0001	2.8 (2.0–3.9)	3.0 (2.2–4.2)	4.5 (3.0–6.9)	32%	35%	25%
dFAST (+)	1245	100%	12.0 ±0.7	7.0 ±0.3	P<.0001	2.4 (1.8–3.2)	2.4 (1.8–3.2)	2.9 (2.1–3.9)	37%	40%	30%
HR ≥120 bpm	1218	98%	9.9 ±0.6	7.3 ±0.3	P<.0001	1.5 (1.2–2.0)	1.6 (1.2–2.1)	1.8 (1.3–2.4)	29%	31%	23%
Penetrating	1242	100%	9.0 ±0.6	7.7 ±0.3	P=0.04	1.0 (0.8–1.4)	1.1 (0.8–1.4)	1.5 (1.1–2.0)	24%	26%	21%
Temp <35.5° C	630	51%	7.7 ±0.8	6.4 ±0.4	P=.11	1.5 (0.9–2.4)	1.6 (1.0–2.5)	1.5 (0.9–2.6)	22%	28%	28%

Modified from Callcut RA, Cotton BA, Muskat P, et al; PROMMTT Study Group: Defining when to initiate massive transfusion: a validation study of individual massive transfusion triggers in PROMMTT patients. *J Trauma Acute Care Surg* 74(1):59–65, 67–68; discussion 66–67, 2013.

BD, Base deficit; bpm, beats per minute; CI, confidence interval; FAST, focused assessment with sonography in trauma; g/dL, grams per deciliter; Hb, hemoglobin; HR, heart rate; INR, internal normalized ratio; MT, massive transfusion; OR, odds ratio; PPV, positive predictive value; RBC, red blood cell; SBP, systolic blood pressure; temp, temperature.

*MT 24 h, 10+ units RBCs in 24 hours; MT 24 h+, 10+ units RBCs in 24 hours plus hemorrhagic deaths within 24 hours; MT6h+, 10+ units RBCs at 6 hours plus hemorrhagic deaths within 6 hours.

failure to achieve hemodynamic stability with 2 L of crystalloid solution. Because emergent transfusions are typically needed before identifying a patient's specific blood type, uncrossmatched RBC (URBC) products are commonly used. Rh-positive blood is commonly used in male trauma patients, with minimal transfusion-related complications, and a low rate of seroconversion of Rh-negative patients.

Rh-negative blood should be used in women of childbearing age if possible. A prompt transition to the use of type-specific (ABO, Rh-matched) blood should be accomplished as quickly as possible (approximately 10 minutes for type-specific RBCs), and use is continued until fully crossmatched units of blood are available (approximately 30 to 40 minutes for full crossmatching). Once a trauma patient has been administered more than one blood volume and the initial antibody screen is negative, there is no point attempting compatibility testing except for ABO matching.

Fresh Frozen Plasma

Fresh frozen plasma (FFP) is administered to trauma patients with hemorrhage in an attempt to correct the ACOT. A systematic review of 37 observational studies documented that in patients undergoing MT, plasma infusion at high FFP:RBC ratios was associated with a significant reduction in the risk of death (OR, 0.38; 95% CI, 0.24 to 0.60) and multiorgan failure (OR, 0.40; 95% CI, 0.26 to 0.60). However, the quality of this evidence was very low due to significant unexplained heterogeneity and several other biases. In patients undergoing surgery without MT, plasma infusion was associated with a trend toward increased mortality rate (OR, 1.22; 95% CI, 0.73 to 2.03). Plasma transfusion was associated with increased risk of developing acute lung injury (OR, 2.92; 95% CI, 1.99 to 4.29). The study conclusion was that very low quality evidence confirms that FFP infusion in the setting of MT for trauma patients is associated with a reduction in the risk of death and multiorgan failure but a threefold increased risk of acute lung injury. We therefore keep thawed plasma available in the emergency department for use in hemostatic/damage control resuscitation in trauma.

Although FFP is widely available as a potential source of fibrinogen, it has multiple shortcomings such as extended administration time, transfusion-related complications, and limited efficacy. Blood group matching is required, and because FFP is stored at −20° C it needs to be thawed before administration. The average concentration of fibrinogen in FFP is around 2.5 g/L, although there is considerable variation. The low concentration of fibrinogen in FFP limits the extent to which the fibrinogen level can be raised. FFP is not typically subjected to viral inactivation procedures, so there are risks of viral transmission. Treatment with methylene blue or solvent detergent unfortunately reduces the level of fibrinogen in the end product (particularly in the case of methylene blue treatment, in which the reduction is around 30%). Finally, numerous publications have documented serious adverse events following FFP transfusion including volume overload and transfusion-related acute lung injury (TRALI).

Platelets

Platelet transfusion is administered early, along with RBCs and FFP, as a part of hemostatic/damage control resuscitation, particularly in patients requiring MT. Platelets should be transfused in bleeding trauma patients with a goal to keep the platelet count higher than 100,000 to establish a stable clot.

The impact of platelet transfusion in trauma patients undergoing MT was evaluated in a retrospective single-institution study. For injured patients requiring MT, as the apheresis Plt:RBC ratio increased, a stepwise improvement in survival was seen. Similar to recently published military data, transfusion of Plt:RBC ratios of 1:1 was associated with improved early and late survival, decreased hemorrhagic death, and a concomitant increase in MOF-related mortality rate in a large multicenter retrospective study. Based on these data, increased and early use of platelets may be justified, pending the results of prospective randomized transfusion trials in trauma.

Similar to data with RBC transfusion, increased storage age of platelets has been associated with adverse outcome. In a study of 380 critically ill trauma patients who received platelet transfusions, there was a stepwise increase in complications, in particular sepsis, with exposure to progressively older platelets. Further evaluation of the underlying mechanism and methods for minimizing exposure to older platelets is warranted, as is further prospective evaluation of the role of platelet transfusion in massively transfused patients.

Cryoprecipitate

Cryoprecipitate contains a higher concentration of fibrinogen than FFP, typically around 15 g/L. However, it shares many of the disadvantages of FFP. The risk of viral transmission is similar to that of FFP, but the risk is enhanced by the fact that each pool of cryoprecipitate contains human plasma from multiple donors. Despite internal quality control protocols in blood banks, the fibrinogen concentration is variable and blood group matching is needed. Finally, time is also required for thawing cryoprecipitate. Cryoprecipitate was withdrawn from most European countries some years ago on the basis of safety concerns, though it remains available in Scandinavia, the United Kingdom, and the United States. Cryoprecipitate is unsuitable for pathogen-reduction steps, but it can be produced from plasma that has undergone treatment.

Fibrinogen Concentrate

Current therapeutic options for supplementing plasma fibrinogen are FFP, cryoprecipitate, and FC. FC is currently indicated for the treatment of acute bleeding episodes in patients with congenital fibrinogen deficiency, including afibrinogenemia and hypofibrinogenemia. FC is increasingly being used in severe trauma patients with hemorrhagic shock, but there is significant controversy regarding its efficacy. The first large multicenter study to examine the effect of FC in traumatic hemorrhage is the retrospective study of the German Trauma Registry. A matched-pairs analysis with two cohorts was used, comparing patients who received FC to those who did not ($n = 294$ in each group). Trauma patients had severe injury (mean ISS of 37 ± 14), hypotension (SBP less than or equal to 90 mm Hg) occurred in 50%, and base excess was -7.5 ± 6 mmol/L on admission, and they received approximately 12 ± 12 PRBC units. The overall hospital mortality rate was 28.6% versus 25.5% ($P = .40$), respectively. The early use of FC was associated with a significantly lower 6-hour mortality rate (10.5% vs. 16.7% [$P = .03$]) and an increased time to death (7.5 ± 14.6 vs. 4.7 ± 8.6 days [$P = .006$]), but also an increased rate of MOF. A reduction of overall hospital mortality rate was not observed in patients receiving FC.

In a study including 128 bleeding trauma patients, goal-directed coagulation management with FC as first-line treatment together with prothrombin complex concentrate was evaluated retrospectively. Observed mortality rate was significantly lower in these patients compared with the mortality rate predicted by the Trauma and Injury Severity Score and the Revised Injury Severity Classification score. Stinger et al reported the association of fibrinogen and fatality in 252 injured soldiers receiving MT at an army combat support hospital. For each patient the amount of fibrinogen transfused (through plasma and cryoprecipitate) was registered and a fibrinogen:RBC ratio was calculated. An increased fibrinogen:RBC ratio was independently associated with improved survival.

A systematic review of studies to date compared efficacy of FFP and FC in trauma or perioperative patients. The weight of evidence does not appear to support the clinical effectiveness of FFP for surgical and massive trauma patients and suggests that it can be detrimental. Perioperatively, FC was generally associated with improved outcome measures, although more high-quality, prospective studies are required before any definitive conclusions can be drawn.

Thromboelastography (TEG) functional fibrinogen assay studies indicate that fibrinogen is critical in correcting abnormal clot strength following trauma. in vitro studies demonstrated that the addition of

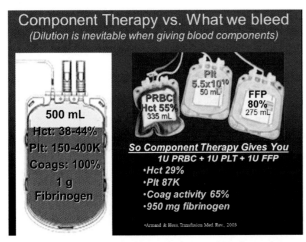

FIGURE 2 Composition of whole blood versus blood component therapy. Note that dilution will be inevitable with transfusion of stored blood components. FFP, Fresh frozen plasma; Plt, platelets; RBC, red blood cell. *(Data from Armand R, Hess JR: Treating coagulopathy in trauma patients.* Transfus Med Rev *17:223–231, 2003, pp 223–231.)*

FC resulted in an increase in functional fibrinogen, clot strength, and percent of fibrinogen contribution to clot strength. These data suggest that fibrinogen should be addressed early in trauma patients manifesting ACOT, but additional studies are warranted to determine dose and timing.

Blood Component Therapy: Fresh Frozen Plasma, Platelets, and Cryoprecipitate

Dilution is inevitable when giving blood component therapy (Fig. 2). The administration of 1 unit each of PRBC, FFP, and platelets does not reconstitute into the amount of coagulation factors in a unit of whole blood. Therefore, dilutional coagulopathy and dilutional thrombocytopenia are common even with early aggressive transfusion of blood components, even with hemostatic/damage control 1:1:1 RBC:FFP:Plt blood component resuscitation, particularly in patients requiring MT.

The administration of early balanced resuscitation of RBCs, plasma, and platelets (hemostatic resuscitation, damage control resuscitation) has been shown in numerous retrospective investigations to have a mortality benefit for patients ultimately requiring MT. Increasing evidence suggests that high FFP:PRBC and Plt:PRBC transfusion ratios may prevent or reduce the morbidity associated with early coagulopathy, which complicates MT. Despite studies demonstrating an advantage for hemostatic/damage control resuscitation in severely injured patients, it remains difficult to readily identify those most likely to benefit from this approach early after injury.

Coagulopathy and thrombocytopenia are a common occurrence during major trauma resuscitation, and hemorrhage remains a major cause of traumatic deaths. Current coagulation factor replacement practices vary, and some may be inadequate. A recent pharmacokinetic model was used to simulate the dilutional component of coagulopathy during hemorrhage and compared various FFP transfusion strategies for the prevention or correction, or both, of dilutional coagulopathy. This study documented that once excessive deficiency of factors has developed and bleeding is unabated 1 to 1.5 units of FFP must be given for every unit of PRBCs transfused. If FFP transfusion should start before plasma factor concentration drops below 50% of normal, an FFP:PRBC transfusion ratio of 1:1 would prevent further dilution. They concluded that during resuscitation of a patient who has undergone major trauma the equivalent of whole-blood transfusion is required to correct or prevent dilutional coagulopathy.

Ultimately, additional blood product administration for the treatment of dilutional and consumptive coagulopathy and

thrombocytopenia in trauma must be guided by blood coagulation testing, with regular monitoring of hemoglobin, platelet count, prothrombin time (PT), partial thromboplastin time (PTT), and fibrinogen levels (see Table 3) and consideration of the use of TEG and thromboelastometry (ROTEM) for more detailed analysis of the ACOT.

The Prospective Observational Multicenter Major Trauma Transfusion Study

PROMMTT, the first multicenter (10 centers) prospective study to examine transfusion practices during active resuscitation of bleeding trauma patients ($n = 1245$, received at least 1 unit RBCs within 6 hours of admission), examined 905 patients who received at least 3 units of RBCs, FFP, or platelets within 24 hours. Plasma:RBC and Plt:RBC ratios were not constant during the first 24 hours. In a multivariable time-dependent Cox model, increased ratios of plasma:RBCs (adjusted hazard ratio 0.31; 95% CI, 0.16 to 0.58) and Plts:RBCs (adjusted hazard ratio 0.55; 95% CI, 0.31 to 0.98) were independently associated with decreased 6-hour mortality rate, when hemorrhagic death predominated. In the first 6 hours, patients with ratios less than 1:2 were three to four times more likely to die than patients with ratios of 1:1 or higher. After 24 hours, plasma and platelet ratios were unassociated with fatality, when competing risks from nonhemorrhagic causes prevailed. This first prospective study documented that higher plasma and platelet ratios early in resuscitation were associated with decreased mortality rate in patients who received transfusions of at least 3 units of blood products during the first 24 hours after admission. Among survivors at 24 hours, the subsequent risk of death by day 30 was not associated with plasma or platelet ratios.

The Pragmatic Randomized Optimal Platelets and Plasma Ratios Trial

The Pragmatic Randomized Optimal Platelets and Plasma Ratios (PROPPR) trial is a phase III trial being conducted at Level I adult trauma centers in the United States and Canada. PROPPR is designed to evaluate the difference in 24-hour and 30-day mortality rate among trauma patients predicted to receive MT, defined as receiving 10 units or more RBCs within the first 24 hours. The goal of PROPPR is to improve the basis on which clinicians make decisions about transfusion protocols for massively bleeding patients. PROPPR is a Resuscitation Outcomes Consortium (ROC) protocol, and is funded by the National Heart, Lung, and Blood Institute, the U.S. Department of Defense, and the Defence Research and Development Canada. Group 1 will be randomized to receive the 1:1:1 ratio of plasma:Plts:RBCs; group 2 will be randomized to receive the 1:1:2 ratio of plasma: Plts:RBCs. Inclusion criteria for the PROPPR trial are subjects who (1) require the highest trauma team activation at each participating center, (2) are estimated to be age 15 years or older or greater than or equal to weight of 50 kg if age unknown, (3) were received directly from the injury scene, (4) underwent initiated transfusion of at least 1 unit of blood component within the first hour of arrival or during prehospital transport, and (5) were predicted to receive an MT by exceeding the threshold score of either the ABC score or the attending trauma physician's judgment criteria. Results of this important study will certainly assist in determination of the ideal blood component resuscitation strategy for trauma patients with hemorrhage.

RESTRICTIVE TRANSFUSION STRATEGIES IN TRAUMA

Once hemorrhage control has been established and the patient has completed resuscitation from hemorrhagic shock, all efforts to restrict RBC transfusion in trauma are advisable. Anemia is common in critically injured trauma patients and persists throughout the duration of critical illness, as documented in a post hoc analysis of a subset of trauma patients ($n = 576$) from a prospective multicenter observational cohort study in the United States. While in the intensive care unit (ICU), 319 (55.4%) trauma patients received a total of 1858 units of blood (or 5.8 ± 5.5 units of blood each on average). The majority (87.1%, $n = 278$) of all ICU trauma patients requiring transfusions received them within the first 4 days, accounting for almost half of all ICU transfusions. However, 5% to 10% of patients continued to receive blood transfusions. Importantly, this study documented that a large number of blood transfusions were administered when the Hb concentration was greater than 10 g/dL.

National guidelines regarding blood transfusion differ, such that the American Society of Anesthesiology recommends maintaining Hb greater than 6 g/dL—whereas the National Institutes of Health (NIH) recommends maintaining Hb greater than 7 g/dL for patients who are critically ill. A Cochrane Database Systematic Review concluded that the limited published evidence (10 trials, $n = 1780$ patients) supports the use of restrictive transfusion triggers (RBC transfusion if Hb <7 g/dL) in patients who are free of cardiac disease. The two most recent guidelines from Society of Critical Care Medicine (SCCM), Eastern Association for the Surgery of Trauma (EAST), and the American Association of Blood Banks (AABB) advocate restrictive transfusion strategies (RBC transfusion if Hb is less than 7 g/dL).

An analysis from the prospective multicenter randomized controlled trial (Transfusion Requirements in Critical Care, TRICC) compared the use of restrictive (transfuse if Hb is less than 7 g/dL) and liberal (transfuse if Hb is less than 10 g/dL) transfusion strategies in resuscitated critically ill trauma patients ($n = 203$). The average hemoglobin concentrations (8.3 ± 0.62 g/dL vs. 10.4 ± 1.2 g/dL, $P <.0001$) and the RBC units transfused per patient (2.3 ± 4.4 vs. 5.4 ± 4.3, $P < .0001$) were significantly lower in the restrictive group than in the liberal group. No differences in mortality rate, multiple-organ dysfunction, or ICU or hospital length of stay (LOS) were identified—suggesting that a restrictive RBC transfusion strategy appears to be safe for critically ill multiple trauma patients if not bleeding or hemodynamically unstable.

RISKS OF BLOOD TRANSFUSION

The blood supply in the United States has never been as safe as it is now. During the past several decades, there have been dramatic progressive reductions in the risk of transfusion-transmitted clinically significant bloodborne infections.

Although there has been a 10,000-fold reduction in the risk to patients from transfusion-transmitted infectious diseases in recent decades, there has been little progress in reducing the risk of noninfectious hazards of transfusion. An analysis of 366 spontaneously reported deaths and major complications of transfusion in the United Kingdom and Ireland identified that the majority (53%) of these adverse events were related to the incorrect blood component being transfused (i.e., a clerical or human-related error). As a result, patients today are harmed from noninfectious serious hazards of transfusion at a rate that exceeds infectious hazards by 100-fold to 1000-fold (Table 6).

Emerging risks of blood transfusion include West Nile virus (WNV) transmission via blood transfusion. Between August 2002 and January 2003, there were 23 confirmed cases of transfusion-associated WNV from 14 donors. Experimental WNV nucleic acid amplification test assays were implemented for blood donor testing in July 2003. Reports through September 2003 indicated that more than 600 infected units of blood were identified from 2.5 million donations during a period of 4137 known WNV infections reported to the Centers for Disease Control and Prevention (CDC). Although nucleic acid amplification testing of blood donations prevented hundreds of cases of WNV infection, it failed to detect units with a low level of viremia—some of which were antibody negative and infectious. These data support the use of targeted nucleic acid amplification testing of individual donations in high-prevalence WNV regions, a strategy that was implemented successfully in 2004.

TABLE 6: Risks Associated with Transfusion

Type of Risk	Incidence
Noninfectious Risks	
Depressed erythropoiesis	Universal
Volume overload, pulmonary edema	10%–40%
Febrile reaction	1/10–1/100
Urticarial reaction	1/33–1/100
Transfusion-related acute lung injury (TRALI)	1/1120–1/5000
Delayed hemolytic transfusion reaction	1/2500
Hemolytic transfusion reactions	1/38,000–1/70,000
Fatal hemolytic transfusion reactions	1/600,000
Anaphylactic shock	1/500,000
Immunosuppression	Unknown
Graft-versus-host disease	1/400–1/10,000
Alloimmunization (RBCs)	1/100
Alloimmunization (platelets)	1/10

ABO-Rh mismatch
  Occurrence
  Mortality
	1/6000–1/20,000
	1/100,000–1/600,000

Infectious Risks	
Cytomegalovirus conversion	7%
Epstein-Barr virus	0.5%
Bacterial contamination (PRBCs + platelets)	1/2000
Hepatitis B transmission	1/220,000
PRBC-related bacterial sepsis	1/500,000–1/786,000
Hepatitis A transmission	1/1,000,000
West Nile virus transmission	1/1,400,000
Hepatitis C transmission	1/1,600,000
HIV transmission	1/1,800,000

Modified from Klein HG: Allogenic transfusion risks in the surgical patient. *Am J Surg* 170;6A:21S–26S, 1995; Silliman CC, Moore EE, Johnson JL, et al: Transfusion in the injured patient: proceed with caution. *Shock* 21 (4):291–299, 2004; Busch MP, Kleinman SH, Nemo GJ: Current and emerging infectious risks of blood transfusions. *JAMA* 289(8):959–962, 2003; and Spiess BD: Risk of transfusion: outcome focus. *Transfusion* 44:4S–14S, 2004.
HIV, Human immunodeficiency virus; PRBC, packed red blood cell; RBC, red blood cell.

There is increasing evidence that the duration of RBC storage negatively impacts outcomes. In the multicenter, double-blind prospective ABLE (Age of Blood Evaluation) study, adult patients admitted to the ICU are randomly assigned to receive leukoreduced RBCs stored for less than 7 days or issued according to standard procedure (expected average storage time of 19 days). The primary end point of this study is 90-day all-cause mortality rate. The target number of patients is 2510 (for an expected improvement in primary end point greater than 5%) with patient recruitment completed January 2013; longterm followup is ongoing.

Although our blood supply is safe, emerging data from the last 2 decades has identified significant risks associated with RBC transfusion, including increased mortality and morbidity rates (SIRS, TRALI, infection, MOF). The largest systematic review of the efficacy of RBC transfusion in critically ill patients included 45 observational cohort studies including 272,596 patients. In 42 of the 45 studies the risks of RBC transfusion outweighed the benefits; the risk was neutral in two studies with the benefits outweighing the risks in a subgroup of a single study (elderly patients with an acute myocardial infarction and a hematocrit less than 30%). Seventeen of 18 studies demonstrated that RBC transfusions were an independent predictor of death; the pooled OR (12 studies) was 1.7 (95% CI, 1.4 to 1.9). Twenty-two studies examined the association between RBC transfusion and nosocomial infection; in all these studies RBC transfusion was an independent risk factor for infection. The pooled OR (nine studies) for developing an infectious complication was 1.8 (95% CI, 1.5 to 2.2). RBC transfusions similarly increased the risk of developing multiorgan dysfunction syndrome (three studies) and acute respiratory distress syndrome (ARDS) (six studies). The pooled OR for developing ARDS was 2.5 (95% CI, 1.6 to 3.3). Despite the inherent limitations in the analysis of cohort studies, this analysis suggests that in adult, ICU, trauma, and surgical patients, RBC transfusions are associated with increased morbidity and mortality risks and therefore current transfusion practices may require reevaluation. The risks and benefits of RBC transfusion should be assessed in every patient before transfusion.

Transfusion-Related Acute Lung Injury

TRALI is a life-threatening complication of blood transfusion. TRALI is now the leading cause of transfusion-related fatality, even though it is probably still underdiagnosed and underreported. The National Heart, Lung and Blood Institute of the NIH convened a working group on TRALI, and a common definition has been established: new acute lung injury occurring during or within 6 hours after a blood transfusion. TRALI, like the ARDS, may be a two-event phenomenon—with both recipient predisposition and factors in the stored blood units playing major roles. The overall prevalence has been reported as 1 in 1120 cellular components transfused.

A recent prospective cohort study documented a significant independent association between the amount of transfused blood and the development of ARDS and hospital fatality. The association between the amount of transfused blood and the development of ARDS remained significant in a multivariable logistic regression model accounting for differences in severity of illness, type of trauma, race/ethnicity, gender, and BD. A larger study in 5260 blunt trauma patients documented that delayed blood transfusion (defined as no blood transfusion received within the initial 48 hours after admission) was independently associated with ventilator-associated pneumonia, ARDS, and death in trauma regardless of injury severity. Similarly, an additional study that examined clinical predictors of ARDS identified that PRBC transfusion was an independent risk factor for increased development of ARDS and increased mortality risk in ARDS. All of these studies mandate a judicious transfusion policy after trauma resuscitation and emphasize the need for safe and effective blood substitutes and transfusion alternatives.

Blood Transfusion and Postinjury Multiple-Organ Failure

Blood transfusion was first identified as an independent risk factor for MOF in a 3-year single-institution prospective cohort study (n = 394)

aimed at finding a predictive model for postinjury MOF. Trauma patients (n = 394) with ISS greater than 15 and survival over 24 hours were examined. The following variables were identified as early independent predictors of MOF: age greater than 55 years, ISS 25 or higher, and more than 6 units of RBCs in the first 12 hours after admission. In addition, BD greater than 8 mEq/L (0 to 12 hours) and lactate greater than 2.5 mmol/L (12 to 24 hours) were independent predictors of MOF in the subgroup of patients who had these measurements obtained. Whether blood transfusion was simply a surrogate measure of severity of hemorrhagic shock in this study was not fully explored.

A subsequent prospective study by this group confirmed that blood transfusion was an independent risk factor of postinjury MOF, controlling for other indices of shock—including BD and lactate. This study had a similar experimental design, with 513 trauma patients with ISS greater than 15 admitted to the ICU who survived longer than 48 hours. A dose–response relationship between early blood transfusion and postinjury MOF was identified, and blood transfusion was confirmed as an independent risk factor in 13 of the 15 multiple logistic regression models tested. The ORs were high, especially in the early MOF models.

Most recently, this group identified that the incidence, severity, and attendant mortality risk of postinjury MOF has decreased over the last 12 years despite an increased MOF risk. This progress is related to improvements in trauma and critical care and to the decreased use of blood transfusion during resuscitation.

Blood Transfusion and Systemic Inflammatory Response Syndrome/Mortality

Blood transfusion (in the first 24 hours) in trauma was associated with an increased incidence of SIRS (defined as SIRS score greater than or equal to 2) in 7602 trauma patients studied at a single institution. Blood transfusion within the first 24 hours was administered to 954 patients, making up 10% of the study cohort. Blood transfusion and increased total volume of blood transfusion was a significant independent predictor of SIRS, ICU admission, and fatality in trauma patients by multinomial logistic regression analysis after stratification for ISS, Glasgow Coma Scale (GCS) score, and age. Trauma patients who received blood transfusion had a twofold to nearly sixfold increase in SIRS (P <.0001) and more than a fourfold increase in ICU admission (OR 4.62) and fatality (OR 4.23, P < .0001), as well as significantly longer ICU and hospital LOS compared to nontransfused trauma patients.

A recent prospective study confirmed that trauma patients are heavily transfused with allogeneic blood throughout the course of their hospital stay and transfusions are administered at relatively high pretransfusion hemoglobin levels (mean of 9 g/dL). One hundred and four patients (87%) received a total of 324 transfusions, 20 (6%) of which were given in the emergency room, 186 (57%) in the SICU (surgical ICU), 22 (7%) post-SICU, and 96 (30%) in the operating room. The mean volume of blood per patient transfused was 3144 mL (±2622 mL). Transfusion of more than 4 units of blood was an independent risk factor for SIRS. Strategies for limiting blood transfusions should be investigated in this population.

BLOOD TRANSFUSION AND MORTALITY

A follow-up study assessed the effect of blood transfusion within the first 24 hours after injury on outcome in trauma in a larger sample size (n = 15,534, 3-year study, 1998–2000). The study controlled for all potential confounding shock variables (including BD, serum lactate, and shock index [HR/SBP]) on admission, as well as stratification by age, gender, race/ethnicity, GCS score, and ISS. Blood transfusion was a strong independent predictor of mortality rate (OR 2.83, 95% CI 1.82 to 4.40, P <.001), ICU admission (OR 3.27, 95% CI 2.69

to 3.99, $P <.001$), ICU LOS ($P <.001$), and hospital LOS (coefficient 4.37, 95% CI 2.79 to 5.94, $P <.001$) when stratified by indices of shock (BD, serum lactate, shock index, and anemia). Patients who underwent blood transfusion were almost three times more likely to die. Blood transfusion early after injury (within the first 24 hours) was therefore confirmed as an independent predictor of fatality, ICU admission, ICU LOS, and hospital LOS in trauma after controlling for severity of shock by admission BD, lactate, shock index, and anemia.

We also examined blood transfusion and outcome in trauma, dependent on whether patients were transfused less than or more than 24 hours after injury. This retrospective study confirmed our trauma registry data with blood bank data, and delineated the association of blood transfusion and fatality—which was higher (OR 4.13 vs. OR 3.10) when patients were transfused early (less than 24 hours) after injury.

A retrospective 4-year single-institution review of all adults with blunt hepatic or splenic injuries admitted to a Level I trauma center recently examined blood transfusion as an independent risk factor for outcome. Of 316 patients presenting with blunt hepatic or splenic injuries, 143 (45%) received blood transfusion within the first 24 hours. Of the total, 230 patients (72.8%) were selected for nonoperative management, of whom 75 (33%) required transfusion in the first 24 hours. Transfusion was an independent predictor of fatality in all patients (OR 4.75, 95% CI 1.37 to 16.4, $P = .014$) and in those managed nonoperatively (OR 8.45, 95% CI 1.95 to 36.53, $P = .0043$) after controlling for indices of shock and injury severity. The risk of death increased with each unit of PRBCs transfused (OR per unit 1.16, 95% CI 1.10 to 1.24, $P < .0001$). Blood transfusion was also an independent predictor of increased hospital LOS (coefficient 5.45, 95% CI 1.64 to 9.25, $P = .005$). Transfusion-associated mortality risk was highest in the subset of patients managed nonoperatively. The authors suggested that prospective examination of transfusion practices in treatment algorithms of blunt hepatic and splenic injuries is warranted.

Another single-institution study examined whether elderly patients are disproportionately affected by blood transfusion in trauma. To determine the possible interaction among age, PRBC transfusion volume, and mortality risk after injury, a 6-year retrospective review (January 1995 through December 2000) of adult patients who received blood transfusion within the first 24 hours after injury was completed. Of the 1312 patients who received PRBCs in the first 24 hours after injury, 1028 (78%) were aged 55 years and younger and 284 (22%) were over 55—and overall mortality rate was 21.2%. Age, ISS, GCS score, and PRBC transfusion volume emerged as independent predictors of fatality. Mean PRBC transfusion volume for elderly survivors (4.6 units) was significantly less than that of younger survivors (6.7 units). No patient aged over 75 years with a PRBC transfusion volume greater than 12 units survived. The authors concluded that age and PRBC transfusion volume act independently, yet synergistically, to increase mortality rate following injury.

Most recently, a 5-year single-institution study confirmed that low hemoglobin, abnormal prothrombin and PTT, and physiologic signs of shock (low SBP and elevated BD) were independent predictors of fatality in trauma. Currently, the only treatment available for low hemoglobin and signs of hemorrhagic shock in a trauma patient is the transfusion of stored RBCs. Blood transfusions are also associated with increased mortality rate in two large prospective multicenter studies quantifying the incidence of anemia and the use of RBC transfusions in critically ill patients.

BLOOD TRANSFUSION AND INFECTION

Immunosuppression is a consequence of allogeneic blood transfusion in humans and is associated with an increased risk in cancer recurrence rates after potentially curative surgery, as well as with an increase in the frequency of postoperative bacterial infections. A meta-analysis examined the relationship of allogeneic blood transfusion to postoperative bacterial infection. Twenty peer-reviewed articles published from 1986 to 2000 were included in a meta-analysis.

Criteria for inclusion included a clearly defined control group (nontransfused) compared with a treated (transfused) group and statistical analysis of accumulated data that included stepwise multivariate logistic regression analysis. In addition, a subgroup of publications that included only the traumatically injured patient was included in a separate meta-analysis.

The total number of subjects included in this meta-analysis was 13,152 (5215 in the transfused group and 7937 in the nontransfused group). The common OR for all articles included in this meta-analysis evaluating the association of allogeneic RBC transfusion to the incidence of postoperative bacterial infection was 3.45 (range 1.43 to 15.15), with 17 of the 20 studies demonstrating a value of $P = .05$. These results provide overwhelming evidence that allogeneic RBC transfusion is associated with a significantly increased risk of postoperative bacterial infection in the surgical patient.

The common OR of the subgroup of trauma patients was 5.263 (range 5.03 to 5.43), with all studies showing a value of $P < .05$ (range 0.005 to 0.0001). These results demonstrate that allogeneic RBC transfusion is associated with a greater risk of postoperative bacterial infection in the trauma patient when compared with those patients receiving allogeneic RBC transfusions during or after elective surgery.

A single-institution study documented that blood transfusions (within the first 28 hours after admission) correlate with infections in trauma patients in a dose-dependent manner. All adult patients ($n = 1593$) admitted to the trauma service of a Level I trauma center from November 1996 to December 1999 were studied. Of these, 12.6% developed at least one infection. The overall transfusion rate was 19.4%. The infection rate in patients who received at least one transfusion was significantly higher ($P < .0001$), at 33.0% versus 7.6% in patients receiving no blood transfusion. Transfusions per patient ranged from 0 to 46 units. There was a clear exponential correlation in patients receiving between 0 and 15 transfusions ($R^2 = 0.757$). Multivariate logistic regression, which was used to identify risk factors for the development of infection, confirmed that transfusion of PRBCs was an independent risk factor for infection (OR 1.084, 95% CI 1.028 to 1.142, $P = .0028$). This study documented a clear dose-dependent correlation between PRBC transfusion and the development of infection in trauma patients. Similarly, studies in critically ill patients have documented increased rates of nosocomial infection in transfused patients compared to nontransfused patients after stratification of severity of illness and age.

POTENTIAL MECHANISMS FOR TRANSFUSION-ASSOCIATED ADVERSE OUTCOME

A number of potential mechanisms have been delineated regarding adverse effects of blood transfusion, including increased storage time of blood, decreased RBC deformability resulting in reduced microcirculatory perfusion, increased inflammatory response, immunosuppression and microchimerism (related to donor leukocytes in nonleukocyte-reduced blood), and increased free hemoglobin with nitric oxide binding. Discussion of each of these potential mechanisms is beyond the scope of this chapter.

A recent review of blood transfusion in the critically ill concluded the following: (1) RBC transfusion does not improve tissue oxygen consumption consistently in critically ill patients, either globally or at the level of the microcirculation; (2) RBC transfusion is not associated with improvements in clinical outcome in the critically ill and may result in worse outcomes in some patients; (3) specific factors that identify patients who will improve from RBC transfusion are difficult to identify; and (4) lack of efficacy of RBC transfusion is likely related to storage time, increased endothelial adherence of stored RBCs, nitric oxide binding by free hemoglobin in stored blood, donor leukocytes, host inflammatory response, and reduced RBC deformability.

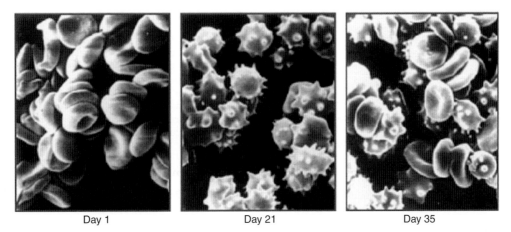

Day 1   Day 21   Day 35

FIGURE 3 Changes in the shape of stored red blood cells (RBCs) using scanning electron microscopy. During storage, the RBC shape changed gradually from normal discoids to echinocytes. Differential counting showed that echinocytic RBC accounted for 80% of the cell population after 3 weeks, and for over 95% at the end of the storage period. *(From Hovav T, Yedgar S, Manny N, Barshstein G: Alteration of red cell aggregability and shape during blood storage. Transfusion 39[3]:277–281, 1999.)*

FIGURE 4 Changes in endogenous red blood cell (RBC) shape and deformability in trauma patients. *Top panels* are postinjury days 3 *(left)* and 7 to 10 *(right)* in survivors. *Bottom panels* are postinjury days 3 *(left)* and 7 to 10 *(right)* in nonsurvivors. Trauma nonsurvivors demonstrated a high percentage of irreversibly changed RBCs, including degenerated RBCs. *(From Berezina TL, Zaets SB, Machiedo GW: Alterations of red blood cell shape in patients with severe trauma. J Trauma 57[1]:82–87, 2004.)*

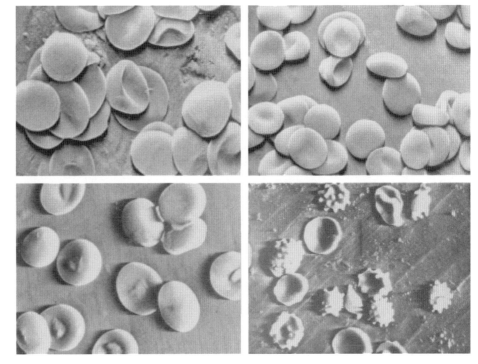

Red Blood Cell Storage Lesion

Erythrocyte aggregation parameters and deformability and shape descriptors were analyzed in blood stored for 35 days. RBC deformability was reduced up to 5% compared with that of fresh samples. Hovav et al reported that blood storage induced changes in RBCs associated with a continuous increase in their aggregability (Fig. 3). Another recent study demonstrated that human RBC deformability decreased by 34% after 4 weeks of storage. During storage, erythrocytes underwent a time-dependent echinocytic shape transformation in another investigation. This transformation increased the suspension viscosity at high and low shear rates. These investigators also confirmed that prestorage leukocyte depletion decreased these effects.

Traumatic injury is also accompanied by a decrease in RBC deformability. RBC shape was examined by scanning electron microscopy in 43 patients with multisystem trauma. Blood samples were taken at admission and every 24 hours afterward for 4 to 10 days. A significant decrease in the percentage of discoid erythrocytes, compared with the volunteers, was observed in both groups of patients at admission ($P < .01$). The percentage of irreversibly changed RBC (spherostomatocytes, spherocytes) was lower in survivors ($12.9 \pm 2.0\%$ vs. $20.3 \pm 9.4\%$, $P < .01$). This study confirmed that RBC shape alterations appear within the first hours after trauma and persist for at least 7 to 10 days (Fig. 4), and these changes are more severe in patients with secondary septic complications.

MANAGEMENT OF COMPLICATIONS RELATED TO BLOOD TRANSFUSION

The aim of massive blood transfusion treatment is to restore adequate blood volume, support hemostasis, maintain oxygen-carrying capacity, and restore or maintain oncotic pressure. Although survival with MT in trauma has improved, a number of complications related to blood transfusion may occur. Physicians caring for patients who require MT must anticipate, identify, and rapidly treat these complications to ensure optimal patient outcome.

Thrombocytopenia

Dilutional thrombocytopenia is inevitable following MT because platelet function declines to zero after only a few days of storage. It has been shown that at least 1.5 times blood volume must be replaced for this to become a clinical problem. However, thrombocytopenia can occur following smaller transfusions if disseminated intravascular coagulation (DIC) occurs or there is preexisting thrombocytopenia.

Coagulation Factor Depletion

Stored blood contains all coagulation factors except V and VIII. Production of these factors is increased by the stress response to trauma. Therefore, only mild changes in coagulation are due to the transfusion per se, and supervening DIC is more likely to be responsible for disordered hemostasis. DIC is a consequence of delayed or inadequate resuscitation and is the usual explanation for abnormal coagulation indices out of proportion to the volume of blood transfused.

Hypocalcemia

Each unit of blood contains approximately 3 g citrate, which binds ionized calcium. The healthy adult liver will metabolize 3 g citrate

A **Transfusion Guideline for Trauma Patient***

Inflammation and the Host Response to Injury

1. Identify critically ill patient with hemoglobin < 7 gm/dL (or Hct < 21%).
2. If hemoglobin < 7 gm/dL transfusion of PRBCs is appropriate.
   a. For patients with severe cardiovascular disease, a higher transfusion trigger may be appropriate.
3. If hemoglobin > 7gm/dL assess the patient for hypovolemia.
   a. If the patient is hypovolemic, administer IV fluids to achieve normovolemia.
   b. If the patient is not hypovolemic, determine whether there is evidence of impaired oxygen delivery (low S_vO_2, persistent/worsening base deficit, presence/worsening of lactic acidosis).
4. If impaired O_2 delivery present, consider pulmonary artery catheter placement, measure cardiac output, and optimize O_2 delivery.
5. If impaired O_2 delivery not present, monitor hemoglobin as clinically indicated.

This protocol assumes that acute hemorrhage has been controlled, the initial resuscitation has been completed, and the patient is stable in the ICU without ongoing hemorrhage.

B **Transfusion Guidelines for Trauma Patient** (excludes immediate resuscitation)

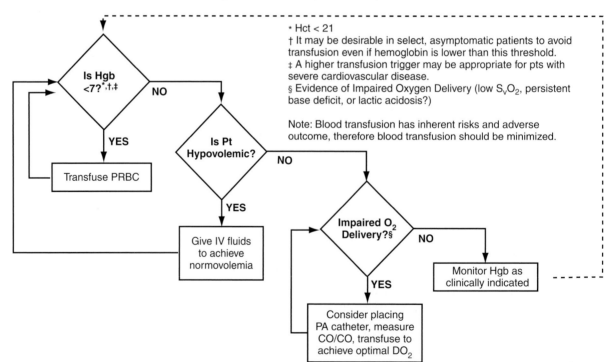

FIGURE 5 Trauma transfusion guideline. Summary of protocol for bedside use. IV, Intravenous; PA, pulmonary artery; PRBCs, packed red blood cells; Pt, patient. *(From West MA, Shapiro MB, Nathens AB, et al: Inflammation and the host response to injury, a large-scale collaborative project: Patient-oriented research core-standard operating procedures for clinical care. IV. Guidelines for transfusion in the trauma patient. J Trauma 61[2]:436–439, 2006.)*

every 5 minutes. Transfusion at rates higher than 1 unit every 5 minutes or impaired liver function may thus lead to citrate toxicity and hypocalcemia. Hypocalcemia does not have a clinically apparent effect on coagulation, but patients may exhibit transient tetany and hypotension. Calcium should only be given if there is biochemical, clinical, or electrocardiographic evidence of hypocalcemia.

Hypokalemia and Hyperkalemia

The plasma potassium concentration of stored blood increases during storage and may be greater than 30 mmol/L. Hyperkalemia is generally not a problem unless very large amounts of blood are given quickly. On the contrary, hypokalemia is more common as RBCs begin active metabolism and intracellular uptake of potassium restarts.

Acid–Base Disturbances

Lactic acid levels in the blood pack give stored blood an acid load of up to 30 to 40 mmol/L. This, along with citric acid, is usually metabolized rapidly. Indeed, citrate is metabolized to bicarbonate, and a profound metabolic alkalosis may ensue. The acid–base status of the recipient is usually of more importance, final acid–base status being dependent on tissue perfusion, rate of administration, and citrate metabolism.

Hypothermia

Hypothermia leads to reduction in citrate and lactate metabolism (leading to hypocalcemia and metabolic acidosis), increase in affinity of hemoglobin for oxygen, impairment of RBC deformability, platelet dysfunction, and an increased tendency to cardiac dysrhythmias.

CONCLUSIONS

Transfusion of the injured patient with stored PRBCs requires careful vigilance during the acute resuscitative and recovery phases after injury. At present, blood transfusion is the only option for treatment of severe hemorrhagic shock and is lifesaving. Hemostatic or damage control resuscitation, with RBC:FFP:Plt blood component resuscitation in nearly a 1:1:1 ratio, has been associated with increased survival, but also with risk for increased acute lung injury related to higher plasma transfusions. MT protocols should be used to facilitate prompt blood component resuscitation in hemorrhagic shock patients at high risk for MT. During the past 2 decades, however, safety concerns have emerged, with data documenting increased morbidity and mortality risks in patients who receive blood transfusions. Therefore, once hemorrhage control is achieved, a more conservative approach to blood transfusion should be used in the trauma patient with stable asymptomatic anemia. Development of institutional protocols for transfusion of blood (Fig. 5) to facilitate a restrictive approach in hemodynamically stable trauma patients can assist in appropriate use of this scarce resource. The decision to transfuse blood should be individualized, based on physiologic and hemoglobin values. In an effort to minimize adverse events, immunosuppression, and hyperinflammation, all attempts to minimize the use of blood transfusion in trauma patients is warranted.

For the chapter's Suggested Readings list, please visit the book at www.ExpertConsult.inkling.com.

CRITICAL CARE II: SPECIAL ISSUES AND TREATMENTS

ACUTE RESPIRATORY DISTRESS SYNDROME

Matthew C. Bozeman, Keith R. Miller, Nicholas A. Nash, and Jorge L. Rodríguez

Since the advent of the mechanical ventilator and the modern era of critical care medicine many topics have been the subject of intense debate and investigation. The acute respiratory distress syndrome (ARDS), first described over 40 years ago by Asbaugh, a surgeon, has been such a subject. Despite multiple trials and attempted strategies, a broad range of mortality rates can be attributed to this disease process. ARDS is often a final common pathway of a myriad of disease processes as diverse as blunt chest trauma and sepsis to transfusion-mediated pulmonary damage, ending often in multisystem organ failure (MSOF). Progress has been made in the treatment of ARDS, however. Recent advances in ventilation strategies and earlier diagnosis, as well as a better understanding of the underlying pathophysiology, have combined to improve diffusion of gases and decrease iatrogenic lung injury, both critical components in managing patients with ARDS. These advances, among others, have contributed to a reported decline in mortality rates from greater than 60% 20 years ago to the now commonly reported 30% to 35%.

DEFINITION, PRESENTATION, AND CLINICAL DIAGNOSIS

Acute lung injury (ALI) and ARDS have been described in the literature since the days of the Vietnam War when civilian physicians noted a disease state characterized by bilateral lung infiltrates, hypoxia, central and peripheral cyanosis, and respiratory infiltrates. Broadly applicable definitions concerning ARDS were not established for 20 years, however, hampering research into the epidemiology and treatment of the disease. New definitions produced in 1988, then refined by the American-European Consensus Conference on ARDS in 1994, defined specific clinical criteria needed to establish the diagnosis of ALI/ARDS.

Both ALI and ARDS are defined by the acute presence of bilateral infiltrates consistent with pulmonary edema without elevated left atrial pressures ($\leq$18 mm Hg) as measured by the pulmonary capillary wedge pressure (PCWP).

Hypoxemia differentiates ALI and ARDS based on the ratio of arterial oxygen tension to the fraction of inspired oxygen (Pao_2/Fio_2).

ARDS is defined by having a Pao_2/Fio_2 ratio of less than 200 and ALI has a higher threshold of Pao_2/Fio_2 ratio less than 300 (Table 1).

It should be noted that the positive end-expiratory pressure (PEEP) is not used when calculating the Pao_2/Fio_2 ratio; however, evidence exists to suggest that a more accurate diagnosis can be obtained when using standard amounts of $PEEP/Fio_2$. The difference in hypoxia between ALI and ARDS is important in that a higher percentage of patients meeting criteria will progress to the need for mechanical ventilation (MV). The degree of hypoxemia is determined by sampling of arterial blood, but in some patients obtaining arterial blood may not be feasible. A reasonable approach in these cases may be to substitute the oxyhemoglobin saturation obtained by pulse oximetry (Spo_2) ratio to Fio_2.

Patients presenting with ARDS initially present with a combination of respiratory compromise and an inciting event. Over 60 different disease states are associated with the onset of ARDS, but only a few make up the bulk of the identifiable causes. Sepsis, pneumonia, pulmonary contusions, multiple transfusions, and aspiration are common causes. Pulmonary contusions and transfusion-related acute lung injury (TRALI) are often associated with trauma patients.

Dyspnea, tachypnea, and hypoxemia often occur fairly early in the clinical course, sometimes within a few hours of the event, but normally within 72 hours. Rapid worsening is also typical in the early course, often leading to the need for mechanical intubation. Laboratory studies can show a metabolic alkalosis, hypoxemia, and an elevated alveolar-arteriolar gradient secondary to shunting of pulmonary blood flow. Other laboratory abnormalities are usually secondary to the underlying disease state. As noted earlier, chest radiographs show diffuse bilateral pulmonary infiltrates, which are acute in nature. The degree or amount of infiltrate has no bearing on the diagnosis. The absence of markings consistent with pulmonary edema is confirmatory. Chest computed tomography (CT) early in the disease demonstrates dependent areas of consolidation with accompanying atelectasis.

The clinical features of ALI/ARDS often have considerable overlap with a variety of other diseases, making ARDS a diagnosis of exclusion. Cardiogenic pulmonary edema and other causes of hypoxemic respiratory failure must be excluded for a diagnosis of ARDS. Cardiogenic pulmonary edema can be quite difficult to distinguish from ARDS because the presentation can be identical clinically. In addition to clinical assessment of fluid balance, cardiac function testing can often be necessary. Measuring plasma B-type natriuretic peptide (BNP) levels, as well as transthoracic or transesophageal echocardiography, can give a picture of cardiac performance; however, echocardiography is often of limited benefit in patients with acute renal failure and fluid overload. Multiple studies have not shown a benefit in the use of a pulmonary artery catheter (PAC) in the diagnosis or management of ARDS; however, right-sided heart catheterization can still be considered if other evaluation techniques are unable to differentiate ARDS from cardiogenic pulmonary edema.

TABLE 1: Defining ARDS and ALI

Feature	ARDS	ALI
Hypoxia	Pao_2/Fio_2 ratio <200	Pao_2/Fio_2 ratio >200 and <300
Acute, diffuse, bilateral infiltrates	Yes	Yes
Left atrial pressure	≤18 mm Hg	≤18 mm Hg

ALI, Acute lung injury; ARDS, acute respiratory distress syndrome.

Other causes of hypoxemic respiratory failure such as various types of pneumonia, cancers, military tuberculosis (TB), alveolar hemorrhage, and pulmonary contusion can be differentiated on the basis of history, clinical and laboratory findings, bronchoscopy, and in a highly selected group of patients, open lung biopsy.

EPIDEMIOLOGY

The incidence of ARDS has been described in several population studies, first in 1972, with a reported incidence of 75 cases per 100,000 person-years. This correlates with 150,000 cases per year. Other studies have demonstrated an increased incidence up to 190,000 cases per year with an associated 3.6 million hospital days. Up to 20% of ventilated patients, and approaching 10% of ICU patients overall, will meet clinical criteria for diagnosis with ARDS.

Fatality related to ARDS is most often not related directly to hypoxemia. Early adequate oxygenation appears to be beneficial, but the degree of hypoxemia derived from the Fio_2/Pao_2 relationship has no bearing on eventual fatality. Predictors for fatality are patient specific, disease specific, and treatment specific. Patients older than 85 years of age portend a worse survival rate than the young. Disease-specific variables include pulmonary vascular dysfunction, dead space, infection, multiorgan dysfunction, and inciting event, and a growing body of evidence suggests that biomarkers and gene polymorphisms are associated with outcome and susceptibility to ARDS. Treatment-specific goals include limiting transfusions, avoidance of fluid overload, and early identification of infectious agents, as well as using other intensive care strategies to be discussed later.

Early fatality is most often secondary to the inciting event; sepsis, usually of a pulmonary source, remains the leading cause of late fatality.

PATHOPHYSIOLOGY

Normal, healthy lungs contribute to a wide variety of processes that aid the body as a whole in maintaining homeostasis including oxygen absorption, carbon dioxide release, and acid-base balance, as well as other functions. Gas exchange, in particular, is dependent on open, dry pulmonary alveoli located in close proximity to a functioning capillary bed. Fluid balance in the lung, just as in other semipermeable tissues, is dependent on a gradient described by the Starling equation. Fluid movement across vessels and the interstitium is therefore directed by a relationship between hydrostatic and oncotic forces, including intracellular proteins. This balance allows a small amount of fluid out of the capillaries, and three main mechanisms prevent the formation of alveolar edema and disruption of gas exchange. The mechanisms include maintenance of tight junctions between alveolar epithelial cells, intracellular proteins favoring reabsorption, and interstitial lymphatics returning lost quantities of fluid to the circulation.

ALI/ARDS is a disease process in which alveolar surfaces are damaged, including the alveolar cell membrane, resulting in the loss of the carefully constructed forces favoring reabsorption and resulting in loss of inflammatory rich fluid into the lung itself. This process is set in motion, either by direct lung injury (pneumonia, aspiration, pulmonary contusions, surgical procedures) or by indirect causes (sepsis, shock, transfusions, or other medical illnesses such as acute pancreatitis).

ALI/ARDS results from this loss of alveolar epithelium. Local injury gives rise to an increase in proinflammatory cytokines such as tissue necrosis factor (TNF), interleukin (IL) 1, IL-6, and IL-8. These cytokines play an important role in neutrophil and macrophage attraction, encouraging these arriving cells to activate and release toxic mediators such as proteases, elastase, and reactive oxygen metabolites, causing increased cell damage. Once the capillary endothelium and alveolar epithelium are bathed in these substances, the resulting cell damage causes release of the formerly intracellular proteins, destroying the oncotic gradient driving fluid reabsorption. Some evidence also exists that lymphatic reabsorption is downregulated as well. Damage to the alveolar epithelium along with fluid overload result in the loss of pulmonary compliance seen in ALI/ARDS.

ALI/ARDS can be separated into three histologically distinct phases with some association to their clinical manifestations. These phases are the exudative, proliferative, and fibrotic stages. Early in the course of disease, the exudative phase, localized alveolar damage and loss of type 1 pneumatocytes become widespread, driven by the arriving neutrophils and macrophages. Hypoxemia and reduced gas exchange are often seen in this early stage. Generally this exudative stage lasts approximately a week to 10 days, and is replaced by a proliferative stage. The proliferative stage is marked histologically by replacement of type 1 pneumatocytes cells with type 2 cells, deposition of collagen, myofibroblasts infiltrating the interstitium, and squamous metaplasia. Surfactant production increases, and pulmonary edema begin to resolve. The clinical course of patients often differs from this second stage of ALI/ARDS for reasons still poorly understood. Some patients progress to resolution of their disease, some decline quickly to death, and still others continue to a fibrotic stage characterized by obliteration and replacement of normal lung tissue with mesenchymal cells, diffuse fibrosis, and duct formation. Histologically, this stage appears to be a fibrosing alveolitis and portends a worse outcome.

THERAPY AND SUPPORTIVE MEASURES

Management strategies in ARDS are broadly divided into either therapeutic or supportive measures. Therapeutic attempts designed to address the proinflammatory properties of the underlying lung injury have been extensively investigated. Supportive strategies are designed through the identification of successful ventilator strategies that maintain oxygenation and ventilation in order to allow time for the resolution of the insult. Unfortunately, therapeutic strategies have proved largely disappointing thus far and care remains supportive. The causes of ARDS are many (trauma, sepsis, pancreatitis, pneumonia, etc.) and the primary insult must be addressed in an efficient and effective manner. This is analogous to the concept of source control in the management of septic shock and cannot be overemphasized. As the disease process evolves through the phases discussed previously, supportive measures and ventilator strategies must be adjusted to the response of the individual patient. Ultimately, refractory hypoxemia and hypercapnia represent the end points of progressive disease with potential progression to MSOF and death.

Fluid Resuscitation and Management

Fluid resuscitation and the determination of overall volume status are cornerstones of the care of any critically ill patient and the same is true in the patient with ARDS. Conceptually, minimizing volume overload in the setting of underlying pulmonary diffusion impairment should be beneficial. Conversely, the complications of underresuscitation add significant morbidity and should be avoided. Noninvasive and invasive hemodynamic monitoring are essential tools that aid in the guidance of appropriate fluid resuscitation. A post hoc subgroup analysis of 244 surgical patients with ARDS conducted by the Acute Respiratory Distress Syndrome Network (ARDSnet) group compared conservative (central venous pressure [CVP] less than 4 mm Hg, pulmonary artery occlusion pressure [PAOP] less than 8 mm Hg) to liberal (CVP 10 to 14 mm Hg, PAOP 14 to 18 mm Hg) fluid resuscitation strategies. Either a PAC or a central venous catheter (CVC) was used to assess volume status. This trial demonstrated no difference in mortality rate but increased ventilator-free days and reduced intensive care unit (ICU) lengths of stay in patients managed with goal-directed conservative fluid management. There was no difference in mortality rate, but patients with PACs received significantly more fluid and had fewer ventilator-free days and longer ICU stays when compared to patients with CVCs.

Noninvasive Mechanical Ventilation Versus Mechanical Ventilation

During the initial assessment, the clinician must decide if the patient with ARDS requires invasive MV or can be managed with less invasive strategies. MV remains the clinician's most reliable ally in managing the patient with severe ARDS. The same criteria used to assess the need for endotracheal intubation and MV in other critically ill patients are generally applied to patients with ARDS. The growing popularity of noninvasive ventilator (NIV) techniques in the treatment of other causes of critical illness has raised the question of applicability in these patients. Scattered case reports have described success with noninvasive continuous positive airway pressure ventilation but a multicenter study examining NIV in all types of respiratory failure identified ARDS as an independent predictor of failure. A small prospective cohort of 31 patients treated with NIV by Ding et al achieved greater than 70% success in avoiding intubation and those who did eventually require intubation deteriorated in the first few hours. This limited data suggests that NIV can be reasonably attempted in select patients who do not clearly require intubation. However, this strategy mandates increased clinical vigilance and the willingness to abandon NIV early if improvement is not observed in the first few hours.

Mechanical Ventilation Techniques

Most patients with moderate to severe forms of ARDS will ultimately require MV. The goal of MV is to maintain adequate oxygenation and ventilation without inducing further iatrogenic lung injury. MV is not a benign supportive measure and it has become increasingly apparent over the last 2 decades that significant lung injury can result from positive-pressure ventilation. Ventilator-induced lung injury (VILI) can be the result of multiple variables including volutrauma (volume), barotrauma (pressure), atelectrauma (cyclic recruitment/derecruitment), and biotrauma (systemic inflammatory mediators). Changes in compliance, either thoracic or pulmonary, during disease progression or resolution requires constant attention from the clinician in order to prevent further injury. Furthermore, despite homogeneous changes in pulmonary vascular permeability, there remains significant heterogeneity in the pulmonary mechanics of different regions of the lung. From a practical standpoint, the concept of three distinct regions of lung functionality can be theoretically useful. These regions include remaining functional parenchyma, nonfunctioning but recruitable parenchyma, and nonrecruitable and nonfunctional parenchyma. This principle underscores the aim to appropriately ventilate normal lung, recruit amenable lung, and avoid VILI in nonrecruitable regions.

Because of the relatively high mortality rate and clinical complexity with which ARDS can present, this disease process has been the subject of many more definitive randomized controlled trials (RCTs) performed in critically ill patients. No single ventilator mode has been shown to be superior to another in patients with ARDS. Conventional ventilation including synchronized intermittent mandatory ventilation (SIMV) and assist-control ventilation (ACV) will suffice in the majority of patients and the choice is largely dictated by institutional preference. In patients with persistently elevated mean airway pressures despite reasonable tidal volumes, pressure-controlled ventilator techniques are often used. More advanced ventilator modes such as airway pressure release ventilation (APRV) and high-frequency oscillatory ventilation (HFOV) are reserved for patients who fail conventional modes. Although no differences in outcome have been demonstrated through the use of different modes of ventilation, three ventilator variables—PEEP, tidal volume, and mean airway pressure—have been the focus of randomized trials and have been purported as targets that may affect outcomes. Again, modifications of these variables likely improve outcomes primarily as a result of minimizing additive iatrogenic lung injury rather than by addressing the underlying disease.

The landmark trial to date in delineating optimal ventilator management in patients with ARDS compared low tidal volume (6 mL/kg, plateau pressures less than 30 cm H_2O) to high tidal volume (12 mL/kg, plateau pressures less than 50 cm H_2O) ventilation and demonstrated substantially reduced risk in the low tidal volume group. This well-designed trial involved more than 800 patients and was stopped early when significant differences were observed in mortality rate, ventilator-free days, and nonpulmonary organ failure demonstrating benefit in the low-volume group. Low-volume ventilation has since become the standard of care in patients with ARDS, and traditional high-volume ventilatory techniques have largely been abandoned. A study using dynamic CT demonstrated that, when allowing for constant PEEP, patients ventilated at 12 mL/kg have better aeration at end-expiration but increased cyclic recruitment and derecruitment when compared to 6 mL/kg. Cyclic recruitment and derecruitment has been identified as a key variable in atelectrauma as the repeated opening and closing of delicate alveoli results in shearing and destruction of normal alveolar geometry that can ultimately impair function. In animal studies, low tidal volume and high PEEP work together to best prevent shear injury in susceptible lung, but PEEP appears to be the more important of the two variables. This appeared to be a mechanical phenomenon in one study as bronchoalveolar washings and serum assays revealed little change in inflammatory markers, refuting the involvement of biotrauma. Despite rather definitive evidence to support low tidal volume ventilation, the appropriate or "optimal" PEEP still remains under some debate. A useful estimation can be derived from an Fio_2/PEEP ratio of 5:1 and correlates well with the PEEP tables used in the ARDSnet trials. With regard to tidal volume, the heterogeneity of the disease process as discussed earlier results in significant regional differences in aeration when nonaffected areas with adequate compliance are hyperinflated and diseased areas with poor compliance are underinflated. This may be one factor contributing to the superiority of low tidal volume ventilation as the portion of "normal lung" is left undamaged and can maintain adequate oxygenation and ventilation as the remaining impaired lung parenchyma recovers. In the ARDSnet trial, plateau pressures were targeted at less than 30 cm H_2O, and respiratory rate and PEEP were adjusted to optimize oxygenation and ventilation, respectively. Given this strategy, ventilation often remains the limiting factor and respiratory rates must be increased to maintain adequate minute ventilation. The concept of permissive hypercapnia in which Pco_2 values as high as 70 mm Hg are generally well tolerated, has limitations as well. Should hypercapnia be allowed, an understanding of the physiologic effects including impaired myocardial contractility and increased intracranial pressures must be addressed and considered in the individual patient.

Evidence-based guidelines that are currently applied to patents with ARDS are accrued from large populations. They are useful in guiding the clinician, but many of these strategies fail in individual patients in the acute setting and require clinicians to adapt their strategies based on continuous reassessment.

Alternative Therapies

Inhaled nitric oxide (INO) is a therapy for ARDS that has been used since the early 1990s. The effect is two pronged: (1) INO acts as a potent, selective vasodilator of the pulmonary vasculature, thereby increasing the perfusion of ventilated lung areas (improved $\dot{V}/\dot{Q}$ mismatch), improving oxygenation, and decreasing pulmonary hypertension; (2) INO has anti-inflammatory properties that combat the progression of ARDS. The typical treatment dose ranges from 1 to 40 parts per million. Although some studies have shown improved oxygenation early in the course of INO therapy, they have failed to demonstrate improvement in hospital mortality rate, duration of ventilation, and ventilator-free days. Furthermore, it appears that that the dose-response curve for INO changes over time in ARDS. Therefore, the prior studies of INO had dosing regimens that likely led to nitric oxide toxicity, resulting in clinical deterioration for the patient. New dosing strategies for each individual based on the studies of Gerlach et al may lead to better clinical outcomes for the patient. Adverse effects of INO therapy include renal dysfunction and methemoglobinemia.

Prone positioning of patients has recently become more popular after Gattinoni et al showed improved oxygenation in the setting of ARDS in 2001. Prone positioning offers the benefit of improving $\dot{V}/\dot{Q}$ mismatch by using gravity to increase the recruitment of alveoli and decrease the compression of other mediastinal structures on the lungs. Recent meta-analysis of RCTs on prone positioning have shown significant reductions in mortality rate when patients with true ARDS (Pao_2/Fio_2 less than 200) are separated from those with ALI (Pao_2/Fio_2 201 to 300). Therefore, in select populations including those with severe hypoxemia (especially those with Pao_2/Fio_2 less than 100), prone positioning is a useful adjunct and should be considered early in these situations. Adverse effects of this therapy include the accidental dislodgement of necessary tubes, drains, and catheters; the development of pressure sores; and the labor demands of patient care in such a specialty bed.

HFOV is another alternative therapy that has shown promise with improving oxygenation, especially in the first 24 hours of use. This mode of ventilation works by delivering small tidal volumes (1 to 5 mL/kg) at a high frequency (300 to 900 breaths per minute), resulting in constant higher mean airway pressures in an effort to prevent cyclic alveolar derecruitment and decrease volutrauma. Unfortunately, the largest randomized control trial to date (the MOAT trial [Multicenter Oscillatory Ventilation for ARDS Trial]) failed to show any survival benefit. Continued research trials are being pursued in this area and HFOV may prove to be of greater benefit in the future, especially when used early in the course of ARDS in patients with refractory hypoxemia.

Partial liquid ventilation is a nontraditional form of therapy for ARDS that has fallen out of favor, but is included here for completeness sake. It involves filling the lungs with perfluorocarbons, which act to improve oxygen gas exchange in prior unventilated portions of the lung due to its higher affinity for oxygen. This strategy showed promise in animal models, but has failed to show any benefit in human RCTs. In addition, there were more reported pneumothoraces, hypoxic episodes, and hypotensive episodes as compared with conventional MV. Thus, it is currently not recommended as treatment for ARDS.

Extracorporeal membrane oxygenation (ECMO) is a reemerging technique that initially fell out of favor in the 1990s after initial RCTs showed no significant mortality rate difference. Technological advances have led to improvement in its application including venovenous circuits, heparin-coated tubing, lower dosing heparin strategies (decrease bleeding risks), and improved ventilation regimens. Roller pumps circulate blood from the femoral vein through a mechanical membrane oxygenator that allows gas exchange and the blood returns to the patient via the internal jugular vein. This extracorporeal oxygenation mechanism allows the damaged lungs to be supported with even lower tidal volumes and airway pressures. The CESAR trial (Conventional Ventilatory Support vs. Extracorporeal Membrane Oxygenation for Severe Adult Respiratory Failure) conducted in the United Kingdom is the most promising RCT to date, showing significantly greater survival at 6 months without disability in the ECMO group. Complications of ECMO are stratified into mechanical or patient-related medical problems. The mechanical complications include oxygenator failure, tubing/circuit disruption, pump or heat exchanger malfunction, and problems associated with cannula placement or removal. Patient-related medical problems include bleeding, neurologic complications, MSOF, barotraumas, infection, and metabolic disorders. The treatment strategy is labor intensive and typically only performed in specialty centers, but does show promise in those patients refractory to other methods of treatment.

Surfactant offered theoretical promise for ARDS given its application and beneficial effects in neonatal respiratory distress syndrome. Unfortunately, RCTs and meta-analyses have not shown improved survival benefit or increased ventilator-free days, and have shed light on the inconsistency of exogenous surfactant as a therapeutic modality. This can be explained by the variable surfactant preparations, dosing regimens, delivery methods, and specific timing of treatment. Further research to determine optimal timing of surfactant therapy and patient-specific dosing strategies may improve its applicability, but currently it has no role in ARDS management of adults.

Steroid use in ARDS remains controversial. Blocking the inflammatory cascade associated with the progression of ARDS has always been a goal of therapy. Steroid use in ARDS has been studied in high-dose and low-dose strategies, and it seems based on the ARDSnet study published in 2006, that low-dose methylprednisolone (2 mg/kg) tapered over time (25 total days of treatment with tapering of the dose over the last 4 days) is the optimal strategy. The results showed this strategy improved oxygenation, improved pulmonary compliance, increased ventilator-free days, increased shock-free days, and decreased vasopressor requirements. There was no increase in infectious complications; however, there was a higher rate of neuromuscular weakness. Furthermore, there was no improvement in 60- or 180-day mortality rates, and there was a significantly increased mortality rate in those patients enrolled in the study 14 days after the onset of ARDS. Authors of the most recent meta-analysis on this issue proposed that low-dose methylprednisolone was associated with improved mortality and morbidity outcomes without increased significant adverse reactions, and advocated its use in ALI and ARDS.

CONCLUSION

ARDS remains a challenging problem with a heterogeneous mix of causes. Current treatment paradigms should be based on identifying and treating the cause of ARDS, using strategies to avoid iatrogenic lung injury using low-volume lung ventilation, and continuing sound overall ICU care for these critically ill patients. Prone positioning and the use of steroids to minimize the inflammatory cascade should be used, especially in those patients difficult to oxygenate/ventilate. APRV and HFOV ventilator strategies should be reserved for those patients refractory to conventional modes until further data prove a definitive benefit over current treatment regimens. Patients who survive ARDS can recover and lead fully functional lives, and further research in this disease process is mandatory to improve morbidity and survival rates in this difficult-to-treat disease.

For the chapter's Suggested Readings list, please visit the book at www.ExpertConsult.inkling.com.

Systemic Inflammatory Response Syndrome and Multiple-Organ Dysfunction Syndrome: Definition, Diagnosis, and Management

Gregory Tiesi, Leonard Mason, Benjamin Chandler, Anthony Watkins, David Palange, and Edwin A. Deitch

In 1973, Tilney et al described 18 patients who developed "sequential system failure" following surgery for ruptured abdominal aneurysms. It was at this time that the idea that severe physiologic insults could lead to multiple-organ failure (MOF) was first established. Several decades later, MOF (or multiple-organ dysfunction syndrome [MODS]) remains a major source of postinjury morbidity and a leading cause of death in surgical intensive care units (SICUs). Although the pathogenesis of this syndrome remains to be fully defined, it is evident that sepsis, systemic inflammatory response syndrome (SIRS), acute respiratory distress syndrome (ARDS), and MODS are closely related phenomena. Consequently, the goal of this chapter is to review SIRS and MODS, focusing on current strategies for diagnosing, managing, and (most importantly) preventing these syndromes.

INCIDENCE

The concept that death from trauma has a trimodal distribution (with these deaths being caused by hemorrhage, head injury, and sepsis/organ failure) is well established. Because MODS is the most common cause of late trauma deaths, it has been the subject of intense investigation. It is now clear that certain clinical risk factors can be used to predict the likelihood of a patient developing MODS. These factors include age, Injury Severity Score (ISS), number of blood transfusions, and lactate/base deficit levels. However, it is only over the last decade that the incidence of MODS in high-risk trauma patients appears to have decreased. This decrease appears to be due to a better knowledge of the factors predisposing patients to its development, as well as to the immunoinflammatory response to shock and trauma. For example, a 12-year prospective study examining 1344 trauma patients noted that the actual incidence of MODS (25%) was lower than its predicted rate.

The authors concluded that this decrease was likely due to the concomitant drop in the liberal use of blood transfusions, which have been shown to be an independent predictor of MODS, SIRS, and mortality rate. Not only does the incidence of MODS appear to be decreasing but there is emerging data to suggest that the mortality rate of patients with MODS is also declining—as reflected in a retrospective study of MODS-related death after blunt multiple trauma during a 25-year period. This study revealed an approximately 50% reduction in MODS-related mortality rate, from 29% to 14% over this time period. As will be discussed later in this chapter, several therapeutic interventions have been developed that have been shown to reduce mortality rate or to attenuate organ dysfunction, which would help explain this decline in mortality rate. In spite of these improvements, once MODS has become established the risk of death is significant—with the patient's prognosis being more closely related to the number of organs that have failed than to any other variable, including the underlying processes that initiated the MODS.

MECHANISMS OF MODS

The clinical picture of MODS is indicative of a generalized systemic inflammatory response, which typically occurs as a result of infection or uncontrolled inflammation in the patient with severe trauma. Several distinct and often conflicting hypotheses have been proposed to explain the mechanisms underlying MODS. Nonetheless, MODS can be viewed as a systemic process involving the excessive stimulation of certain inflammatory responses mediated by circulating factors whose effects contribute to injury or dysfunction in organs not involved in the initial insult. To a large extent, the cascade of events culminating in MODS is likely to be mediated by the same factors irrespective of the exact nature of the triggering insult. In fact, it is the host's inflammatory response to injury or infection that is probably more important in the genesis of SIRS, ARDS, and MODS than the microbial agent or the initiating insult. Thus, an appreciation of the role of the inflammatory response of the host in the pathogenesis of MODS is vital in order to develop new and effective modalities for the prevention and treatment of this syndrome.

The earliest reports of postinjury MODS identified occult intra-abdominal infection as the cause in approximately half of the cases. However, the recognition that more than 50% to 70% of patients with MODS do not have an identifiable focus of infection meant that uncontrolled infection could not be the universal cause of MODS. From this early work came the recognition that only a fraction of septic-appearing patients were infected and that the host's own response to tissue injury or shock could result in a noninfectious septic state. In turn, this recognition that the host's immunoinflammatory response to microbial infection, tissue injury, necrotic tissue, or shock was similar led to the hypothesis that immune cell products, such as cytokines, contributed to the development of MODS.

The overall hypothesis was based on the concept that an excessive immunoinflammatory response due to activated macrophages and other immune cells led to cytokine-mediated tissue injury and thereby the development of SIRS and MODS. This hypothesis was supported by several experimental and clinical observations. For example, cytokine levels were increased in trauma patients and the administration of tumor necrosis factor alpha (TNF-α) to humans elicited a clinical response similar to SIRS, whereas preclinical animal studies documented that TNF-α neutralization improved survival in animals receiving a lethal dose of endotoxin. However, things were not this simple—as soon became apparent from multiple failed clinical trials of anti-inflammatory agents and the results of more complex preclinical animal studies. In fact, it is now recognized that cytokines have many beneficial functions, such as the control of infection. It is also recognized that elevated cytokine levels appear to be more markers or predictors of the host response than inducers of MODS.

Another mechanism by which hemorrhagic shock and trauma could predispose to the developments of MODS is through an ischemia-reperfusion injury or damage to the microcirculation. Because shock is essentially a total-body ischemia-reperfusion insult and the microcirculation of various tissues and organs are highly susceptible to ischemia-reperfusion–mediated insults, this process has been termed the microcirculatory hypothesis of MODS. Physiologically, circulatory shock could contribute to MODS through inadequate global oxygen delivery, the ischemia-reperfusion phenomenon, or the promotion of deleterious endothelial cell–leukocyte interactions.

Although prolonged tissue hypoxia leads to inadequate adenosine triphosphate (ATP) generation and potentially irreversible cell damage, under most clinical conditions the shock period is not long enough for this process to occur. Thus, in clinical situations it appears that most of the tissue damage occurs after ischemia is relieved by reperfusion and that this damage is due to the production of reperfusion-induced oxygen radicals and proinflammatory factors (such as oxidants, nitric oxide, chemokines, cytokines). In fact, studies show that the combination of reperfusion-induced increased levels of nitric oxide and superoxide anion synergistically increase cell injury via the production of peroxynitrite, which is a long-lasting and potent oxidant that causes direct cell injury through lipid peroxidation. This notion that increased nitric oxide production is important in the pathogenesis of MODS is supported by clinical studies showing that serum nitrate levels (an index for the systemic production of nitric oxide) correlated well with MODS scores in critically ill patients. Most recently, this paradigm of ischemia-reperfusion injury has revealed that the products of injured or killed cells, such as high-mobility group box 1 (HMGB1) and other ischemia-reperfusion-modified host-derived molecules, can also cause cellular and tissue injury and promote the inflammatory response. These host-derived proinflammatory and tissue injurious molecules have been termed "danger signals" or "alarmins" and are an active area of investigation.

Endothelial cell–leukocyte interactions leading to tissue injury also seem to be a key step in the pathogenesis of SIRS, ARDS, and MODS. Many factors related to shock and tissue injury, including cytokines, necrotic tissue, endotoxins, and oxidants, can convert endothelial cells from a quiescent state to a proinflammatory procoagulant one and can activate neutrophils. The combination of these changes in endothelial cell phenotype and neutrophil activation has been documented to lead to increased neutrophil adherence to the microcirculatory endothelium, thereby promoting neutrophil-mediated microvascular injury. Experimentally, inhibition of neutrophil–endothelial cell interactions has been shown to limit shock- and sepsis-induced injury to a number of organs, including the lung. Furthermore, neutrophil activation in trauma patients has been identified as a predictor of the development of SIRS, ARDS, and MODS. Therefore, endothelial cell–neutrophil interactions, whether induced by shock, sepsis, or an augmented inflammatory response, appear to be an important effector mechanism in the development of ARDS and MODS.

The gut hypothesis of MODS has been used to explain why no identifiable focus of infection can be found in as many as 30% of bacteremic patients who die from MODS. An extensive body of experimental as well as clinical studies supports this hypothesis. For example, clinical studies indicate that intestinal permeability is increased in patients with sepsis after major thermal injury or trauma and that loss of intestinal barrier function correlates with the development of systemic infection, ARDS, and MODS. Although both clinical and experimental studies implicated intestinal injury and bacterial translocation in the development of SIRS and MODS, a study by Moore et al began to cast doubt on the clinical relevance of bacterial translocation.

These investigators failed to find bacteria or endotoxin in the portal blood of severely injured patients, including a subgroup of patients developing MODS. One potential explanation for this failure to find endotoxin or bacteria in the portal blood was that the gut-derived factors contributing to SIRS, ARDS, and MODS were exiting the gut via the lymphatics. Studies testing this possibility have documented that nonbacterial factors exiting the ischemic gut contribute to acute ARDS, MODS, neutrophil activation, and endothelial cell injury/activation in both rodent and primate models of trauma-hemorrhagic shock and have led to the gut-lymph hypothesis of MODS. This gut-lymph hypothesis of MODS proposes that nonbacterial noncytokine factors released from the stressed gut via the lymphatic system activate neutrophils and endothelial cells, thereby leading to organ dysfunction. Thus, over the last several years the gut hypothesis has expanded beyond bacterial translocation and now also implicates gut-derived nonbacterial proinflammatory and tissue-injurious factors in the pathogenesis of SIRS, ARDS, and MODS.

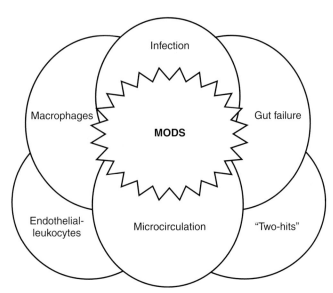

FIGURE 1   Overlapping nature of multiple hypotheses believed to be responsible for causing multiple organ dysfunction syndrome (MODS).

Although each of the various MODS hypotheses was presented individually, in patients many of these pathways overlap and the induction of one pathway can lead to activation of others. For example, severe bacterial infection activates the immunoinflammatory response, which in turn leads to microcirculatory dysfunction and gut ischemia. Likewise, nonbacterial gut-derived factors have been shown to activate neutrophils, lead to an augmented inflammatory response, and promote microcirculatory dysfunction. Furthermore, shock states are associated with microcirculatory failure, gut injury, induction of an inflammatory response, and augmented neutrophil–endothelial cell interactions. In addition, in many patients who develop MODS no one major insult seems to have occurred. Instead, it appears that the development of MODS is related to the summation of several minor insults rather than one major event.

This clinical observation has led to the "two-hit" hypothesis of MODS, in which potentially clinically modest events prime the host so that the host's response to subsequent secondary events becomes exaggerated, culminating in SIRS, ARDS, and MODS. Additionally, there is an immunosuppressed state that develops after shock, termed the compensatory anti-inflammatory response syndrome (CARS); CARS is thought to contribute to the increased incidence of infection seen with critically ill patients. Although this two-hit theory needs to be further understood, it is a feasible explanation of how trauma or burn injury can convert a nonlethal infectious or hypoxic challenge into a lethal insult. In fact, as illustrated in Figure 1 it is clear that the difficulty in finding an effective therapy to prevent or treat MODS relates to the overlapping nature of the multiple systems activated by shock and trauma as well as the ability of one system to prime other systems for an exaggerated physiologic response to secondary insults. Nonetheless, the knowledge gained from these basic studies of the physiology of inflammation and MODS have provided important therapeutic insights. For example, they highlight the importance of prompt and adequate volume resuscitation and microcirculatory blood flow to prevent organ ischemia, the need for early excision of nonviable tissue to limit systemic inflammation, and the need for therapies to better preserve gut barrier dysfunction and limit uncontrolled inflammation.

DIAGNOSIS

A key step in the treatment of a disease process is the establishment of an accurate diagnosis. To that end, a number of consensus

TABLE 1: Definition of Systemic Inflammatory Response Syndrome

Temperature $>38°$ C or $<36°$ C
Heart rate >90 bpm
RR > 20 or $Paco_2$ <32 mm Hg (<4.3 kPa)
WBC count of $>12,000$ or $<4,000$ cells/mm^3; $>10\%$ immature forms

bpm, Beats per minute; RR, respiratory rate; WBC, white blood cell.

conferences have been held in an attempt to provide classification schemes that allow SIRS, ARDS, and MODS to be accurately diagnosed. SIRS was defined as the response to a variety of severe clinical insults, which is manifested by two or more of the four conditions listed in Table 1. However, although these SIRS criteria are considered too sensitive and nonspecific to be of clinical use in individual patients, SIRS should be viewed as an evolved dynamic process that has adaptive survival value for the host under most circumstances because it signals the body to respond to injury or to an external threat such as a bacterial infection. However, if this protective inflammatory response becomes uncontrolled or excessive it has maladaptive consequences that result from its potential to injure the host's own tissues.

The term "MODS" was introduced by a consensus conference of the American College of Chest Physicians (ACCP) and the Society of Critical Care Medicine (SCCM) in 1991. Prior to that time, this syndrome had many different names, including *sequential organ dysfunction syndrome* and *multiple-organ failure syndrome*. Several MODS scoring systems have been established that grade the severity of MODS and emphasize the concept that there exists a continuous spectrum from mild to full-blown dysfunction that correlates, on a patient population level, with mortality and morbidity rates (Table 2).

These systems, much like the sequential organ failure assessment (SOFA) score developed by Vincent et al, score organ failure by assigning a numerical scale in which more points are given to the higher degree of organ dysfunction in several organ systems. These scores can be calculated daily, allowing the clinician to track net clinical improvement or deterioration over time and to assess the progression or resolution of organ dysfunction. Thus, although not developed to predict fatality in individual patients, such scoring systems can be beneficial in the assessment and treatment of critically ill patients. This benefit includes their use in the daily clinical evaluation of a patient's response, in research involving epidemiologic studies, and in the assessment of new therapies in clinical trials. Although

these scoring systems use slightly different parameters to grade organ failure, most studies have found that the clinical use of these scoring systems is comparable.

MANAGEMENT

At the current time, the treatment of patients with established MODS is largely symptomatic and dedicated to supporting organs and systems that have failed. Because there is no "cure" for MODS, once it is present—and because the mortality rate of patients with established MODS is high—prevention becomes a key strategy in the care of the high-risk trauma patient. Therefore, it is important to understand and use certain strategies and approaches that have been shown to reduce the risk for developing MODS. In trauma patients, prevention begins in the field, with rapid transport to a medical facility, and extends throughout the resuscitative, operative, and ICU phases of care (Table 3). Because the approaches and strategies used at different phases of patient care may vary to some extent, each of these phases is discussed individually—although in actual clinical practice these phases often overlap.

Resuscitative Phase

The resuscitative phase has as its central goal the restoration of an effective blood volume, optimization of microcirculatory blood flow (and hence tissue perfusion), and the prevention/limitation of ischemia-reperfusion injury. Recognition that shock causes a global ischemia-reperfusion injury, which directly and indirectly leads to cellular and hence organ injury, has led to an increasing emphasis on the adequacy of volume resuscitation as well as a search for more effective resuscitation fluids. The primary end point of resuscitation, however, remains controversial. Parameters such as base deficit and lactate levels, oxygen delivery, gastric intramucosal pH (pHi), and invasive monitoring using pulmonary artery catheters have all been used in an attempt to optimize volume resuscitation.

Because blood pressure and urine output may not reflect the adequacy of volume resuscitation in the severely injured trauma patient, arterial blood base deficit and serum lactate levels have been shown to be useful markers with which to monitor the response to resuscitation. A worsening base deficit or serum lactate has been shown to correlate with ongoing blood loss or inadequate volume resuscitation, whereas improvements in these parameters are indicative of adequate volume resuscitation. Because in severely injured patients the period of volume resuscitation may last up to 48 hours, serial measurements are important. Based on prospective studies demonstrating that patients who cleared their base deficit or lactate levels within 48 hours

TABLE 2: Comparison of Scores Evaluating Multiple-Organ Dysfunction

System	Brussels Score	MODS Score	LOD Score	SOFA Score
Respiratory	Pao_2/Fio_2 ratio	Pao_2/Fio_2 ratio	Pao_2/Fio_2 ratio	Pao_2/Fio_2 ratio
Cardiovascular	Arterial pressure Response to fluids Acidosis	Pressure-adjusted heart rate	Arterial pressure Heart rate	Arterial pressure Vasoactive drugs
Renal	Creatinine	Creatinine	Creatinine, urea, UO	Creatinine, UO
Hematologic	Platelets	Platelets	Platelets, leukocytes	Platelets
Hepatic	Bilirubin	Bilirubin	Bilirubin, PT	Bilirubin
Neurologic	GCS	GCS	GCS	GCS

GCS, Glasgow Coma Scale; LOD, logistic organ dysfunction; MODS, multiple-organ dysfunction syndrome; PT, prothrombin; SOFA, sequential organ failure assessment; UO, urine output.

TABLE 3: Prevention of Multiple Organ Failure

Resuscitative Phase

Shock resuscitation

Base deficit and lactate monitoring

Restrictive strategy for blood transfusion

Operative Phase

Vigilance in preventing missed injuries

Damage-control laparotomy

Early fracture fixation

ICU Phase

Infection-related issues

Early nutritional support and glucose control

Specific organ support

Recognition of abdominal compartment syndrome

Pharmacologic therapy

ICU, Intensive care unit.

had a reduced incidence of ARDS and MODS plus a higher survival rate than those who did not, the resuscitative goal should be to reduce and keep the base deficit below –2 mmol/L and the serum lactate less than 1.5 mEq/L.

The choice of resuscitative fluid has become a more controversial subject with the recognition that Ringer's lactate is proinflammatory and thus may exacerbate the inflammatory response and contribute to the development of organ injury in shock states. Given these concerns, plus the recent recognition that large-volume resuscitation with crystalloid solutions contributes to the development of the abdominal compartment syndrome (ACS), attention has refocused on the early resuscitation of trauma patients with alternative resuscitative fluids (Dextran, hypertonic saline, and colloids). At the current time, owing to the paucity of positive clinical trials, there is not enough data to determine whether or not any of these is superior to appropriate crystalloid volume resuscitation of the trauma patient. Another approach is the use of resuscitation fluids containing antioxidants, with three clinical trials, including a prospective randomized trial, showing that splanchnic-directed antioxidant therapy helps prevents MODS in trauma patients. As investigations into novel resuscitation fluids with pharmacologic actions (i.e., gut-protective, immunomodulatory) continues, it is likely that the initial resuscitative approach of the trauma patient will evolve from Ringer's lactate to include new fluid formulas.

The role of blood transfusions in trauma patients has also undergone an intense reevaluation based on clinical studies showing that blood is immunosuppressive and that blood transfusions are an independent predictor of MODS, especially when blood older than 2 weeks is administered. These observations, plus the fact that ICU patients as well as trauma patients can be safely managed with hemoglobin levels in the range of 7 g/dL, has led to the emergence of a selective transfusion policy in which prophylactic transfusions for anemia are no longer routinely administered. In fact, the Transfusion Requirements in Critical Care (TRICC) trial demonstrated a significant reduction in the severity of new organ dysfunction in a critical care setting when transfusion was withheld unless the hemoglobin concentration was less than 7 g/dL. Thus, based on the existing literature regarding the clinical efficacy of prophylactic red blood cell (RBC) transfusions

for anemia in the critically ill, two general conclusions can be made: (1) prophylactic RBC transfusions to raise the hemoglobin above 7 g/dL does not improve tissue oxygen consumption consistently in critically ill patients, either globally or at the level of the microcirculation, and (2) prophylactic RBC transfusion is not associated with improvements in clinical outcome in the critically ill and may result in worse outcomes in several patient subgroups. Lastly, in patients with massive hemorrhage, the liberal use of transfusion is clearly indicated and a systematic and organized approach for the delivery of large amounts of blood products via massive transfusion protocols (MTPs) has been shown to be clinically beneficial. For further in-depth discussion on MTPs see the chapter entitled "Transfusion: Management of Blood and Blood Products in Trauma."

Operative Intervention

In an early landmark article on MODS, Eiseman et al described a series of 42 surgical patients with MODS, 24 of whom developed MODS as a result of intraoperative error or postoperative mismanagement. This study emphasizes one of the key elements in the perioperative care of trauma patients: missed injuries are relatively common in trauma patients and are important risk factors in the development of ARDS, MODS, and death. Although the specifics of the operative care of the trauma patient are covered elsewhere, certain aspects are important in the context of MODS. An example is the judicious use of damage-control laparotomy (DCL) to limit both acute and delayed MODS. Although a 2010 Cochrane review on DCL found no randomized controlled trials that compared DCL with immediate, definitive repair in patients with major abdominal trauma, today the standard of care remains avoiding extensive procedures on unstable patients in favor of planned, staged reoperation after successful resuscitation in the ICU. Avoiding the "lethal triad" of acidosis, hypothermia, and coagulopathy prevents an irreversible physiologic insult and the subsequent development of MODS, with an apparent survival benefit in some studies.

A second example of operative intervention to reduce the incidence of ARDS and MODS is early fixation of long-bone fractures. Numerous prospective and retrospective clinical trials have documented that so-called, "damage control orthopedics" with early fixation of long-bone fractures compared with delayed fracture fixation is associated with early patient mobility, improved pulmonary toilet, decreased systemic inflammation, decreased thromboembolic events, and decreased morbidity and mortality rates, as well as decreased hospital resource use. Although operative fixation may expose the patient to an additional insult that can precipitate ARDS in patients with chest injuries or worsening of a traumatic brain injury in a susceptible patient, even in these high-risk patients, early definitive stabilization appears to be associated with acceptably low rates of complications when compared with delayed fixation.

Intensive Care Unit Management Phase

Postoperative and postinjury MODS can be prevented through strategies such as continued resuscitation, management of infectious complications, and early nutritional and specific organ support. Although some organs (such as the pulmonary system) have randomized prospective data supporting certain therapies that improve outcome, other systems (such as the hepatic system) rarely require specific treatment. In this section we focus on preventive and therapeutic strategies that appear to have reduced the incidence of MODS or improved outcome in patients with MODS (Tables 3 and 4).

Because infections can contribute to the development of MODS and can increase mortality rate, several key concepts must be kept in mind to limit infection-related MODS. The use of early empiric antibiotics in patients suspected of having pneumonia is important because the use of early adequate empiric antibiotic has been shown

TABLE 4: ICU Interventions That Reduce Mortality Rate or Attenuate Organ Dysfunction

Objective	Intervention
Resuscitation	Early goal-directed resuscitation
Prophylaxis	SDD/SOD
ICU support	Restrictive transfusion strategy Low tidal volume ventilation Daily awakening Glucose control Enteral feeding Selenium supplementation
Mediator-targeted therapy	Activated protein C Low-dose corticosteroids (+/−)

ICU, Intensive care unit; SDD, selective decontamination of digestive tract; SOD, selective oropharyngeal decontamination.

to reduce pneumonia-related fatality. A second approach is the use of prophylactic antibiotic regimens involving selective decontamination of the digestive tract (SDD) and selective oropharyngeal decontamination (SOD). The process of SDD includes the oropharyngeal application of a nonabsorbable topical antimicrobial paste and the oral administration of nonabsorbable antibiotics into the gastrointestinal tract, along with the systemic administration of antibiotics targeting gram-positive organisms. In contrast to SDD, SOD does not involve the administration of systemic antibiotics. Although not used frequently in the United States it appears that both regimens reduce infectious complications as well as fatality in critically ill trauma and other surgical patients. The concept behind both methods of bacterial decontamination is that the oropharynx and gut are major reservoirs for organisms causing pneumonias and bacteremias. Thus, by controlling oropharyngeal and intestinal bacterial overgrowth, the incidence of infections and hence fatality will be reduced. In a large randomized multicenter study, the use of SOD along with SDD was associated with improved survival and a lower incidence of ICU-acquired bacteremia; however, SOD is preferred because it does not include systemic antibiotics. The reason for failure to employ selective decontamination appears to relate to the fact that this therapy is very labor intensive and has only recently been shown to improve survival.

In situations in which MODS develops in the postoperative or posttrauma period, a meticulous search for a source of infection should be made, with particular attention to wounds, incisions, sites of previous injury or surgery, and intravenous (IV) catheter sites because the development of ARDS or MODS is not an uncommon manifestation of an occult infection. Despite extensive research involving various pharmacologic therapies of severe sepsis, with the exception of activated protein C, the results of clinical trials of immunomodulatory agents have been distressing. In contrast, a prospective randomized trial documented that the recombinant form of activated protein C improved 28-day survival and led to a more rapid resolution of cardiovascular, respiratory, and hematologic dysfunction in patients with severe sepsis. The reason activated protein C was effective when other agents were not may relate to the fact that it has both anticoagulant and anti-inflammatory activity, thereby protecting the microcirculation as well as limiting the inflammatory response. Lastly, the use of prolonged low-dose steroids continues to be an effective therapy to restore blood pressure in patients with septic shock refractory to vasopressor and fluid therapy. Early studies indicating that this approach improved survival have not been validated in recent prospective clinical trials. Thus, while low-dose steroid

therapy in patients with refractory septic shock continues to be used, its ultimate effect on overall survival may be limited. In addition to infectious issues, other non-organ-specific therapies that appear to be beneficial include early enteral alimentation, glucose control, elevation of the head of the bed, and daily cessation of sedative infusions in ventilated patients. The notion of early enteral feeding is based on the concept of limiting gut-origin sepsis because the fed gut is more resistant to stress-induced injury and parenteral alimentation is associated with gut atrophy, increased permeability, and loss of barrier function. Based on the results of multiple prospective randomized trials, early enteral nutrition has been found to effectively reduce infectious complications, ICU days, and total hospital length of stay, although it does not appear to improve survival. Thus, in an attempt to further improve the beneficial effects of enteral feedings, a number of immune-enhancing enteral formulas were produced and tested in trauma and ICU patients. Although some studies comparing standard to immune-enhancing enteral formulas suggested that immune-enhancing diets are associated with a further decrease in infectious complications, others did not. When the exact composition of the diets and dietary supplements are analyzed, certain clinical recommendations emerge, which are based on randomized clinical studies showing that these nutritionally based strategies improve morbidity and mortality rates in high-risk patients. These clinical strategies include the IV use of selenium (400–1000 µg/day) with or without vitamin C (1.5–3.0 g/day) and vitamin E (500 mg/day orally [PO]) supplementation; parenteral glutamine as the alanyl-glutamine dipeptide (0.50 g/kg/day); and the use of IV omega-3 fats or PO enteral diets containing high omega-3 fatty acid levels. Although all of the mechanisms by which these nutrients improve survival remain to be determined, they have been documented to limit oxidant-mediated tissue injury and support the immune system. Thus, the combination of early enteral feeding plus the administration of selenium, vitamin C, vitamin E, IV glutamine, and omega-3 fats appears to be a successful approach to limiting the development and severity of MODS.

A second metabolic approach has been the institution of tight glucose control in which insulin is liberally used to keep the serum glucose level less than 120 mg/dL. Since the original prospective randomized controlled study showing that tight glucose control (<120 mg/dL) was associated with a survival advantage compared to a more liberal glucose control regimen (<215 mg/dL), other studies including several systematic reviews and meta-analyses have led to differing conclusions on tight glucose control using intensive insulin therapies. Recently, one of the largest randomized international multicenter trials demonstrated an increase in 90-day mortality rate and severe hypoglycemia using the intensive insulin regimen. Thus, it appears that the concept of maintaining strict normoglycemia (81 to 108 mg/dL) may not be as beneficial to critically ill patients as previously thought. On the basis of these recent results documenting the adverse effects of tight glucose control, recommendations have emerged suggesting the use of lower targets of glucose control (<180 mg/dL).

Other easily instituted ICU therapies have been shown to reduce complications. For example, daily interruption of sedative infusions in critically ill patients undergoing mechanical ventilation reduces ICU length of stay and morbidity, whereas elevation of the head of the bed of ventilated patients reduces the incidence of pneumonia and helps to preserve pulmonary function.

In addition to elevating the head of the bed and daily sedative cessation, other advances in the care of the patient with respiratory failure have been made over the last several years. The most important of these was the recognition that high tidal volumes and increased airway pressures cause, rather than prevent, lung injury by inducing lung inflammation. This process has been termed *ventilator-induced lung injury* (VILI). Consistent with this physiologic concept, multicenter randomized controlled trials confirmed that mechanical ventilation of patients with acute lung injury and ARDS with a lower tidal volume (i.e., 6 mL/kg) than traditionally used results in decreased mortality rate and attenuates the local and systemic release of proinflammatory mediators. In addition, further clinical trials documented that outcomes in patients with acute lung injury or ARDS are similar whether lower or higher positive end-expiratory pressure (PEEP) levels are used when an end-inspiratory plateau-pressure limit of 30 cm H_2O is maintained.

Although oxygenation is maintained with low tidal volumes and permissive hypercapnia, and increased CO_2 levels may develop as a result of decreased ventilation, this does not appear to be harmful. Thus, the use of low tidal volume ventilation that maintains the inspiratory plateau pressure below 30 cm H_2O is effective both in the prevention and treatment of acute lung injury and ARDS. A number of other ventilatory strategies (inhaled nitric oxide and high-frequency oscillatory ventilation) have demonstrated their use in improving oxygenation in patients with ARDS; however, this has not translated into a survival benefit. In a recent meta-analysis, prone positioning in patients with ALI and severe hypoxemia was found to provide a significantly improved survival benefit. Therefore, the use of prone positioning has been suggested as a form of rescue strategy in patients with severe refractory hypoxemia, particularly in centers with limited resources in other specialized therapies.

Renal replacement therapy has been effective in treatment of critically ill patients with MODS by allowing regulation of fluid and electrolytes. Renal replacement therapy also has the potential to remove toxins and circulating mediators of inflammation. Methods of supporting renal function, such as the prophylactic use of low-dose dopamine, have not been found to be effective. Thus, currently the best way to limit renal failure is to avoid underresuscitation and to promptly diagnose and treat infectious complications. Once renal failure has occurred, continuous venovenous hemodialysis appears to be superior to hemodialysis because it avoids the need for systemic anticoagulation and is less likely to cause hypotensive episodes in the fragile patient.

A recently recognized and important treatable cause of MODS is the abdominal compartment syndrome (ACS). The ACS can be viewed as a reversible mechanical cause of MODS that is related to increased intraabdominal pressure. As the intraabdominal pressure rises, abdominal visceral perfusion decreases, ventilation is impaired, and cardiac output declines. Clinically, the ACS is manifested as a decreasing urine output, inadequate ventilation associated with elevated peak airway pressures, and hypotension. Patients at highest risk of developing ACS are those suffering from multiple trauma, massive hemorrhage, and prolonged operations with massive volume resuscitation, as well as those requiring intraabdominal packing to control bleeding.

ACS can also develop in patients after severe hemorrhagic shock without an abdominal or retroperitoneal injury, and this phenomenon is known as secondary ACS. Secondary ACS is due to progressive visceral and retroperitoneal edema in shocked patients with the capillary leak syndrome who receive massive crystalloid fluid resuscitation. The diagnosis of ACS is made or confirmed by measuring the abdominal pressure through a Foley catheter placed in the bladder, with ACS being defined as the combination of a urinary bladder pressure more than 25 mm Hg, progressive organ dysfunction (urinary output less than 0.5 mL/kg/hour or Pao_2/Fio_2 ratio less than 150 or peak airway pressure greater than 45 cm H_2O or cardiac index less than 3 L/minute/m^2 despite resuscitation), and improved

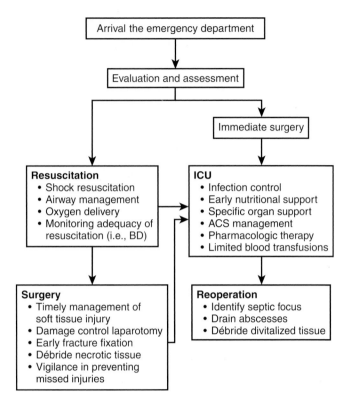

FIGURE 2 Algorithm for preventing and managing multiple organ dysfunction syndrome. ACS, Abdominal compartment syndrome; BD, base deficit; ICU, intensive care unit.

organ function after surgical abdominal decompression. Surgical treatment, consisting of opening the abdomen, leads to rapid and profound correction of the physiologic abnormalities in most cases; whereas if untreated, the ACS is highly lethal, with a mortality rate approaching 100%.

CONCLUSIONS AND ALGORITHM

The development of SIRS and MODS in trauma patients remains relatively common. However, owing to advances in understanding the biology of the host's immunoinflammatory system as well as the mechanisms involved in the pathogenesis of SIRS, ARDS, and MODS, progress in the treatment and prevention of these syndromes has occurred. This progress is reflected both as a decrease in the incidence of MODS and an improvement in the survival of patients with MODS. The strategies used to accomplish these goals involve both preventive and therapeutic approaches that begin in the resuscitative phase of the operative care of these patients and continue through the operative and ICU phases (Fig. 2).

For the chapter's Suggested Readings list, please visit the book at www.ExpertConsult.inkling.com.

Sepsis, Septic Shock, and Its Treatment

Corrado Paolo Marini, Gary Lombardo, Anthony Policastro, and Dimitryi Karev

In the United States, each year there are approximately 750,000 cases of bacteremia causing approximately 275,000 events of severe sepsis and septic shock with an associated mortality rate that ranges between 20% and 30%. Sepsis remains the leading cause of death in intensive care units (ICUs), and unfortunately, the incidence of sepsis is increasing due to a variety of reasons, including the increasing age of the population, the increased number of comorbid conditions present in patients experiencing sepsis, the increased use of cytotoxic and immunosuppressive drugs, and more importantly, the emergence of antibiotic-resistant organisms. The increased incidence of severe sepsis and septic shock applies also to trauma patients due to the presence of several incremental risk factors, including the presence of significant comorbid conditions secondary to aging of the trauma population and more patients surviving their initial injuries from improved medical and surgical care and therefore at risk of developing subsequent infections. Additionally, trauma patients have an increased risk of developing severe sepsis and septic shock due to the presence of central nervous system injuries, pulmonary contusions from blunt chest injuries, preoperative shock, and the frequent administration of blood transfusions with its immunosuppressive effects.

Septic shock is the final stage of a continuum along a pathway that may progress in a stepwise fashion from infection to bacteremia, sepsis, severe sepsis, and ultimately, septic shock. This continuum is characterized by the progression from signs associated with the systemic inflammatory response syndrome (SIRS)—temperature higher than 38° C or lower than 36° C, heart rate more than 90 beats per minute, respiratory rate more than 20/minute or $Paco_2$ 32 mm Hg, white blood cell (WBC) count greater than 12,000 cells/mm^3 or less than 4000 cells/mm^3 or more than 10% bands—to the development of organ dysfunction, hypotension, and hypoperfusion manifested by an increase in lactate level, oliguria, and changes in mental status. Ultimately, patients manifest sustained hypotension (systolic blood pressure [SBP] less than 90 mm Hg) despite adequate fluid resuscitation or patients may be normotensive with inotropic or vasopressor support. The transition from SIRS to severe sepsis and septic shock is accompanied by imbalances between oxygen supply and demand causing varying degrees of perfusion deficits in different organs, eventually resulting in global tissue hypoxia characterized by the increase in lactate levels. New concepts in the pathophysiology of oxygen metabolism during sepsis.

Although only 4% of patients with SIRS progress to full septic shock, 71% of patients with culture proven septic shock are initially identified as being in one of the milder categories. It is for this reason that it is extremely important to identify at an early stage those patients who are at risk of progression from the milder forms of sepsis to severe sepsis and septic shock. It is unclear at this time which biomarkers have the best predictive value in helping to stratify patients with sepsis at risk of progression to severe sepsis and septic shock in order to implement an early goal-directed therapy (EGDT) aimed at preventing the development of the full-blown late distributive shock, which, in our opinion, most of the time is less amenable to successful treatment.

There are at least three areas in which early diagnosis and implementation of time-sensitive therapies have been shown to improve significantly outcome from the standpoint of overall mortality rate and functional outcome of the patients: myocardial infarction, stroke, and trauma. There is a consensus that the timely treatment of these patients is the most essential component of the treatment strategy itself. An important question pertaining to patients with severe sepsis and septic shock is whether there is evidence to suggest their therapy should follow a time-sensitive approach similar to that used to treat patients with myocardial infarction and stroke and whether there is mechanistic evidence at the cellular and molecular level to support the findings of Dr. Rivers and his associates regarding the role of EGDT. Does EGDT affect the inflammatory response independent of antimicrobial treatment? Is the availability of cytosolic and mitochondrial oxygen through an approach that emphasizes targeting oxygen transport and output variables, such as venous oxygen saturation (Svo_2) and lactate, the "key" to the successful treatment of patients with severe sepsis and septic shock? It is our opinion that septic patients should receive a time-sensitive approach not dissimilar to that used to treat patients with stroke, myocardial infarction, and trauma. Although the time window for the treatment of patients with stroke, myocardial infarction, and trauma has been clearly identified, it remains ill defined for septic patients. In this chapter, we will focus on strategies useful to identify septic patients, not necessarily trauma patients, at risk of progression toward severe sepsis and septic shock, on the cellular and molecular reasons that justify the use of EGDT in septic patients using a very narrow time-sensitive approach, and finally, on a specific treatment algorithm applicable to all septic patients.

DIAGNOSIS

The early diagnosis of infection, severe sepsis, and septic shock is more difficult to make in trauma patients because of the almost universal presence of signs of SIRS in noninfected trauma patients secondary to the activation of the proinflammatory response from the injury itself. The most common causes of sepsis in trauma patients include ventilator-associated pneumonia from prolonged mechanical ventilation, catheter-related bloodstream infections, and intra-abdominal infections in patients who have undergone laparotomy for injuries to the gastrointestinal tract or solid organ. An important question regarding patients at risk of infection and sepsis is whether hypotension alone is a sufficiently sensitive screening marker for tissue perfusion deficits to identify the transition of patients from infection/sepsis to severe sepsis and septic shock. Many studies support the superiority of serial measurement of lactate levels over other markers, including hypotension, from the standpoint of identifying the progression of patients from sepsis to severe sepsis and septic shock and from the standpoint of prediction of sepsis-related fatality. Although anion gap and base deficits are routinely used to risk-stratify trauma patients, they have been shown to be insensitive in septic patients. Normal anion gaps and base deficits have been observed in 22% and 25% of patients with mean lactate levels of 4 and 7 mmol/L, respectively. The difference between anion gap, base deficits, and lactate levels in sepsis disappears only when lactate levels exceed 10 mmol/L. Lactate represents a useful and clinically obtainable surrogate marker of tissue hypoxia and disease severity, independent of blood pressure. Previous studies have shown that a lactate concentration greater than 4 mmol/L in the presence of SIRS criteria significantly increases ICU admission rates and mortality rate in normotensive patients. Lactate can be measured in the ICU as well as in the emergency department using point of care devices with a turnaround time of 2 minutes and because peripheral venous lactate levels can be used in substitution of arterial lactate as long as tourniquet times are short, arterial or venous lactate levels should be obtained in septic patients to identify septic patients who should be treated with EGDT to prevent the development of multiple organ dysfunction syndrome (MODS).

Persistently elevated lactate has been shown to be better than oxygen transport variables (oxygen delivery, oxygen consumption, and oxygen extraction ratio) as an indicator of mortality rate. Bakker and his associates defined "lactime" as the time during which lactate remains above 2 mmol/L and observed this duration of lactic acidosis was predictive of organ failure and survival. Trauma patients whose lactate normalized in 24 hours (lactime more than 24 hours) were shown to have 100% survival rate, whereas lactate elevation longer than 6 hours is associated with increased mortality rate. Additionally, elevated lactate concentrations up to 48 hours are associated with higher mortality rate in postoperative hemodynamically stable patients. Our own experience suggests that prolongation of lactate clearance is associated with increasing mortality rate in surgical patients. In fact, failure of a patient to normalize lactate is associated with 100% mortality rate. When infection is suspected, the patient should be pan-cultured, namely, should undergo culture of urine, body fluids, sputum, and cerebrospinal fluid as indicated, including two sets of blood cultures and have either arterial or venous blood drawn for measurement of lactate. If the lactate level is increased, the patient should be assumed to be at risk of progression from

infection to severe sepsis and septic shock; therefore, following the administration of broad-spectrum empiric antibiotics, EGDT should be initiated to minimize lactime.

Lactate Production in Sepsis

To understand the role of using lactate levels to risk-stratify septic patients and to monitor the response to therapy by measuring serial lactate levels, as well as to understand the pathogenetic mechanisms causing the increased lactate levels in septic patients, one must understand the biochemical pathways responsible for its production. In normal conditions, a cytosolic oxygen tension of 6 mm Hg and a mitochondrial oxygen tension of 1.2 mm Hg are associated with normal aerobic glycolysis; therefore, the pyruvate derived from the anaerobic glycolysis enters the Krebs cycle as acetyl-CoA (acetyl coenzyme A) in the mitochondrion. In the absence of sepsis, the microcirculation is regulated through many mechanisms, including functional capillary density, to match at organ level oxygen supply to oxygen demand.

As shown in Figure 1, during anaerobic glycolysis there are three rate-limiting, energy-using steps; they involve the activity of glucose exokinase, phosphofructokinase (PFK), and pyruvate kinase. PFK is the "pacemaker" of the anaerobic glycolysis because it exerts the

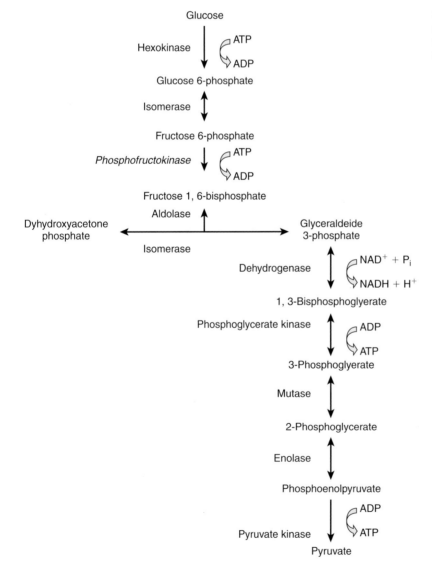

FIGURE I   The pathway of glycolysis with rate-limiting steps. ADP, Adenosine diphosphate; ATP, adenosine triphosphatase; NAD, nicotinamide adenosine dinucleotide; NADH, reduced form of NAD.

major rate-limiting effect. It is the first irreversible reaction of the glycolytic pathway, called the *committed step*; it involves the phosphorylation of fructose 6-phosphate to fructose 1,6-bisphosphate. Therefore, PFK is the primary control site or the pacemaker of the anaerobic glycolysis. Its function is affected by the energy state of the cell (level of adenosine triphosphatase [ATP]), the pH in the cytosol, the level of available citrate, heat-shock proteins, endotoxin, and specific genes. Although there is an ongoing debate regarding whether in sepsis the increased lactate level is the result of dysoxia or of a hyperactive glycolytic pathway causing a production of pyruvate in excess of the enzymatic ability of the pyruvate dehydrogenase complex to produce acetyl-CoA, the net effect is an increased production of lactate due to the transformation of pyruvate, which cannot be stored, into lactate. Depicted in Figure 2 are the two more effective biochemical

pathways that shuttle pyruvate: (1) the pyruvate conversion to lactate on an equimolar basis by lactate dehydrogenase with conversion of lactate to glucose in the liver and renal cortex via the Cori cycle; and (2) the transamination of pyruvate to alanine by the acceptance of an amino group by pyruvate so that they may enter the Krebs cycle. Typically, the proportional conversion of pyruvate to lactate is not associated with a change in cytosolic pH, hence cellular acidosis. It is important to understand the difference between lactate excess with and without acidosis (Fig. 3).

Lactic acid is a weak acid with a low pK_a (3.86); it is only partially dissociated in water, resulting in ion lactate and H^+. Depending on the environmental pH, lactic acid is either present as the acid in its undissociated form at low pH or as the ion salt at higher pH. Under physiologic circumstances the pH is generally higher than the pK_a, so the majority of lactic acid in the body will be dissociated and be present as lactate. One should think of the lactate/pyruvate (L/P) ratio as the mirror image of the NADH/NAD ratio, where NAD = nicotinamide adenosine dinucleotide. In normal conditions when the energy state of the cell is within normal range, that is, when the NADH/NAD ratio is normal, the L/P ratio is less than 20. In the setting of an increase in lactate level proportional to pyruvate with a ratio less than 20, there is enough energy to provide synthesis of ATP from adenosine diphosphate (ADP) and inorganic phosphate (Pi) and hydrogen ions; therefore, there is no net increase in cytosolic hydrogen ions and no change in pH. In contrast, when the L/P ratio is greater than 20, the energy state of the cell is compromised; therefore, there is hydrolysis of ATP in ADP, Pi, with an increase in the hydrogen ion concentration, hence cellular acidosis. The subsequent hydrolysis of ADP to adenosine monophosphate (AMP) and then adenosine is aimed at inducing a relaxation of the precapillary sphincters in order to increase functional capillary density, and hence local blood flow and oxygen availability at cellular level to restore the redox potential and cellular pH.

Shown in Figure 4 is the relationship between oxygen delivery, extraction, and consumption. In normal conditions, oxygen consumption remains supply independent as oxygen delivery decreases due to increased extraction. However, when the extraction ratio approaches 60%, the anaerobic threshold, oxygen delivery, and oxygen consumption become linearly dependent; therefore, the patient is now in a state of supply-dependent oxygen consumption and lactate production. Any further increase or decrease in oxygen delivery will be accompanied by a respective increase or decrease in oxygen consumption. Although the anaerobic threshold, when lactate is produced, is reached at an extraction ratio of 60%, this does not correspond to the maximal body extraction ratio, which is 80%. The question of whether the slope of the Do_2/Vo_2 curve changes in sepsis, shifting the critical level of oxygen delivery to the right, has been debated for years without achieving a consensus. Further controversy exists surrounding the need to normalize oxygen extraction in critically ill

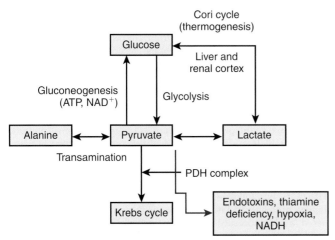

FIGURE 2 Pathways of pyruvate metabolism. If the pyruvate dehydrogenase (PDH) complex is inhibited by endotoxins, thiamine deficiency, or cellular hypoxia, there is an increase in pyruvate, which independent of its causes, will activate different shuttling mechanisms because it cannot be stored. Pyruvate can be converted to lactate by lactate dehydrogenase, and the lactate will then be converted to glucose in the liver and renal cortex via the Cori cycle. This is a futile biochemical reaction that does not use or produce energy and therefore must produce heat. Typically, the proportional conversion of pyruvate to lactate will not be associated with a change in cytosolic pH. Another mechanism used to shuttle pyruvate is the transamination of amino acids that donate the amino group to pyruvate forming alanine so that they can enter Krebs cycle. ATP, Adenosine triphosphate; NAD, nicotinamide adenosine dinucleotide; NADH, reduced form of NAD.

FIGURE 3 Lactate excess with and without acidosis. ADP, Adenosine diphosphate; AMP, adenosine monophosphate; ATP, adenosine triphosphate; L/P, lactate/pyruvate; NAD, nicotinamide adenosine dinucleotide; NADH, reduced form of NAD; Pi, inorganic phosphate.

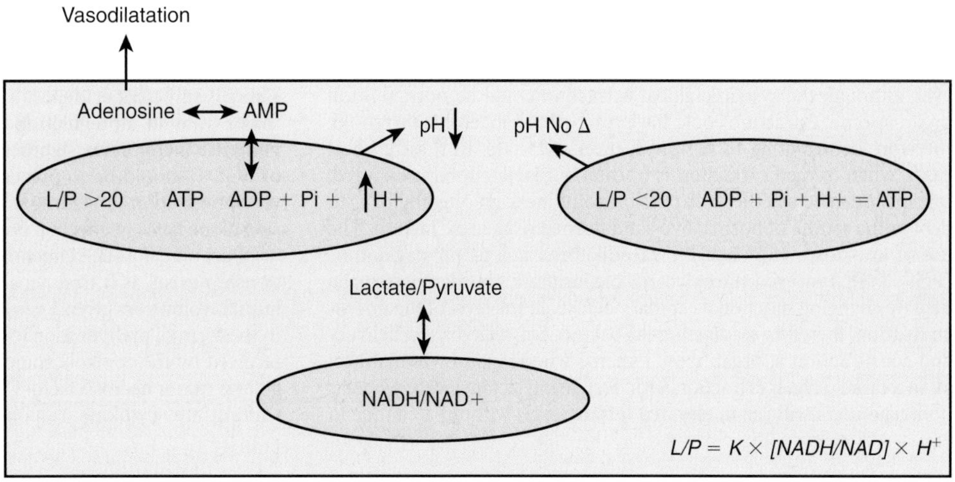

Vasodilatation

Adenosine ⟷ AMP

L/P >20   ATP   ADP + Pi + ↑H+   pH↓

pH No Δ

L/P <20   ADP + Pi + H+ = ATP

Lactate/Pyruvate

NADH/NAD+

$L/P = K \times [NADH/NAD] \times H^+$

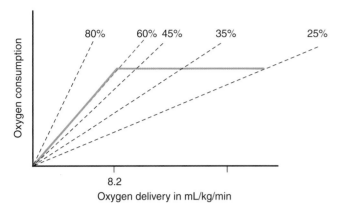

FIGURE 4 The relationship between oxygen delivery, extraction, and consumption. In normal conditions, oxygen consumption remains supply independent as oxygen delivery decreases due to increased extraction. However, when the extraction ratio approaches 60%, the anaerobic threshold, which occurs when oxygen delivery is 8.2 mL/kg/minute, oxygen delivery and consumption become linearly dependent, and therefore, the patient is now in a state of supply-dependent oxygen consumption and lactate production. Any further increase or decrease in oxygen delivery will be accompanied by an increase or decrease in oxygen consumption.

patients. As shown in Figure 4, supply-independent oxygen consumption can be maintained by increased extraction up to 60%. Is the patient whose oxygen consumption is supply independent through an increased extraction at higher risk of developing MODS than the patient whose extraction has been normalized by a targeted therapy aimed at restoring the oxygen extraction to a normal level? Organs, such as the heart, with a high extraction ratio at baseline can maintain oxygen consumption constant only through increased flow, as opposed to organs with low extraction ratios, such as the kidneys, that can maintain oxygen consumption constant through increased extraction. Is an increased global oxygen extraction ratio pathogenetically related to organ-specific supply/demand imbalance that can activate an inflammatory response causing MODS?

Normal Extraction Ratio and Elevated Lactate

The presence of elevated lactate level with a normal oxygen extraction in the setting of sepsis can be seen when there is an ongoing imbalance between oxygen supply and demand at the microcirculatory level of districts contributing lactate production. Typically this distributive abnormality, characterized by a hyperdynamic hemodynamic profile with increased oxygen delivery to low demand regions and conversely, decreased oxygen delivery to high demand regions, is seen late in sepsis. A normal extraction ratio is typically not associated with increased lactate due to the fact that the an extraction ratio of 25% is below the anaerobic threshold coupled with lactate production; however, although the systemic global extraction could be normal, local organ-specific extraction could have reached the anaerobic threshold, therefore contributing to the production of lactate. In these clinical cases, when oxygen extraction is normal but lactate level is elevated, one must decide whether it is possible to unmask an ongoing oxygen debt in the setting of normal Svo_2 and normal oxygen extraction. The use of low-dose, short half-life vasodilators, such as prostaglandins (PGI_2, PGE_2) or even nitroglycerin can unmask an ongoing oxygen debt by changing functional capillary density at the level of the microcirculation, therefore readjusting the balance between oxygen delivery and consumption at organ level. Patients who respond will manifest an increased oxygen extraction with decreasing lactate levels, whereas nonresponders will retain elevated lactate levels without a change in

venous oxygen saturation, indicating there is an irreversible defect in oxygen use at mitochondrial level.

Hypoxic Chemotransduction and Upregulation of Inflammation

The question of whether there are specific pathophysiologic mechanisms that could explain the beneficial effects of EGDT targeted to specific oxygen transport variable end points remains unanswered. However, if one thinks of molecular oxygen availability at the cellular level as a major modulator of cytokine response, then one could hypothesize that an imbalance between Do_2 and Vo_2 in certain microcirculatory districts can be associated with upregulation of the inflammatory response through activation of intracytosolic pathways that favor a sustained proinflammatory state. Is there direct or indirect clinical or laboratory evidence showing a relationship between achievement and failure to achieve specific oxygen transport end points, hence appropriate cellular oxygen tension, and decreased or increased cytokine response either in animal models or in humans?

All humans have oxygen-sensing mechanisms that help them to adapt to hypoxia. Among the mechanisms used to sense oxygen there is the hypoxia-inducible transcription factor (HIF). HIF is a heterodimer composed of a constitutive HIF-1β subunit and one of three different oxygen-dependent and transcriptionally active α subunits, of which HIF-1α and HIF-2α are identified as the promoters of adaptation to hypoxia. In normoxic conditions, HIF-1α subunits are constantly produced but they do not accumulate because they are hydroxylated by prolyl 4-hydroxylases (PHDs) and factor inhibiting HIF (FIH) and following capture by the ubiquitin ligase von Hippel-Lindau protein (vHL) is targeted for proteosomal degradation or rendered transcriptionally less active (Fig. 5). Conversely, in hypoxic conditions, the enzymatic activity of PHDs is significantly reduced because the availability of its cosubstrate, α-ketoglutarate, from the Krebs cycle is limited due to impairment of the mitochondrial respiratory chain; therefore, HIF-1α and HIF-1β subunits accumulate and translocate to the nucleus where they bind as heterodimers to a hypoxia response element (HRE), inducing transcription of genes, such as those of nuclear factor κB (NF-κB) and toll-like receptors (TLRs) (Fig. 6). Hypoxia upregulates the NF-κB pathway by increasing the expression and signaling of TLRs, which in turn enhance the production of cytokines and inflammation. Vascular leakage, leukoaggregation in multiple organs, and elevated serum cytokines have already been documented in mice after a very short exposure to low oxygen concentrations. It is also already known that increased levels of proinflammatory cytokines, such as interleukin 6 (IL-6), IL-6 receptor, and C-reactive protein are observed in people exposed to elevation greater than 3400 m. Furthermore, periods as short as 2 to 4 hours of hypoxic stress upregulate the expression of TLR4 in macrophages via HIF-1, contributing to an amplified inflammatory response to bacterial infection, and potentially, predisposing patients to a protracted inflammatory response, which may cause the development of MODS. There is sufficient evidence to suggest that cellular hypoxia may play a major role in upregulating the inflammatory response in septic patients; therefore, a significant or probably the major component of EGDT should be to prevent the development of cellular hypoxia via optimization of volume status of the patient. Does volume expansion alone have an effect on the pro- or anti-inflammatory response via its effect on cytosolic/mitochondrial oxygen availability? If such a relationship exists, is it time sensitive? There is experimental evidence in human volunteers given *Escherichia coli* endotoxin that volume loading in the form of prehydration followed by hydration at a rate double that received by the control group decreases symptom score and downregulates tumor necrosis factor (TNF-α) but not affecting IL-10, therefore shifting the cytokine response toward a more anti-inflammatory

FIGURE 5 Pathway of hypoxia inducible factor and nuclear factor kappa B (NF-κB) in normoxic conditions. In normoxic conditions, hypoxia-inducible transcription factor (HIF)-1α subunits are constantly produced but they do not accumulate because they are hydroxylated by prolyl 4-hydroxylases and factor inhibiting HIF (FIH) and following capture by the ubiquitin ligase von Hippel-Lindau proteins are targeted for proteosomal degradation or rendered transcriptionally less active. HRE, Hypoxia response element; IKK, IκB kinase; OH, hydroxide; TLR, toll-like receptor.

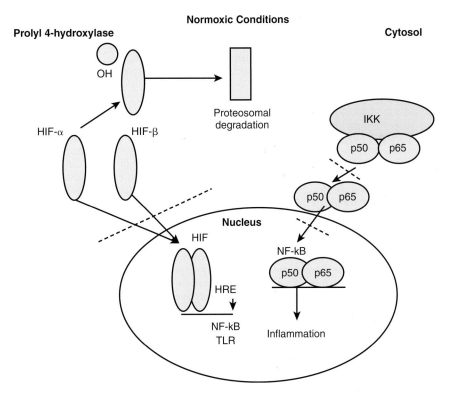

FIGURE 6 Pathway of hypoxia inducible factor and nuclear factor (NF)-κB in hypoxic conditions. Hypoxia activates both hypoxia-inducible transcription factor (HIF) and NF-κB pathways, although it regulates differentially the activity of HIF and NF-κB pathways. There is cross-talk between these two pathways at a number of levels. The enzymatic activity of prolyl 4-hydroxylases (PHDs) is significantly reduced because the availability of its cosubstrate, α-ketoglutarate, from the Krebs cycle is limited because of impairment of the mitochondrial respiratory chain; therefore, HIF-1α and HIF-1β subunits accumulate and translocate to the nucleus where they bind as heterodimers to a hypoxia response element (HRE), inducing transcription of genes, such as those of NF-κB and toll-like receptors (TLRs). The hypoxia-sensitive component of the NF-κB pathway is at the level of the IKK (IκB kinase) complex. OH, Hydroxide.

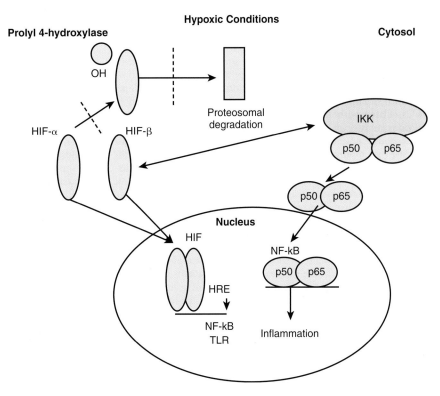

balance without having any effect on systemic blood pressure and heart rate. Based on the available evidence, it is our opinion that septic patients should undergo very early aggressive fluid resuscitation in order to modulate the hypoxic upregulation of the inflammatory response. Ideally, fluid resuscitation should be accomplished within 2 to 6 hours of the diagnosis of sepsis.

TREATMENT

There is a growing body of evidence showing that the treatment of sepsis should be implemented with a time-sensitive approach not dissimilar to that employed for patients with stroke, myocardial infarction, and traumatic injuries. As shown by Rivers and his coworkers, the first 6 hours of early sepsis are the most important from the therapeutic perspective. Based on the proven temporal relationship between an aggressive goal-directed therapy and the decreased levels of proinflammatory cytokines, it is likely that early resuscitation with aggressive fluid therapy targeted to specific end points, such as Svo_2 and normalization of lactate, coupled with the control of the septic source may avert the transition of the patient from severe sepsis and septic shock to overt MODS and its associated high mortality rate by modulating the inflammatory response.

The question of the potential increased morbidity associated with very aggressive fluid therapy from the standpoint of pulmonary complications, including prolongation of mechanical ventilation, the development of intra-abdominal hypertension, as well as worsened neurologic status must be viewed in light of the decreased sepsis-related fatality associated with a time-sensitive approach to EGDT based predominantly on volume expansion. The use of aggressive volume therapy started only 24 to 48 hours after the onset of sepsis, when the patient may have already developed acute lung injury (ALI), will probably be associated with prolonged mechanical ventilation compared with a more conservative fluid strategy started within the same time frame. However, an aggressive fluid resuscitation strategy started within 2 hours of the onset of the diagnosis of sepsis and aimed at achieving normal lactate levels with normal oxygen extraction ratio (resuscitation phase) will likely limit the inflammatory response triggered by the septic source and the subsequent development of ALI and or acute respiratory distress syndrome (ARDS), the intra-abdominal hypertension from bowel wall edema and third spacing, and organ dysfunction; therefore, it is unlikely to be associated with the detrimental consequences observed in a previous study.

Obviously, once the diagnosis of sepsis has been made there must be a stepwise approach to the resuscitation of the patient using a progressive therapeutic strategy that starts with aggressive volume resuscitation, the administration of a broad-spectrum antibiotic, and, if necessary, a timely surgical intervention or percutaneous drainage of the septic source. We believe that once the diagnosis of sepsis has been made, if the patient is not already in the ICU, he/she should be transferred to the ICU to be instrumented with an arterial line preferentially placed in one of the radial arteries to monitor blood pressure and an oximetric central venous line. We advise against the use of noninvasive blood pressure monitoring even in patients who are not in overt shock (SBP less than 90 mm Hg) because of its limitations in patients with compensated shock. We agree with the limitations of using static central venous pressure (CVP) values instead of some more accurate dynamic indices of volume responsiveness such as inferior vena cava diameter as measured by ultrasonography, pulse pressure variation (PPV), or stroke volume variation (SVV) to assess volume responsiveness and guide fluid therapy. Because PPV and SVV are dependent on the cyclic changes in intrathoracic pressure induced by positive-pressure ventilation, they are not applicable to spontaneously breathing patients; therefore, when treating patients

who are breathing spontaneously, fluid therapy should be targeted to normalization of Svo_2. In septic patients requiring mechanical ventilation, we prefer to use SVV to determine preload responsiveness to guide fluid therapy.

With respect to using only a 10% lactate clearance and normalization of lactate instead of normalization of $Scvo_2$ for patients with severe sepsis and septic shock as shown by the noninferiority trial of Jones and his associates in the study that compared lactate clearance versus central venous oxygen saturation as goals of early sepsis therapy, we continue to prefer monitoring $Scvo_2$ in addition to lactate clearance. We prefer $Scvo_2$ monitoring as opposed to the use of lactate monitoring in isolation because, in our opinion, it allows a more rapid achievement of hemodynamic optimization. The goal of therapy is to provide adequate oxygen delivery by optimizing cardiovascular function to allow optimization of oxygen consumption at tissue level as measured indirectly by normalization of lactate level in the setting of a $Scvo_2$ 70% or higher.

Fluid Resuscitation

The choice of the resuscitation fluid remains controversial because of the conflicting results of multiple trials that have compared crystalloids and colloids. Although some studies have shown increased mortality rate related to the use of colloids, namely, albumin, other studies have suggested a potential beneficial effect associated with the use of colloids. In fact, a subgroup analysis of patients with severe sepsis enrolled in the SAFE (Saline versus Albumin Fluid Evaluation) trial suggests that resuscitation with albumin may be superior to resuscitation with saline from the standpoint of risk of death at 28 days; of the 603 patients with severe sepsis who received albumin as resuscitation fluid, 185 (30.7%) died as opposed to 217 of 615 (35.3%) patients who were resuscitated with saline (relative risk, 0.87; 95% confidence interval, 0.74 to 1.02; $P = .09$). Based on the available evidence, we advise against the use of hydroxyethylstarches as resuscitation fluid because it is now established that the use of hydroxyethylstarch as resuscitation fluid in sepsis is associated with an increased risk of acute renal failure and the subsequent need for renal replacement therapy. It is our opinion that resuscitation with crystalloids is more cost effective, at the same time acknowledging that the infusion of colloids provides an advantage from the standpoint of the smaller volume of resuscitation fluid required and the shorter time needed to achieve the same hemodynamic end points. With respect to the choice between normal saline (NS) versus lactated Ringer's (LR) solution, although we acknowledge the immunologic issues associated with the use of LR, we continue to prefer LR instead of NS to avoid the hyperchloremic acidosis associated with the use of large amounts of NS. Our strategy in septic patients on mechanical ventilation with tidal volume greater than 7 mL/kg is to initially monitor SVV and to infuse LR until SVV is less than 13% while monitoring $Scvo_2$ and arterial lactate. Preload recruitment of stroke volume with volume loading, when done correctly, imposes the least increase in myocardial oxygen consumption compared with the use of inotropes and vasopressors and it is not associated with the increased systemic oxygen consumption caused in particular by epinephrine.

Inotropic and Vasopressor Support

If patients do not meet the end points of therapy while undergoing volume resuscitation guided by SVV, we insert an oximetric continuous cardiac output pulmonary artery catheter to optimize cardiovascular function and to guide inotropic and vasopressor therapy. The choice of available inotropic and vasopressor agents includes dopamine, dobutamine, milrinone, epinephrine, norepinephrine, phenylephrine, and vasopressin. Hypotensive patients who have been properly volume resuscitated who have decreased systemic vascular resistance index are treated with norepinephrine to increase the afterload to match not more than half of the myocardial contractility by optimizing the effective left ventricular end-systolic elastance between 1.5 and 2.0 mm Hg/mL based on lean body weight ranging from 60 kg to 80 kg. Patients with hypotension refractory to the infusion of norepinephrine in the setting of an arterial pH greater than 7.30 are treated with hydrocortisone 50 mg every 6 hours after having drawn blood to measure cortisol level. If the cortisol level is greater than 25 µg/dL, we discontinue the administration of hydrocortisone; if conversely, the level is less than 25 µg/dL, we administer hydrocortisone for 7 days with a slow tapering over 3 days. We do not use vasopressin in septic patients with recent gastrointestinal anastomosis due to the decreased splanchnic blood flow associated with its use and the resulting potential detrimental effect on gastrointestinal healing observed in our own institution. Furthermore, recent evidence does not support a beneficial clinical effect of vasopressin in conjunction with norepinephrine in septic patients. We preferentially use dobutamine starting at 7.5 µg/kg/minute over epinephrine in normotensive, volume resuscitated patients requiring higher cardiac output to achieve therapeutic end points. In contrast, we use epinephrine instead of dobutamine in hypotensive patients requiring inotropic support. We reserve the use of milrinone for those patients with decreased right ventricular function from increased right ventricular afterload.

Blood Transfusion

We do not believe there is adequate evidence to justify the transfusion of packed red blood cells in an attempt to increase oxygen delivery in order to increase Scvo₂ in septic patients unless fresh blood is used. In fact, because of a variety of reasons, including the increased risk of infections, ARDS, and death in critically ill patients, we believe that the transfusion of packed red blood cells, which typically are older than 14 days with an age that varies between 21 to 24 days

at the time of transfusion, should not be part of the treatment protocol unless fresh blood is used. It is well known that the p50 of stored red blood cells is very low, 6 mm Hg instead of the normal 27 mm Hg; therefore, red blood cells unload less oxygen. Furthermore, they become less deformable with storage and therefore in low-shear rate districts, such as the splanchnic district, may actually impair the microcirculation, compromise tissue oxygenation, and increase the production of lactate. In addition, stored blood is proinflammatory and prothrombotic. The transfusion of packed red blood cells in patients with sepsis may therefore impair microcirculatory flow and further compromise tissue oxygenation. However, in the event that fresh blood is used, we believe that a hematocrit of 30% to 35% is ideal from the standpoint of restoring oxygen extraction to normal level.

CONCLUSIONS

The incidence of sepsis, severe sepsis, and septic shock is increasing because of a variety of reasons and the mortality rate associated with it remains high, ranging from 20% to 30%, and reaching 80% when complicated by the development of MODS. The best approach to decreasing the mortality rate associated with sepsis is to understand that its treatment should follow a time-sensitive approach not dissimilar to that employed to treat stroke, myocardial infarction, and trauma patients. Therefore, early diagnosis, prompt initiation of antimicrobial therapy, source control, and an early goal-directed approach targeted to normalization of mixed venous oxygen saturation and lactate should be implemented as soon as possible (Fig. 7). The hallmark of EGDT is restoration of volume status and optimization of cardiovascular function to provide adequate oxygen delivery to meet the oxygen demand to prevent the progression of patients from sepsis to severe sepsis and septic shock in order to improve the overall mortality rate of septic patients (Fig. 8).

For the chapter's Suggested Readings list, please visit the book at www.ExpertConsult.inkling.com.

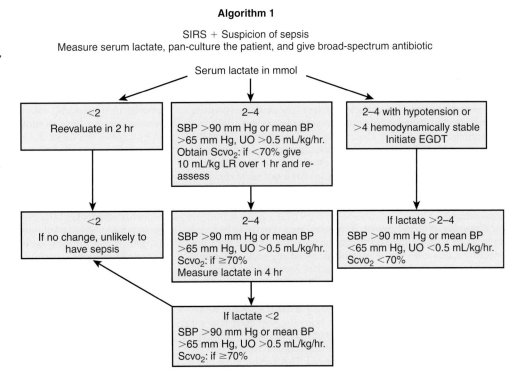

FIGURE 7 Algorithm for systemic inflammatory response syndrome (SIRS) + suspicion of sepsis. BP, Blood pressure; EGDT, early goal-directed therapy; LR, lactated Ringer's solution; SBP, systolic blood pressure; UO, urinary output.

Algorithm 1

SIRS + Suspicion of sepsis
Measure serum lactate, pan-culture the patient, and give broad-spectrum antibiotic

Serum lactate in mmol

<2
Reevaluate in 2 hr

2–4
SBP >90 mm Hg or mean BP >65 mm Hg, UO >0.5 mL/kg/hr. Obtain Scvo₂: if <70% give 10 mL/kg LR over 1 hr and re-assess

2–4 with hypotension or >4 hemodynamically stable
Initiate EGDT

<2
If no change, unlikely to have sepsis

2–4
SBP >90 mm Hg or mean BP >65 mm Hg, UO >0.5 mL/kg/hr. Scvo₂: if ≥70%
Measure lactate in 4 hr

If lactate >2–4
SBP >90 mm Hg or mean BP <65 mm Hg, UO <0.5 mL/kg/hr. Scvo₂ <70%

If lactate <2
SBP >90 mm Hg or mean BP >65 mm Hg, UO >0.5 mL/kg/hr. Scvo₂: if ≥70%

Algorithm of EGDT

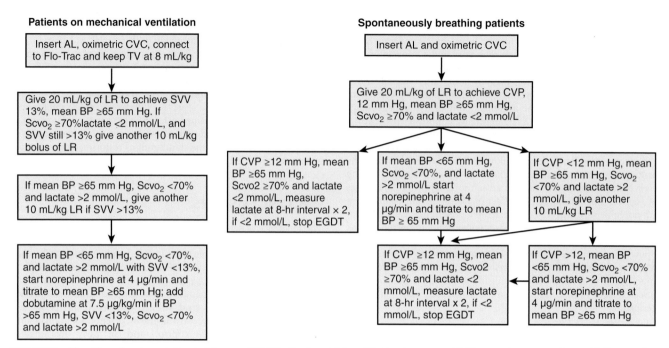

FIGURE 8   Algorithm of early goal-directed therapy (EGDT). AL, Arterial line; BP, blood pressure; CVC, central venous catheter; CVP, central venous pressure; LR, lactated Ringer's; SVV, stroke volume variation; TV, tidal volume.

IMMUNOLOGY OF TRAUMA

Christine S. Cocanour and S. Rob Todd

The immune response to injury is mediated by the innate and adaptive arms of the immune system. The innate response is nonspecific and includes polymorphonuclear leukocytes (PMNLs), eosinophils, natural killer (NK) cells, and complement, but the adaptive response is pathogen- and antigen-specific and is exemplified by T and B cells. Evolutionarily primitive pattern recognition receptors (PRRs) recognize and bind conserved microbial constituents called pathogen-associated molecular patterns (PAMPs). PAMPs allow for differentiation between infectious and noninfectious antigens.

Classically, immune-mediated responses were thought to be based on self and nonself interactions, but because this concept does not adequately describe other immunologic situations such as tumors, autoimmunity, or trauma, another model has been proposed by Matzinger et al. The danger model theorizes that danger, not "foreignness," is what initiates an immune response. The mechanism by which a cell dies determines whether an immune response is initiated. Normally occurring apoptotic cells are scavenged and no immune response occurs. When injury or infection causes cell damage (lysis or apoptosis with release of intracellular contents) both innate and adaptive responses are triggered. These endogenous controlling signals are termed alarmins. They are the alarm signals that emanate from stressed or injured tissues. Both PAMPs (which respond to exogenous signals) and alarmins (which respond to endogenous signals) have similar conserved hydrophobic portions that are able to engage the same PRRs and elicit a comparable inflammatory response. Because of their similarities, PAMPs and alarmins are classified as danger-associated (or sometimes damage-associated) molecular patterns (DAMPs).

The immune response to trauma is markedly similar to that seen with a microbial infection (Fig. 1). The PAMPs/DAMPs released in response to trauma and infection elicit an intrinsic inflammatory immune response through similar PRRs such as the toll-like receptor (TLR) family. The TLRs are a key molecular link between tissue injury, infection, and inflammation. TLRs are membrane-bound receptors that are known to activate two distinct signaling pathways in inflammation. The first is a myeloid differentiation factor 88 (MyD88)-dependent pathway that is activated by all TLRs with the exception of TLR3. This signaling cascade is propagated through a number of interleukin 1 (IL-1) receptor–associated kinases with subsequent quick activation of nuclear factor kappa B (NF-κB) cells and mitogen-activated protein kinase (MAPK), leading to the production of proinflammatory cytokines (IL-1α/β, IL-6, IL-8, macrophage inflammatory protein [MIP]-1α/β, tumor necrosis factor [TNF]-α). The second signaling pathway is a MyD88-independent pathway and is activated through binding of TLR3 and TLR4. This pathway culminates with the induction of interferon (IFN).

Because there are numerous TLRs (12 human TLRs are currently described), and each recognizes PAMPs/DAMPs through diverse mechanisms, functional responses differ depending upon the TLR signaling pathway activated. Following trauma, tissue injuries, hypoxia, and hypotension, as well as secondary insults such as

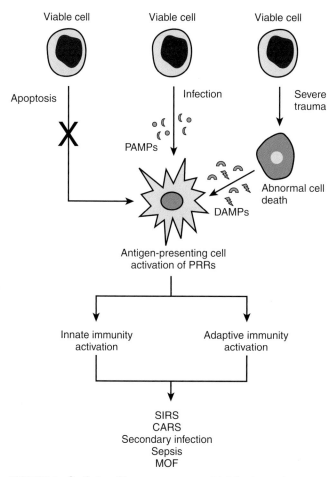

FIGURE 1 Similarity of immune response with infection and trauma. CARS, Compensatory anti-inflammatory syndrome; DAMPs, damage-associated molecular patterns; MOF, multiple organ failure; PAMPs, pathogen-associated molecular patterns; PRRs, pattern recognition receptors; SIRS, systemic inflammatory response syndrome.

ischemia/reperfusion, compartment syndromes, operative interventions, and infections, all TLRs contribute to a response that is characterized by local and systemic release of proinflammatory cytokines, arachidonic acid metabolites, activation of complement factors, kinins, and coagulation factors as well as release of hormonal mediators. Clinically, this is the systemic inflammatory response syndrome (SIRS). Paralleling SIRS is an anti-inflammatory response referred to as the compensatory anti-inflammatory response syndrome

(CARS). The injured patient must strike a fine balance between SIRS and CARS for healing and recovery to occur. When these processes are unbalanced, the patient is at risk for increased susceptibility to infection and multiple organ failure (MOF) (Fig. 2).

In this chapter we will discuss the main components of the immune response following trauma including examples of specific DAMPs: cytokine response; leukocyte recruitment; protease and reactive oxygen species; complements, kinins, and coagulation; acute phase reactants; SIRS; CARS; and the two-hit model.

DANGER (DAMAGE)-ASSOCIATED MOLECULAR PATTERNS

Many of the molecules identified as DAMPs are proteins released from the cell following injury. Intracellular proteins include high-mobility group box 1 (HMGB1) and heat shock proteins (HSPs); extracellular matrix proteins include hyaluronan fragments. Nonprotein DAMPs include deoxyribonucleic acid (DNA), adenosine 5′-triphosphate (ATP), and uric acid. Two examples of DAMPs are discussed next.

High-Mobility Group Box 1

HMGB1 is a nuclear, nonhistone chromosomal DNA-binding protein that functions as a structural cofactor for proper DNA transcriptional regulation and gene expression. When released extracellularly from injured or necrotic cells, it stimulates both innate and adaptive immune responses. It drives the initiation and potentiation of proinflammatory mediators, inducing a cell-mediated (T helper [T_H]1 type) response and serves as a chemoattractant for immature dendritic cells. In apoptotic cells, HMGB1 is irreversibly bound to the chromatin and does not stimulate an immune response. If large numbers of apoptotic cells are cleared by macrophages, then HMGB1 is passively released. Active secretion of HMGB1 occurs from a variety of cell types following an inflammatory stimulus, thus potentiating the inflammatory response to trauma, burn, and infection while initiating tissue regeneration.

Heat Shock Proteins

HSPs are highly conserved intracellular proteins that are constitutively expressed and function as molecular chaperones that facilitate the synthesis and folding of proteins. Under stressful conditions such as heat shock, pH shift, or hypoxia, their expression is increased, protecting the cell by stabilizing unfolded proteins and allowing the cell to repair or synthesize replacement proteins. When HSP production is upregulated or they are released extracellularly, they act as danger signals and elicit immune responses, at least some of which are mediated through the interaction with TLRs.

FIGURE 2 Postinjury multiple organ failure (MOF) occurs as a result of a dysfunctional inflammatory response. CARS, Compensatory anti-inflammatory response syndrome; SIRS, systemic inflammatory response syndrome.

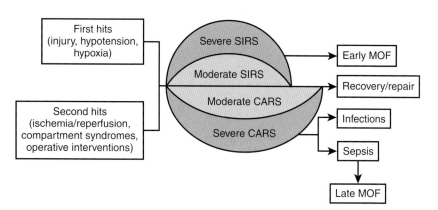

CYTOKINE RESPONSE

Once the immune response is initiated a multitude of mediators are released. Cytokines exert their effects in both a para- and autocrine manner. Proinflammatory cytokines TNF-α and IL-1β are released within 1 to 2 hours. Secondary proinflammatory cytokines are released in a subacute fashion and include IL-6, IL-8, macrophage migratory factor (MMF), IL-12, and IL-18. Clinically, IL-6 levels correlate with Injury Severity Score (ISS) and the development of MOF, acute respiratory distress syndrome (ARDS), and sepsis.

IL-6 also acts as an immunoregulatory cytokine by stimulating the release of anti-inflammatory mediators such as IL-1 receptor antagonists and TNF receptors, which bind circulating proinflammatory cytokines. IL-6 also triggers the release of prostaglandin E$_2$ (PGE$_2$) from macrophages. PGE$_2$ is potentially the most potent endogenous immunosuppressant. Not only does it suppress T-cell and macrophage responsiveness, it also induces the release of IL-10, a potent anti-inflammatory cytokine that deactivates monocytes. Serum IL-10 levels correlate with ISS as well as the development of posttraumatic complications.

Following trauma, IL-12 production is decreased, stimulating a shift in favor of T$_H$2 cells and the subsequent production of anti-inflammatory mediators IL-4, IL-10, IL-13, and transforming growth factor beta (TGF-β). This decrease in IL-12 and resultant increase in T$_H$2 cells correlates with adverse outcomes. A listing of pro- and anti-inflammatory mediators may be found in Tables 1 and 2.

TABLE 1: Proinflammatory Mediators

Mediator	Action
IL-1	IL-1 is pleiotropic. Locally, it stimulates cytokine and cytokine receptor production by T cells as well as stimulating B-cell proliferation. Systemically, IL-1 modulates endocrine responses and induces the acute phase response.
IL-6	Il-6 induces acute phase reactants in hepatocytes and plays an essential role in the final differentiation of B cells into Ig-secreting cells. Additionally, IL-6 has anti-inflammatory properties.
IL-8	IL-8 is one of the major mediators of the inflammatory response. It functions as a chemoattractant and is also a potent angiogenic factor.
IL-12	IL-12 regulates the differentiation of naïve T cells into T$_H$1 cells. It stimulates the growth and function of T cells and alters the normal cycle of apoptotic cell death.
TNF-α	TNF-α is pleiotropic. TNF-α and IL-1 act alone or together to induce systemic inflammation as mentioned previously. TNF-α is also chemotactic for neutrophils and monocytes, as well as increasing neutrophil activity.
MIF	MIF forms a crucial link between the immune and neuroendocrine systems. It acts systemically to enhance the secretion of IL-1 and TNF-α.

IL, Interleukin; Ig, immunoglobulin; MIF, migration inhibitory factor; T$_H$1, T helper lymphocyte; TNF, tumor necrosis factor.

TABLE 2: Antiinflammatory Mediators

Mediator	Action
IL-4	IL-4, IL-3, IL-5, IL-13, and CSF2 form a cytokine gene cluster on chromosome 5q, with this gene particularly close to IL-13.
IL-10	IL-10 has pleiotropic effects in immunoregulation and inflammation. It downregulates the expression of T$_H$1 cytokines, MHC class II antigens, and costimulatory molecules on macrophages. It also enhances B-cell survival, proliferation, and antibody production. In addition, it can block NF-κB activity, and is involved in the regulation of the JAK-STAT signaling pathway.
IL-11	IL-11 stimulates the T-cell–dependent development of immunoglobulin-producing B cells. It is also found to support the proliferation of hematopoietic stem cells and megakaryocyte progenitor cells.
IL-13	IL-13 is involved in several stages of B-cell maturation and differentiation. It upregulates CD23 and MHC class II expression, and promotes IgE isotype switching of B cells. It downregulates macrophage activity, thereby inhibiting the production of proinflammatory cytokines and chemokines.
IFN-α	IFN-α enhances and modifies the immune response.
TGF-β	TGF-β regulates the proliferation and differentiation of cells, wound healing, and angiogenesis.
α-MSH	α-MSH modulates inflammation by way of three mechanisms: (1) direct action on peripheral inflammatory cells; (2) actions on brain inflammatory cells to modulate local reactions; and (3) indirect activation of descending neural anti-inflammatory pathways that control peripheral tissue inflammation.

CSF, Colony-stimulating factor; IFN, interferon; Ig, immunoglobulin; IL, interleukin; JAK-STAT, Janus kinase/signal transducers and activators of transcription; MHC, major histocompatibility complex; MSH, melanocyte-stimulating hormone; TGF, transforming growth factor; T$_H$, T helper.

CELL-MEDIATED RESPONSE

Trauma alters the ability of splenic, peritoneal, and alveolar macrophages to release IL-1, IL-6, and TNF-α leading to decreased levels of these proinflammatory cytokines. Kupffer cells, however, have an enhanced capacity for production of proinflammatory cytokines. Cell-mediated immunity not only requires functional macrophage and T cells but also intact macrophage–T cell interaction. Following injury, human leukocyte antigen (HLA-DR) receptor expression is decreased, leading to a loss of antigen-presenting capacity and decreased TNF-α production. PGE$_2$, IL-10, and TGF-β all contribute to this "immunoparalysis."

T helper cells differentiate into either T$_H$1 or T$_H$2 lymphocytes. T$_H$1 cells promote the proinflammatory cascade through the release of IL-2, IFN-γ, and TNF-β, and T$_H$2 cells produce anti-inflammatory mediators. Monocytes/macrophages, through the release of IL-12, stimulate the differentiation of T helper cells into T$_H$1 cells. Because IL-12 production is depressed following trauma, there is a shift toward T$_H$2 cells, which has been associated with an adverse clinical outcome.

Adherence of the leukocyte to endothelial cells is mediated through the upregulation of adhesion molecules. Selectins such as leukocyte adhesion molecule-1 (LAM-1), endothelial leukocyte adhesion molecule-1 (ELAM-1), and P-selectin are responsible for PMNLs "rolling." Upregulation of integrins such as the CD11/18 complexes or intercellular adhesion molecule-1 (ICAM-1) is responsible for PMNL attachment to the endothelium. Migration, accumulation, and activation of the PMNLs are mediated by chemoattractants such as chemokines and complement anaphylatoxins. Colony-stimulating factors (CSFs) likewise stimulate monocytopoiesis or granulocytopoiesis and reduce apoptosis of PMNLs during SIRS. Neutrophil apoptosis is further reduced by other proinflammatory mediators, thus resulting in PMNL accumulation at the site of local tissue destruction.

LEUKOCYTE RECRUITMENT

Proinflammatory cytokines enhance PMNL recruitment, phagocytic activity, and the release of proteases and oxygen free radicals by PMNLs. This recruitment of leukocytes represents a key element for host defense following trauma, although it allows for the development of secondary tissue damage. It involves a complex cascade of events culminating in transmigration of the leukocyte, whereby the cell exerts its effects. The first step is capture and tethering, mediated via constitutively expressed leukocyte selectin denoted L-selectin. L-selectin functions by identifying glycoprotein ligands on leukocytes and those upregulated on cytokine-activated endothelium.

Following capture and tethering, endothelial E-selectin and P-selectin assist in leukocyte rolling or slowing. P-selectin is found in the membranes of endothelial storage granules (Weibel-Palade bodies). Following granule secretion, P-selectin binds to carbohydrates presented by P-selectin glycoprotein ligand (PSGL-1) on the leukocytes. In contrast, E-selectin is not stored, yet it is synthesized *de novo* in the presence of inflammatory cytokines. These selectins cause the leukocytes to roll along the activated endothelium, whereby secondary capturing of leukocytes occurs via homotypic interactions.

The third step in leukocyte recruitment is firm adhesion, which is mediated by membrane expressed β_1- and β_2-integrins. The integrins bind to ICAM resulting in cell-cell interactions and ultimately signal transduction. This step is critical to the formation of stable shear-resistant adhesion, which stabilizes the leukocyte for transmigration.

Transmigration is the final step in leukocyte recruitment following the formation of bonds between the aforementioned integrins and Ig-superfamily members. The arrested leukocytes cross the endothelial layer via bicellular and tricellular endothelial junctions in a process coined diapedesis. This is mediated by platelet-endothelial cell adhesion molecules (PECAM), proteins expressed on both the leukocytes and intercellular junctions of endothelial cells.

PROTEASES AND REACTIVE OXYGEN SPECIES

Polymorphonuclear lymphocytes and macrophages are not only responsible for phagocytosis of microorganisms and cellular debris but can also cause secondary tissue and organ damage through degranulation and release of extracellular proteases and formation of reactive oxygen species or respiratory burst. Elastases and metalloproteinases that degrade both structural and extracellular matrix proteins are present in increased concentrations following trauma. Neutrophil elastases also induce the release of proinflammatory cytokines.

Reactive oxygen species are generated by membrane-associated nicotinamide adenine dinucleotide phosphate (NADPH) oxidase, which is activated by proinflammatory cytokines, arachidonic acid metabolites, complement factors, and bacterial products. Superoxide anions are reduced in the Haber-Weiss reaction to hydrogen peroxide by superoxide dismutase located in the cytosol, mitochondria, and cell membrane. Hydrochloric acid is formed from H_2O_2 by myeloperoxidase, while the Fenton reaction transforms H_2O_2 into hydroxyl ions. These free reactive oxygen species cause lipid peroxidation, cell membrane disintegration, and DNA damage of endothelial and parenchymal cells. Oxygen radicals also induce PMNLs to release proteases and collagenase as well as inactivating protease inhibitors.

Reactive nitrogen species cause additional tissue damage following trauma. Nitric oxide (NO) is generated from L-arginine by inducible nitric oxide synthase (iNOS) in PMNLs or vascular muscle cells and by endothelial nitric oxide synthase (eNOS) in endothelial cells. NO induces vasodilatation. iNOS is stimulated by cytokines and toxins, whereas eNOS is stimulated by mechanical shearing forces. Damage by reactive oxygen and nitrogen species leads to generalized edema and the capillary leak syndrome.

COMPLEMENT, KININS, AND COAGULATION

The complement cascade, kallikrein-kinin system, and coagulation cascade are intimately involved in the immune response to trauma. They are activated through proinflammatory mediators, endogenous endotoxins, and tissue damage. The classical pathway of complement is normally activated by antigen-antibody complexes (immunoglobulin [Ig] M or G) or activated coagulation factor XII (FXII), and the alternative pathway is activated by bacterial products such as lipopolysaccharide. Complement activation following trauma is most likely from the release of proteolytic enzymes, disruption of the endothelial lining, and tissue ischemia. The degree of complement activation correlates with the severity of injury. The cleavage of C3 and C5 by their respective convertases results in the formation of opsonins, anaphylotoxins, and the membrane attack complex (MAC). The opsonins C3b and C4b enhance phagocytosis of cell debris and bacteria by means of opsonization. The anaphylotoxins C3a and C5a support inflammation via the recruitment and activation of phagocytic cells (i.e., monocytes, polymorphonuclear cells, and macrophages), enhancement of the hepatic acute phase reaction, and release of vasoactive mediators (i.e., histamine). They also enhance the adhesion of leukocytes to endothelial cells which results in increased vascular permeability and edema. C5a induces apoptosis and cell lysis through the interaction of its receptor and the MAC. Additionally, C3a and C5a activate reparative mechanisms. C1-inhibitor inactivates C1s and C1r, thereby regulating the classical complement pathway. However, during inflammation, serum levels of C1-inhibitor are decreased via its degradation by PMNL elastases.

The plasma kallikrein-kinin system is a contact system of plasma proteases related to the complement and coagulation cascades. It consists of the plasma proteins FXII, prekallikrein, kininogen, and factor XI (FXI). The activation of FXII and prekallikrein is via contact activation when endothelial damage occurs, exposing the basement membrane. FXII activation forms factor XIIa (FXIIa), which initiates the complement cascade through the classical pathway; whereas prekallikrein activation forms kallikrein, which stimulates fibrinolysis through the conversion of plasminogen to plasmin or the activation of urokinase-like plasminogen activator (uPA). Tissue plasminogen activator (tPA) functions as a cofactor. Additionally, kallikrein supports the conversion of kininogen to bradykinin. The formation of bradykinin also occurs through the activation of the tissue kallikrein-kinin system, most likely through organ damage as the tissue kallikrein-kinin system is found in many organs and tissues including the pancreas, kidney, intestine, and salivary glands. The kinins are potent vasodilators. They also increase vascular permeability and inhibit the function of platelets.

The intrinsic coagulation cascade is linked to the contact activation system via the formation of factor IXa (FIXa) from factor XIa (FXIa). Its formation leads to the consumption of FXII, prekallikrein, and FXI, and plasma levels of enzyme-inhibitor complexes are increased. These complexes include FXIIa-C1 inhibitor and kallikrein-C1 inhibitor. C1 inhibitor and α1-protease inhibitor are both inhibitors of the intrinsic coagulation pathway.

Although the intrinsic pathway provides a stimulus for activation of the coagulation cascade, the major activation following trauma is via the extrinsic pathway. Increased expression of tissue factor (TF) on endothelial cells and monocytes is induced by the proinflammatory cytokines TNF-α and IL-1β. The factor VII (FVII)-TF complex stimulates the formation of factor Xa (FXa) and ultimately thrombin (FIIa). Thrombin-activated factor V (FV), factor VIII (FVIII), and FXI result in enhanced thrombin formation. Following cleavage of fibrinogen by thrombin, the fibrin monomers polymerize to from stable fibrin clots. The consumption of coagulation factors is controlled by the hepatocytic formation of antithrombin (AT) III. The thrombin-antithrombin complex inhibits thrombin, FIXa, FXa, FXIa, and FXIIa. Other inhibitors include TF pathway inhibitor (TFPI) and activated protein C in combination with free protein S. Free protein S is decreased during inflammation due to its binding with the C4b binding protein.

Disseminated intravascular coagulation (DIC) may occur following trauma. After the initial phase, intravascular and extravascular fibrin clots are observed. Hypoxia-induced cellular damage is the ultimate result of intravascular fibrin clots. Likewise, there is an increase in the interactions between endothelial cells and leukocytes. Clinically, coagulation factor consumption and platelet dysfunction are responsible for the diffuse hemorrhage. Consumption of coagulation factors is further enhanced via the proteolysis of fibrin clots to fibrin fragments. The consumption of coagulation factors is further enhanced through the proteolysis of fibrin clots to fibrin fragments by the protease plasmin.

ACUTE PHASE REACTION

The acute phase reaction describes the early systemic response following trauma and other insult states. During this phase, the biosynthetic profile of the liver is significantly altered. Under normal circumstances, the liver synthesizes a range of plasma proteins at steady-state concentrations. However, during the acute phase reaction, hepatocytes increase the synthesis of positive acute phase proteins (i.e., C-reactive protein [CRP], serum amyloid A [SAA], complement proteins, coagulation proteins, proteinase inhibitors, metal-binding proteins, and other proteins) essential to the inflammatory process at the expense of the negative acute phase proteins. The acute phase proteins are listed in Table 3.

The acute phase response is initiated by hepatic Kupffer cells and the systemic release of proinflammatory cytokines. IL-1, IL-6, IL-8, and TNF-α act as inciting cytokines. The acute phase reaction typically lasts for 24 to 48 hours prior to its downregulation. IL-4, IL-10, glucocorticoids, and various other hormonal stimuli function to downregulate the proinflammatory mediators of the acute phase response. This modulation is critical. In instances of chronic or recurring inflammation, an aberrant acute phase response may result in exacerbated tissue damage.

The major acute phase proteins include CRP and SAA, the activities of which are both poorly understood. CRP was so named secondary to its ability to bind the C-polysaccharide of *Pneumococcus*. During inflammation, CRP levels may increase by up to 1000-fold over several hours depending on the insult and its severity. It acts as an opsonin for bacteria, parasites, and immune complexes; activates complement via the classical pathway; and binds chromatin. Binding chromatin may minimize autoimmune responses by disposing of nuclear antigens from sites of tissue debris. Clinically, CRP levels are relatively nonspecific and are not predictive of posttraumatic complications. Despite this fact, serial measurements are helpful in trending a patient's clinical course.

SAA interacts with the third fraction of high-density lipoprotein (HDL3), thus becoming the dominant apolipoprotein during acute inflammation. This association enhances the binding of HDL3 to

TABLE 3: Acute Phase Proteins

Protein Group	Individual Proteins
Positive Acute Phase Proteins*	
Major acute phase proteins	C-reactive protein, serum amyloid A
Complement proteins	C2, C3, C4, C5, C9, B, C1 inhibitor, C4 binding protein
Coagulation proteins	Fibrinogen, prothrombin, von Willebrand factor
Proteinase proteins	α₁-Antitrypsin, α₁-antichymotrypsin, α₂-antiplasmin, heparin cofactor II, plasminogen activator inhibitor I
Metal-binding proteins	Haptoglobin, hemopexin, ceruloplasmin, manganese superoxide dismutase
Other proteins	α₁-Acid glycoprotein, heme oxygenase, mannose-binding protein, leukocyte protein I, lipoprotein (a), lipopolysaccharide-binding protein
Negative Acute Phase Proteins	Albumin, prealbumin, transferrin, apolipoprotein AI, apolipoprotein AII, α₂-Heremans-Schmid glycoprotein, inter-α-trypsin inhibitor, histidine-rich glycoprotein, protein C, protein S, antithrombin III, high-density lipoprotein

*Positive acute phase proteins increase production during an acute phase response. Negative acute phase proteins are those that have decreased production during an acute phase response.

macrophages, which may engulf cholesterol and lipid debris. Excess cholesterol is then used in tissue repair or excreted. Additionally, SAA inhibits thrombin-induced platelet activation and the oxidative burst of neutrophils, potentially preventing oxidative tissue destruction.

SYSTEMIC INFLAMMATORY RESPONSE SYNDROME

The release of mediators results in what we know as SIRS. In 1991, a consensus conference of the American College of Chest Physicians and the American Society of Critical Care Medicine (ACCP/SCCM) defined SIRS as a generalized inflammatory response triggered by a variety of infectious and noninfectious events. They arbitrarily established clinical parameters through a process of consensus. Table 4 summarizes the diagnostic criteria for SIRS. At least two of the four

TABLE 4: Clinical Parameters of the Systemic Inflammatory Response Syndrome

1.	Heart rate >90 beats/minute
2.	Respiratory rate >20 breaths/minute, or $Paco_2 < 32$ mm Hg
3.	Temperature >38° C or <36° C
4.	Leukocytes >12,000/mm³ or <4,000/mm³ or ≥10% juvenile neutrophil granulocytes

$Paco_2$, Arterial CO_2 partial pressure.

criteria must be present to fulfill the diagnosis of SIRS. Note, this definition emphasizes the inflammatory process regardless of the presence of infection. The term *sepsis* is reserved for SIRS when infection is suspected or proved. Subsequent studies have validated these criteria as predictive of increased intensive care unit (ICU) mortality risk, and that this risk increases concurrent with the number of criteria present.

SIRS is characterized by the local and systemic production and release of multiple mediators, including proinflammatory cytokines, complement factors, proteins of the contact phase and coagulation system, acute phase proteins, neuroendocrine mediators, and an accumulation of immunocompetent cells at the local site of tissue damage. The severity of trauma, duration of the insult, genetic factors, and general condition of the individual determine the local and systemic release of proinflammatory cytokines and phospholipids.

COMPENSATORY ANTI-INFLAMMATORY RESPONSE SYNDROME

Trauma not only stimulates the release of proinflammatory mediators, but also the parallel release of anti-inflammatory mediators. This compensatory anti-inflammatory response is present concurrently with SIRS (see Fig. 2). When these two opposing responses are appropriately balanced, the traumatized individual is able to effectively heal the injury without incurring secondary injury from the autoimmune inflammatory response. However, overwhelming CARS appears responsible for posttraumatic immunosuppression, which leads to increased susceptibility to infections and sepsis. With time, SIRS ceases to exist and CARS is the predominant entity.

TWO-HIT MODEL

In the two-hit model, the inciting injury induces a systemic inflammatory response (Fig. 3). This "first hit" primes the immune system for an exaggerated and potentially lethal inflammatory reaction to a secondary, otherwise nonlethal, stimulus ("second hit"). This secondary stimulus may be either endogenous or exogenous. Endogenous second hits include cardiovascular instability, respiratory distress, metabolic derangements, and ischemia/reperfusion injuries.

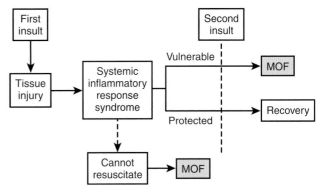

FIGURE 3   Pathogenesis of postinjury multiple organ failure (MOF).

In contrast, exogenous second hits include surgical interventions, blood product transfusions, and missed injuries. The two-hit model proposes that this second hit results in destructive inflammation leading to MOF and potentially death. This model has been supported by the work of Moore and colleagues who linked postinjury opportunistic infections to SIRS and MOF.

SUMMARY

Injury triggers a tremendously complex response involving a multitude of systems. The individual's immune system must balance the proinflammatory response, which is necessary to clear injured tissue, yet not cause overwhelming endogenous injury with a necessary downregulation of the inflammatory process in order to provide an environment of minimal inflammation that can nurture the cell proliferation and tissue remodeling needed for healing. A loss of this balance can cause additional tissue injury from the immune response itself or leave the individual susceptible to infection and sepsis. As our understanding of the immune response following injury grows, our ability to monitor and effectively manage the traumatized, critically ill patient will hopefully result in improved outcomes.

For the chapter's Suggested Readings list, please visit the book at www.ExpertConsult.inkling.com.

OVERVIEW OF INFECTIOUS DISEASES IN TRAUMA PATIENTS

Donald E. Fry

Infection is the major threat to recovery among most trauma patients who survive the successful resuscitation and intervention of the initial 24 hours following severe injury. The infectious risk may occur from environmental contamination that attended the injury process, or from endogenous microflora of disrupted organ structures within the patient. Infection may complicate the surgical site

employed for injury repair. Similarly, the trauma patient receives a large measure of care in the critical care unit with multiple invasive tubes and monitoring devices and each serves as a portal for microbial entry and potential life-threatening infection. From injury until recovery, the trauma patient is exposed to pathogens at the site of injury and everywhere "the hands of man" have been in the process of treatment.

Not only are there abundant opportunities for infection, but the trauma patient sustains a remarkable compensatory suppression of immune responses. Virtually every measurable component of the innate and adaptive immune response is suppressed. The exact benefit for the suppressed host is often hard to rationalize from an evolutionary perspective, but modulation of the wholesale systemic activation of the innate inflammatory response that is activated by major tissue injury must provide some protection for the injured host. However, the millennia of evolution did not anticipate aggressive resuscitation, surgical interventions, and critical care units. The contemporary end result is survival through incredible multisystem injury, only to have a recovering host that is a human Petri dish.

The critical care unit becomes the common ground of immunosuppression and infection risk that is shared by all trauma/critically ill patients. It is a wonder that all do not die of infection after major injury.

This overview will briefly discuss a model of common clinical issues that cause infection in the care of trauma patients. This will not be a detailed discussion of each anatomic site of infection or a detailed discussion of pathogens and antibiotic choices because most are discussed in detail in other chapters. It will highlight the common features that are associated with the important infections of the trauma patient, and will use examples of specific infections and specific pathogens to emphasize these features. This overview will hopefully give a perspective to the many areas that deserve continued attention and investigation.

DETERMINANTS OF INFECTION

All injuries and all patients are not at the same risk for the development of infection. Infection occurs as a result of the complex interaction of numerous variables of the pathogen and the host (Fig. 1).

Microbial Inoculum

One of the most commonly studied areas of infection is the number of microbes that contaminate an anatomic site, and the critical threshold that is required for infection to result. All injured sites, all surgical incisions, and all invasive medical devices will have recoverable bacteria when cultured. Our environment is not sterile, and the human being has more microbial colonists than eukaryotic cells. The presence of bacteria does not uniformly determine infection, but the numbers of bacteria per gram of tissue or unit of surface area of tissue are predictive.

Classic studies of experimental and clinical wounds have created the magical 10^5 organisms per gram of tissue as the necessary microbial threshold for infection as an outcome. The 10^5 threshold is held as the standard in the definition of infection in the urinary tract. A threshold of 10^4 bacteria is considered the defining limit of bacteria in bronchoalveolar lavage samples of lung secretions in the critical care unit patient. There must be a definable limit of *Clostridium difficile* spores that are ingested to create the colitis syndrome. Although there is some biologic variability around the 10^5 threshold, the supporting research has clearly defined that there is a limit to the magnitude of contamination that can be handled without resultant infection by the host at each anatomic site (Fig. 2).

Microbial Virulence

Bacteria have individual profiles of virulence characteristics. Virulence factors include structural components of the bacterial cell (e.g., endotoxin), secreted protein products that damage tissues or specifically retard phagocytic cell function, and antimicrobial resistance factors that impair the effectiveness of treatment strategies.

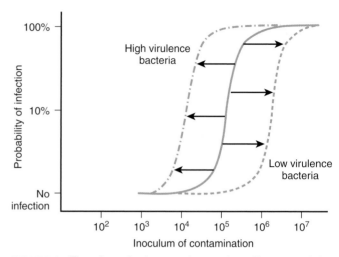

FIGURE 2   The relationship between the inoculum of bacteria and the probability of infection. With conventional pathogens, the probability of infection tends to cluster around the magical "10^5" bacteria per gram of tissue. With bacteria that have increased virulence factors, the curve shifts to the left. Less virulent bacteria shift the curve to the right and require a larger density of bacteria (or an impaired host) to cause infection.

The presence of lipid A in gram-negative endotoxin, potent exotoxins produced by *Clostridium perfringens*, superantigens from *Streptococcus pyogenes*, and coagulase from *Staphylococcus aureus* means that selected bacteria pose a greater infectious risk. It means that fewer microbes are required to cause infection than the traditional view of 10^5 bacteria per gram.

Conversely, many bacterial species lack potent virulence factors but still pose infection risks. *Pseudomonas aeruginosa*, *Staphylococcus epidermidis*, *Enterococcus* spp., and *Candida albicans* are microbes that demonstrate poor virulence characteristics in experimental models, but have proved to be very real pathogens in the clinical setting. They share the capacity to resist the antimicrobial activity of many drugs and emerge as major pathogens in the immunosuppressed critical care patient when prior treatment has eliminated the more susceptible common bacterial pathogens. Intrinsically low virulence organisms in terms of structural or secreted protein products can assume major importance in critically ill patients because of resistance. In the critical care unit, virtually any microbe can assume a role as a pathogen when competing microflora have been eliminated, and the host response is suppressed.

Adjuvant Factors

At the end of his spectacular scientific career, Pasteur is alleged to have said, "The microbe is nothing, the terrain is everything." Although bordering on hyperbole, the comment by Pasteur emphasizes the importance of the local environment surrounding the bacterial contaminant in the trauma patient as being paramount in determining infection as an outcome. The presence of hemoglobin

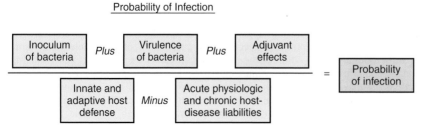

FIGURE 1   This schematic represents a hypothetical equation of variables that predict infection in the trauma patient. The "numerator" represents the three major groups of variables that are additive or even synergistic in the development of infection in the trauma patient. The "denominator" of host defense offsets the proinfection events of the numerator. Acute physiologic and chronic medical conditions impair the response of the host and increase the probability that infection will occur.

and hematoma in the traumatic wound or surgical site provides a rich source of nutrients and critical amounts of iron to promote microbial growth. Necrotic tissue provides a haven for bacterial proliferation that is poorly accessible by host phagocytic cells.

Foreign bodies assume importance as adjuvant variables in the development of infections in all surgical patients, but especially following injury. Traumatic injury may result in foreign debris from the injury process, or fecal material from colonic disruption that is laden with microbes that promote infection. The surgical site will have suture material that is well documented to lower the required bacterial inoculums to cause infection. Endotracheal tubes, urinary catheters, drains, and indwelling intravascular devices provide foreign body surfaces for bacteria to colonize and become the nidus for infection. The foreign body surface retards the phagocytic function of the host, but also provides a surface for biofilm production as a unique virulence expression of bacteria to promote infection.

Not only do indwelling devices compromise host functions, but they may directly damage the nonspecific primary epithelial and endothelial barriers of the patient. Endotracheal tubes defeat the normal barrier of the glottis and provide a direct conduit from the external environment into the lower airway passages. Foley catheters not only create an avenue for microbial access, but erode the protective transitional cell lining of the bladder. Similarly, the indwelling intravascular device creates access for treatment, but clot and endothelial damage at the site of entrance must have a role in infection.

Host Defenses

The impaired host defense of the injured and critically ill patient may be the most important determinant of infection. Each patient has a unique, genetically programmed innate and adaptive immune response. Each patient has a genetic vulnerability for death from infection. The magnitude of functional differences in the intrinsic polymorphism of host responsiveness between patients has been difficult to quantify. All patients do not have the same efficiency in the eradication of soft tissue contamination, or in the physiologic response to infection.

Acquired immune influences are of great significance to the trauma patient. The systemic perturbations of the injured patient have been well chronicled and their immune effects are well appreciated. Hemorrhage, shock, hypoxemia, and extensive soft tissue injury have profound consequences for host responsiveness. The influences of hypothermia and hyperglycemia are contributors to the impaired host. Preexisting diabetes, chronic renal failure, poor nutritional status, and chronic medications (e.g., corticosteroids) impact immune functions. Even the treatments employed in the care of injured patients (e.g., transfusion) have adverse host effects. It is likely that acquired influences upon immune efficiency are far more clinically relevant than individual genetic variability.

Thus, a generic model can be proposed to predict infection as a clinical event in the trauma patient. Whether it is infection in the soft tissues, the peritoneal or pleural spaces, the lung, the urinary tract, or *C. difficile* infection, the determinants of infection are the same. Infection risk is the biologic summation of the quantity of bacteria that access the anatomic site, the virulence characteristics of the microbial contaminants, and net effects of microenvironmental factors. These proinfection variables are then offset by the nonspecific and specific mechanisms of host defense. Host responsiveness is then impacted by acute and chronic conditions. Our current prevention and therapy for infection in the trauma patient is to minimize the liabilities leading to infection and to optimize the effectiveness of the host (see Fig. 1).

PREVENTION OF INFECTION

Infection prevention begins at the time of presentation of the trauma patient. Failures in preventive strategies during resuscitation and

surgical management will have long-term consequences in infection as an outcome. Although the initial 24 hours of care are dedicated to the acute survival of the patient, a keen sense of awareness about prevention from the very beginning and through the following days of care will pay dividends.

Reduction of the Microbial Inoculum

Infection prevention begins with gowns and gloves in the resuscitation room. Occlusive dressings are applied after hemostasis is achieved to avoid further contamination of open wounds. Indwelling intravascular lines are placed with expediency, but should all be changed under appropriate infection control conditions once the frenzy of initial management has subsided. The replacement of central lines should follow accepted guidelines for placement. The Foley catheter is a necessary evil in the management of these patients and is placed with appropriate antiseptic preparation. As care progresses from the acute phase to the critical care unit, infection control practices must avoid needless contamination of indwelling catheters and access lines. It is very important to remove lines, catheters, and drains once their primary function is completed.

Excessive duration of Foley catheters is a commonly repeated event in the care of trauma patients. Bacteria will gain access to the pericatheter space within the urethra and will gain access to the bladder. Appropriate efforts are made to keep the perineum clean, but the human reality is that dense microbial colonization is a given and the probability of infection will increase as the duration of catheterization increases. Although maintaining the closed drainage system and avoiding the "sump" effects of the catheter movement by anchoring it in place are important, the best prevention of urinary tract infection in the trauma patient is removal of the Foley catheter once its purpose has been served.

Following the acute management of life-threatening priorities, soft tissue wounds should be managed. Environmental contamination from the mechanical injury requires débridement of the dead tissues and removal of foreign bodies. Precise débridement will reduce the microbial burden and the dead tissue that will support infection. Pulsed lavage with saline may remove the bacterial-laden fibrin peel that is present in all of these injuries, and appropriate occlusive dressings are applied to avoid secondary contamination. In the long-term care of open soft tissue wounds, desiccation creates additional dead tissue and needs to be avoided with moist dressings. The use of most topical antiseptics will likely damage exposed soft tissues and should not be used. Topical antibiotics are not of value in the prevention of infection in traumatic wounds. Topical burn management agents such as mafenide acetate or silver sulfadiazine are appropriate topical considerations for infection prevention in especially large wounds until skin grafting or flap closure can be entertained.

Prevention of infection at the site of surgical intervention is an important objective. All of the usual preventive strategies of the operating room environment continue to be important in the trauma patient. Hair is removed with electrical clippers. Hair removal may be avoided in selected patients because it has not been demonstrated to reduce rates of infection. Hair removal will obviously be necessary for craniotomy and for hirsute patients. The proposed surgical site is cleansed with an antiseptic scrub. Topical antiseptic preparation of the skin will reduce contamination of the wound and is probably best done with chlorhexidine application.

Preventive systemic antibiotics have become an important measure to prevent infection at the surgical site. Although there are no placebo-controlled clinical trials that have documented a reduction in surgical site infection (SSI) in trauma patients, there is a wealth of evidence in many other areas to validate the appropriate use of preoperative antibiotics for these patients. The experimental principles of the importance for preincisional administration and of using antibiotics appropriate for the anticipated pathogens have been well documented. The antibiotic must be present in the tissues at the time of

704 OVERVIEW OF INFECTIOUS DISEASES IN TRAUMA PATIENTS

contamination, and postcontamination initiation of antibiotics does not change the incidence of SSI. For sites other than the surgical site, contamination of the tissues from severe soft tissue injury or intestinal disruption will have already occurred. However, the débridement and management of these injuries will entail dissection and the opening of fresh tissue planes; thus, it is reasonable to believe that antibiotics in the tissues at the time of débridement of soft tissues or management of intestinal injuries will serve a positive purpose.

Antibiotic selection should focus upon the likely pathogens to be encountered at the surgical site. For orthopedic, neurosurgical, and thoracic interventions, cutaneous colonization of the patient and the operating room environment are the major sources of bacteria to access the incision. Preoperative cefazolin (1 to 2 g intravenously before the incision) is still recommended to cover *S. aureus*. Gram-negative and anaerobic coverage should also be included with farm injuries or incisions in proximity to the perineum. Laparotomy for trauma should include coverage for both enteric gram-negative rods (*Escherichia coli*) and gut anaerobes (e.g., *Bacteroides fragilis*). Specific indications for preventive antibiotics in the trauma setting are not provided by the Food and Drug Administration (FDA). Applications of antibiotics in the trauma setting are considered by the FDA to be presumptive therapy, and preventive drugs in laparotomy are those used for the treatment of intra-abdominal infection. Studies of

potential choices are identified in Table 1. It should be noted that no randomized clinical trials for preventive antibiotics in abdominal trauma can be identified since the year 2000.

Massive contamination of the soft tissues or the abdominal incision is seen often in major trauma centers. Following débridement of the injury or source control of the offending gastrointestinal injury, the surgeon is left with a traumatic or surgical site that is laden with an enormous bacterial inoculum. Infection appears to be a virtual certainty. Delayed primary or secondary closure is a traditional and important option in these circumstances. The cleansed wound is left open with occlusive dressings and daily management. Topical mafenide acetate or silver sulfadiazine is an appropriate topical consideration. Selected wounds may be amenable to delayed primary closure. Negative-pressure management has been a significant addition to managing these open wounds. Open soft tissue injuries may require skin grafting or flap closure, and abdominal incisions commonly are managed by secondary intention. Continued systemic antibiotics are not an appropriate option for the prevention of infection in the open soft tissue or surgical wound.

The sustained care of the trauma patient requires continued vigilance in the avoidance of exposure to pathogenic microbes in the critical care unit environment. An attitude of prevention must be the objective. Methicillin-resistant *S. aureus* (MRSA), resistant

TABLE 1: Characteristics of Randomized Clinical Trials Involving Laparotomy of Trauma Patients*

Author (year)	Patient Population	Antibiotics	No. of Patients	No. of Infections (SSIs)	Comments
Kirton, 2000	Laparotomy, penetrating injury	Ampicillin-sulbactam: 5 days	159	16 (10%)	No advantage to prolonged antibiotics beyond 24 hours
		Ampicillin-sulbactam: 1 day	158	13 (8%)	
Cornwell, 1999	Laparotomy, penetrating injury	Cefoxitin: 1 day	31	6 (19%)	Underpowered study, but no advantage for longer course of antibiotics
		Cefoxitin: 5 days	32	12 (38%)	
Schmidt-Matthiesen, 1999	Penetrating Trauma	Ceftriazone: 1 dose	97	4 (4%)	Heterogeneous population of injuries, but no advantage to longer course of antibiotics
		Cefoxitin: 3 days	98	5 (5%)	
Bozorgzadeh, 1999	Penetrating abdominal injury	Cefoxitin: 1 day	148	24 (16%)	No advantage to longer course of antibiotics
		Cefoxitin: 5 days	152	26 (17%)	
Tyburski, 1998	Penetrating abdominal injury	Ciprofloxacin/metronidazole	35	7 (20%)	1 day of antibiotics if stomach or small bowel injury; 4 days for colon injury; underpowered study
		Gentamicin/metronidazole	33	5 (15%)	
Sims, 1997	Penetrating abdominal injury	Cefoperazone	101	6 (6%)	Duration of administration varied with severity of injury; no benefit to using multiple antibiotics
		Ceftriaxone/metronidazole	95	2 (2%)	
		Gentamicin/ampicillin/metronidaole	95	5 (5%)	
Fabian, 1994	Penetrating abdominal injury	Aztreonam/clindamycin	37	1 (3%)	*P* < .03 in favor of aztreonam/clindamycin; underpowered study
		Gentamicin/clindamycin	36	7 (19%)	
Weigelt, 1993	Laparotomy for abdominal injury	Cefoxitin	309	22 (7%)	*P* < .004 in favor of ampicillin-sulbactam
		Ampicillin-sulbactam	283	6 (2%)	

SSIs, Surgical site infections.

*The drugs employed, results, and commentary are provided. Clinical trials of newer antibiotics have not been undertaken over the last decade.

gram-negative bacteria, and *C. difficile* spores are transmitted from patient to patient by lapses in infection control practices. Gloves and gowns for each patient contact are essential. Handwashing is important to avoid transmission of resistant bacteria and *C. difficile* spores. Mechanical cleansing of the hands remains the best strategy to avoid microbial transmission. Infection control in suctioning ventilator-dependent patients and in the manipulation of all indwelling lines/catheters remains important. Vigilance in removing all drains, tubes, and lines remains the best preventive strategy.

Selective gut decontamination (SGD) has been a method employed to reduce infections in trauma and critically ill patients. Because the gastrointestinal lumen is felt to be the source of many nosocomial infections, the concept of SGD has been to give oral antibiotics which are poorly absorbed and hopefully reduce the microbial reservoir of pathogenic bacteria. Aerobic bacteria are targeted and efforts are made to preserve the anaerobic colonization and maintain colonization resistance. Most studies have demonstrated some reductions in infections, but mortality rates in trauma patients have not been impacted with this method.

Managing Microbial Virulence

Obviously, the surgeon has no control over the virulence characteristics of the would-be pathogens that contaminate the patient with injury. However, if one accepts the premise that microbial resistance is an important component of microbial virulence, the management decisions in antibiotic use will influence virulence.

The single most problematic consideration in the prevention of infection in trauma patients is the continuation of systemic preventive antibiotics into the postinjury period. Prevention of infection at the surgical site is not achieved with postoperative preventive antibiotics. Hospital-acquired pneumonia, intravascular device infections, catheter-associated urinary tract infections, and *C. difficile* infection are not prevented by systemic antibiotics. The argument that antibiotics must be continued to "cover" indwelling drainage tubes or catheters or open wounds is without validity. The continuation of the systemic antibiotics ensures that subsequent nosocomial infections will be with organisms that are resistant to the chosen preventive drug.

The management of open fractures is a case in point. There is no question that concerns about infection in the open fracture are valid because these infections result in substantial morbidity and potential loss of extremities. The management should be appropriate systemic antibiotics at the time of débridement of the fracture, use of pulse lavage to further reduce microbial colonization, appropriate infection control in the management of the open wound, and wound closure when clinical evidence indicates that it is safe to do so. After all, a fracture is a soft tissue injury with a broken bone within it. The same concepts govern the use of preventive antibiotics in open fracture wounds that are applied in the management of other soft tissue wounds. Prolonged systemic antibiotics result in colonization of the patient with resistant organisms. These resistant organisms infect the open fracture wound, and they infect the patient at other anatomic sites.

The national epidemic of *C. difficile* infection affects trauma patients, and has largely been driven by the generalized deployment of antibiotics. Systemically administered antibiotics adversely affect the ecology of the human colon, adversely influence the normal anaerobic species, and permit the ingested *C. difficile* spores to make the transition to the vegetative form of the organism. The vegetative gram-positive rod adheres to the colonocyte and produces the toxin A and toxin B enterotoxins, with damaging enterocolitis as the result. Furthermore, hypervirulent strains of *C. difficile* are identified which produce 20 times the amount of enterotoxin and cause a fulminant infection that may lead to toxic megacolon and the need for surgical colectomy. Prevention of this enterocolitis syndrome requires a reduction in spore transmission to the patient with improved compliance to handwashing protocols. Alcohol-based hand rubs have been less effective than traditional soap and water washing. Overall infection control policies must be enhanced, especially in the critical care units, but a reduction in unnecessary antibiotic use such as is seen in prolonged postoperative preventive use is likewise important for prevention.

The antimicrobial resistance of hospital-acquired infections among trauma patients is progressively increasing. MRSA, vancomycin-resistant enterococci (VRE), expanded-spectrum β-lactamase (ESBL) producing gram-negative rods, and *Klebsiella pneumoniae* carbapenemases (KPC) in gram-negative organisms have become all too common and are directly the consequences of the generalized use of antimicrobial agents. First, the prevention of resistance requires that antibiotic therapy cover the identified pathogen(s) in appropriate doses. Subtherapeutic dosing is a recipe for bacterial resistance. Second, deescalate antibiotic therapy once culture evidence is available. Obviously, antibiotic combinations will be initially started prior to culture evidence of the infection. Unfortunately, antibiotic therapy with redundant or unnecessary drugs is continued when culture evidence indicates that fewer drugs or less toxic (or costly) alternatives could be used. It makes no sense to get cultures and then ignore the results. Finally, shorter therapeutic courses of antibiotics are being documented to be as effective as longer courses. Shorter courses for pneumonia and intra-abdominal infection are as effective. There is a clinical price to be paid for the patient being treated when excessive antibiotics are used.

Management of Adjuvant Factors

Elimination of adjuvant factors requires appropriate technique and judgments in patient care. Hematomas should be evacuated, hemothoraces are drained, and effective hemostasis avoids subsequent risk of blood accumulation in tissues. Dead tissue is débrided, and wisdom and constraint in the use of the electrocautery will avoid the "scorched earth" that becomes the breeding ground for bacteria within wounds. Parsimony in the overall use of suture material, avoidance of braided materials, and preferences for monofilaments is encouraged.

The use of indwelling foreign bodies is necessary in the trauma patient for clinical monitoring, therapeutic intervention, and evacuation of dead space. All catheters, lines, and drains are two-way streets that make wounds and body cavities open to the external environment. The foreign surface permits microbial growth. All indwelling lines deserve adherence to infection control practices and removal as soon as their purpose has been fulfilled. Although antibiotic and silver impregnation of indwelling devices has been advocated, the effectiveness of these catheters remains unproved and they are expensive for standard application. The best infection prevention is prompt removal.

Enhancement of the Host

Although efforts to enhance or modulate the host response to infection have largely been unsuccessful, considerable progress has been made with the concept that optimization of the normal physiologic state of the host can enhance effectiveness in the prevention of infection. Oxygen is essential for leukocyte function in intracellular killing of pathogens. Considerable experimental evidence makes a strong case for optimization of oxygen delivery to prevent infection, and some elective surgical experience makes a similar case. Host defense doubtlessly benefits from an ample supply of tissue oxygen. That may not make the case for supranormal oxygen concentrations.

Maintenance of core body temperature has long been recognized as important in trauma patients to avoid preventable coagulopathy. Experimental evidence identifies slowed biologic reactions and impaired leukocyte mobility into injured and infected tissues with even slight degrees of hypothermia. Elective surgical experience in colon surgery has demonstrated benefits to maintaining core temperatures. The support of core body temperature during resuscitation, operation, and early critical care management with various mechanical heating devices needs to be employed in that early phase of patient management. The best temperature control method remains to be defined.

A controversial issue in support of host defenses has been glycemic control. A large clinical trial demonstrated reductions in multiple organs dysfunction and deaths in critically ill surgical patients with rigorous glycemic control (80 to 110 mg/dL). More recent clinical trials have challenged the value of this degree of glycemic control and have identified negative consequences to patients with episodes of hypoglycemia. Hyperglycemia is a reality in trauma patients because of underlying glucose intolerance among injured patients, excess exogenous administration of glucose, and the accelerated gluconeogenesis that is characteristic of the hypermetabolic response to injury and sepsis. Appropriate glycemic control is likely to be beneficial to the trauma patient, but the degree of management remains undefined. A lesson from preventive strategies in cardiac surgery might indicate that an upper threshold of 200 mg/dL is appropriate. Real-time glucose monitoring will be a technology that needs to evolve to permit answering the question of the limits of benefit in glucose management.

Nutritional support for injured patients is generally recommended to hopefully prevent protein depletion and prevent infection. Effective protein delivery (1.5 g/kg/day) with an appropriate administration of nonprotein calories (100 to 150 calories/g protein) is generally recommended. Evidence supports the use of specific components of glutamine, arginine, nucleotides, omega-3 fatty acids, antioxidants, and trace minerals. This nutritional support should be delivered by the alimentary tract whenever possible.

Finally, improved vigilance in the treatment methods that suppress host responsiveness is necessary. Blood transfusion is necessary but immunosuppressive, and reappraisal of transfusion requirements is always useful. Histamine blockage and proton-pump inhibitors have generally been employed in the critically ill trauma patient to prevent stress mucosal bleeding. However, acid inhibition has been associated with nosocomial pneumonia and with *C. difficile* infection because gastric acidity is a recognized nonspecific defense mechanism. Nonsteroidal anti-inflammatory drugs have similarly been associated with *C. difficile* infection.

DIAGNOSIS OF INFECTION

The traditional hallmarks for the diagnosis of infection are to recognize the appropriate signs and symptoms and to document the infection by culturing the responsible pathogen to provide guidance in therapy. The classical signs of inflammation, induration, and purulent discharge from wounds and incisions indicate infection. The presence of fever and leukocytosis are not perfect indicators, but are generally of value. Chest roentgenograms and computed tomography are well-accepted methods to visualize sites of clinical infection. Cultures of exudates, blood, intravascular catheters, and urine are standards for diagnosis. Detection of toxins in the stool is the diagnostic method for *C. difficile* infection. However, some issues remain in the diagnosis of infection.

Inadequate sampling of the infection site can give misleading information about the infectious pathogen. Superficial swabs of infected wounds may miss the deep-seated pathogens especially in polymicrobial infections of soft tissues. Deeper tissue biopsies that are processed for culture will give more reliable results. Pus and infected tissues in the abdominal cavity need rapid culturing to capture anaerobes and facultative organisms, and these pathogens may best be isolated when samples are directly inoculated into the culture medium at the time of sampling. Tracheal aspirates as opposed to bronchoalveolar sampling will identify colonization and perhaps not the pathogens.

Blood cultures are frequently performed in trauma patients, but have a low yield of isolated pathogens. Many infections in soft tissues and in the abdominal cavity are polymicrobial and pyogenic in character, and are infrequently associated with bacteremia. Similarly, pulmonary infection is not commonly bacteremic. However, intravascular device infection has bacteremia as its signature, and blood cultures are of value when these infections are suspected. A positive blood culture for *S. aureus* in a trauma patient is an intravascular device infection until proved otherwise.

Catheter-associated urinary tract infections remain a problematic area for trauma patients. The traditional diagnosis of 10^5 organisms/mL of urine was derived from community-acquired cystitis patients. It was not derived from patients who currently had a Foley catheter in place. The catheter surface is a platform for microbial growth and shedding into the urine. Bacteriuria may or may not be reflective of invasive infection or of foreign body effect. Positive urinary tract cultures may not be the source for fever in trauma patients. Additional research into the diagnosis of urinary tract infection in catheterized patients seems warranted.

TREATMENT OF INFECTION

When infection occurs, the treatment of the trauma patient requires the mechanical interventions of containment, drainage, and débridement at the local site of infection. Infected wounds must be opened, dead tissue débrided, foreign bodies removed, pus drained, and fibrin/inflammatory debris must be eliminated from infected soft tissue injuries and surgical incisions. The source of pathogens from perforations and suture line leaks within the abdominal cavity must be contained. Abscesses and empyemas must be drained. Purulent bronchopulmonary secretions and potential plugs to airways must be suctioned and evacuated. Infected indwelling intravascular devices have to be removed. Suppurative thrombophlebitis must be excised. Only when the infected focus is mechanically controlled can the next steps in management be successful.

The supportive measures that are necessary in the management of the infected trauma patient are extensive and have been well detailed elsewhere. The Surviving Sepsis Campaign provides an excellent presentation of the supportive measures of the severely infected patient. The critical points are to maintain effective oxygenation and tissue perfusion by all support methods and pharmacologic interventions that are necessary. Monitoring the response of the patient by simple measures of pulse, respirations, pulse oximetry, and urine output prove to be a poor man's valid method of gauging supportive care. With multisystem injury, nutritional support must be initiated early and effectively to avoid the extremes of the catabolic responses that follow injury and invasive infection.

Antibiotic therapy is a two-edged sword in the care of trauma patients. Therapy should be directed at the anticipated pathogens of the wounded structure when infection emerges in the early days (3 to 5) of care. Blunt soft tissue injuries will be susceptible to gram-positive cocci; farm accidents will involve polymicrobial gram-positive organisms, gram-negative organisms, and gut anaerobes; and infections following missiles and penetrating weapons will correspond to the structures that were transgressed with injury. In intra-abdominal infection in the trauma patient, the clinical presumption is that both enteric gram-negative and enteric anaerobic pathogens require initial treatment until refinement with culture evidence (Table 2).

C. difficile infections must be treated promptly and appropriate antibiotics should be given orally if at all possible (Table 3). Abdominal exploration and subtotal colectomy may be necessary for the patient with the *C. difficile* infection when an acute abdomen is present, for severe systemic inflammatory response syndrome, and for the patient with pneumatosis coli. Ileostomy with colonic irrigation with vancomycin has recently been reported as an innovative intervention that may obviate the need for colectomy.

TABLE 2: Antibiotic Choices, Biologic Elimination Half-Life (t$_{1/2}$), Dosing, and Commentary on Choices Available for Treatment of Intra-abdominal Infection in Trauma Patients*

Antibiotic Choice	Half-life (t$_{1/2}$)	Adult Dosing	Comments on Intra-abdominal Infection
Piperacillin-tazobactam	1 h	3.375 g every (q) 6 h	The most popular agent; has both aerobic and anaerobic coverage; single agent therapy
Cefazolin	1.7 h	1–2 g q8h	Must have metronidazole added for treatment; usually reserved for prevention in trauma patients
Cefoxitin	0.75 h	2 g q6h	Short t$_{1/2}$; has been used for 30 years; aerobic and anaerobic activity but resistance is a problem
Cefotetan	4 h	1–2 g q12h	Has aerobic and anaerobic activity but resistance to gram-negative organisms is a current issue
Cefuroxime	2 h	1.5 g q8h	Must have metronidazole added; limited use in this indication
Cefotaxime	1 h	1–2 g q6–8 h	Marginal anaerobic activity for use without metronidazole; it has a bioactive metabolite
Ceftazidime	2 h	2 g q8h	Must have metronidazole added; most commonly used for gram-negative infections
Ceftriaxone	7–8 h	1 g q12h	Long t$_{1/2}$ antibiotic; marginal anaerobic activity; metronidazole is commonly added; most commonly used in community pneumonia
Cefepime	2 h	2 g q8–12 h	No anaerobic coverage; must have metronidazole added; most commonly used for gram-negative, hospital-acquired infections
Ciprofloxacin	4 h	400 mg q12h	No anaerobic activity; must have metronidazole added
Levofloxacin	6–8 h	750 mg q24h	No anaerobic activity; must have metronidazole added
Moxifloxacin	12 h	400 mg q24h	Only quinolone with anaerobic activity; can be used as single agent
Metronidazole	8 h	500 mg q8h	Exclusively an anaerobic agent; must have enteric gram-negative coverage added
Gentamicin	2 h	1 mg/kg q8h; 5–7 mg/kg q24h	Excellent gram-negative coverage; requires pharmacokinetic dosing; must have metronidazole added
Tobramycin	2 h	1 mg/kg q8h; 5–7 mg/kg q24h	Excellent gram-negative coverage; requires pharmacokinetic dosing; must have metronidazole added
Amikacin	2 h	7.5 mg/kg q12h; 15–20 mg q24h	Excellent gram-negative coverage; requires pharmacokinetic dosing; must have metronidazole added
Doripenem	1 h	500 mg q8h	Comprehensive aerobic and anaerobic coverage; more commonly used for hospital-acquired infections
Ertapenem	4 h	1 g q24h	Comprehensive enteric aerobic and anaerobic coverage; long t$_{1/2}$ carbapenem
Imipenem-cilastatin	2 h	500 mg q6h; or 1 g q8h	Comprehensive aerobic and anaerobic coverage; more commonly used for hospital-acquired infections
Meropenem	1 h	1 g q8h	Comprehensive aerobic and anaerobic coverage; more commonly used for hospital-acquired infections
Aztreonam	1.7 h	1–2 g q6–8 h	Must have metronidazole added for anaerobic coverage
Tigecycline	40 h	50 mg q12h	Comprehensive coverage of aerobic and anaerobic coverage

*All doses are for intravenous administration. The drug choice or choices should target gram-negative enteric bacteria and enteric anaerobes (*Bacteroides fragilis*). Cultures are very important with infection at reoperation and prior antibiotic therapy, because pathogens under these circumstances will likely be with resistant bacteria. When drains have been used previously, methicillin-resistant *Staphylococcus aureus* will emerge as a pathogen in reoperation or percutaneous drainage patients.

TABLE 3: Current Choices for Treatment
of *Clostridium Difficile* Infection*

Antibiotic	Dosage	Comments
Metronidazole	250–500 mg qid for 10 days; or 500–750 mg tid for 10 days	Considered the treatment of choice for mild-to-moderate infections
Vancomycin	125–500 mg qid for 10 days	Recommended for the treatment of severe cases
Fidaxomicin	200 mg bid for 10 days	FDA approved for treatment of initial infections
Rifampicin (Rifampin)	300 mg bid for 10 days	Expensive agent used with metronidazole for recurrent infections
Bacitracin	25,000 units qid for 10 days	Poorly absorbed, good in vitro activity; expensive and not readily available
Fusidic acid	250 mg tid for 7–10 days	Limited clinical experience; significant systemic absorption
Tigecycline	50 mg intravenously bid until clinical resolution	Anecdotal reports at this time; used only in refractory cases

bid, Twice a day; FDA, Food and Drug Administration; qid, four times a day;
tid, three times a day.
*Metronidazole and vancomycin remain the choices for initial infection.
Fidaxomicin was approved in May 2011. Other choices are considered only
with infections refractory to initial treatment or for patients with recurrent
infections. All drugs are given orally except for tigecycline.

If infection emerges after 5 days in the critical care unit, then infection will likely be with hospital-acquired pathogens. If cultures are not yet available, then antibiotic coverage needs to be consistent with the known antibiogram of pathogens from the critical care unit. Empirical choices should be deescalated as specific organisms are identified to include only the necessary antibiotic choice(s). Specific antibiotics are used to address the sensitivity of recovered isolates that are addressed in other chapters.

Key Points

Pointers in using antibiotics and other management issues of infections in the trauma patient are as follows:

- SSIs seldom require systemic antibiotics without evidence of a perimeter cellulitis or wound necrosis. Effective local management with drainage and débridement are key treatments.
- Open surgical site wounds and open traumatic wounds will all have positive cultures, but are commonly not infected if adequately drained and débrided. Antibiotics should be used to treat infection, not colonization.
- Cultures of intra-abdominal abscess and empyema following drains, tubes, and prior antibiotics will have hospital-acquired pathogens. Sensitivities of isolated pathogens are critical.
- Antibiotic dosing should be aggressive. Infected trauma patients have an expanded volume of distribution and a

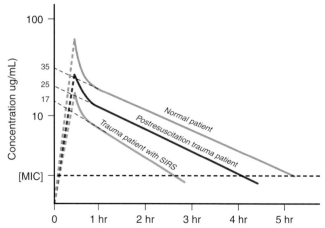

FIGURE 3   This graph illustrates the clearance from serum of a hypothetical antibiotic that has a half-life ($t_{1/2}$) of approximately 6 hours in a "normal patient." The administered dose was 1 g intravenous. The concentration target for the minimum inhibitory concentration (MIC) is illustrated as 1 µg/mL. The peak concentration is about 60 µg/mL. The equilibrated time-zero (t_0) concentration is 35 µg/mL (the intercept on the y-axis). In the postresuscitation trauma patient, the volume of distribution is expanded and is evidenced by the decline in the t_0 concentration of 25 µg/mL. The duration of antibiotic concentration above the MIC is reduced by a full hour. In the systemic inflammatory response syndrome (SIRS) trauma patient, the volume of distribution is further expanded (t_0 concentration = 17 µg/mL) by twofold over the normal patient, and the $t_{1/2}$ is reduced for the drug because of the hyperdynamic circulation and faster drug elimination. The time to the critical MIC is now less than 3 hours. Antibiotics in postresuscitated or infected trauma patients must have more aggressive drug dosing or more frequent drug administration.

hyperdynamic circulation. Larger doses of antibiotics that are given more frequently are the best way to assure adequate drug delivery in established infection. Expanded program of pharmacokinetic dosing of antibiotics in critically ill trauma patients needs to be considered in the future (Fig. 3).

- Shorter duration of antibiotics will be in the patient's best interest. If they have not responded in 7 days, then there is likely pus to drain or you must reevaluate the diagnosis or pathogen of concern.
- Diarrhea is *C. difficile* infection until proved otherwise. When diarrhea occurs in the critical care unit, do not use antiperistaltic agents. Antiperistaltic drugs promote toxic megacolon and colonic necrosis. The new hypervirulent strains of *C. difficile* produce large amounts of toxin rapidly and can lead to rapidly evolving disease (and toxic megacolon) even without diarrhea. With elderly critical care trauma patients and evolving abdominal distention, think of *C. difficile* infection.
- Disruption of the gut microecology is fundamental to infections with *C. difficile* and *Candida* spp. Discontinuation of other antibiotics not specifically used in the treatment of these two pathogens should be discontinued if possible. Furthermore, the gut is the likely reservoir for microbial translocation, endotoxin release, and cytokine dissemination from gut-associated lymph tissues that become drivers of the septic response and organ dysfunction.
- Beware of assigning postinjury fever and leukocytosis to urinary tract infection, especially in the well-drained urinary tract. There is commonly infection elsewhere.
- Documented bacteremia with *Staphylococcus* spp. is presumed to be from indwelling intravascular devices. All lines must be changed and intravenous antistaphylococcal

antibiotic therapy should be extended a full 14 days to avoid complications with endocarditis.

■ Although vancomycin has been effective in the treatment of infection with MRSA, it has been demonstrated to be suboptimal in the coverage of methicillin-sensitive *S. aureus* (MSSA) for both prevention and treatment. Early generation β-lactams remain appropriate choices (nafcillin, cefazolin) for MSSA.

■ Fever is a positive response of the host. In trauma patients, antipyretics may be a liability. Infection should be treated, not fever.

SUMMARY

Infection in the trauma patient will continue to be a challenge for the future. The last 40 years has witnessed an amazing change in the virulence characteristics of bacteria and in microbial resistance. It is likely that these trends will continue. Furthermore, progress in overall management has resulted in improved acute survival of patients who would have died in years past. Thus, more virulent and resistant bacteria will be encountered in severely immunosuppressed hosts.

What will be the changes in the management of these patients in the upcoming decades? Will antibiotic technology continue to produce new agents with activity against the new generation of pathogens? The numbers of new antibiotics for the treatment of gram-negative infections are few. No one would doubt that *S. aureus* will continue to develop new patterns of resistance and new virulence factors. Gram-negative resistance has progressed over the last 2 decades and shows no evidence of stopping. It is alarming to see the decline in the number of randomized trials of new antibiotics over the last decade. The antibiotic era may be coming to a close.

New treatments may focus upon antivirulence strategies to treat infection in the trauma patient. This may include antibody therapy to neutralize specific toxins, interference with adherence mechanisms, or genetic regulation of virulence genes. Manipulation of the ionic environment has been demonstrated to modulate microbial virulence and is yet another potentially new strategy. Perhaps probiotic therapy will neutralize microbial virulence by restoring the normal colonization of the host and letting competitive inhibition eliminate the pathogens. Until newer innovations are developed, the prevention and management of infection of the trauma patients will continue to be efforts to refine infection control practices, eliminate the pathogen when infection occurs, and enhance the host response.

For the chapter's Suggested Readings list, please visit the book at www.ExpertConsult.inkling.com.

NOSOCOMIAL PNEUMONIA

Paul M. Maggio and David A. Spain

Two broad classes of pneumonia are community-acquired pneumonia (CAP) and nosocomial pneumonia. Nosocomial pneumonia includes patients with hospital-acquired pneumonia (HAP), ventilator-associated pneumonia (VAP), and health care–associated pneumonia (HCAP). HAP is defined as pneumonia occurring more than 48 hours after hospital admission that was not incubating at the time of admission. If the infection develops after the patient has undergone intubation and mechanical ventilation for longer than 48 hours the condition is termed VAP. HCAP can occur inside or outside the hospital and refers to pneumonia in patients who are at high risk for multidrug-resistant (MDR) pathogens from prior health care exposure. VAP is a common and serious infections occurring in critically ill or injured surgical patients and is associated with a significant increase in hospital mortality rate and resource use (i.e., ventilator days, intensive care unit (ICU) length of stay, and costs). Thus, prevention is the best strategy.

INCIDENCE, MORBIDITY, AND MORTALITY

Pneumonia remains the most common nosocomial infection in the ICU and the leading cause of death due to a hospital-acquired infection. HAP accounts for 25% to 48% of all nosocomial infections and the mortality rate ranges from 20% to 50%. The incidence of VAP varies depending on risk factors, patient population, and the diagnostic approach. In the United States, the incidence of VAP ranges from 2.2 cases per 1000 mechanical ventilation days among medical ICU patients to 8.1 and 10.7 cases per 1000 mechanical ventilation days for patients in a trauma or burn ICU, respectively, where surgical procedures, multiple blood transfusions, spinal cord injury, and high device use influence the risk of infection. Mechanical ventilation remains the most significant risk factor for developing VAP and there is approximately a 1% cumulative associated risk of developing VAP per day of mechanical ventilation. The risk is greatest during the initial 5 days of mechanical ventilation (3% per day) and then it steadily decreases. Patients who develop HAP have higher mortality rate, have longer ICU and hospital stays, and incur higher costs. Nosocomial pneumonia increases the overall hospital stay by approximately 9 to 12 days, and for critically ill patients, it increases ICU stay by 4 to 6 days.

RISK FACTORS AND PREVENTIVE MEASURES

Modifiable and Nonmodifiable Risk Factors

Although the greatest risk factor for VAP is duration of mechanical ventilation, there are many other risk factors (Table 1). These are directly related to the pathogenesis of VAP. As the lower respiratory tract is sterile under basal conditions, the introduction of pathogens into the lungs and the impairment of traditional host defenses (both at the local and systemic levels) are necessary to cause infection. There is growing evidence that aspiration of pathogens colonizing or contaminating the oropharynx or gastrointestinal tract results in lower respiratory tract infection. Colonization of the endotracheal tube itself also may lead to alveolar infection during suctioning or bronchoscopy. Other less frequent sources include bacteremia and hematogenous spread or inhalation of infected aerosols.

Mechanical Ventilation

Mechanical ventilation is the single greatest risk factor for HAP and is associated with a 6- to 20-fold increase in the risk of lung infection. Intubation itself increases the risk of pneumonia because of its

TABLE 1: Risk Factors for Ventilator-Associated Pneumonia

Nonmodifiable	Modifiable
Age ≥60	Mechanical ventilation ≥3 days
Male gender	Self-extubation
History of COPD	Reintubation
Presence of	Tracheostomy
significant	Bronchoscopy
comorbid	Nasogastric tube
conditions	Endotracheal cuff pressure of 20 cm H_2O
Steroid use	Supine positioning
Admitting	Antacids or histamine type 2 antagonists
diagnosis of	Elevated gastric pH
burns	Aspiration
Admitting	Use of paralytic agents
diagnosis of	GCS score ≤9
trauma	Septic shock
Head trauma and	Hypoalbuminemia
other CNS	No prophylactic antibiotics administered in
disease	first 48 hours of ICU stay
Emergency or field	Patient transport out of ICU
intubation	Hemodialysis
Emergency surgery	Blood transfusions
	APACHE II score

APACHE, Acute Physiology and Chronic Health Evaluation; CNS, central nervous system; COPD, chronic obstructive pulmonary disease; GCS, Glasgow Coma Scale; ICU, intensive care unit.

potential for direct inoculation of pathogens into the lungs during the procedure. Therefore, intubation should be avoided when possible. Noninvasive positive-pressure ventilation to avoid intubation, when clinically feasible, may be a preferred alternative. A prospective study of noninvasive ventilation versus mechanical ventilation showed that, after adjusting for severity of illness, both the risk of VAP and nosocomial infections in general were reduced. Other invasive procedures such as tracheostomy, bronchoscopy, placement of a nasogastric (NG) tube, and chest tube thoracostomy also increase the risk. Thoracic trauma and chest operations lead to a disproportionately higher incidence of VAP.

In a trauma or surgical unit, the majority of patients are mechanically ventilated secondary to chest injury or postoperative respiratory failure. All efforts to decrease sedation and wean the patient postoperatively should be made. This is best accomplished by a daily assessment of sedation needs and an assessment for weaning and extubation. Numerous studies in a variety of patient populations have demonstrated that when this approach is incorporated into the care of patients, there is a significant reduction in time on the ventilator.

Oropharyngeal secretions that accumulate above the endotracheal cuff and subsequently leak into the lower respiratory tract are a potential source of infection. Specially designed endotracheal tubes are now available that allow in-line intermittent removal of secretions. A recent meta-analysis of five studies (896 patients) found that aspiration of subglottic secretions reduced the incidence of early-onset VAP by nearly half (risk ratio 0.51, 95% confidence interval [CI] 0.37 to 0.71) in patients expected to require 72 hours of mechanical ventilation. However, they appear to be less effective in preventing late-onset VAP; there is a risk of mucosal injury, and the suction lumen frequently occludes. As a result, the use of subglottic suction endotracheal tubes has been slow to enter clinical practice.

The ventilator circuit can also become contaminated from condensation and patient secretions and these should be removed

promptly to avoid aspiration and VAP. Routine ventilator circuit changes may promote aspiration and the risk of VAP and should only be made when the circuit is damaged or visibly soiled. The endotracheal tube cuff pressures should also be maintained at 20 cm H_2O to prevent tracking of bacterial pathogens around the cuff and into the lower respiratory tract. This should be monitored, as it is known that endotracheal cuff pressures of 25 cm H_2O or greater can cause decreases in tracheal mucosal blood flow and thus cause tracheal injury. There has also been the recent introduction of modified endotracheal tubes (e.g., silver-coated endotracheal tubes) to help fight infection. Although there are some early encouraging data, routine use has not been established.

Impaired Host Defenses

Markers of impaired host defenses, such as increased age, the presence of lung disease and other comorbid conditions including sepsis, steroid use, and a history of multiple blood transfusions, have been shown to be risk factors. Patients with these risk factors should be carefully monitored with all precautionary measures implemented to prevent pneumonia.

Oropharyngeal Colonization

Although the oropharynx is not normally colonized by enteric gram-negative bacteria, such colonization occurs in 75% of the ICU population within 48 hours of admission. Oropharyngeal colonization can be reduced by aggressive oral hygiene and the use of the oral antiseptic chlorhexidine. Oral inspections, tooth brushing, and mouth swabs should all be used on a regular basis. Multiple randomized trials have shown up to a 60% decrease in VAP in postoperative patients with the use of chlorhexidine, but most studies demonstrate a more modest reduction.

Aspiration

Factors that increase the risk of aspiration such as continuous sedation, a low Glasgow Coma Scale (GCS) score, use of paralytic agents, and the supine position have all been shown to increase the risk of VAP. All efforts should be made to reduce the aspiration of gastric and oropharyngeal contents. The supine position results in increased aspiration and VAP compared to the semirecumbent position. Therefore, patients should be semirecumbent with the head of the bed elevated to 30 to 45 degrees whenever possible. This is a simple, low-cost maneuver that significantly reduces the risk of VAP and should be implemented routinely. For patients with confirmed or suspected spine injuries, the reverse Trendelenburg position can be used. Continuous lateral rotation of ICU patients has also shown a protective effect and is another possibility but is more costly, as it requires a specialized bed. Transporting patients out of the ICU for procedures also increases the risk of VAP, potentially due to supine positioning during transportation. Thus, patients should be kept semirecumbent during transport whenever possible.

Although it was been postulated that enteral nutrition, due to aspiration, would result in increased VAP compared to parenteral nutrition, the evidence suggests the opposite. VAP is less common with enteral nutrition as long as the initial rate is kept modest for 48 to 72 hours (approximately half) and then increased to goal rate by 72 to 96 hours. Feeding in the semirecumbent position is preferable. Other data suggest a benefit to smaller nasogastric tubes as well as postpyloric or small intestine feeding. However, neither of those techniques has been proved to consistently decrease the risk of VAP.

Gastrointestinal Tract Bacterial Overgrowth

Antacids and histamine type 2 antagonists predispose the gastrointestinal tract to bacterial overgrowth and have been associated with increased risk of VAP, presumably due to aspiration. Although there have been controversial results on the effect of sucralfate on VAP, the latest large randomized trial showed that although sucralfate resulted in a significantly lower rate of VAP compared to ranitidine and antacids, it is associated with a higher incidence of gastrointestinal bleeding. Therefore, no method of stress ulcer prophylaxis is clearly superior.

Selective decontamination of the digestive tract (SDD) may be effective in reducing the incidence of VAP. It attempts to reduce oropharyngeal and gastric colonization with aerobic gram-negative bacilli and *Candida* species, without affecting anaerobic flora. Most regimens include a combination of an aminoglycoside, amphotericin B, or nystatin, and a nonabsorbable antibiotic such as polymyxin. Systemic antimicrobials are also added in many trials. Multiple randomized controlled trials have shown that SDD results in reduced incidence of VAP, decreased hospital mortality rate, and a decrease in MDR infections as well. However, these preventive effects were inversely related to study quality, and were much less pronounced in hospitals with high levels of antibiotic resistance. Finally, recent data suggest that prolonged use of SDD leads to an increase in bacterial resistance. Therefore, SDD is not recommended for routine use, particularly for patients with risk factors for resistant pathogens. It has been postulated that the intravenous antibiotic component of SDD is the main cause of improved survival. However, at this point, intravenous antibiotics are not currently recommended for prophylaxis.

Resistant Organisms

There has recently been an increase in the incidence of VAP caused by resistant organisms. Methicillin-resistant *Staphylococcus aureus* (MRSA), in particular, is now responsible for 15% to 27% of VAP. Risk factors for infection with one of these pathogens include a recent history of antibiotic use, hospitalization of 5 days or more, admission from an allied health facility, immunosuppressive disease or therapy, presence of a severe, chronic comorbid condition, and a high frequency of antibiotic resistance in that particular hospital or community. Another recent study also showed that aspiration, emergency intubation, and a GCS score of 9 or less are specific risk factors for early-onset VAP that is caused by resistant organisms.

Putting All Risk Factors Together

A probability of VAP following trauma can be calculated using the formula:

$$\text{probability of VAP}\ (P_{VAP}) = e^{f(x)} / \left(1 + e^{f(x)}\right)$$

where f(x) = –3.08 – 1.56 (mechanism of injury, penetrating = 1, blunt = 0) – 0.12 (GCS score) + 1.37 (spinal cord injury where yes = 1, no = 0) + 0.30 (chest abbreviated injury score) + 1.87 (emergency laparotomy where yes = 1, no = 0) + 0.67 (units of blood transfused in the resuscitation room) + 0.05 (Injury Severity Score) + 0.66 (intubation in either the field or the resuscitation room, where yes = 1, no = 0). This formula was 95% accurate in predicting subsequent development of VAP.

General Prophylaxis

Maximizing hand hygiene protocols and barrier precautions is crucial in preventing the spread of nosocomial infections. Compliance with hand hygiene protocols has improved with the introduction of alcohol foams and gels. These products have improved efficacy and take substantially less time to use compared to thorough handwashing. Health care personnel should use these products before and after any contact with patients who are being mechanically ventilated. Gowns and gloves should also be used appropriately in any situation in which contamination with respiratory secretions or other bodily fluids is possible.

Effectiveness of Preventive Measures—"Bundles"

There is increasing evidence that routine use of protocols or bundles aimed at preventing VAP may be successful. A bundle is a method of improving patient care using a set of evidence-based practices that when performed collectively have been proved to improve patient outcomes. One institution showed that the prevalence rate of VAP decreased by 51% after an educational session emphasizing positioning (head of bed elevated 30 degrees or more), appropriate use of sedation, routine oral hygiene, and management of respiratory devices. As VAP routinely results in increased hospital stays and therefore cost, this program was very cost effective and the estimated savings were over $400,000.

DIAGNOSIS

Pneumonia is suspected when a patient develops new or progressive radiographic lung infiltrates (Fig. 1), along with a clinical scenario of pulmonary infection (i.e., fever, leukocytosis, purulent sputum, respiratory distress, and a worsening of oxygenation) (Table 2). Of note, in patients diagnosed with acute respiratory distress syndrome (ARDS), the suspicion of pneumonia should be especially high. Several studies have noted a higher incidence of pneumonia in patients with ARDS. For example, one study showed a pneumonia rate of 55% in patients with ARDS compared to 28% in those without. Another study noted a 60% incidence of pneumonia in patients with severe ARDS (PaO_2/FIO_2 ratio less than 150 mm Hg).

Diagnostic Strategies

Gram stain of sputum suctioned from the endotracheal tube plays little role in the diagnosis or treatment of suspected pneumonia in trauma patients. Ventilated trauma ICU patients often have

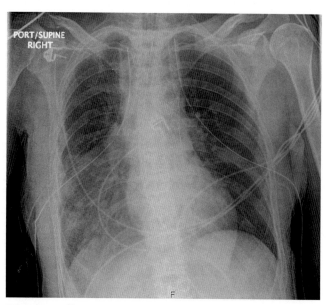

FIGURE 1 Chest radiograph with right lower lobe consolidation.

TABLE 2: Centers for Disease Control and Prevention Criteria for Defining Hospital-Acquired Pneumonia

Radiology	Signs/Symptoms	Laboratory
Two or more serial chest radiographs with at least one of the following: New or progressive and persistent infiltrate Consolidation Cavitation Pneumatoceles, in infants <1 year old *Note:* In patients without underlying pulmonary or cardiac disease (e.g., respiratory distress syndrome, bronchopulmonary dysplasia, pulmonary edema, or chronic obstructive pulmonary disease), one definitive chest radiograph is acceptable.	*At least one of the following:* Fever (>38 °C or >100.4 °F) with no other recognized cause Leukopenia (<4000 WBCs/mm^3) or leukocytosis (>12,000 WBCs/mm^3) For adults ≥70 years old, altered mental status with no other recognized cause *and* *At least one of the following:* New onset of purulent sputum, or change in character of sputum or increased respiratory secretions, or increased suctioning requirements New onset or worsening cough, or dyspnea, or tachypnea Rales or bronchial breath sounds Worsening gas exchange (e.g., O$_2$ desaturations [e.g., Pao$_2$/Fio$_2$ ratio <240], increased oxygen requirements, or increased ventilation demand)	*At least one of the following:* Positive blood culture not related to another source of infection Positive growth in pleural fluid culture Positive quantitative culture from minimally contaminated specimen (e.g., BAL or PSB) ≥5% BAL-obtained cells contain intracellular bacteria on direct microscopic examination (e.g., Gram stain) *Histopathologic examination shows at least one of the following evidences of pneumonia:* Abscess formation or foci of consolidation with intense PMN accumulation in bronchioles and alveoli Positive quantitative culture of lung parenchyma Evidence of lung parenchyma invasion by fungal hyphae or pseudohyphae

BAL, Bronchoalveolar lavage; PMN, polymorphonuclear leukocytes; PSB, protected specimen brush; WBC, white blood cell.

radiographic infiltrates, fever, and thick respiratory secretions in the absence of pneumonia. The presence of organisms on Gram stain is unreliable, both in diagnosing pneumonia and in identifying the causative organism. To assess the diagnostic efficacy of clinical criteria alone for VAP, one study reviewed 25 patients who died while on mechanical ventilation and used lung histologic findings plus quantitative lung culture as the standard for pneumonia. The presence of radiographic chest infiltrates plus two of three clinical criteria (leukocytosis, purulent secretions, fever) had a sensitivity of 69% and a specificity of 75%. Thus, it is important to obtain sputum cultures to confirm the diagnosis of VAP; additionally, identifying the causative organism(s) aids in selecting appropriate antibiotics.

The use of obtaining a sputum culture was illustrated in a study of 43 trauma patients undergoing mechanical ventilation and demonstrating symptoms of pneumonia, namely fever, leukocytosis, purulent sputum, and changing radiographic infiltrates. Of this group, 20 had positive cultures with greater than or equal to 10^5 colony-forming units (CFUs) per milliliter. Antibiotics were discontinued in the other 23 patients, and 65% showed improvement after stopping the antibiotics. Overall, there was no difference in mortality rate between the two groups.

Methods of Obtaining Sputum Cultures

Samples for sputum culture may be obtained noninvasively, via tracheal aspiration, or invasively with bronchoscopy and either bronchoalveolar lavage (BAL) or a protected specimen brush (PSB). Positive tracheal cultures may reflect simple tracheal colonization and overestimate the rate of pneumonia. Invasive cultures are more accurate in diagnosing pneumonia. In one multicenter randomized trial, those receiving invasive bronchoscopic management had a lower mortality rate at day 14, but not at day 28, and lower mean sepsis-related organ failure assessment scores on days 3 and 7. At 28 days, the invasive management group had significantly more antibiotic-free days (11 ± 6 vs. 7 ± 7). A multivariate analysis showed a significant difference in mortality rate (hazard ratio 1.54, 95% CI 1.10 to 2.16). Both BAL and PSB have sensitivities and specificities greater than 80%. Studies have shown that these two techniques yield similar results (Table 3). Most studies involving BAL have used 10^4 or 10^5 CFUs/mL as the threshold for a positive culture. The presence of intracellular organisms can be detected by Gram stain and is particularly useful as it provides a rapid result with high predictive value (see Table 3). If bronchoscopic sampling is not immediately available, nonbronchoscopic techniques can reliably obtain lower respiratory

TABLE 3: Quantitative Cultures and Microscopic Examination of Lower Respiratory Tract Secretions in Diagnosis of Ventilator-Associated Pneumonia

Diagnostic Techniques	Sensitivity (%)	Specificity (%)	Positive Predictive Value (%)	Negative Predictive Value (%)
PSB cultures (>10^3 CFUs/mL)	82	89	90	89
BAL cultures (>10^4 CFUs/mL)	91	78	83	87
Microscopic examination of BAL fluid (>5% intracellular organisms)	91	89	91	89

BAL, Bronchoalveolar lavage; CFUs, colony-forming units; PSB, protected specimen brush.

tract quantitative cultures. Blinded bronchial sampling, mini-BAL, and blinded PSB involve blindly wedging a catheter into a distal bronchus and obtaining a sample. Sensitivities and specificities of these techniques are similar to those involving fiberoptic bronchoscopy. Bronchial sampling techniques aside, when there is a high suspicion of pneumonia, or the patient is clinically unstable or septic, antibiotic therapy should be initiated promptly regardless of whether bacteria is detected from the distal respiratory tract.

Value of Clinical Pulmonary Infection Score in Trauma Patients

The clinical pulmonary infection score (CPIS) is an attempt to optimize a noninvasive diagnostic approach by pooling several clinical indicators of pneumonia (Table 4). A CPIS greater than 6 has been shown to be highly suggestive of pneumonia and correlates with a high concentration of bacteria from invasive cultures. The main criticisms of the CPIS are that all elements are weighted equally even though some are stronger predictors of pneumonia and some elements are necessarily subjective, such as the interpretation of chest radiographs. Furthermore, most of the components of the CPIS may be altered by trauma, and therefore simply reflect the systemic inflammatory response syndrome (SIRS). A recent study of trauma patients found the average CPIS to be 6.9 in those with VAP confirmed by BAL versus 6.8 in those with a negative BAL. The sensitivity

and specificity of a CPIS greater than 6 to diagnose VAP were only 61% and 43%, respectively.

MANAGEMENT

Adequate Initial Antibiotics

Effective treatment for nosocomial pneumonia depends on the rapid institution of appropriate antimicrobial therapy. Mortality rate almost doubles when the initial choice of antibiotics is inadequate. The initial antibiotic coverage must be sufficiently broad to cover the most likely organisms. Patients receiving appropriate initial antibiotics, but with a delay of more than 24 hours from time of meeting diagnostic criteria, had a VAP-attributable mortality rate of 39% compared to 11% in those receiving timely antibiotics.

Hospitalization for 5 days or longer and recent antibiotic or health care exposures are common risk factors for developing MDR pneumonia (Table 5). After determining the likelihood of antibiotic resistance, an appropriate initial therapy is selected. If the likelihood of antibiotic resistance is low, there are several potential choices (Table 6). If the patient has risk factors for MDR pneumonia, initial antibiotics should include coverage for gram-negative organisms and MRSA. The necessity of double coverage for gram-negative organisms is controversial and evidence of synergy has been inconsistent. One potential advantage of double coverage is simply to increase the odds that at least one of the drugs will have activity against the suspected MDR organism. For MRSA coverage, it is important to remember that vancomycin has relatively poor lung penetration, and serum drug levels should be monitored to ensure adequate dosage. Daptomycin binds avidly to pulmonary surfactant, and therefore cannot be used in the treatment of pneumonia. Linezolid is another option, and two retrospective analyses comparing vancomycin to linezolid in treating MRSA nosocomial pneumonia showed improved survival and clinical cure rates with linezolid therapy (Table 7).

Appropriate and rapid initiation of broad-spectrum antibiotics against the most likely causative organism(s) is vital for good clinical treatment of VAP. For any clinical scenario, there are numerous antibiotic regimens that would be a sufficient first choice. Hospital-specific or even ICU-specific patterns of antibiotic resistance are particularly useful in guiding antibiotic decisions.

TABLE 4: Calculation of Clinical Pulmonary Infection Score

Variable	Finding	Points
Temperature (°C)	>36.5 and ≤38.4	0
	>38.5 and ≤38.9	1
	>39 or <36	2
Blood leukocytes (n/mm³)	>4000 and ≤11,000	0
	≤4000 or >11,000	1
	Plus band forms >50%	Add 1
Tracheal secretions	Absent	0
	Nonpurulent secretions present	1
	Purulent secretions present	2
Oxygenation (Pao_2/Fio_2)	≥240 or ARDS*	0
	<240 and no ARDS	2
Pulmonary radiography	No infiltrate	0
	Diffuse (or patchy) infiltrate	1
	Localized infiltrate	2
Progression of pulmonary infiltrates	No radiographic progression	0
	Radiographic progression (after CHF and ARDS excluded)	2
Culture of tracheal aspirate	Pathogenic bacteria cultured in very low to low quantity or not at all	0
		1
	Pathogenic bacteria cultured in moderate or high quantity	Add 1
	Same pathogenic bacteria seen on Gram stain	

ARDS, Acute respiratory distress syndrome; CHF, congestive heart failure; Fio_2, fraction of inspired oxygen; Pao_2, arterial oxygen tension; PAWP, pulmonary arterial wedge pressure.
*Defined as Pao_2/Fio_2 ratio ≥200 and pulmonary arterial wedge pressure ≥18 mm Hg, with acute bilateral infiltrates.

TABLE 5: Risk Factors for Multidrug-Resistant Pathogens Causing Hospital-Acquired Pneumonia and Ventilator-Associated Pneumonia

Antimicrobial therapy in preceding 90 days

Current hospitalization of 5 days or more

High frequency of antibiotic resistance in community or the specific hospital unit

Recent health care exposure

Hospitalization for 2 days or more in the preceding 90 days

Residence in a nursing home or extended care facility

Home infusion therapy (including antibiotics)

Chronic dialysis within 30 days

Home wound care

Family member with multidrug-resistant pathogen

Immunosuppressive disease and/or therapy

TABLE 6: Initial Empiric Antibiotic Therapy for Hospital-Acquired Pneumonia or Ventilator-Associated Pneumonia in Patients with No Known Risk Factors for Multidrug-Resistant Pathogens

Potential Pathogens	Recommended Initial Antibiotics
Streptococcus pneumonia	Ceftriaxone
Haemophilus influenzae	*or*
Methicillin-sensitive *Staphylococcus aureus* (MSSA)	Levofloxacin or Moxifloxacin
Enteric gram-negative bacilli	*or* Ampicillin/sulbactam
Escherichia coli	*or* Ertapenem
Klebsiella pneumoniae	
Enterobacter sp.	
Proteus sp.	
Serratia marcescens	

Impact of Prior Antibiotic Use on Diagnosis and Treatment

Prior antibiotic therapy can impair the ability to obtain accurate culture results. The key factor appears to be the duration of antibiotics. Initiation of antibiotic therapy within the preceding 24 hours decreases the chances of obtaining a positive sputum culture, although this impact is less pronounced for BAL than other methods. However, in patients receiving antibiotics for longer than 72 hours, the sensitivity and specificity of BAL and PSB are essentially unaffected. Thus, these modalities are still useful for diagnosing pneumonia in those patients in the midst of a course of antibiotics. They can also help identify treatment failures in patients who remain critically ill despite apparent adequate antibiotic coverage.

Deescalation of Antibiotics

Although starting broad-spectrum antibiotics for VAP is necessary to ensure adequate coverage, it is inappropriate to routinely continue these agents for the duration of therapy. Sputum culture from the lower respiratory tract should be obtained at the time of diagnosis. The results should be used to tailor antibiotic therapy based upon the sensitivities when available (36 to 48 hours). All final decisions should be based culture results. The question remains, however, how to manage antibiotics when the cultures are negative. These patients are often categorized into two groups: those with clinical improvement on therapy and those with deterioration or lack of improvement. In the former group, you are likely treating some other infection you are yet to diagnose. In the latter, regardless of the cause, the treatment is inadequate. In either case, a diligent search should be made for another source of sepsis. If none is found, then the antibiotic should be discontinued and the patient reassessed clinically in 24 to 36 hours.

Duration of Therapy

To help determine the optimal duration of therapy, a prospective, randomized trial assessed 401 patients with VAP. Antibiotics were

TABLE 7: Initial Empiric Therapy for Hospital-Acquired Pneumonia and Ventilator-Associated Pneumonia in Patients with Late-Onset Disease or Risk Factors for Multidrug-Resistant Pathogens

Potential Pathogens	Combination Antibiotic Therapy
Pathogens listed in Table 6 and multidrug-resistant (MDR) pathogens	Antipseudomonal cephalosporin (cefepime, ceftazidime)
Pseudomonas aeruginosa	*or*
Klebsiella pneumoniae extended-spectrum β-lactamase (ESBL+)*	Antipseudomonal carbepenem (imipenem or meropenem)
	or
Acinetobacter species*	β-Lactam/β-lactamase inhibitor (piperacillin–tazobactam)
	plus
	Antipseudomonal fluoroquinolone (ciprofloxacin or levofloxacin)
	or
	Aminoglycoside (amikacin, gentamicin, or tobramycin)
	plus
Methicillin-resistant *Staphylococcus aureus* (MRSA)	Linezolid or vancomycin
Legionella pneumophila†	

*If an ESBL+ strain, such as *Klebsiella pneumoniae*, or an *Acinetobacter* species is suspected, a carbepenem is a reliable choice.
†If *Legionella pneumophila* is suspected, the combination antibiotic regimen should include a macrolide (e.g., azithromycin) or a fluoroquinolone (e.g., ciprofloxacin or levofloxacin) should be used rather than an aminoglycoside.

discontinued at either 8 or 15 days of therapy, regardless of the patient's condition, except in the situation of a documented pneumonia recurrence. The two groups had similar results regarding ventilator-free days, length of stay, and 60-day mortality rate. The only apparent disadvantage to the shorter course of therapy was a higher recurrence rate in those with nonfermenting gram-negative bacilli (e.g., *Pseudomonas aeruginosa*). Otherwise, pneumonia recurrence rates were similar between the two groups. For most patients, treatment should be 8 days.

Antibiotic Therapy Protocol

When a critically ill or injured patient is suspected of having VAP:

1. Broad-spectrum antibiotic coverage should be initiated when the diagnosis is suspected. Antibiotic(s) choice should be driven mainly by patient characteristics (time in hospital, prior antibiotic exposure) and unit-specific antibiotic resistance patterns. The principle is to have sufficient, initial antibiotic coverage against the most likely organisms.

2. Sputum sample for culture should be obtained from the lower respiratory tract as soon as possible after the diagnosis is suspected (essentially coincident with initiation of antibiotics). A variety of techniques can be used but the hallmark is a specimen from the deep respiratory tract.
3. Cultures results should be checked at 36 to 48 hours and antibiotic coverage tailored (deescalated) to the causative organism(s).
4. For most patients, treatment should be 8 days. Patients with nonfermenting gram-negative bacilli (e.g., *Pseudomonas aeruginosa*) should be considered for 15 days of treatment.

Antibiotic Prophylaxis and Tube Thoracostomy

The Eastern Association for the Surgery of Trauma (EAST) practice group has recommended 24 hours of therapy with a first-generation cephalosporin after tube thoracostomy. The calculated number needed to treat to prevent a pulmonary infection is six. As chest tube placement is a known risk factor for VAP, such treatment may well decrease the incidence of VAP as well as empyema and should be practiced on a regular basis.

For the chapter's Suggested Readings list, please visit the book at www.ExpertConsult.inkling.com.

ANTIBIOTIC USE IN THE INTENSIVE CARE UNIT: THE OLD AND THE NEW

Philip S. Barie

Not only are surgeons involved with infections that require invasive measures for treatment (e.g., complicated intra-abdominal infections [cIAIs] and complicated skin/soft tissue infections [cSSTIs]), but surgical patients are particularly vulnerable to nosocomial infections. Therefore, the surgeon must be concerned with the prevention and treatment of all infections that affect surgical patients, including surgical site infections (SSIs), central line–associated bloodstream infections (CLABSIs), urinary tract infections (UTIs), and hospital-acquired pneumonia or ventilator-associated pneumonia (HAP/VAP). Trauma patients are particularly vulnerable to infections of injured tissue as well as nosocomial infections related to environmental factors (e.g., hypothermia), host immunosuppression (e.g., inadequate glycemic control), and therapeutic interventions (e.g., multiple incisions and catheters, blood transfusion).

Recognizing and minimizing risk goes hand in hand with an aggressive approach to diagnosis and treatment. Infection is preventable to some degree, and every acute care surgeon must do his or her utmost toward prevention. An ensemble of tactics is required, because no single method, including antibiotic prophylaxis, is effective itself. Infection control is paramount. Surgical illness and injury are immunosuppressive, as are many critical care therapies. Surgical incisions and traumatic wounds must be handled gently, inspected daily, and dressed if necessary using strict asepsis. Drains and catheters must be avoided if possible, and removed as soon as practicable. Prophylactic and therapeutic antibiotics, whether empiric or directed against a known infection, must be used optimally so as to minimize antibiotic selection pressure on the development of multidrug-resistant (MDR) pathogens.

PHARMACOKINETICS AND PHARMACODYNAMICS

Pharmacokinetics (PK) describes the principles of drug absorption, distribution, and metabolism. Dose-response relationships are influenced by dose, dosing interval, and route of administration. Plasma and tissue drug concentrations are influenced by absorption, distribution, and elimination, which in turn depend on drug metabolism and excretion. Relationships between local drug concentration and effect are described by pharmacodynamic (PD) principles (see following discussion).

Bioavailability, the percentage of drug dose that reaches the systemic circulation after oral administration, is affected by absorption, intestinal transit time, and hepatic metabolism. *Half-life* ($t_{1/2}$), the time required for the serum drug concentration to reduce by one half, reflects both *clearance* and *volume of distribution* (VD). The VD is used to estimate the plasma drug concentration achievable from a given dose. VD varies substantially according to pathophysiology; reduced VD may cause a higher plasma drug concentration for a given dose, whereas fluid overload and hypoalbuminemia (which decrease drug binding) increase VD, making dosing more complex.

Clearance refers to the volume of fluid from which drug is eliminated completely per unit of time, regardless of the mode of elimination (e.g., metabolism, excretion, or dialysis); knowledge of drug clearance is important to determine the dose of drug necessary to maintain a steady-state concentration (Fig. 1). Most drugs are metabolized by the liver to polar compounds for eventual renal excretion, which may occur by filtration or either active or passive transport. In general, if 40% or more of active drug (including active metabolites) is eliminated unchanged in the urine, a dosage adjustment is required if renal function is decreased.

Pharmacodynamics are unique for antibiotic therapy, because drug-patient, drug-microbe, and microbe-patient interactions must be accounted for. Microbial physiology, inoculum characteristics (i.e., size, quorum sensing, presence of a device-related biofilm), microbial growth phase, mechanisms of resistance, the microenvironment (e.g., local pH), and the host's response must be considered. Because of microbial resistance, mere administration of the "correct" drug may not be microbicidal if an adequate dose/concentration is not achieved. in vitro results may be irrelevant if bacteria are inhibited only by drug concentrations that cannot be achieved clinically.

Antibiotic PD parameters determined by laboratory analysis include *the minimal inhibitory concentration* (MIC), the lowest serum drug concentration that inhibits bacterial growth (MIC_{90} refers to 90% inhibition) (Fig. 2). However, some antibiotics may suppress bacterial growth at subinhibitory concentrations (*postantibiotic effect*, PAE). Sophisticated analytic strategies use both PK and PD, for example, by determination of the peak serum concentration/MIC ratio, the duration of time (fT) that plasma concentration remains above the MIC (fT > MIC), and the area of the plasma concentration-time curve above the MIC (the *area under the curve*, or AUC) (Fig. 3). Accordingly, aminoglycosides exhibit concentration-dependent killing, whereas β-lactam agents exhibit efficacy determined by time above the MIC. For β-lactam antibiotics with short $t_{1/2}$, it may be efficacious to administer by continuous infusion, although prolonged

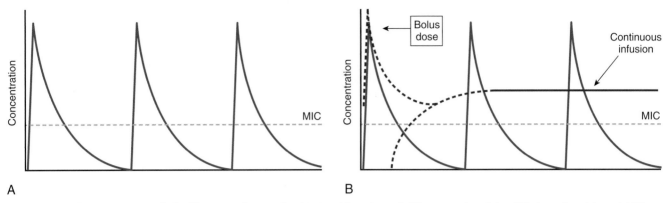

A

B

FIGURE 1 **A,** Elimination curve of bolus 30-minute infusions of antibiotic at 6-hour intervals. The proportion of time (fT) above the minimum inhibitory concentration (MIC) must be at least 40% for bactericidal activity in most cases. If the MIC is low, this can be achieved with conventional dosing, but not for organisms with higher MICs. **B,** Continuous infusion of antibiotic after an initial loading dose (whether bolus or not; *dotted lines*) is depicted. Not only is the fT/MIC ratio higher, but the antibiotic becomes effective against organisms with higher MICs, depending on the rate of continuous infusion. Lower total daily doses of antibiotic may be used against bacteria with low MICs. For drugs that exhibit time-dependent bactericidal activity (e.g., β-lactams), this is the ideal mode of administration, provided vascular access is sufficient.

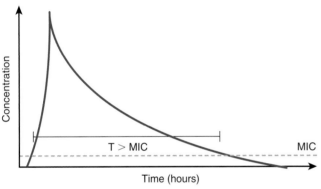

FIGURE 2 An elimination curve is shown for a single bolus dose of a parenteral antibiotic. Some drugs (e.g., aminoglycosides) exhibit concentration-dependent bactericidal activity; a peak concentration/minimum inhibitory concentration (MIC) ratio greater than 10 is optimal for bacterial killing. β-Lactam agents exhibit time-dependent bactericidal activity; the proportion of time above the MIC should be at least 40% for optimal killing. Efficacy of still other drugs (e.g., vancomycin, fluoroquinolones) is reflected by the area under the concentration curve (AUC), a method of measurement of the bioavailability of a drug based on a plot of blood concentrations sampled at frequent intervals. The AUC is directly proportional to the total amount of unaltered drug in the patient's blood. A ratio of AUC/MIC greater than 125 is associated with optimal antibacterial effect and minimization of the development of resistance.

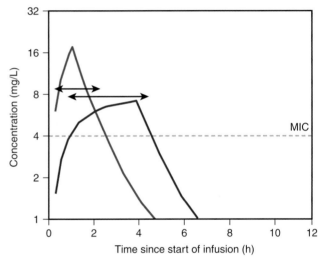

FIGURE 3 A concentional bolus dose of antibiotic with a 30-minute infusion and a 6-hour dosing interval is compared with the same drug given as a 4-hour infusion over the same dosing interval. The fT/MIC (minimum inhibitory concentration) ratio is doubled (compare the lengths of the *short* and *long double arrows*), but organisms with higher MICs can still be treated. The interruption allows the intravenous line to be used for fluid or other medication during the hiatus, without compromising bactericidal action.

intermittent infusion may accomplish the same while freeing up vascular access for other medications. Some agents (e.g., fluoroquinolones, vancomycin) exhibit both properties; bacterial killing increases as drug concentration increases up to a saturation point, after which the effect becomes concentration-independent. A 24-hour AUC/MIC ratio greater than 125 is associated with optimal effect.

ANTIBIOTIC PROPHYLAXIS

Prophylactic antibiotics are used most often to prevent SSIs, for which the benefit is demonstrated. However, if not administered properly, antibiotic prophylaxis is ineffective and may even be harmful. Antibiotic prophylaxis does not prevent postoperative nosocomial infections, which actually occur at an increased rate after prolonged prophylaxis, selecting for more resistant pathogens when infection does develop.

Four principles guide the administration of antimicrobial agent for prophylaxis: (1) safety; (2) an appropriate narrow spectrum of coverage of relevant pathogens; (3) little or no therapeutic use; and (4) timely administration prior to incision and for a defined, brief period of time thereafter (no more than 24 hours [48 hours for cardiac surgery]; ideally, a single dose). The optimal time for administration is within 1 hour prior to incision. Agents given sooner, or after the incision is closed, are ineffective. Antibiotics with a short $t_{1/2}$ (more than 2 hours, e.g., cefazolin or cefoxitin) should be redosed every 3 (cefoxitin) or 4 hours (cefazolin) during prolonged or bloody operations.

Most SSIs are caused by gram-positive cocci, and therefore, prophylaxis should be directed primarily against staphylococci for clean cases and high-risk clean-contaminated upper abdominal surgery. A first-generation cephalosporin is preferred in most circumstances, with clindamycin used for penicillin-allergic patients. If gram-negative or anaerobic coverage is required (e.g., penetrating abdominal trauma), cefoxitin or cefazolin plus metronidazole are the regimens of first choice. Vancomycin prophylaxis is generally not recommended, except in institutions where the incidence of methicillin-resistant *Staphylococcus aureus* (MRSA) infection is high (more than 20% of all SSIs caused by MRSA).

Skin closure of a contaminated or dirty incision increases the risk of SSI, but few good studies evaluate the multiplicity of wound closure techniques used by surgeons. "Open abdomen" techniques of temporary abdominal closure for management of trauma or severe peritonitis are used increasingly. Antibiotic prophylaxis of the open abdomen is not indicated, although an inability to achieve primary abdominal closure is associated with several nosocomial infections (pneumonia, bloodstream infection, and SSI) and substantially increased cost from prolonged length of stay, but not higher mortality rate.

For trauma, antibiotic prophylaxis may be required for operative management or prevention of infection of traumatic wounds. Moreover, many surgical procedures performed for trauma are likely to be in a contaminated field (e.g., penetrating trauma, open reduction/internal fixation of open fractures). The evidence is robust for penetrating abdominal trauma, for which no more than 24 hours of prophylaxis with a second-generation cephalosporin (or equivalent) is recommended, even for colon injury. Likewise, although most traumatic wounds are contaminated somewhat, and the likelihood of infection increases when contamination is greater, prolonged antibiotic prophylaxis is not indicated.

PRINCIPLES OF ANTIBIOTIC THERAPY

Antimicrobial therapy is a mainstay of the treatment of infections, but widespread overuse and misuse of antibiotics have led to an alarming increase in MDR pathogens (Table 1). New agents and innovative ways to administer existing antibiotics may allow shorter courses of therapy, which is desirable for cost savings and microbial ecology. Effective therapy with no toxicity requires a careful but expeditious search for the source of infection and an understanding of the principles of PK (see previous discussion).

Evaluation of Possible Infection

Fever is usually the trigger for an evaluation for the presence of infection (hence, "fever workup"). However, some infected patients (e.g., elderly patients; those with open abdominal wounds, end-stage liver disease, or chronic kidney disease; and patients taking anti-inflammatory or antipyretic drugs) do not manifest fever and may be even be hypothermic. Absent a fever, any sign of hypotension, tachycardia, tachypnea, confusion, rigors, skin lesions, hypoxemia, oliguria, lactic acidosis, leukocytosis, leukopenia, immature neutrophils (i.e., bands greater than 10%), or thrombocytopenia may indicate the need for an evaluation for infection and immediate empiric therapy. Moreover, fever in the early postoperative period (before postoperative day 4) often has a noninfectious cause and hence does not equate with infection (Table 2). In addition, noninfectious and infectious causes of fever may coexist, and an infected patient may harbor more than one discrete focus of infection.

Antibiotics should not be given until evaluation has occurred, including the collection of specimens for culture. Therefore, evaluation must be expeditious, as delay in antibiotic administration is associated with an increased risk of death. Inspection of all incisions is mandatory. If an incision is opened and cultured, a deep culture specimen should be collected rather than swabbing the open wound superficially or collecting fluid from drains (the likelihood of colonization is high). A chest radiograph is optional for evaluation of postoperative fever unless mechanical ventilation, physical examination, abnormal blood gases, or pulmonary secretions suggest a high yield. Urinalysis/urine culture is not mandatory in the early postoperative period unless there is reason by history or examination to suspect a UTI. However, on or after postoperative day 4, nosocomial infection becomes much more likely; evaluation should be comprehensive, and the threshold for empiric therapy decreased.

Empiric Antibiotic Therapy

Empiric antibiotic therapy must be administered judiciously and expeditiously. Injudicious therapy could result in undertreatment of established infection, or unnecessary therapy in the setting of sterile

TABLE 1: Causes and Consequences of Bacterial Resistance as Related to Antibiotic Selection

Initial Therapeutic Agent	Emergent Resistant Bacteria	Treatment of Resistant Bacteria
Fluoroquinolones	MRSA	Vancomycin, others
	MDR gram-negative bacilli*	Carbapenem or polymyxin or tigecycline (not for *Pseudomonas*)
	Clostridium difficile	Vancomycin or metronidazole or fidaxomycin
Vancomycin, daptomycin	VRE	Tigecycline, linezolid
	VISA	Ceftaroline, tigecycline, linezolid, daptomycin
Cephalosporins, daptomycin	VRE	Tigecycline, linezolid
	MDR gram-negative bacilli*	Carbapenem or polymyxin or tigecycline (not for *Pseudomonas*)
	C. difficile	Vancomycin or metronidazole or fidaxomycin
Carbapenems	MDR gram-negative bacilli*	Carbapenem or polymyxin or tigecycline (not for *Pseudomonas*)
	Stenotrophomonas maltophilia	Trimethoprim/sulfamethoxazole
	C. difficile	Vancomycin or metronidazole or fidaxomycin

MDR, Multi-drug resistant; MRSA, methicillin-resistant *Staphylococcus aureus*; VISA, vancomycin-intermediate *Staphylococcus aureus*; VRE, vancomycin-resistant *Enterococcus*.
*MDR gram-negative bacilli include producers of extended-spectrum β-lactamases, metallo-β-lactamases, and carbapenemases.

TABLE 2: Miscellaneous Causes of Fever Related to Noninfectious States

Acalculous cholecystitis

Acute myocardial infarction

Acute respiratory distress syndrome (fibroproliferative phase)

Adrenal insufficiency

Cytokine release syndrome

Fat embolism

Gout

Hematoma

Heterotopic ossification

Immune reconstitution inflammatory syndrome (IRIS)

Infarction of any tissue

Intracranial hemorrhage (trauma or vascular cause)

Myocardial infarction

Pancreatitis

Pericarditis

Pulmonary infarction

Stroke

Thyroid storm

Transfusion of blood or blood products

Transplant rejection

Tumor lysis syndrome

Venous thromboembolic disease

Withdrawal syndromes (e.g., drug, alcohol)

TABLE 3: Factors Influencing Antibiotic Choice

Activity against known/suspected pathogens

Disease believed responsible

Distinguish infection from colonization

Narrow-spectrum coverage most desirable

Antimicrobial resistance patterns

Patient-specific factors

Location prior to presentation: home vs. health care facility

Recent prior antibiotic therapy

Severity of illness

Age

Immunosuppression

Organ dysfunction

Allergy

Institutional guidelines/restrictions: institutional preapproval required

Agent on formulary

Logistics: onset, dose, and dosing interval; single or multiple agents

Duration of infusion and course of therapy

TABLE 4: Antibacterial Agents for Empiric Use

Antipseudomonal Agents

Piperacillin-tazobactam

Cefepime, ceftazidime

Imipenem-cilastatin, meropenem, doripenem

Ciprofloxacin, levofloxacin (depending on local susceptibility patterns)

Aminoglycoside

Polymyxins (polymyxin B, colistin [polymyxin E])

Targeted-Spectrum Agents

Gram-Positive Organisms

Glycopeptide (e.g., vancomycin, telavancin)

Lipopeptide (e.g., daptomycin; not for known/suspected pneumonia)

Oxazolidinone (e.g., linezolid)

Gram-Negative Organisms

Third-generation cephalosporin (not ceftriaxone)

Monobactam

Polymyxins (polymyxin B, colistin [polymyxin E])

inflammation or bacterial colonization; either may be deleterious. Inappropriate therapy (e.g., delay more than 1 hour, therapy misdirected against usual pathogens, failure to treat MDR pathogens) leads unequivocally to increased mortality rate.

Antibiotic choice is based on several interrelated factors (Table 3). Paramount is activity against identified or likely (for empiric therapy) pathogens, presuming infecting and colonizing organisms can be distinguished, and that narrow-spectrum coverage is always desired. Important factors include the disease process believed responsible; whether the infection is health care–associated or community- or hospital-acquired; and whether MDR organisms are present, or likely to be. Local knowledge of antimicrobial resistance patterns is essential. Patient-specific factors of importance include age, debility, intrinsic organ function, immunosuppression, prior allergy or other adverse reaction, and recent antibiotic therapy. Institutional factors of importance include guidelines, formulary availability, outbreaks of infections caused by MDR pathogens, and antibiotic control programs.

Choice of Antibiotic

Numerous agents are available for therapy (Table 4). Agents may be chosen based on spectrum, whether broad or targeted (e.g.,

TABLE 4: Antibacterial Agents for Empiric Use—Cont'd

Broad-Spectrum Agents

Piperacillin-tazobactam

Carbapenems

Fluoroquinolones (depending on local susceptibility patterns)

Tigecycline (plus an antipseudomonal agent)

Trimethoprim-sulfamethoxazole (used primarily for CA-MRSA, *Stenotrophomonas*)

Antianaerobic Agents

Metronidazole

Carbapenems

β-Lactam/β-lactamase combination agents

Tigecycline

Anti-MRSA Agents

Ceftaroline

Daptomycin (not for use against pneumonia)

Minocycline

Linezolid

Telavancin

Tigecycline (not in pregnancy or for children under age 8 years)

Vancomycin

CA-MRSA, Community-associated MRSA; MRSA, methicillin-resistant *Staphylococcus aureus*.

antipseudomonal, antianaerobic), in addition to the previous factors. If a nosocomial gram-positive pathogen is suspected (e.g., wound or SSI, CLABSI, HAP/VAP) or MRSA is endemic, empiric vancomycin (or linezolid) is appropriate. Some authorities recceommend dual-agent therapy for serious *Pseudomonas* infections (i.e., an antipseudomonal β-lactam drug plus an aminoglycoside), but evidence of efficacy is mixed. Regardless of the choice that is made, initial empiric therapy of any infection caused potentially by either a gram-positive or gram-negative bacterium (e.g., HAP/VAP, hospital-acquired intra-abdominal infection) must include activity against all likely pathogens.

Optimization of Therapy

Conventional antibiotic dosing may not apply to the critically ill or injured patient. Higher doses may be required for MDR isolates, increased extracellular volume, decreased serum albumin concentration, or increased glomerular filtration rate (e.g., burns, traumatic brain injury, multiple trauma). Underdosing of antibiotics is a major factor for the development of resistance during therapy and failure thereof. By contrast, lower doses may be required with multiple organ dysfunction syndrome, acute kidney injury, and chronic kidney disease. Dosing of vancomycin and aminoglycosides may be monitored via measurement of drug concentrations in serum.

Continuous or prolonged infusion of β-lactam agents may be the optimal way to administer these drugs. Lengthened fT that is greater than MIC is achieved, increasing the likelihood of therapeutic success, especially against organisms with higher MICs, and minimizing the development of resistance. Prolonged infusions may accomplish the same without monopolizing an intravenous line. Continuous-infusion vancomycin has been described but is not recommended currently.

Vancomycin has been a mainstay of therapy of infections of critically ill patients, but MICs for vancomycin against MRSA have been increasing, even within the susceptible range. As a result, MIC cut-points for resistance of *S. aureus* have been revised downward to minimize the chance of ineffective therapy, and higher doses of vancomycin are recommended, although at a greater risk of nephrotoxicity. The use of vancomycin therapy in patients with MRSA infections caused by isolates with MICs between 1 and 2 mg/mL should be undertaken with caution. Adequate therapeutic conncetrations may not be achievable for *S. aureus* isolates with MICs greater than 2 µg/mL, so alternative therapy should be considered. Linezolid retains generally excellent activity, but resistance to daptomycin is being reported.

Aminoglycoside therapy is resurgent owing to limited options for treatment of MDR pathogens that have resulted from the increasing prevalence of extended-spectrum β-lactamase (ESBL)-producing strains and the emergence of carbapenemases, although use as part of an empiric therapy regimen remains debated. Single daily-dose aminoglycoside therapy ensures that a peak serum concentration/MIC ratio greater than 10 will be achieved to optimize therapy. A dose of gentamicin or tobramycin (7 mg/kg) or amikacin (20 mg/kg) is administered and a trough concentration is determined at 23 hours after dose (some protocols call for an intermediate determination as well, at ~16 hours after dose, so that the elimination curve can be determined with greater precision). A trough concentration of 0.5 to 2 µg/mL is sought for gentamicin or tobramycin, whereas a trough concentration of 5 to 10 µg/mL is ideal for amikacin. Outcomes are comparable or better compared with conventional dosing, with decreased toxicity. Single daily-dose aminoglycoside therapy has not been validated for children, during pregnancy, with burns, in patients older than age 70, or with treatment of bacterial endocarditis.

Infections caused by highly resistant ("panresistant") gram-negative bacilli pose a major problem. Carbapenems, tigecycline, and polymyxins (see later) retain useful activity against ESBL-producing organisms. MDR nonfermenting gram-negative bacilli (e.g., *Pseudomonas aeruginosa*, *Acinetobacter* spp., *Stenotrophomonas* spp.) and carbapenemase-producing Enterobacteriaceae may require therapy with a polymyxin, high-dose carbapenem by prolonged infusion, or unusual combinations of agents that have demonistrated synergy in vitro but remain of uncertain clinical use.

Duration of Therapy

The end point of antibiotic therapy is largely undefined, because quality data are few. If cultures are negative, empiric antibiotic therapy should be stopped in most cases after no more than 48 to 72 hours. Unnecessary antibiotic therapy increases the risk of MDR infection; therefore, prolonged therapy with negative cultures is usually unjustifiable. The morbidity of antibiotic therapy also includes allergic reactions; development of nosocomial superinfections (e.g., fungal, enterococcal, and *Clostridium difficile*-related infections); organ toxicity; reduced yield from subsequent cultures; and vitamin K deficiency with coagulopathy or accentuation of warfarin effect.

If infection is evident, treatment is continued as indicated clinically, but the microbiology data should be examined to see if the antibiotic regimen can be deescalated to a narrower regimen (e.g., choosing a narrower-spectrum agent, changing multidrug therapy to monotherapy). If empiric therapy has been appropriate, escalation of therapy (e.g., choosing a more broad-spectrum agent, changing monotherapy to multidrug therapy, adding antifungal therapy) should be seldom needed.

Every decision to start antibiotics must be accompanied by an *a priori* decision regarding duration of therapy. A reason to continue therapy beyond the predetermined end point must be compelling. Bacterial killing is rapid in response to effective agents, but the host response may not subside immediately. Therefore, the clinical response of the patient should not be the sole determinant. There is increasing belief that shorter courses of antibiotic therapy that were used previously are equally effective with fewer side effects, and that therapy should continue to a predetermined end point, after which it should be stopped.

Procalcitonin has been evaluated extensively (11 randomized prospective trials) as a biomarker to guide duration of therapy (to initiate therapy [three trials], to end therapy [four trials], and as a guide to both [four trials]). Without exception, clinical outcomes were unchanged (nine trials) or length of stay was reduced (two trials). Also without exception, procalcitonin monitoring was antibiotic-sparing, reducing prescriptions of antibiotics by 32% to 72% in three trials, and duration of therapy by 1.7 to 7.1 days in eight trials.

There are few data and no guidelines for the clinical approach to the patient who has failed a course of antibacterial therapy. There is not even a clear definition of what constitutes failure. Has the patient failed if the systemic inflammatory response persists after 3 days, or 5, or 7? When should antibiotics be changed? Is the antibiotic therapy well chosen, but the patient has inadequate source control and requires operation (or reoperation)? If a patient still has systemic inflammatory response syndrome (SIRS) at the predetermined end point, it is more useful to stop therapy and reevaluate for persistent or new infection, MDR pathogens, and noninfectious causes of SIRS than to continue therapy uninformed or to add or change antibiotics without additional data?

SPECTRA OF ANTIBIOTIC ACTIVITY

Susceptibility testing of specific organisms is necessary for management of serious infections (including all nosocomial infections). This chapter will focus on the agents most useful for the treatment of serious/nosocomial infections; not every agent within the class will receive mention. Recommended agents for specific organisms are given as guidelines only, because in vitro susceptibilities may not correlate with clinical efficacy.

Cell Wall–Active Agents

β-Lactam Antibiotics

The β-lactam antibiotic group consists of penicillins, cephalosporins, monobactams, and carbapenems. Within this group, several agents have been combined with β-lactamase inhibitors to broaden the spectrum of activity. Several subgroups of antibiotics are recognized within the group, notably penicillinase-resistant penicillins and several "generations" of cephalosporins.

Penicillins

Penicillinase-resistant semisynthetic penicillins include methicillin, nafcillin, and oxacillin. These agents are the treatments of choice for sensitive strains of staphylococci, but not as empiric agents, because of high rates of MRSA. Virtually all enterococcal species are resistant.

Except for carboxypenicillins and ureidopenicillins, penicillins retain little or no activity against gram-negative bacilli. Carboxypenicillins (ticarcillin and carbenicillin) and ureidopenicillins (azlocillin, mezlocillin, and piperacillin; sometimes referred to as acylampicillins) are no longer used without a β-lactamase inhibitor in combination (BLIC) such as, tazobactam, clavulanic acid, sulbactam), which enhances the effectiveness of the parent β-lactam agent (piperacillin > ticarcillin > ampicillin) and to a lesser extent the inhibitor (tazobactam > sulbactam ∼ clavulanic acid). Piperacillin-tazobactam has the widest spectrum of activity against gram-negative bacteria, and

reasonable potency against *P. aeruginosa*. Ampicillin-sulbactam is unreliable against *Escherichia coli* and *Klebsiella* (resistance rate ∼50%), but it has some activity against *Acinetobacter* spp. owing to the sulbactam moiety. All of the BLIC agents have excellent antianaerobic activity.

Cephalosporins

The 20+ agents of the class vary widely; thus, the clinician should have broad familiarity with all of these drugs. First- and second-generation agents are useful only for prophylaxis, for uncomplicated infections, or for deescalation when results of susceptibility testing are known. "Third-generation" agents have enhanced activity against gram-negative bacilli (some have specific antipseudomonal activity), but only ceftriaxone is active against gram-positive cocci (but not MRSA), and none are effective against anaerobes. Cefepime, a "fourth-generation" cephalosporin, has antipseudomonal activity and activity against most gram-positive cocci, but not MRSA. Ceftaroline (usual dose, 600 mg intravenously every 12 hours) has not been classified, but has anti-MRSA activity unique among the cephalosporins while retaining modest activity comparable to first-generation agents against gram-negative bacilli. None of the cephalosporins are useful against enterococci. Third-generation cephalosporins, particularly ceftazidime, have been associated with the induction of ESBL production among many of the Enterobacteriaceae.

The potential of cefepime for induction of ESBL production is less than that of ceftazidime, but it, too, has no activity against either enterococci or enteric anaerobes. Cefepime is intrinsically more resistant to hydrolysis by β-lactamases, but not enough to be reliable against ESBL-producing bacteria.

Monobactams

Aztreonam, the single agent of this class, has activity against gram-negative bacilli comparable to that of the third-generation cephalosporins, but no activity against gram-positive organisms or anaerobes. Aztreonam is not a potent inducer of β-lactamases. Resistance to aztreonam is widespread, but the drug remains useful for directed therapy against susceptible strains, and for penicillin-allergic patients because the incidence of cross-reactivity is low.

Carbapenems

Imipenem-cilastatin, meropenem, doripenem, and ertapenem are available in the United States. Imipenem-cilastatin, meropenem, and doripenem have the widest (and generally comparable) antibacterial spectrum of any antibiotics, with excellent activity against aerobic and anaerobic streptococci, methicillin-sensitive staphylococci, and virtually all gram-negative bacilli except *Acinetobacter* spp., *Legionella* spp., *Pseudomonas cepacia*, and *Stenotrophomonas maltophilia*. All carbapenems are effective antianaerobic agents, and thus, there is no reason to combine a carbapenem with metronidazole. Meropenem and doripenem have less neurotoxicity than imipenem-cilastatin, which is contraindicated in patients with active central nervous system disease or injury (excepting the spinal cord), because of the rare (∼0.5%) appearance of myoclonus or generalized seizures in patients who have received high doses (with normal renal function) or inadequate dosage reductions with renal insufficiency. Ertapenem is not useful against *Pseudomonas* spp., *Acinetobacter* spp., *Enterobacter* spp., or MRSA, but its long $t_{1/2}$ permits once-daily dosing. Ertapenem is active against ESBL-producing Enterobacteriaceae and has low potential for neurotoxicity. With all carbapenems, disruption of the host microbiome may lead to superinfection (e.g., fungi, *C. difficile*, *S. maltophilia*, resistant *Enterococcus* spp.).

Lipoglycopeptides

Vancomycin, a soluble lipoglycopeptide, is bactericidal, but tissue penetration is poor, which limits its effectiveness (Table 5). Both

TABLE 5: Situations in Which Use of Vancomycin Is Discouraged

Routine surgical prophylaxis in the absence of life-threatening allergy to β-lactam antibiotics

Empiric therapy of febrile neutropenia in the absence of evidence for a gram-positive infection

Continued empiric use when microbiologic data suggest a reasonable alternative

Systemic or local (i.e., catheter flush) prophylaxis of indwelling vascular catheters

Selective decontamination of the digestive tract

Eradication of colonization of methicillin-resistant staphylococci

Primary treatment of antibiotic-associated colitis due to *Clostridium difficile*

Routine prophylaxis for patients on hemodialysis or continuous ambulatory peritoneal dialysis

Use for topical irrigation or application

S. aureus and *Staphylococcus epidermidis* are usually susceptible to vancomycin, although MICs for *S. aureus* are increasing, requiring higher doses for effect, and leading to rates of clinical failure that exceed 50% in some reports. *Streptococcus pyogenes*, group B streptococci, *S. pneumoniae* (including penicillin-resistant *S. pneumoniae* [PRSP]), and *C. difficile* are susceptible. Most strains of *Enterococcus faecalis* are inhibited (but not killed) by attainable concentrations, but *Enterococcus faecium* is increasingly resistant to vancomycin.

Telavancin, a synthetic vancomycin derivative, is approved only for treatment of cSSTI. Telavancin exhibits a dual mechanism of action, including cell membrane disruption and inhibition of cell wall synthesis. The drug is active against MRSA, susceptible and penicillin-resistant pneumococci, and vancomycin-susceptible enterococci with MICs less than 1 μg/mL. The most common side effects are taste disturbance, nausea, vomiting, and headache. There may be a small increased risk of acute kidney injury. The usual dose is 10 mg/kg, infused intravenously over 60 minutes, every 24 hours for 7 to 14 days; dosage reductions are necessary in renal insufficiency. No information is available regarding dosing during renal replacement therapy.

Cyclic Lipopeptides

Daptomycin has potent, rapid bactericidal activity against most gram-positive organisms. The mechanism of action is via rapid membrane depolarization; potassium efflux; arrest of DNA, RNA, and protein synthesis; and cell death. Daptomycin exhibits concentration-dependent killing and has a long $t_{1/2}$ (8 hours). The recommended dose is 4 mg/kg for cSSTI, versus 6 mg/kg/day for bacteremia. The dosing interval should be increased to 48 hours when creatinine clearance is less than 30 mL/minute. Daptomycin is active against most aerobic and anaerobic gram-positive bacteria, including *Peptostreptococcus* spp., *Clostridium perfringens*, and *C. difficile* and MDR strains such as MRSA, methicillin-resistant *Staphylococcus epidermidis* (MRSE), and vancomycin-resistant enterococci (VRE). Resistance to daptomycin has been reported for both MRSA and VRE. Importantly, daptomycin must not be used for the treatment of pneumonia or empiric therapy when pneumonia is in the differential diagnosis, even when caused by a susceptible organism, because daptomycin penetrates lung tissue poorly and is inactivated by pulmonary surfactant.

Polymyxins

Polymyxins are cyclic, cationic peptides that have fatty acid residues; polymyxins B and E (polymixin E=colistimethate or colistin) are used clinically. Polymyxins bind to the anionic bacterial outer membrane, leading to a detergent effect that disrupts membrane integrity. High affinity binding to the lipid A moiety of lipopolysaccharide may have a endotoxin-neutralizing effect. Commercial preparations of polymyxin B are standardized, but those of colistimethate (the less toxic prodrug of colistin that is administered clinically) are not, so dosing depends on which preparation is being supplied. Most recent reports describe colistimethate use, but the drugs are therapeutically equivalent.

Dosing of polymyxin B is 1.5 to 2.5 mg/kg (15,000 to 25,000 U/kg) daily in divided doses, whereas dosing of colistimethate (polymyxin E) ranges from 2.5 to 6 mg/kg/day, also in divided doses. The diluent is voluminous, adding substantially to daily fluid intake. Excellent activity persists despite the widespread emergence of MDR pathogens. Data on PK are scant, but the drugs exhibit rapid concentration-dependent bacterial killing against a wide variety of gram-negative bacilli, including most isolates of *E. coli*, *Klebsiella* spp., *Enterobacter* spp., *P. aeruginosa*, *S. maltophilia*, and *Acinetobacter* spp. Combination of either polymyxin plus rifampin exhibits synergistic activity in vitro. Tissue uptake is poor, but administration intrathecally and by inhalation are possible.

Polymyxins fell out of favor originally due to nephro- and neurotoxicity, but the emergence of MDR pathogens has restored their use. The incidence of acute kidney injury is 40% for colistimethate-treated patients and 5% to 15% for polymyxin B. Neurotoxicity (5% to 7% for both) usually becomes manifest as muscle weakness or polyneuropathy.

Protein Synthesis Inhibitors

Aminoglycosides

Aminoglycoside use is resurgent owing to development of resistance to newer antibiotics (especially third-generation cephalosporins and fluoroquinolones). Gentamicin, tobramycin, and amikacin remain in use. Aminoglycosides bind to the bacterial 30S ribosomal subunit, inhibiting protein synthesis. Gentamicin has modest activity against gram-positive cocci; otherwise, the spectrum of activity of the agents is nearly identical. Prescribing decisions should be based upon toxicity and local resistance patterns. Owing to potential toxicity, aminoglycosides are used seldom for first-line therapy, except synergistically to treat a serious *P. aeruginosa* infection, enterococcal endocarditis, or an infection caused by a MDR gram-negative bacillus. Aminoglycosides are less active against *Acinetobacter*, and limited against *P. cepacia*, *Aeromonas* spp., and *S. maltophilia*.

Aminoglycosides kill bacteria most effectively with a concentration peak/MIC greater than 10, therefore a loading dose is necessary and serum drug concentration monitoring is performed. Marked dosage reductions are necessary in renal insufficiency, but the drugs are dialyzed and a maintenance dose should be given after each hemodialysis treatment.

Tetracyclines

Tetracyclines bind irreversibly to the 30S ribosomal subunit, but they are bacteriostatic only. Widespread resistance limits their use in the hospital setting (with the exceptions of doxycycline, minocycline, and tigecycline [intravenously only]). Tetracyclines are active against anaerobes; *Actinomyces* can be treated successfully. All tetracyclines are contraindicated in pregnancy and for children under the age of 8 years, owing to dental toxicity.

Tigecycline is a novel glycylcycline derived from minocycline. With the exceptions of *Pseudomonas* spp. and *P. mirabilis*, the spectrum of activity is broad, including many MDR gram-positive and gram-negative bacteria, including MRSA, VRE, ESBL-producing strains, and *Acinetobacter* spp. Antianaerobic activity is excellent.

Concern has been raised recently by a post hoc analysis that the mortality rate of tigecycline-treated patients is higher in pooled phase 3 and 4 clinical trials, including unpublished registration trials. The adjusted risk difference for all-cause mortality rate based on a random effects model stratified by trial weight was 0.6% (95% confidence interval [CI] 0.1–1.2) between tigecycline and comparator agents, but trials were included for which the drug is not indicated. An independent meta-analysis found no such survival disadvantage in an analysis of eight published randomized controlled trials (4651 patients). Overall, no difference was identified for the pooled clinically (odds ratio [OR] 0.92, 95% CI 0.76–1.12) or microbiologically evaluable populations (OR 0.86, 95% CI 0.69–1.07) from the trials.

Oxazolidinones

Linezolid, the only member of the class available commercially, binds to the ribosomal 50S subunit, preventing complexing with the 30S subunit, thereby preventing translation of mRNA and blocking assembly of the functional initiation complex for protein synthesis. Linezolid is bacteriostatic against susceptible organisms (pneumococci excepted). With minor exceptions, gram-negative bacteria are linezolid-resistant because the drug is excreted from bacterial cells by efflux pumps.

Linezolid is active against MRSA, vancomycin-susceptible and -resistant enterococci, and penicillin-susceptible and -resistant pneumococci. *Bacteroides* spp. are susceptible. Linezolid requires no dosage reduction in renal insufficiency and exhibits excellent tissue penetration. Meta-analysis suggests that linezolid is equivalent to vancomycin for HAP/VAP, but some clinicians believe that linezolid should supplant vancomycin as first-line therapy for serious infections caused by gram-positive cocci.

The Macrolide-Lincosamide-Streptogramin Family

Clindamycin

The only lincosamide in active use in surgical practice is clindamycin, which also binds to the 50S ribosome. Clindamycin has modest antianaerobic activity and reasonably good activity against susceptible gram-positive cocci (not MRSA or VRE). Clindamycin inhibits exotoxin production in vitro and has been advocated preferentially to penicillin as first-line therapy of invasive *S. pyogenes* infections. Clindamycin is used occasionally for anaerobic infections and is preferred over vancomycin for prophylaxis of clean surgical cases in penicillin-allergic patients.

Drugs That Disrupt Nucleic Acids

Fluoroquinolones

Fluoroquinolones inhibit bacterial DNA synthesis by inhibiting DNA gyrase, which folds DNA into a superhelix prior to replication. Fluoroquinolones exhibit excellent oral bioavailability, a diminishihg spectrum of activity, and numerous toxicities (e.g., photosensitivity, cartilage [especially in children] and tendon damage, prolongation of the QTc interval). These agents have a marked propensity to induce resistance. Ciprofloxacin, levofloxacin, and moxifloxacin (which has some antianaerobic activity) are available parenterally and orally.

Fluoroquinolones are modestly active against enteric gram-negative bacteria, particularly the Enterobacteriaceae and *Hemophilus* spp. There is some activity against *P. aeruginosa*, *S. maltophilia*, and gram-negative cocci. Activity against sensitive gram-positive cocci is variable, being least for ciprofloxacin and best for moxifloxacin.

However, rampant overuse of fluoroquinolones is rapidly causing resistance that has diminished their usefulness, including *E. coli*, *Klebsiella* spp., *P. aeruginosa*, and MRSA. Fluoroquinolones prolong the QTc interval and may precipitate the ventricular dysrhythmia *torsades de pointes*, so electrocardiographic measurement of the QTc interval before and during fluoroquinolone therapy is important. Also, fluoroquinolones interact with warfarin to cause a rapid, marked prolongation of the international normalized ratio (INR), so warfarin anticoagulation must be monitored closely during therapy.

Cytotoxic Antibiotics

Metronidazole

Metronidazole has potent bactericidal activity against nearly all anaerobes, and many protozoa that parasitize human beings, although it is ineffective in actinomycosis. Resistance remains rare and of negligible clinical importance. Metronidazole causes DNA damage after intracellular reduction of the nitro group of the drug. The drug penetrates well nearly all tissues, including neural tissue, making it effective for deep-seated infections and bacteria that are not multiplying rapidly. Absorption after oral or rectal administration is rapid and nearly complete. The $t_{1/2}$ of metronidazole is 8 hours, owing to an active hydroxy metabolite. Intravenous metronidazole is usually administered every 8 to 12 hours, but once-daily dosing is possible. No dosage reduction is required for renal insufficiency, but the drug is dialyzed effectively and administration should be timed to follow dialysis. In marked hepatic insufficiency, a dosage reduction of 50% is suggested.

Trimethoprim-Sulfamethoxazole

Sulfonamides exert bacteriostatic activity by interfering with bacterial folic acid synthesis, necessary for DNA synthesis. Resistance is widespread, limiting use. The addition of sulfamethoxazole to trimethoprim, which prevents the conversion of dihydrofolic acid to tetrahydrofolic acid by the action of dihydrofolate reductase, accentuates the activity of trimethoprim.

The combination of *trimethoprim-sulfamethoxazole* (TMP-SMX) is active against *S. aureus*, *S. pyogenes*, *S. pneumoniae*, *E. coli*, *P. mirabilis*, *Salmonella* and *Shigella* spp., *Yersinia enterocolitica*, *S. maltophilia*, *Listeria monocytogenes*, and *Pneumocystis jirovecii*. The drug is a treatment of choice for infections caused by *S. maltophilia*, and outpatient (and sometimes inpatient) treatment of infections caused by CA-MRSA (community-associated MRSA).

A fixed-dose combination of TMP-SMX in a ratio of 1:5 is available for parenteral administration. The standard oral formulation is 80 mg/400 mg, but lesser and greater strength tablets are available. Oral absorption is rapid and bioavailability is nearly 100%. Tissue penetration is excellent. Ten milliliters of the parenteral formulation contains 160 mg/800 mg drug. Full doses (150 to 300 mg TMP in three or four divided doses) may be given if creatinine clearance is more than 30 mL/minute, but the drug is not recommended when the creatinine clearance is less than 15 mL/minute.

ANTIBIOTIC TOXICITIES

β-Lactam Allergy

Allergic reaction is the most common toxicity of β-lactam antibiotics. The incidence is approximately 7 to 40/1000 treatment courses of penicillin, and is more likely with parenteral therapy. Most serious reactions occur in patients with no history. Patients with a prior reaction have a four- to sixfold increased risk of another reaction compared to the general population, but the risk decreases with time, from 80% to 90% skin test reactivity at 2 months to 20% reactivity at 10 years. The risk of cross-reactivity between penicillins and other β-lactams (carbapenems and cephalosporins) is approximately 5%, being highest for first-generation cephalosporins. There is negligible cross-reactivity to monobactams.

Red Man Syndrome

Tingling and flushing of the face, neck, or thorax may occur with parenteral vancomycin therapy, but is less common than fever, rigors, or local phlebitis. *Red man syndrome* is believed to be mediated by histamine release due to local hyperosmolality. Red man syndrome has a clear association with too-rapid infusion of vancomycin (less than1 hour for a 1 g dose, or less than 1.5 to 2 hours for a larger dose) and is not a true allergy. Too-rapid infusion can also cause hypotension. A maculopapular rash due to hypersensitivity occurs in about 5% of patients.

Nephrotoxicity

All aminoglycosides are nephrotoxic, with little to distinguish among them. Aminoglycosides do not provoke inflammation, and thus there is no allergic component to any manifestation of aminoglycoside toxicity. Toxicity is mediated by ischemia of the renal proximal tubular cell. Kidney injury manifests as a reduction of the glomerular filtration rate and decreased creatinine clearance, but is usually reversible; a need for renal replacement therapy is rare. Factors that may accentuate aminoglycoside nephrotoxicity are frequent dosing, older age, sodium or volume depletion, acidemia, hypokalemia, hypomagnesemia, and coexistent liver disease. The risk is ameliorated by single daily-dose therapy. If renal function deteriorates, it is advisable to discontinue therapy unless treatment is for a life-threatening infection.

Vancomycin nephrotoxicity is on the increase, owing to higher dosing and concurrent administration of other nephrotoxins. Nephrotoxicity of polymyxins may be unavoidable; the need to use an agent with known nephrotoxic potential to treat serious infections caused by MDR gram-negative bacilli exists when alternatives are few or none.

Ototoxicity

Aminoglycosides cause cochlear or vestibular toxicity that is usually irreversible and may develop after the cessation of therapy. Repeated exposures create cumulative risk. Most patients develop either cochlear toxicity or a vestibular lesion, but rarely both. Cochlear toxicity can be subtle, because few patients have baseline audiograms, and fewer still undergo formal screening. Few patients complain of hearing loss, yet when sought, the incidence of cochlear toxicity may be more than 60%. Clinical hearing loss may occur in 5% to 15% of patients. Ototoxicity due to vancomycin is most common when coadministered with another ototoxin (e.g., aminoglycoside, furosemide). There is no correlation between ototoxicity and nephrotoxicity for drugs that cause either (e.g., aminoglycosides, vancomycin).

Avoiding Toxicity: Adjustment of Antibiotic Dosage

Hepatic Insufficiency

The liver metabolizes and eliminates drugs that are too lipophilic for renal excretion. The cytochromes P-450 (a gene superfamily consisting of more than 300 different enzymes) oxidize lipophilic compounds to water-soluble products. Oxidation is disrupted in particular when liver function is impaired. Other enzymes mediate

TABLE 6: Antimicrobials Requiring Dosage Reduction in Hepatic Disease

Aztreonam
Cefoperazone
Chloramphenicol
Clindamycin
Erythromycin
Isoniazid
Metronidazole
Nafcillin
Quinupristin/dalfopristin
Rifampin
Tigecycline

conjugation with sugars, amino acids, sulfate, or acetate to facilitate biliary or renal excretion,

Drug dosing in hepatic insufficiency is complicated by insensitive clinical assessments of liver function (Table 6), and changing metabolism as the degree of impairment fluctuates (e.g., resolving cholestasis). Changes in renal function with progressive hepatic impairment add considerable complexity. The effect of liver disease on drug disposition is thus difficult to predict for individual patients. Generally, a dosage reduction of up to 25% of the usual dose is considered if hepatic metabolism is 40% or less and renal function is normal. Greater dosage reductions (up to 50%) are advisable if the drug is administered chronically, there is a narrow therapeutic index, protein binding is significantly reduced, or the drug is excreted renally and renal function is severely impaired.

Renal Insufficiency

Renal drug elimination depends on glomerular filtration, tubular secretion, and reabsorption, any of which may be altered with renal dysfunction. Kidney disease or acute kidney injury may affect hepatic as well as renal drug metabolic pathways. Drugs whose hepatic metabolism is likely to be disrupted in renal insufficiency include aztreonam, penicillins, several cephalosporins, macrolides, and carbapenems (Table 7).

Accurate estimates of renal function are important in patients with mild-to-moderate renal dysfunction, because the clearance of many drugs by renal replacement therapy actually makes management easier. Factors influencing drug clearance by hemofiltration include molecular size, aqueous solubility, plasma protein binding, equilibration kinetics between plasma and tissue, and the apparent V_D. The need to dose patients during or after a renal replacement therapy treatment must be borne in mind (Table 8); during continuous renal replacement therapy, the estimated creatinine clearance is approximately 15 to 25 mL/minute in addition to the patient's intrinsic clearance. For sustained low-efficiency dialysis (SLED) clearance rates of 60 to 100 mL/minute may be achieved. Cefaclor, cefoperazone, ceftriaxone, chloramphenicol, clindamycin, cloxacillin and dicloxacillin, doxycycline, erythromycin, linezolid, methicillin/nafcillin/oxacillin, metronidazole, rifampin, and tigecycline do not require dosage reductions in renal failure. Prolonged infusion of β-lactam agents is not precluded.

For the chapter's Suggested Readings list, please visit the book at www.ExpertConsult.inkling.com.

TABLE 7: Dosage Reductions for Selected Antimicrobials in Renal Insufficiency

Drug (Usual Dose)	Dose for Ccr 10–50 mL/min	Dose for Ccr < 10 mL/min	Dialyzed?
Aminoglycosides	Individualize	Individualize	Yes
Ampicillin (1–2 g q4h)	0.5–1 g q6h	0.5–1 g q12h	Yes
Aztreonam (1 g q8h)	0.5 g q8h	0.5 g q12h	HD only
Cefamandole (1–2 g q6h)	1–2 g q8–12 h	1–2 g q8–24 h	HD/CAVHD
Cefazolin (1 g q8h)	1 g q12–24 h	1 g q48h	HD only
Cefepime (2 g q12h)	1 g q12h	1 g q24h	Yes
Cefotaxime (1 g q6h)	1 g q8–12 h	1 g q24h	HD only
Cefotetan (1 g q12h)	1 g q24h	0.5–1 g q24h	No
Cefoxitin (1–2 g q6h)	1–2 g q8–12 h	1–2 g q24h	HD/CAVHD
Ceftazidime (1 g q8h)	1 g q24h	1 g q48h	Yes
Ceftizoxime (1 g q8h)	1 g q12–24 h	1 g q48h	HD only
Ciprofloxacin (0.4 g q8–12 h)	0.4 g q8h	0.4 g q16h	No
Imipenem/ cilastatin (0.5 g q6h)	0.25–0.5 g q6–8 h	0.25–0.5 g q12h	HD only
Levofloxacin (0.5–0.75 g q12h)	0.5 g q24h	0.5 g q24h	CAVHD only
Piperacillin (2–4 g q4h)	2–4 g q6h	2–3 g q8h	HD/CAVHD
Vancomycin (1 g q12h)	Individualize	Individualize	High-flux HD only

CAVHD, Continuous arteriovenous or venovenous hemodialysis; Ccr, creatinine clearance; HD, hemodialysis; PD, peritoneal dialysis; q, every.
Notes: Formula for estimation of creatinine clearance (Ccr): $(140 - age \times [1.00 \text{ (male) or } 0.85 \text{ (female)}] \times weight \text{ [kg]})$. Ccr (mL/min) = serum Cr concentration (mg/dL) $\times 72$.

TABLE 8: Dosing of Selected Parenteral Antibiotics Applied After Dialysis

Antibiotic	Dose
Amikacin	2.5–3.75 mg/kg
Ampicillin	1 g
Azlocillin	3 g
Aztreonam	0.125 g
Cefamandole	0.5–1 g
Cefepime	0.5 g
Cefoxitin	1 g
Ceftazidime	1 g
Ceftizoxime	1–3 g
Cefuroxime	0.75 g
Chloramphenicol	1 g
Gentamicin	1.0–1.7 mg/kg
Imipenem/cilastatin	0.25–0.5 g
Meropenem	0.5 g
Mezlocillin	2–3 g
Netilmicin	2 mg/kg
Piperacillin	2 g
Piperacillin/ tazobactam	2.25 g
Ticarcillin	3 g
Ticarcillin/clavulanic acid	3.1 g
Tobramycin	1.0–1.7 mg/kg
Trimethoprim/ sulfamethoxazole	5 mg/kg trimethoprim
Vancomycin	0.5 g if using polysulfone dialysis membrane; otherwise no supplement

FUNGAL COLONIZATION AND INFECTION DURING CRITICAL ILLNESS

Marc J. Shapiro, Eduardo Smith-Singares, Soumitra R. Eachempati, Jared M. Huston, and Philip S. Barie

KEY POINTS

- Fungal infections are an increasing cause of nosocomial infections in patients, in particular those residing in the intensive care unit (ICU).
- Risk factors for developing fungal infections include diabetes mellitus, immunosuppression, previous antibiotic use, prolonged ICU length of stay, malignancy, parenteral nutrition, neutropenia, and prolonged central line catheterization.
- Although *Candida albicans* is the most common fungus infection seen, other mycoses including other *Candida* subspecies such as *Candida glabrata* and *Candida krusei* and other mycoses such as *Aspergillus* create challenges as to identification and early appropriate treatment.
- There are a number of classes of antifungal agents available. Being familiar with their sensitivities and resistance is crucial to selecting the proper agent(s).

HISTORY AND PREVALENCE

Invasive mycoses have emerged as a major cause of morbidity and mortality in hospitalized surgical patients. It is estimated that the incidence of nosocomial candidemia in the United States is about 8 per 100,000 inhabitants and imposes an excess in health care cost of approximately $1 billion per year. Medical costs per candidemia episode have been estimated at $34,123 per Medicare patient and $44,536 per private insurance patient. In the United States, *Candida* is the fourth most common cause of catheter-related infection, and a recent prospective, observational study reported the incidence of fungemia in the surgical intensive care unit (SICU) at nearly 10 cases per 10,000 admissions with unadjusted mortality rates in these patients of 25% to 50%. Fungemia is the fourth most common type of septicemia in the United States, and every year about 20 new opportunistic pathogenic species of fungi are discovered. Outside the United States, several studies have reported a rise in candidemia and other forms of *Candida* infections. In the EPIC II (Extended Prevalence of Infection in Intensive Care) study of 7087 infected ICU patients in 75 countries, the *Candida* spp. were the third most frequent organism cultured, accounting for 17% of all isolates. In Canada, there has been a rise in the number of *Candida* isolates since 1991, and currently it constitutes 6% of all blood cultures in a single institution experience. In general, the rates reported from European hospitals are slightly less than those from North America. However, in the National Taiwan University Hospital, *Candida* has been the most common type of nosocomial blood infection since 1993. In a meta-analysis of randomized, placebo-controlled trials with fluconazole prophylaxis the incidence of fungal infections was significantly reduced, but there was no survival advantage, raising the issue of the value of prophylaxis. The first clinical description of *Candida* infection can be traced to Hippocrates with Parrot recognizing a link to severe illness and Lagenbeck implicating fungus as a source of infection and Berg establishing causality

between this organism and thrush by inoculating healthy babies with aphthous "membrane material." The first description of a deep infection by *C. albicans* was made by Zenker in 1861, even though it was not named until 1923 by Berkout. On the other hand, the genus *Aspergillus* was first described in 1729 by Michaeli, and the first human cases of aspergillosis were described in the mid-1800s. With the introduction of antibiotics and the subsequent appearance of ICUs, new instances of opportunistic fungal infections began to emerge. The use of immunosupression, organ transplantation, implantable devices, and the human immunodeficiency virus (HIV) has also radically changed the spectrum of fungal pathogenicity.

Fungi are ubiquitous heterotrophic eukaryotes, quite resilient to environmental stress and able to thrive in the most unusual places. They may belong to either kingdom Chromista or kingdom Eumycota. For identification purposes, the separation of taxa is based on the method of spore production, assisted by molecular biology techniques (rRNA and rDNA) that further refine fungi phylogeny and establish new relationships between groups. The most important human pathogens are the yeasts and the molds (from the Norse *mowlde*, fuzzy). The dual modality of fungal propagation (sexual/teleomorph and asexual/anamorph states) has meant that since the last century there has been a dual nomenclature.

PREDICTORS FOR FUNGAL INFECTIONS

The National Healthcare Safety Network began collecting voluntary reported data in 2005. Its first report showed *Candida* spp. are the fourth most common infection in overall pathogenic isolates in all cases of healthcare associated infections (HAI). They are the third most common central line associated blood stream infection and the second most common catheter associated urinary tract infection. In addition, several conditions (both patient-dependent and disease-specific conditions) have been recognized (using multiple logistic regression analysis) as independent predictors for invasive fungal complications during critical illness. By univariate logistic regression analysis, the degree of morbidity and the duration of mechanical ventilation were independent predictive factors for death, but infection with *Candida* spp. was not. ICU length of stay was associated with *Candida* infection as were the degree of morbidity, alterations of immune response, and the number of medical devices involved. Neutropenia, diabetes mellitus, new-onset hemodialysis, total parenteral nutrition (TPN) use, broad-spectrum antibiotic administration, bladder catheterization, azotemia, diarrhea, use of corticosteroids, and cytotoxic drug use are also associated with candidemia.

Diabetes Mellitus

Diabetes is an independent predictor for mucosal candidiasis, invasive candidiasis, and aspergillosis. Uncontrolled diabetes and ketoacidosis has a strong association with rhinocerebral mucor (produced by *Zygomycetes*), and other atypical fungal infections, with hyperglycemia being the strongest predictor of candidemia after liver transplantation and cardiac bypass. It has been postulated that hyperglycemia produces several alterations in the normal host response to infection and in the fungus itself, increasing its virulence. Some of the models proposed involve the glycosylation that facilitates fungal binding and subsequent internalization and apoptosis of the targeted cells, glycosylation of opsonins that render them unable to recognize the fungal antigens, the diminished capacity of diabetic serum to bind iron (therefore making it available to the pathogen), altered T_H1 lymphocyte recognition of fungal targets (therefore impairing the production of interferon gamma), and evidence that *Candida* spp. overexpresses a C3-receptor-like protein that facilitates fungal adhesion to endothelium and mucosal surfaces. Dendritic cells and other antigen-presenting cells have been postulated as crucial in the induction of cell-mediated responses to fungi, and diabetic patient vaccination studies have showed an impaired antigen–T cell interaction.

Neutropenia

There's a direct correlation between the degree of neutropenia and the risk for developing invasive fungal infections. Although a recent meta-analysis has concluded that there is little benefit from prophylaxis or preemptive treatment in neutropenic cancer patients, this is a regular practice in the United States. Empirical antifungal therapy is the standard of care for febrile severely neutropenic patients after undergoing chemotherapy or bone marrow transplantation. When profound neutropenia exists, the risk for breakthrough candidemia (during antifungal therapy) is significantly higher, and the response to voriconazole (and likely other antifungals) is decreased. Novel therapies for the treatment of invasive fungal infections in neutropenic patients include granulocyte transfusions and interferon gamma infusions.

Organ Transplantation and Immunosuppressant Medication

The two most common opportunistic fungal infections in transplant patients are *Candida* spp. and *Aspergillus* spp., generally by the inhalation route (*Aspergillus*) or from gastrointestinal sources (*Candida*). Interestingly the risk of fungal infection decreases 6 months after transplantation, unless a rejection episode requires intensification of the immunosuppressant regimen. In the solid organ recipient, the graft is often affected. In liver transplant, the risk of fungemia increases with the duration of the surgery and the number of transfusion requirements. Other risk factors include the type of bile duct anastomosis (Roux-en-Y), the presence of ischemic tissue, infection with cytomegalovirus (CMV), and graft-versus-host disease. The most common place of occurrence for *Aspergillus* tracheobronchitis in lung transplant patients is at the bronchial anastomosis and the presence of anastomotic colonization is both a risk factor for subsequent disruption or hemorrhage and a predictor for rejection and diminished graft survival. Surveillance bronchoscopies are recommended in this setting. *Aspergillus* is also the main organism responsible for fungemia after heart transplantation and second only to CMV as the cause of pneumonia in the first month after operation.

Infectious complications are the main cause of morbidity and mortality in pancreas and pancreas-kidney transplantation. The most common organisms are gram-positive cocci, closely followed by gram-negative rods and *Candida*. Risk factors for fungal infections include bladder drainage and use of OKT-3 for rejection treatment. Kidney recipients have, of all the other solid organ transplants, the least amount of infectious complications. In the New York–Presbyterian SICU, fungal prophylaxis (with fluconazole) is indicated only in recipients of solid organ grafts.

Solid and Hematologic Malignancy

Cancer patients are susceptible to opportunistic infections. Cancer and the chemotherapy needed to treat it produce three types of immune dysfunctions that render the patient vulnerable to opportunistic infections: (1) neutropenia (see earlier), (2) deficits in lymphocyte-mediated immunity (as in Hodgkin disease and during corticosteroid treatment), and (3) humoral immunodeficiency (e.g., multiple myeloma, Waldenström macroglobulinemia, and after splenectomy). The first two types are the most relevant in terms of fungal vulnerability. Up to one third of the cases of febrile neutropenia after chemotherapy for malignant diseases are due to invasive fungemia (see Treatment later).

The type of lymphopenia is as important as the nadir of the lymphocyte count: although T_H1 type responses (tumor necrosis factor

[TNF]-α, interferon-γ, and interleukin 12) confer protection against fungal infections, T_H2 (interleukin 4 and interleukin 10) are associated with progression of disease. Corticosteroids have anti-inflammatory properties, related to their inhibitory effects on the activation of various transcription factors, in particular, nuclear factor kappa B (NF-κB) cells. In a murine model, steroid treatment increased the production of interleukin 10 in response to a fungal insult, and decreased the recruitment of mononuclear cells to the site of infection. It does not, however, inhibit recruitment of neutrophils to the inflammatory sites (interleukin 8 mediated).

Long-Term Use of Central Venous Catheters

Numerous studies have shown that many, if not most, episodes of candidemia are catheter related; and one of the largest prospective treatment studies of fungemia implicated a catheter 72% of the time. The isolation of *Candida parapsilosis* from blood cultures is strongly associated with central venous catheter infection, hyperalimentation, and prosthetic devices. The source of the fungal contaminants is different in neutropenic patients when compared with their non-neutropenic counterparts. In non-neutropenic subjects the most common portal of entry for catheter contamination (and subsequent infection) is the skin during catheter placement, manipulation of an existent catheter, and cross infection among ICU patients attributed to hand carriage of biologic flora from health care workers. Other possible sources for primary catheter colonization include contaminated hyperalimentation, multiple medication administration which violated the catheter, and the presence of other medical devices. The secondary route of contamination for intravascular catheters and other foreign bodies in direct contact with the bloodstream, such as pacemakers, cardiac valves, and orthopedic joints, is candidemia originating via translocation from the gastrointestinal tract. This is the most common route in neutropenic and other immunosuppressed patients. Once the catheter becomes contaminated, a well-studied series of events take place: the yeast adheres to the surface of the catheter and develops hyphal forms that integrate into a matrix of polysaccharides and proteins that increase in size and tridimensional complexity. This is called biofilm and is the main reservoir for candidemia secondary to contaminated medical devices. Biofilm confers the fungi resistance to antimycotic medication and against the protective immune response.

In general, the removal of all central venous catheters is indicated following the diagnosis of systemic fungal infections and fungemia. Removal may not be necessary in neutropenic patients in whom the fungi originated from the gastrointestinal tract. Antifungals in general are continued after the catheter is removed, and it is recommended that *Candida* ocular dissemination be ruled out (see Endophthalmitis later).

Candida Colonization

The overgrowth and recovery of *Candida* sp. from multiple sites (without clinical symptoms of disease) has been linked to a high likelihood of invasive candidiasis, and the cumulative risk of death in these two conditions is very similar. Risk factors for the development of *Candida* colonization include prior use of antibiotics or a bacterial infection prior to ICU admission, a prolonged stay in the ICU, and multiple gastrointestinal surgeries. Until the 1980s, *C. albicans* was responsible for the vast majority of fungal infections. However, currently about one half of these infections are due to non-*albicans* species, with *C. glabrata* being the second most common isolate recovered in North America and much of Europe and having a higher lethality rate, in part due to a 10% to 15% fluconazole resistance rate and taking up to 5 days to identify in culture. In the ICU setting six independent risk factors have been identified for *C. glabrata* fungemia: age over 60 years, recent abdominal surgery, 7 or more days from

ICU admission to first blood culture, recent use of cephalosporins, presence of a solid tumor, and absence of diabetes mellitus. Similarly *C. parapsilosis* is increasing in incidence. The source of most of the outbreaks of systemic candidiasis in the context of colonization can frequently be traced to the gastrointestinal tract.

Because colonization with *Candida* sp. in the context of critical illness is not a benign occurrence, it is desirable to identify and further characterize patients in terms of risk for invasive candidiasis. Screening techniques include routine surveillance cultures in ICU patients. The modified method originally proposed by Pittet (the modified colonization index) has been validated in surgical patients. A threshold index of 0.4 has been proposed for the initiation of empiric antifungal therapy in critically ill individuals (see Treatment later), although some authorities consider the presence of multiple *Candida* isolates in such dire situations an epiphenomenon.

Use of Broad-Spectrum Antibiotics

Although the use of broad-spectrum antibiotics is one of the best documented risk factors for fungal overgrowth and invasive infections, the precise mechanism for such a risk is not completely understood. When pondering the effect of antibiotic use one must consider first the complex interrelations between bacteria and fungi in human disease.

At least three experimental models have been created to investigate and characterize the possible interactions between bacterial and fungal pathogens. In a mouse model ticarcillin-clavulanic acid and ceftriaxone (antianaerobic therapy) are associated with substantial increases in the yeast flora of the gut. On the other hand, antibiotics with poor anaerobic activity are less likely to produce this effect (e.g., ceftazidime and aztreonam) and were validated in a clinical review of the quantitative colonization of stool in immunocompromised patients treated with those antibiotics. However, this interaction between fungi overgrowth and anaerobic suppression is different from the well-studied model of *Escherichia coli* and *Bacteroides fragilis* in intraabdominal abscess formation. The work of Sawyer et al has showed that *C. albicans* induces bacterial translocation into abscesses, but the relationship is one of direct competency, rather than synergy or cooperation. This process is different from the cooperation between *C. albicans* and *Staphylococcus aureus*, *Serratia marcescens,* and *Enterococcus faecalis*, in which an amplification type interaction has been documented. A number of immunomodulatory and immunosuppressive viruses have been shown to facilitate superinfections with opportunistic fungi, the most notable examples being CMV and human herpesvirus (HHV)-6, because they induce the production of immunosuppressive cytokines. It seems the case that *C. albicans* thrives in situations in which immunocompromise is present and adds virulence and fatality to existent bacterial infections in a species-specific scenario; this has been validated from clinical observations, in which the treatment with antifungals adds little to the therapeutic effect of antimicrobials alone.

Thus, the use of antibiotics (three or more), especially those with antianaerobic properties, constitute a risk factor for fungal colonization and overgrowth, which in turn is a predictor for systemic fungal infections. The precise mechanism of action for this observation is unknown but probably related to fungi-to-microbe competence and growth suppression. *Candida* may enhance the pathogenicity of certain bacteria, but not others, and this interaction remains to be elucidated.

Candida Peritonitis

Candida spp. can be isolated in almost 20% of postoperative intraabdominal samples, primarily in cases of upper gastrointestinal perforation and nosocomial infections. Mortality rate can be significant with risk factors including an Acute Physiology and Chronic Health Evaluation (APACHE) II score over 17 on admission, respiratory failure on admission, upper gastrointestinal source of peritonitis, and presence of *Candida* on direct examination of the peritoneal fluid. Thus, in the scenario of severe sepsis or septic shock and peritonitis, a sample positive for yeast suggests serious consideration of systemic treatment for yeast.

ICU and invasive mechanical ventilation duration are related: epidemiologic observation correlating the length of mechanical ventilation and the amount of intensive care required correlates with the occurrence of both systemic fungal infections and fungal colonization.

Other factors involved in the pathogenesis and susceptibility of systemic candidiasis are TPN, use of H_2 blockers, acquired immunodeficiency syndrome (AIDS), radiation therapy, previous bacteremia, abdominal surgery, hemodialysis, extremes of age, recurrent mucocutaneous candidiasis, and duration of cardiopulmonary bypass greater than 120 minutes.

PATHOGENIC ORGANISMS

Candida albicans

The most common fungal pathogen both in the United States and abroad, and ranked as one of the most common sources of ICU sepsis, *C. albicans* is a common offender in human disease. *C. albicans* accounts for 59% of *Candida* species, followed by *C. glabrata,* at 15% to 25% of all fungal infections. Colonization occurs with evidence of yeast in a single location sample without signs of dissemination. Invasive candidiasis can be multifocal or disseminated. Multifocal candidiasis is the simultaneous isolation of *Candida* in two or more of the following locations: respiratory system, digestive tract, urinary tract, wounds, or drainage. Disseminated candidiasis is microbiologic evidence of yeast in fluids from normally sterile sites such as cerebrospinal, pleural, pericardial, or peritoneal or histologic samples from deep organs or diagnosis of endophthalmitis or candidemia with negative catheter-tip cultures. The incidence of candidemia has increased over the past 30 years with mortality rates reported in some series to be as high as 80%. The NNIS system of the Centers for Disease Control and Prevention found *Candida* species responsible for 8% to 15% of all nosocomial bloodstream infection episodes in the United States in 1993 and ranked as the fourth most commonly isolated pathogen in patients with bloodstream infections.

It is well established that a morphologic transition in *C. albicans,* from yeast to hyphal forms, is the most important determinant of dissemination because the mycelial phase is invasive. Both host and pathogen play a role on this dimorphism. During the hyphal transition the fungus produces several proteins, which are currently the focus of research. The thiol-specific antioxidant 1 (TSA1) has shown an increased survival capability in an antioxidant environment created by host cells. Host recognition molecules (adhesins), secreted aspartyl proteases and phospholipases, and phenotypic switching accompanied by changes in antigen expression, colony morphologic transition, and tissue affinities are other recognized virulence factors. The inducer mechanisms and the multiple stimuli that trigger this change are presently unknown.

From the host side, the presence of the enzyme indoleamine 2,3-dioxygenase (IDO) has been linked to antifungal defense mechanisms, acting by blocking this morphologic transition. The enzyme is induced in infectious sites and in dendritic cells by interferon-γ. Interferon serves in a pivotal position in immunity from *C. albicans* invasion. Other immune mechanisms blocking the transformation include salivary histidine, other gastrointestinal inhibitory peptides, and the resident population of dendritic cells. The dimorphic change produces in susceptible hosts disseminated candidiasis (also known as hepatosplenic candidiasis) and specific end-organ involvement. Of those metastatic infections, the most interesting from the clinical point of view has traditionally been fungal endophthalmitis.

Disseminated candidiasis and fungemia can lead to septic shock, similar to that seen with other microorganisms. Research suggests that the dimorphic transition generates shock and end-organ failure in susceptible individuals, and these events are independent of TNF-α. The diagnosis of fungemia as the cause of a patient's sepsis depends on a strong clinical suspicion. Only 50% of the blood cultures for invasive candidiasis are positive, and bacterial pathogens may interfere with the recovery of *Candida*. There are no reliable laboratory tests to differentiate between *Candida* colonization and invasive candidiasis, and no single site of isolation was superior to others in predicting which patients are likely to have developed systemic infection. The diagnostic criteria for fungemia are a combination of positive tissue cultures (including burn excision cultures, and peritoneal cultures), endophthalmitis, osteomyelitis, and candiduria. Purpura fulminans and unexplained myalgias are suggestive of candidiasis with the right clinical history. The presence of three or more colonized sites or two positive blood cultures at least 24 hours apart with one of them obtained after the removal of the central line are strong indicators for fungemia. Although asymptomatic recovery of *Candida* in urine rarely requires therapy, candiduria should be treated in symptomatic, neutropenic renal transplant patients and after instrumentation. The removal or at least changing of the Foley catheter is required.

Fungal endophthalmitis usually occurs as a result of hematogenous spread from systemic fungemia. *Candida* spp. are the most common offenders, although *Aspergillus*, *Cryptococcus*, *Fusarium*, *Scedosporium*, and others have been reported to lead to endophthalmitis. Retinal involvement has been diagnosed in between 28% and 45% of all known candidemic patients and may actually be the first sign of clinically undetected fungemia. The early initiation of systemic treatment for deep tissue fungal infection appears to dramatically decrease the incidence of endogenous fungal endophthalmitis. It is mandated for all individuals with systemic candidiasis and fungemia to have a formal ophthalmologic assessment to rule out eye involvement. The observation of a classic three-dimensional retina-based vitreal inflammatory process is virtually diagnostic of endogenous endophthalmitis due to *Candida* spp.

Treatment consists of aggressive intravenous antifungals and it may require intraocular injections of amphotericin B, caspofungin, or voriconazole. In cases in which extension to the vitreous or pars anterior is evident, surgical débridement or vitrectomy will be required. Delays in treatment frequently lead to blindness.

Non–*Candida albicans* Yeast

The incidence of non–*Candida* fungemia and septic syndrome has been increasing in recent years, accounting for up to half of non-*albicans Candida* adult ICU infections. The reasons for this are likely multifactorial. Undoubtedly, one explanation for the emergence of *C. glabrata* and *C. krusei* is the selection of less susceptible species by the pressure of antifungal agents. Other species of yeast are related to specific events, such as the presence of a central indwelling catheter and *C. parapsilosis*. The increased incidence of *Candida tropicalis* in oncology patients is secondary to the increased invasiveness of the organism, especially in damaged gastrointestinal mucosa. The clinical features of this infection are indistinguishable from *C. albicans*.

Aspergillus

The noninvasive types of aspergillosis include allergic bronchopulmonary aspergillosis (a form of hypersensitivity reaction in asthmatics) and aspergilloma. These entities, without tissue invasion, usually do not require antifungal therapy. Invasive aspergillosis has experienced an increased incidence over the last decade and has become a major cause of death among hematologic malignancy patients. Although invasive *Aspergillus* infections usually occur via inhalation of conidia, the fungus is also frequently present on food

(i.e., pepper, regular and herbal tea bags, fruits, corn, and rice). The thermotolerant spores of *Aspergillus* and other fungi present are difficult to eradicate, and represent a port of entry in the immunocompromised host. The conidia that fail to get cleared by the alveolar macrophages germinate in the alveolar space and hyphal forms invade the pulmonary tissues, with prominent vascular invasion and early dissemination (Figs. 1 to 3).

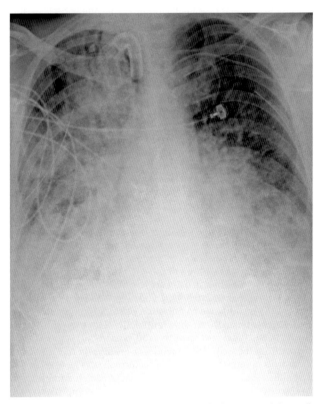

FIGURE 1 Chest radiograph of a patient with disseminated *Aspergillus* infection and pneumonia. The image is identical to that of acute respiratory distress syndrome. *(Courtesy of E. Smith-Singares, P.S. Barie, and S.R. Eachempati, The Anne and Max A. Cohen Surgical Intensive Care Unit, New York–Presbyterian Hospital, Weill Cornell Medical College, New York.)*

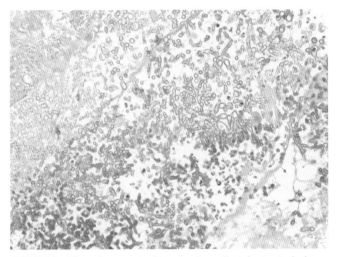

FIGURE 2 Microphotograph of invasive *Aspergillus* infection in the lungs of the patient in Figure 1. *(Courtesy of C.R. Minick, E. Loyd, and B. Amin, Department of Pathology and Laboratory Medicine, New York Hospital, Weill Cornell Medical College, New York.)*

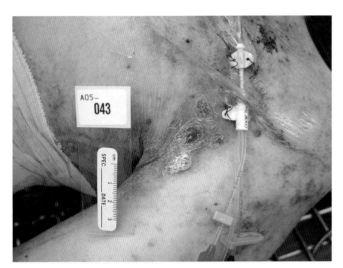

FIGURE 3 Purpura fulminans in a victim of hepatosplenic candidiasis. *(Courtesy of C.R. Minick, E. Loyd, and B. Amin, Department of Pathology and Laboratory Medicine, New York Hospital, Weill Cornell Medical College, New York.)*

Other Emerging Fungal Pathogens

Zygomycetes (mucor) are becoming increasingly important in ICU patients. The port of entry in the immunocompromised host is usually inhalation of aerosolized, thermotolerant spores, although percutaneous exposure (i.e., surgical or traumatic wounds and burns) has been reported. The source of these spores is usually decaying organic matter in the soil, but they can be found in hospital food: fruit, bread, sweet biscuits, regular and herbal tea, and pepper. The major risk factors for mucormycosis are diabetic ketoacidosis, neutropenia, iron overload, deferoxamine therapy, and protein-calorie malnutrition. Treatment includes surgical débridement, depending on the extent of the disease.

PRINCIPLES OF THERAPY

Although there has been a major expansion in the repertoire of antifungals with the introduction of less toxic formulations of amphotericin, improved triazoles, echinocandin development, and agents that target the fungal cell wall, a study on U.K. ICUs and fungal therapy demonstrated that most do not have a documented treatment protocol and that there is a low threshold to empirically treat at-risk patients with antifungal drugs. As described by Flanagan and Barnes, the therapy for fungal infections in the ICU can be directed using four different strategies: prophylactic, preemptive, empiric, and definitive. Some data have suggested a decrease in invasive fungal infections with prophylactic antifungal therapy in non-neutropenic critically ill surgical patients with *Candida* isolates from sites other than blood and the presence of risk factors mentioned earlier. Others have suggested that the prophylactic use of anti-*Candida* regimens in unselected SICU patients increases mortality rate, length of stay, and the appearance of resistance in previously susceptible fungi, not to mention the increase in ICU care cost generated by this approach. Prophylactic fluconazole treatment in the SICU leads to secondary mycoses infections with up to 80% of these infections resistant to the original agent. Tables 1 and 2 and Figures 4 and 5 show one schema used in the SICU at New York–Presbyterian Hospital's SICU. Independent of the species, fluconazole resistant *Candida* doubles the mortality rate. A colonization index developed by Pittet et al and Ostrosky-Zeichner has been retrospectively validated and suggests that high-risk patients are those who remain in the ICU for 4 or more days and who either have a central line in place or are treated with antibiotics in addition to two of the following: use of parenteral total nutrition, need for dialysis, recent major surgery, diagnosis of pancreatitis, and treatment with systemic corticosteroids or other immunosuppressive agents. Studies have documented the lack of benefit for fluconazole therapy in unselected trauma patients and in ICU patients in whom the contribution of candidemia to mortality rate is surpassed by that of age and severity of illness.

Table 3 presents a list of available antifungals. Amphotericin B is a natural polyene macrolide that primarily binds to ergosterol, the principal sterol in the fungi cell membrane, leading to ion channels and apoptosis. It also produces oxygen free radicals. It is active against most fungi, including those in the cerebrospinal fluid. Because of its high level of protein binding, levels are not usually affected by hemodialysis. Infusion-related reactions can occur in up to 73% of patients with the first dose and often diminish during continued therapy. Amphotericin-associated nephrotoxicity can lead to azotemia and hypokalemia, although acute potassium release with rapid infusion can occur and lead to cardiac arrest. Amphotericin B lipid formulations allow for higher dose administration with lesser side effects of nephrotoxicity. Nystatin is a polyene similar in structure to amphotericin and is currently used topically for *C. albicans*. A parenteral formulation is currently undergoing studies. Flucytosine is a fluorinated pyrimidine analog that is converted to 5-fluorouracil, which causes RNA miscoding and inhibits DNA synthesis. It is available in the United States in oral form only and has been used with amphotericin B for synergism against *Candida* spp.

TABLE 1: Usual Susceptibilities of *Candida* Species to Selected Antifungal Agents

Candida spp.	Fluconazole	Itraconazole	Voriconazole (not standardized)	Amphotericin B	Caspofungin (not standardized)
C. albicans	S	S	S	S	S
C. tropicalis	S	S	S	S	S
C. parapsilosis	S	S	S	S	S to I (?R)
C. glabrata	S-DD to R	S-DD to R	S to I	S to I	S
C. krusei	R	S-DD to R	S to I	S to I	S
C. lusitaniae	S	S	S	S to R	S

Modified from Pappas PG, Rex JH, Sobel JD, et al: Guidelines for treatment of candidiasis. *Clin Infect Dis* 38(2):161–189, 2004.
I, Intermediate; R, resistant; S, susceptible; S-DD, susceptible-dose dependent (increased minimal inhibitory concentration may be overcome by higher dosing, such as 12 mg/kg/day fluconazole).

TABLE 2: Approximate Antifungal Daily Costs, 2005

Antifungal	Approximate Cost/Dose	Usual Adult Dose	Approximate Cost/Day
Fluconazole 400 mg IV	$14	400 mg IV daily	$14
Fluconazole 400 mg PO	$1	400 mg PO daily	$1
Itraconazole 200 mg PO solution	$43	200 mg PO twice daily	$86
Voriconazole 400 mg IV	$230	400 mg IV twice daily (load)	$460
Caspofungin 70 mg IV	$421	70 mg IV daily (load)	$421
Caspofungin 50 mg IV	$405	50 mg IV daily (maintenance)	$405
Amphotericin B conventional 70 mg IV	$12	70 mg IV daily	$12
Amphotericin B lipid (Abelcet)	$300	350 mg IV daily	$300

Courtesy Marc R. McDowell, PharmD, Advocate Christ Medical Center, Oak Lawn, Ill.
IV, Intravenous; PO, orally.

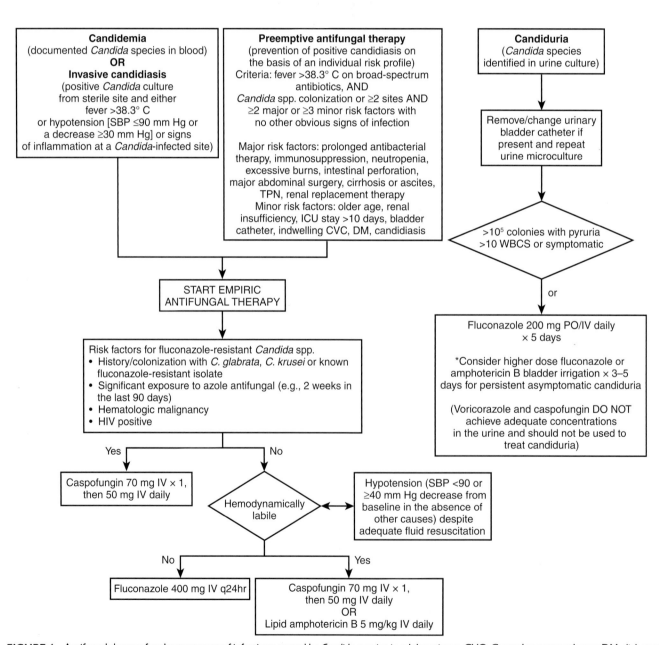

FIGURE 4 Antifungal therapy for the treatment of infections caused by *Candida* species in adult patients. CVC, Central venous catheter; DM, diabetes mellitus; HIV, human immunodeficiency virus; ICU, intensive care unit; IV, intravenously; PO, orally; q, every; SBP, systolic blood pressure; TPN, total parenteral nutrition; WBC, white blood cell.

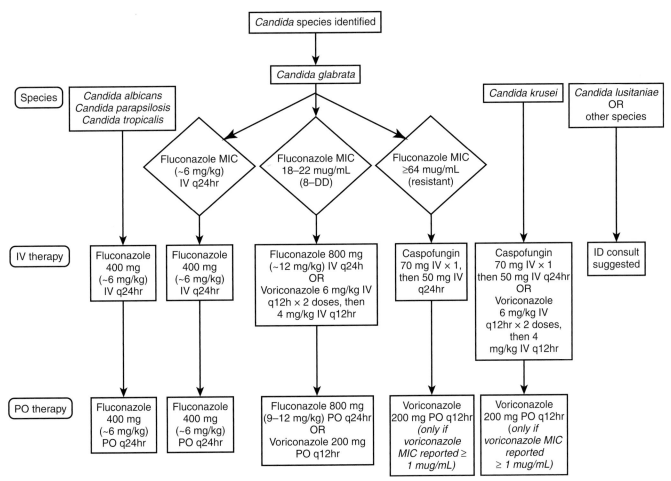

FIGURE 5 Treatment algorithm when *Candida* spp. are identified. ID, Infectious diseases; IV, intravenous; MIC, minimal inhibitory concentration; PO, orally; q, every.

TABLE 3: Antifungal Agents

Antifungal Agent	Organisms	Routes/Dosage

Amphotericin B	*Candida albicans* (>95%)
	C. glabrata (95%), *C. parapsilosis* (>95%)
	C. krusei (>95%), *C. tropicalis* (99%)
	C. guillermondi; *C. lusitaniae*
	Variable activity: *Aspergillus* spp., ferrous *Trichosporon*
	    beigelii,
	Fusarium spp., *Blastomyces dermatidis*
		IV: 0.3–1 mg/kg/day over 2–6 hours
		Oral: 1 mL oral suspension, swish and swallow 4 ×
		    daily, times 2 weeks

Amphotericin B liposomal (less nephrotoxicity)	*C. albicans* (>95%), *C. glabrata* (>95%) *C. parapsilosis* (>95%), *C. krusei* (>95%) *C. tropicalis* (99%), *C. guillermondi*, *C. lusitaniae* Variable activity: *Aspergillus*	IV: 3–5 mg/kg/day
Amphotericin B colloidal dispersion (more infusional)	*C. albicans* (>95%), *C. glabrata* (>95%) *C. parapsilosis* (>95%), *C. krusei* (>95%) *C. tropicalis* (99%), *C. guillermondi*; *C. lusitaniae* Variable activity: *Aspergillus*	IV: 3–4 mg/kg/day
Amphotericin B lipid complex	*C. albicans* (>95%), *C. glabrata* (>95%) *C. parapsilosis* (>95%), *C. krusei* (>95%) *C. tropicalis* (99%), *C. guillermondi*, *C. lusitaniae* Variable activity: *Aspergillus*	IV: 5 mg/kg/day

Continued

TABLE 3: Antifungal Agents—Cont'd

Antifungal Agent	Organisms	Routes/Dosage
Ketoconazole	*C. albicans*	PO: 200–400 mg/daily
Voriconazole	*Aspergillus, Fusarium* spp., *C. albicans* (99%) *C. glabrata* (99%), *C. parapsilosis* (99%) *C. tropicalis* (99%), *C. krusei* (99%), *C. guillermondi* (>95%) *C. lusitaniae* (95%)	IV: 6 mg/kg q12h × 2, then 4 mg/kg IV q12h PO: >40 kg, 200 mg q12h; <40 kg, 100 mg q12h
Fluconazole	*C. albicans* (97%) *C. glabrata* (85–90% resistant/intermediate) *C. parapsilosis* (99%) *C. tropicalis* (98%) *C. krusei* (5%) Fungistatic against *Aspergillus*	Candidiasis: Prophylaxis (IV or oral): 200–400 mg/day Invasive: 400–800 mg/day Oropharyngeal: 200 mg day 1, then 100 daily × 2 weeks
Itraconazole	Fungicidal to *Aspergillus, C. albicans* (93%) *C. glabrata* (50%), *C. parapsilosis* (45%), *C. tropicalis* (58%), *C. krusei* (69%), *C. guillermondi, C. lusitaniae* Blastomycoses, histoplasmosis, chromomycosis	IV: Load 200 mg IV 2 × daily × 4 doses, then 200 mg 4 × daily maximum 14 days Oral: 200 mg daily or q12h Life threatening: load 600–800/day × 3–5 days then 400–600 mg/day
Caspofungin	*C. albicans, C. glabrata, C. parapsilosis, C. tropicalis, C. krusei, C. guillermondi, C. lusitaniae*	IV: 70 mg IV, then 50 mg IV every day
Flucytosine	Not effective for *C. krusei* Effective for *C. albicans, C. tropicalis, C. parapsilosis, C. lusitaniae*	PO: 50–150 mg/kg/day divided q6h
Nystatin	*C. albicans*	100,000 units swish and swallow qid
Clotrimazole	Thrush	Oral troches 5 × daily × 14 days

IV, Intravenously; PO, orally; q, every; qid, four times a day.

The azoles inhibit the cytochrome P-450 dependent enzymes and alter fungal cell membranes. Ketoconazole comes only in tablet form and is indicated for candidiasis, thrush, and candiduria. Fluconazole and itraconazole are active against *Candida* spp. except *C. krusei* and *C. fusarium*. Itraconazole is active against *Aspergillus* spp. As mentioned earlier, *C. glabrata* and *C. krusei* resistance has been seen with fluconazole, which however can be useful in cryptococcal and coccidioidomycosis meningitis. Both drugs also have levels influenced by many agents such as antacids, H2-antagonists, isoniazid, phenytoin, and phenobarbitol.

Second-generation antifungal triazoles include posaconazole, ravuconazole, and voriconazole. They are active against *Candida*, fungi with fluconazole resistance, and *Aspergillus* spp.

The echinocandins include caspofungin, which is a third-line treatment for invasive aspergillosis. Owing to their distinct mechanism of action, the echinocandins can be used in combination with the more standard antifungal agents. The IDSA (Infectious Disease Society of America) favors the use of an echinocandin for primary therapy of candidemia in patients who are moderately to severely ill.

Invasive fungal infections in non-neutropenic ICU patients are treated if histologic or cytopathologic examination shows yeast cells or pseudohyphae from a needle aspiration or biopsy excluding mucous membranes; a positive culture obtained aseptically from a normally sterile and clinically or radiologically abnormal site consistent with infection, excluding urine, sinuses, and mucous membranes; or a positive percutaneous blood culture in patients with temporally related clinical signs and symptoms compatible with the relevant organism.

Neutropenic Patients and Preemptive Therapy

A novel approach in the use of antifungal therapy in patients who do not exhibit clinical evidence of systemic candidiasis is the concept of preemptive therapy. Being more than just a semantic difference, prophylaxis is defined as treatment triggered by risk stratification (thus directed at patients with "possible" fungal infection), but preemptive therapy is the treatment of early identified infection, without clinical signs, detected by the use of surrogate markers or non–culture-based methods. The appeal of preemptive therapy (for patients with "probable" fungal infection) is that theoretically it combines the best of the evidence for fungal prophylaxis with the benefits of early treatment, and the confidence of targeted strategies, putting at ease those critics that point to the increase in fungal resistance and the recovery of resistant strains. Because there is evidence that the prophylactic use of fluconazole confers little benefit in the management of nonfebrile neutropenic patients, the development of new protocols using frequent surveillance and screening (instead of therapy) for patients at high risk is imperative.

Prophylactic Antifungal Therapy in Solid Organ Transplant Recipients

Invasive fungal infections remain a frequent complication among the recipients of solid organs. The risk is greater during the early posttransplant period, decreasing after 6 months from the date of the operation. Liver transplantation carries the highest risk, followed by heart and lung transplantation. Other risk factors have been identified, including liver and renal dysfunction, retransplantation, rejection, surgical complications, and CMV infections. A recent review of the best evidence available showed that fluconazole is effective for prevention of invasive fungal infections, but without any reduction in mortality rate. In liver transplant patients, the number necessary to treat (NNT) in order to prevent one infection is 14, given an incidence of 10%. The meta-analysis also concluded that for lower-risk recipients (i.e., renal recipients) the NNT increases to 28. Prophylaxis should be reserved for those patients with a higher stratified risk and in settings where fungal complications are found to be more prevalent. For those immunosuppressed patients who have experienced a noncandidal systemic fungal infection, prolonged suppressive antifungal therapy may be required to prevent a relapse.

Acquired Immunodeficiency Syndrome and Empiric Antifungal Therapy

The incidence of invasive candidiasis is low, a surprising fact when considering the almost ubiquitous presence of mucocutaneous candidiasis in HIV-infected patients. This underscores that the host defense mechanisms required for resistance against mucocutaneous and invasive candidiasis are different. Therefore, patients who develop AIDS and associated *Candida* infections frequently have additional risk factors, such as TPN, catheters, broad-spectrum antibiotics, or neutropenia due to HIV-related lymphoma or cytotoxic therapy. The use of empiric fluconazole for these patients is not cost effective, and should be discouraged.

Therapy Tailored to Specific Risk Factors and Likely Offending Organisms

The New York–Presbyterian Hospital has developed algorithms and guidelines for the use of antifungal agents (see Tables 1 and 2 and Figs. 4 and 5) based on epidemiologic considerations. Table 3 lists the antifungal drugs most commonly in use in the United States. Several studies have demonstrated that azole antifungals have immunosuppressive activity in that imidazoles interfere with neutrophils and lymphocyte function. Ketoconazole has been used to attempt to reduce the frequency of the acute respiratory distress syndrome in high-risk patients, possibly as a thromboxane A_2 synthetase inhibitor. Itraconazole and miconazole are potent inhibitors of 5-lipoxygenase. Fluconazole, which has no effect on plasma thromboxane and leukotriene levels, has been shown in animals and in vitro to augment the bactericidal activity of neutrophils, suggesting a positive role in treating septic patients.

FUNGI AS AN EPIPHENOMENON

Recent advances in critical care have produced a selected population of very ill individuals who in previous years would have succumbed to their disease processes. Many of these improvements in survival have preceded (and in some cases paralleled) the explosive outgrowth in fungal colonization and infection in ICU patients and the availability of antifungal therapy. As antibiotic availability has become more complex and resistance has developed, so too has the complexity of fungal infections and the multimodality therapy expanded. Although there's little argument that invasive fungal infections are associated with an increased mortality rate, morbidity, and length of stay (both ICU and hospital), the precise amount of the mortality rate attributable to these infections remains controversial. More problematic is the fact that, although antifungal prophylaxis is effective in preventing fungal colonization and invasive infections, this does not translate into a difference in mortality rate. Data on length of stay is also contradictory, with staunch supporters for both sides. Localized fungal infections and colonization have different natural histories depending on the severity of illness, although they remain predictors of invasive infection in the very ill as determined by higher APACHE scores.

SUMMARY

Fungal infections are increasingly prevalent among ICU patients. The most common offending fungi are *C. albicans*, other *Candida* species, and *Aspergillus*. Therapy should be directed toward specific risk factors, but the use of empiric antifungal therapy is discouraged in non-neutropenic patients as well as the treatment of isolated nonblood positive cultures.

For the chapter's Suggested Readings list, please visit the book at www.ExpertConsult.inkling.com.

PREOPERATIVE AND POSTOPERATIVE NUTRITIONAL SUPPORT: STRATEGIES FOR ENTERAL AND PARENTERAL THERAPIES

Patricia Marie Byers, S. Morad Hameed, and Stanley J. Dudrick

Nutritional support is an integral part of trauma and critical care management, and its role has undergone a dramatic evolution over the last two decades of the twentieth century as a better, more comprehensive understanding of the complex inflammatory and metabolic pathways that accompany surgical stress has been gained. The manipulation of this stress response and its inherent catabolic reaction is a primary focus of emerging nutritional therapies.

MALNUTRITION

Malnutrition may be defined as a state of relative nutrient deprivation and metabolic disturbance that compromises host defenses and increases the risks of complications and death. For years, protein-calorie malnutrition has been characterized by weight loss, hypoalbuminemia, decreased skeletal muscle mass, reduced fat stores, and decreased total lymphocyte counts. In 1936, Hiram O. Studley first identified preoperative malnutrition as a specific operative risk factor in patients with peptic ulcer disease. He noted a 10-fold increase in mortality rate in patients who had lost over 20% of their body weight, and wondered if this might be reversible with a preoperative method for overcoming this deficit. Multiple studies performed since his time have confirmed that malnutrition results in poor wound healing, increased infection rates, prolonged postoperative ileus, lengthened hospital stays, and increased mortality.

METABOLIC STRESS

Patients who are injured or submitted to extensive and complicated surgery manifest a pronounced acute phase reaction in response to tissue injury, reperfusion, and hemodynamic disturbances. A metabolic environment of increased catecholamines and cortisol orchestrates an increase in energy expenditure and protein turnover. The resultant insulin resistance is responsible for the decreased peripheral use of glucose and an increase in the rates of lipolysis and proteolysis for the provision of amino acids and fatty acids as fuel substrates. The conversion of peripherally mobilized amino acids (primarily alanine) to glucose by gluconeogenesis is not suppressed by hyperglycemia or the infusion of glucose solutions in this environment. The amino acid pool rapidly becomes depleted of essential amino acids as the branched chain amino acids are used preferentially as fuel in skeletal muscle while large amounts of the conditionally essential amino acid glutamine are required for metabolic processes, especially in the intestinal mucosa. Decreased protein synthesis in skeletal muscle and in the gastrointestinal tract is accompanied by increased protein breakdown, with the shuttling of amino acids to lung, cardiac, liver, and splenic tissue, where protein synthesis is better maintained. As this catabolic process is perpetuated by cytokine activation, the critically ill and injured patient remains catabolic and consumes skeletal and visceral muscle and fat reserves rapidly. All these disturbances can deplete important trace elements and vitamins, and their deficiencies may be associated with end-organ dysfunction.

In the stress state, malnutrition may be manifest as a functional deterioration in organ system function along with poor wound healing or wound breakdown. Respiratory muscle weakness can predispose to atelectasis, pneumonia, and prolonged ventilator dependence. In addition, all aspects of the immune response may be impaired by malnutrition. Host barrier function may be compromised together with cell-mediated and humoral immunity as cell growth and turnover are diminished.

PREOPERATIVE NUTRITION

There are two notable circumstances in which preoperative nutritional support should be considered a high priority. The first involves patients who will require major operative intervention, but cannot undergo immediate surgery and will likely have a prolonged fast for more than 5 days. In the other circumstance operative intervention must be delayed to rehabilitate patients with significant nutritional deficits that could increase postoperative morbidity if not ameliorated or corrected (Fig. 1).

In the preoperative patient, the response to starvation is associated with a redistribution of substrate flow from peripheral tissues to meet metabolic demands. The falling level of insulin promotes the release of fatty acids and amino acids from adipose tissue and skeletal muscle. Although most peripheral tissues can use fatty acids as fuel, proteolysis continues to fuel gluconeogenesis in order to support the fuel requirements of the glucose-dependent tissues (Fig. 2). Over time, adaptation to starvation occurs as the brain metabolism adapts to use ketones for 50% of its fuel needs. As fat-derived fuel sources are used more, the dependence on protein catabolism decreases from 85% to 35% (Figs. 2 and 3).

Patients with upper gastrointestinal tract malignancies have the highest incidence of protein-calorie malnutrition, with over 30% of patients demonstrating significant nutritional deficits. Preoperative chemotherapy and radiation, combined with cancer cachexia, obstruction, increased nutrient losses, and abnormal substrate metabolism, increase nutritional risk.

Prospective studies have shown a decrease in major complications such as anastomotic leak and wound disruption when surgery is delayed and preoperative parenteral nutrition is administered to

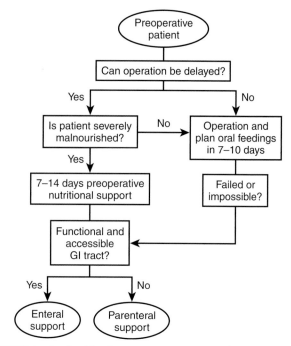

FIGURE 1   An algorithm for preoperative nutritional support.

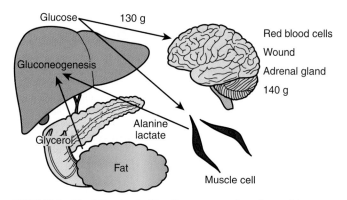

FIGURE 2   The falling level of insulin promotes the release of fatty acids and amino acids from adipose tissue and skeletal muscle. Although most peripheral tissues can use fatty acids as fuel, proteolysis continues to fuel gluconeogenesis in order to support the fuel requirements of the glucose-dependent tissues.

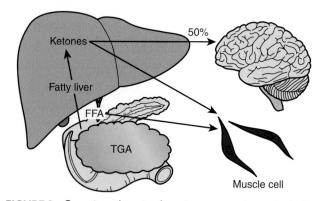

FIGURE 3   Over time, there is adaptation to starvation as the brain becomes able to use ketones for 50% of its fuel needs. As fat-derived fuel sources are used more, the dependence on protein catabolism decreases from 85% to 35%. FFA, Free fatty acids; TGA, triglycerides.

severely malnourished patients. However, an increase in infectious complications can occur without apparent clinical benefit when preoperative parenteral nutrition is administered to patients who are well nourished or only mildly malnourished. It is important, therefore, to define malnutrition precisely to select patients appropriately for this treatment modality.

The diagnosis of severe malnutrition can be established using a clinical nutritional evaluation tool, such as the Subjective Global Assessment. In 1982, Baker demonstrated the validity of a clinical assessment relative to one made on the basis of more objective laboratory values. The clinician uses historical information about recent food intake or unintentional weight loss and examines the patient for signs of nutritional depletion. Patients with multiple or severe stigmata of malnutrition or more than 15% weight loss within 6 months would be considered as seriously depleted. However, in patients with biopsy-proven carcinoma, a weight loss of only 10% in 6 months constitutes a high-risk group who would likely benefit from a course of preoperative nutritional support.

After selection of a patient for preoperative nutrition, it is necessary to select an appropriate formulation and treatment course. Although the optimal duration of therapy has yet to be determined, preoperative nutritional therapy for 7 to 15 days is standard. Total nonprotein calories should be calculated at 150% of basal energy expenditure as measured using indirect calorimetry or derived from the Harris-Benedict equations (Table 1). It is prudent to initiate a nutritional program in patients with severe malnutrition and starvation at a basal energy rate for a few days to prevent refeeding syndrome before increasing nutritional support to goal levels. After 3 days, support may be increased to 125% of basal requirements and then increased to goal as tolerated under close metabolic surveillance.

Preoperative Total Parenteral Nutrition

Total parenteral nutrition (TPN) should be administered to patients who are severely malnourished and have compromised or nonfunctioning gastrointestinal tracts. Dextrose and fat emulsion formulas are used to provide nonprotein calories, usually in a 70:30 ratio. The caloric values of TPN substrates can be found in Table 2. The amount of dextrose administered should range between 4 and 6 mg/kg/minute. However, in patients with chronic obstructive pulmonary disease or diabetes, it is recommended that dextrose administration be

TABLE 1: Harris-Benedict Equations

BEE Women = 655 + (9.6 × weight in kg) + (1.7 × height in cm) – (4.7 × age in years)

BEE Men = 66 + (13.7 × weight in kg) + (5 × height in cm) – (6.8 × age in years)

From Van Way CW 3rd: Variability of the Harris-Benedict equation in recently published textbooks. *J Parenteral Enteral Nutr* 16:566–68, 1992. BEE, Basal energy expenditure.

TABLE 2: Caloric Value of Parenteral and Enteral Nutrients

Nutrient	Parenteral (kcal/g)	Enteral (kcal/g)
Carbohydrate	3.4	4.0
Fat	9.0	9.0
Protein	3.4	4.0

maintained at 4 mg/kg/minute or less. Blood sugar levels must be monitored and kept tightly controlled between 100 and 140 mg/dL.

Fat emulsions can be used to supplement nonprotein calories; however, data suggest that preoperative intravenous lipid therapy should be limited to less than 30% of the total calories. Lipids are usually administered as a 20% emulsion, and depending upon caloric needs, quantities of 100 to 250 mL may be prescribed daily.

Protein is administered as a free amino acid solution at dosages of 1.5 g/kg of body weight daily to promote protein anabolism, and should not be included in calculations as a source of calories. Adequate nonprotein calories must be administered to support protein synthesis in a 150:1 calorie to nitrogen ratio, along with multivitamins and trace elements as part of the comprehensive nutritional regimen.

Although providing preoperative parenteral nutrition for patients with gastrointestinal dysfunction, it is important to consider fluid requirements. A more dilute, high-volume solution may be needed in patients with large fluid deficits or losses, although more concentrated, lower volume solutions will be necessary in patients who have volume restrictions secondary to heart failure, renal failure, or hepatic insufficiency.

With protein-calorie malnutrition, intracellular losses of potassium, magnesium, and phosphorus occur simultaneously with gains in sodium and water. During injudicious refeeding, sodium balance may become markedly positive and result in water retention. Potassium, phosphorus, and magnesium plasma levels may drop precipitously upon initiation of nutritional support, as these ions are transported intracellularly together with the infused macronutrients and micronutrients. It is important to monitor electrolytes and fluid balance meticulously to avoid the risk of refeeding syndrome. In addition, potassium, phosphorus, and magnesium deficiencies must be corrected if optimal anabolism is to occur (Table 3).

Trace minerals are inorganic compounds and vitamins are complex organic compounds that regulate metabolic processes (Table 4). The majority of these micronutrients act as coenzymes or as essential elemental constituents of enzyme complexes regulating the biotransformation of carbohydrates, proteins, and fats. Iron, zinc, copper, chromium, selenium, iodine, and cobalt are known to be necessary for normal health and function in human beings. Furthermore, in malnourished and seriously ill patients, requirements for zinc and selenium should be especially assessed and supplemented as is necessary.

If the patient's fluid and electrolyte status stabilizes during parenteral support, together with blood glucose levels under good control, the patient may be discharged home on cyclic overnight feedings for continuity of nutritional rehabilitation while awaiting surgery. The parenteral cycle is gradually decreased from 24 hours to 18 hours and then to 14 to 16 hours daily as tolerated to allow the patient some freedom from the infusion apparatus. A permanent central venous access port customarily is indicated for maximally safe and effective home parenteral nutrition.

Preoperative Enteral Nutrition

Enteral nutritional support is the delivery of nutrients into the gastrointestinal tract which may require a temporary or permanent feeding tube. Enteral feeding is the preferred route of nutritional support and should be used whenever possible. Surgical patients can benefit from enteral nutrition due to maintenance of the gut-associated lymphoid tissue (GALT), enhancement of mucosal blood flow, and maintenance of the mucosal barrier.

The initial gastrointestinal barrier function is provided by mucus-containing lactoferrin and lysozyme, both of which are effective, non-specific inhibitors of microbial growth. Normal, undisturbed bacterial flora exerts a similar effect. Epithelial tight junctions form the next line of nonspecific defense, with junctional integrity being energy dependent, and at least partially reliant on the presence of intraluminal energy substrates. Specific intestinal immunity is governed by the GALT. The inductive sites in the Peyer patches provide an interface

TABLE 3: Electrolyte Requirements, Compartments, and Sequelae of Abnormal Levels

Electrolyte	Daily Requirement	Fluid Compartment	Effects of Excessive Levels	Effects of Diminished Levels
Sodium (Na^+)	60–120 mEq	Extracellular	Dry mucous membranes, maniacal behavior	Seizures, altered mental status
Potassium (K^+)	40–120 mEq	Intracellular	Cardiac arrest, peaked T waves, wide QRS complex on electrocardiogram	Cardiac dysrhythmias, muscle weakness
Magnesium (Mg^{2+})	10–20 mmol	Intracellular	Cardiac dysrhythmias, hypotonia	Hypokalemia, hypocalcemia, seizures
Phosphorus (PO_4^{2-})	14–20 mmol	Intracellular	Calcium phosphate salt deposits	Altered mental status, muscle weakness, hemolysis, paresthesias
Calcium (Ca^{2+})	5 mg	Intracellular	Lethargy, constipation	Tetany, hyperreflexia, seizures, cardiac dysrhythmias

TABLE 4: Daily Dietary Requirements for Vitamins and Minerals

Vitamin or Mineral	Function	Daily Requirement
Biotin	Coenzyme of carboxylase	60 µg
Chromium	Insulin use	10–20 µg
Copper	Enzyme systems and ceruloplasmin	0.1–0.5 µg
Folic acid	Nucleic acid synthesis	600 µg
Iron	Porphyrin-based compounds, enzymes, mitochondria	0–2 mg
Niacin	Component of nicotinamide adenine dinucleotide and its phosphate (NADP)	50 mg
Pantothenate	Component of coenzyme A	15 mg
Pyridoxine	Coenzyme of amino acid metabolism	5 mg
Riboflavin	Coenzymes in redox enzyme system	5 mg
Selenium	Component of glutathione perioxidase	20–200 µg
Thiamine (vitamin B_1)	Cocarboxylase enzyme system	5 mg
Vitamin A	Epithelial surfaces, retinal pigments	2500 IU
Vitamin B_{12}	Nucleic acid synthesis	12 µg
Vitamin C	Redox reactions, collagen, immune function	1000 mg
Vitamin D	Bone metabolism	25–100 mcg
Vitamin E	Membrane phospholipids	50 IU
Vitamin K	Coagulation factors, bone health	1–2 mg
Zinc	Enzyme systems	1–15 µg

between antigen presenting cells and circulating lymphocytes. Some animal studies have demonstrated improved immunity in enterally fed groups compared with the parenterally fed groups, but this finding has not been confirmed uniformly or unequivocally to date in controlled, prospective, randomized human studies.

Patients may have inadequate appetite or gastrointestinal function to maintain optimal nutrition on oral intake alone. Enteral feeding has been used successfully to meet the nutritional needs of such patients with a wide range of surgical problems including cancer, inflammatory bowel disease, and pancreatic disorders. However, its use is contraindicated in cases of bowel obstruction, persistent intolerance of feedings, hemodynamic instability, major gastrointestinal bleeding, and inability to access the gastrointestinal tract effectively and safely.

Once it has been decided to administer enteral nutrition, the optimal type of enteral access must be selected. Factors that determine the choice of enteral access include which components of the gastrointestinal tract are available, how long a course of enteral therapy is planned, whether the patient is at risk for aspiration, and finally, the nutritional status of the patient. When available, the gastric route is usually preferred. Postpyloric feeding into the duodenum or jejunum may be indicated in the presence of early satiety, gastric disease, or risk of aspiration. Nasogastric and nasoenteral tubes are recommended for short-term feeding because of their ease of placement, low cost, and low complication rate, whereas percutaneous endoscopic gastrostomy has become one of the most common methods for placing gastrostomy tubes for longer term feeding. Interventional radiology personnel can also place feeding tubes percutaneously into the stomach as well as into the jejunum. If these less invasive techniques are not successful, feeding tubes may be placed by open or laparoscopic techniques; however, this approach is less desirable in the preoperative patient with severe malnutrition.

The appropriate selection of enteral formulation requires knowledge of the physiologic mechanisms of the digestion and absorption of each macronutrient. Sources of carbohydrate found in enteral formulas range from simple sugars to complex starches. The larger molecular weight starches exert less osmotic pressure in the intestinal lumen, are less sweet, and require more time for digestion prior to absorption. Different enteral formulas contain variable amounts of carbohydrates, which can range from 28% to 70% of total calories. Patients with diabetes or carbon dioxide retention due to chronic obstructive pulmonary disease should be given formulas with lower percentages of carbohydrate calories. (See previous discussion under "Preoperative Total Parenteral Nutrition.")

Many enteral formulas now contain fiber, which may be soluble or insoluble. Insoluble fiber improves colonic function and bowel transit

following surgery or injury. However, hemodynamic stability should always be attained first in order to avoid a low flow state in the mesenteric circulation and secondary intestinal necrosis from ischemia. Administration of continuous tube feedings usually is initiated at 10 to 20 mL/hour and may be increased by the same volume every 8 to 24 hours depending on the clinical scenario and patient tolerance. Abdominal distention should prompt the immediate decrease in the tube feeding rate by half and should mandate cessation of feedings if distention persists. Bolus feedings into the stomach of 200 to 300 mL every 2 to 6 hours may also be given and may help to maintain adequate amounts of feeding despite the interruption in feedings related to other requirements of daily care and diagnostic tests. Note that it is important to continue enteral feedings until it has been documented that the patient is taking an adequate volitional oral diet.

Natural foods can be blended to provide complete nutrition either orally or by tube directly into the stomach (nasogastric tube, percutaneous endoscopic gastrostomy [PEG], gastrostomy); or polymeric solutions are available, which are formulations of macronutrients in the form of isolates of intact protein, triglycerides, and carbohydrate polymers designed to provide complete nutrition into the stomach. Monomeric (elemental) solutions are mixtures of protein moieties in the form of peptides and amino acids; fat as long-chain triglycerides (LCT), or a combination of LCT and medium-chain triglycerides (MCT); and carbohydrates as partially hydrolyzed starch maltodextrins and glucose oligosaccharides, and are designed primarily for tube feeding below the duodenum into the jejunum, or for patients with abnormalities of digestion or absorption.

Special metabolic solutions are also available and are designed for patients having unique metabolic requirements related, or secondary, to renal failure, liver failure, heart failure, pulmonary insufficiency, and trauma. (See discussion under "Preoperative Enteral Nutrition.") Some examples of these special nutrients include enriched branched-chain amino acids for some patients with multiple systems organ failure, stress, and sepsis; and immune-modulating solutions consisting of omega-3 fatty acids, RNA, and arginine which have been shown to be associated with reduction of infections, wound complications, and hospital stays by decreasing inflammation and the resultant tendency toward multisystem organ dysfunction. Other nutrients that have been identified as potentially important components of immune-modulating nutrient solutions include carnitine, taurine, glutamine, *N*-acetylcysteine, antioxidant vitamins, and trace elements. Wound-healing formulas have been shown to be especially helpful in burn patients and contain higher levels of zinc, vitamin C, and vitamin A. Although some studies have demonstrated improved outcomes in infectious morbidity and length of hospital stay with the use of immunonutrition, no effect has been shown on mortality rate outcomes (see "Nutritional Support Challenges and Controversies" next).

NUTRITIONAL SUPPORT CHALLENGES AND CONTROVERSIES

Accentuated intense interest in providing optimally safe and effective nutritional support has spawned thousands of basic and clinical investigations and subsequent reports. However, interest has been focused primarily on three dynamic areas of utmost importance: (1) the role, rationale, and results associated with tight glycemic control; (2) immunonutrition; and (3) the route, timing, and combination of feedings most appropriate for meeting target nutritional requirements for critically ill patients.

The treatment of hyperglycemia in the ICU has major implications for the use of nutritional support, and is a topic that has been, and currently is, the focus of a variety of multiple conflicting clinical trials. An emerging body of data suggests that it is virtually impossible to separate intensive insulin therapy from optimal nutritional management in the ICU. However, this most important issue has not attracted sufficient attention in the literature, in training programs, in clinical practice, or in research endeavors. Glycemic control is certainly important in several categories of patients, but getting the patients adequately fed is probably at least as important. In their most recent versions, the ASPEN (American Society for Parenteral and Enteral Nutrition) and SCCM (Society of Critical Care Medicine) clinical guidelines do not direct sufficient attention to energy delivery, and this omission may actually unintentionally promote malnutrition from routine underfeeding. Indeed, malnutrition remains a major threat to ICU patients, and the combined nutritional support of early enteral and parenteral nutrition appears to be a reasonable answer to this problem. Committing to tight glycemic control while simultaneously underfeeding the patients does not seem prudent, given the existent data and our understanding of the physiology of ICU patients, and may explain the increased mortality rate in the tight glycemic control groups studied subsequent to the original Leuven trials. Although both situations are important to avoid, the pendulum recently has swung too far from overfeeding to underfeeding, and greater efforts must be made to achieve optimal or ideal feeding targets, which lie somewhere between these two extremes.

Immune function has been shown to be altered following major trauma and surgical procedures ever since the early days of nutritional support. More recently, acquired impaired immunity has been demonstrated by T-cell proliferation, cutaneous anergy, decreased production of interleukin 2 and interferon-γ, and abnormalities in the T-cell receptor complex. Immunonutrition is a nutritional therapeutic approach in which these pathologic alterations in innate and acquired immunity can purportedly be modulated beyond the capability of the usual standard diet, by a feeding formula supplemented with immune-enhancing or immune-modulating nutrients.

Multiple clinical studies have confirmed the beneficial effects of various "immune formulas" in surgical patients; however, not all populations have been shown to benefit equally. The most favorable responses, consisting of decreased infectious wound complications and reduced length of hospitalization, have been observed in studies of high-risk, malnourished patients undergoing upper and lower gastrointestinal surgery for cancer.

Most of the uncertainty with the use of immunonutrition lies in its use in the critically ill population, in whom a number of studies have been conducted with diverse results. Indeed, the two largest well-controlled studies showed radically different outcomes (one positive and one without effect) on infectious complications. Attempts at resolution of the immunonutrition controversy through meta-analysis have not been definitive but have suggested that although this therapy can lower rates of infection, it does not lower the overall mortality rate. The current recommendation that has evolved is that immunonutrition should be avoided in seriously ill patients, especially those with sepsis. Attempting to modulate the immune system in such patients most likely requires use of stronger forms of therapy such as pharmacologic agents or antibodies that block cytokine production or action. Accordingly, it is the immunologically vulnerable patients with underlying malnutrition and less life-threatening illnesses in which nutritional support, including immunonutrition, is most likely to improve outcome. Exactly what the optimal content of the immunonutritional support should be has not yet been satisfactorily resolved, and perhaps many ICU patients are too ill or metabolically compromised to benefit from immunonutrition as a means of disease manipulation. Additional prospective, adequately powered, randomized, controlled trials are required to define the composition, timing, and use of immunonutrition feedings, and the evolution of this vital area will inevitably continue to advance and to define its use and effectiveness.

Finally, the questionable adage that enteral nutrition is *always* preferable and superior to parenteral nutrition is continuing to be evaluated and modulated as data accumulate from studies worldwide, indicating that the aggressive use of early enteral feeding might improve outcome for patients and that the combination of early enteral feeding to its maximum tolerance, combined with sufficient early parenteral nutrition supplementation to meet the patients' nutrition needs precisely and adequately, is the most rational, practical, and effective approach for the optimal feeding of critically ill patients.

Early enteral nutrition remains the recommended feeding route in ICU patients; however, it is often unable to meet nutritional needs totally. Therefore, parenteral nutrition, whether alone or in combination with enteral nutrition, is recommended if enteral nutrition is not feasible or is insufficient to meet target requirements. Most intensive care nutritionists aim at providing 25 kcal/kg/day, administering enteral nutrition by nasogastric tube, gastrostomy, or jejunostomy. Ample evidence exists in the literature that achieving targeted nutritional goals exclusively with enteral nutrition is difficult, especially during the early phase after admission to the ICU. These studies emphasize further that the inability to deliver adequate nutrition early has been associated ultimately with increased morbidity and mortality rates. The investigators list difficulties in providing early optimal nutrition as being related to a number of factors, which include gastrointestinal dysfunction such as vomiting and diarrhea, repeated procedures and surgical operations associated with interruption of the enteral feedings, displacement of the feeding tube, inadequate nursing procedures with delayed administration of the enteral feedings, or premature withdrawal of enteral nutrition support.

In 14 collaborating Canadian hospitals, survival in ICU patients was improved when evidence-based guidelines for nutrition were followed assiduously and larger amounts of nutrition were delivered more consistently. Other studies have reported that only 58% of ICU patients included in an enteral nutrition protocol achieved their nutritional targets. On the other hand, when good compliance to the enteral nutrition protocol was maintained, more than 80% of the prescribed volume was administered by the third day. Despite several corrective measures proposed during recent years, exclusive enteral nutrition in ICU patients has remained associated with nutritional deficiencies that are correlated ultimately with impaired short-term and long-term clinical outcomes. Thus, although malnutrition in critically ill patients is known to be associated with higher ICU morbidity and mortality rates, and although underfeeding is recognized as a factor in increased morbidity, a significant number of ICU patients receiving enteral nutrition still fail to reach their prescribed nutrient goals. Supplemental parenteral nutrition should be considered in order to meet the energy and protein targets when enteral nutrition alone fails to achieve the targeted goals. Whether such combined nutritional support can provide additional benefit to the overall clinical outcome, however, remains to be proved in future prospective studies.

TECHNICAL ASPECTS OF PARENTERAL AND ENTERAL ACCESS

Central Venous Access

Insertion of central venous access catheters should be performed by an experienced operator with full aseptic precautions, including surgical gown, gloves, mask, and cap after antibacterial handwashing. These antimicrobial catheters may be placed into patients either temporarily at the bedside or permanently in an operative suite. In addition, the catheters may be placed by accessing a central vein directly or indirectly by using a peripheral venous access route. The routine use of venous Doppler devices has been demonstrated to decrease complications related to venipuncture. Peripherally inserted central venous catheters (PICC) can be placed by trained clinical specialists. These catheters may be made of silicone or polyurethane and are available with single or double lumens in gauges from 16 to 23. A flexible stylet or guidewire is provided in the commercially available kit to help with insertion using a Seldinger technique with a peel-away sheath or by using a catheter-over-the-needle technique. Veins at

or below the antecubital space are used for venipuncture. A supine position with the arm abducted at a 90-degree angle from the body is recommended. Catheter advancement should be halted if any resistance is encountered. A radiograph of the chest following the procedure is required to document that the catheter tip is appropriately positioned in the central venous system.

Femoral vein cannulation is relatively safe and may not necessarily be associated with increased risk of infection. However, it is not a preferred site for long-term catheter venous access due to the increased susceptibility to thrombosis and its associated complications and morbidity. Superior vena cava access can be obtained and, if tolerated, should be performed with the patient in Trendelenburg position in order to dilate the intended target veins maximally. The internal jugular vein is a preferred site of short-term central venous access, especially when required intraoperatively by anesthesiologists or in other acute situations, with three different approaches available: anterior to the sternocleidomastoid muscle, centrally between the two bellies of the sternocleidomastoid muscle, and posterior to the sternocleidomastoid muscle. The external jugular vein may also be used; however, successful cannulation of the superior vena cava by this route is achieved only 50% of the time or less. Due to the anatomic dependability and stability of location, the subclavian vein route, although potentially the most treacherous, is the preferred site for long-term central venous access with subcutaneously tunneled catheters and infusion port catheters. The subclavian approach should be attempted only by skilled, experienced, and certified clinicians who have been trained in, and rigidly adhere to, the established technical, aseptic, and antiseptic principles and practices in order to assure maximal safety and efficacy for the patient.

Gastrointestinal Access

In patients with adequate gastric emptying, nasogastric feedings infused through small-bore, flexible, inert, weighted tubes are usually adequate. These tubes range from 5 to 8 F in diameter, are ordinarily made of polyurethane, and often are provided with a stylet for insertion. Prior to insertion, the tube should be lubricated, and the patient should have a topical anesthetic applied in the nostril. The tube is inserted through the nostril, and advanced through the nasopharynx, pharynx, and esophagus for a distance of approximately 50 cm. Next, 50 to 100 mL of air is injected gently, and the tube is advanced further along the greater curvature toward the pylorus. An abdominal radiograph should always be obtained to confirm appropriate position of the tube prior to initiating feedings.

With some modifications, this technique can also be used for postpyloric feeding tube placement. First, the patient is given intravenous metoclopramide prior to the procedure. Second, the tube is advanced a bit further along the greater curvature of the stomach, until a point of resistance is met at the pylorus. Third, gentle pressure is maintained on the tube until the pylorus opens and the tube advances into the duodenum, and an abdominal radiograph is obtained to confirm the position of the tube in the duodenum.

If long-term gastrointestinal access is indicated, a more invasive approach will be required. The endoscopic placement of percutaneous gastrostomy tubes is now standard and can be performed with the patient in bed in the ICU. If special precautions are taken, this procedure can also be performed safely in patients with a history of previous abdominal surgery. Above all, it is important to know if any gastrointestinal anatomic changes have resulted from the previous surgery. It is important to obtain abdominal films and review prior scans to be certain that the stomach is approachable through a safe abdominal wall window. During endoscopy, a bright light should be seen transabdominally in an area accessible for tube placement. A finder needle should be inserted through the abdominal wall into the stomach to ensure that as air is aspirated into the syringe, the needle is visualized endoscopically in the lumen of the stomach. Gastrostomy tubes may be placed either by a push or a pull technique and should have a bolster holding them in place after insertion. Combination tubes are available having an inner jejunostomy portion of the gastrostomy tube that can be placed transpylorically. These tubes can also be placed in the radiology suite by a specially trained interventional radiology team. It is important to remember that tubes placed transabdominally, under fluoroscopic guidance alone, puncture and enter the stomach, but are not secured to the abdominal wall as with the open techniques. When using the radiologic approach, it is recommended that a postpyloric tube is used and that feeding is infused distally, to guard against gastric distention and leakage, until a tract has formed around the tube, usually in approximately 5 to 7 days following puncture.

Patients should have enteral access established during the primary operative abdominal procedure whenever it is anticipated that nutritional support will be needed postoperatively (see Figs. 4 and 5). The type of access selected depends on the primary surgical procedure performed and the gastrointestinal function anticipated. A gastrostomy can be easily placed in the left upper quadrant when the size of the gastric remnant is sufficient to do so. Stamm sutures should be placed to secure the stomach to the abdominal wall. An inner jejunostomy tube can be placed if postpyloric feedings are desired along with proximal gastric drainage. A separate jejunostomy tube can also be placed directly in the jejunum, but may be associated with torsion of the bowel and potential volvulus. It is important to note that all cases of reported jejunal necrosis following enteral feeding have been associated with this type of jejunal access. To avoid this risk, it is advisable to access the jejunum via the stomach with long gastrojejunostomy catheters whenever possible.

MORBIDITY AND COMPLICATIONS MANAGEMENT

Metabolic Complications

Some complications can occur which are directly related to injudicious administration of exogenous substrates. Malnourished patients may develop electrolyte derangements and congestive heart failure when fed too aggressively. This can be avoided by limiting fluids and sodium, and carefully monitoring serum phosphorus, potassium, and magnesium levels while hypocaloric feedings are initially administered. In addition, feeding with excessive carbohydrate dosages can cause the development of hyperglycemia with secondary glycosuria, osmotic diuresis, electrolyte derangements, dehydration, and an increased incidence of infectious complications. Patients with compromised respiratory function may develop hypercarbia and respiratory failure secondary to an excessive carbohydrate load.

Complications of Parenteral Nutrition

It is important to be aware of complications that may occur while obtaining central venous access for TPN. If adequate precautions are not observed, air embolus may occur and present with catastrophic hemodynamic collapse. If the air embolism has occurred or is suspected, the patient should be immediately placed in deep Trendelenburg position with the right side up. If possible, an attempt may be made to aspirate air from the right atrium through the catheter. This complication can be minimized by hydrating the patient to fill the venous compartment and creating venous hypertension in the upper body with Trendelenburg position, prior to attempting central venous catheterization; and by securing all connections of the infusion line from the bag to the indwelling catheter to minimize or prevent inadvertent disconnections allowing air into the system throughout the course of therapy. Anatomic structures adjacent to the subclavian vein may be injured; subclavian and internal jugular

line placements may result in the development of hemothoraces or pneumothoraces, due to vascular or lung injuries. Access on the left side may be associated with thoracic duct injury with clear lymph drainage from the insertion site or chylothorax formation. After catheter removal, the pleural space must be evacuated until lymphatic drainage ceases. Misplacements of the catheter into the pleural space or mediastinum are other complications that may occur, and result in hydromediastinum or hydrothorax. Malposition of a catheter tip into the atrium may cause dysrhythmias, injury, or infected thrombosis and has been associated with atrial perforation and pericardial tamponade. All of the catheter complications are technical in nature and preventable with adequate training, experience, and adherence to established principles and practices.

Line sepsis is the most common complication of indwelling central venous catheters and necessitates catheter removal. Primary catheter infections are usually characterized by the development of fever, flu-like symptoms, and positive blood cultures. In the presence of bacteremia, the catheter should be removed, but may be changed over a guidewire, with a semiquantitative culture of the intracutaneous portion of the catheter if there is doubt about the diagnosis. A semiquantitative tip culture is diagnostic when there are 15 or more colony-forming units reported. Usually, removal of the catheter results in resolution of symptoms; however, intravenous antibiotic therapy may be required for up to 2 weeks with documented bacteremia due to *Streptococcus* line sepsis, or with other organisms as necessary.

Another common complication of indwelling central venous catheters is venous thrombosis, which may be manifested by thrombophlebitis and extremity edema. This can usually be treated by catheter removal and extremity elevation. Patients with subclavian vein thrombosis have a risk of up to 30% for the development of nonlethal pulmonary embolism and should receive anticoagulation therapy. Catheter thrombosis is another potential complication and may be treated successfully with the instillation of thrombolytic agents.

Complications of Enteral Nutrition

It is important to be aware of complications that can be associated with the double-edged sword of enteral access. A 45% incidence of dislodgement of nasoenteral tubes occurs in ICUs. Dislodgement of percutaneous enteral access catheters from the lumen of the intestine into the peritoneum is a much more serious complication and may be associated with severe peritoneal soilage, peritonitis, and death. Radiographic confirmation of appropriate tube placement or replacement using contrast studies should be obtained to help avoid this complication. Another problem that may occur with gastrointestinal access is catheter occlusion. Care of these catheters must include frequent flushes with water to maintain patency of the catheter lumen. Enteral feeding tubes that have remained in situ long term may leak and cause skin breakdown. The placement of a smaller catheter and decreasing the infusion volume for a day or two will usually allow the catheter exit site to contract around the replacement catheter and thus correct the problems of leaking that had developed around the original catheter.

Adynamic ileus may occur in postoperative patients due to decreased splanchnic perfusion, injury, manipulation, impaired sympathetic tone, inflammatory response, and high-dose opiates. Gastrointestinal tract dysmotility can also result in aspiration and pneumonia. Aspiration can be minimized by keeping the head of the bed and the head of the patient elevated 30 degrees whenever clinically feasible.

Nonocclusive intestinal necrosis can occur when splanchnic perfusion is severely compromised by low blood flow states. (See discussion under "Gastrointestinal Access.") The most common signs include tachycardia, fever, leukocytosis, and abdominal distention. Tolerance of tube feeding may be optimized by minimizing opioid use, by using epidural anesthetics to blunt sympathetic nervous system activity, and by using promotility agents. However, abdominal distention must be addressed by decreasing the infusion rate or stopping the feedings. When intestinal necrosis occurs, early intervention and definitive surgical therapy for this potentially highly lethal combination has a survival rate of about 56%.

Frequent interruption of tube feedings for various reasons obviously impairs adequate delivery of nutritional support and results in malnutrition. In one series, only 52% of the feeding goal was able to be administered in a 24-hour period. Feedings are often stopped due to intercurrent procedures, diagnostic tests, and nursing care protocols. New advanced feeding pumps allow nursing personnel to record the exact amount of feedings administered during each shift so that this problem can be recognized promptly and treated or corrected.

SUMMARY AND ALGORITHMS

Preoperative parenteral nutrition should be provided to patients who are severely malnourished and require a major operative intervention in which healing complications are likely to pose a major risk, as long as enteral support is not an option, and a course of 7 to 15 days of support is considered safe and feasible (see Fig. 1). Postoperative parenteral nutrition should be used when the postoperative or postinjury period without adequate or feasible oral or enteral nutrition is expected to surpass 7 to 10 days, when the patient has received preoperative nutrition preparation and is not a candidate for postoperative enteral feedings, and when surgical complications develop in the postoperative period that are associated with gastrointestinal dysfunction. Careful serum glucose control is critical to successful use of this therapy with minimal morbidity and maximal effectiveness. Enteral feeding is the preferred method of providing nutrients to patients with a functional gastrointestinal tract if it is judiciously and expertly administered at goal dosages, and is feasible in the majority of patients, especially by dedicated nutrition support teams. Enteral feeding preserves the structure and function of the intestine and is associated with fewer infectious and metabolic complications (see Fig. 4). Finally, feeding critically ill surgical patients is a dynamic and constantly changing process, which must be thoughtfully conceived and planned, conscientiously and competently administered, and responsively and specifically tailored to each individual patient. It must be modified, adjusted, and augmented by expert applications of the multiple and complex nutritional support techniques, technologies, and substrates available for the optimal provision of the most efficacious nutrients for the maximal metabolic benefits and outcomes of the patients.

Key Points

- Enteral feedings should be started within 24 hours of admission to the ICU once resuscitation has been completed and hemodynamic stability has been achieved.
- TPN should be started with tight glucose control in all patients who are predicted not to be likely to tolerate enteral feedings within 10 days of injury or surgery.
- In critically ill and injured patients, 25 kcal/kg and 1.5 to 2 g/kg of protein are ordinarily sufficient during the injury phase. Benefits of enteral feeding accrue if 50% of these needs are met.
- Fluid imbalance and deficiencies in magnesium, potassium, and phosphorus must be treated aggressively in patients with energy deficits to avoid refeeding syndrome.
- In patients who are receiving less than 4 mg/kg/minute of carbohydrates, CO_2 retention should not be exacerbated.
- Renal failure is a catabolic state in which protein should not be restricted; patients need full, balanced nutritional support and aggressive dialysis.
- Bronchopulmonary aspiration of enteral feedings most often occurs during patient transfer.
- Glutamine is a conditionally essential amino acid in the metabolic environment of stress.
- Diarrhea that occurs with intestinal atrophy should respond to a more monomeric elemental formula. If it does not, *Clostridium difficile* infection must be considered and treated.

For the chapter's Suggested Readings list, please visit the book at www.ExpertConsult.inkling.com.

Venous Thromboembolism: Diagnosis and Treatment

Susan Evans and Ronald Sing

Venous thromboembolism (VTE) is a challenge in the management of injured patients. The mainstay of management requires thoughtful decision making regarding prevention, diagnosis, and therapy, all of which have inherent risks. For this reason, many institutions have moved to using algorithms for decision making in specific patient populations. However, the trauma population, in particular, has a varied risk tolerance (e.g., immobility, hemorrhage, intracranial hemorrhage), which makes general algorithms difficult to apply. Despite this variability, we will provide an algorithm that provides structure yet allows flexibility to address the specifics of each patient. Ultimately, it is important to determine which patients fit easily into an algorithm pathway and which patients require a multidisciplinary team to determine a management plan.

INCIDENCE

Venous thrombosis occurs in as many as 58% of injured patients who do not receive prophylaxis, and most of these thromboses (98%) are initially asymptomatic. Patients with lower extremity fracture (69%), spinal cord injury (62%), and traumatic brain injury (TBI, 54%) have the highest incidences of VTE. Furthermore, other factors such as older age (odds ratio [OR] = 1.05), blood transfusion (OR = 1.74), and surgery (OR = 2.3) contribute to the risk of VTE development. A 2004 review of the National Trauma Data Bank (NTDB) showed that VTE and pulmonary embolism (PE) occurred in 0.36% and 0.13%, respectively, of all patients admitted with injury. Importantly, VTE can occur early after injury, with 6% of PE episodes occurring within 24 hours of injury and 25% within the first 3 days. Although thromboprophylaxis, specifically, has contributed to a decrease of VTE in the past 2 decades, other aspects of patient management such as early mobility and decreased time in the operating room have improved patient outcomes overall and likely the incidence of VTE.

PATHOPHYSIOLOGY

Trauma incorporates all three aspects of Virchow's triad (stasis, endothelial injury, hypercoagulable state), which explains the prevalence of VTE after injury. Immobility of the patient as a whole or of injured extremities leads to stasis within the venous system. Stasis is more pronounced in the intensive care unit (ICU), particularly in patients requiring neuromuscular blockade. This is the premise by which intermittent pneumatic compression (IPC) devices were initially created, although their contribution to fibrinolysis extends beyond their local effect. Direct injury to the venous system can occur with and without hemorrhage. Patients with vascular injury have insult to the endothelium causing release of tissue factor. Stretch, compression, and crush injury from impacts, fractures, and shear stress from cavitation due to gunshot wounds can cause intimal injury to the venous system without disruption of the vein. However, direct venous injury is not required to put injured patients at increased risk of thrombosis. Posttraumatic cytokine release from injury at a remote location causes activation of procoagulant factors, reduction in anticoagulant factors, and a relative hypercoagulable state. As the body recognizes the need to stop bleeding, the development of thrombus begins, and VTE can form within minutes of the trauma. In fact, in a group of 200 critically injured patients without vascular injury, greater than one third of the 26 patients who developed deep venous thromboses (DVTs) developed them within the first week, and 10% developed them on the first day.

DIAGNOSIS

The diagnosis of DVT is made using duplex ultrasound (DUS), which has supplanted venography as a diagnostic tool for this disease. DUS should be performed when signs of thrombus occur (unilateral extremity edema). Routine screening of asymptomatic patients is not supported by the American College of Chest Physicians (ACCP) or Eastern Association for the Surgery of Trauma (EAST). However, screening in patients who are at the highest risk and have received insufficient prophylaxis is supported by both ACCP and EAST. It is important to recognize that DUS is insufficient to diagnose VTE in pelvic vessels. Therefore, if a central thrombus is suspected, venous phase CT angiography is the diagnostic modality of choice and has also succeeded venography in most institutions. CT angiography has also surpassed conventional angiography and ventilation-perfusion scanning for the diagnosis of PE. Although computed tomography (CT) angiography is limited by a relative contraindication in patients with low creatinine clearance or with intravenous contrast allergies, it is not surpassed by the alternative modalities in these conditions. The decision to use intravenous contrast for CT angiography in these patients requires an analysis of risks and benefits to determine the need for the information provided by the study. Additionally, medical prophylaxis for patients with contrast allergies can be administered prior to the study.

MANAGEMENT

Risk Assessment

Not all patients who have a diagnosis of injury are at an increased risk of developing VTE. This is demonstrated by the extremely low

TABLE 1: Risk Factors for Venous Thromboembolism in Trauma Patients

Spinal cord injury*
Lower extremity or pelvic fracture
Need for surgical procedure
Venous injury/venous catheterization
Older age*
Prolonged immobility
Delay in thromboprophylaxis

*Consistent in meta-analyses.

incidence of VTE in NTDB reviews of injured patients. Although some of the low incidence was due to factors that prevent VTE, much of the low incidence can be attributed to the number of minimally injured patients who had a risk of VTE equal to the uninjured population. Therefore, establishing a formula for injured patients who are at an increased risk of developing VTE would be helpful. Although such a formula is not available, certain injuries and conditions are associated with higher risk (Table 1). Therefore, thromboprophylaxis should be considered for patients with these injuries.

Prevention

Prevention of VTE is the mainstay in management, and simultaneously, the most controversial aspect of the disease. Specifically, low-molecular-weight heparin (LMWH, enoxaparin 30 mg subcutaneously twice daily) and low-dose unfractionated heparin (LDUH, 5000 units subcutaneously every 8 hours) are the most effective interventions to decrease the incidence of DVT, yet have the risk of contributing to hemorrhage in a patient population that is already among the highest risk for bleeding. The use of heparin (LMWH or LDUH) is supported by the ACCP guidelines, which state, "For major trauma patient, we suggest use of LDUH (Grade 2C), LMWH (Grade 2C), preferably with intermittent pneumatic compression (IPC, Grade 2C)," and by the EAST guidelines, which state, "Trauma patients with an ISS greater than 9, who can receive anticoagulants, should receive LMWH as their primary mode of VTE prophylaxis (Level III)." Importantly, although LDUH was previously considered to be inferior to LMWH for VTE chemoprophylaxis in trauma patients, the current edition of the ACCP guidelines consider them to be equal. In patients who have a low creatinine clearance (less than 20 to 30 mL/minute) prohibiting the use of LMWH, LDUH is the preferred agent. Additionally, dalteparin (Table 2) is a LMWH that has demonstrated efficacy in VTE prophylaxis and therapy after the publication of the 9th edition of the ACCP guidelines.

For patients with temporary limitations to the use of VTE chemoprophylaxis (e.g., patients with solid-organ injury, hemorrhage from long-bone fractures, TBI), mechanical prophylaxis should be used. This includes IPC and graded compression stockings. Additionally, foot pumps can be used as an alternative to IPC in patients with external fixators or casts. ACCP guidelines state, "For trauma patients in whom LMWH and LDUH are contraindicated, we suggest mechanical prophylaxis, preferably with IPC, over no prophylaxis (Grade 2C) when not contraindicated by lower-extremity injury. We suggest adding pharmacologic prophylaxis with either LMWH or LDUH when the risk of bleeding diminishes or the contraindication to heparin resolves (Grade 2C)." The obvious remaining question is, When is the risk of bleeding diminished? Determining parameters that assess the degree of ongoing hemorrhage is helpful to establish patterns of management. In the authors' institution, a decrease in hemoglobin (Hb) of less than 1 g/dL over a 24-hour period is considered cessation of hemorrhage and the indicator to initiate chemoprophylaxis. An exception to this practice is an injury to the central nervous system, specifically TBI, spine fracture, and spinal cord injury. Initiation of chemoprophylaxis in this population requires greater caution. Relatively minimal additional hemorrhage into the brain or spinal cord can cause catastrophic changes in outcomes.

Duration

The duration of thromboprophylaxis necessary for injured patients is not yet defined. It is reasonable to continue chemoprophylaxis throughout the hospitalization and rehabilitation. Both ACCP and EAST guidelines support this practice. It is likely that some patients with prolonged immobility remain at high risk of developing VTE even after discharge. Although there are no data to provide guidance for extended VTE prophylaxis, it is certainly worthwhile to consider extended LMWH or a vitamin K antagonist (VKA, e.g., warfarin) until the patient is mobile.

Anticoagulation Therapy

When VTE occurs, the appropriate intervention is therapeutic anticoagulation with LMWH (2 mg/kg subcutaneously daily or 1 mg/kg subcutaneously twice daily), fondaparinux (see Table 2 for dosing), preferentially, over intravenous LDUH (with targeted activated partial thromboplastin time $\approx$ 50 to 80 seconds), unless contraindicated. Additionally, these agents should be started in patients for whom there is an intermediate or high suspicion for VTE while awaiting diagnostic tests to confirm VTE. Parenteral anticoagulation should continue a minimum of 5 days through initiation of a VKA and until international normalized ratio (INR) reaches 2.0 for a total of 3 months of therapy. Unlike previous recommendations, the current ACCP guidelines state that 3 months is appropriate for both DVT and PE in this posttrauma setting. Furthermore, distal leg (below knee) thrombosis should be treated as proximal leg thrombosis if there are severe symptoms or there is a high risk of extension.

Thrombolysis and Thrombectomy

For patients who are highly symptomatic from PE, interventions to address the clot burden should be considered, in order of increasing invasiveness. Specifically, if the patient is hypotensive (e.g., systolic blood pressure [SBP] less than 90 mm Hg), ACCP suggests "systemically administered thrombolytic therapy (Grade 2C) for a 2-hour infusion through a peripheral vein (Grade 2C). Furthermore, they suggest catheter-assisted thrombus removal in patients with (1) contraindication to thrombolysis, (2) failed thrombolysis, or (3) shock that is likely to cause death before systemic thrombolysis can take effect (Grade 2C). In patients (1) who are refractory to catheter-assisted

embolectomy or (2) shock is progressing more rapidly than can be treated with thrombolysis, surgical pulmonary embolectomy is suggested (Grade 2C)." The ACCP strongly recommends that the invasive procedures only be performed "in patients who have a low risk of bleeding ... [and] if appropriate surgical expertise and resources are available (Grade 2C)." Additionally, these procedures should only be performed in patients with good overall functional status and prognosis other than the VTE. In either thrombolysis or thrombectomy, continuation of anticoagulation is necessary for the same duration as patients who do not undergo thrombolysis/thrombectomy.

Vena Cava Filters

The conventional indications for vena cava filters (VCFs) are (1) proximal (popliteal vein or above) DVT or a PE with a contraindication to therapeutic anticoagulation and (2) recurrent PE despite full anticoagulation. Extended indications have evolved over the past several decades and include the following conditions: (1) large free-floating thrombus in the iliac vein or inferior vena cava (IVC), (2) following massive PE in which recurrent emboli may prove fatal, and (3) during/after surgical embolectomy. Opinions regarding the need for a VCF during thrombolysis are varied. However, most interventionalists insert VCFs following pharmacomechanical thrombolysis.

The insertion of VCFs in trauma patients remains controversial. Rogers et al, in the mid-1990s, demonstrated a benefit to selected high-risk trauma patients for a "prophylactically" inserted VCF. The term "prophylactic" was used because these patients had VCFs inserted without an identified DVT or PE. Since these early reports, a number of other trials (level II and level III evidence) have shown a benefit to VCFs in high-risk trauma patients which led to a cautious support of VCFs from the EAST guidelines for VTE. The Spinal Cord Injury Consortium (SCI Consortium) statement supports the consideration of using a VCF when prophylactic doses of anticoagulation are not safe within 72 hours from injury. In contrast, the 9th edition of the ACCP guidelines states, "For trauma patients, we suggest that an IVC filter should not be used for primary VTE prevention (Grade 2C)." It is important to address the term, "prophylactic" as it relates to VCFs. In fact, all VCFs are prophylactic in that they have no therapeutic impact on DVT or PE, but they simply prevent subsequent embolization of thrombus to the heart and lungs. Therefore, VCFs should *not* be used exclusively for the prophylaxis of DVT. However, in high-risk patients who have extended contraindications to VTE chemoprophylaxis, a VCF may at least decrease the incidence of PE, a fatal complication of VTE. EAST provides some guidance with regard to these difficult to manage patients, "Insertion of a 'prophylactic' vena caval filter should be considered in very high risk trauma patients who cannot receive anticoagulation because of increased bleeding risk, and have one or more of the following injury patterns: severe closed head injury (GCS less than 8), incomplete spinal cord injury with para or quadriplegia, complex pelvic fractures with associated long-bone fractures, multiple long-bone fractures (Level III)."

TABLE 2: Low-Molecular-Weight Heparin

Heparin	Dose	Indications	Contraindications
Enoxaparin (Lovenox)	Prophylaxis: 30 mg SC bid or 40 U SC daily* Therapy: 1 mg/kg SC bid	Appropriate for VTE prophylaxis and treatment as well as unstable angina and MI	High risk of bleeding Daily dosing recommended in spinal and epidural anesthesia
Dalteparin (Fragmin)	Prophylaxis: 5000 U SC daily Therapy: 100 anti–factor Xa U/kg SC bid	Appropriate for VTE prophylaxis and treatment as well as unstable angina and MI	High risk of bleeding

bid, Twice a day; MI, myocardial infarction; SC, subcutaneously; VTE, venous thromboembolism.
*Increase dosing to 40 mg subcutaneously twice a day in patients > 150 kg.

Similarly, the SCI Consortium recommends to, "Consider placing a vena cava filter only in those patients with active bleeding anticipated to persist for more than 72 hours and begin anticoagulants as soon as feasible (Level III/IV Grade C)." The use of VCF outside the conventional or extended indications should be based on a risk/benefit analysis for each patient. In our practice, this is frequently a multispecialty discussion regarding PE risk and prophylactic anticoagulant risk.

There has been much discussion regarding the French PREPIC (Prévention du Risque d'Embolie Pulmonaire par Interruption Cave) trial, the only randomized controlled study of VCFs. In this trial, in patients with DVT and appropriate anticoagulation, there was no difference in mortality rate and an increased rate of DVT in patients who had VCFs placed (in addition to VTE anticoagulation). The results of this trial are commonly quoted and have likely impacted the use of VCFs in the United States. However, a thorough review of this report reveals many flaws and misinterpretations. First, the patients who were randomized (filter or no filter) were *all* therapeutically anticoagulated. It is not the practice in the United States to insert VCFs in patients who can be anticoagulated. Because the mortality rate after DVT and PE with anticoagulation is low, a mortality rate benefit of adding a VCF would not be expected. The most frequently used VCF in this trial was the B. Braun Vena Tech LGM, which has had reported IVC thrombosis rates as high as 25%. Another device used was the Bard Cardial filter, which was not approved for use in the United States. In addition, all of the VCFs in the PREPIC trial were permanent devices; thus, the advantage of retrieving the device when the PE risk resolved could not be examined. For these reasons, the PREPIC trial is not applicable to current devices, standards, and practice.

Vena Cava Filter Insertion Procedure

Over the past several years, the science surrounding the insertion and retrieval of VCFs has evolved dramatically. Initially placed via laparotomy and venotomy, VCFs are now percutaneously inserted with a variety of devices, some that use insertion sheaths as small as 6 F. This technological advancement, developed for the placement of a filter in the IVC, has now been adopted by other disciplines such as interventional radiology and interventional cardiology, which perform insertion and retrieval procedures outside the operating room, in the cardiac catheterization or interventional radiology suite. Furthermore, the percutaneous nature of the VCF insertion and retrieval procedures has made it portable even to the bedside in the ICU.

The equipment needs for VCF insertion are fairly simple. Sterile technique is used with personal protection consisting of cap, eye protection, sterile gown, and gloves. Most VCFs are commonly packaged with insertion sheaths that use dilators that be used as injection catheters for caval imaging. These catheters have multiple side ports to enhance mixing of contrast agent with the blood. Premeasured radiopaque markers assist in measurement of the IVC diameter (Fig. 1). The patient is widely prepped and draped based on the planned access (similar to central venous catheterization). Venous access is most commonly the right femoral vein, but the jugular veins can also be used. Several small-profile devices can be inserted using other veins such as the subclavian, axillary, and even the antecubital and popliteal veins. Access should avoid a vein that has a known DVT. Imaging is required for the safe insertion of VCFs. In our practice, imaging is accomplished with fluoroscopy; thus, appropriate lead shielding of the torso and thyroid is necessary. Others have demonstrated the safety and efficacy of intravascular ultrasound (IVUS) and DUS. Bedside insertion in the ICU using fluoroscopy requires a fluoroscopy-capable bed. Road mapping or imaging of the vena cava is standard of care and has been demonstrated to greatly decrease insertion complications. With fluoroscopy, a contrast agent is used, either iodinated contrast, gadolinium, or carbon dioxide gas. Carbon dioxide (CO_2) gas has the advantage of having no allergic or nephrotoxic effects but does require digital subtraction, and the image quality can be negatively affected by obesity and bowel gas. Notably, the CO_2 used in fluoroscopy is not the same as that used for laparoscopy: laparoscopic grade CO_2 is 99.90% pure, whereas vascular grade CO_2 is 99.99% pure.

Once venous access is obtained, a long guidewire (typically 150 cm [length] or greater, 0.035 inch size [width]) is advanced into the IVC. Imaging of the IVC is performed to determine the IVC anatomy and the deployment site and to measure the IVC diameter (Fig. 2). We typically use 30 mL of nonionic iodinated contrast agent, injected over 2 seconds using a pressure injector. The infrarenal location is preferred, but anatomic anomalies or thrombus in this region may require suprarenal deployment. VCFs are manufactured with a range of maximum diameters, though most are 28 to 30 mm, so measurement of the vena cava diameter is important. It should be noted that there are no optional (retrievable) devices approved in the United States for diameters greater than 30 mm. Once the IVC anatomy and diameter are determined, the insertion sheath is advanced to the appropriate position for deployment in the IVC. In order to prevent perforation, it is important that no sheath or dilator is advanced without a guidewire. We commonly insert the insertion sheath beyond the planned deployment site and withdraw the sheath into position for exact placement. The actual release/deployment of the filter may be specific to the individual devices; however, conceptually they are all deployed using an "unsheathing" technique rather than "pushing out" into the IVC. A completion cavagram is made with

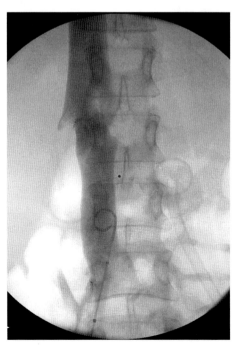

FIGURE 2   Contrast inferior vena cavagram.

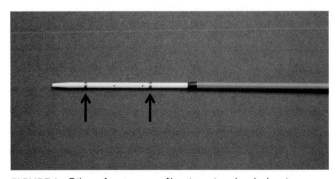

FIGURE 1   Dilator for vena cava filter insertion sheath showing radiopaque measuring guides and side holes *(arrows)*.

a hand injection through the insertion sheath to document the orientation and placement of the filter. Prior to and during the procedure, we flush all catheters, dilators, and tubing with saline to avoid thrombus formation within the catheters and to avoid air embolism. The insertion sheath is removed and gentle pressure is held for 10 minutes (15 minutes if the patient is anticoagulated), and an adhesive dressing is applied to the site.

There are several caveats to consider in the bedside insertion of VCFs, in particular when using fluoroscopy. First, radiation safety is a priority. Following the three tenets of radiation safety—time, distance, and shielding—this procedure can be performed safely at the bedside. Fluoroscopy time should be kept to a minimum (commonly less than 60 seconds). Anyone not directly involved should maintain a minimum distance of 3 meters from the patient, where scatter exposure is negligible. Those involved with the procedure should be appropriately lead shielded, both torso and thyroid. The second caveat to bedside VCF insertion is *not* to lower the side bed rail, as the sterile drapes can be fashioned into a "valley" for catheters, syringes, etc. Furthermore, the raised rail can perform its function of keeping the patient from rolling onto the floor!

Vena Cava Filter Retrieval Procedure

In 2003, the first Food and Drug Administration (FDA)-approved device for removal in the United States was the Bard Recovery IVC filter (Fig. 3). This device was removed using a proprietary retrieval cone. Since that time, a number of other "optional" devices have been approved (Fig. 4). These all have a hook in either the cephalad or caudal ends, allowing them to be ensnared with an endovascular snare.

Most retrievals are performed as an outpatient procedure that allows a period of time for the PE risk to subside. Patients who can be therapeutically anticoagulated can have their VCF removed once they have demonstrated no evidence of bleeding for 7 days. A preoperative, lower extremity DUS is performed within 72 hours of the retrieval to determine stability of known DVT or to identify new DVT. Obviously, a new DVT in the face of not being anticoagulated will contraindicate retrieval unless the patient is anticoagulated.

Anesthesia is based on patient preference and tolerance. We perform most procedures with conscious sedation and local anesthesia at the site of the retrieval-sheath insertion. VCFs that have had long implant durations (more than 12 months) are more uncomfortable when being disengaged from the IVC, and in these cases, we tend

to use deep sedation or general anesthesia. We also use general anesthesia for brain-injured patients as they tend to move too much and are typically inconsolable.

Retrieval is accomplished by "ensnaring" a hook on the filter using a gooseneck or multiloop endovascular snare. The majority of the currently available removable devices are retrieved via the jugular system, except for the OptEase (Cordis Endovascular), which is retrieved via the femoral approach and the Crux (Volcano Corp), which can be retrieved via the jugular or the femoral approach. Once venous access is achieved, a 5 F injection catheter is positioned caudad to the VCF. Contrast cavagraphy is performed in both the anteroposterior (AP) and lateral projections to determine the orientation of the filter within the IVC and to determine the presence or absence of thrombus within the filter. The presence of trapped thrombus within the filter in a non-anticoagulated patient is an indication that the procedure should be aborted and the patient started on therapeutic anticoagulation with a plan for a later attempt at retrieval. If the patient is anticoagulated, small clots (less than 25% of the depth of the cone) can be removed with the filter. After review of the cavagram, the injection catheter is removed over a guidewire, and a large sheath is inserted. We use a dual sheath system with a 12 F outer sheath over a 9 F inner sheath. Once the sheaths are in place, a snare is inserted to "lasso" the hook. The hook of the VCF is snared, the inner sheath is advanced over the tip of the filter while maintaining tension with the snare and prior to pulling the filter into the sheath (Fig. 5). The filter is withdrawn into the inner sheath and to avoid dragging the filter through the sheath, the entire inner sheath is removed (see Fig. 5). Different devices may have slightly differing retrieval techniques. A short tug is usually required to disengage the struts from the wall of the IVC. The VCF is removed and examined on the back table to document that the filter is intact. The injection catheter is reinserted, and a completion cavagram is performed to document no extravasation and the integrity of the IVC. Pressure is held for 10 minutes after the sheath is removed (minimum of 15 minutes if the patient is anticoagulated). It is not necessary to correct the INR for retrieval. The patients are discharged from the recovery room after a 2-hour observation period.

LIMITATIONS TO GUIDELINES

Although the recommendations for prevention and management of VTE are helpful for a segment of the population, many injured patients have conditions that place them outside the scope of these recommendations. Often these are the most critically ill patients for whom medical decision making is challenging in many aspects. We have included discussion of these patients in the following sections.

Hemorrhaging Patients

Patients with ongoing hemorrhage have a clear contraindication to chemoprophylaxis. Interestingly, it is not evident that the associated coagulopathy protects hemorrhaging patients from VTE. Hemorrhagic control is the mainstay of management. During hemorrhage, pneumatic compression devices are the reasonable option for VTE prophylaxis. When the hemorrhage is controlled, initiation of chemoprophylaxis is appropriate. Physiologic parameters such as Hb drift are appropriate determinants of cessation of hemorrhage. As mentioned previously, parameters such as an Hb decrease of less than 1 g/dL over a 24-hour period can be considered cessation of hemorrhage and the indicator for beginning chemoprophylaxis.

Multitrauma with Drifting Hemoglobin

A common clinical scenario following trauma is a patient with multiple injuries without active hemorrhage but with drifting Hb levels. This can often persist for many days, depending on the number

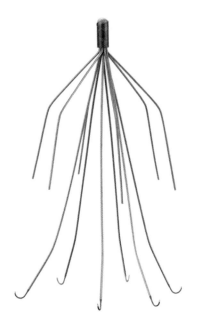

FIGURE 3   The Bard Recovery vena cava filter. *(© 2015 C.R. Bard, Inc. Used with permission.)*

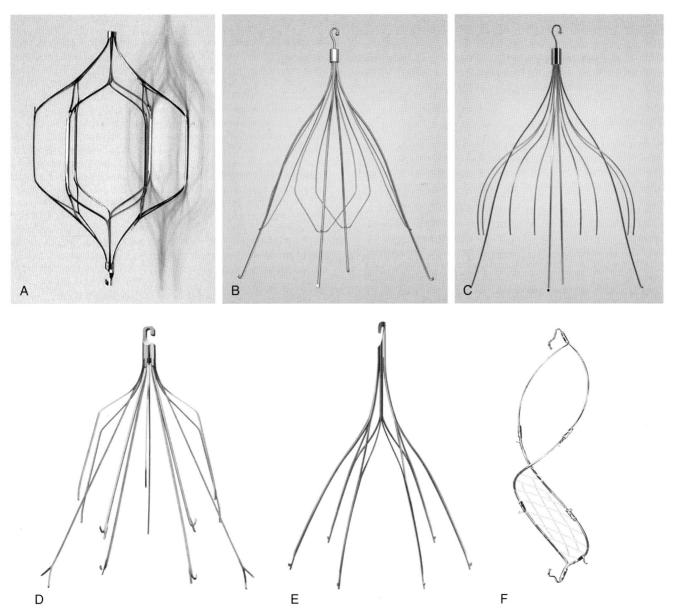

FIGURE 4   Several optional vena cava filters. **A,** OptEase (Cordis Endovascular). **B,** Tulip (Cook Medical). **C,** Celect (Cook Medical). **D,** Denali (© 2015 C.R. Bard, Inc. Used with permission). **E,** Option Elite (Argon Medical). **F,** Crux (Volcano Medical).

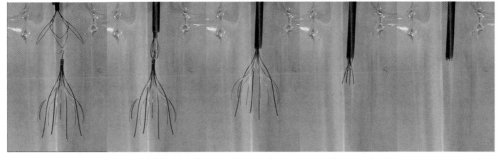

FIGURE 5   Snare technique for vena cava filter retrieval.

of injuries, the timing of stabilization (e.g., splenic embolization, fixation of long-bone fractures), the nutritional status, and the catabolic state of the patient. Often these patients will have a decrease in Hb of nearly 1 g/dL on subsequent days. Although the daily small decreases are not contraindications to chemoprophylaxis, the cumulative change can contribute to the need for transfusion, delays to the operating room while stability is somewhat compromised, and an unwillingness to initiate chemoprophylaxis. Additionally, the use of pneumatic compression devices may be inhibited by splints, casts, or traction.

In these patients, it is often necessary to determine if physiologically indicated blood transfusions are an acceptable risk of the initiation of VTE chemoprophylaxis. If not and chemoprophylaxis is withheld, insertion of a VCF may be considered. Importantly, multiply injured patients are among those with the highest risk of VTE and have the poorest ability to tolerate such an insult.

Traumatic Brain Injury

Patients with traumatic brain injury are probably the most controversial patient population with regard to VTE prophylaxis. This is understandable because this widely diverse population is at high risk for VTE, is substantially compromised from the development of VTE, and can be neurologically devastated from the hemorrhagic complications of VTE chemoprophylaxis. Interestingly, the governing bodies recommending prevention of VTE provide little to no guidance with regard to patients with TBI. The ACCP has no recommendation, and EAST states that "LMWH has not been sufficiently studied in the head-injured patient with intracranial bleeding to justify its use at this time (Level III), and the Brain Trauma Foundation acknowledges that, no reliable data can support a recommendation regarding when it is safe to begin pharmacological prophylaxis (Level III)." Authors of a recent prospective observational study suggested that it is safe to begin enoxaparin within 48 hours after admission with a TBI and strongly encouraged its use in patients with TBI and additional high-risk traumatic injuries. However, 1.1% of their patients had clinically significant progression of cerebral hemorrhage following administration of enoxaparin, and one patient died from this progression of cerebral hemorrhage as a direct result of the enoxaparin use. Additionally, many patients with brain injury (e.g., intracerebral hematomas or contusions more than 2 cm in diameter, multiple small contusions within one region of the brain, subdural or epidural hematomas more than 8 mm thick, persistent intracranial pressure greater than 20 mm Hg, increased size or number of brain lesions on 24-hour follow-up CT scan, and neurosurgeon or trauma surgeon reluctance to initiate prophylaxis) were excluded. This highly specific group substantially limits the population to which this recommendation can be applied.

In contrast to the patients who hemorrhage from intra-abdominal sources, it is clear that progression of hemorrhage from brain injury is not an acceptable "compromise" to the benefit of protection from VTE. Caution in this patient population should be focused on prevention of hemorrhage rather than prevention of VTE. Decision making in TBI patients should focus on the extent of the initial injury, the risk of progression, and the risk of compromise from VTE. For example, the patient with a few punctate frontal contusions and a Glasgow Coma Scale (GCS) score of 15 has a different VTE and hemorrhage risk than the patient with a 2-cm frontal contusion and a GCS score of 6. Similarly, the awake patient with a subarachnoid hemorrhage has a lower risk of compromise from hemorrhage than the comatose patient with a 1-cm subarachnoid hemorrhage that requires evacuation. Beginning VTE prophylaxis should be a multispecialty discussion. The decision-making group should include the neurosurgeon, the trauma surgeon, and (depending on the institution) the intensivist managing the patient. Guides such as repeat CT scans to determine the stability of hemorrhage before starting prophylaxis are useful tools.

Spinal Cord Injury

Patients with spinal cord injury are another unique patient population. They have the highest risk of developing VTE with or without thromboprophylaxis, and their risk extends longer than for most other patients because of their prolonged immobility. ACCP, EAST, and the SCI Consortium all recommend early chemoprophylaxis. However, in patients with spinal hematomas, chemoprophylaxis should be delayed until hemostasis is evident.

Obesity

Obesity leads to increased complications in many facets of care. With regard to VTE, the overall risk is higher simply due to obesity, dosing regimens are not defined, and interventions such as VCF placement are much more difficult in this patient population. Owing to the increased risk of VTE, all obese patients admitted with injury, even with minor injuries, should be treated in a high-risk category. Additionally, traditional doses of prophylactic and therapeutic LMWH and LUFH are likely to be insufficient for obese patients. Recent studies addressing LMWH safety using anti–factor Xa levels suggest that most patients are underdosed with current dosing regimens, and the obese patients are most frequently underdosed. The ACCP recommends, "For patients undergoing inpatient bariatric surgery, we suggest that higher doses of LMWH or LDUH than usual for non-obese patients be used (Grade 2C)." Although this recommendation is ambiguous, it is consistent with the concern that traditional doses are insufficient. Until these doses are well defined, anti–factor Xa may be the most helpful guide to therapy. Increasing enoxaparin dosing to 60 mg twice a day or 0.5 mg/kg daily is a reasonable option to consider.

Extensive Immobility

Although extensive immobility is often associated with spinal cord injury, it can often be related to multiple lower extremity fractures with limitations to weight bearing that exceed 12 weeks. Thromboprophylaxis started during hospitalization should ideally continue in some form after discharge in these patients. Although randomized controlled trials are not available to guide this management, we can extrapolate from the current ACCP and EAST guidelines that the VTE prophylaxis should continue for the extent of the immobility. In such situations, VKAs are preferable to LMWH.

Epidural Catheters

The only organization to make a recommendation regarding epidural catheters is EAST, which states, "LMWH should not be in use when epidural catheters are placed or removed (Level III)." However, the use of LMWH in conjunction with epidural catheters has now been accepted by many anesthesia societies when specific criteria are achieved. A consortium of guidelines from multiple national anesthesiology organizations (including the American Society of Regional Anesthesia and Pain Medicine) provides recommendations for the use of LMWH in conjunction with epidural catheters (Table 3).

Heparin-Induced Thrombocytopenia

Thrombocytopenia is a frequent finding following trauma and surgery. Common causes include platelet consumption from

---

TABLE 3: Epidural Catheters and Low-Molecular-Weight Heparin

LMWH should be administered using once daily dosing.

Dosing should be prophylactic only.

LMWH should be administered a minimum of 10–12 hours *before* the insertion or removal of the catheter.

LMWH should be administered a minimum of 2–4 hours *after* the insertion or removal of the catheter.

LMWH, Low-molecular-weight heparin.

TABLE 4: Alternative Anticoagulants for Heparin-Induced Thrombocytopenia

Agent	Dose	Monitoring	Notes
Argatroban (Argatroban)	Bolus: none Infusion: 2 µg/kg/min	Goal aPTT = 1.5–3.0 × baseline	Dose reduction in hepatic failure
Bivalrudin (Angiomax)	Bolus: none Infusion: 0.15 mg/kg/hr	Goal aPTT = 1.5–2.5 × baseline	
Fondaparinux	<50 kg: 5 mg SC daily 50–100 kg: 7.5 mg SC daily >100 kg: 10 mg SC daily	May adjust to peak anti–factor Xa activity of 1.5 fondaparinux U/mL	Limited or contraindicated in renal impairment
Lepirudin* (Refludan)	Bolus: 0.4 mg/kg Infusion: 0.15 mg/kg/hr	Goal aPTT = 1.5–2.5 × baseline In absence of thrombus, omit bolus and use aPTT goal of 1.5–2.0 × baseline	Dose reduction in renal failure

aPTT, Activated partial thromboplastic time; SC, subcutaneously.
*Not currently available in the United States.

hemorrhage and lack of thrombopoiesis due to malnutrition and acute illness. However, for those patients receiving heparin (unfractionated or low-molecular-weight heparin), heparin-induced thrombocytopenia (HIT) must be considered as a cause, when thrombocytopenia occurs. For patients with thrombocytopenia due to causes other than heparin, heparin administration still remains the preferred prophylaxis for VTE. Therefore, identifying those patients in whom the thrombocytopenia is due to heparin administration is critical. The common presentation of HIT includes patients with a 50% decrease in platelet count between 5 and 14 days of initial heparin dose, and a nadir above 20,000 platelets per milliliter. Alternatively, if the patient has recently (past 30 days) been exposed to heparin, heparin antibodies may have previously been formed and may contribute to an immediate decrease in platelet count.

HIT can be divided into two types. HIT type I results in platelet counts below $150,000 \times 10^9$/L, but above $100,000 \times 10^9$/L, and is not associated with an immune reaction. Although HIT type I can result in exacerbation of the thrombocytopenia from other causes, cessation of heparin is not necessary. In contrast, HIT type II is associated with an IgG antibody formation to platelet factor 4 (PF4) resulting in platelet, heparin immune complex formation, and local thrombus formation. This subset of HIT is present in 5% of patients receiving heparin and can result in much more substantial thrombocytopenia (platelet counts of $20,000 \times 10^9$/L to $100,000 \times 10^9$/L) as well as severe complications and even death from thrombi. Additionally, the thrombocytopenia can potentiate ongoing hemorrhage. The definitive diagnosis for HIT type II is through identifying the heparin-PF4 antibodies through enzyme-linked immunosorbent assay (ELISA) and flow cytometry. Cessation of heparin administration is necessary to allow resolution of immune activation and recovery of platelet concentration. Additionally, alternative thromboprophylactic agents must be provided to limit the thrombosis. Argatroban and lepirudin are the two FDA-approved agents for treatment of patients with HIT (Table 4). A Clinical Practice Guideline on the Evaluation and Management of Adults with Suspected Heparin-induced Thrombocytopenia, created by the American Society of Hematology in conjunction with the ACCP, provides helpful information on diagnosis and management of HIT in surgical and nonsurgical patients.

Upper Extremity/Thoracic Deep Venous Thrombosis and Superficial Venous Thrombosis

Management of upper extremity and thoracic DVTs is essentially the same as that of lower extremity DVTs. The vessels considered deep veins of the upper extremity and thoracic cavity include the axillary, subclavian, internal jugular, and innominate veins. For upper extremity DVTs associated with central venous catheters, the ACCP suggests that the "catheter not be removed if it is functional if there is an ongoing need for the catheter (Grade 2C)." Anticoagulation should be continued for 3 months (grade 1B) or as long as the catheter remains (grade 1C).

Superficial venous thromboses (SVTs) of the lower limb that are at least 5 cm in length should be treated with prophylactic doses of fondaparinux (2.5 mg daily) or LMWH for 45 days (grade 2B). There are no recommendations for SVTs of the upper extremities.

MORBIDITY AND COMPLICATIONS MANAGEMENT

The consequences of VTE are dependent on the location of the thrombus. In the extremity, long-term thrombus results in venous stasis with loss of integrity of venous valves, vasodilation, and extremity edema. This can ultimately lead to skin changes and limitation to wound healing. Although much of the venous stasis is not evident in the acute setting, it can lead to a lifetime of morbidity.

The morbidity of PE can be much more dramatic and, consequently, is identified in the acute setting. The onset of hypoxia and even hemodynamic instability require immediate intervention beginning with physiologic support and extending to thrombectomy.

CONCLUSIONS AND ALGORITHM

All injured patients should be evaluated for the risk of VTE. Because of the low risk of placement of sequential depression devices, these devices should be considered in all patients. Patients stratified to moderate- or high-risk categories for VTE should receive LMWH for the duration of their hospitalization or until their mobility normalizes. For patients with contraindications to LMWH for more than 72 hours following injury, VCFs *may* be considered. The determination of contraindication should be made with a multispecialty approach. The algorithm in Figure 6 can be followed as a guide for these challenging and crucial decisions.

For the chapter's Suggested Readings list, please visit the book at www.ExpertConsult.inkling.com.

VTE Prophylaxis Algorithm

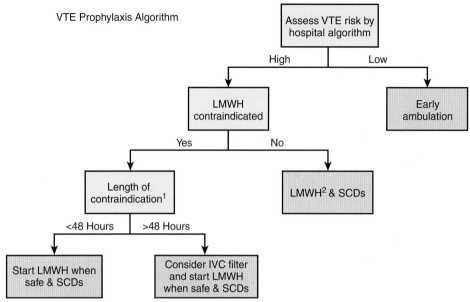

FIGURE 6 Venous thromboembolism (VTE) prophylaxis algorithm. *1*, Contraindications to low-molecular-weight heparin (LMWH): (a) Unstable hemoglobin. (b) Solid organ injury. Patients can be started on LMWH when the patient has had less than 1 g/dL decrease in hemoglobin over 24 hours and there are no other contraindications. (c) Intracranial bleed and spinal cord injury. Neurologic injuries have high incidence of VTE and also high morbidity associated with further bleeding. LMWH should be started as soon as possible as determined by neurosurgical/neuropedic consultation. (d) Coagulopathy defined as a platelet count less than $50,000 \times 10^9/mm^3$ or an international normalized ratio (INR) or activated partial thromboplastin time more than 1.5 times normal. (e) Creatinine higher than 1.6. These patients should be started on subcutaneous heparin 5000 units every 8 hours if there are no other contraindications to chemoprophylaxis. 2, LMWH should be dosed 30 mg every 12 hours. If the patient weighs more than 150 kg, the dosing should be increased to 40 mg every 12 hours. IVC, Inferior vena cava; SCD, sequential compression device.

HYPOTHERMIA AND TRAUMA

Larry M. Gentilello and R. Lawrence Reed II

Human beings, as homeotherms, maintain their temperature within a narrow range around a core temperature of 37° C. Hypothermia is associated with an increase in fatality in trauma patients. However, because it occurs more frequently in more seriously injured patients, there has been uncertainty over whether this increase in fatality is primarily attributable to the hypothermia itself, or to the severity of the underlying injuries. Some have proposed that hypothermia is protective during shock, and mortality rates would not be higher when injury severity and other risk factors are taken into account. However, recent prospective studies have documented an adverse effect of hypothermia on outcome and a significantly improved likelihood of successful resuscitation when hypothermia is aggressively treated.

DETRIMENTAL EFFECTS OF HYPOTHERMIA

Effects on Coagulation

Perhaps the most serious effects of hypothermia are its impact on coagulation (Fig. 1). The extent to which hypothermia causes coagulation problems is often underestimated because of the multiplicity of potential causes for coagulation impairment that are usually present.

These patients often have acidosis, tissue trauma, shock, dilution of circulating blood volume, and reduced concentrations of clotting factors. Normal coagulation requires adequate platelet count and function and adequate clotting factor levels and activity. Theoretically, hypothermia could affect blood coagulation in each of these domains.

EFFECTS ON PLATELET COUNT AND FUNCTION

Experimental studies in dogs have demonstrated a reversible thrombocytopenia associated with systemic hypothermia. However, this only occurs at levels of hypothermia well below that typically seen in a trauma setting (<30° C).

Platelets experience a reversible inhibition of function during hypothermia, mediated at least in part through the temperature dependence of thromboxane B_2, a potent vasoconstrictor that stimulates platelet aggregation. The effect of hypothermia was demonstrated by Valeri and associates, who induced hypothermia in baboons, but kept one arm normothermic by using heating blankets and radiant warmers. Simultaneous bleeding time measurements in the warm and cold arm were 2.4 and 5.8 minutes, respectively. Owing to the effect of hypothermia on platelet function, transfusions in hypothermic patients may not be effective at reducing blood loss without concomitant, effective core rewarming.

EFFECTS ON CLOTTING FACTOR LEVELS AND FUNCTION

Studies suggest that alterations in clotting factor activity do not occur except at temperatures below 33° C. Yet, clinical experience suggests

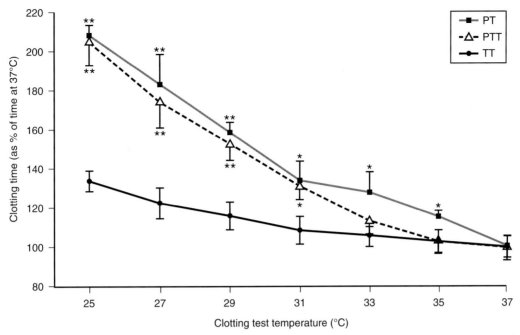

FIGURE 1   Comparison of effects of clotting test temperature with progressive degrees of hypothermia. Clotting times were performed on standard concentrations of assayed reference plasma using a fibrometer modified to enable control of the temperature at which the clotting test was conducted. PT, Prothrombin time; PTT, partial thromboplastin time; TT, thrombin time. *$P < .001$ vs. thrombin time prolongation. **$P < .0001$ vs. thrombin time prolongation. *(Modified from Reed R, Bracey A, Hudson J, et al: Hypothermia and blood coagulation: dissociation between enzyme activity and clotting factor levels. Circ Shock 32:141–152, 1990.)*

otherwise. This apparent discrepancy was highlighted in a study of the kinetic effects of hypothermia on clotting factor function undertaken by Reed et al. Standard hospital fibrometers are temperature standardized to 37° C, and do not measure clotting times at the patient's actual core temperature. In this study, an external digital temperature controller was connected to the heat block to enable measurement of clotting times at the range of hypothermic temperatures typically encountered in trauma patients.

Measurement of the prothrombin time, partial thromboplastin time, and thrombin time was performed on human plasma containing normal levels of all clotting factors at temperatures ranging from 25° to 37° C. The significant slowing of clotting factor function, with a prolongation of all three coagulations tests, was proportional to the degree of hypothermia. A subsequent study demonstrated that hypothermia could produce a coagulopathy functionally equivalent to a severe clotting factor deficiency, even at intermediate levels of hypothermia, and even though there was no actual deficiency of clotting factors (Fig. 2).

These results were confirmed by Gubler and colleagues in a study using a similar modified fibrometer that demonstrated an additive effect of hypothermia on dilutional coagulopathy (Fig. 3). A recent analysis indicates that at mild temperature reductions between 33° and 37° C, platelet activity and aggregation are more profoundly affected than are clotting factors, and are more responsible for hypothermia-related coagulopathy, although clotting factor dysfunction becomes increasingly severe as temperature cools further.

FIGURE 2   Relative clotting factor activities at various temperatures expressed as percentage of normal clotting factor activity. *(Data from Johnston T, Chen Y, Reed R: Functional equivalence of hypothermia to specific clotting factor deficiencies. J Trauma 37:413–417, 1994.)*

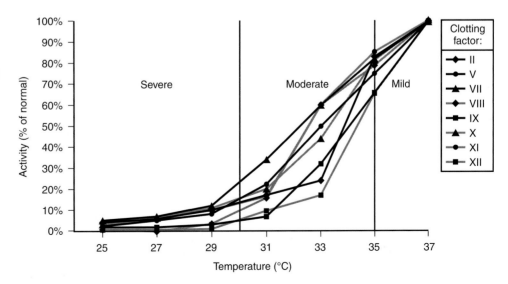

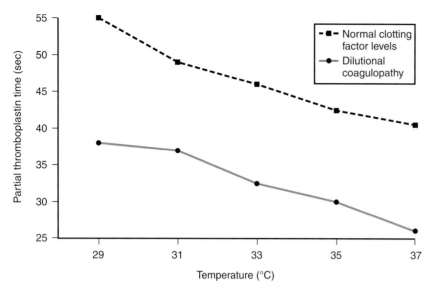

FIGURE 3 Prolongation of partial thromboplastin time (PTT) that results from cooling of the blood in samples with normal clotting factor levels, and in samples of blood with diluted clotting factor levels. *(Data from Gubler K, Gentilello L, Hassantash S, Maier R: The impact of hypothermia on dilutional coagulopathy. J Trauma 36:847–851, 1994.)*

In summary, hypothermia does little to affect platelet and clotting factor levels, but it does a great deal to affect the function of these coagulation components.

EFFECTS ON OTHER ORGANS

The organ systems that are most commonly affected by hypothermia include the circulatory, immunologic, neurologic, and coagulation systems. Cardiac function can be affected by hypothermia in the form of bradydysrhythmias, and at a core temperature below 28° to 30° C, ventricular fibrillation often occurs. Shivering, the body's attempt at restoring normothermia, results in a significant elevation of oxygen consumption, which exacerbates the effects of inadequate oxygen delivery on core organs, and increases the risk of cardiac complications in elderly patients.

The potential immunologic consequences of hypothermia have been extensively studied. Because of the enzymatic nature of most immunologic functions, it makes sense that hypothermia would inhibit many of these processes. Moreover, our immunologic system is often pitted against bacteria that are not homeothermic, and may therefore not suffer as severe a functional deterioration in the presence of a hypothermic environment. Some well-done clinical studies provide evidence that even mild hypothermia is associated with an increased risk for surgical site infection.

Neurologically, hypothermia can be detrimental and produces mental status changes when temperature drops below 33° C. Respiratory drive is increased during the early stages of hypothermia, but below 33° C progressive respiratory depression occurs, resulting in a decline in minute ventilation. Reduction in blood pressure and cardiac output decreases glomerular filtration rate, but urinary output is maintained due to an impairment in renal tubular Na^+ reabsorption (cold diuresis). Vasoconstriction also results in an initial increase in central blood volume, which prompts a diuresis.

MANAGEMENT

Humans produce heat by combustion, as a byproduct of oxygen consumption. In considering management options it is important to consider the underlying mechanism of the hypothermia. Primary accidental hypothermia occurs in patients with normal heat production who are submerged in cold water or stranded in a cold environment. These patients initially have increased heat production due to shivering, but temperature preservation is eventually overwhelmed by the degree of cold stress.

Hypothermia in trauma patients occurs through a different mechanism, and is referred to as secondary accidental hypothermia. The definition of shock is a decrease in systemic oxygen delivery to a point at which normal oxygen consumption can no longer be maintained. This decrease in heat production makes the patient vulnerable to even mild cold stresses, such as occur in the emergency department or operating room environment. Through this mechanism, all seriously injured patients in shock are at high risk of developing hypothermia.

Passive Rewarming

The specific heat of the body is 0.83 kcal/kg/° C. This means that 0.83 kcal are required to raise the temperature of 1 kg of body mass by 1° C. Thus, a 70-kg patient must gain 58.1 kcal to raise average body temperature by 1° C. Because basal heat production is approximately 1 kcal/kg/hour, endogenous heat production in a 70-kg patient will produce a rewarming rate of roughly 1.2° C/hour if the patient is sufficiently insulated to prevent further heat loss (Fig. 4).

Compared to the patient's endogenous heat production, most rewarming methods add little additional thermal energy to the patient. Clinically observed rewarming is most often a result of the patient's own heat production, coupled with the use of insulative techniques to prevent further heat losses. The most important principle in the treatment of hypothermia is to correct the underlying shock, which will restore oxygen consumption and heat production to normal levels, while aggressively preventing further heat loss.

Active External Rewarming

Heat flows from an area of higher temperature to one of lower temperature as a function of the laws of thermodynamics (entropy). Because the temperature of the skin is generally 10° C cooler than the core in a vasoconstricted, hypothermic patient, the skin must first be warmed to a temperature greater than that of the core before heat transfer to the core can occur. Therefore, external rewarming has little immediate effectiveness, and should not be relied upon as the principal means of rewarming patients who are suffering adverse effects of hypothermia.

Convective air rewarmers provide a large surface area for heat exchange. However, the density of air is so low that it contains very little thermal energy. For example, a human can tolerate a 150° F sauna for 10 minutes, but inserting a hand in 150 ° F water for 10 seconds will result in a serious burn injury.

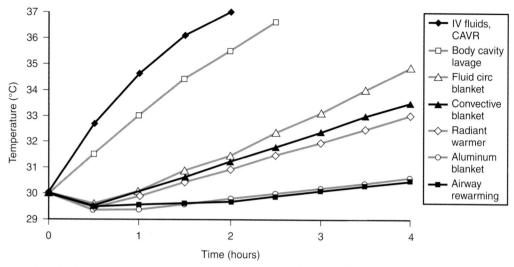

FIGURE 4   Computerized simulation of rewarming rates using various clinical techniques. CAVR, Continuous arteriovenous rewarming; circ, circulating; IV, intravenous. *(Modified from Gentilello LM, Moujaes S: Treatment of hypothermia in trauma victims: thermodynamic considerations. J Intensive Care Med 10:5–14, 1995.)*

The low heat-carrying capacity of air means that very little heat can be transferred to a patient by blowing warm air over the skin. However, an additional consequence of entropy is that when two masses are in contact with one another, heat always flows from the area of higher temperature to the area of lower temperature. The purpose of a convective warmer is to establish a layer of air around the patient that is warmer than skin temperature. Although this transfers little heat to the patient, the law of entropy prevents all further heat loss from the covered skin (except through sweating).

These devices may be used to minimize heat loss from covered areas, but are ineffective means of treating hypothermia, and most of the actual warming that is observed is due to the patient's own heat generation. In a randomized treatment study hypothermic patients did not warm faster with a convective heating blanket than with a standard cotton hospital blanket.

Aluminum space blankets are made of material often used as a lining in survival apparel, and are designed to minimize radiant heat loss by reflecting emitted photons back to the patient. The distance between the emitting and reflective surface is an important determinant of effectiveness. Proper use requires wrapping the blanket relatively tightly over the patient, and placement of an additional standard blanket on top of the space blanket to minimize underlying air movement. Because scalp vessels do not vasoconstrict even in hypothermic patients, a large amount of radiant heat loss occurs above the neck. Wrapping the head or covering it with a reflective cap may prevent cephalic heat loss.

Active Core Rewarming

Airway rewarming using humidified air at 41° C is a frequently used core rewarming technique. Fully saturated 41° C air can hold 0.05 mL H_2O/L. At 30° C air can only hold only 0.03 mL H_2O/L. If a 30° C patient inspires a liter of saturated 41° C air, then 0.02 mL H_2O condenses within the airway when the air cools down to 30° C within the lung space. Thus, with a minute ventilation of 10 L/minute, 12 mL of H_2O will condense each hour. When water condenses, heat is liberated at a rate of 0.58 kcal/mL H_2O (latent heat of vaporization). Therefore, the amount of heat contributed by airway rewarming under these conditions will only achieve a maximum of 7 kcal/hour (0.58 kcal/mL H_2O × 12 mL H_2O/hour). An additional 1 to 2 kcal will be transferred by the warming effect of the inspired air, independent of condensation. Because 58 kcal is required to increase core temperature by 1° C in a 70-kg patient,

as with external rewarming techniques, airway rewarming has limited effectiveness.

Pleural or peritoneal lavage is sometimes considered for use in unstable patients with a deleterious response to hypothermia. The amount of heat transferred depends on the difference between the inlet and outlet water temperature, and the water flow rate. Because the specific heat of water is 1 kcal/kg/° C, if 1 L of 42° C water infused into a body cavity exits at 35° C, 7 kcal of heat will have been left in the body. However, prolonging operative time in order to irrigate an open peritoneal cavity with warm fluids is counterproductive, as most of the heat that is lost from the water will be transferred to the 21° C operating room environment, rather than to the patient.

The high specific heat of water makes it important to warm cold intravenous (IV) fluid prior to administration. A patient will have to generate 16 kcal to warm 1 L of crystalloid infused into the body at room temperature (21° C). When patients are under anesthesia, their metabolic rate is relatively fixed. If they cannot increase their metabolic rate to generate this additional heat, the loss of 16 kcal will decrease the body temperature of a 70-kg patient by 0.28° C, which is enough to cause vigorous shivering.

The need to have an effective means of warming blood products is evident, as they are typically frozen or kept at temperatures as low as 4° C. The specific heat of blood is close to that of water. Thus, an infusion of 1 L of 4° C blood is sufficient to reduce body temperature by 0.56° C. Inadequately warmed IV fluids and blood products in patients in shock or under anesthesia, who cannot increase their heat production, are a major cause of hypothermia in trauma patients.

When IV fluids are adequately warmed, they provide a simple means of transferring significant amounts of heat to patients requiring large volume fluid resuscitation. Fluids administered into the body equilibrate with body temperature, liberating heat in the process. Given the specific heat of water, a 1-L infusion of 40° C crystalloid infused into a 32° C patient is, in effect, equivalent to a transfusion of 8 kcal. Because hypothermic trauma patients frequently require massive fluid resuscitation, warm IV fluids can provide a significant quantity of heat, depending upon the difference in temperature between the body and the infused fluid.

MORTALITY

Current recommendations for treatment of injured patients call for strict efforts to prevent hypothermia, and for aggressive treatment to reverse it once it has occurred. These recommendations are based

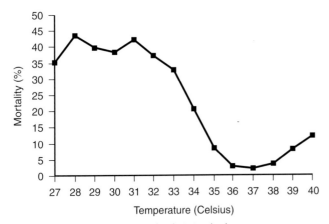

FIGURE 5 Mortality rate at each admission body temperature determined from the National Trauma Data Bank (NTDB).

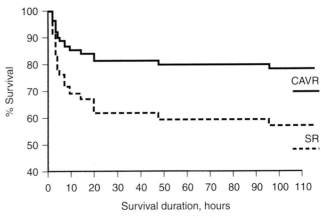

FIGURE 6 Cumulative survival (Kaplan-Meier) comparing patients treated with standard rewarming (SR) methods, or with continuous arteriovenous rewarming (CAVR), an extracorporeal technique performed by placing a catheter into the femoral artery and vein, connecting them to a heat exchanger, and using the patient's blood pressure to create a fistula through a fluid warming device. CAVR patients rewarmed significantly faster ($P < .001$). Differences in mortality rate occurred primarily during resuscitation ($P = .047$). *(From Gentilello LM, Jurkovich GJ, Stark MS, et al: Is Hypothermia in the major trauma victim protective or harmful? A randomized, prospective study. Ann Surg 226:439-449, 1997.)*

on clinical studies demonstrating that mortality rate is significantly higher in trauma patients who develop hypothermia. One study controlled for magnitude of injury using the Injury Severity Score (ISS), the presence or absence of shock, and fluid and blood product requirements. Patients who became hypothermic had significantly higher mortality rates than similarly injured patients who remained normothermic. Mortality rate was 100% if core body temperature dropped to 32° C, even in mildly injured patients.

A study analyzing the NTDB (National Trauma Data Bank) found that hypothermia was an independent predictor of mortality rate by using stepwise logistic regression (odds ratio 1.54, 95%; confidence interval [CI] 1.40– to 1.71) (Fig. 5). An additional NTDB analysis spanning 8 years stratified hypothermic and normothermic patients by Injury Severity Score and shock, and used logistic regression to control for multiple potential confounders including age; sex; mechanism of injury; severity of head, chest, and abdominal injuries; Glasgow Coma Scale score; and base deficit. Although hypothermia was more common in more seriously injured patients, hypothermia remained a strong, independent predictor of mortality rate (odds ratio, 1.19; 95% CI, 1.05 to 1.35).

A prospective study compared the mortality rate of hypothermic patients (<35° C) admitted over a 10-month period who were treated with a combination of airway rewarming, fluid circulating or convective heating blankets, an aluminized head covering, and warm IV fluids, with a consecutive sample of patients who were rapidly rewarmed with continuous arteriovenous rewarming (CAVR). Time to rewarming (T >35° C) was 3.23 hours with standard rewarming techniques and 39 minutes with CAVR. Rapid rewarming with CAVR resulted in a 57% decrease in blood product requirements, a 67% decrease in crystalloid requirements, and a reduction in mortality rate in trauma patients (Fig. 6).

In a prospective randomized clinical trial comparing slow versus rapid rewarming in critically injured patients, significantly more patients in the rapid rewarming (CAVR) group were able to be successfully resuscitated ($P < .01$).

INDUCED HYPOTHERMIA

There is a long history of research on the use of induced hypothermia to reduce ischemic injury in various clinical contexts. Initial laboratory studies suggested that hypothermia after traumatic brain injury appeared promising, with virtually every study demonstrating neuroprotective effects. However, induced hypothermia with the intention of providing a therapeutic effect in trauma patients has resulted in an increase in complications and harm in certain patient subgroups, without any convincing evidence of benefit.

Clifton conducted a National Institutes of Health (NIH) sponsored randomized, multicenter clinical trial, the North American

Acute Brain Injury Study (NABIS). A total of 392 patients were enrolled, making it the largest study to date of induced hypothermia in trauma patients. The investigation was terminated early because of futility, with 56% of patients in both groups having a poor outcome and similar mortality rate (28% and 27%). Patients in the hypothermia group had more complications, including hypotensive episodes and infections. Poor outcomes with hypothermia were more common in patients over the age of 45 (88% vs. 69%, $P = .08$).

The investigators also conducted NABIS II, a similar randomized trial, with earlier, more aggressive cooling. Despite rapid induction of hypothermia, the outcome was poor in 31 of 52 hypothermia patients (60%), and 25 of 45 control patients (55%). Twelve patients in the hypothermia group died, compared to eight in the normothermia group. This study was also terminated owing to futility. The investigators concluded that there is no further basis for testing the idea that hypothermia is protective after diffuse brain injury, and that further research is needed to determine if it is protective in patients with a hematoma.

The detrimental effects of induced hypothermia appear to be more severe in children. In a multicenter trial of hypothermia in 225 children (ages 1 to 17) with traumatic brain injury, the unfavorable outcome rate was 31% in hypothermia patients, and 22% in patients managed with normothermia ($P = .08$). In patients 7 years of age or older, the risk of an unfavorable outcome was even higher with hypothermia (relative risk, 1.71; 95% CI, 0.96 to 3.06; $P = .06$). Hypothermia was associated with significantly higher mortality rate in patients with normal intracranial pressure (relative risk, 2.12; 95% CI, 1.07 to 4.19; $P = .03$).

There have been investigations on the use of rapid induction of hypothermia with cardiopulmonary bypass in patients with cardiac arrest after penetrating trauma. Animal models have shown feasibility. However, logistic obstacles remain before clinical trials can be undertaken. Plans for reaping any potential benefit of induced hypothermia in trauma patients have yet to be realized.

Complications associated with its use include rebound intracranial hypertension, infections, hypotension, frequent need for vasopressors, bradycardia, decubitus ulcers due to cutaneous vasoconstriction, ileus, hypokalema, acid-base disturbances, and other electrolyte complications.

CONCLUSIONS

The relatively high specific heat of the body makes hypothermia very difficult to treat. Prompt control of hemorrhage and elimination of shock to restore normal heat production, coupled with early attention to the mechanisms of heat loss outlined previously, is the best form of therapy. Based on current data, hypothermia has an adverse effect on outcome, and every attempt should be made to aggressively treat it once it has occurred.

For the chapter's Suggested Readings list, please visit the book at www.ExpertConsult.inkling.com.

SURGICAL PROCEDURES IN THE SURGICAL INTENSIVE CARE UNIT

Ziad C. Sifri and Alicia M. Mohr

Please visit the book at www.ExpertConsult.inkling.com to read this chapter in full.

ANESTHESIA IN THE CRITICAL CARE UNIT AND PAIN MANAGEMENT

Andrew Loukas, Shawn M. Cantie, and Edgar J. Pierre

Please visit the book at www.ExpertConsult.inkling.com to read this chapter in full.

DIAGNOSTIC MANAGEMENT OF BRAIN DEATH IN THE INTENSIVE CARE UNIT AND ORGAN DONATION

Darren Malinoski and Ali Salim

Please visit the book at www.ExpertConsult.inkling.com to read this chapter in full.

REHABILITATION AND QUALITY OF LIFE AFTER TRAUMA AND OTHER ISSUES

PALLIATIVE CARE IN THE TRAUMA INTENSIVE CARE UNIT

Anastasia Kunac and Anne C. Mosenthal

Please visit the book at www.ExpertConsult.inkling.com to read this chapter in full.

TRAUMA REHABILITATION

Wayne Dubov, Joseph J. Stirparo, and Michael D. Pasquale

Please visit the book at www.ExpertConsult.inkling.com to read this chapter in full.

TRAUMA OUTCOMES

Glen Tinkoff and Michael Rhodes

Please visit the book at www.ExpertConsult.inkling.com to read this chapter in full.

Note: A Page numbers followed by *b* indicates boxes, *f* indicates figures, and *t* indicates tables.